Quick Reference to Standard Protocols for All Nursing Interventions

All nursing skills must include certain basic steps for the saftey and well-being of the client and the nurse. To save space and prevent repetition, *these steps are not included in each skill unless it is necessary to clarify them as applied for that skill.* Remember that these steps are essential and must be followed to deliver appropriate and responsible nursing care.

A logo is used in this text to identify circumstances when the use of clean gloves is recommended. Clean gloves are used to protect both caregivers and the clients. By wearing clean, disposable gloves before contact with mucous membranes, non-intact skin, or moist body substances, most microorganisms are kept off the caregiver's hands. However, gloves are not 100% effective and can have invisible small holes or tears. Handwashing after removing the gloves effectively prevents transfer of microorganisms to other clients. The following logo is used to indicate situations in which the likelihood of contact with mucous membranes, non-intact skin, or moist body substances is increased:

Effective handwashing, as well as changing clean gloves, is required between clients and between activities with the same client or when gloves become excessively soiled (Centers for Disease Control, CDC, 1992).

EQUIPMENT

Armband for client identification
Consent form (if required by agency policy)
Clean disposable gloves (if contact with body secretions or excretions is anticipated)

BEFORE THE SKILL

1. Verify physician's orders if skill is a dependent or collaborative nursing intervention. Independent nursing interventions may be verified with the nursing care plan, Kardex, or primary nurse.
2. Identify client by checking armband and having client state name (if able to do so).
3. Introduce yourself to client, including both name and title or role, and explain what you plan to do.
4. Explain the procedure and the reason it is to be done in terms client can understand.
5. Assess client to determine that the intervention is still appropriate. (Each skill has an assessment section that includes appropriate specific findings.)
6. Gather equipment and complete necessary charges.
7. Wash hands for at least 10-15 seconds before each new client contact (see Skill 3.1 on p. 50).
8. Adjust the bed to appropriate height and lower side rail on the side nearest you.
9. Provide privacy for client. Position and drape client as needed.

DURING THE SKILL

10. Promote client involvement if possible.
11. Assess client tolerance, being alert for signs of discomfort and fatigue.

COMPLETION PROTOCOL

12. Assist client to a position of comfort, and place needed items within reach. Be certain client has a way to call for help and knows how to use it.
13. Raise the side rails and lower the bed to the lowest position.
14. Store or remove and dispose of soiled supplies and equipment.
15. After client contact, remove gloves, if used.
16. Wash hands for at least 10 seconds.
17. Document client's response and expected or unexpected outcomes. Inability to tolerate a procedure is described in the nurses' notes.

To my children and grandchildren whose love constantly reminds me of the most important things in life,
To my partner, Mary Ann, whose love, patience, and encouragement empowered
me throughout the many long hours of manuscript preparation, and
To the many nursing students who have provided valuable input into this edition from the unique viewpoint of learners.

Martha Keene Elkin

To professional nurses who incorporate care and compassion into their competent nursing practice.

Anne Griffin Perry

Thanks to my doctoral student colleagues: Amy, Cathy, Charlotte, Jerri, Julie, Myra, Patti, and Rita for the most rewarding, enlightening, and challenging two years of my life.

Patricia A. Potter

DATE DUE

2ND EDITION

Nursing Interventions & Clinical Skills

Martha Keene Elkin, RN, MSN
Faculty
Central Maine Technical College
Auburn, Maine

Anne Griffin Perry, RN, MSN, EdD
Professor and Coordinator, Adult Health Specialty
Saint Louis University School of Nursing
Saint Louis University Health Sciences Center
St Louis, Missouri

Patricia A. Potter, RN, MSN
Research Scientist
Barnes-Jewish Hospital
St Louis, Missouri

With over 900 illustrations

M Mosby

St. Louis Baltimore Boston Carlsbad Chicago Minneapolis New York Philadelphia Portland
London Milan Sydney Tokyo Toronto

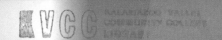

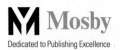

Mosby
Dedicated to Publishing Excellence

Editor-in-Chief: Sally Schrefer
Senior Editor: Susan Epstein
Developmental Editors: Billi Carcheri, Sharon Malchow
Project Manager: John Rogers
Senior Production Editor: Kathleen L. Teal
Design Manager: Kathi Gosche
Designer: John Rokusek, Rokusek Design
Photography: Rick Brady

Composition by Graphic World, Inc.
Printing/binding by Von Hoffmann Press

Mosby, Inc.
A Harcourt Health Sciences Company
11830 Westline Industrial Drive
St. Louis, Missouri 63146

Printed in the United States of America

International Standard Book Number 0-323-00802-X
99 00 01 02 03 / 9 8 7 6 5 4 3 2 1

CONTRIBUTORS

V. Christine Champagne, RN, CS, BSN, MSN(R), ANP
Adult Nurse Practitioner, Pulmonary
Midwest Chest Consultants, PC
St Charles, Missouri

Eileen Costantinou, RN, BSN
Professional Practice Consultant
Barnes-Jewish Hospital
St Louis, Missouri

Sheila A. Cunningham, BSN, MSN
Assistant Professor
Neumann College
Aston, Pennsylvania

Wanda Dubuisson, RN, BSN, MN
Assistant Professor
University of Southern Mississippi
Hattiesburg, Mississippi

Deborah Oldenburg Erickson, BSN, MSN
Instructor
Methodist Medical Center School of Nursing
Peoria, Illinois

Susan Jane Fetzer, BA, BSN, MSN, MBA, PhD
Assistant Professor
University of New Hampshire
Manchester, New Hampshire

Melba J. Figgins, MSN, BSN
Associate Professor
The University of Tennessee at Martin
Martin, Tennessee

Janet B. Fox-Moatz, RN, BSN, MSN
Assistant Professor
Neumann College
Aston, Pennsylvania

Lynn C. Hadaway, MEd, RNC, CRNI
Principal
Hadaway and Associates
Milner, Georgia

Susan Hauser Jeffers, RN, BSN, BA, MS
Instructor
Mansfield General Hospital School of Nursing
Mansfield, Ohio

Linda L. Kerby, RNC, BSN, MA, BA
Educational Consultant
Leawood, Kansas

Marilee Kuhrik, BSN, MSN, PhD
Associate Professor
Colorado Mountain College
Glenwood Springs, Colorado

Nancy Kuhrik, BSN, MSN, PhD
Associate Professor
Colorado Mountain College
Glenwood Springs, Colorado

Amy Lawn, BSN, MS, CIC
Infection Control Coordinator
Spectrum Health
Grand Rapids, Michigan

Mary MacDonald, RN, MSN
Staff Educator
Spectrum Health
Grand Rapids, Michigan

Mary Kay Knight Macheca, MSN(R), RN, CS, ANP, CDE
Adult Nurse Practitioner/Certified Diabetes Educator
The Bortz Diabetes Control Center
Richmond Heights, Missouri

Cynthia L. Maskey, MS
Professor of Nursing
Lincoln Land Community College
Springfield, Illinois

Barbara McGeever, RN, RSM, BSN, MSN, DNSc
Assistant Professor
Neumann College
Aston, Pennsylvania

Marsha Evans Orr, RN, MS
Owner
CreativEnegy, LLC Healthcare Consultants
Mesa, Arizona

Deborah Paul-Cheadle, RN
Registered Nurse, Infection Control
Spectrum Health
Grand Rapids, Michigan

Jacqueline A. Raybuck, CS, RN, PhD
Assistant Professor
Jewish Hospital College of Nursing and Allied Health
St Louis, Missouri

Roberta J. Richmond, MSN, RN, CCRN
Cardiac Case Manager
Central Maine Medical Center
Lewiston, Maine

Linette M. Sarti, RN, BSN, CNOR
Senior Coordinator
University Community Hospital
Tampa, Florida

Phyllis G. Stallard, BSN, MSN, ACCE
Assistant Professor
Neumann College
Aston, Pennsylvania

Victoria Steelman, PhD, RN, CNOR
Advanced Practice Nurse, Intensive and Surgical Services
University of Iowa Hospitals and Clinics
Iowa City, Iowa

Sue G. Thacker, RNC, BSN, MS, PhD
Professor
Wytheville Community College
Wytheville, Virginia

Stephanie Trinkl, BSN, MSN
Instructor, Department of Nursing
Immaculata College
Immaculata, Pennsylvania

Kathryn Tripp, BSN
Nursing Instructor
Southeastern Community College
Keokuk, Iowa

Pamela Becker Weilitz, MSN(R), RN, CS, ANP
Adult Nurse Practitioner
Washington University School of Medicine, University Care
St Louis, Missouri

Trudie Wierda, RN, MSN
Staff Educator
Spectrum Health
Grand Rapids, Michigan

Laurel A. Wiersema-Bryant, MSN, RN, CS
Clinical Nurse Specialist, Adult Nurse Practitioner
Barnes-Jewish Hospital
St Louis, Missouri

REVIEWERS

Sylvia Baird, RN, BSN, MM
Quality Improvement Program Manager
Spectrum Health
Grand Rapids, Michigan

Julie K. Baylor, RN, MSN
Assistant Professor
Bradley University
Peoria, Illinois

Margaret W. Bellak, BSN, MN
Associate Professor
Indiana University of Pennsylvania
Indiana, Pennsylvania

Teri Boese, BSN, MSN
Learning Resources Coordinator
University of Iowa College of Nursing
Iowa City, Iowa

Janice Boundy, RN, PhD
Professor/Coordinator
Saint Francis Medical Center College of Nursing
Peoria, Illinois

Sister Mary Rosita Brennan, CSSF, MSN, DSNc
Chair, Department of Associate Nursing
Felician College
Lodi, New Jersey

Victoria M. Brown, BSN, MSN, PhD
Professor
Georgia College and State University School of Health
　Sciences
Milledgeville, Georgia

Susan Burchiel, BSN, MSN, RN, C
Instructor of Nursing
Cuesta College, Nursing Division
San Luis Obispo, California

Susan Burkett, RN, MAS, CPNP, CPN
Administrator, TCTCH and Erlanger Woman's Services
Erlanger Medical Center
Chattanooga, Tennessee

Jeanie Burt, RN, BSN, MA, MSN
Assistant Professor of Nursing
Harding University School of Nursing
Searcy, Arkansas

Darlene Nebel Cantu, BSN, MSN, RNC
Director
Baptist Health System School of Professional Nursing
San Antonio, Texas

Gale Carli, RN, BSN, MHed, MSN
Associate Profesor
Ohlone College
Fremont, California

Kathlyn Carlson, RN, BSN, MA, CPAN
RN, Surgical Services
Abbott Northwestern Hospital
Minneapolis, Minnesota

Judith Chovanec-Toy, BSN, MS, RN
Assistant Professor
Kauai Community College
Lihue, Hawaii

Laura H. Clayton, RN, MSN, FNP
Assistant Professor
Shepherd College, Department of Nursing Education
Shepherdstown, West Virginia

Scotty Louise Connolly, RN, BS, CIC
Infection Control Coordinator
Spectrum Health—East Campus
Grand Rapids, Michigan

Lynne Alison Dearing, ARNP, MSN, MA
Clinical Specialist in Psychology and Mental Health
   Nursing
Cascade Counseling
Olympia, Washington

Karen Delrue, RN, BSN, CEN
Educator
Spectrum Health
Grand Rapids, Michigan

Patricia A. Eagan, RN, BSN, MSN
Retired
Pine Bluff, Arkansas

Patti A. Ellison, BSN, MSN, CEN, CFNP
Family Nurse Practitioner
Franciscan Health System of the Ohio Valley, Inc.
Cincinnati, Ohio

Carol Feingold, BS, BSN, MS
Senior Lecturer
University of Arizona College of Nursing
Tuscon, Arizona

Leah W. Frederick, RN, MS, CIC
Infection Control Practitioner
Infection Control Consultants
Phoenix, Arizona

Denise Goldy, BS, MS, MAE, MSN, CFNP
Associate Professor
Morehead State University
Morehead, Kentucky

Heidi Hahn, MHS, PT
Physical Therapist
Barnes-Jewish Hospital
St Louis, Missouri

Thelma Halberstadt, BS, MS, EdD
Professor of Nursing
Northern Essex Community College, Lawrence Campus
Lawrence, Massachusetts

Amy Hall, RN, MS
Assistant Professor
Saint Francis Medical Center College of Nursing
Peoria, Illinois

Lois C. Hamel, BSN, MS, ANP
University of New England, Westbrook College Campus
Portland, Maine

Adrienne Hentemann, BSN, MS
Administrative Associate
Spectrum Health
Grand Rapids, Michigan

Mary A. Herring, BSN, MSN, COHN-S
Wellness Program Specialist
Motorola, Inc. and University of Phoenix
Phoenix, Arizona

Janice Hoffman, BSN, MSN, CCRN
Assistant Professor
Anne Arundel Community College
Arnold, Maryland

Patricia M. Jacobson, RN, BSN, MSN
Nursing Instructor
Bullard Havens Rvts, State of Connecticut
Bridgeport, Connecticut

Judith Ann Kilpatrick, MSN, RNC, ANCC
Lecturer
Widener University
Chester, Pennsylvania

Christine Kuntz, ADN
Registered Respiratory Therapist
Memorial Medical Center
Springfield, Illinois

Virginia Lester, RN, BSN, MSN
Assistant Professor, Clinical Nurse Specialist
Angelo State University Department of Nursing
San Angelo, Texas

Frances E. Love, RN, MSN, CDE
Diabetes Education Coordinator
Mercy Fitzgerald Hospital
Darby, Pennsylvania

Rita G. Mertig, MS, BSN, RNC
Associate Professor
John Tyler Community College
Chester, Virginia

Ramona Reiber Midamba, RN, BS, CNM, MS
Director of Nursing Programs
Valley Grande College
Weslaco, Texas

Claudia Louth Mitchell, RN, BS, MS
Professor and Director, Associate Degree Nursing Program
Santa Barbara City College
Santa Barbara, California

Catherine Moore, RN, BS, CIC
Infection Control Nurse
Spectrum Health–East Campus
Grand Rapids, Michigan

Mary E. Newell, RN, MSN
Nursing Program Director
Highline Community College
Des Moines, Washington

Kathryn Nold, MSN
Assistant Professor
Jewish Hospital College of Nursing and Allied Health at
   Washington University Medical Center
St Louis, Missouri

Bonnie Ozarow, RN, BSN
Clinical Improvement Systems Specialist
Spectrum Health–Downtown Campus
Grand Rapids, Michigan

Melissa Powell, RN, MSN
Assistant Professor
Eastern Kentucky University
Richmond, Kentucky

Patricia Reese, RN, BSN, MSN
Nursing Skills Lab Supervisor
Penn Valley Community College Division of Nursing
Kansas City, Missouri

Catherine A. Robinson, RN, BA
Clinical Nurse Manager, Professional Practice and Systems
Barnes-Jewish Hospital
St Louis, Missouri

Nancy Semenza, RN, MS
Adjunct Faculty
MacMurray College, Department of Nursing
Jacksonville, Illinois

April Sieh, MSN
Assistant Professor of Nursing
Delta College
Flushing, Michigan

Julie S. Snyder, RNC, BSN, MSN
Freshman Faculty
Louise Obici School of Professional Nursing
Suffolk, Virginia

Kathleen G. Stilling, RN, C, BSN, MS
Assistant Professor
Essex Campus, The Community College of Baltimore
   County
Baltimore, Maryland

Patricia A. Stockert, BSN, MS
Associate Professor
Saint Francis Medical Center College of Nursing
Peoria, Illinois

Sylvia Tatman, RN, BSN, MSN, CS
Associate Instructor
Mt San Jacinto College, Menifee Campus
Menifee, California

Rowena Tessman, DCur, RN, CNS
Assistant Professor
University of Maine at Fort Kent
Fort Kent, Maine

Susanne M. Tracy, BSN, MN, MA
Associate Professor of Nursing
Rivier-St Joseph School of Nursing
Nashua, New Hampshire

Kathleen Upham, MS(N), ONC
Assistant Professor
Coastal Georgia Community College
Brunswick, Georgia

Anne Falsone Vaughn, BSN, MSN, CCRN, ACLS-I
former Lecturer
University of Washington School of Nursing
Seattle, Washington

Lois L. VonCannon, BSN, MSN
Clinical Assistant Professor
University of North Carolina, Greensboro, School of
Nursing
Greensboro, North Carolina

Melinda A. Warfield, BSN, CNA
Quality Improvement Director
Commjnity Mental Health Services for Ionia
Ionia, Michigan

PREFACE TO THE STUDENT

This text was designed to be clear and easy to follow. The 5-step nursing process provides the overall framework that you will find is also used in most of your nursing books. Each section and every feature was carefully developed to help you learn both how to perform the skills and how to effectively care for your clients. We've developed checklists to enable you to evaluate your performance for each of the skills in the text. These checklists can be accessed and printed by going to our Web site at <www.mosby.com/Nursing/Elkin/>.

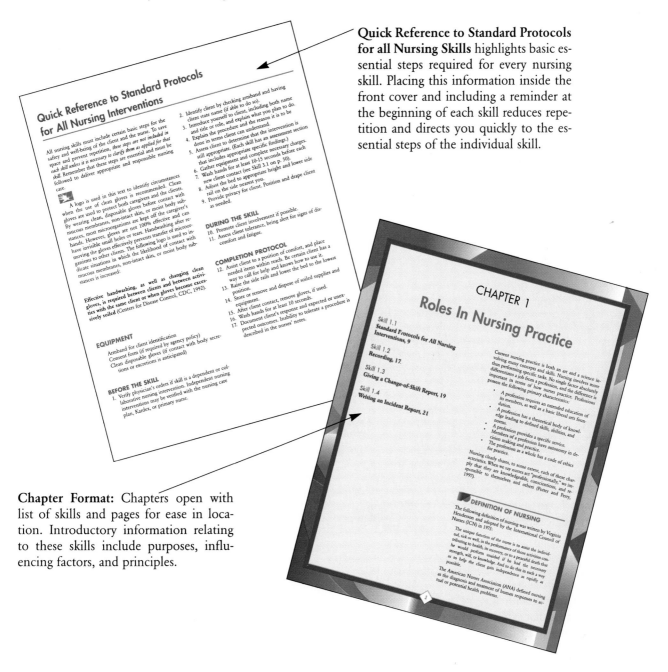

Quick Reference to Standard Protocols for all Nursing Skills highlights basic essential steps required for every nursing skill. Placing this information inside the front cover and including a reminder at the beginning of each skill reduces repetition and directs you quickly to the essential steps of the individual skill.

Chapter Format: Chapters open with list of skills and pages for ease in location. Introductory information relating to these skills include purposes, influencing factors, and principles.

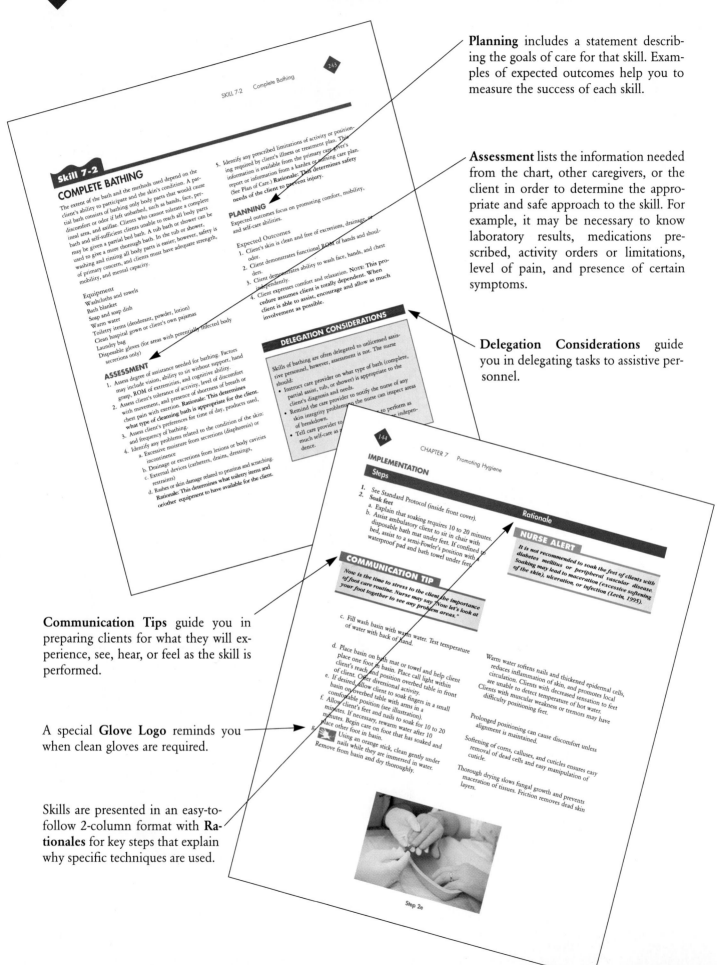

Planning includes a statement describing the goals of care for that skill. Examples of expected outcomes help you to measure the success of each skill.

Assessment lists the information needed from the chart, other caregivers, or the client in order to determine the appropriate and safe approach to the skill. For example, it may be necessary to know laboratory results, medications prescribed, activity orders or limitations, level of pain, and presence of certain symptoms.

Delegation Considerations guide you in delegating tasks to assistive personnel.

Communication Tips guide you in preparing clients for what they will experience, see, hear, or feel as the skill is performed.

A special **Glove Logo** reminds you when clean gloves are required.

Skills are presented in an easy-to-follow 2-column format with **Rationales** for key steps that explain why specific techniques are used.

Nurse Alerts help you remember important safety issues.

Nearly 1000 full-color photographs and drawings clearly show how steps are performed.

Unexpected Outcomes and Related Interventions describe how to assess for complications related to each skill and take the appropriate action.

Recording and Reporting lists information to chart.

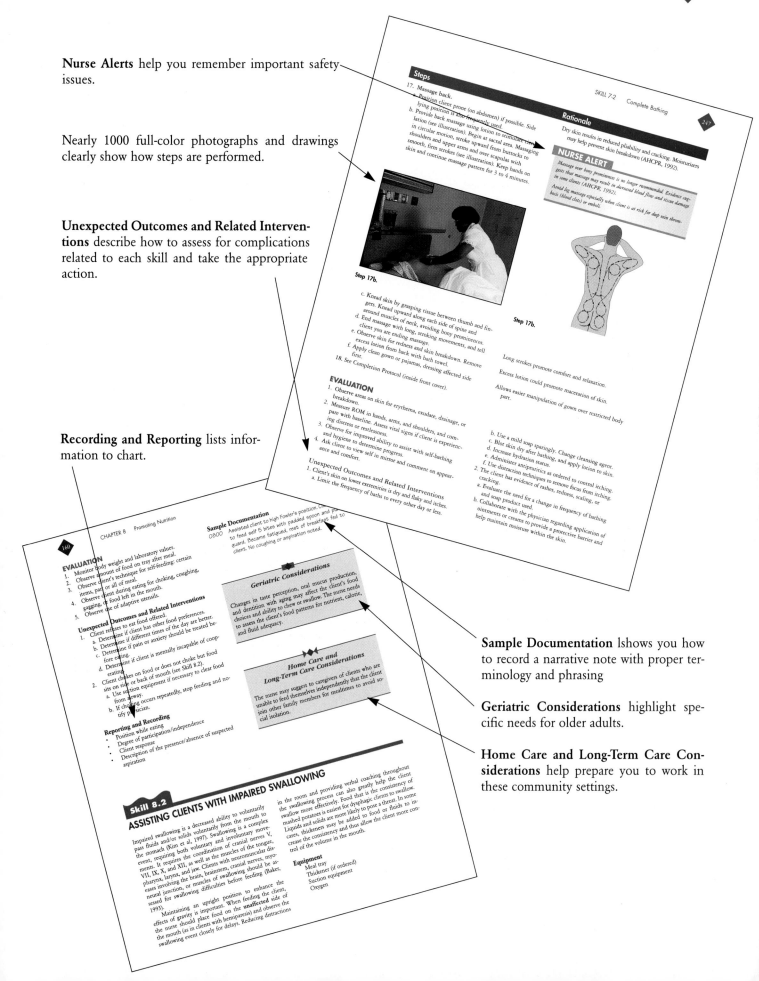

Sample Documentation shows you how to record a narrative note with proper terminology and phrasing

Geriatric Considerations highlight specific needs for older adults.

Home Care and Long-Term Care Considerations help prepare you to work in these community settings.

PREFACE TO THE INSTRUCTOR

We are grateful for the enthusiastic responses to the first edition of *Nursing Interventions and Clinical Skills* and have carefully preserved the features that made it unique: its streamlined and concise approach, language easily understood by beginning nursing students, generous use of color photographs to illustrate skills, and integration of skills in accordance with the way they are best learned and performed.

The revision builds on the basic organization and format of the first edition. Early chapters include basic skills typically introduced prior to, or during, initial clinical experiences, such as infection control and vital signs. Later chapters focus on more complex skills often encountered in medical-surgical nursing, such as gastric intubation and enteral nutrition. All chapters include a brief introduction including a unique segment that describes related nursing diagnoses in a way that helps students identify their intended use. Skills are presented in the nursing process format. Steps of the skills include parallel rationales to explain underlying scientific principles. Hundreds of close-up, full-color photographs facilitate learning.

We have responded to the increasing demands of faculty and students to teach and learn in an environment flooded with enormous amounts of changing information, limited clinical facilities, and less time. The second edition incorporates new features that introduce delegation considerations, communication tips, and home care and long-term care considerations.

We have enlisted contributions from nurses throughout the country who have provided their expertise in revising and updating each chapter. We carefully reviewed and refined the contributors' material ourselves to maintain a consistent organization and writing level to help beginning nursing students effectively grasp essential information.

KEY FEATURES FROM THE FIRST EDITION

- Nearly 1000 **full color photographs** are conveniently placed near the accompanying text.
- **Standard Protocols** for beginning and completion of each skill emphasize safety and infection control practices.

- A **Glove Logo** is used to visually highlight the circumstances when the use of **clean** gloves is recommended.
- **Sample Documentation** provides examples of clear, concise narrative documentation.

NEW FEATURES

- **Delegation Considerations** are included in the planning section for each skill to help the learner identify when delegation to assistive personnel is appropriate and what to include to clarify expectations regarding performance of the task.
- **Communication Tips** provide guidelines for explaining to clients what they may see, hear, or feel as the steps are performed. In addition, there are tips that help students know when to offer valuable instruction.
- **Recording and Reporting** provides a concise, bulleted list of information to be documented and reported.
- **Special Considerations** include guidelines for adaptation of skills in various settings, including home care and long-term care.
- More detailed **Table of Contents** facilitates location of skills within the text.

NEW CHAPTERS AND SKILLS

- **Professional Nursing Practice** presents an overview of the nursing profession and identifies nursing roles. Concepts introduced include standards of care, the nursing process, delegation, standard protocols, recording, reporting, and incident reports.
- **Basic Infant Care** includes skills related to maintaining physiologic stability as well as bathing and feeding of infants.

- **Preparation for Medication Administration** discusses the underlying principles and concepts of administering medications, including responsibilities related to understanding the effects of drugs, routes of administration, physician's orders, systems of administration, and dosage calculations. The "5 rights" prevention of medication errors and client and family teaching are also addressed.
- **Clients with Special Needs** includes skills on Mechanical Ventilation, Central Venous Lines, Hemodialysis, and Peritoneal Dialysis.
- **Communication** adds skills on Establishing Therapeutic Relationships, Communication with Anxious Clients, Deescalating a Potentially Violent Client, and Client Teaching.
- **Safety** includes new skills on Designing a Restraint-Free Environment and Safety with Radioactive Materials
- **Laboratory and Diagnostic Tests** adds skills on Collecting Blood Specimens and Care of Clients undergoing Contrast Media Studies, Nuclear Imaging, and Cardiac Studies.
- Each Chapter concludes with all new **Critical Thinking Exercises** and a list of current references. Answers to the critical thinking exercises are provided in the Instructor's Resource Manual.

TEACHING-LEARNING PACKAGE

The comprehensive teaching and learning package includes the following:

- **Instructor's Resource Manual with Testbank** includes learning objectives and teaching strategies, learning activities, and a NEW test bank in the NCLEX format.
- **Skills Checklists** for each skill accessible to both you and your students from the Mosby Web site <www.mosby.com/Nursing/Elkin/>
- **Mosby's Nursing Skills Video Series** provides valuable visual reinforcement for learning.
- **Interactive videodiscs** produced by Mosby/FITNE, *Applying Critical Thinking to Nursing Skills*, provide visual interactive reinforcement to enhance learning of critical thinking in relation to the performance of basic skills. For information or to order, please contact FITNE, Inc. At 800-337-4107.

We hope that each chapter will help students develop a solid base on which to build the knowledge and ability to use critical thinking and the nursing process to provide nursing care for clients safely, effectively, and with an awareness of why, as well as how, the steps of each skill are performed.

ACKNOWLEDGMENTS

We are especially grateful to the students who have provided valuable input into the revision of this book from the unique viewpoint of the learner; the many nursing faculty members and practitioners who have offered their comments, recommendations, and suggestions; the contributors who revised selected chapters of this edition; and the reviewers for the insightful feedback.

Thanks to Rick Brady, Diana Kleidon, and Michael Clement, M.D. for the expert color photography and to John and Kim Rokusek of Rokusek Designs for the creative design that provides attractive and unique visual appeal. These contributions significantly enhance the process of learning.

Thanks also to the talented and dedicated professionals at Mosby: Suzi Epstein, Senior Editor, who provided leadership, energy, and enthusiasm for the revision process; Billi Carcheri, Developmental Editor, who greatly enhanced the quality of this book by her organizational skills, persistent and courteous communications, and dedication to accuracy and quality; Shari Malchow, Developmental Editor, who saw the project through the final production stages; Graquel Hutchinson, Editorial Assistant, who cheerfully assisted with a myriad of details; Kathy Teal, whose careful editing and thoughtful handling ensured an accurate, consistent book; Jeanne Genz, who made up each page to flow clearly and logically. Special thanks go to Mary Hamby and Tom Wilhelm for their unique, collaborative efforts in helping us create a new edition that meets the needs of today's nursing students.

Finally, thanks to our friends and families for their understanding, patience, and encouragement.

Martha "Marty" Keene Elkin
Anne Griffin Perry
Patricia A. Potter

CONTENTS

UNIT ONE
Professional Nursing

1 **Roles in Nursing Practice, 2**
Marty Elkin, RN, MSN
Skill 1.1 Standard Protocols for All Interventions, 9
Skill 1.2 Recording, 17
Skill 1.3 Giving a Change-of-Shift Report, 19
Skill 1.4 Writing an Incident Report, 21

UNIT TWO
Fundamental Concepts

2 **Facilitating Communication, 25**
Jacqueline Raybuck, CS, RN, PhD
Skill 2.1 Establishing Therapeutic Communication, 29
Skill 2.2 Comforting, 32
Skill 2.3 Active Listening, 34
Skill 2.4 Interviewing, 36
Skill 2.5 Communicating with an Anxious Client, 40
Skill 2.6 Verbally Deescalating a Potentially Violent Client, 42
Skill 2.7 Client Teaching, 44

3 **Promoting Infection Control, 47**
Deborah Paul-Cheadle, RN
Skill 3.1 Handwashing, 50
Skill 3.2 Using Disposable Clean Gloves, 53
Skill 3.3 Caring for Clients under Isolation Precautions, 55
Skill 3.4 Special Tuberculosis Precautions, 60

4 **Basic Sterile Technique, 63**
Linette M. Sarti, RN, BSN, CNOR
Skill 4.1 Creating and Maintaining a Sterile Field, 63
Skill 4.2 Sterile Gloving, 69

5 **Promoting a Safe Environment, 73**
Amy Lawn, BSN, MS, CIC
Skill 5.1 Safety Equipment and Fall Prevention, 76
Skill 5.2 Designing a Restraint-Free Environment, 81
Skill 5.3 Applying Restraints, 85
Skill 5.4 Seizure Precautions, 91
Skill 5.5 Safety Measures for Radioactive Materials, 92

UNIT THREE
Activities of Daily Living

6 **Promoting Activity and Mobility, 96**
Shiela A. Cunningham, BSN, MSN
Skill 6.1 Assisting with Moving and Positioning Clients in Bed, 97
Skill 6.2 Minimizing Orthostatic Hypotension, 106
Skill 6.3 Transferring from Bed to Chair, 107
Skill 6.4 Using a Mechanical (Hoyer) Lift for Transfer from Bed to Chair, 112
Skill 6.5 Transferring from Bed to Stretcher, 115
Skill 6.6 Assisting Ambulation, 117

7 **Promoting Hygiene, 121**
Cynthia Maskey, MS
Skill 7.1 Complete Bathing, 123
Skill 7.2 Oral Care, 130
Skill 7.3 Hair Care, 135
Skill 7.4 Foot and Nail Care, 140
Skill 7.5 Bedmaking, 147

8 **Promoting Nutrition, 155**
Marsha Evans Orr, RN, MS
Skill 8.1 Feeding Dependent Clients, 156
Skill 8.2 Assisting Clients with Impaired Swallowing, 160
Skill 8.3 Obtaining Body Weights, 163

9 **Assisting with Elimination, 167**
Melba J. Figgins, MSN, BSN
Skill 9.1 Monitoring Intake and Output, 168
Skill 9.2 Providing a Bedpan and Urinal, 173
Skill 9.3 Caring for Incontinent Clients, 177
Skill 9.4 Applying an External Catheter, 181
Skill 9.5 Administering an Enema, 185

10 **Promoting Comfort, Sleep, and Relaxation, 190**
Kathryn Tripp, BSN
Skill 10.1 Comfort Measures that Promote Sleep, 191
Skill 10.2 Relaxation Techniques, 195

11 **Basic Infant Care, 203**
Sue Thacker, RNC, BSN, MS, PhD
Skill 11.1 Thermoregulation Using a Radiant
Warmer, 204
Skill 11.2 Infant Feeding, 206
Skill 11.3 Infant Bathing, 212
Skill 11.4 Changing a Diaper, 215
Skill 11.5 Swaddling and Use of a Mummy
Restraint, 218

UNIT FOUR
Assessment Skills

12 **Vital Signs, 222**
Susan Jane Fetzer, BA, BSN, MSN, MBA, PhD
Skill 12.1 Assessing Temperature, Pulse, Respirations,
and Blood Pressure, 231
Skill 12.2 Tympanic Temperature, 242
Skill 12.3 Electronic Blood Pressure Measurement, 245
Skill 12.4 Measuring Oxygen Saturation with Pulse
Oximetry, 249

13 **Shift Assessment, 255**
Marty Elkin, RN, MSN
Skill 13.1 General Survey and Inspection of
Integument, 257
Skill 13.2 Auscultating Lung Sounds, 262
Skill 13.3 Auscultating Apical Pulse, 266
Skill 13.4 Assessing the Abdomen, 269
Skill 13.5 Assessing Extremities and Peripheral
Circulation, 274

14 **Comprehensive Health Assessment, 280**
Pamela Becker Weilitz, MSN(R), RN, CS, ANP
Skill 14.1 Assessing the Head, Face, and Neck, 283
Skill 14.2 Assessing the Nose, Sinuses, and
Mouth, 288
Skill 14.3 Assessing the Eyes and Ears, 293
Skill 14.4 Assessing the Thorax, Lungs, and
Breasts, 299
Skill 14.5 Assessing the Heart and Circulation, 309
Skill 14.6 Assessing the Abdomen, 317
Skill 14.7 Assessing the Genitalia and Rectum, 322
Skill 14.8 Assessing Neurological Function, 327
Skill 14.9 Assessing Musculoskeletal Function, 339

15 **Laboratory and Diagnostic Tests, 344**
Marilee Kuhrik, BSN, MSN, PhD
Nancy Kuhrik, BSN, MSN, PhD
Skill 15.1 Specimen Collection (Urine, Stool, Sputum,
Cultures), 346
Skill 15.2 Blood Specimens (Venipuncture; Vacuum
Tube; Blood Cultures), 360
Skill 15.3 Unit Specimen Testing (Glucose,
Chemstrip/Multistix, Hemoccult,
Gastroccult), 368
Skill 15.4 Contrast Media Studies (Arteriogram,
Computed Tomography, Intravenous
Pyelogram), 376
Skill 15.5 Nuclear Imaging Studies (Bone Scan, Brain
Scan, Thyroid Scan), 380
Skill 15.6 Asisting with Diagnostic Studies (Aspirations
[Bone Marrow, Lumbar Puncture,
Paracentesis, Thoracentesis, Liver Biopsy],
Bronchoscopy, Endoscopy, Magnetic
Resonance Imaging), 383
Skill 15.7 Cardiac Studies (Electrocardiogram, Exercise
Stress Test, Dobutamine Stress
Echocardiography, Cardiac Nuclear Scanning,
Cardiac Catheterization), 396

UNIT FIVE
Administration of Medication

16 **Preparation for Medication
Administration, 404**
Marty Elkin, RN, MSN

17 **Non-Parenteral Medications, 420**
Marty Elkin, RN, MSN
Skill 17.1 Administering Oral Medications, 422
Skill 17.2 Applying Topical Medications, 429
Skill 17.3 Instilling Eye and Ear Medications, 433
Skill 17.4 Using Metered-Dose Inhalers, 438
Skill 17.5 Inserting Rectal and Vaginal
Medications, 442

18 **Administration of Injections, 447**
Patricia A. Potter, RN, MSN
Skill 18.1 Subcutaneous Injections (Includes
Insulin), 457
Skill 18.2 Intramuscular Injections, 464
Skill 18.3 Intradermal Injections, 469

UNIT SIX
Perioperative Nursing Care

19 Preparing the Client for Surgery, 475
Victoria Steelman, PhD, RN, CNOR
Skill 19.1 Preoperative Assessment, 476
Skill 19.2 Preoperative Teaching, 480
Skill 19.3 Physical Preparation, 485

20 Intraoperative Techniques, 492
Linette M. Sarti, RN, BSN, CNOR
Skill 20.1 Surgical Hand Scrub, 493
Skill 20.2 Donning Sterile Gown and Closed
Gloving, 497

21 Caring for the Postoperative Client, 503
Janet B. Fox-Moatz, RN, BSN, MSN
Skill 21.1 Providing Immediate Postoperative Care in
Postanesthesia Care Unit, 506
Skill 21.2 Providing Comfort Measures During Phase II
(Convalescent Phase), 512
Skill 21.3 Providing Surgical Wound Care, 516
Skill 21.4 Monitoring and Measuring Drainage
Devices, 520
Skill 21.5 Removing Staples and Sutures (Including
Applying SteriStrips), 534

22 Pain Management, 530
Deborah Oldenburg Erickson, BSN, MSN
Skill 22.1 Nonpharmacological Pain Management, 533
Skill 22.2 Pharmacological Pain Management, 537
Skill 22.3 Patient-Controlled Analgesia (PCA), 539
Skill 22.4 Epidural Analgesia, 544

23 Therapeutic Use of Heat and Cold, 551
Susan Hauser Jeffers, RN, BSN, BA, MS
Skill 23.1 Moist Heat, 553
Skill 23.2 Dry Heat, 556
Skill 23.3 Cold Compresses and Ice Bags, 559

UNIT SEVEN
Managing Immobilized Clients

**24 Pressure Ulcers and Wound Care
Management, 565**
Anne Perry, RN, MSN, EdD
Skill 24.1 Pressure Ulcer Risk Assessment and
Prevention Strategies, 568
Skill 24.2 Treatment of Pressure Ulcers and Wound
Management, 576
Skill 24.3 Applying Dressings, 585
Skill 24.4 Changing Transparent Dressings, 592
Skill 24.5 Applying Binders and Bandages, 594

25 Special Mattresses and Beds, 601
Laurel A. Wiersema-Bryant, MSN, RN, CS
Skill 25.1 Using a Support Surface Mattress, 602
Skill 25.2 Using an Air-Suspension Bed, 605
Skill 25.3 Using an Air-Fluidized Bed, 608
Skill 25.4 Using a Rotokinetic Bed, 611
Skill 25.5 Using a Bariatric Bed, 614

26 Promoting Range of Motion, 617
Anne Perry, RN, MSN, EdD
Skill 26.1 Range-of-Motion Exercises, 618
Skill 26.2 Continuous Passive Motion (CPM)
Machine (for Client with Total Knee
Replacement), 632

27 Traction, 636
Wanda Dubuisson, RN, BSN, MN
Skill 27.1 Maintaining Skin Traction, 639
Skill 27.2 Skeletal Traction Assessment and Pin Site
Care, 642

28 Cast Care, 648
Phyllis G. Stallard, BSN, MSN, ACCE
Skill 28.1 Cast Application, Assessment, and
Care, 650
Skill 28.2 Cast Removal, 655

29 Assistive Devices for Ambulation, 659
Eileen Costantinou, RN, BSN
Skill 29.1 Preventing Falls, 662
Skill 29.2 Teaching Use of Cane, Crutches, and
Walker, 665
Skill 29.3 Caring for the Client with an Orthotic Device
(Brace/Splint), 677

UNIT EIGHT
Managing Complex Nursing Interventions

30 Intravenous Therapy, 683
Lynn C. Hadaway, MEd, RNC, CRNI
Skill 30.1 Basic IV Insertion Techniques (Intermittent and Continuous Infusion), 684
Skill 30.2 Regulating Flow Rates, 696
Skill 30.3 Maintenance of IV Site, 703
Skill 30.4 Administering IV Medications, 711
Skill 30.5 Transfusion with Blood Products, 720

31 Promoting Oxygenation, 727
V. Christine Champagne, RN, CS, BSN, MSN(R), ANP
Skill 31.1 Oxygen Administration, 728
Skill 31.2 Airway Management: Noninvasive Interventions, 735
Skill 31.3 Airway Management: Suctioning, 739
Skill 31.4 Airway Management: Endotracheal Tube and Tracheostomy Care, 747
Skill 31.5 Managing Closed Chest Drainage Systems (Including Managing Postoperative Autotransfusions), 754

32 Gastrointestinal Intubation, 765
Marsha Evans Orr, RN, MS
Skill 32.1 Inserting Nasogastric Tube (Includes Checking Placement of Nasal Tube), 766
Skill 32.2 Irrigating Nasogastric Tube, 770
Skill 32.3 Removing Nasogastric Tube, 772

33 Enteral Nutrition, 775
Barbara McGeever, RN, RSM, BSN, MSN, DNSc
Skill 33.1 Intubating the Client with a Small-Bore Nasogastric or Nasointestinal Feeding Tube, 776
Skill 33.2 Administering Medication Through a Feeding Tube, 787

34 Altered Bowel Elimination, 791
Trudie Wierda, RN, MSN
Mary MacDonald, RN, MSN
Skill 34.1 Removing Impactions, 792
Skill 34.2 Pouching an Enterostomy, 794
Skill 34.3 Irrigating a Colostomy, 803

35 Altered Urinary Elimination, 809
Stephanie Trinkl, BSN, MSN
Patricia A. Potter, RN, MSN
Skill 35.1 Urinary Catheterization: Male and Female, 810
Skill 35.2 Urinary Diversions (Continent and Incontinent), 818
Skill 35.3 Continuous Bladder Irrigation, 825
Skill 35.4 Suprapubic Catheter, 828

36 Altered Sensory Perception, 832
Patricia A. Potter, RN, MSN
Skill 36.1 Caring for Clients with Contact Lenses, 833
Skill 36.2 Caring for an Eye Prosthesis, 839
Skill 36.3 Eye Irrigations, 842
Skill 36.4 Caring for Clients with Hearing Aids, 845
Skill 36.5 Ear Irrigations, 848

37 Fluid, Electrolyte, and Acid-Base Balance, 852
Marty Elkin, RN, MSN
Skill 37.1 Monitoring Fluid Imbalance, 856
Skill 37.2 Monitoring Electrolyte Imbalance, 859
Skill 37.3 Monitoring Acid-Base Imbalance, 864

38 Emergency Measures for Life Support in the Hospital Setting, 869
Roberta J. Richmond, MSN, RN, CCRN
Skill 38.1 Resuscitation, 870
Skill 38.2 Code Management, 877
Skill 38.3 Care for the Body after Death, 882

39 Care of the Client with Special Needs, 888
Linda L. Kerby, RNC, BSN, MA, BA
Skill 39.1 Managing Central Venous Lines, 889
Skill 39.2 Administration of Total Parenteral Nutrition, 898
Skill 39.3 Mechanical Ventilation, 901
Skill 39.4 Care of Clients Receiving Hemodialysis, 907
Skill 39.5 Peritoneal Dialysis, 911

40 **Discharge Teaching and Home Health Management, 917**
Mary Kay Knight Macheca, MSN(R), RN, CS, ANP, CDE
Skill 40.1 Risk Assessment and Accident Prevention, 918
Skill 40.2 Teaching Self-Administration of Non-Parenteral Medications, 922
Skill 40.3 Teaching Self-Injections, 926
Skill 40.4 Teaching Home Self-Catherization, 932
Skill 40.5 Using Home Oxygen Equipment, 936
Skill 40.6 Teaching Home Tracheostomy Care, 941

Appendixes

A   **Sample Forms, 948**
Admission Patient Profiles, 949
Diabetic Management Record, 954
Patient/Visitor Incident Report, 955
Routine Nursing Assessment, 956
Critical Care Path, 958
Vital Signs, 959

B   **Abbreviations and Equivalents, 960**

C   **Nursing Diagnoses: (1999-2000) North American Nursing Diagnosis Association (NANDA) and Functional Health Patterns, 962**

D   **Norms for Common Laboratory Tests, 965**

E   **Height and Weight Table: Weights for Persons 29 to 59 Years According to Build, 967**

Glossary, 968

Index, 975

UNIT ONE

Professional Nursing

Chapter 1
Roles in Nursing Practice

CHAPTER 1

Roles In Nursing Practice

Skill 1.1
Standard Protocols for All Nursing Interventions, 9

Skill 1.2
Recording, 17

Skill 1.3
Giving a Change-of-Shift Report, 19

Skill 1.4
Writing an Incident Report, 21

Current nursing practice is both an art and a science involving many concepts and skills. Nursing involves more than performing specific tasks. No single factor absolutely differentiates a job from a profession, and the difference is important in terms of how nurses practice. Professions possess the following primary characteristics:

- A profession requires an extended education of its members, as well as a basic liberal arts foundation.
- A profession has a theoretical body of knowledge leading to defined skills, abilities, and norms.
- A profession provides a specific service.
- Members of a profession have autonomy in decision making and practice.
- The profession as a whole has a code of ethics for practice.

Nursing clearly shares, to some extent, each of these characteristics. When we say nurses act "professionally," we imply that they are knowledgeable, conscientious, and responsible to themselves and others (Potter and Perry, 1997).

DEFINITION OF NURSING

The following definition of nursing was written by Virginia Henderson and adopted by the International Council of Nurses (ICN) in 1973:

> The unique function of the nurse is to assist the individual, sick or well, in the performance of those activities contributing to health, its recovery, or to a peaceful death that he would perform unaided if he had the necessary strength, will, or knowledge. And to do this in such a way as to help the client gain independence as rapidly as possible.

The American Nurses Association (ANA) defined nursing as the diagnosis and treatment of human responses to actual or potential health problems.

ROLES OF THE PROFESSIONAL NURSE

Nurses perform many roles simultaneously. Nurses are caregivers who are perceptive and sensitive to their clients' needs. Nurses are teachers, who facilitate learning as an interactive process that results in knowledge to improve, maintain and promote health. Nurses are counselors, who help individuals to recognize and cope with problems and improve relationships. Nurses are client advocates, who defend client rights and encourage caregivers to provide what is best for them. Nurses are leaders attempting to influence others to improve the health status of individuals and groups and improve the systems of delivery of health care in a variety of settings. Nurses are managers, responsible for planning, and developing health care policies. They coordinate and supervise the delivery of nursing care including delegation of nursing tasks to others. Nurses may become generalists, able to function in a variety of settings, or specialize in medical-surgical nursing, gerontologic nursing (care of older adults), pediatric nursing (care of children and adolescents), perinatal nursing (care of families before, during, and after childbirth), community health nursing, and psychiatric and mental health nursing.

Nursing practice involves four areas: health promotion, health maintenance, health restoration, and care for dying clients and their families. Health promotion focuses on helping people maintain wellness and enhance their health. Health maintenance helps clients maintain a stable health status and use their abilities to the greatest extent possible. Health restoration assists clients toward wellness after illness, injury, or surgery. Care of the dying provides support and comfort for clients and their families in homes, hospitals, extended-care facilities, or hospices specifically designed for this purpose.

STANDARDS OF CARE

Standards of care are guidelines that establish expectations for the provision of safe and appropriate nursing care. The law defines the standards of care in each state in the form of Nurse Practice Acts. These state laws regulate the scope of nursing practice and specify educational requirements. Professional organizations also define standards of care. The American Nurses Association (ANA) has established standards of nursing practice that correlate to the nursing process (Figure 1-1). It is important for professional nurses to be involved in establishing and maintaining standards of practice, because these standards define the responsibility and accountability for the profession.

TRENDS IN HEALTH CARE

Consumers of health care have increased their knowledge and awareness of health promotion, illness prevention, and treatment practices. They are concerned about access to cost-effective, quality health care. The United States Department of Health and Human Services (USDHHS) has developed a national strategy to promote health called *Healthy People 2000* (USDHHS, 1991). The objectives of this program include increasing the span of healthy life by risk reduction, health services and protection, and research. Another major change in health care has been development of diagnosis-related groups (DRGs). The DRG categories allow pretreatment billing for hospitals reimbursed by Medicare. With hospitals now financially responsible if clients exceed the allotted hospital stay, more clients are discharged at earlier stages of recovery. This has increased the need for home care and increased the need for skilled care in long-term care settings.

Case management is a health care delivery system that was created in response to pressure to provide care in a more cost-effective way. This model includes established timelines and standards called *critical pathways*, guidelines for care, or CareMaps. Critical pathways are multidisciplinary plans that include the aspects of care for an illness or surgery and the expected outcomes. Aspects of care are developed by professionals from all disciplines who care for a specific type of client and incorporate expected outcomes each day over a projected length of stay, including the day of discharge. Each day includes clinical assessments, treatments, dietary interventions, activity and exercise, client education, and other plans that promote a normal recovery process.

In addition, professional and government organizations have developed clinical practice guidelines for management of certain symptoms of diseases. These guidelines reflect research which support changes in practice. For example, the Agency for Health Care Policy and Research (AHCPR) has initiated guidelines in the areas of pain management and pressure ulcer prevention and treatment.

DELEGATION

As a result of the changing demands in health care systems and increasing need for accessible, affordable, quality health care, there is a trend toward utilization of a variety of health care workers with different levels of education and training. In addition, professional nurses are finding themselves in situations that require more support to perform the daily, repetitive tasks of care. The registered nurse (RN) is needed to assess, diagnose, plan, and evaluate client needs and responses to care; coordinate care delivery for groups of clients; make the professional judgments

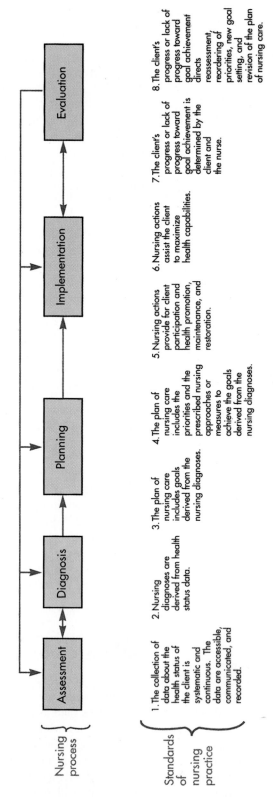

Figure 1-1 Nursing process compared with standards of nursing practice. *Modified from American Nurses Association: Nursing's social policy statement, Washington, DC, 1995, American Nurses Foundation/American Nurses Association. Reprinted with permission.*

necessary to adjust therapies and deliver care; deliver complex therapies; and provide client education and counseling. The best use of the RN's time requires wise and efficient use of ancillary personnel.

Ancillary staff include both licensed and unlicensed personnel. The licensed practical or vocational nurse (LPN/LVN), who works under the supervision of a professional nurse, has 12 to 18 months of basic nursing education. Although the LPN/LVN uses the nursing process under the direction of the RN, there are some limitations based on the scope of practice determined by the Nurse Practice Acts in each state (Box 1-1). In many states the LPN administers medications and with additional education may initiate intravenous (IV) therapy. Certified nursing assistants have 2 to 3 months of basic nursing care training with a focus on basic skills administered in long-term care facilities. Assistive personnel (AP) have on-the-job training of specific tasks in a particular health care setting.

Delegation is the transferring of responsibility for the performance of an activity or task while retaining accountability for the outcome (ANA, 1995). In delegating there is a decision-making process that must take into account which tasks can be delegated and in what situations, according to the Nurse Practice Act. The nurse needs to know the qualifications of the caregiver, including the caregiver's education, skills, and experience, as well as the caregiver's demonstrated and documented evidence of current competency. Delegation requires assessment of each situation, as well as effective prioritization of client needs and therapies. In addition, the professional nurse must provide direction and clear expectations regarding performance of the task and evaluate the effectiveness of the performance in relation to established standards. Ancillary staff are important members of the health care team and can be very productive when their contributions are

recognized and valued. Box 1-2 lists the Five Rights of Delegation recommended by the National Council of State Boards of Nursing (1995).

Throughout this text, boxes are included to assist learners in identifying delegation considerations that should be taken into account as RNs decide which tasks can be delegated and how to safely delegate tasks to AP. The LPN is responsible for assessing the needs of the client and the skills of the AP to determine if the two match. Part of delegation includes specific instructions regarding under what circumstances the AP should consult the licensed nurse, as well as what should be reported. Delegation of any given task may be appropriate in some situations and inappropriate in others. The licensed nurse must decide whether the client's response to the performance of the task is reasonably predictable and whether the AP will achieve results similar to those the licensed nurse will achieve in performing that task.

DELEGATION GUIDELINES

When the RN determines that someone who is not licensed to practice nursing can safely provide a selected nursing task for a client and delegates that task, the nurse remains responsible and accountable for the care provided (Wong and Perry, 1997).

NURSING PROCESS

The nursing process is an approach that enables a nurse to organize and deliver nursing care. This process involves critical thinking that allows decision making and

---

Box 1-1 Role of the LPN/LVN in the Nursing Process

Assessing: Observe and report significant cues (e.g., signs, symptoms) to RN or physician.
Diagnosing: Assist in validating current nursing diagnoses.
Planning: Assist with goal identification and priority setting; suggest nursing interventions.
Implementing: Carry out physician and nursing orders.
Evaluating: Assist with evaluation of progress toward goals and suggest alternative nursing interventions when necessary.

Modified from Christensen B, Kockrow E: *Foundations of nursing,* ed 3, St Louis, 1999, Mosby.

Box 1-2 Five Rights of Delegation

Right Task: One that can safely be delegated for a specific client, such as repetitive tasks that require little supervision and that are relatively noninvasive.
Right Circumstances: Appropriate client, setting, and resources.
Right Person: Right person delegates the right task to the most appropriate person, to be performed on the right client.
Right Direction/Communication: Clear, concise description of the task, including its objective, limits, and expectations.
Right Supervision: Appropriate monitoring, evaluation, intervention, as needed, and feedback.

Modified from National Council of State Boards of Nursing: *Delegation: concepts and decision making process. Reprinted with permission of the National Council of State Boards of Nursing, Inc., Chicago, Ill.*

judgments based on knowledge and experience. The nursing process is dynamic and continuous. It is a creative organizational structure, yet it is flexible and useful in any setting. The purposes of the nursing process are to identify health care needs, determine priorities, establish goals, communicate the plan of care, provide nursing interventions designed to meet client needs, and evaluate the effectiveness of nursing care. The nursing process includes the following steps: assessment, nursing diagnosis, planning, implementation, and evaluation (Table 1-1).

Assessment

The diagnostic process begins with assessment, as the nurse collects information about the client (see Box 1-3). This includes interviewing the client and others significant to the situation, conducting a physical assessment, conferring with health team members, and reviewing information in the client record.

Diagnosis

Data are analyzed and organized into clusters of related cues, which then lead to the formulation of a nursing diagnosis. Clusters of subjective and objective cues support the selection of the nursing diagnosis (Table 1-2). Numerous resources are available to assist nurses with identifying characteristics that may be included in cue clusters for a given nursing diagnosis. Many agencies have initial nursing assessment forms that facilitate identification of nursing diagnoses (see Appendix A).

A nursing diagnosis is composed of problem and etiology statements:

- The problem statement describes a physiological or psychological response to a health problem.
- The etiology statement describes contributing factors that influence development of the response.

Identifying the First Part of the Diagnostic Statement

The North American Nursing Diagnosis Association's (NANDA) list of accepted nursing diagnoses can also be categorized into the 11 functional patterns listed in Appendix C. For each of the 11 patterns, the nurse assesses clients by organizing patterns of behavior and physiological responses that pertain to a functional pattern category. The assessment of each of the 11 patterns represents the interaction of the client and the environment, and each pattern interacts with other patterns (Gordon, 1997).

Box 1-3 Creating a Nursing Diagnosis

Step 1
Start with information from a client assessment.

a. Make a comprehensive list of all significant cues, such as symptoms, laboratory data, subjective data, and other information. This would *not* include medical diagnosis, physician orders, treatments, or interventions.
b. Group cues according to ways that make sense to you.
c. Each group of cues then provides supporting defining characteristics for a nursing diagnosis label.

Step 2
Determine the etiology or contributing factors for the diagnosis. (This becomes the *"related to"* part of the statement.)

a. "What makes or maintains the client's unhealthy response?"
b. The related factor should clearly indicate what nurses can independently do to help alleviate the problem.
c. Compare with *contributing factors* or related factors as listed in references. NOTE: Watch out for medical diagnoses that may be there and may *not* be used in this step except by using the phrase ". . . secondary to. . . ."
d. The related factor directs the nursing interventions and becomes the second part of the diagnostic statement.
e. In some cases the contributing factors are "unknown."

Step 3
Identify the client *problem* or *response* from the NANDA listing.

a. This becomes the *stem* or *label* and the first part of the diagnostic statement.
b. For this part you must use the exact NANDA words.

The first part of the statement, the problem or stem, may be an actual or high-risk nursing diagnosis. A high-risk nursing diagnosis indicates the client is at risk for this response, although it is not yet present. Most nursing diagnosis labels can be used as either actual or high-risk nursing diagnoses. For example, a client may have a nursing diagnosis of actual **Impaired Physical Mobility** or **High Risk for Impaired Physical Mobility.**

Table 1-1

Summary of the Nursing Process

Component	Purpose	Steps
Assessment	To gather, verify, and communicate data about a client so that a database is established	1. Collecting nursing health history 2. Performing physical examination 3. Collecting laboratory data 4. Validating data 5. Clustering data 6. Documenting data
Nursing diagnosis	To identify health care needs of a client, to formulate nursing diagnoses	1. Analyzing and interpreting data 2. Identifying client problems 3. Formulating nursing diagnoses 4. Documenting nursing diagnosis
Planning	To identify a client's goals; to determine priorities of care, to determine expected outcomes, to design nursing strategies to achieve goals of care	1. Identifying client goals 2. Establishing expected outcomes 3. Selecting nursing actions 4. Delegating actions 5. Writing nursing care plan 6. Consulting
Implementation	To administer nursing actions necessary for accomplishing the care plan	1. Reassessing client 2. Reviewing and modifying existing care plan 3. Performing nursing actions
Evaluation	To determine the extent to which goals of care have been achieved	1. Comparing client response to criteria 2. Analyzing reasons for results and conclusions

Table 1-2

Example of the Diagnostic Process

Assessment	Data Clusters	Analysis	Nursing Diagnosis
Inspection of skin	Open lesion on sacrum 1 × 1 cm Red area 3 × 3 cm around coccyx	Pressure on coccyx	
Palpation of skin	Skin moist from diaphoresis	Skin moisture promotes breakdown	
	Tenderness noted around lesion		**Impaired Skin Integrity** related to immobility secondary to traction
Historical data	Fractured left leg on 5/3	Immobility	
	Positioned on back for traction to leg for 2 weeks; anticipate 4 more weeks minimum		

Identifying the Second Part of the Diagnostic Statement

Etiology or contributing factors for a nursing diagnosis are the second part of the statement and are linked with the connecting phrase "related to." It is essential that the related factor communicates something that nurses can address within the domain of nursing practice. Interventions are selected based primarily on this part of the nursing diagnosis. The contributing factors would be validated with the client when possible. For example, the diagnosis **Impaired Physical Mobility** could be related to "pain, weakness, or lack of balance." One can understand that interventions for pain are very different than those for weakness or lack of balance. In some cases the contributing factors are unknown. The statement could read, ". . . related to unknown factors," and interventions involve assessment for contributing factors. More than one contributing factor may be identified for a single nursing diagnosis.

When the primary nursing focus needs to be client teaching, the second part of the nursing diagnosis is "lack of knowledge of (specific topic)." Example: **High Risk for Injury** related to lack of knowledge of safe transfer and crutch-walking techniques.

When assessment reveals that a client has significant risk factors that could contribute to a nursing diagnosis, the second part of the statement includes identified risk factors, and the focus becomes prevention. Example: **High Risk for Impaired Skin Integrity** related to immobility and diaphoresis. In this case, interventions are directed toward promoting mobility, positioning, and dry skin, all of which prevent skin breakdown.

Because physicians are responsible for the treatment of medical diagnoses, it is not appropriate to use a medical diagnosis in a nursing diagnosis statement. When it is difficult to identify an etiology or contributing factor different from the medical diagnosis, the client's response to the medical problem may be the contributing factor. For example, **Impaired mobility** related to fractured femur would be incorrect. However, the nurse might ask "What is this client's response to the fracture?" **Impaired mobility** related to pain secondary to fracture would be accurate.

It is also ineffective to repeat the same concept in different words for the first and second parts of the nursing diagnosis; for example, **Fluid Volume Deficit** related to dehydration. This statement does not identify contributing factors, which could include either increased losses or decreased intake. Knowing the contributing factors directs the nurse toward identifying appropriate interventions.

This text includes information in each chapter that identifies nursing diagnoses that are related to the interventions and skills for that chapter. This information includes a description of the diagnostic statement, related factors that may be pertinent, and the focus for related nursing care. By reviewing this information, the reader is able to compare applicable data and determine which diagnosis would best communicate a client's particular needs.

Planning

Planning includes identifying goals and expected outcomes derived from the nursing diagnosis, determining priorities, and selecting nursing actions that will facilitate goal achievement. Goals and expected outcomes are specific statements of client behaviors or responses that the nurse anticipates from nursing care. Each must be realistic, observable, client centered, and mutually set with the client. Goals reflect the client's highest level of wellness, for example, client practices self management techniques for diabetes. Expected outcomes are specific, step-by-step achievements that help the client achieve the goals of care and resolution of the etiology for the nursing diagnosis. Expected outcomes must be measurable and specify a time frame. An example of an expected outcome is as follows: Client will demonstrate insulin self-injection by 3/20. At the time specified, progress toward achievement is evaluated, and if necessary, the plan of care is revised. For the purpose of this text, outcomes will be described behaviorally; to avoid redundancy, expected time frames will not be included.

Implementation

Implementation involves putting the plan into action. To be most effective, the care plan will include nursing interventions that are individualized to the client's needs. These include what, when, how much, how far, how long, how often, where, by whom, and with what. For example, "Encourage ambulation" is not adequate. Acceptable nursing interventions may include "Assist to walk to bathroom two times on 5/9"; "Assist to ambulate in hall at least 20 feet two times on 5/9"; and "Assist to ambulate 50 feet three times on 5/10."

Evaluation

The nursing process is dynamic and continuous. Whether or not outcomes were achieved by the target date should be well documented. If not achieved, the interventions or expected outcomes should be revised. Often, changing the target date is all that is required. When expected outcomes are achieved, the goals of care are met and the nursing diagnosis can be documented as "resolved." Evidence of systematic evaluation of the nursing process is one of the standards of the Joint Commission on Accreditation of Healthcare Organizations (JCAHO, 1993).

Skill 1.1

STANDARD PROTOCOLS FOR ALL NURSING INTERVENTIONS

All nursing skills must include certain basic steps for the safety and well-being of the client and the nurse. To save space and prevent repetition, *these steps are not included in each skill unless it is necessary to clarify them as applied for that skill.* Remember that these steps are essential and must be followed to deliver appropriate and responsible nursing care.

A logo is used in this text to identify circumstances when the use of clean gloves is recommended. Clean gloves are used to protect both caregivers and the clients. By wearing clean, disposable gloves before contact with mucous membranes, nonintact skin, or moist body substances, most microorganisms are kept off the caregiver's hands. However, gloves are not 100% effective and can have invisible small holes or tears. Handwashing after removing the gloves effectively prevents transfer of microor-

ganisms to other clients. The following logo is used to indicate situations in which the likelihood of contact with mucous membranes, nonintact skin, or moist body substances is increased.

Effective handwashing, as well as changing clean gloves, is required between clients and between activities with the same client when gloves become excessively soiled (Centers for Disease Control (CDC), 1992).

Equipment
Armband for client identification
Consent form (if required by agency policy)
Clean disposable gloves (if contact with body secretions or excretions is anticipated)

IMPLEMENTATION

Steps	Rationale

Before the skill

1. Verify physician's orders if skill is a dependent or collaborative nursing intervention. Independent nursing interventions may be verified with the nursing care plan, Kardex, or primary nurse.

Dependent and collaborative interventions include most invasive procedures, such as medications and urinary catheterization. Check agency policy.

2. Identify client by checking armband and having client state name (if able to do so).

Armbands are standard for client identification in most agencies. Clients who have difficulty hearing or have an altered level of consciousness may answer to a name other than their own. Some agencies use armbands to communicate special safety concerns, such as allergies.

3. Introduce yourself to client, including your name and title or role, and explain what you plan to do.

Clients have the right to know what will be done and by whom, as well as when those involved are students (American Hospital Association, 1992; see Box 1-4 on pp. 10-11).

4. Explain the procedure and the reason it is to be done in terms client can understand.

Understanding what is being done enhances client's ability and willingness to cooperate. Client has the right to relevant, current, and understandable information (American Hospital Association, 1992).

5. Assess client to determine that the intervention is still appropriate. (Each skill has an assessment section that includes appropriate specific findings.)

Clients have the right to make decisions about the plan of care before and during the course of treatment (American Hospital Association, 1992).

6. Gather equipment and complete necessary charges.

Some equipment is reusable and is kept at the bedside. Some equipment is disposable and charged to the client as used. Check agency policy.

7. Wash hands for at least 10 to 15 seconds before each new client contact (see Skill 3.1 on p. 50).

Handwashing is the most important technique in prevention and control of the transmission of microorganisms (CDC, 1992).

8. Adjust the bed to appropriate height and lower side rail on the side nearest you.

Minimizes muscle strain on caregivers and helps prevent injury and fatigue.

Box 1-4 A Patient's Bill of Rights

Introduction

Effective health care requires collaboration between patients and physicians and other health care professionals. Open and honest communication, respect for personal and professional values, and sensitivity to differences are integral to optimal patient care. As the setting for the provision of health services, hospitals must provide a foundation for understanding and respecting the rights and responsibilities of patients, their families, physicians, and other caregivers. Hospitals must ensure a health care ethic that respects the role of patients in decision making about treatment choices and other aspects of their care. Hospitals must be sensitive to cultural, racial, linguistic, religious, age, gender, and other differences, as well as the needs of persons with disabilities.

The American Hospital Association presents *A Patient's Bill of Rights* with the expectation that it will contribute to more effective patient care and be supported by the hospital on behalf of the institution, its medical staff, employees, and patients. The American Hospital Association encourages health care institutions to tailor this bill of rights to their patient community by translating and/or simplifying the language of this bill of rights as may be necessary to ensure that patients and their families understand their rights and responsibilities.

Bill of Rights*

1. The patient has the right to considerate and respectful care.
2. The patient has the right to and is encouraged to obtain from physicians and other direct caregivers relevant, current, and understandable information concerning diagnosis, treatment, and prognosis.

    Except in emergencies when the patient lacks decision-making capacity and the need for treatment is urgent, the patient is entitled to the opportunity to discuss and request information related to the specific procedures and/or treatments, the risks involved, the possible length of recuperation, and the medically reasonable alternatives and their accompanying risks and benefits.

    Patients have the right to know the identity of physicians, nurses, and others involved in their care, as well as when those involved are students, residents, or other trainees. The patient also has the right to know the immediate and long-term financial implications of treatment choices, insofar as they are known.

3. The patient has the right to make decisions about the plan of care prior to and during the course of treatment and to refuse a recommended treatment or plan of care to the extent permitted by law and hospital policy and to be informed of the medical consequences of this action. In case of such refusal, the patient is entitled to other appropriate care and services that the hospital provides or transfer to another hospital. The hospital should notify patients of any policy that might affect patient choice within the institution.

4. The patient has the right to have an advance directive (such as a living will, health care proxy, or durable power of attorney for health care) concerning treatment or designating a surrogate decision maker with the expectation that the hospital will honor the intent of that directive to the extent permitted by law and hospital policy.

    Health care institutions must advise patients of their rights under the state law and hospital policy to make informed medical choices, ask if the patient has an advance directive, and include that information in patient records. The patient has the right to timely information about hospital policy that may limit the hospital's ability to implement fully a legally valid advance directive.

5. The patient has the right to every consideration of privacy. Case discussion, consultation, examination, and treatment should be conducted so as to protect each patient's privacy.

6. The patient has the right to expect that all communications and records pertaining to care will be treated as confidential by the hospital, except in cases such as suspected abuse and public health hazards when reporting is permitted or required by law. The patient has the right to expect that the hospital will emphasize the confidentiality of this information when it releases it to any other parties entitled to review information in these records.

7. The patient has the right to review the records pertaining to medical care and to have the information explained or interpreted as necessary, except when restricted by law.

Box 1-4 A Patient's Bill of Rights—cont'd

8. The patient has the right to expect that, within its capacity and policies, a hospital will make reasonable response to the request of a patient for appropriate and medically indicated care and services. The hospital must provide evaluation, service, and/or referral as indicated by the urgency of the case. When medically appropriate and legally permissible, or when a patient has so requested, a patient may be transferred to another facility. The institution to which the patient is to be transferred must first have accepted the patient for transfer. The patient must also have the benefit of complete information and explanation concerning the need for, risks, benefits, and alternatives to such a transfer.

9. The patient has the right to ask and be informed of the existence of business relationships among the hospital, educational institutions, other health care providers, or payors that may influence the patient's treatment and care.

10. The patient has the right to consent to or decline to participate in proposed research studies or human experimentation affecting care and treatment or requiring direct patient involvement, and to have those studies fully explained prior to consent. A patient who declines to participate in research or experimentation is entitled to the most effective care that the hospital can otherwise provide.

11. The patient has the right to expect reasonable continuity of care when appropriate and to be informed by physicians and other caregivers of available and realistic patient care options when hospital care is no longer appropriate.

12. The patient has the right to be informed of hospital policies and practices that relate to patient care, treatment, and responsibilities. The patient has the right to be informed of available resources for resolving disputes, grievances, and conflicts, such as ethics committees, patient representatives, or other mechanisms available in the institution. The patient has the right to be informed of the hospital's charges for services and available payment methods.

The collaborative nature of health care requires that patients, or their families/surrogates, participate in their care. The effectiveness of care and patient satisfaction with the course of treatment depend, in part, on the patient fulfilling certain responsibilities. Patients are responsible for providing information about past illnesses, hospitalizations, medications, and other matters related to health status. To participate effectively in decision making, patients must be encouraged to take responsibility for requesting additional information or clarification about their health status or treatment when they do not fully understand information and instructions. Patients are also responsible for ensuring that the health care institution has a copy of their written advance directive if they have one. Patients are responsible for informing their physicians and other caregivers if they anticipate problems in following prescribed treatment.

Patients should also be aware of the hospital's obligation to be reasonably efficient and equitable in providing care to other patients and the community. The hospital's rules and regulations are designed to help the hospital meet this obligation. Patients and their families are responsible for making reasonable accommodations to the needs of the hospital, other patients, medical staff, and hospital employees. Patients are responsible for providing necessary information for insurance claims and for working with the hospital to make payment arrangements, when necessary.

A person's health depends on much more than health care services. Patients are responsible for recognizing the impact of their life-style on their personal health.

Conclusion

Hospitals have many functions to perform, including the enhancement of health status, health promotion, and the prevention and treatment of injury and disease; the immediate and ongoing care and rehabilitation of patients; the education of health professionals, patients, and the community; and research. All these activities must be conducted with an overriding concern for the values and dignity of patients.

Steps	Rationale
9. Provide privacy for client. Position and drape client as needed.	Respect for privacy is basic for preserving human dignity. Clients have the right to privacy (American Hospital Association, 1992).
During the skill	
10. Promote client involvement if possible.	Participation enhances client motivation and cooperation.
11. Assess client tolerance, being alert for signs of discomfort and fatigue. Inability to tolerate a procedure is described in the nurses' notes.	Clients' ability to tolerate interventions varies depending on severity of illness and disability. Nurses need to use judgment in providing the opportunity for rest and comfort measures.
Completion protocol	
12. Assist client to a position of comfort and place needed items within reach. Be certain client has a way to call for help and knows how to use it.	Clients may attempt to reach items and risk falling or injury.
13. Raise the side rails and lower the bed to the lowest position.	This minimizes the risk of clients getting out of bed unattended. Nursing judgment may allow alert, cooperative clients to have side rails down during the day without risking injury (see Chapter 5).
14. Store or remove and dispose of soiled supplies and equipment.	See CDC guidelines for handling and disposal of contaminated supplies/equipment (see Chapter 3).
15. Wash hands for at least 10 seconds after client contact.	Wearing gloves does not eliminate the need to wash hands. Handwashing is the most important technique in prevention and control of the transmission of microorganisms (CDC, 1988).
16. Document client's response and expected or unexpected outcomes.	Quality documentation enhances continuity of nursing care.

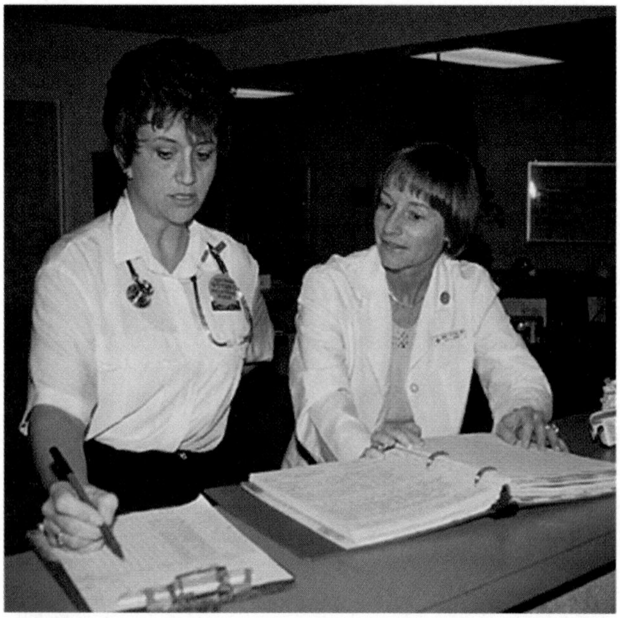

Figure 1-2 Nurses collaborate with the health care team.

COMMUNICATION WITHIN THE HEALTH CARE TEAM

Records and reports communicate specific information about a client's health care. Reports include oral and written information shared between caregivers in several ways. Nurses give a verbal or taped report when responsibility for care is being transferred (Figure 1-2). A physician may call a nursing unit to receive a verbal report on a client's progress. The laboratory provides written reports or results of diagnostic tests.

Because the nursing process shapes a nurse's approach and direction of care, good reporting and recording reflects the nursing process. Assessment results are recorded to offer to all health care members a database from which to draw conclusions about the client's problems. Information describing the client's concerns or condition assists caregivers to choose an appropriate care plan. Evaluation of client responses to nursing care determines the client's success in achieving expected outcomes of care.

Nurses involved in the direct care of clients are responsible for recording thorough assessments of a client's condition, descriptions of changes in a client's condition, a detailed accounting of nursing interventions, and an evaluation of the client's response to care. Various methods are used for nursing progress notes. Regardless of the method, certain basic guidelines must be followed (see Box 1-5, p. 13).

Box 1-5 Guidelines for Effective Documentation

Factual: includes descriptive, objective, and pertinent subjective data

Accurate: uses precise terms that facilitate comparisons

Complete: includes significant data and describes progress toward wellness

Concise: eliminates unnecessary words and repetitive information

Current: entries are made as soon as possible after completion of task

Organized: sequence of events is readily apparent

Case Management and Critical Pathways

The case management model of delivering care may use its own documentation format. This model uses a multidisciplinary plan of care that is often summarized into critical pathways. These are usually one- to two-page formats that include key interventions and expected outcomes that allow the health care team to follow integrated care plans for client problems specific to a medical condition or surgical procedure (see Appendix A).

The critical paths are used on each shift of care to direct and monitor the flow of client care. Because of the nature of human responses, there are variances in outcomes as the client deviates from the critical path plan. These variances refer to either the positive or negative changes in a client's progression toward expected outcomes (Acord-Szczesny, 1994). A variance analysis is necessary to review the data for trends and developing and implementing an action plan to respond to the identified client problems.

Computerized Records

Computers are used in health care facilities in a variety of ways, including computerized documentation systems. There are many benefits to computerized documentation, such as reduction of transcription errors, standardization of nursing care, increasing nursing productivity and efficiency, and easier monitoring of quality improvement. Computerization of data results in complete legibility and offers a structure through software design that reinforces standards of nursing care.

Computerized documentation continues to change drastically with the increased use of new technological interfaces (Chu, 1993). Notebook-sized computers with pen-based reading functions, handwriting recognition capabilities, and automated speech-recognition systems are examples of technology that is influencing nursing documentation.

Acuity Systems

Acuity of care refers to the time required for client care based on the number and type of nursing interventions required and the length of time needed for each. Calculation of the acuity of care for clients on a given unit assists administrators to determine staff requirements for the next shift. In many agencies this is a computerized process.

THE MEDICAL RECORD

The medical record is a legal document. Through accurate documentation the record serves as a description of exactly what happened in the health care system. The purpose of the record is to provide information for communication, education, assessment, research, financial billing, auditing, and legal accountability. Nursing care actually provided may have been excellent; however, in a court of law, "care not documented is care not done."

Agencies use a variety of forms to make documentation of medical and nursing interventions easy, quick, and comprehensive. Ideally, forms are designed to make data easy to find and interpret, and to avoid unnecessary duplication. Most of the forms have a place for client identification, date and times, and a key to indicate the meaning of abbreviations/entries used and the type of information required. Because of legal requirements, certain guidelines for correct recording must be followed (Table 1-3). Medical record forms that nurses have traditionally used for documentation include nursing admission history, physical assessment and vital signs graphic, medication administration records, nurses' notes, and nursing care flow sheets (see Appendix A).

In addition, many agencies have a variety of worksheets that are useful for routine client care and that are not a permanent part of the record (Box 1-6). An example includes the nursing Kardex, which is kept at the nurses' station as a resource for caregivers regarding current orders for activities of daily living (ADLs), diagnostic tests ordered, and in some cases standard or individualized nursing care plans. The Kardex is being replaced in many agencies with a computerized client care summary, which is automatically updated when any new orders are entered and provides a current summary of physicians' and nurses' orders (Figure 1-3).

GUIDELINES FOR EFFECTIVE REPORTING AND RECORDING

Factual

A factual record or report contains descriptive objective information about what a nurse sees, hears, feels, or smells. An objective description (e.g., pulse 54, strong and irregular) is the result of physical assessment skills. Words such as *good, adequate, fair,* or *poor* are subject to interpretation and should be avoided. Inferences are conclusions based

Table 1-3

Guidelines for Correct Recording

Guideline	Correct Action
Do not erase, apply correction fluid, or scratch out errors made while recording.	Draw a single line through the error, write the word "error" above it, and sign your name or initials. Then record the note correctly.
Do not leave blank spaces in nurses' notes.	Draw a line horizontally through the space and sign your name at its end.
Record all entries legibly and permanently.	Use black or blue ink for all entries (check agency policy for type of ink preferred); never use pencil, which can be erased.
Begin each entry with the time and end with your signature and title (students may be required to sign an abbreviation of their school).	Sign using first initial, complete last name, and title (C. Robinson, RN *or* T. Wallace, SN, U of I).

Box 1-6 Nursing Documentation Forms and Worksheets

Nursing History Forms

Completed when a client is admitted to a nursing unit. Includes basic biographical data (e.g., age, method of admission, physician), admitting medical diagnosis or chief complaint, a brief medical-surgical history (e.g., previous surgeries or illnesses, allergies, medication history, client's perceptions about illness or hospitalization, physical assessment of all body systems). Encourages a systematic complete assessment and identification of relevant nursing diagnoses. Provides baseline data to compare with changes in the client's condition. The JCAHO (1993) requires a nursing assessment be completed for each client at the time of admission to a health care agency.

Graphic Sheets and Flow Sheets

Include routine observations on a repeated basis using a check mark (e.g., when bath is given, client is turned). When completing a flow sheet, the nurse should review previous entries to identify changes.

Computerized Patient Care Summary

Includes pertinent information about clients and their on-going care plans, such as the following:

1. Basic demographic data (e.g., age, physician's name, religion)
2. Primary medical diagnosis
3. Current physician's orders to be carried out routinely
4. Nursing orders or interventions
5. Scheduled tests or procedures
6. Safety precautions to be used in the client's care
7. Factors related to ADLs

Nursing Kardex (Worksheet)

Includes information needed for daily care on a flip card or in a notebook. Usually kept at the nurses' station. Information can be used for change-of-shift report and facilitates access to information without referring to the client record. Includes demographic data, tests ordered, therapies, and information related to ADLs. May include standardized or individualized nursing care plans.

---

on factual data. For example, an inference might be, "The client has a poor appetite." The factual data is, "The client ate only two bites of toast for breakfast." Suppose that in one case the client was nauseated, whereas in another case the client was hungry but did not like the food on the tray. If nurses document inferences or conclusions without supportive factual data, misinterpretations about the client's health status occur.

Subjective data include clients' perceptions about their health problems. Documentation using the client's words in quotes; for example: The client states she is "nauseated" or The client states she "does not like the food choices," is factual and acceptable. In both cases, it would be helpful to document the actual food intake, as well as the subjective data.

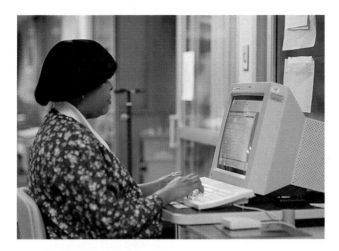

Figure 1-3   Data entry using a computer.

A comparison of a concise and lengthy note follows:

Concise, factual entry	**Lengthy entry using vague terms**
0900 L toes cool and pale; capillary return > 5 sec; L pedal pulse 1+; R pedal pulse 4+. Describes pain as dull, aching 4 (scale 0–10).	0900 The client's left toes are cool, with pale color. There is no inflammation. There is slow capillary return present exceeding 5 seconds. Dorsalis pedis pulse in left foot is weak, and the client complains of some discomfort. The pain is described as aching at a level of 4 on a scale of 0–10.

Accurate

Accurate documentation uses reliable, precise measurements as a means to determine when a client's condition has changed. Charting that an "abdominal wound is 5 cm in length, without redness or edema" is more accurate and descriptive than "large abdominal wound is healing well." To avoid misunderstandings, use only approved agency abbreviations and write out all terms that may be confusing. For example, o.d. (once daily) could be misinterpreted to mean OD (right eye). Correct spelling is essential, because terms can easily be misinterpreted (e.g., accept or except, dysphagia or dysphasia). When observations are reported to another caregiver and interventions are performed by someone else, clearly indicate that fact (e.g., "Surgical dressings removed by Dr. Kline. Pulse of 104 reported to J. Kemp, RN"). End each entry with first name or first initial, last name, and title. Nursing students include the approved abbreviation for the school and level.

Complete

Complete and concise information is essential. Consider the following example of what may occur when a note has not been recorded completely.

A nurse does not document or report the teaching session about giving insulin injections. During the next shift, another nurse spends time assessing Mrs. Blake's learning needs because the previous teaching was not communicated. Time is wasted, and Mrs. Blake becomes frustrated with the unnecessary repetition.

Current

To be current, the following activities or findings need to be communicated at the time of occurrence:

1. Critical changes in vital signs
2. Administration of medications and treatments
3. Preparation for diagnostic tests or surgery
4. Critical change in status
5. Admission, transfer, discharge, or death of a client

Refer to the client's concern, nursing interventions provided, and client response as soon as possible after the occurrence. Writing scratch notes at the time of the event helps ensure accuracy in documentation. Many agencies use military time, a 24-hour system that uses digit numbers to indicate morning, afternoon, and evening times (Table 1-4).

Table 1-4

Comparison of Military and Civilian Times

Military	Civilian
0100	1:00 AM
0200	2:00 AM
0415	4:15 AM
1200	Noon
1420	2:20 PM
1800	6:00 PM
2400	Midnight
0001	12:01 AM

Organized

The following compares a well-organized note with a disorganized note:

Organized note	Disorganized note
7/17 0630 Client reports sharp pain 9 (scale 0–10) in left lower quadrant of abdomen, worsened by turning onto right side. Positioning on left side decreases pain to 8 (scale 0–10). Abdomen is tender to touch and rigid. Bowel sounds are absent. Dr. Phillips notified. To x-ray for CT scan of abdomen. T. Reis, RN	7/17 0630 Client experiencing sharp pain in lower quadrant of abdomen. MD notified. Abdomen tender to touch, rigid, with bowel sounds absent. Positioning on left side offers minimal relief of pain. CT scan ordered of the abdomen. J. Adams, RN

CONFIDENTIALITY

Nurses are legally and ethically obligated to keep information about clients confidential. When health care professionals have reason to use records for data gathering, research, or education, there is no break in confidentiality as long as the records are used with permission and according to established guidelines.

HOME HEALTH CARE DOCUMENTATION

In the home setting, documentation is the crucial element for continuity of nursing care; it provides evidence of achieving nursing standards and is the basis for reimbursement for home health care services. Because Medicare has specific guidelines for eligibility for reimbursement, documentation that fulfills these guidelines is essential. Both quality of care and justification for financial reimbursement depend on effective documentation (Braunstein, 1993). Because some parts of the record are needed in the home and other parts are needed in the caregiver's office, methods are being developed to include the use of modems and laptop computers (Miller, 1995).

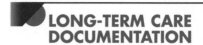

LONG-TERM CARE DOCUMENTATION

The challenges of caring for residents in long-term care are very different from the acute care setting, which creates significant differences in documentation (Iyer and Camp, 1995). For example, acute care charting includes frequent physical assessment findings (e.g., vital signs, head-to-toe assessment), in some cases using an hourly format, or at least every shift. For stable long-term care residents, these entries may be made weekly or monthly. Outside agencies such as the state department of health determine the standards and policies for long-term care documentation. The RN is responsible for identifying episodic changes that may require more intensive nursing intervention and documentation for residents who become ill.

Charting by Exception

Charting by exception is an innovative approach to streamline documentation by reducing repetition and time spent in charting (Iyer and Camp, 1995). It is a shorthand method for documenting normal findings and routine care based on clearly defined standards of practice and predetermined criteria for nursing assessments and interventions. With standards integrated into documentation forms, such as predefined normal assessment findings or predetermined interventions, a nurse needs to document only significant findings or exceptions to the predefined norms. In other words, the nurse writes a variance note only when the standardized statement on the form is not met. Assessments are standardized on forms so that all caregivers evaluate and document findings consistently.

Because the standard assessments are located in the chart, client data are already present on the permanent record, so nurses do not have to keep temporary notes for later transcription. In addition, caregivers have easy access to current data. The assumption with charting by exception is that all standards are met with a normal or expected response unless otherwise documented. When nurses see entries in the chart, they know that something out of the ordinary has been observed or has occurred.

Skill 1.2

RECORDING

Because the nursing process shapes a nurse's approach to client care, good documentation reflects the nursing process. Assessment data are recorded to provide all health care team members with a database from which to make decisions about the client's needs and problems. After a plan of care is developed, with goals and expected outcomes established, documentation needs to include a description of nursing care provided. Evaluation of care communicates the client's degree of progress toward wellness and success in meeting expected outcomes of care.

Progress notes are a form of recording that document a client's progress. A variety of formats may be used for progress notes, including SOAP (acronym for Subjective data, Objective data, Assessment or Analysis, and Plan); SOAPE (which adds Evaluation to the previous acronym); PIE (acronym for Problem, Intervention, and Evaluation); APIE (acronym for Assessment, Plan, Intervention, and Evaluation); and DAR (Data, Action, and Response) used in focus charting (Box 1-7). Any caregiver needs to be able to read a progress note and understand what type of problem a client has, the level of care provided, and the results of the interventions.

Box 1-7 Formats for Recording

PIE: Acronym for Problem, Intervention, and Evaluation. Problem-oriented system in which progress notes are written based on a list of identified problems, and detailed data may be entered by any member of the health care team. For example:

P: Problem—Client states, "I am dreading this surgery because last time I had a terrible reaction to the anesthesia and had such terrible pain when they made me get out of bed." Noted muscle tension and loud, agitated voice.

I: Intervention—Notified anesthesiologist, Dr. Moore of experience. Discussed alternatives for anesthesia and pain-control options. Stressed importance of activity for circulation and healing. Encouraged to keep nurses informed of pain level and need for medication and told client that pain usually is present, but manageable.

E: Evaluation—Client stated she was "very relieved." Stated she would tell the nurses about pain.

SOAP: Acronym for Subjective data, Objective data, Assessment or Analysis, and Plan. Usually based on a numbered list of problems or nursing diagnoses. For example:

S: Subjective data—The client's statements regarding the problem. (e.g. Client states, "I am dreading this surgery because last time I had a terrible reaction to the anesthesia and had such terrible pain when they made me get out of bed.")

O: Objective data—Observations that support or are related to subjective data. (e.g. Noted muscle tension and loud, agitated voice.)

A: Assessment/Analysis—Conclusions reached based on data. Intense fear related to pain/anesthesia.

P: Plan—The plan for dealing with the situation. (e.g. Notified anesthesiologist, Dr. Moore, of experience. Dis-

cussed alternatives for anesthesia and pain-control options. Stressed importance of activity for circulation and healing. Encouraged to keep nurses informed of pain level and need for medication and told client that pain usually is present, but manageable.)

Focus Charting: A way to organize progress notes to make them more clear and organized. For example:

D: Data—Client states, "I am dreading this surgery because last time I had a terrible reaction to the anesthesia and had such terrible pain when they made me get out of bed." Noted muscle tension and loud, agitated voice.

A: Action—Notified anesthesiologist, Dr. Moore, of experience. Discussed alternatives for anesthesia and pain-control options. Stressed importance of activity for circulation and healing. Encouraged to keep nurses informed of pain level and need for medication and told client that pain usually is present, but manageable.

R: Response—Client stated she was "very relieved." Stated she would tell the nurses about pain.

Narrative Note: Describes client data in a narrative paragraph. For example:

Client states, "I am dreading this surgery because last time I had a terrible reaction to the anesthesia and had such terrible pain when they made me get out of bed." Noted muscle tension and loud, agitated voice. Notified anesthesiologist, Dr. Moore, of experience. Discussed alternatives for anesthesia and pain-control options. Stressed importance of activity for circulation and healing. Encouraged to keep nurses informed of pain level and need for medication and told client that pain usually is present, but manageable.

Equipment
Forms (manual or computer)

ASSESSMENT

1. Review assessments, goals and expected outcomes, interventions, and client responses as soon as possible after contact with each client. **Rationale: This facilitates use of documentation as a method of reviewing and evaluating the effectiveness of the nursing care provided and the need for a change in the plan.**

PLANNING

Planning documentation includes reviewing the nursing process as it has been utilized and clarifying pertinent subjective and objective data that communicate progress toward goals.

DELEGATION CONSIDERATIONS

Charting progress notes requires problem solving and knowledge unique to a professional nurse. Delegation to AP is inappropriate. Some documentation may be delegated, including vital signs, intake and output (I&O), and routine care related to ADLs. It is essential to give clear information regarding what should be reported for appropriate follow-up.

IMPLEMENTATION

Steps	Rationale

1. Identify the forms you are expected to maintain and where they are located.
  a. Forms at the bedside or on a rack just outside the door may include a graphic chart for vital signs, Intake and Output (I&O) record, checklist of flow sheet for routine care or CareMap, medication administration record, and nurses' progress notes (see sample forms in Appendix •).
  b. Other nursing forms that may be included under certain circumstances are IV flow sheets; diabetic record; pain-management flow sheet; admission, transfer, and discharge forms; and teaching documentation.
	Provides information about where to look for information, as well as what information is required.

2. After each client contact, identify information that needs to be documented. Consider:
  a. Abnormal findings
  b. Changes in status
  c. New problems identified
	Prompt documentation increases accuracy and promotes effective communication to other members of the health care team.

3. Document in a timely fashion, without leaving open spaces between notes, and include date and time.	Prompt documentation provides accurate record of client status and prevents omissions resulting from unexpected events.

4. Using agency format, determine the most effective way to include significant changes, including:
  a. Pertinent, factual, objective data
  b. Selected subjective data that validates or clarifies
  c. Nursing actions taken
  d. Client responses to actions taken
  e. Additional plans that should be implemented
  f. To whom the information has been reported, including name and status
	When additional follow-up is needed, documenting to whom this has been reported shares responsibility with that individual.

Steps	Rationale
5. Sign progress note with full name or first initial and last name and status according to agency policy. Students are usually required to indicate their level of education and school affiliation.	Identifies persons responsible for client care.

Skill 1.3

GIVING A CHANGE-OF-SHIFT REPORT

In addition to written documentation, nurses report information about their assigned clients to the nurses working on the next shift. The purpose of the report is to provide continuity of care for the client. A change-of-shift report may be given orally in person, by audiotape recording, or with rounds from client to client (Figure 1-4). Oral reports are given in a conference room with nurses from both shifts participating. When an audiotape is used, the report is recorded before the end of the shift. This allows the nurses who are preparing to leave to finish last-minute tasks while the oncoming staff listens to the report. It is beneficial to allow time for clarification or updates before the previous nurses leave the unit. Reports given in person or on rounds allow immediate feedback when questions are raised. Confidentiality must be maintained.

Equipment
> Worksheets, nursing Kardex or client care profile, nursing care plan, critical pathway or multidisciplinary treatment plan
> Tape recorder (according to agency policy)

ASSESSMENT

1. Review information on worksheets, get report from co-workers to whom care has been delegated, and gather other relevant information (e.g., pertinent assessment data, laboratory reports, physicians' orders). **Rationale: Data reported needs to reflect changes during the shift and be pertinent, specific, and accurate. Preparation enhances a clear, well-organized report with fewer pauses.**

PLANNING

Expected outcomes focus on identifying appropriate information to report to the nurses on the next shift.

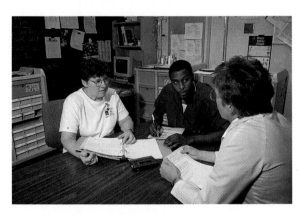

Figure 1-4 Giving a change-of-shift report.

DELEGATION CONSIDERATIONS

The skill of change-of-shift report requires problem solving and knowledge application unique to a professional nurse. For this skill, delegation is inappropriate. However, AP should know what to report to a nurse (e.g., apparent change in client's level of pain, reduction in level of consciousness, change in vital signs) so that the nurse may include any pertinent information (after validation) in the report.

IMPLEMENTATION

Steps	Rationale
1. Develop an organized format for delivering report that provides a description of the client's needs and concerns.	Organizes data based on priorities and individualized by the reporting nurse.
2. For each client, include:	
a. *Background information*—Include client's name, gender, age, current primary reason for hospitalization, and brief history. Also include any known allergies, code status (i.e., do not resuscitate), and special needs as related to any physical challenges (e.g., blind, hearing deficit, amputee).	A more in-depth background report may be needed if a nurse new to a unit or an inexperienced nurse will be working the next shift.
b. *Assessment data*—Provide objective observations and measurements made by the nurse during the shift. Describe client's condition and emphasize any recent changes. Include any *relevant* information reported by client, family, or health care team members, such as laboratory data and diagnostic test results.	Oncoming nurse will use data as a baseline for comparison during next shift.
c. *Nursing diagnoses*—Explain clearly the nursing diagnoses appropriate for client.	
d. *Interventions and evaluation*—(steps can be combined in a report).	Clarifies client's current responses to health problems.
(1) Describe therapies or treatments administered during shift and expected outcomes (e.g., medication changes, laboratory results, consultation visits). Specify how interventions are uniquely given for this client. Explain client's response and whether outcomes are met. The format of evaluation could take the format of a critical pathway and the utilization of variance documentation. Do not explain basic steps of procedure.	Staff learn the effect interventions are having on client's recovery and progress.
(2) Describe instructions given in teaching plan and client's ability to demonstrate learning.	Ensures continuity of teaching, minimizing repetition, but communicating any needs for reinforcement.
e. *Family information*—Report on family visitation or involvement, specifically as it influenced client. Explain if family members were included in care procedures or instruction.	Informs staff as to level of involvement family members have assumed in client's care.
f. *Discharge plan*—The client's progress in reaching discharge is reviewed on an ongoing basis during each change-of-shift report. Discuss status of educational progress, communication with referral agencies, and preparation of family members for clients who are being discharged. This plan also identifies the roles and responsibilities of the multidisciplinary team and their follow-up visits.	All team members collaborate to follow the plan of care that promotes discharge. The discharge plan identifies the interventions and outcomes needed to allow the client to have a smooth transition from hospital or health care facility to home.
g. *Current priorities*—Explain clearly the priorities to which oncoming nurse must attend.	
(1) Report on the immediate treatment planned for a newly admitted client.	
(2) Explain the status of specific preparatory activities for clients who are going for diagnostic or treatment procedures.	

Steps	Rationale

(3) Describe current physical status of clients returning from diagnostic or operative procedures.

• • •

EVALUATION

1. Ask staff from the oncoming shift if they have questions regarding information reported.
2. When using a tape recorder, periodically self-evaluate for clarity, organization, rate of speaking, and volume level.

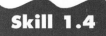

Skill 1.4

WRITING AN INCIDENT REPORT

An incident is any event that is not consistent with the routine operation of the health care unit or routine care of a client. Clients, visitors, and employees may be at risk when unusual occurrences take place. Examples of incidents include client falls, needle-stick injuries, and medication errors. Incidents may involve both actual and potential injuries.

When an incident occurs, the nurse involved or who witnesses the incident completes an incident report, which helps identify circumstances or system problems that may be correctable. The report is essential even when an injury is not apparent. The information helps identify ways to prevent repeated occurrences.

Equipment

Incident report form (see Appendix A)

ASSESSMENT

1. Use critical-thinking skills to systematically and carefully determine exactly what was involved in the incident and factors that may have contributed to the situation. **Rationale: The best reporting includes objective, accurate, and detailed information in chronological order. The person(s) who witnessed the incident or who discovered it files the report.**

2. The first priority is the safety and well-being of the client. Assess the need to notify the physician immediately. Visitors or employees may need to go to the emergency room or employee health department for follow-up care.

PLANNING

Planning an incident report includes reviewing the details involved in the situation and clarifying contributing factors and potential outcomes.

DELEGATION CONSIDERATIONS

Incident reporting often involves AP who actually find the client situation requiring the report. Caregivers need to know what actions to take, as well as the importance of specific details when reporting to the nurse. Writing the incident report requires the problem solving and knowledge unique to a professional nurse. Therefore, delegation is inappropriate.

IMPLEMENTATION

Steps	Rationale
1. Complete the incident report form as quickly as possible, completely, and accurately.	An incident can result in a lawsuit.
2. Describe objectively what was observed when the incident was discovered, taking care to avoid personal opinions and feelings. Include times, witnesses (names and status), condition of individual, and who was notified at what time (Table 1-5).	Establishes a factual basis for comparison with later developments.
3. Describe measures taken by any caregivers at the time of the incident, including assessment of body systems.	
4. Sign the report and obtain additional signatures (e.g., physician, nursing supervisor) as required by agency.	Provides a mechanism for keeping all appropriate persons informed.
5. Document factual data on the client's medical record, including the incident and related assessments and interventions. Do not include details contrary to agency policy, and do not include any reference to having completed an incident report.	Client's medical records are legally recoverable and can be used in court. Incident reports are the property of the institution. Incident reports can be recoverable through a subpoena if information in the medical record validates that a report was completed.

• • •

EVALUATION

1. Seek to identify actions that could help prevent similar occurrences, and collaborate with the appropriate persons to institute new or revised policies. Risk-management programs and quality-improvement programs are enhanced by involvement of professional nursing staff.

Table 1-5

Example of Incident Report Entries

Proper Entry	Incorrect Entry
6 PM Client found on floor at foot of bed; able to respond to name when called. 2-cm abrasion noted across left forehead. Vital signs stable. Dr. Smith notified and arrived on floor at 6:15 PM. Placed client on fall-prevention protocol.	Client found on floor at foot of bed, probably fell on way to bathroom. Small abrasion over left forehead. Dr. Smith notified. Client instructed to use call light when needing to go to bathroom.
1600 Morphine 10 mg given IM. Dr. Jones notified.	Administered 10 mg morphine sulfate at 4 PM.
1615 Vital signs stable. Will monitor q15min every 4 hrs.	When 6 mg was ordered because order on medication record was unclear. Client resting quietly.
2000 Vital signs stable. Client alert and oriented. Right index finger punctured by 18-gauge angiocath while turning client. Minimal bleeding. Reported to employee health department for follow-up.	Needle-stick injury to right index finger caused by RN who left 18-gauge needle in bed after starting IV 1 hour earlier.

CRITICAL THINKING EXERCISES

1. The nurses in charge in some long-term care units are responsible for delegating certain tasks to other caregivers. The AP reports that a client has abdominal pain and is asking for a laxative. The nurse is aware that the client has a history of constipation. What is necessary before deciding to delegate administration of a prescribed laxative to the client? What follow-up would be indicated?

2. After a nursing diagnosis is established for a client, the nurse is responsible for planning nursing care. What are three aspects of planning that should be included?

3. A nursing diagnosis of **Anxiety** related to unknown factors manifested by restlessness, shakiness, hyperventilation, and withdrawal is established for a 72-year-old female client who has never been hospitalized before. When planning nursing interventions, what would be the focus for dealing with the anxiety?

REFERENCES

Acord-Szczesny J: Computer tracking of critical path variations, *Inside Case Manage* 1(2):1, 1994.

American Hospital Association: *A patient's bill of rights*, Catalog No 157759, Chicago, 1992, The Association.

American Nurses Association: *Nursing's social policy statement*, Washington, DC, 1995, American Nurses Foundation/American Nurses Association.

Braunstein ML: The electronic patient records solution, *Caring* 12(7):30, 1993.

CDC: Universal precautions for prevention of human immunodeficiency virus, hepatitis B virus, and other bloodborne pathogens in health care settings, *MMWR* 37:377, 1988.

CDC: Surveillance, prevention and control of nosocomial infections, *MMWR* 41:783, 1992.

Christensen B, Kockrow E: *Foundations of nursing*, ed 2, St Louis, 1995, Mosby.

Gordon M: *Nursing diagnosis: process and application*, ed 3, St Louis, 1997, Mosby.

Iyer PW, Camp NH: *Nursing documentation: a nursing process approach*, ed 2, St Louis, 1995, Mosby.

International Council of Nurses (1973). The 1973 code for nurses. Geneva: Impimeries Populaires.

Joint Commission on Accreditation of Healthcare Organizations: *Accreditation manual for hospitals*, Chicago, 1993, The Commission.

Miller K: Home health care update 95, *Nursing 95*:7, 1995.

National Council of State Boards of Nursing: *Delegation: concepts and decision making process*, Chicago, 1995, The Council.

Potter PA, Perry AG: *Fundamentals of nursing: concepts, process, and practice*, St Louis, 1997, Mosby.

USDHHS, PHS: *Healthy people 2000: national health promotion and disease prevention objectives*, Washington DC, 1990, US Government Printing Office.

Wong DL, Perry SE: *Maternal child nursing care*, St Louis, 1998, Mosby.

UNIT TWO

Fundamental Concepts

Chapter 2
Facilitating Communication

Chapter 3
Promoting Infection Control

Chapter 4
Basic Sterile Techniques

Chapter 5
Promoting a Safe Environment

CHAPTER 2

Facilitating Communication

Skill 2.1
Establishing Therapeutic Communication, 29

Skill 2.2
Comforting, 32

Skill 2.3
Active Listening, 34

Skill 2.4
Interviewing, 36

Skill 2.5
Communicating with an Anxious Client, 40

Skill 2.6
Verbally Deescalating a Potentially Violent Client, 42

Skill 2.7
Client Teaching, 44

Communication is a basic human need and the foundation for establishing a caring relationship between the nurse and the client. Communication involves the expression of emotions, ideas, and thoughts through verbal (words or written language) and nonverbal (e.g. behaviors) exchanges. Verbal communication includes both the spoken and written word. Nonverbal communication includes body movement, physical appearance, personal space, touch, and facial expression. The interaction between the nurse and the client then progresses to a therapeutic level in which the nurse offers goal-directed activities to help the client feel comfortable sharing ideas and feelings. With practice, nurses can develop skills that limit social interactions and maintain a congenial and warm style that helps clients feel comfortable in sharing ideas and feelings.

The basic elements of communication include a message, a sender, a receiver, and feedback (Figure 2-1). The message is the information expressed, which can be motivated by experience, emotions, ideas, or actions. The message may be sent through visual, auditory, and tactile senses. Generally, the more channels used, the better the message is understood.

For communication to be effective, the receiver must be aware of the sender's message. The message received is understood as filtered through perceptions shaped from previous experiences. People tend to interpret life experiences through general assumptions and values they hold; in essence, this is the concept of filtering. The more aware people are of how these assumptions influence how they perceive the world and others, the more open they can be when interacting with others.

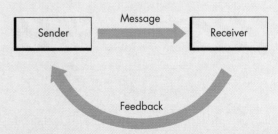

Figure 2-1 Communication is a two-way process.

Feedback, verbal or nonverbal, is a response to the sender that can indicate the meaning of the message that was received. Because communication is a two-way process, the nurse must give feedback to clients and seek feedback from clients to validate clients' understanding of the messages conveyed.

Communication is a complex process that is influenced by many factors (see Box 2-1). Each person is unique and associates different ideas with a message and interprets it differently than any other person. For example, a facial expression may convey anger to one person and pain to another. It is essential for nurses to clarify messages so that incorrect inferences and miscommunication with the client are avoided (Figure 2-2).

Silence can be therapeutic. It gives the nurse and client time to think. It is important for the nurse to notice the client's inner feelings. It is also important to pay attention to a client's nonverbal behavior for cues that suggest what the client is feeling and to reflect the nurse's impressions to validate what the client is experiencing. If silence lasts too long or becomes uncomfortable for the client, it can be helpful to say, "You seem very quiet," or "Could you tell me what you need right now?" or "How are you feeling?"

Preoccupation with the techniques of communication can interfere with rather than enhance the process; however, effective communication can be learned and requires practice, as does any other skill. An attitude of acceptance is helpful to promote open communication. To listen effectively, it helps to face clients, maintain eye contact, pay attention to what is being conveyed, and give feedback to verify accurate understanding. Even though the nurse may

not agree with clients, the nurse can accept clients' rights to their opinions. It is best to avoid arguing with clients. The nurse simply reflects an understanding of what clients are communicating without agreeing or disagreeing. Ineffective communication may not halt conversation, but it tends to inhibit clients' willingness to express concerns openly. The nurse needs to find an appropriate place, allow sufficient time, and facilitate communication according to clients' circumstances and needs. Table 2-1 summarizes techniques that facilitate and inhibit communication.

Cultural considerations relating to communication

It is important to recognize cultural diversity and to demonstrate respect for people as unique individuals. Culture is just one factor that influences communication between two persons. It is imperative that nurses be aware of cultural norms or values to enhance understanding of nonverbal cues. The nurse must consider any potential communication differences to effectively communicate with persons from other cultures (see Box 2-2).

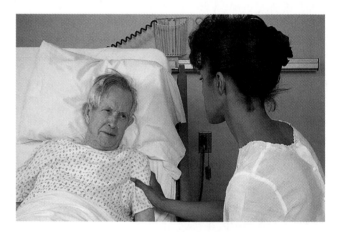

Figure 2-2 Clarify nonverbal body language.

Box 2-1 Factors That Influence Communication

Perceptions: personal views based on past experiences
Values: beliefs a person considers important in life
Emotions: subjective feelings about a situation (e.g., anger, fear, frustration, pain, anxiety, personal appearance)
Sociocultural background: language, gestures, and attitudes common for a specific group of people relating to family origin, occupation, or lifestyle
Knowledge level: level of education and experience that influences a person's knowledge base
Roles and relationships: conversation between two nurses differs from that between nurse and client
Environment: noise, lack of privacy, and distractions influence effectiveness
Space and territoriality: distance of 18 inches to 4 feet is ideal for sitting with a client for an interaction. Clients may have different needs for personal space

---

Box 2-2 Cultural Considerations for Effective Communication

- Vocal emphasis of words; avoid overly technical words or jargon
- Eye contact; may be improper to make with authority figure
- Use of touch may be inappropriate for some cultures, whereas others embrace tactile relationships
- Personal space; client may have no boundaries or may be aloof and distant
- Nonverbal behaviors; use gestures with shared meanings

Table 2-1

Facilitating and Inhibiting Communication

Technique	Examples	Rationale
INITIATING AND ENCOURAGING INTERACTION		
Giving information	"It is time for me to . . ." "I will be here until . . ."	Informs client of facts needed to understand situation. Provides a means to build trust and develop a knowledge base for client to make decisions.
Stating observations	"You are smiling." "I see you are up already."	By calling client's attention to what is observed, nurse encourages client to be aware of behavior.
Open questions/ comments	"What is your biggest concern?" "Tell me about your health."	Allows client to choose the topic of discussion according to circumstances and needs.
General leads	"And then?" "Go on . . ." "Say more . . ."	Encourages client to continue talking.
Focused questions/ comments	"Tell me about your pain." "What did your doctor say?" "How has your family reacted?" "What is your biggest fear?"	Encourages client to give more information about specific topic of concern.
HELPING CLIENT IDENTIFY AND EXPRESS FEELINGS		
Sharing observations	"You look tense." "You seem uncomfortable when . . ."	Promotes client's awareness of nonverbal behavior and feelings underlying the behavior. Helps clarify meaning of the behavior.
Paraphrasing	Client:"I could not sleep last night." Nurse: "You've had trouble sleeping?"	Encourages client to describe the situation more fully. Demonstrates that nurse is listening and concerned.
Reflecting feelings	"You were angry when that happened?" "You seem upset . . ."	Focuses client on identified feelings based on verbal or nonverbal cues.
Focused comments	"That seems worth talking about more." "Tell me more about . . ."	Encourages client to think about and describe a particular concern in more detail.
ENSURING MUTUAL UNDERSTANDING		
Seeking clarification	"I don't quite follow you . . ." "Do you mean . . . ?" "Are you saying that . . . ?"	Encourages client to expand on a topic that is not yet clear or that seems contradictory.
Summarizing	"So there are three things you are upset about, your family being too busy, your diet, and being in the hospital so long."	Reduces the interaction to three or four points identified by nurse as significant. Allows client to agree or add other concerns.
Validation	"Did I understand you correctly that . . . ?"	Allows clarification of ideas that nurse may have interpreted differently than intended by client.
INHIBITING COMMUNICATION		
"Why" questions	"Why did you eat that when you know it gives you stomach pain?" "Why did you go back to bed?"	Asks client to justify reasons. Implies criticism and makes client feel defensive. Better to focus on what happened and encourage telling the whole story.
Sidestepping or changing subject	Client: "I'm having a hard time with my family." Nurse: "Do you have any grandchildren?"	This eases nurse's own discomfort. It avoids exploring topic identified by client.
False reassurance	"Everything will be okay." "Surgery is no big deal."	This is vague and simplistic and tends to belittle client's concerns. It does not invite a response.
Giving advice	"You really should exercise more." "You shouldn't eat fast food every day."	This keeps client from actively engaging in finding a solution. Often client knows what should/should not be done and needs to explore alternative ways of dealing with issue.
Stereotyped responses	"You have the best doctor in town." "All clients with cancer worry about that."	This does not invite client to respond.
Defensiveness	"The nurses here work very hard." "Your doctor is extremely busy."	Moves focus away from client's feelings without acknowledging concerns.

- Who is the nurse from a cultural perspective?
- Who is the client from a cultural perspective?
- What is the nurse's heritage?
- What is the client's heritage?
- What are the health traditions of the nurse's heritage?
- What are the health traditions of the client's heritage?

Transcultural communication is most effective when each person attempts to understand the other's point of view from that person's cultural heritage.

Use of language, gestures, and vocal emphasis of words: Take care to determine if understanding was achieved.

Eye contact: Direct eye contact is valued in some cultures, whereas other cultures find it improper and intrusive.

Use of touch/personal space: Some cultures are "noncontact" cultures and have needs for clear boundaries; other cultures value close contact, handshakes, and embracing.

Time orientation: Many cultures are oriented to the present; some cultures value planning for the future.

Nurses need to adopt an attitude of flexibility, respect, and interest to bridge any communication barriers imposed by cultural differences.

If a client does not speak the nurse's language, a translator is needed. Often, however, the client speaks the nurse's language with limited ability or uses language with meaning different from the nurse's meaning. For example, the client may know customary greetings such as "How are you?" but not understand "pain" or "nausea." When communication fails, nurses tend to speak louder, stop talking

and concentrate on the tasks, or begin doing things for, rather than with, the client. This can result in painful isolation, anger, or misunderstanding for the client and inability of the client to cooperate. Special approaches that can help avoid these outcomes are described (see Box 2-3).

Gerontologic Considerations

Older adults with sensory losses require communication techniques that maximize existing sensory and motor functions (see Chapter 36). Some clients are unable to speak because of physical or neurological alterations, such as paralysis, a tube in the trachea to facilitate breathing (Figure 2–3), or a stroke resulting in aphasia. When a client experiences receptive aphasia, neither the sounds of speech nor its meaning can be distinguished, and comprehension of both written and spoken language is impaired. Expressive aphasia affects the motor function of speech so that the client has difficulty speaking and writing; however, the client can hear and understand. Hearing loss affects one's quality of life and may be easily overlooked by health care providers. Older adults are at higher risk for hearing impairments than the younger population. Communication is impaired when a message is lost or misinterpreted because the message is not heard due to the client's hearing loss (Lindblade and McDonald, 1995). Communication aids can facilitate communication (see Box 2-4 on p. 29).

NURSING DIAGNOSIS

Communication, involving an exchange of information, is a basic human need. **Impaired Verbal Communication** is the state in which an individual experiences a decreased or absent ability to use or understand language in human interaction (Kim, McFarland, and McLane, 1997). If a client has difficulty communicating, either sending or receiving information, several factors should be considered. Perhaps

---

Box 2-3 Special Approaches for Client Who Speaks a Different Language

Use a caring tone of voice and facial expression to help alleviate the client's fears.

Speak slowly and distinctly, but not loudly.

Use gestures, pictures, and play acting to help the client understand.

Repeat the message in different ways if necessary.

Be alert to words the client seems to understand and use them frequently.

Keep messages simple and repeat them frequently.

Avoid using medical terms that the client may not understand.

Use an appropriate language dictionary or have interpreter or family make flash cards to communicate key phrases.

Modified from Giger J. Davidhizar R: *Transcultural nursing,* St Louis, 1995, Mosby.

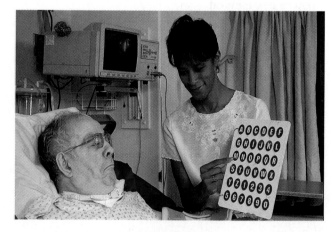

Figure 2-3 Tracheostomy interferes with speech.

Box 2-4 Communication Aids

Pad and felt-tipped pen or magic slate
Board with words, letters, or pictures denoting basic
    needs (e.g., water, bedpan, pain medication)
Call bells or alarms
Sign language
Use of eye blinks or movement of fingers for simple re-
    sponses (e.g., "yes" or "no")
Flash cards with pictures rather than words

there are language barriers; sensory/perceptual deficits; or psychological barriers such as anxiety, fear, or loneliness that are interfering with the communication process. **Anxiety, Ineffective Individual Coping,** or **Risk for Violence: Directed at Others** may be an appropriate nursing diagnosis when the focus is to help the client deal with a crisis, facilitating the expression of anxiety or anger. **Sensory/Perceptual Alterations: Auditory** or **Visual** may be an appropriate nursing diagnosis when the focus is to help enhance the client's altered communication patterns. **Social Isolation** or **Impaired Social Interaction** may be an appropriate nursing diagnosis when the client experiences loneliness or has an insufficient quantity or ineffective quality of social exchange (Kim, McFarland, and McLane, 1997).

When clients have no knowledge of an important health topic or their knowledge is deficient, **Knowledge deficit** is a possible diagnosis. The diagnosis must specify the deficit (e.g., Regarding diabetic self-care or low fat diet management) in order for the nurse to select teaching strategies.

There are two other nursing diagnoses related to client teaching. **Health-Seeking Behaviors Related to Knowledge Deficit** may be an appropriate nursing diagnosis when a client in stable health seeks ways to alter personal health habits and/or the environment in order to move toward optimal health. **Risk for Altered Health Maintenance** may be an appropriate nursing diagnosis when the client is unable to identify, manage, or seek help to maintain health. Related factors may include an alteration in communication, cognitive impairment, or lack of material resources. (Kim, McFarland, and McLane, 1997).

Skill 2.1

ESTABLISHING THERAPEUTIC COMMUNICATION

The primary goal of effective therapeutic communication for the nurse is to promote wellness and growth in clients. Therapeutic communication empowers clients to make decisions. Therapeutic communication differs from social communication in that it is client centered and goal directed with limited disclosure from the professional. However, an important aspect of therapeutic communication is the nurse's ability to show caring for the client. Caring establishes trust and creates an openness on the part of the client to communicate.

Nurses avoid sharing intimate details of their personal lives with clients. This personal self-disclosure by the nurse (e.g., if they have any children; what nursing school they attended) may occur if it may be of help to the client, such as helping the client focus on key issues. The nurse should answer questions and return the focus to the client. This may assist the nurse to establish a professional relationship with the client. Social communication that involves equal opportunity for personal disclosure and in which both participants seek to have personal needs met is not appropriate between nurses and clients (Keltner, Schwecke, and Bostrom, 1991). Factors that influence communication include the client's perceptions, values, sociocultural background, and knowledge level. See Table 2-1 on p. 27 on facilitating and inhibiting communication.

ASSESSMENT

1. Determine client's need to communicate (e.g., client who constantly uses call light, client who is crying, client who does not understand an illness, client who has just been admitted to the hospital or nursing home).
2. Assess reason client needs health care.
3. Assess factors about self and client that normally influence communication: perceptions, values and beliefs, emotions, sociocultural background, severity of illness, knowledge, age level, verbal ability, roles and relationships, environmental setting, physical comfort, and discomfort. **Rationale: Communication is a dynamic process influenced by interpersonal and intrapersonal processes. By assessing factors that influence communication, the nurse can more accurately assess the experiences of the client.**
4. Assess client's language and ability to speak. Does the client have difficulty finding words or associating ideas with accurate word symbols? Does the client have difficulty with expression of language and/or reception of messages? What is the client's primary language?

5. Observe client's pattern of communication and verbal or nonverbal behavior (e.g., gestures, tone of voice, eye contact). **Rationale: Client's patterns of communication may determine the type of and manner of communication used by the nurse.**

6. Encourage the client to ask for clarification at any time during the communication. **Rationale: This gives the client a sense of control and keeps the channels of communication open.**

PLANNING

Expected outcomes focus on using therapeutic communication skills to obtain information about the client's ideas, fears, and concerns.

Expected Outcomes

1. Client expresses ability to communicate with the nurse without feeling threatened or defensive.
2. Client expresses thoughts and feelings to the nurse through verbal and nonverbal communication.

DELEGATION CONSIDERATIONS

Effective communication is a goal of all client interactions. Although establishing therapeutic communication is a professional nursing skill, often assistive personnel (AP) are able to facilitate effective communication because of the extended length of time they are with the client. It is essential for AP to be aware of the following guidelines:

- All information discussed must be considered confidential.
- Client concerns, including anger and anxiety, should be communicated to the professional nurse to determine if additional nursing interventions are needed.
- All interactions need to be respectful and kind, including special considerations for clients who have cognitive or sensory impairment.

IMPLEMENTATION

Steps	Rationale
1. See Standard Protocol (inside front cover).	
2. Create a climate of warmth and acceptance. Consider the need to alter the environment by lowering noise level and providing privacy and comfort. Also consider timing in relation to visitors or personal routines.	Environmental factors can promote open communication.
3. Provide an introduction by addressing the client by name and introducing self and role. For example: "Hello, my name is Jane, and I am the nurse who will take care of you today."	
4. Be aware of nonverbal cues that are both sent and received (e.g., eye contact, facial expression, posture, body language). Be particularly alert to behaviors that are incongruent with the client's verbal message.	Incongruence is an indication that something may be interfering with open communication. Behaviors are often more accurate than words, and clarification may be indicated before proceeding.
5. Explain purpose of the interaction when information is to be shared.	
6. Encourage the client to ask for clarification at any time during the communication.	
7. Use questions carefully and appropriately. Ask one question at a time and allow sufficient time to answer. Use direct questions. Avoid asking questions about information that may not have yet been disclosed to the client (e.g., medical diagnosis). Avoid asking "why" questions.	"Why" questions may cause increased defensiveness in the client and may hinder communication.
8. Use clear and concise statements with a client who experiences altered levels of consciousness and cognition; repeat information, orient to surroundings, and offer reassurance.	
9. Focus on understanding the client, providing feedback and assisting in problem solving, and providing an atmosphere of warmth and acceptance.	Clients experiencing emotionally charged situations may not comprehend the message.

Steps	Rationale
10. Adjust the amount and quality of time for communicating depending on clients' needs.	Flexibility and adaptation of techniques may be necessary to encourage client's self-expression.
11. Be aware of cultural and gender differences when interacting with clients. Plan for identified communication difficulties associated with culture, language, age, and gender. Be alert to literacy status.	
12. Summarize with clients what was discussed during the interaction. Ask clients to state their understanding of the information shared or conclusion reached if the nurse suspects clients may in any way have misunderstood the communication.	
13. See Completion Protocol (inside front cover).	

• • •

EVALUATION

1. Observe client's verbal and nonverbal responses toward your communication.
2. Ask client for feedback regarding message communicated. Verify if information obtained from client is accurate regarding client's ideas, fears, and concerns.

Unexpected Outcomes and Related Interventions

1. Client continues to verbally and nonverbally express feelings of anxiety, fear, anger, confusion, distrust, and helplessness.
   a. Assess client's level of anxiety, fear, and distrust.
   b. Come back at another time to repeat the message.
2. Feedback between nurse and client reveals a lack of understanding.
   a. Assess for and remove barriers to communication.
   b. Repeat the message.
3. Nurse is unable to acquire information about client's ideas, fears, and concerns.
   a. Use alternative communication techniques to promote client's willingness to communicate openly.
   b. Offer another professional for the client to talk with to obtain the necessary information.

Recording and Reporting

- Report pertinent information, subjective data, and nonverbal cues, including:
  Response to illness
  Response to therapy
  Questions
  Concerns
- Record information and interventions and client responses.

Sample Documentation

0800 Client with expressive aphasia communicated with the nurse through the use of a pad and felt-tipped pen as communication aids. He reported anxiety and fear about his inability to communicate verbally.

Geriatric Considerations

- Be aware of any cognitive or sensory impairment.
- Each client needs to be assessed individually. Avoid stereotyping older adults as having cognitive or sensory impairments.
- The nurse should speak face-to-face with the hard-of-hearing client articulate clearly in a moderate tone of voice, and assess whether the client hears and understands the words.
- Encourage clients with visual impairments to use assistive devices such as eyeglasses and large-print reading material to aid in communication.

Home Care and Long-Term Care Considerations

- Identify a primary caregiver for the client. This individual may be a family member, friend, or neighbor.
- Assess level of understanding of the client and primary caregiver regarding the client's condition.
- Incorporate the client's usual daily habits and routines into the communication event (e.g., bathing and dressing client).

Skill 2.2

COMFORTING

It is quite common for a nurse to encounter a client who needs comfort and support while experiencing threatening situations. A newly diagnosed illness, separation from family, the discomfort of surgery or diagnostic and treatment procedures, grief, and loss are just a few examples of health-related situations that may require this skill.

ASSESSMENT

1. Observe interactions between client and others in the environment, including family or persons who provide the support system.
2. Identify medications that may alter speech. **Rationale: Medications such as antidepressants, antipsychotics, or sedatives may cause a client to slur words or use incomplete sentences.**
3. Identify body language that conveys positive or negative responses.

PLANNING

Expected outcomes focus on helping clients and families communicate effectively.

Expected Outcomes

1. Client verbalizes feelings regarding identified threat or concern.
2. Client identifies factors that provide support and comfort.
3. Client contacts one or more support systems.

(For Delegation Considerations, Geriatric Considerations, and Long-Term Care Considerations, see boxes on pp. 30-31.)

IMPLEMENTATION

Steps	Rationale
1. See Standard Protocol (inside from cover).	
2. Provide a private, quiet, and calm environment.	Environmental factors can promote open communication.
3. Acknowledge and respond to physical discomfort by positioning, medication, or other comfort measures. Consider individual preferences and expressed needs.	Physical discomfort, difficulty breathing, or pain interferes with communication.
4. Convey interest by maintaining eye contact and using open, relaxed posture (see illustration).	

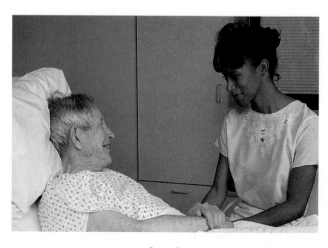

Step 4

Steps	Rationale
5. Convey acceptance without judgment. Avoid facial expressions or gestures that suggest disapproval.	Acceptance is not the same as agreement but is a willingness to hear the person without conveying doubt or disagreement.
6. Provide empathy, which involves a sensitive and accurate awareness of client's feelings.	Empathy helps clients explain and explore their feelings so that problem solving might occur.
7. Remain centered on the current concern. Avoid introducing new information.	Clients may be overwhelmed by additional information. Talking about self, other people, or events shifts the focus away from clients.
8. Guide client's description of the situation to include what happened, thoughts about the experience, and feelings about the experience (e.g., "What happened then?" "How did you feel after that?").	This assists the process of clarifying the experience.
9. Communicate understanding by repeating what you understand the message to be (e.g., "I understand you . . .," "I hear you saying . . .," "I sense that . . .").	Communicating understanding tends to decrease the intensity of feelings.
10. Use open questions to explore possible alternatives.	Open questions cannot be answered by "yes" or "no" and encourage expression of ideas or thoughts.
11. Offer honest reassurance to the extent possible (e.g., that someone cares, that there is hope, that client is not alone).	
12. Explore support services available and what services client has previously utilized. Refer as appropriate.	
13. See Completion Protocol (inside front cover).	

• • •

EVALUATION

1. Ask for feedback about effectiveness of support and comfort provided.
2. Observe client's response (e.g., body language, verbal statements) after discussion of feelings and circumstances that have been identified.
3. Ask in what way support systems are expected to become available and helpful.

Unexpected Outcomes and Related Interventions

1. Client is unable or unwilling to express feelings or circumstances.
   a. Consider the level of trust that has been established. If appropriate, facilitate greater level of trust in relation to other matters, such as providing for physical needs.
   b. Respect client's need, and offer opportunity to discuss the situation at another time or with another person.
2. Client expresses continued anger or discontent with alternatives available.
   a. Suggest taking more time to explore possibilities.
   b. Avoid telling client how to feel or what to think.
   c. Acknowledge and name the expressed feelings.

3. Client is unable to identify family or friends that can provide support. Family is too far away or estranged and unwilling to become involved.
   a. Identify community resources that may be helpful (e.g., church, neighbors, support groups).
   b. Facilitate a telephone support system.

Recording and Reporting

Document summary of client concerns. Include the following:

- Subjective data (e.g., significant quote)
- Objective data (e.g., body language)

Sample Documentation

1900   Client states, "The doctor said I have months, not years, to live." She and her family have talked about this. Tearful when stating her son is on his way from out of state to see her today because he is worried about her. Talked about wanting to be able to finish a quilt for her daughter, but not having felt well enough to work on it lately. Requested to talk more about this later because this conversation was helpful.

Skill 2.3

ACTIVE LISTENING

Active listening is one of the most effective ways to facilitate communication. It conveys interest in the client's needs, concerns, and problems and requires complete attention to understand the entire verbal and nonverbal message. A synonym for active listening is empathy. Empathy is the act of communicating to other persons that we have understood their feelings and what makes them feel that way. This requires acceptance of the individual in need of help. Once people know they have been understood and accepted, they do not have to struggle to explain or justify their reactions (Smith, 1992).

Listening techniques are learned behaviors. At first they seem awkward and time consuming, and as with any skill, become more comfortable with practice. It is essential that the nurse appear natural, relaxed, and at ease while listening.

ASSESSMENT

1. Assess patterns of communication with caregivers:
   a. Does client initiate conversation and ask appropriate questions?
   b. Does body language support and complement the verbal message?
   c. Does client talk excessively and control the topic of conversation?
   d. Does client avoid expressing feelings or thoughts and confine conversation to necessary facts? **Rationale: Awareness of communication patterns facilitates planning for the interaction.**
2. Identify sensory and neurological factors that affect the client's ability to communicate. **Rationale: Altered vision or hearing or expressive aphasia (in which words cannot be formed or expressed) or receptive aphasia (in which language is not understood) interferes with communication.**

3. Identify cultural influences that affect communication (Giger and Davidhizar, 1995). What language does client predominantly use in thinking? Does client need an interpreter? Is client able to read and/or write in English? What verbal or nonverbal communication shows respect (e.g., tempo, eye/body contact, topic restrictions)?

PLANNING

The expected outcomes focus on achieving clear understanding of client's communication.

Expected Outcomes

1. Client demonstrates comfort and willingness to communicate, stating that the nurse is listening to identified needs.
2. Client verbalizes a sense of feeling understood.

DELEGATION CONSIDERATIONS

Effective communication is a goal of all client interactions. The RN can encourage AP to improve listening skills, using these guidelines:

- When performing procedures, pay attention to what client has to say and do not ignore questions or concerns that may cause a temporary delay.

- Eye contact is critical in showing interest in the client.

- Do not anticipate what the client wants to say. Let him finish.

- Report client concerns to the RN.

IMPLEMENTATION

Steps	Rationale
1. See Standard Protocol (inside front cover).	
2. Use physical attending to convey interest by sitting within 4 feet of client, maintaining eye contact, and using open, relaxed posture (arms and legs not crossed).	This nonverbal language conveys interest and concern.
3. Ask one related open-ended question at a time following a logical sequence that encourages client to tell the whole story.	Open questions encourage client to elaborate and provide more accurate and detailed descriptions.

IMPLEMENTATION

Steps	Rationale
4. Listen without interrupting until a natural break occurs.	This avoids interference with client's flow of thoughts.
5. Offer feedback that lets client know what you understood. Paraphrase by restating client's message using fewer words.	
6. If the message is unclear, back up the conversation and clarify. Admit confusion and ask for more information.	Without clarification, valuable information is lost.
7. Focusing eliminates vagueness in communication by limiting the area of discussion. Avoid numerous direct questions and "why" questions that may result in defensiveness.	When focusing, nurse asks questions that encourage full understanding of one aspect rather than allowing the focus to shift before understanding is achieved.
8. Identify when a verbal message conflicts with nonverbal cues. Stating observations gives feedback that helps increase awareness of whether client communicated the intended message.	People may be unaware of the way the message was received unless the impressions created by the nonverbal cues are described.
9. Allow silence, which can be an effective means of allowing the organization of thoughts and processing of information. When client becomes emotionally upset or cries, a quiet period can be helpful.	Silence shows that nurse is accepting and willing to wait for client to be ready to continue.
10. At the conclusion of the interaction, summarize by giving a concise review of the key aspects of the main ideas.	Client is able to review information and make additions or corrections.

• • •

EVALUATION

1. Ask client what facilitates or interferes with communication of needs.
2. Ask if the communication was accurately interpreted by caregivers.

Unexpected Outcomes and Related Interventions

1. Client shifts conversation back to the nurse rather than discussing own issues.
   a. Answer questions briefly if appropriate, then state your need to focus on client issues.
   b. Ask what client is most concerned about at this time.
2. Client has difficulty hearing the questions.
   a. Reduce or remove background noise.
   b. If client has a hearing aid, be sure it is clean, inserted properly, and has a functioning battery.
   c. Adjust volume of hearing aid to a comfortable level.
   d. Speak slowly and articulate clearly.
   e. Face client to provide opportunity for lip reading.
   f. Talk toward client's best ear.

3. Client has dysarthria (difficult, poorly articulated speech from interference in control of muscles of speech) or expressive aphasia.
   a. Ask simple closed questions. Client can answer "yes" or "no" or nod or shake head in response.
   b. Allow time for understanding and a response.
   c. Use visual cues (pictures, objects, gestures).
   d. Encourage continued efforts to speak.
   e. Allow time and demonstrate an interested and patient attitude.
   f. Refer to speech therapist as needed.

Recording and Reporting

Document summary of client concerns. Include the following:

- Subjective data (e.g., significant quote)
- Objective data (e.g., body language)

Sample Documentation

1000 Client expressed concern about being able to regain ability to "do things like gardening and golf." Acknowledged being overwhelmed and discouraged. Talked at length about active lifestyle in past year. Expressed desire to work hard in physical therapy to build muscle strength as quickly as possible.

Skill 2.4

INTERVIEWING

The interview involves communication initiated for a specific purpose and focused on a specific content area, such as the initial assessment of newly admitted clients or obtaining a health history in a health care provider's office. In nursing, the interviewer obtains information about the client's health state, lifestyle, support systems, patterns of illness, patterns of adaptation, strengths and limitations, and resources. This information can be used for an admission database or health history and provides data for identifying the client's expectations and for responding appropriately to individualized client needs (see Box 2-5).

The interview can facilitate a positive nurse-client relationship, which makes it easier for clients to ask questions about the health care environment and expectations regarding daily routines and procedures. It is important to indicate to clients that they may ask questions at any time. They also have the right *not* to answer questions. Indicating the purpose of the interview helps to establish trust and to put the client at ease.

The interview involves phases of orientation, working, and termination. The interview may be scheduled at a time when interruptions will be minimal and visitors are not present. In some cases it is possible to include family members in the interview while the focus is clearly kept with identifying the client's needs.

Orientation phase. Before beginning, the nurse tells the client the purpose for the interview and the types of data to be obtained. Then time is spent becoming acquainted with the client. Establish a time frame for the interview, and honor this commitment to the client.

Working phase. The nurse asks questions to form a database from which a care plan can be developed (see box below). The nurse observes for evidence of discomfort and is willing to stop the interview when appropriate.

A direct-question technique is a structured format requiring one- or two-word answers and is frequently used to clarify previous information or obtain basic routine information (e.g., allergies, marital status). The open-question technique is used to promote a more complete description of identified areas of concern. Examples of open questions/comments include "What are your health concerns?" "How have you been feeling?" and "Tell me about your problem."

Termination phase. The client is given an indication that the interview is coming to an end a few minutes before conclusion is anticipated. This allows the client to ask questions and keeps the client aware of what to expect. The interview is terminated in a friendly manner, indicating specifically if there will be further contact. It is helpful to ask if anything else is needed before leaving the client's bedside.

Box 2-5 Interview Database

Health-Related Concerns
Perception of health status, past health problems and therapies, effect of health status on role, influence on relationship with members of household, influence on occupation, ability to complete activities of daily living (ADLs)

Emotional Concerns
Support system, significant losses, major life changes or stressors (divorce, death, job change, victim of traumatic event), changes related to sexuality, sense of self-esteem or self-worth (What makes you feel good about yourself?)

Knowledge Level/Learning Needs
Long-term and recent memory, intellectual abilities, education, environmental risk factors, understanding of illness, medications, treatment plans

Cultural and Spiritual Factors
Religious background, important religious practices, cultural background, values and beliefs (how this illness affects plans [goals/dreams])

ASSESSMENT

1. Review available information, which may include admission information such as name, address, age, marital status, employment, and reason for admission or reason for office visit.
2. Consider factors that may influence ability or willingness of client or significant other to respond to the questions, such as physical pain, discomfort, or anxiety. **Rationale: These factors may need to be alleviated before the interview. Intellectual level affects the choice of words used in the questions.**
3. Determine if client is alert and oriented. Assess for hearing and speech difficulties (see Chapter 36). If these factors interfere with the interview, another source of information will be needed.

PLANNING

Expected outcomes focus on gathering information for a database to develop an appropriate plan of care.

Expected Outcomes

1. Client (or signifciant other) is able to describe health concerns.
2. Verbal and nonverbal messages are congruent.

Interviewing is a professional-level skill and is not appropriately delegated to AP.

IMPLEMENTATION

Steps	Rationale

Orientation phase

1. Greet client and significant others and introduce yourself by name and job title (see illustration). Tell client why the interview is being done. Tell client you need to ask some questions that will require about 15 to 20 minutes. Assure client that this information will be kept confidential.

This allays anxiety about divulging information to a stranger and encourages participation.

2. Provide privacy and eliminate distractions, unnecessary noise, and interruptions by going to a quiet unoccupied room and/or closing the door. If others are present, ask client if they should stay.

Controlling environmental factors is especially important when a client is anxious, angry, or depressed (White, Kaas, and Richie, 1996).

3. Sit facing client at approximately the same eye level.

This facilitates active listening and places client more at ease.

4. If client is alert enough to state name, where he or she is, and what day it is, proceed with the interview.

If a client is disoriented or confused or information does not seem reliable, seek validation by other responsible persons (Domarad and Buschman, 1995).

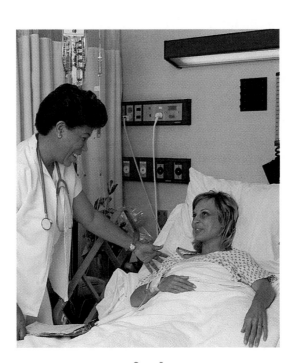

Step 1

Steps	Rationale

Working phase

5. If client is talkative, refocus the interview when client strays from the topic.

6. Ask what led client to seek health care. Attempt to obtain a descriptive account of all the events in the order in which they occurred.

Active listening encourages the exchange of information (see Skill 2.3). Conducting an interview by only asking questions may make client feel like a subject of interrogation.

This provides a focus for collecting more specific data related to the primary areas of concern.

7. Observe and clarify nonverbal behaviors. Listen to client responses.

8. For each symptom, determine when, where, and under what circumstances it occurred. Also determine location; quality; quantity; duration; and aggravating, alleviating, and associated factors (Table 2-2).

9. Within each symptom, also clarify the absence of other symptoms that are generally associated with the problem.

10. Identify past hospitalizations, past surgical procedures and complications, and previous major health problems.

Table 2-2

Dimensions of a Symptom

Dimensions	Questions to Ask	Dimensions	Questions to Ask
Location	"Where do you feel it?" "Does it move around?" "Show me where."	Timing	"When did you first notice it?" "How long does it last?" "How often does it happen?"
Quality or character	"What is it like? Sharp, dull, stabbing, aching?"	Setting	"Does it occur in a particular place or under certain circumstances?"
Severity	"On a scale of 0 to 10, with 10 the worst, how would you rate what you feel right now?" "What is the worst it has been?" "In what ways does this interfere with your usual activities?"	Aggravating or alleviating factors	"What makes it better?" "What makes it worse?" "When does it change?" "Have you noticed other changes associated with this?"

Steps	Rationale
11. Determine whether client regularly takes medications and, if so, for what period of time. Ask the name, reason for taking, dosage, and frequency. Specifically ask about over-the-counter (OTC) medications such as aspirin, acetaminophen, ibuprofen, laxatives, sleeping pills, or diet pills.	Clients may not think of over-the-counter (OTC) medications, because these do not require prescriptions.
12. Also ask if client takes narcotics, insulin, digitalis, contraceptives, steroids, or hormone replacements.	Clients may not mention these if such drugs seem unrelated to the reason for admission or when they think that the physician would have previously conveyed this information.
13. Identify risk factors related to lifestyle that influence the client's health, knowledge level, and awareness of the risk.	Risk factors include smoking, alcohol use, drug abuse, lack of exercise, stress, nutritional factors (e.g., fluids, cholesterol, carbohydrates, fiber, salt), exposure to violence, and sexual activity that is unprotected.
14. Continue with additional areas of interest or concern according to the focus of the interview (see box on p. 36).	
Termination phase	
15. Give information that tells client you are nearly finished.	This offers client a chance to ask final questions before nurse is finished.
16. Summarize your understanding of client's health concerns.	

• • •

EVALUATION

1. Ask if client or significant other has had an adequate opportunity to describe health concerns.
2. Observe client's nonverbal expressions during interview. Do they match verbal statements?

Unexpected Outcomes and Related Interventions

1. Family or significant other answers for client, even when client is capable of answering.
   a. Direct the question to client, using client's name.
   b. Avoid giving eye contact to family member.
   c. Acknowledge the answer given by a family member, then state you are interested specifically in what client has to say about it.
   d. Conclude the interview, and resume again after the family members are gone. If necessary, you may suggest that family take a break for a while, get coffee or a meal, or walk outside briefly for some fresh air.

2. Client is unable to communicate and family members are present.
   a. Interview family member as you would client.
   b. Explore the needs of family and client.

Recording and Reporting

List what is to be included in the admission profile:

- Reason for admission
- Medical-surgical history; family history
- Allergies
- Health habits
- Current prescribed therapies

Sample Documentation

Documentation involves use of a standard format for a database (see Admission Patient Profile, Appendix A).

Skill 2.5

COMMUNICATING WITH AN ANXIOUS CLIENT

Clients in the health care setting may experience anxiety for a variety of reasons. A newly diagnosed illness, separation from loved ones, threat associated with diagnostic tests or surgical procedures, a language barrier, and expectations of life changes are just a few factors that can cause anxiety. How successfully a client copes with anxiety depends in part on previous experiences, the presence of other stressors, the significance of the event causing anxiety, and the availability of supportive resources. The nurse can be a support to the client. The nurse can help to decrease anxiety through effective communication. Communication methods reviewed in this skill assist the nurse in helping the anxious client clarify factors causing anxiety and cope more effectively. There are stages of anxiety with corresponding behavioral manifestations: mild, moderate, severe, and panic (see box below).

ASSESSMENT

1. Assess for physical, behavioral, and verbal cues that indicate the client is anxious, such as dry mouth, sweaty palms, tone of voice, frequent use of call light, difficulty concentrating, wringing of hands, and statements such as "I am scared." **Rationale: Anxiety can interfere with usual manner of communication and thus interfere with client's care and treatment. Extreme anxiety can interfere with comprehension, attention, and problem-solving abilities.**
2. Assess for possible factors causing client anxiety (e.g., hospitalization, fatigue).
3. Assess factors influencing communication with the client (e.g., environment, timing, presence of others, values, experiences, need for personal space because of heightened anxiety).
4. Assess own level of anxiety as nurse, and make a conscious effort to remain calm. **Rationale: Anxiety is highly contagious, and one's own anxiety can exacerbate the client's anxiety.**

PLANNING

Expected outcomes focus on reducing the client's anxiety through the use of effective communication techniques.

Expected Outcomes

1. Client establishes rapport, achieves a sense of calm, and discusses coping and decision making about current situation.
2. Client's physical and emotional discomforts are acknowledged.
3. Client discusses factors causing anxiety.

Behavioral Manifestations of Anxiety: Stages of Anxiety

Mild Anxiety
- Increased auditory and visual perception
- Increased awareness of relationships
- Increased alertness
- Able to problem solve

Moderate Anxiety
- Selective inattention
- Decreased perceptual field
- Focus only on relevant information
- Muscle tension; diaphoresis

Severe Anxiety
- Focus on fragmented details
- Headache; nausea; dizziness
- Unable to see connections between details
- Poor recall

Panic State of Anxiety
- Does not notice surroundings
- Feeling of terror
- Unable to cope with any problem

DELEGATION CONSIDERATIONS

Therapeutic communication is a goal of all client interactions, delegated or not. Communicating effectively with an anxious client is a skill that can be delegated to AP. However, before delegation of this skill, the nurse should adhere to the following guidelines:

- Inform assistive care provider in proper way to interact verbally and nonverbally with the client.
- Review skills with assistive personnel for communicating with the anxious client.

IMPLEMENTATION

Steps	Rationale
1. See Standard Protocol (inside front cover).	
2. Provide brief, simple introduction; introduce yourself and explain purpose of interaction.	Anxiety may limit amount of information client may understand.
3. Use appropriate nonverbal behaviors (e.g., relaxed posture, eye contact) and active listening skills, such as staying with the client at the bedside.	Clients experiencing emotionally charged situations may not comprehend the delivered message. Focus on understanding the client, providing feedback and assisting in problem solving, and providing an atmosphere of warmth and acceptance.
4. Use appropriate verbal techniques that are clear and concise to respond to the anxious client.	Coping mechanisms provide the foundation for effective communication so that the client can explore causes of anxiety and steps to alleviate anxious feelings.
5. Help client acquire alternative coping strategies, such as progressive relaxation, slow deep-breathing exercises, and visual imagery (see Chapter 10).	A less-stimulating environment can create a calming, stress-free atmosphere that reduces anxiety (White, Kaas, and Richie, 1996).
6. Minimize noise in physical setting.	
7. Adjust the amount and quality of time for communicating depending on clients' needs.	Flexibility and adaptation of techniques may be necessary based on clients' ability to communicate, level of anxiety, and need for more time to establish trust.

• • •

EVALUATION

1. Have client discuss ways to cope with anxiety in the future and make decisions about current situation.
2. Observe for continuing presence of physical signs and symptoms or behaviors reflecting anxiety.
3. Ask client to discuss factors causing anxiety.

Unexpected Outcomes and Related Interventions

1. Physical signs and symptoms of anxiety continue.
   a. Utilize refocusing or distraction skills, such as re-laxation and imagery, to reduce anxiety (see Skill 10. 2).
   b. Be direct and clear when communicating with client, to avoid misunderstanding.
   c. Touch, when used appropriately, may help control feelings of panic.
   d. Administering an antianxiety medication may be necessary.

Recording and Reporting

Record in nurses' notes the following:

- Cause of anxiety
- Nonverbal behaviors
- Methods used to relieve anxiety
- Client response (verbal and nonverbal)

Sample Documentation

0400   Client pacing back and forth in room. Stated, "I've got to go home. I can't stand it here any longer." Tremors of hands noted. Discussed family situation and reasons for hospitalization for 15 minutes.

0500   Client lying in bed. Client stated he feels less distress now that he has a plan for dealing with his concerns.

Skill 2.6

VERBALLY DEESCALATING A POTENTIALLY VIOLENT CLIENT

Anger is the common underlying factor associated with a potential for violence. The degree and frequency of anger ranges from everyday mild annoyance, to anger related to feelings of helplessness and powerlessness, and ultimately to rage when usual coping methods are no longer effective to manage the situation. There are positive functions of anger, including anger as an energizing behavior, anger to protect positive image, and anger to give a person greater control over a situation. A client can become angry for a variety of reasons. The anger may be directly related to a client's experience with illness, or it can be associated with problems that existed before the client entered the health care system. In the health care setting, the nurse has frequent contact with a client and thus may become the target of the client's anger when the client cannot express it toward a significant other. It is important for the nurse to understand that in many cases the client's ability to express anger is important to recovery. For example, when a client has experienced a significant loss, anger becomes a means to help cope with grief. A client may express anger toward the nurse, but the anger often hides a specific problem or concern. For example, a client diagnosed as having cancer may voice displeasure with the nurse's care instead of expressing a fear of dying.

It can be stressful for a nurse to deal with an angry client. Anger can represent rejection or disapproval of the nurse's care. A nurse's efforts at satisfying the needs of one angry client can result in a failure to meet the priorities of other clients. The nurse needs to allow the client to express anger openly and not feel threatened by the client's words (Maier, 1996).

The client's anger cannot be allowed to compromise care. Skills for communicating with an angry client or a potentially violent client will allow a nurse to assist the client in dealing with anger constructively and in refocusing emotional energy toward effective problem solving. Deescalation skills are useful techniques that can be used to manage the potentially violent client; these skills range from using nonthreatening verbal and nonverbal messages to safely disengaging and controlling the aggressor physically (Fortinash and Holoday-Worret, 1996).

ASSESSMENT

1. Observe for behaviors that indicate the client is angry (e.g., pacing, clenched fist, loud voice, throwing objects) and/or expressions that indicate anger (e.g., repeated questioning of the nurse, irrational complaints about care, nonadherence to requests, belligerent outbursts, threats). **Rationale: Anger is a normal expression of frustration or a response to feeling threatened. However, its expression can interfere with or block communication and interactions.**

2. Assess factors that influence communication of the angry client, such as refusal to comply with treatment goals, use of sarcasm or hostile behavior, having a low frustration level, or being emotionally immature.

3. Consider resources available to assist in communicating with the potentially violent client, such as members of the health care team and family members.

PLANNING

Expected outcomes focus on promoting effective and socially appropriate verbal and nonverbal expressions of anger.

1. Client's feelings of anger subside without harm to self or others.
2. Client's anger is diffused, and problem solving is initiated.

DELEGATION CONSIDERATIONS

Therapeutic communication is a goal of all client interactions. Communicating effectively with the potentially violent client is a skill that should be taught to all AP who may need to use it (e.g., security personnel, AP who work in psychiatric units).

IMPLEMENTATION

Steps	Rationale
1. See Standard Protocol (inside front cover).	
2. Create a climate of client acceptance. Maintain nonthreatening verbal and nonverbal communication skills when interacting with the angry or potentially violent client.	A relaxed atmosphere may prevent further escalation.
3. Respond to the potentially violent client with therapeutic silence, and allow client to ventilate feelings.	These techniques often deescalate anger, because anger expends emotional and physical energy; client runs out of momentum and energy to maintain anger at a high level.
4. Answer questions; if client presents a power-struggle type of question (e.g., "Who said you were in charge; I don't have to listen to you"), redirect and set limits by giving clear, concise expectations. Inform client of potential consequences, and follow through with consequences if behaviors are not altered. Do not argue with client, because arguing will escalate anger. Do not get defensive with client.	By setting limits on power-struggle questions, structure is provided and anger is diffused (Gibson, 1997).
5. Encourage client to write about negative thoughts.	
6. Encourage physical exercise as a means of directing energy in an acceptable way (Potter and Perry, 1997).	
7. If the client is making verbal threats to harm others, remain calm yet professional and continue to set limits with inappropriate behavior. If a strong likelihood of imminent harm to others is present, the nurse should notify the proper authorities (e.g., nurse manager, security).	Angry clients lose the ability to process information rationally and therefore may impulsively express themselves through intimidation.
8. Maintain personal space and safety with the client who is making verbal threats of violence directed at others. It may be necessary to have someone with you and to keep the door open. Maintain nonthreatening nonverbal behaviors, including body language (e.g., relaxed posture, arms open and hands not in pockets, not invading the client's personal space).	Clients experiencing emotionally charged situations may not comprehend the message. Focus on understanding the client, providing feedback and assisting in problem solving, and providing an atmosphere of warmth and acceptance.

NURSE ALERT

The potentially violent client can be impulsive and explosive, and therefore it is imperative the nurse keep personal safety skills in mind. In this case, avoid touch.

Steps	Rationale
9. Adjust the amount and quality of time for communicating depending on the client's needs. Try to deescalate the client's anger first, then return later to deliver the message.	It is futile to try to communicate a complicated message to a client in the height of anger.
10. If the client appears to be calm and anger is diffused, explore alternatives to the situation or feelings of anger.	May prevent future explosive outbursts and teach the client effective ways of dealing with anger.
11. See Completion Protocol (inside front cover).	

• • • •

EVALUATION
1. Ask client if feelings of anger have subsided.
2. Determine client's ability to answer questions and solve problems.

Unexpected Outcomes and Related Interventions
1. Client continues to demonstrate behaviors or verbal expression of anger or violence. Nurse is unable to assist the client in relieving source of anger or in expressing anger openly without violent acts.
   a. If anger continues to escalate, reassess factors contributing to anger.
   b. Remove or alter factors contributing to anger.

Recording and Reporting
- Observations related to factors precipating anger
- Use exact quotes
- Threats of violence made and who was notified
- Nursing action for deescalation and limit setting
- Response

Sample Documentation
2100 Client has been verbally assaultive to staff since refusing medications at 2000. Attempts at verbal deescalation and limit setting have been successful. Client was escorted by staff to the seclusion room to decrease sensory stimulation. Client is currently resting quietly and is no longer making verbal threats to staff. Client accepted missed dose of medications at this time.

Geriatric Considerations
- Clients who have cognitive impairments may exhibit tantrumlike behaviors in response to real or perceived frustration. The nurse can use distraction techniques to remove the cognitively impaired adult client from the disturbing stimuli, or the nurse can use redirection to an activity that is pleasurable to the client.

Home Care and Long-Term Care Considerations
- Personal safety is a major concern in settings in which there is no access to additional support from other health care personnel. The nurse should not enter an unsafe environment. In all settings, the nurse needs to be aware of both verbal and nonverbal cues that indicate escalating anger. In settings in which additional support is not readily available, it is also important to be aware of physical surroundings, possible exits, and communication systems to call for assistance (e.g., telephone, emergency call system). A quick exit is appropriate if efforts to deescalate are not successful.
- Allow adequate personal space, and use a firm and calm tone of voice at a moderate pace. The level of speech should be clearly audible, avoiding both shouting and timid tones.
- The nurse needs to use a nonthreatening posture (e.g., avoid standing over the individual, shaking a finger, putting hands on hips).

Skill 2.7

CLIENT TEACHING

Health teaching is an important role of the professional nurse. Health teaching takes place in a variety of settings, such as the hospital, classroom, and community. One of the most important goals in health care today is to engage clients and families in maintaining health and managing health problems. General nursing practice standards require that client education be included as a part of the treatment plan (Blair and Ramones, 1997). The purposes of health teaching include shattering myths, quelling fears, and conveying information. Nurses provide information to clients that will help prevent complications and promote self-care and independence (Katz, 1997). During each interaction with a client, the nurse has an opportunity to teach knowledge and skills needed to promote more healthy living and an improved level of health. Much health teaching is informal and integrated into daily routines.

Teaching uses basic principles to promote participation and follows steps similar to the steps of the nursing process (i.e., assessment, analysis, planning, implementation, and evaluation). Teaching priorities must be established based on the client's needs. The content and teaching methods are individualized for the client. Incorporating the client's cultural beliefs about health information into the teaching plan promotes better acceptance. Health teaching includes active involvement of the learner and possibly other significant persons from the client's support network.

ASSESSMENT

1. Assess client's readiness to learn. **Rationale: Several factors affect learner readiness, such as motivation to learn and stability of physical condition.**
2. Assess the presence of any barriers to learning. **Rationale: To enhance the client's learning, capabilities must be assessed and the teaching style must be adapted to meet the individualized needs of the client.**

PLANNING

Expected outcomes focus on the client's successful learning experience and on a change in client behavior related to health issues.

1. The client demonstrates skills needed for self-care.
2. The client identifies strategies for illness prevention or early detection of disease.

DELEGATION CONSIDERATIONS

The skill of client teaching requires problem solving and knowledge application unique to a professional nurse.

IMPLEMENTATION

Steps	Rationale
1. See Standard Protocol (inside front cover).	
2. Select setting that is conducive to learning with minimal interruptions, comfortable temperature, and good lighting.	
3. State objectives for what the learner needs to accomplish and how achievement will be measured.	Objectives are client oriented and reflect what the learner will be able to do after completion of the instruction (Rega, 1993).
4. Select media, methods of teaching, and aids (e.g., hands-on equipment, pamphlets, audio-visual materials) appropriate to client's needs.	One of the most effective teaching methods is to verbally deliver information, leave written information, and ask the client for follow-up questions after the client hears and reads the information. Videos work well with clients who cannot read. The emphasis is on repetition.
5. Vary the tone of voice to convey interest in the teaching process, and use simple, clear language.	
6. Be specific about what the client needs to know; repeat and highlight key points.	
7. Use demonstration and return demonstration to practice manual skills.	Active participation enhances the learning process (Rega, 1993).
8. Be a role model for techniques, such as handwashing, posture, injection techniques, and dressing change techniques.	People learn best by modeling the behaviors of others (Katz, 1997).
9. Use opportunities to teach while providing care. See every interaction with client as an opportunity to communicate or impart knowledge.	
10. Involve family and friends in the teaching process.	
11. Review material over time.	Teaching small amounts of information over time is most effective, and constant repetition leads to compliance (Katz, 1997).
12. Give clients praise for return demonstrations that are accurate or for behavior changes resulting from information given.	
13. See Completion Protocol (inside front cover).	

• • •

EVALUATION

1. Observe ability to demonstrate skills needed for self-care and compliance with therapeutic regimen.
2. Ask client to describe strategies for illness prevention or early detection of disease.

Unexpected Outcomes and Related Interventions

1. Client is able to correctly verbalize or demonstrates desired skills or behaviors, but evidence suggests lack of compliance.
   a. Identify factors that interfere with desired behavior, such as expense of equipment or time/place inconvenience.
   b. A written chart may be helpful if client is forgetful, rather than intentionally neglecting desired behaviors.
   c. Encourage follow-up support system (family or other provider) to develop additional strategies to enhance compliance.
   d. Consider need for referral for home health follow-up visits.

Recording and Reporting

- Objectives or topic being taught
- Methods used
- Client response to teaching/learning

Sample Documentation

0830　Client and husband reviewed videotape on how to measure blood glucose for the management of diabetes. Demonstrated to client and husband procedure for monitoring blood glucose. Return demonstration successful.

CRITICAL THINKING EXERCISES

1. Mr. Jones was recently admitted for complications from diabetes mellitus. He was diagnosed 10 years ago, and in the past few weeks he has experienced numbness and tingling in both legs. The nurse attempts to gather information to develop an appropriate plan of care. He is very anxious about his condition, is fearful about the hospitalization, and suffers from a hearing loss. Identify possible barriers to effective communication, and state the techniques to be used during the client interview to initiate interaction and facilitate communication.

2. You are attempting prenatal teaching with a client who is 8 months pregnant with her first child. She is wringing her hands and continually states, "I don't know what to do when this baby arrives; I'm so nervous." How would you implement client teaching with this person?

3. Mr. Moore has been a client on the nursing division for 3 weeks. You see him in the hall, talking in a loud voice and making threats to physically hurt the staff. How would you communicate effectively with this client?

REFERENCES

Blair DT, Ramones VA: Education as psychiatric intervention: the cognitive-behavioral context, *J Psychosoc Nurs* 12(35):29–35, 1997.

Domarad BR, Buschman MT: Interviewing older adults: increasing the quality of the interview data, *J Gerontol Nurs* 14–19, 1995.

Fortinash K, Holoday-Worret P: *Psychiatric-mental health nursing*, St Louis, 1996, Mosby.

Gibson M: Differentiating aggressive and resistive behaviors in long-term care, *Gerontol Nurs* 21–27, 1997.

Giger J, Davidhizer R: *Transcultural nursing*, St Louis, 1995, Mosby.

Katz JR: Back to basics: providing effective patient teaching, *Am J Nurs* 5:33–36, 1997.

Keltner N, Schwecke L, Bostrom C: *Psychiatric nursing: a psychotherapeutic management approach*, St Louis, 1991, Mosby.

Kim MJ, McFarland GK, McLane AM: *Pocket guide to nursing diagnoses*, ed 7, St Louis, 1997, Mosby.

Lindblade DD, McDonald M: Removing communication barriers for the hearing-impaired elderly, *Med Surg Nurs* 5(4):379–385, 1995.

Maier GJ: Managing threatening behavior: The role of talk down and talk up, *J Psychosoc Nurs* 6(34):25–30, 1996.

Potter P, Perry A: *Fundamentals of nursing*, ed 4, St Louis, 1997, Mosby.

Rega MD: A model approach for patient education, *Med Surg Nurs* 6(2):477–495, 1993.

Smith S: *Communications in nursing*, ed 2, St Louis, 1992, Mosby.

White MK, Kaas MJ, Richie MF: Vocally disruptive behavior, *J Gerontol Nurs* 23–28, 1996.

CHAPTER 3

Promoting Infection Control

Skill 3.1
Handwashing, 50

Skill 3.2
Using Disposable Clean Gloves, 53

Skill 3.3
Caring for Clients Under Isolation Precautions, 55

Skill 3.4
Special Tuberculosis Precautions, 60

Infections present a significant hazard in all health care settings. Although protection of the client is an obvious priority, health care workers, including nurses, are at risk for contact with infectious material or exposure to a communicable disease. Knowledge of the infectious process and how a disease is transmitted, as well as the critical thinking involved in how to use and when to use aseptic technique and barrier protection, cannot be overemphasized. Today's nurse plays a vital role in the prevention and control of infection.

Risk factors for hospital-acquired, or nosocomial, infections are greatly increased for clients in health care settings. In acute care or ambulatory care facilities, clients can be exposed to new or different microorganisms. Some of these microorganisms may be resistant to most antibiotics. In all settings, clients may have procedures or treatment modalities that lower their resistance to infections. For example, clients' immune systems may be altered if they are receiving radiation or chemotherapy treatments; therefore, they are more susceptible to infections, even from their own normal flora. Additionally, invasive procedures, such as the insertion of intravenous (IV) or urinary catheters, disrupt the body's natural defense barriers. In all health care settings, the nurse is responsible for teaching clients and their families about the source and transmission of infections, reason for susceptibility, and infection control principles.

Clients or health care workers do not have to develop an infection or acquire a disease with every exposure to a microorganism. This process depends on the chain of infection, which is a model for the events that can lead to an infection (Figure 3-1). There are six links in the chain of infection: (1) an infectious agent or pathogen; (2) the reservoir or place where the organisms reside; (3) the portal of exit from the reservoir; (4) a method or mode of transmission; (5) the portal of entrance into the host; and (6) the susceptibility of the host. Breaking any one of these links prevents an infection. For example, a nurse may prevent the client from acquiring an IV line infection by breaking the chain in several places. The reservoir or the microorganisms present on the skin can be altered by properly preparing the site before needle insertion. The mode of transmission can be reduced by handwashing and using proper aseptic techniques.

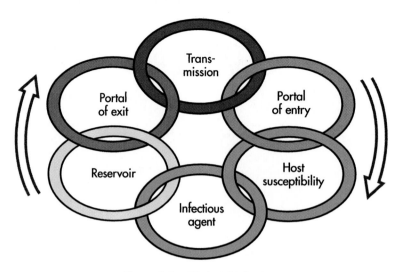

Figure 3-1   Chain of infection.

Another example of breaking the infection chain includes alteration of a host response after a vaccination. A vaccine activates antibodies and protects the person from infection. By using infection prevention principles and client education, nurses can break the chain of infection.

Infections can be prevented or minimized by the use of aseptic technique. *Aseptic technique* is the purposeful prevention of the transfer of infection (Crows, 1989). Medical and surgical asepsis are the two types of techniques; both can be used in any health care setting. *Medical asepsis,* or *clean technique,* includes procedures (e.g., handwashing, barrier techniques, routine environmental cleaning) that reduce the number of microorganisms. Principles of medical asepsis are commonly followed in the home, such as handwashing before preparing food or disinfecting a surface after contact with body fluids.

Medical aseptic techniques are not as rigid as surgical asepsis. *Surgical asepsis* refers to practices designed to render and maintain objects or skin maximally free from microorganisms (see Chapter 4). This practice also is referred to as *sterile technique.* Sterile technique must be practiced by nurses in operating rooms or during invasive procedures in which sterile supplies are used. Sterile supplies have undergone a process called *sterilization,* whereby all microorganisms, including spores, have been destroyed. Sterile technique protects the client from the health care worker and/or the environment (e.g., the operating room).

Barrier protection protects the health care worker from the client's blood and body fluids and helps prevent the transfer of organisms to other clients and to the environment. This is the basis for Standard Precautions, as well as other isolation practices. Barrier protection includes use of gowns, masks, protective eyewear, and gloves. Some form of personal protective equipment (PPE) is indicated for all clients who potentially have an infection that can be transmitted to others. Because of the increased attention to the prevention of certain diseases, such as hepatitis B, acquired immunodeficiency syndrome (AIDS), and tuberculosis (TB), the Centers for Disease Control and Prevention (CDC) and the U.S. Occupational Safety and Health Administration (OSHA) have stressed the importance of the use of barriers and precautions.

In 1983 the CDC published guidelines for isolation precautions that encouraged decision making by the user. First, hospitals were given the choice of selecting between two systems: category-specific or disease-specific isolation. Second, personnel placing a client under precautions were encouraged to make decisions regarding need for a private room and necessity for certain types of barrier protection (Garner and Simmons, 1984). Thus, some clients were "overisolated," whereas others were "underisolated."

As new data regarding disease transmission became available, several portions of the guidelines were updated by the CDC. For example, the CDC has modified the isolation recommendation for clients with TB (Garner, 1996b) and those with suspected hemorrhagic fever (CDC, 1988b).

In 1988, the *Body Substance Isolation* (BSI) system was developed and focused personnel on selecting barrier protection whenever there was risk of contacting body substances (e.g., blood, saliva, feces, urine, wound drainage) rather than only on the basis of isolation category or diagnosis. The rationale for BSI was that any client may be a source for infection. For example, nurses would wear gowns and gloves when changing the bed of an incontinent client.

When using BSI, workers should put on clean gloves just before contact with mucous membranes or nonintact skin of all clients. Furthermore, protective barriers should be used when it is likely that the worker will come in contact with a body substance that might soil skin or clothing. These precautions are intended to interrupt transmission of the most common source for organisms: colonized body substances.

Another system, *Universal Precautions* (UP), recommended barriers and procedures that limit an individual's exposure to infectious bloodborne agents such as the human immunodeficiency virus (HIV), which causes AIDS, and the virus that causes hepatitis (CDC, 1988a). OSHA (1991) published regulations that required facilities to utilize UP as the minimum standard of practice. UP requires workers to assume that all clients are potentially infected with HIV or other bloodborne agents and to use PPE to prevent exposure.

Hospitals then incorporated UP or BSI into their existing isolation systems. This produced confusion and inconsistent application of isolation precautions. There was much discussion and continued lack of agreement about major issues, such as which procedures required glove usage, and many local variations in the interpretation of recommendations. There was also inconsistent recognition of emerging multidrug-resistant microorganisms and application of appropriate precautions that would contain them. In the 1990s the CDC recognized that isolation had become an infection control dilemma. As a result of this turmoil, in 1996 the CDC developed a new system of isolation that would provide guidelines for preventing the spread of infections.

This new system takes the major features of BSI and UP and combines them into a set of precautions known as *Standard Precautions* (see Box 3-1). These precautions are designed to reduce the risk of transmission of bloodborne and other pathogens. They should become habit and be observed in every client encounter.

Microorganisms are transmitted by several routes, the five main routes being contact, droplet, airborne, common vehicle, and vectorborne. The developed guidelines are aimed at using barrier precautions to interrupt the mode of transmission (see Box 3-3 on p. 55).

The early 1990s also saw an increase in the number of outbreaks of TB in clients and health care workers, and the CDC issued proposed guidelines that have been challenged and revised over the past 8 years. A draft is currently undergoing the review process, and a final rule is not expected until at least 1999. This standard involves medical screening and requires that all health care workers be fit-tested and trained in the wearing and storage of a high-efficiency particulate air (HEPA) respirator or N95 particulate respirator mask that meets or exceeds the standard. Other requirements include annual TB skin testing for health care workers and the isolation of any clients suspected of having TB (see Box 3-2 on p. 50). This is the most important precaution that the health care worker can take, because the greatest risk of exposure is before a diagnosis is made and precautions are implemented. It is essential that the health care worker has good assessment

Box 3-1 Standard Precautions (Tier One)*

- Standard precautions apply to blood, all body fluids, secretions, excretions (except sweat), nonintact skin, and mucous membranes.
- Hands are washed between client contact after contact with blood, body fluids, secretions and excretions and after contact with equipment or articles contaminated by them; and immediately after gloves are removed, and when indicated to prevent transfer of microorganisms between other clients or environment.
- Gloves are worn when touching blood, body fluid, secretions, excretions, nonintact skin, mucous membranes, or contaminated items. Gloves should be removed and hands washed between client care.
- Masks, eye protection, or face shields are worn if client care activities may generate splashes or sprays of blood or body fluid.
- Gowns are worn if soiling of clothing is likely from blood or body fluid. Hands are washed after removing gown.
- Client care equipment is properly cleaned and reprocessed, and single-use items are discarded.
- Contaminated linen is placed in leak-proof bag and handled so as to prevent skin and mucous membrane exposure.
- All sharp instruments and needles are discarded in a puncture-resistant container. CDC recommends that needles be disposed of uncapped or that a mechanical device for recapping be used.
- A private room is unnecessary unless the client's hygiene is unacceptable. Check with infection control professional or facility manual.

skills and can determine which clients are potential risks. The symptoms of TB include fatigue, weight loss, fever and night sweats, and cough that can sometimes be productive of blood. The physician or nurse in charge should be notified whenever the health care worker feels that a client is a potential risk for TB so that appropriate tests can be ordered and precautions implemented. TB isolation will be further discussed in Skill 3.4.

Powerlessness and social isolation can be heightened in the geriatric population; these are already potential problems for this population. This can cause noncompliance with isolation in the geriatric client, rather than lack of understanding. Reassurance that isolation will not keep health care workers from entering the client's room is essential, as well as reassurance to family and friends regarding visitations. PPE worn by the health care worker can also add to confusion and disorientation, and closed doors can interfere with client safety. Special problems or con-

Box 3-2 TB Isolation

- TB isolation should be practiced for all clients with known or suspected TB. (Suspected TB is defined by agency policy and generally means any client with a positive AFB smear, a cavitating lesion seen on chest x-ray study, or identified as high risk by a screening tool.)
- Isolation must be in a single-client room designated as negative airflow and having at least six air exchanges per hour. Room air must be vented to the outside. The door must be closed to maintain negative pressure.
- Health care workers must wear an N95 particulate respirator mask or HEPA respirator when entering an AFB isolation room. (Check agency's policy for type of mask.)
- Workers must be fit-tested* before using a respirator for the first time. This ensures type and size of respirator appropriate for an individual.
- Workers must fit-check† the respirator's fit before each use.
- Respirator may be reused and stored according to agency policy.

AFB, Acid-fast bacillus.
*Fit test: Procedure to determine adequate fit of respirator, usually by qualitative measure (wearers are exposed to a concentrated saccharin solution and asked if they can detect taste wearing respirator).
†Fit check: Procedure in which worker uses negative pressure to see if mask is properly sealed to face.

cerns should be discussed with the health care team for appropriate, consistent intervention.

Young children are not always able to comprehend the need for isolation. Protective equipment can be decorated and made less frightening, but it is a challenge to help them understand why they cannot leave their room and join the others in the playroom. Explanations should be simple, and parents/family members need to be included. Toys and games that are brought into the room should be ones that can be effectively cleaned with an approved germicide.

Long-term care facilities are considered the client's home, and part of the community. Hospitals/acute care facilities differ in that the client population is generally sicker, with lowered immune responses. For this reason, isolation is indicated in the acute care facility, but not necessarily indicated for the same microorganism in the client at home or residing in a long-term care facility.

NURSING DIAGNOSES

Several nursing diagnoses may be appropriate when using infection control measures. **Risk for Infection** relates to clients who may have specific risk factors that may increase their potential for acquiring an infection. These include pathological conditions (immunosuppression, chronic disease, obesity), treatments (surgery, invasive procedures, steroids), situational factors (disease exposure, inadequate immunizations, lack of handwashing by caregiver), or maturation (client's age).

A diagnosis of **Knowledge Deficit** regarding infection prevention is appropriate when the nurse teaches individuals, families, or groups information about infection control measures. Clients can experience **Fear** or a feeling of **Powerlessness** when restricted to a respiratory isolation type of environment or when required to use protective barriers. **Social Isolation** may also be appropriate when use of protective barriers and environmental restrictions are required.

Skill 3.1

HANDWASHING

Handwashing is the single most important means of controlling and preventing the spread of infections. The purpose of handwashing is to remove soil and transient microorganisms from the hands and to reduce total microbial count over time (Larson, 1996). The decision to wash hands depends on three factors: (1) the intensity or degree of contact with the client or infectious material, (2) the extent of contamination that may occur with the contact, and (3) the client's susceptibility to infection (Larson, 1996). Larson further describes that for most general client care, a plain nonantimicrobial soap is acceptable in any convenient form (bar, leaflets, liquid, powder). In most health care settings, liquid or foam soap is used for handwashing. Some agencies have sinks with foot controls or an electric eye for turning the water supply on and off. This system reduces the transmission of microorganisms that can occur when touching a contaminated faucet after handwashing. An antimicrobial soap should be used when performing invasive procedures, working in special care units, or dealing with immunosuppressed clients.

Care must be taken to protect all clients from bacteria present on the nurse's hands. This is especially important if clients have an immune deficiency.

Equipment

Liquid or foam soap (antimicrobial soap under certain conditions)
Warm running water
Paper towels or air dryer

ASSESSMENT

1. Assess client's risk for or extent of infection (e.g., immunosuppressed, invasive procedure, open wound).
2. Inspect surface of nurse's hands for breaks or cuts in skin or cuticles. Cover lesions before providing client care.
3. Inspect hands for heavy soiling and nails for length.

PLANNING

Expected outcomes focus on preventing the transmission of infection.

Expected Outcomes

1. Client's signs and symptoms demonstrate absence of infection.

DELEGATION CONSIDERATIONS

Handwashing and infection control using isolation precautions are basic skills that must be performed correctly by all caregivers. When delegating these skills it is important for the registered nurse to be knowledgeable about the mode of transmission of microorganisms involved.

- Observe handwashing techniques, including both consistency and thoroughness used.
- Instruct caregivers on mode of transmission of microorganisms and the appropriate PPE needed.

IMPLEMENTATION

Steps	Rationale
1. Push wristwatch and long uniform sleeves above wrists. Avoid wearing rings. If worn, remove during washing.	Wearing of rings increases number of microorganisms on hands (Garner, 1996a).
2. Stand in front of sink, keeping hands and uniform away from sink surface. (If hands touch sink during hand washing, repeat.)	Inside of sink is a contaminated area. Reaching over sink increases risk of touching edge, which is contaminated.
3. Turn on water. Turn facuet on or push knee pedals laterally or press pedals with foot to regulate flow and temperature.	
4. Avoid splashing water against uniform.	Microorganisms travel and grow in moisture.
5. Regulate flow of water so that temperature is warm.	
6. Wet hands and wrists thoroughly under running water. Keep hands and forearms lower than elbows during washing.	Hands are the most contaminated parts to be washed. Water flows from least to most contaminated area, rinsing microorganisms into sink.
7. Apply a small amount of soap or antiseptic, lathering thoroughly (see illustration). Soap granules and leaflet preparations may be used.	The use of antiseptic exclusively can be drying to the hands and can cause skin irritations. The decision whether to use an antiseptic should depend on the procedure to be performed and the client's immune status.
8. Wash hands using plenty of lather and friction for at least 10 to 15 seconds. Interlace fingers and rub palms and back of hands with circular motion at least 5 times each. Keep fingertips down to facilitate removal of microorganisms.	

Steps	Rationale

9. Areas underlying fingernails are often soiled. Clean them with fingernails of other hand and additional soap or clean orangewood stick.

Area under nails can be highly contaminated, which will increase the risk of infections for the nurse or client.

NURSE ALERT

Do not tear or cut skin under or around nail.

10. Rinse hands and wrists thoroughly, keeping hands down and elbows up (see illustration).
11. Optional: repeat steps 1 through 9 and extend period of washing if hands are heavily soiled.
12. Dry hands thoroughly from fingers to wrists and forearms with paper towel, single-use cloth, or warm air dryer.
13. If used, discard paper towel in proper receptacle.
14. Turn off water with foot or knee pedals. To turn off hand faucet, use clean, dry paper towel; avoid touching handles with hands.
15. If hands are dry or chapped, a small amount of lotion or barrier cream can be applied.

Rinsing mechanically washes away dirt and microorganisms.

Drying from cleanest (fingertips) to least clean (forearms) area avoids contamination. Drying hands prevents chapping and roughened skin.

Wet towel and hands allow transfer of pathogens by capillary action.

Use small individual-use container of lotion because large, refillable containers have been associated with nosocomial infections.

• • •

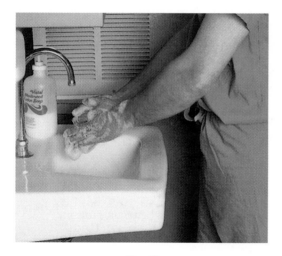

Step 7

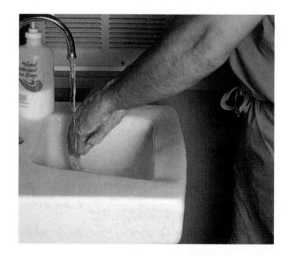

Step 10

EVALUATION
1. Inspect surfaces of hands for obvious signs of soil or other contaminants.
2. Inspect hands for dermatitis or cracked skin.

Unexpected Outcomes and Related Intervention
Client(s) develop infection transmissable through hand contact.

Skill 3.2

USING DISPOSABLE CLEAN GLOVES

Disposable gloves must be worn before coming in contact with mucous membranes, nonintact skin, blood, body fluids, or other infectious material. Additionally, gloves are indicated when there are cuts; abrasions; or oozing, draining wounds on the caregiver's hands (Larson, 1996). Gloves should be inspected before use for cuts, tears, or holes. Gloves found with any of these deficiencies will not provide proper barrier protection.

There are many types of gloves available to the health care worker. It is important that individuals choose gloves that suits their needs. Latex allergies are occurring with more frequency in the health care field, not only in health care workers but also in clients. Often, health care workers suspect a latex allergy when their hands are actually reacting to the powder in the gloves or to the soap they are using. If redness, inflammation, extreme dryness, or vesicles appear on the hands, an evaluation by a physician should be performed. Synthetic vinyl gloves are just as effective a barrier as latex gloves and are an excellent alternative to latex.

Clients need to be questioned regarding allergies, and it is imperative that they be specifically asked about latex allergies. A latex allergy can precipitate a respiratory arrest, which is a life-threatening event, and must not be ignored or forgotten. The health care worker should not wear latex gloves when caring for clients with latex allergies.

Hand lotion is most beneficial just after washing and lightly drying your hands. Avoid using lotions that contain mineral oil or petroleum as their main ingredients, because these impair the integrity of latex and the effectiveness of gloves. When choosing a lotion, remember that it should be compatible with the ingredients in antimicrobial soaps. Lotion can be a culture media for organisms, so do not share a lotion bottle. Also, do not buy the large economy jugs and refill a small portable container, because the longer the lotion sits, the more time microorganisms have to multiply in the lotion.

Equipment
Pair of clean disposable gloves of appropriate size and type (latex or vinyl)

ASSESSMENT
1. Inspect hands for cuts, abrasions, or wounds that indicate need for gloves.
2. Inspect skin for redness, inflammation, extreme dryness, or vesicles that may indicate latex allergy.

PLANNING
Expected outcome focuses on preventing the transfer of microorganisms from nurse's hands to client. Additionally, nurse should be protected from infections.

Expected Outcome
Client's signs and symptoms demonstrate absence of infection.

IMPLEMENTATION

Steps	Rationale
1. See Standard Protocol (inside front cover).	
Application	
2. Put on gloves (no special technique required). If wearing an isolation gown, pull cuffs of gloves over cuffs of gown. If not wearing a gown, pull up the gloves to cover the wrist.	Protects nurse's skin from exposure to microorganisms.
3. Interlink fingers to adjust glove fit.	Ensures proper, comfortable fit.

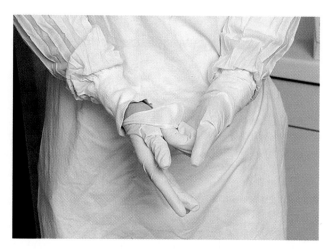

Step 4

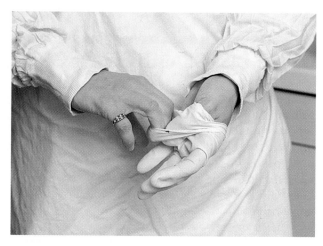

Step 7

Steps	Rationale

Removal

4. Remove first glove by grasping outer surface of lower cuff, taking care to touch only glove to glove (see illustration).

Keeps soiled part of gloves from touching skin of hand or wrist.

5. Pull glove inside out over hand, taking care to touch only inside of glove.
6. Discard glove in receptacle.
7. With ungloved hand, tuck finger inside cuff of remaining glove and pull it off, inside out. Discard in receptacle (see illustration).

Avoids contamination of hands.

8. Wash hands thoroughly for at least 10-15 seconds.
9. See Completion Protocol (inside front cover).

NURSE ALERT

Gloves should be replaced as soon as practical when contaminated and after each procedure, or as soon as feasible if they are torn, punctured, or their ability to function as a barrier is compromised.

EVALUATION

Evaluate client for signs of infection (e.g., temperature elevation, drainage, elevated white blood cell count, chills, malaise, nonhealing wound).

Unexpected Outcomes and Related Interventions

Client develops signs of infection.

a. Notify physician of findings.
b. Provide appropriate therapy (e.g., wound care, hydration to reduce fluid loss, nutritional support).
c. Continue to use good handwashing technique.

Skill 3.3

CARING FOR CLIENTS UNDER ISOLATION PRECAUTIONS

The purpose of isolation and barrier precautions is to protect the client from the nurse, and others from contact with microorganisms. Gowns, gloves, eyewear, and masks are the recommended types of barrier protection. Depending on the potential for exposure, additional items such as shoe covers or hair covers may be necessary (OSHA, 1991). In determining the type of barriers to be used, the following must be considered: the susceptibility of the client or the nurse, the potential for cross-contamination or exposure, the infectiousness of the disease or microorganism, the type and amount of body fluids anticipated, and the facility's policies and procedures for infection control and isolation precautions.

Correct use of barrier protectors still appears to be a problem. Many nurses either overuse or underuse barrier protection. Several studies have found that nurses and other health care workers either forget or choose not to use recommended barriers.

Many nurses tend to use unnecessary barrier protection without exercising critical judgment about controlling transmission of infectious material or without consideration of the cost to their facilities. An example is the AIDS epidemic, which caused many health care workers to question the barrier effectiveness of gloves used in clinical settings. The fear of exposure to contaminated blood or infectious material forced some workers to wear double or even triple gloves. With this in mind, a study by Korniewicz et al. (1994) examined barrier protection with multiple vs. single gloving. They concluded that a single glove offered the same amount of protection as double gloves.

In 1996, the CDC and the Hospital Infection Control Practices Advisory Committee (HICPAC) revised the 1991 *Isolation Precautions in Hospitals*. These guidelines state that all hospitals must put in place a category-specific isolation procedure and educate client care personnel in the correct application and use of barrier equipment (see Box 3-3). It is essential that you are aware of and understand the polices and procedures in your work setting. The concepts are fundamental, although the application varies because of facility-specific criteria.

When a client requires isolation, determine the reason and the mode of transmission. Evaluate the task to be performed to identify the barrier equipment that will be needed. For example, a client in respiratory isolation for measles or pertussis has an organism that can be carried on droplets. A mask is necessary when entering the room for any reason. To hold and feed an infant, it would be appropriate to wear both a mask and gown, to protect your clothing from secretions that the infant could drool or burp onto you. It would be appropriate to add gloves to assist in intubating the infant. When a client is in contact isolation for a resistant organism in sputum, you need to wear gown, gloves, and mask within 3 feet of the client. To introduce yourself to the client, the room may be entered without any protective equipment.

Taking care of a client in isolation can be frightening for health care workers. It is essential to understand the chain of infection and how the organism travels to a receptive host. The most common mode of transmission is your hands. *Wash your hands after every client contact, even when gloves have been worn.* Be aware of unconscious actions

---

Box 3-3 CDC Isolation Guidelines

Transmission Categories (Tier Two)
Category
Airborned precautions
Droplet precautions
Contact precautions
Disease
Droplet nuclei smaller than 5 microns; measles; chickenpox (varicella); disseminated varicella zoster; pulmonary or laryngeal TB
Droplets larger than 5 microns, diphtheria (pharyngeal); rubella; streptococcal pharyngitis, pneumonia, or scarlet fever in infants and young children; pertussis; mumps; mycoplasma pneumonia; meningococcal pneumonia or sepsis; pneumonic plague
Direct client or environmental contact; colonization or infection with multidrug-resistant organism; respiratory syncytial virus; shigella and other enteric pathogens; major wound infections; herpes simplex; scabies, varicella zoster (disseminated)
Barrier Protection
Private room, negative airflow of at least six excahnges per hour, mask or respiratory protection device (see CDC TB Guidelines)
Private room or cohort clients; mask
Private room or cohort clients; gloves, gowns

Modified from Garner JS: Giudlines for isolation precautions for hospitals, *Infect Control Hosp Epideminol* 17(1):54, 1996b.

such as rubbing your eyes or nose, picking teeth, or biting fingernails. For respiratory/droplet-spread organisms, a safe zone 3 to 5 feet from the client can be assumed. Therefore, it is appropriate to walk into the room of a client in isolation, without barrier equipment, to introduce yourself, and be seen without your face covered. This is a good opportunity to inform the client why it is necessary to wear masks, gowns, or gloves while doing certain tasks. The exception to this is when a client is in strict or TB isolation.

Isolation precautions are to prevent the spread of bacteria to compromised hosts. A person who is healthy, gets adequate sleep, maintains a nutritious diet, and practices good hygiene is not a compromised host. Proper use of barrier equipment avoids transmission of organisms to another client who is compromised.

Isolation can be difficult for the client and family. It often fosters a feeling of loneliness. It is also frightening and conjures up horror stories of plagues and epidemics. Clients and families need to be reassured with appropriate education regarding the infectious agent, its mode of transmission, and the purpose of isolation. This education helps maintain the client's self-concept or body image, minimizes feelings of isolation, and facilitates recovery.

Another important consideration is the client's age. The very young and very old have lower immune systems and are more susceptible to colds, flus, and other common viruses such as herpes, which can be life threatening to a newborn. An adolescent or teenage client can provide problems of a different nature, manifested as rebellion against rules. Adolescents do not always comprehend the impact their actions today can have on their life in the future or on others' lives. Age-appropriate education is a key in obtaining client compliance in isolation.

Equipment (Figure 3-2)
    Disposable gloves
    Mask
    Eyewear, protective goggles or glasses, face shield
    Fluid-resistant gown
    Medication
    Hygiene items

ASSESSMENT
1. Review the precautions for the specific isolation system and client's existing condition.
2. Review laboratory reports for results of culture, acid-fast bacillus (AFB) smears, and serology and for changes in white blood cell (WBC) count (see Appendix D).

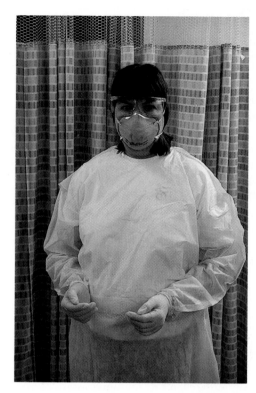

Figure 3-2 Equipment needed varies for isolation precautions.

3. Consider types of care measures to be performed while in client's room. **Rationale: Allows nurse to organize all equipment needed in room.**
4. Determine from chart or significant other if client understands purpose of isolation.

PLANNING
Expected outcomes focus on preventing transmission of infection to nurse and improving client's knowledge of the purpose of isolation.

Expected Outcomes
1. Client and/or family verbalizes purpose of isolation.
2. Infection does not develop in neighboring clients.

IMPLEMENTATION

Steps	Rationale

1. See Standard Protocol (inside front cover).
2. 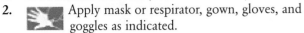 Apply mask or respirator, gown, gloves, and goggles as indicated.
   a. Apply mask or respirator around mouth and nose; tie securely, making sure mask fits snugly.

   Prevents transfer of airborne droplet nuclei. It is the first piece of PPE put on, because it is the most important piece for the health care worker's protection.

   b. Apply gown, being sure it covers all outer garments; pull sleeves down to wrist. Tie securely at neck and wrist (see illustration).

   Reduces possibility of contamination of clothing from splashes or splatters.

   c. Apply disposable gloves. If worn with gown, bring cuffs over edge of gown sleeves.

   Gloves are applied last so that they can be placed over the cuffs of the gown. This prevents wicking of fluids.

   d. Apply goggles or face shield to fit snugly around face and eyes (see illustration).

   Necessary when a possibility of exposure to splashing or splattering of body fluids exists.

COMMUNICATION TIP

Reassure clients and families that isolation is used for diseases that are easily spread, not for diseases that are "extra terrible." It is instituted to protect other clients in the facility from exposure to the mi-croorganism. Be positive, and focus on what they can do (e.g., receive/send mail, watch TV, use the phone, receive visitors). Assure them that the goal is for isolation to be as short and pleasant as possible.

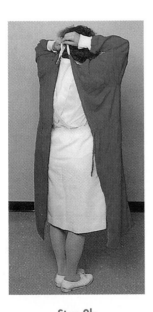

Step 2b

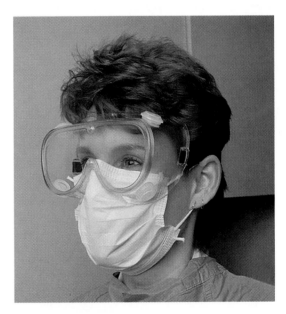

Step 2d

3. Enter client's room. Arrange supplies and equipment. (If equipment will be removed from room for reuse, place on clean paper towel.)

   Minimizes contamination of care items.

4. Explain purpose of isolation and precautions necessary to client, family, and visitors. Offer opportunity to participate in care and to ask questions.

   Improves client's ability to participate in care, and minimizes anxiety.

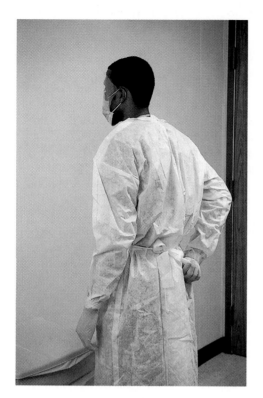

Step 7b

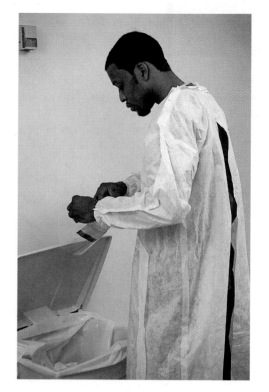

Step 7c

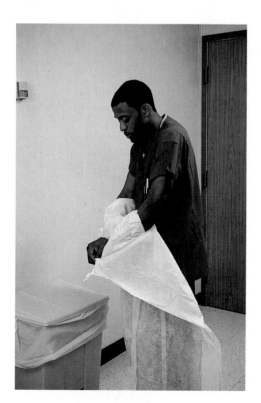

Step 7d

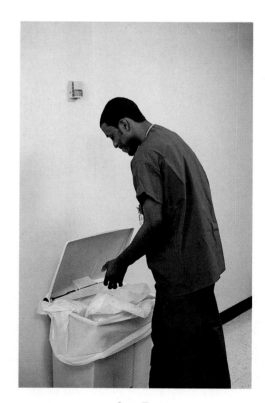

Step 7e

Steps	Rationale
5. Administer care.	
6. Explain to client when you plan to return to room. Ask whether client requires any personal care items.	Includes client in care plan.
7. Prepare to leave isolation room, removing barriers at door of room.	
a. Remove eyewear or goggles without touching hair or face.	Gloved hands are used to remove eyewear or goggles splattered with body fluids.
b. Untie gown at waist (see illustration). Remove one glove by grasping cuff and pulling glove inside out over hand. Discard glove. With ungloved hand, tuck finger inside cuff of remaining glove and pull it off, inside out. Discard in proper receptacle.	Gloves and gown are removed by avoiding further contamination of hands.
c. Without touching outer surface of mask, remove mask; drop mask into trash receptacle (see illustration).	
d. Untie neck strings of gown. Allow gown to fall from shoulders. Remove hands from sleeves without touching outside of gown (see illustration).	
e. Hold gown inside at shoulder seams, and fold inside out. Discard in laundry bag (see illustration).	Clean hands can contact clean items.
f. Wash hands.	
8. Leave room, opening door as little as possible.	Keeping door open too long equalizes pressure in room and can allow organisms to flow out of room.
9. See Completion Protocol (inside front cover).	

• • • •

NURSE ALERT

Needles and syringes should be disposed of un-capped in a puncture-resistant container in client's room (Figure 3-3).

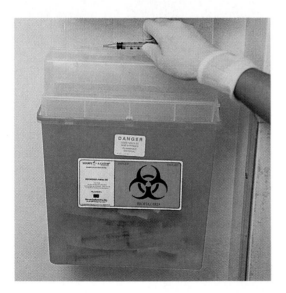

Figure 3-3   Puncture-resistant container for sharps disposal.

EVALUATION

1. Ask client to explain purpose of isolation in relation to diagnosed condition.
2. Monitor clinical status of neighboring clients.

Recording and Reporting

Document the following:

- The type of isolation in use and the microorganism (if known)
- Education given to client/family
- Client/family response to education
- Client/family response to PPE

Sample Documentation

1320   Contact isolation in place for salmonella in stool. Client incontinent of liquid stool. Wife at bedside, asking questions about barrier equipment. Discussed the method by which salmonella is transmitted and explained the purpose of barrier equipment. Wife verbalized good understanding when she requested gloves and gown to assist in cleanup.

Skill 3.4

SPECIAL TUBERCULOSIS PRECAUTIONS

The dramatic upsurge of TB cases in the United States with several outbreaks, some involving drug-resistant strains, has increased concern regarding nosocomial transfer. Guidelines for preventing TB in health care settings stress the importance of early identification and treatment of persons with known or suspected TB and proper isolation in the health care setting. In 1994 the CDC released guidelines for stricter adherence to infection control measures. One should suspect TB in any client with respiratory symptoms lasting longer than 3 weeks. Suspicious symptoms include presence of a productive cough and dyspnea, especially if accompanied by night sweats or unexplained weight loss.

NURSE ALERT

TB transmission often occurs before the client is identified as having TB and before special precautions are taken. If a client complains of night sweats, fatigue, weight loss, loss of apetite, or a chronic cough (that may bring up blood), notify the nurse in charge or the physician. Encourage clients to cover their mouths with tissue when they cough.

Isolation for clients with known or suspected TB includes a special, private isolation room. Such rooms in existing facilities have negative pressure in relation to surrounding areas so that air is exhausted to the outside, having a minimum of six air exchanges per hour. In new construction or renovations, rooms should have at least 12 air exchanges per hour.

In 1993, OSHA issued a mandate requiring health care facilities to follow 1990 CDC guidelines for fitting health care workers potentially exposed to TB with a HEPA respirator (Figure 3-4). As a minimum level of protection, a 0.1-micron filter mask is used with a filter efficiency of 95%. NIOSH-approved HEPA respirators are currently the only model that meets or exceeds that standard. In agencies having major problems with drug-resistant TB, a powered air-purifier respirator (PAPR) has been used. The type of respirator protection depends on agency policy. Research has not substantiated use of any respirators or masks in preventing TB transmission. In December of 1997, OSHA's proposed rule requires an N95 mask (particulate respirator), which filters 0.3-micron particles at 95% efficiency.

NURSE ALERT

Nurses must first check their respirator protection device before entering the room. Doors to TB isolation rooms must be closed to ensure negative pressure. Sign stating proper isolation must be outside door.

There has been much debate regarding the precautions that facilities should take, and it is important to keep up with new guidelines that clarify the most recent thinking for protection of clients and health care workers.

OSHA also requires employers to provide training concerning transmission of TB and proven methods of prevention, especially in areas where risk of exposure is high, such as during bronchoscopy. Health care facilities must provide TB skin tests for all employees and appropriate follow-up evaluation when a previously negative skin test becomes positive (OSHA, 1993).

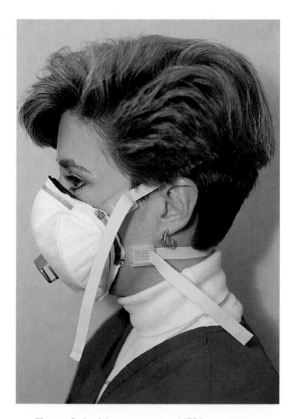

Figure 3-4   Nurse wearing HEPA respirator.

Equipment
   TB isolation room
   Respiratory protective device (check agency policy)

ASSESSMENT

1. Assess client's potential for infectious pulmonary or laryngeal TB (e.g., documentation of positive AFB smear or culture; history of fever, night sweats, or productive cough; cavitation on chest x-ray study; signs or additional symptoms of TB, and history of a recent exposure; physician progress notes indicate plan to rule out TB).

2. Assess effectiveness of isolation room (e.g., check negative airflow using flutter strip or smoke stick, or consult with institution's plant engineering department).

PLANNING

Expected outcomes focus on prevention of transmission of TB and client understanding of TB transmission.

Expected Outcomes
1. Client describes how TB may be transmitted.
2. Neighboring clients or staff do not develop TB.

IMPLEMENTATION

Steps	Rationale
1. See Standard Protocol (inside front cover).	
2. Before entering room, apply recommended mask. Be sure it fits snugly.	Reduces transmission of airborne droplet nuclei.
3. Explain purpose of AFB isolation to client, family, and others.	Improves ability of client to participate in care. TB cannot be transmitted through contact with clothing, bedding, food, or eating utensils.

> **COMMUNICATION TIP**
>
> *TB is transmitted by inhalation of droplets that remain suspended in the air when client coughs, sneezes, speaks, or sings (Boutotte, 1993). Offer opportunity for questions.*

Steps	Rationale
4. Instruct client to cover mouth with tissue when coughing and to wear mask when leaving the room.	Reduces spread of droplet nuclei.

> **NURSE ALERT**
>
> *The particulate respirator that the health care worker wears is not to be placed on the client. The added work of breathing through the respirator is an added stress on an already compromised pulmonary system.*

Steps	Rationale
5. Provide care.	
6. Leave the room, and close the door.	
7. Remove respiratory protective devices such as HEPA respirator.	Most respiratory devices are reusable. The number of times depends on agency policy.
8. Place reusable device in labeled paper bag for storage, being careful not to crush device. (Check agency policy for number of times it can be reused.)	Plastic bags seal in moisture.
9. See Completion Protocol (inside front cover).	

• • • •

EVALUATION

1. Assess client's laboratory data for repeated AFB smears that may be negative.
2. Ask client and/or family to identify method of transmission for TB.

Unexpected Outcomes and Related Interventions

1. Client fails to follow precautions for preventing transmission (e.g., fails to cover mouth when coughing, improperly disposes of soiled tissue).
   a. Reexplain significant risk to family and friends.
   b. Discuss client's concerns/feelings about the disease.

Recording and Reporting

Document the following:
- TB isolation is in place
- Education given to client/family
- Response of client/family to education
- Response of client/family to isolation
- Referrals made

Sample Documentation

0800 AFB isolation maintained. Client instructed on TB transmission and need for isolation. Client verbalized concern about family exposure. Referred to M.D. and local health department.

REFERENCES

Boutotte J: TB the second time around . . . and how you can help control it. *Nursing* 23(5):42-50, 1993.

Centers for Disease Control and Prevention: Universal precautions for prevention of transmission of human immunodeficiency virus, hepatitis B virus, and other blood borne pathogens in health care settings, *MMWR* 37:24, 1988a.

Crow S: Asepsis: an indispensable part of the patient's care plan, *Crit Care Nurs Q* 11(4):11, 1989.

Garner J, Simmons B: CDC guidelines for the prevention and control of nosocomial infections: guideline for isolation precautions in hospitals, *Am J Infect Control* 12(4):103, 1984.

Garner JS: Isolation systems. In Olmstead R, editor: *APIC infection control and applied epidemiology*, St Louis, 1996a, Mosby.

Garner JS: Guidelines for isolation precautions for hospitals. *Infect Control Hosp Epidemiol* 17(1):54, 1996b.

Korniewicz D et al: Barrier protection with examination gloves; double versus single, *Am J Infect Control* 22(1):12, 1994.

Larson E: APIC guideline for the use of topical antimicrobial agents, *Am J Infect Control* 16(6):253, 1996.

Occupational Safety and Health Administration: Bloodborne pathogens, *Federal Register* 56(235):64175, 1991.

Occupational Safety and Health Administration: *Enforcement policies on procedures for occupational exposure to tuberculosis*, Washington DC, 1993, OSHA.

CRITICAL THINKING EXERCISES

1. Last month you were working in an acute care facility and were caring for a client with MRSA (a resistant staphylococcal blood infection) in the sputum and blood. This client was in contact isolation, and you wore a mask, gown, and gloves when you gave personal care. Today you are working at a nursing home and have the same client. You are surprised that there is no sign on the door designating that this is a client in contact isolation. The client's wife recognizes you and asks you to tell the nurses that her husband must be in isolation like he was at the hospital. How would you handle this situation?

2. A client has come into the waiting room of the ambulatory clinic you are staffing. He is coughing and holding a crumpled, blood-tinged tissue. His wife is also coughing. The client tells you that he just can't cough any more, he is tired and can't get any sleep, and he keeps waking up in a cold sweat. He wants to know if he can get some cough syrup for his cold. What is indicated in this situation, and what actions are appropriate for you to take?

CHAPTER 4

Basic Sterile Techniques

Skill 4.1
Creating and Maintaining a Sterile Field, 64

Skill 4.2
Sterile Gloving, 69

Sterile technique, or surgical asepsis, is a method of creating and maintaining an area free of all microorganisms, including spores and pathogens. As in medical asepsis, handwashing with an appropriate soap or antiseptic is essential before the initiation of an aseptic procedure. Microorganisms can be endogenous (from within the body) or exogenous (from outside the body). Strict adherence to the principles of sterile technique limits a client's risk for infection during invasive procedures, although infection can occur because of the presence of endogenous organisms.

Surgical asepsis is routine in the operating room, labor and delivery areas, and some diagnostic areas (e.g., during cardiac catheterization). Nurses use principles of sterile technique (Box 4-1 on p. 64) at the client's bedside in the following three types of situations:

- During procedures that require intentional perforation of a client's skin, such as insertion of an intravenous (IV) catheter.
- When the skin integrity is impaired, such as with surgical incision, trauma, burns, or some advanced pressure ulcers.
- During procedures requiring insertion of devices or instruments into a sterile body cavity, such as urinary catheterization.

A sterile field is an area that provides sterile surfaces draped for placement of sterile equipment. The following basic rules are essential according to the Association of Operating Room Nurses (AORN, 1998):

- A sterile field is established immediately before the procedure, because there is a direct relationship between the time the sterile field is open and the presence of airborne contaminants.
- The sterile field must always be within view of the nurse, to prevent unobserved contamination.
- The sterile field is not covered, because it is too difficult to uncover without contaminating the field.

Principles of sterile technique are used for certain procedures, such as parenteral injections, although a sterile field is not needed because of the use of sterile barriers to cover the needle (see Chapter 18).

Box 4-1 Principles of Surgical Asepsis

1. All items used within a sterile field must be sterile.
2. A sterile barrier that has been permeated by moisture must be considered contaminated.
3. Once a sterile package is opened, the edges are considered unsterile.
4. Gowns, once put on, are considered sterile in front from chest to waist or table level; sleeves are considered sterile from 5 cm (2 inches) above elbows to fingertips of gloved hand. (NOTE: Cuffs are not considered sterile once glove has been removed.)
5. Tables draped as part of sterile field are considered sterile only at table level.
6. If there is any question or doubt of an item's sterility, the item is considered to be unsterile.
7. Persons with sterile barriers (gloves) or sterile items contact only sterile areas/items. Persons without sterile barriers contact only unsterile items.
8. Movement around and in the sterile field must not compromise or contaminate the sterile field.

Nurses must recognize the importance of strict adherence to aseptic principles. Nurses are also expected to play an active role in enforcing these principles with other members of the health care team. The nurse can serve as an excellent role model and client advocate, reinforcing principles when another caregiver breaks technique.

In the operating room, control of aseptic technique is more easily enforced because of the controlled environment. At the bedside it is important for the nurse to explain what a client can do to avoid contaminating sterile items, including avoiding sudden body movement, not touching sterile areas or supplies, and avoiding coughing or talking over a sterile area.

The use of sterile technique is intended to protect the client from exogenous infections. However, there are situations in which this technique is expanded to include the use of Standard Precautions to protect the nurse from potential contact with blood and body fluids. The use of Standard Precautions include the use of masks, eye protection, and gowns when there is risk of being splattered with infectious materials (see Chapter 3).

NURSING DIAGNOSES

The nursing diagnosis most directly related to clients requiring procedures involving sterile technique is **Risk for Infection.** Use of meticulous sterile technique has substantially reduced the incidence of wound infections in surgical clients. However, endogenous microorganisms can cause infections even when the principles of surgical asepsis have been carefully followed.

Skill 4.1

CREATING AND MAINTAINING A STERILE FIELD

A sterile field provides a microorganism-free area in which to perform a procedure. For minor procedures, a sterile kit or bundle of supplies can be opened on a clean surface and used as the sterile field (Figure 4-1). For more complicated procedures or those requiring several supplies, a table can be covered with a sterile, water-repellent drape. Sterile drapes can be linen, paper, or plastic but must be water repellent. Sterile supplies and solutions can then be delivered to the sterile field.

The inside of a sterile kit may also serve as a sterile field. Examples of sterile kits are urinary catheter insertion kits or triple-lumen catheter kits. Some institutions wrap and process their own bundles of equipment for proce

dures such as lumbar punctures or thoracentesis trays. Bundles packaged by the institution generally contain external and internal sterile (chemical) indicators that indicate the item has completed a sterilization process (Figure 4-2).

Equipment

Sterile gloves
Sterile, water-repellent drapes (often included within a kit)
Sterile equipment and solutions (as appropriate)
Sterile gown, cap, mask, and protective eyewear (if required based on type of procedure and agency policy)

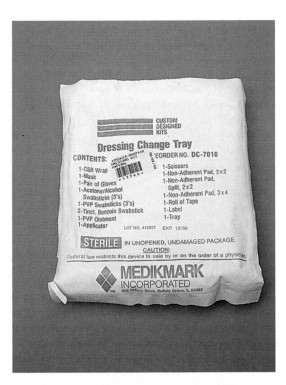

Figure 4-1   Sterile dressing change kit.

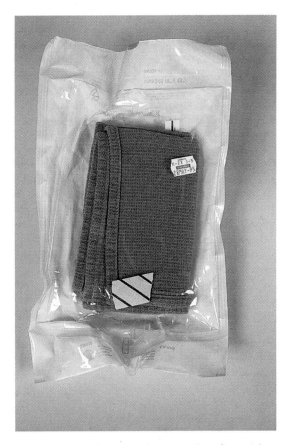

Figure 4-2   Tape with stripes changes color after sterilization.

ASSESSMENT

1. Verify that procedure requires surgical aseptic technique.
2. Assess client's comfort, oxygen requirements, and elimination needs before procedure. **Rationale: Certain sterile procedures may last a long time. The nurse should anticipate the client's needs, enabling the client to relax and avoid any unnecessary movement that might disrupt the procedure.**
3. Assess for latex allergies. **Rationale: A focused review may reveal latex allergies even when no known allergies are indicated during the chart review.**
4. Check commercially packaged kits (often disposable) for package integrity, expiration date, and statement of sterility. **Rationale: Moisture, punctures, tears, and outdated supplies increase the risk of contamination. Supplies considered unsterile must be reprocessed or discarded.**

PLANNING

Expected outcomes focus on prevention of localized or systemic infection.

Expected Outcomes

1. Client remains afebrile 24 to 48 hours after the procedure or during course of repeated procedures.
2. Client displays no signs of localized infection (e.g., redness, tenderness, edema, drainage) 24 hours after the procedure.

DELEGATION CONSIDERATIONS

Procedures requiring sterile technique are generally performed by professional nurses and should not be delegated. In some settings, assistive personnel (AP) (e.g., surgical technicians) are specifically trained to perform sterile technique under the supervision of a professional nurse.

IMPLEMENTATION

Steps	Rationale

1. See Standard Protocol (inside front cover).
2. Prepare a clean, dry work surface at or above waist level.

COMMUNICATION TIP

Instruct the client not to touch the work surface or equipment during the procedure, and to remain still.

3. If using linen-wrapped supply bundle processed by agency:
   a. Place on selected work surface.
   b. Remove sterile (chemical) indicator tape from outside of package discard.
   c. Open outer wrapper layer and inner sterile drape (one at a time).
   d. Locate and grasp outer surface of tip of outermost flap and open away from yourself (see illustration).
   e. Open first side flap in same manner but to the side and without reaching over sterile field (see illustration). Keep arm to side and not over sterile surface.

Once created, sterile field is sterile only at table level.
Linen-wrapped items have two layers and may be enclosed in plastic. The first is a dust cover, and the second layer must be opened to view the sterile (chemical) indicator. If dropped, linen packages are considered contaminated.

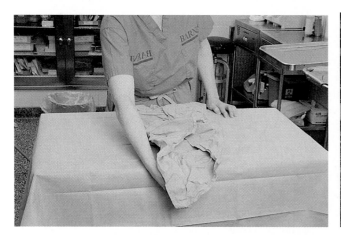

Step 3d

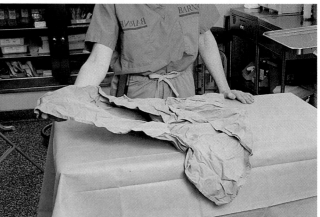

Step 3e

   f. Repeat as above for flap on other side (see illustration).
   g. Carefully grasp outside surface of final and innermost flap corner. Stand away from sterile item and pull flap back, allowing it to fall flat (see illustration).
4. Prepare commercially packaged kit with paper wrap:
   a. Remove kit from outer dust cover.
   b. Place on selected work surface.
   c. Open sterile wrapper layer as with above kit (steps 3a-g).

Steps	Rationale

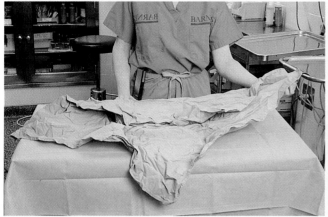

Step 3f

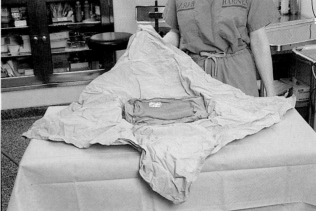

Step 3g

5. Delivering sterile items to the sterile field:
   a. Add packaged items to sterile field (following package directions) by carefully pulling back the edges of the outer wrapper (see illustration).
   b. Gently toss item onto the sterile field while preventing wrapper from touching sterile field.

   Reaching over or touching sterile field contaminates field.

   c. Dispose of outer wrapper.
6. Pouring sterile solutions:
   a. Verify contents and expiration date of solution.
   b. Remove seal and cap from bottle, keeping inside of cap sterile.
   c. Hold bottle with label touching palm. Pour solution slowly into sterile container without splashing and while maintaining safe distance from the sterile field (see illustration).

   Prevents liquid from smearing the label. Splashing liquids causes fluid permeation of the sterile barrier, called *strike through*, resulting in contamination.

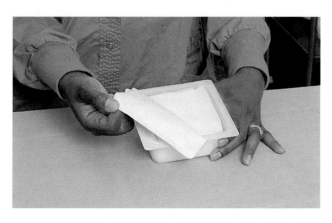

Step 5a

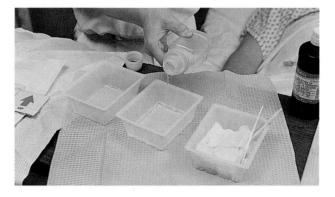

Step 6c

Steps	Rationale

    d. Label container with expiration date and time (see illustration).

7. Proceed with intended sterile procedure.

Solution is considered contaminated 24 hours after opening (check agency policy).

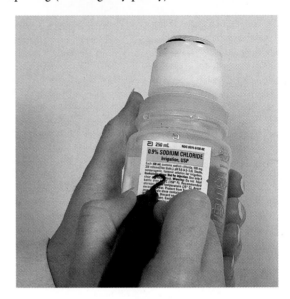

Step 6d

• • • •

EVALUATION

1. Evaluate client for fever for 48 hours after procedure.
2. Inspect treated area for localized signs of infection (e.g., redness, tenderness, edema, warmth, odor, drainage).

Unexpected Outcomes and Related Interventions

1. Client develops signs of infection.
   a. Notify physician of findings.
   b. Continue strict aseptic technique and vigorous handwashing.
   c. Monitor temperature every 4 hours and prn.
   d. Encourage and document client's intake of fluids.

Recording and Reporting

Include procedure performed using sterile technique and client response and ability to cooperate. Depending on the procedure, include the following:

- Optimal position
- Understanding/knowledge of the procedure
- Ability to cooperate
- Number and type of supplies used

Sample Documentation

1400 24 hrs after lumbar puncture, site is without redness, tenderness, or edema. Adhesive bandage is dry and intact. Client denies complaints of discomfort.

Geriatric Considerations

- Older adults may be at greater risk for infection because of compromised circulation, inadequate nutrition, or decreased body defenses caused by chronic illness.
- Memory and sensory deficits may impair client's ability to understand and cooperate with the procedure.

Home Care and Long-Term Care Considerations

- Adaptations may be made for some procedures, such as self-catheterization and home tracheostomy care. In some cases, clients use medical asepsis rather than surgical technique (see Chapter ••).
- If possible, the client/family learns to perform sterile procedures well before discharge from acute care so that skill and adaptations can be worked out with professional assistance.
- Home visits should include cleanliness of the environment, as well as the understanding and ability of client and family to perform procedure safely.

Skill 4.2

STERILE GLOVING

Sterile gloves act as a barrier against the transmission of pathogenic microorganisms and should be put on before performing any sterile procedure, such as a sterile dressing change or urinary catheter insertion. The nurse must remember that sterile gloves do not replace vigorous handwashing.

The open glove method is used for most sterile procedures not requiring a sterile gown. The nurse must take care not to contaminate the gloved hands by touching unsterile items or areas. The hands should remain clasped in front of the body until ready to perform the procedure. If a glove becomes contaminated, it must be changed immediately.

It is important to select the correct type of gloves, because many individuals are developing allergies to powders and latex (APIC, 1996). Studies have shown that individuals who are highly sensitive to latex develop local and systemic reactions when latex gloves are removed and the latex glove powder particles are suspended in the air (Beezold, Kostyol, and Wiseman, 1994). Latex-free and powder-free gloves should be made available in all work settings. It is also important to select the proper size of gloves. Gloves should not stretch too tightly over the fingers, cutting off circulation and increasing the risk of tears, nor should they be too loose and cause difficulty manipulating equipment.

While using sterile gloves the nurse should always be conscious of the position of the hands. If a sterile glove touches a clean, contaminated, or possibly contaminated item, the glove must be considered unsterile. It is helpful to hold the hands together, 10 to 12 inches from the body and just above waist level, except when engaged in the sterile procedure itself. If a glove tears or becomes contaminated, it must be replaced immediately and before touching any other sterile area or item.

Equipment

Package of correctly sized sterile gloves (Figure 4-3)

ASSESSMENT

Verify that the procedure to be performed requires sterile gloves. **Rationale: Some sterile procedures can use a "no-touch" technique.**

PLANNING

Expected outcomes focus on prevention of localized or systemic infection.

Expected Outcomes

1. Client remains afebrile 24 to 48 hours after the procedure or during the course of repeated procedures.
2. Client displays no signs of localized infection (e.g., redness, tenderness, edema, drainage) 72 hours after the procedure.

DELEGATION CONSIDERATIONS

See Delegation Considerations for Skill 4.1.

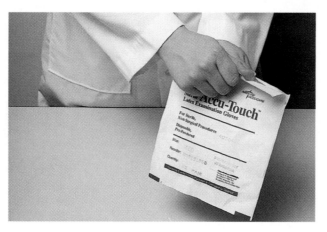

Figure 4-3 Package of sterile gloves.

IMPLEMENTATION

Steps	Rationale

1. See Standard Protocol (inside front cover).
2. Open sterile gloves by peeling back adhered package edges (see illustration).
3. Remove inner wrapper and carefully open without touching the wrapper's inner surface (see illustration).
4. Select glove of dominant hand and grasp folded edge of cuff with nondominant hand. Touch only the inside surface of glove (see illustration).
5. Pull glove over dominant hand, carefully working thumb and fingers into correct spaces. Gently let go of cuff while preventing it from rolling up wrist (see illustration).

NURSE ALERT

Check to see if client has a latex allergy or sensitivity. If so, check agency policy regarding type of sterile gloves to be used.

Inner edge of cuff will touch skin and is no longer considered sterile.

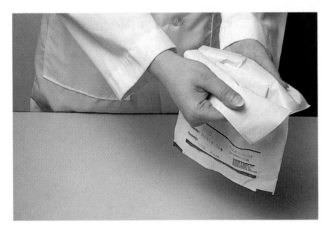

Step 2

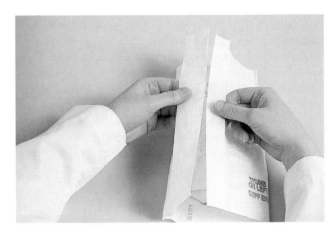

Step 3

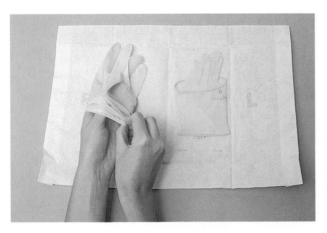

Step 4

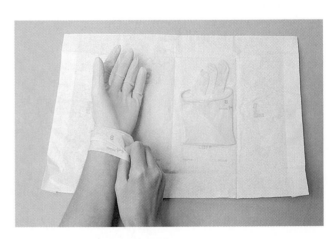

Step 5

Steps	Rationale

6. Slide fingers of gloved hand underneath second glove's cuff (see illustration), and pull over fingers of nondominant hand. Do not touch exposed areas with gloved hands; keep thumb of dominant hand abducted back (see illustration).

Cuff protects gloved fingers; abducting thumb prevents contamination from contact with unsterile surface.

7. Interlock fingers of gloved hands and hold away from body until beginning procedure.

8. Proceed with intended procedure.

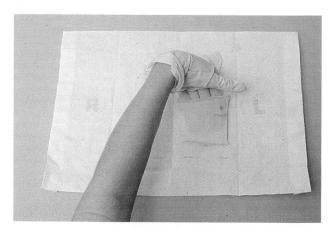 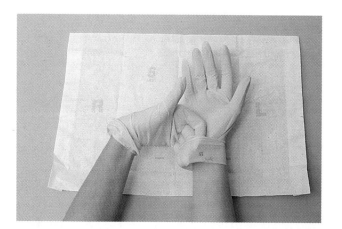

Step 6

Glove disposal

9. Pull off glove of one hand, turning inside out by grasping outside of the cuff with other gloved hand. Discard in proper receptacle.

Minimizes contamination of bare hands.

10. Remove remaining glove by placing fingers of bare hand under cuff, and pull off by turning inside out. Discard in proper receptacle.

11. See completion protocol.

• • •

EVALUATION

1. Evaluate client for fever for 48 hours after the procedure.

2. Inspect treated area for localized signs of infection (e.g., redness, tenderness, edema, warmth, odor, drainage).

Unexpected Outcomes and Related Interventions

1. Client develops signs of infection.
   a. Notify physician of findings.
   b. Continue strict aseptic technique and vigorous handwashing.
   c. Monitor temperature every 4 hours and prn.
   d. Encourage and document client's intake of fluids.

CRITICAL THINKING EXERCISES

1. Mrs. Thomas is 90 years old and very frail. She has a deep RUQ abdominal wound that requires dressing changes 3 times a day that involve irrigation and packing. The procedure is so traumatic for Mrs. Thomas that she has started crying whenever she thinks it is time for her dressing change. What is the best way to handle this situation?

2. Dr. Johnson has requested that you assist him to perform a lumbar puncture on Mr. Smith, who has agreed to the procedure. It takes several minutes to position the client, prepare the area, and inject the local anesthetic. Mr. Smith becomes very restless and complains about feeling very uncomfortable in the required position. Dr. Johnson reaches for the spinal needle but doesn't notice that it is touching the edge of the sterile field. Is this a problem? If so, why? How would you handle the situation?

3. Which of the following procedures require sterile (aseptic) technique? Which require only clean technique?
   a. Urinary catheterization
   b. Insertion of IV catheter
   c. Insertion of rectal suppository
   d. Vaginal douche
   e. Lumbar puncture
   f. Sitz bath

4. You have several dressing changes to perform this morning and have just spent an hour with another client that had to be transferred to the ICU. After first checking on all your clients, you start with Mrs. Martinez, a pleasant but confused lady with an abdominal wound infection. Trying to make up for lost time, you start opening supplies and preparing Mrs. Martinez for the dressing change. You realize you do not have everything you need for the dressing change. As you turn around to look for the missing supplies, Mrs. Martinez sits up in bed, contaminating the sterile field. What preparations could you make ahead of time to avoid this situation?

REFERENCES

APIC: *Infection control and applied epidemiology,* St Louis, 1996, Mosby.

Association of Operating Room Nurses: Recommended practices for aseptic technique. In *AORN standards and recommended practices for perioperative nursing,* Denver, 1998, AORN.

Beezold D, Kostyol D, Wiseman J: The transfer of protein allergens from latex gloves, *AORN J,* 59:30, 1994.

CHAPTER 5

Promoting A Safe Environment

Skill 5.1
Safety Equipment and Fall Prevention, 76

Skill 5.2
Designing a Restraint-Free Environment, 81

Skill 5.3
Applying Restraints, 85

Skill 5.4
Seizure Precautions, 91

Skill 5.5
Safety Measures for Radioactive Materials, 92

Safety is a basic human need often defined as freedom from psychological and physical injury. Nurses in any setting are responsible for identifying and eliminating safety hazards and providing communication and support that promote a feeling of security and allow clients to focus on recovery. Client safety is a priority in health care agencies, in long-term care facilities, and in the home.

Promoting client safety in the acute care setting reduces the length and cost of treatment, the frequency of treatment-related accidents, the potential for lawsuits, and the number of work-related injuries to personnel. There are many safety features that are part of the structure and design of a health care environment, such as specialized equipment including beds, hand rails, call bells, and alarm systems.

ACCIDENTS

Beginning at about age 70, the death rate from falls increases dramatically and continues to increase with age. Falls are a leading cause of injury in older adult clients. Factors that contribute to the risk of falls include being in an unfamiliar environment; difficulty communicating because of impaired vision, hearing, or speech; and impaired cognition. In many agencies a falls risk assessment is routinely completed on admission and may be repeated at specified intervals (Box 5-1 on p. 74). Signs, special armbands, or color-coded footwear may be used to identify clients at risk for falls.

Fire prevention in health care agencies is a basic responsibility of all health care workers. Fires in health care agencies are most often related to electrical safety and anesthesia (Potter and Perry, 1997). Because smoking is both a health hazard and a safety hazard, it is not permitted in the hospital setting without a physician's order. Some clients need supervision while smoking. Fires in health care agencies may result from malfunction or damage to electrical equipment or from anesthesia. Electrical equipment must be maintained in good condition and must be grounded. All health care workers are responsible for inspecting electrical cords and reporting damaged equipment to the maintenance department.

Box 5-1 Risk for Falls Assessment Tools

Tool 1: Risk Assessment Tool for Falls

Directions: Place a check mark in front of elements that apply to your client. The decision of whether a client is at risk for falls is based on your nursing judgment. *Guideline:* A client who has a check mark in front of an element with an asterisk (*) or four or more of the other elements would be identified as at risk for falls.

General Data
__ Age over 60
__ History of falls before admission*
__ Postoperative/admitted for surgery
__ Smoker

Physical Condition
__ Dizziness/imbalance
__ Unsteady gait
__ Diseases/other problems affecting weight-bearing joints
__ Weakness
__ Paresis
__ Seizure disorder
__ Impairment of vision
__ Impairment of hearing
__ Diarrhea
__ Urinary frequency

Mental Status
__ Confusion/disorientation*
__ Impaired memory or judgment
__ Inability to understand or follow directions

Medications
__ Diuretics or diuretic effects
__ Hypotensive or central nervous system suppressants (e.g., narcotic, sedative, psychotropic, hypnotic, tranquilizer, antihypertensive, antidepressant)
__ Medication that increases gastrointestinal motility (e.g., laxative, enema)

Ambulatory Devices Used
__ Cane
__ Crutches
__ Walker
__ Wheelchair
__ Geriatric (Geri) chair
__ Braces

Tool 2: Reassessment is Safe "Kare" (Risk) Tool

Directions: Place a check mark in front of any element that applies to your client. A client who has a check mark in front of any of the first four elements would be identified as at risk for falls. In addition, when a high-risk client has a check mark in front of the element "Use of a wheelchair," the client is considered to be at greater risk for falls.
__ Unsteady gait/dizziness/imbalance
__ Impaired memory or judgment
__ Weakness
__ History of falls
__ Use of a wheelchair

Data from Brians LK et al: *Rehabil Nurs* 16(2):67, 1991.

Table 5-1

Fire Extinguishers and Their Uses

Class of Fire	Fire Extinguisher
Class A: Paper, wood, rubbish	Contains water or a solution with a large percentage of water; quenches and cools
Class B: Flammable liquids (gasoline, oil, grease, or solvents)	Dry chemical, carbon dioxide, foam, and halogenated hydrocarbons cut off oxygen supply
Class C: Electrical	Carbon dioxide or dry chemical cuts off oxygen supply

 FIRE SAFETY

If a fire occurs in a health care agency, the nurse protects clients from injury, reports the location of the fire, and contains the fire. One helpful acronym in the event of a fire is RACE: *rescue* or *remove* the client from immediate danger (Box 5-2 on p. 75) pull the *alarm; confine* the fire by closing all doors and windows; and *extinguish* the fire if manageable by using a blanket, sheet, or water pitcher.

Fire extinguishers are available at specified locations. They are to be used by persons who have been trained and have had the opportunity to practice. The three basic types of fires for which extinguishers are used are paper, wood, and rubbish (type A); grease and anesthetic gas (type B); and electrical (type C). The appropriate extinguisher should be used for each type (Table 5-1).

Box 5-2 Client Removal Methods

Infant and Child Removal

1. Place a blanket or sheet on the floor.
2. Place two infants in each bassinet, using diapers or small blankets for padding.
3. Place the bassinet in the middle of the blanket.
4. Use the baby vest if available or fold the blanket over one end, fold the corners in, then roll the sides in to form a pocket.
5. Grasp the folded corners of the blanket and pull the infants to safety. Two persons (or, if necessary, one person) can drag eight babies to the prescribed area.
6. Alternatively, place as many children as possible in one crib and pull the crib to the prescribed area.

Universal Carry

The universal carry is a method of removing a client from a bed to the floor. It is a quick and effective method for removing a client who is in immediate danger. This carry can be used by anyone, regardless of client size.

1. Spread a blanket, sheet, or bedspread on the floor alongside the bed, placing one third of it under the bed and leaving about 8 inches to extend beyond the client's head.
2. Grasp the client's ankles, and move the client's legs until they fall at the knee over the edge of the bed.
3. Grasp each shoulder, slowly pulling the client to a sitting position.
4. From the back, encircle the client with your arms, place your arms under the client's armpits, and lock your hands over the client's chest.
5. Slide the client slowly to the edge of the bed, and lower the client to the blanket. If the bed is high, instruct the client to slide down one of your legs.
6. Taking care to protect the client's head, gently lower the head and upper torso to the blanket and wrap the blanket around the client.
7. At the client's head, grip the blanket with both hands, one above each shoulder, holding the client's head firmly in the 8 inches of blanket. Do not let the client's head snap back.
8. Lift the client to a half-sitting position, and pull the blanketed client to safety.

Swing Carry

The swing carry requires two trained persons.

1. One carrier, feet together, slides an arm under the client's neck and grasps the client's far shoulder. The carrier's free hand is slipped under the client's other upper arm, grasping it. Taking one step toward the foot of the bed, the carrier brings the client to a sitting position.
2. The second carrier now grasps the client's ankles, bringing the client's legs at the knee over the edge of the bed.
3. Each carrier takes one of the client's wrists and pulls it down over the carrier's shoulder, supporting the client's body.
4. Each carrier reaches across the client's back, placing one carrier's free hand on the other's shoulder.
5. Each carrier reaches under the client's knees to lock hands with the other.
6. Standing close to the client, the carriers bring their shoulders up and remove the client from the bed, carrying the client to a safe area.
7. At the safe area, each carrier drops on the knee closest to the client, leans against the client, and rests the client's buttocks on the floor. The client's torso is lowered to the floor, and the client's head is placed on a pillow or similar protection. The client's head must always be carefully protected.

Blanket Drag

If vertical or downward evacuation by an interior stairway is necessary, in many cases one person can handle a helpless client by using the blanket drag.

1. Double a blanket lengthwise, and place it on the floor parallel and next to the bed, leaving 8 inches to extend above the client's head.
2. Using cradle drop, kneel drop, or other suitable means, remove the client from the bed to the folded blanket on the floor alongside the bed.
3. Grasping the blanket above the client's head with both hands, drag the client headfirst to the stairway.
4. Position yourself one, two, or three steps lower than the client, depending on your height and the client's height. The client's lower body inclines upward.
5. Place your arms under the client's arms, and clasp your hands over the client's chest.
6. Back slowly down the stairs, constantly maintaining close contact with the client, keeping one leg against the client's back.

RESTRAINTS

The optimal goal for all clients is a restraint-free environment. Adults who have altered cognitive ability often are at risk for injury from wandering, falls, and disruptive or agitated behavior. Traditionally, restraints have been used in hospitals to keep clients safe. However, it has more recently been well documented that clients are at high risk for injuries when restrained (Miles and Irvine, 1992). Growing research findings indicate that the hazards of restraints outweigh the apparent benefits. Since the Omnibus Budget Reconciliation Act (OBRA) of 1987, several health care organizations have developed standards and guidelines promoting the development of suitable alternatives to the use of restraints (Stolley, 1995).

A wide variety of electronic options (e.g. bed alarms) have recently been developed to alert staff when clients under supervision need assistance. Nurses are responsible for identifying and using all other alternatives before using mechanical or physical restraints. Sometimes having someone sit and spend time talking with clients helps to reorient them and reduces wandering. When restraints are necessary, documentation must show the reason for restraint and that the restraint is the only appropriate intervention that will maintain a client's safety. Both the client and family need to be informed that the restraint is temporary and protective. Measures to prevent the hazards of immobility and other complications must be initiated.

SEIZURE PRECAUTIONS

Clients who are at risk for seizure activity need to have seizure precautions instituted to protect them from injury during a seizure. Seizures may occur in several forms and result from a variety of conditions. The most alarming form of seizure activity is called *grand mal seizures*, which is characterized by loss of consciousness and alternating rigid and jerking movements. Clients may also have altered breathing and loss of bowel and bladder control. Objects are not to be placed in the client's mouth during a seizure, because this practice has resulted in injury (Ellis, 1993). Clients experiencing a seizure are not restrained and need to be protected from injury.

RADIATION SAFETY

Another source of environmental hazard in health care settings is use of radioactive materials that may be present in radiology departments, nuclear medicine, clinical laboratories, and client care areas. The safe handling, use, and disposal of radioactive materials is under the management of the Nuclear Regulatory Commission (NRC). Regulations require limiting the exposure of employees to radiation, including use of caution signs, personal radiation dose meters, and actions to be taken after accidental exposure.

NURSING DIAGNOSES

Risk for Injury (trauma) is appropriate for clients with safety issues for a variety of reasons. Risk factors may include altered cognitive ability (e.g., disorientation, impaired judgment); unfamiliar setting or inability to use call system; impaired mobility resulting from weakness, paralysis, balance and coordination problems, or dizziness; and sensory/perceptual alterations including vision, hearing, or touch (Gordon, 1998). **Risk for Injury** related to lack of knowledge of safety precautions is appropriate when teaching the client and family about home safety, fire safety, and radiation safety.

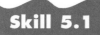

SAFETY EQUIPMENT AND FALL PREVENTION

It is important for nurses and other health care workers to be acutely aware of potential safety hazards in acute care and long-term care settings. Falls account for up to 90% of all reported hospital incidents, with the risk for older adults significantly greater (Brady et al., 1993). Most falls occur within a few feet of the client's bed or en route to the bathroom (Chaff, 1996). Clients at risk for falling need to be identified by a visual system (e.g., sign on the door or bedside, color-coded armband). These clients need to be watched closely under all circumstances.

For clients who need assistance to get out of bed and do not remember to call for assistance, electronic monitoring devices can be used (see Skill 5.2). Hospital units are designed with safety as a major concern. Floor surfaces must be kept dry and free of clutter. Spills of water, food, or urine must be immediately wiped up from the floor or a safety cone placed to alert staff and clients of the hazard. One side of all hallways are to be kept free of equipment and clutter to provide for safe ambulation (Chaff, 1994). Lighting must be adequate, without glaring. Adequate ventilation, stable room temperature, and humidity provide both comfort and safety.

Hospital beds have a frame that can raise or lower the entire bed. The bed is raised when care is being provided, to promote good body mechanics for caregivers. The bed is kept in low position at all other times. Side rails can be raised to remind clients to call for help to get out of bed. Side rails also help clients turn and reposition in bed.

Every client must have a call light or signaling device easily accessible and be given instructions on its use. Call bells or intercom systems at each bedside and in bathrooms and treatment rooms facilitate emergency calls for assistance. Safety features in bathrooms include shower chairs that allow clients to sit safely during the shower. Safety grips and nonskid surfaces are provided in bathrooms and shower areas (Figure 5-1). A raised toilet seat with arms may be used for clients who have difficulty sitting down and standing after having been seated.

Most hospital rooms have a straight-back chair and a lounge chair to be used by the client and visitors. Reclin-

ing chairs with elevated foot support and an attached tray are often used for older clients who are not ambulatory (Figure 5-2).

When preparing clients for discharge to home and when making home care visits, assessment of safety hazards in the home environment is essential. Assessment should include access to the home; general safety concerns (e.g., lighting, floors, furniture, electrical and fire safety); and specific concerns relating to kitchen, bedroom, and bathroom (Box 5-3 on p. 78).

Equipment

> Risk for Falls Assessment Tool
> Hospital bed
> Side rails
> Call bell/intercom system
> Wheelchair (for transport of clients too unsteady or weak to walk)
> Stretcher (for transport of clients unable to safely sit upright)

ASSESSMENT

1. Assess the client's age, level of consciousness, degree of orientation, and ability to follow directions and cooperate.
2. Assess the client's mobility, hearing, and sight.
3. Assess medications and alcohol intake.
4. Assess history of hypotensive episodes and seizures. **Rationale: Assessment determines the degree of assistance needed to maintain safety.**

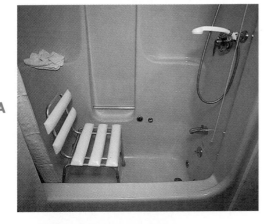

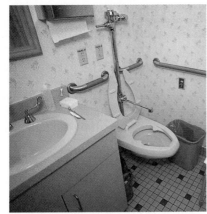

Figure 5-1 A, Nonslip surface in tub prevents falls. Shower chair allows clients to sit while in the shower. **B,** Safety features in bathrooms include safety grip bar and emergency call bell.

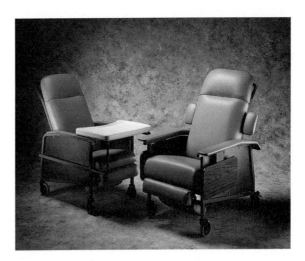

Figure 5-2 A Geri chair with attached tray and elevated foot support may be used for nonambulatory clients. *Courtesy Invacare Corporation, Elyria, Ohio.*

Box 5-3 Home Hazard Assessment

Home Exterior
Are sidewalks uneven?
Are steps in good repair?
Do steps have securely fastened hand rails?
Is there adequate lighting?
Is outdoor furniture sturdy?

Home Interior
Do all rooms, stairways, and halls have adequate lighting?
Are night-lights available?
Are area rugs secured?
Are wooden floors nonslippery?
Is furniture placed appropriately to permit mobility?
Is furniture sturdy enough to provide support for getting up and down?
Are temperature and humidity within normal range?
Are there any steps or thresholds that may pose a hazard?
Are step edges clearly marked with colored tape?
Are hand rails available and secure?
Are extension cords used appropriately?
Are smoke, fire, and carbon monoxide detectors installed?

Kitchen
Are handwashing facilities available?
Is the pilot light on for the gas stove?
Are the dials on the stove readable?
Are storage areas within easy reach?

Are cleaning fluids, bleach, etc., in original containers and stored properly?
Is the water temperature within normal range?
Are there clean areas for food storage and preparation?
Is refrigeration adequate?
Are appliances in good working order?
Are electrical appliances located away from water sources?
Are electrical cords in good condition?

Bathroom
Are handwashing facilities available?
Are there skidproof strips or surfaces in the tub or shower?
Are bath mats secured?
Does the client need grip bars near the bathtub and toilet?
Does the client need an elevated toilet seat?
Is the medicine cabinet well lighted?
Are medications in their original containers?
Have outdated medications been discarded?

Bedroom
Are beds of adequate height to allow getting on and off easily?
Is day and night lighting adequate?
Are floor coverings nonskid?
Does the client have a telephone nearby?
Are emergency numbers visible near the phone?

Data from Tideiksaar R: Home safe home: practical tips for fall-proofing, *Geriatr Nurs* 11(6):284, 1989, and Ebersole P, Hess P: *Toward healthy aging: human needs and nursing process*, ed 4, St Louis, 1994, Mosby.

PLANNING
Expected outcomes focus on recognition of hazards in the environment and appropriate use of safety equipment.

Expected Outcomes
1. Client does not fall or suffer injury while in the health care agency.
2. Client and family demonstrate use of the call bell to obtain assistance.
3. Client and family state reasons safety devices are used.

DELEGATION CONSIDERATIONS

Prevention of falls, fire safety, and promoting safety in a restraint-free environment may be delegated to assistive personnel (AP). However, assessment is not delegated. When delegating safety measures, the professional nurse needs to stress the importance of the following:

- On each contact with the client, check for safety hazards in the environment.
- Before leaving a client, make sure the bed is in low position and the call bell is within reach.
- Safety measures for restrained clients including frequency of checks and release for range of motion, skin care, and repositioning.

IMPLEMENTATION

Steps	Rationale

1. See Standard Protocol (inside front cover).

2. Explain the use of the call bell or intercom (see illustration).
   a. Provide client with hearing aid and glasses if used.
   b. Demonstrate to both client and family how to turn the call bell on and off at bedside.
   c. Have client/family return demonstration.

   d. Inform client and family of expectations for when the call bell/intercom is to be used (i.e., to use the bathroom or get out of bed).
   e. Secure call bell in an accessible location, such as on the side rails or clipped to bedding. Make sure client can reach the device easily and is aware of its location.
3. Use of hospital bed and side rails:
   a. Keep bed in low position with locks on wheels secured whenever care is not being provided (see illustration).

NURSE ALERT

Before using any equipment for the first time, make sure you understand the safety features and proper method of operation.

Reinforces understanding and evaluates ability to manipulate controls.

Minimizes risks if client attempts to get out of bed without help.

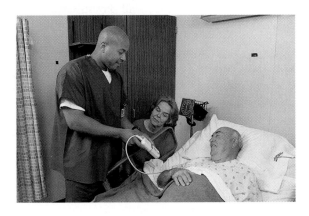

Step 2

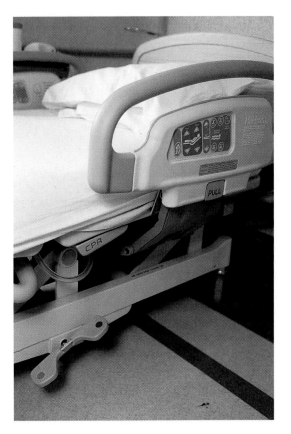

Step 3

Steps	Rationale
b. Teach the client/family that the purpose of side rails is to remind the client to call for assistance before getting out of bed and to assist with moving and turning in bed.	Client and family understanding promote cooperation.
c. Keep side rails in up position if client is an older adult, weak, confused, sedated, or sleeping.	Reminds client upon awakening of unfamiliar environment and to call for assistance.
d. Leave one side rail up and one down (on the side where oriented and ambulatory client gets out of bed).	Client can use up side rail for repositioning in bed.
4. Arrange necessary items (e.g., water pitcher, telephone, reading materials) within the client's easy reach.	Facilitates independence and self-care and prevents falls from attempts to reach too far.
5. Safe transport using a wheelchair (see illustration):	
a. The brakes on both wheels must be locked securely when a client is transferred into or out of a wheelchair (Chapter 6).	Keeps chair steady and secure.
b. Raise the footplates before the transfer; lower them, placing the client's feet on them, after the client is seated.	Promotes client's stability during transfer.
c. Make sure the client is seated with buttocks well back in the seat. Use a seat belt.	Protects client from sliding out of the chair.
d. Back the wheelchair into and out of an elevator, rear large wheels first.	Makes a smoother ride and prevents smaller wheels from catching in the crack between the elevator and the floor.

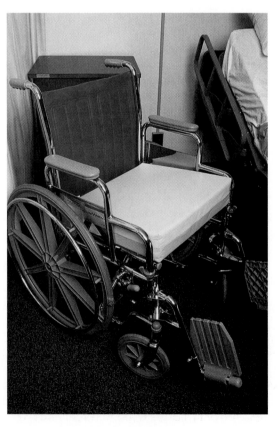

Step 5

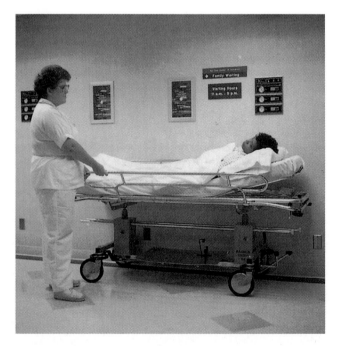

Step 6b

Steps	Rationale
e. When navigating on a ramp or incline, turn so that the chair pushes against your body, which is between the chair and the bottom of the ramp.	Prevents a runaway wheelchair that can pull away and roll faster down ramp than intended.
6. Safe transport using a stretcher:	
a. Lock the wheels during transfer from bed to stretcher or stretcher to bed.	
b. Use a safety belt across the client's upper thighs, or raise side rails (see illustration on p. 80).	
c. Push the stretcher from the end where the client's head rests. Some stretchers may have the head raised for comfort. For stretchers with stationary wheels on one end and swivel wheels on the other, the head of the stretcher has the stationary wheels.	Protects the client's head in case of a collision.
d. Maneuver the stretcher into an elevator head first.	Facilitates entry without bumping the sides.
7. See Completion Protocol (inside front cover).	

NURSE ALERT

Clients are not to be left on a stretcher unattended, especially when medicated or confused.

• • •

EVALUATION

1. Identify risk for falls or injuries in the health care agency.
2. Observe appropriate use of the call bell to obtain assistance.
3. Ask client and family to explain reasons for safety devices.

Recording and Reporting

- Risk for Falls Assessment Tool may be completed on admission and at specified intervals.
- Note that the decision of whether a client is at risk for falls is a nursing judgment.

Sample Documentation

0900   Risk for Falls Assessment Tool completed. Client identified at risk based on weakness and unsteady gait, use of walker, urinary frequency, and use of diuretics.

Skill 5.2

DESIGNING A RESTRAINT-FREE ENVIRONMENT

The standard of care for institutionalized older adults is avoidance of mechanical restraints, except as needed under exceptional circumstances, and only after all other reasonable alternatives have been tried. Physical restraints are devices that limit a client's movement. The immobility resulting from physical restraints can result in serious complications, including death (see Skill 5.3). Care of the person who may be prone to threats to safety and security requires a creative, systematic, and attentive approach to care.

A wide variety of electronic devices have been developed to alert staff to a client's need for assistance. One type is a battery-operated alarm attached to the client's leg. When the client changes position to get out of bed, the alarm sounds and alerts staff to provide assistance. A tether alarm is a device that can be attached to a chair, bed, or doorway and clipped to a client with a 4-foot cotton tape. When a magnet connection is disrupted, the alarm sounds. A weight-sensitive alarm can be placed under the client in bed or in a chair. When the person tries to get up, the alarm sounds (Figure 5-3).

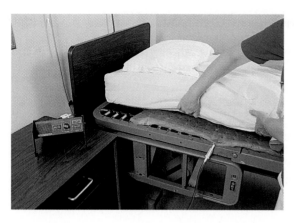

Figure 5-3 Weight-sensitive alarm. *From Sorrentino SA: Assisting with patient care, St Louis, 1999, Mosby.*

Equipment
Calendar
Clock
Radio or television
Audio books, music, videotapes
Wedge pillow
Ambularm or pressure-sensitive bed or chair alarm

ASSESSMENT
1. Ask about the use of restraints before admission to the agency.
2. Identify the history behaviors that increase risk for injury, such as impaired cognition, poor balance, altered gait, impaired vision and hearing, and orthostatic hypotension (dizziness upon arising quickly, because of a fall in blood pressure).
3. Review prescribed medications (e.g., sedatives, hypnotics) for interactions and untoward effects.
4. Assess orientation to time, place, and person.
5. Use one-on-one observation or behavior-monitoring logs to document specific risks related to inability to understand, remember, and follow directions.

PLANNING
Expected outcomes focus on maintaining client safety while avoiding the need for physical restraints.

Expected Outcomes
1. The client will remain free of injury without the use of restraints.
2. The client will not exhibit violence toward others.

DELEGATION CONSIDERATIONS

Monitoring client behavior for risk for injury and promoting a safe environment may be delegated to AP. Assessment of client behaviors and decisions about avoiding use of restraints require the problem solving ability unique to the professional nurse.

IMPLEMENTATION

Steps	Rationale
1. Standard Protocol (inside front cover).	

COMMUNICATION TIP

Approach client in a calm, nonthreatening, professional manner. Orient the client and family to surroundings, introduce staff, and explain all procedures. This may need to be repeated often, especially when the environment has changed from what the client is accustomed to.

2. Encourage family and friends to stay with the client. Sitters and companions can be helpful.	Presence of a consistent companion reduces client anxiety and increases feelings of security.
3. Place the client in a room close to the nurses' station.	Facilitates close observation.

Steps	Rationale
4. Provide visual and auditory stimuli, including a clock, radio, television, and calendar with large print (see illustration).	Assists with orientation to day, time, and physical surroundings.
5. Encourage family to supply family pictures and several personal belongings of sentimental value.	Promotes orientation to person and provides psychological comfort.
6. Provide the same caregivers to the extent possible.	Provides stability of routine care and consistency in approach.
7. Respond promptly to client's needs for toileting, relief of pain, and requests for activity.	Promotes comfort and minimizes anxiety.
8. Organize a predictable daily routine that provides opportunity for stimulation alternated with sleep and rest.	Routine facilitates psychological security and avoids overstimulation.
9. Use a wedge pillow on chair, with the thickest part toward the front of the chair.	Prevents clients with limited mobility from being able to rise to a standing position.
10. Use a pressure-sensitive bed or chair pads with alarms for alerting staff to an unsteady client who is standing without help. To use Ambularm monitoring device:	
a. Explain the use of the device to the client and family.	
b. Measure the client's thigh circumference just above the knee to determine appropriate size (see illustration). For a leg circumference less than 18 inches, use the regular size; use a large size for 18 inches or greater.	A band that is too loose may slip off; a band that is too tight may interfere with circulation or cause skin irritation.

NURSE ALERT

Use of Ambularm is contraindicated in the presence of impaired circulation, swelling, skin irritation, or breaks in the skin.

c. Test battery and alarm by touching snaps to corresponding snaps on leg band.

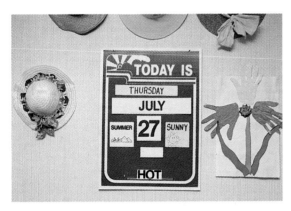

Step 4   *From Sorrentino SA: Assisting with patient care, St Louis, 1999, Mosby.*

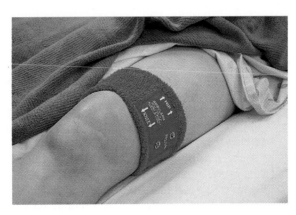

Step 10b   *Courtesy AlertCare, Mill Valley, California.*

Steps	Rationale

   d. Apply the leg band just above the knee and snap
      battery securely in place (see illustration).

   e. Instruct client that alarm will sound unless the leg
      is kept in a horizontal position (see illustration).

   f. To assist client to ambulate, deactivate the alarm
      by unsnapping the device from the leg band.

11. Use stress-reduction techniques such as massage and
guided imagery (see Chapter 10).

12. Use music, audio books, or videotapes chosen
specifically for the client.

                               Provides diversional activities.

13. Consult with physical therapy, speech therapy, and
occupational therapy for appropriate activities to
provide stimulation and exercise.

14. See Completion Protocol (inside front cover).

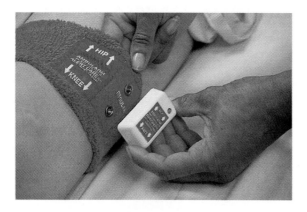

Step 10d *Courtesy AlertCare, Mill Valley, California.*

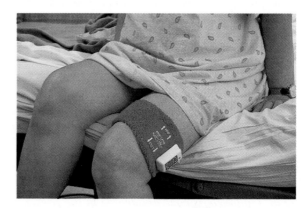

Step 10e *Courtesy AlertCare, Mill Valley, California.*

• • •

EVALUATION

1. Review incidence of behaviors that increase risk for
injury without the use of restraints.

2. Verify absence of violence toward others.

Unexpected Outcomes and Related Interventions

1. Client displays behaviors that substantially increase
risk for injury to self or others.

   a. Review episodes for a pattern (e.g., activity, time
of day) that indicates alternatives that could eliminate the behavior.

   b. Engage in creative thinking with all caregivers and
support service personnel for alternative problem
solving that promotes safe, consistent care.

2. The client sustains an injury or is out of control,
placing others at risk for injury.

   a. Complete an incident report (see Skill 1.4).

   b. Identify alternative measures to promote safety
without a restraint. As a last resort, identify appropriate restraint to use (see Skill 5.3).

Recording and Reporting

Document all behaviors that relate to cognitive status and
ability to maintain safety:

- Orientation to time, place, and person
- Ability to follow directions
- Mood and emotional status
- Understanding of condition and treatment plan
- Medication effects related to behaviors
- Interventions used and client response

Sample Documentation

0900 *Up and dressed, oriented to person but not time or
place. Upset and crying when unable to call wife on
the telephone. Pacing in room.*

1000 *Participated for 15 minutes with ball toss to music
at O.T.; then resting in rocking chair, smiling, and interacting socially with roommate.*

Skill 5.3

APPLYING RESTRAINTS

Although the goal in health care settings today is a restraint-free environment, there are some extreme circumstances in which clients need to be temporarily restrained when other measures have failed (see Skill 5.2). Physical restraint involves the use of any physical or mechanical device that the person cannot remove, that restricts the person's physical activity or normal access to the body, and that is not a usual part of treatment plans indicated by the person's condition or symptoms. Clients needing temporary restraints include those at risk for falls, as well as confused or combative clients at risk for self-injury or violence to self or others. In addition, restraints are used to prevent interruption of therapy such as an intravenous (IV) catheter, Foley or surgical drains, nasogastric tube, traction, or life support equipment.

Restraints are not a solution to a client problem, but rather a temporary means to maintain client safety. The use of restraints is associated with serious complications, including pressure ulcers, constipation, urinary and fecal incontinence, and urinary retention. In some cases restricted breathing or circulation has resulted in death. Loss of self-esteem, humiliation, fear, and anger are additional serious concerns (Weick, 1992). The Food and Drug Administration (FDA), which regulates restraints as medical devices, requires manufacturers to label restraints as prescription only. In most agencies, a specific physician's order is required for their use. Orders may not be on a prn. basis and must include a time limit not to exceed 24 hours. Circumstances are reviewed if the orders need to be extended. When restraints are required, both the client and family should be informed that the restraint is temporary and protective.

Equipment
Appropriate restraint and padding if needed. Restraint options include the following:
    Jacket restraint (vest or Posey)
    Belt restraint
    Extremity (ankle or wrist) restraint
    Mitten restraint

ASSESSMENT
1. Assess the need for restraint when all other measures have failed, and determine the most appropriate type and size to use.
2. Inspect the area where the restraint is to be placed, including the condition of the skin and the adequacy of circulation. **Rationale: Provides baseline to evaluate onset of injury.**

NURSE ALERT

Choice of restraint should include consideration of avoiding interference with therapeutic equipment. Avoid constricting IV access devices, arteriovenous (AV) shunt used for dialysis, and drainage tubes.

PLANNING
Expected outcomes focus on protecting the client from injury and maintaining prescribed therapy.

Expected Outcomes
1. The client will be free of injury.
2. The prescribed therapies will be continued without interruption.

DELEGATION CONSIDERATIONS

Application of restraints may be delegated to AP. However, assessment for when restraints are needed and the appropriate type to use is not delegated. Stress the importance of the following:

*   Correct placement of the restraint
*   Observing for constriction of circulation, skin integrity, and adequate breathing
*   When and how to change position, range of motion, and skin care
*   Providing opportunities for socialization

IMPLEMENTATION

Steps	Rationale

1. See Standard Protocol (inside front cover).
2. Check agency policies regarding restraints and obtain a physician's order for the least restrictive type. The order should be time limited (usually 24 hours) and include client behaviors for which the restraint is needed.
3. Obtain consent for the use of restraints if possible.
4. Place the client in proper body alignment.

5. Review manufacturer's instructions.
6. Pad bony prominences where restraints will be placed.
7. Apply selected restraint.
   a. Jacket restraint: Vestlike garment applied over clothing or hospital gown; used when client is in bed or chair. The front and back of the garment are labeled to facilitate correct application (see illustration).
   b. Belt restraint: Secures client in bed or stretcher. Make sure it is placed at the waist, not the chest, and avoid excessive tightness (see illustration).

COMMUNICATION TIP

Explain to both the client and family the reason for the restraint, and stress that it is temporary and protective. Explain other measures that have been taken to avoid the restraint and that they have failed.

Promotes comfort, prevents contractures, and prevents neurovascular injury.
Promotes client safety by correct use of the device.
Protects the skin from irritation.

Proper application prevents suffocation or choking. Clothing or gown prevents friction against the skin.

Tight application or misplacement can interfere with ventilation.

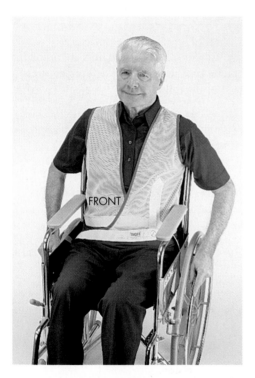

Step 7a   *Courtesy J.T. Posey Co., Arcadia, California.*

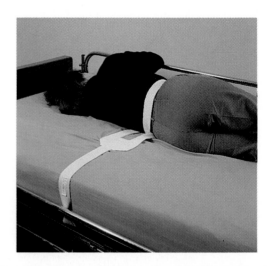

Step 7b   *Courtesy J.T. Posey Co., Arcadia, California.*

Steps	Rationale

c. Extremity/limb restraint (wrist or ankle): With client in the lateral position, may be used to immobilize one or all extremities. Commercial restraints have sheepskin or foam padding. Check that two fingers can be inserted under the restraint (see illustration).

d. In an emergency when a commercial extremity restraint is not immediately available, a clove-hitch restraint can be constructed by making a figure-eight with gauze and placing it over a padded extremity (see illustration).

The lateral position helps prevent aspiration if the client vomits. Tight restraints may constrict circulation or ventilation and cause neurovascular injury or cause therapeutic devices to become occluded.

NURSE ALERT

A clove hitch that is not constructed properly can tighten when ends are pulled. Check after 15 minutes to make sure device has not tightened. If this occurs, it should be removed and applied properly.

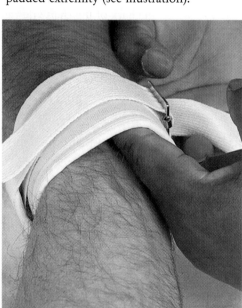

Step 7c   *Courtesy J.T. Posey Company, Arcadia, California.*

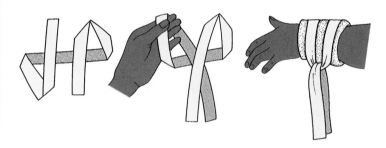

Step 7d

e. Mitten restraint: A thumbless fabric mitten to prevent use of fingers to scratch skin or dislodge equipment, while allowing some movement (see illustration).

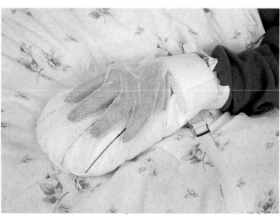

Step 7e   *From Sorrentino SA: Assisting with patient care, St Louis, 1999, Mosby.*

Steps	Rationale
8. Attach restraints to the moveable part of bed frame, which moves when the head of the bed is raised or lowered (see illustration).	When the bed is raised/lowered, the strap will not tighten and restrict circulation.

NURSE ALERT

Do not attach restraints to side rails, which could cause injury when side rail is lowered.

Steps	Rationale
9. When the client is in a chair, the jacket restraint should be secured with the ties under the armrests and tied at the back of the chair (see illustration).	When ties are not under the armrests, clients may be able to slide the ties up the back of the chair and free themselves.
10. Use quick-release ties (see illustration).	Allows quick release in an emergency.
11. Before leaving client, make sure call bell is within reach. Tell the client when you will return, remembering that the restrained client is dependent on caregivers for all basic needs (e.g., fluids, toileting, exercise).	
12. Every 15 to 30 minutes, the restraint should be checked for placement, and the client evaluated for pulses, temperature, color, and sensation of the distal part of the extremities.	Prevents complications from constriction and impaired circulation.

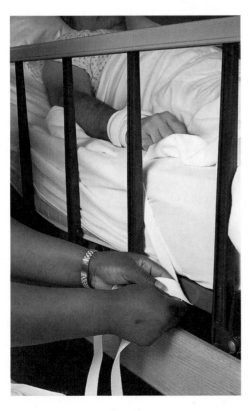

Step 8

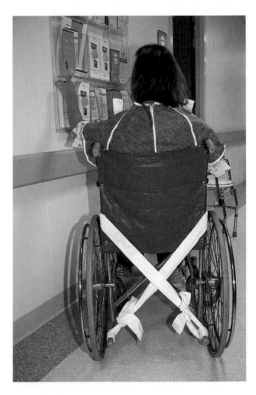

Step 9

Steps	Rationale

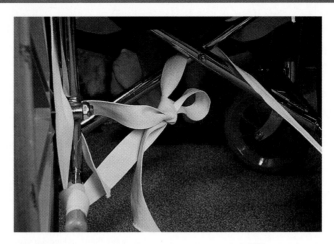

Step 10 *Courtesy J.T. Posey Company, Arcadia, California.*

13. Every 2 hours, release the restraints entirely for 30 minutes and complete active or passive range of motion. Encourage change of position and assess the underlying skin integrity for irritation.
14. See Completion Protocol (inside front cover).

• • •

EVALUATION
1. Observe for effectiveness of chosen restraint in preventing harm to the client.
2. Verify that prescribed therapies are continued without interruption.

Recording and Reporting
Document evidence that client's safety was at risk and specific restraint was warranted, including the following:

- Behavior before restraints were applied
- Level of orientation
- Client/family teaching
- Type of restraint used and time applied
- Client behavior after restraint was applied
- Assessments related to oxygenation, circulation, and skin integrity
- Times of each subsequent assessment and release, range of motion, turning and position
- Time restraints were removed, and client response

Also see behavioral restraint flow sheet (Figure 5-4).

Holy Family Hospital and Medical Center
70 East Street, Methuen, MA 01844

BEHAVIORAL RESTRAINT
FLOW SHEET

Behavior Requiring Restraint: (Check all that apply)

☐ Confusion/disorientation/combative

☐ Self Harm

☐ Harm to others/surroundings

☐ Removing medical devices

☐ Other: _____

Physician order obtained: ☐ Yes; ☐ No

Type of Restraint: (Check all that apply)

☐ Soft wrist/ankle

☐ Halter type vest

☐ Seat Belt

☐ Mitts

☐ Leather

☐ Other: _____

Less Restrictive Measures Attempted: (Check all that apply)

☐ Pain/comfort measures

☐ Schedule position changes

☐ Schedule toileting

☐ Place closer to Nursing Station

☐ Reorient

☐ Encourage family/friends to visit

☐ Other: _____

Patient/Family Informed: ☐ Yes; ☐ No

If no, Comment: _____

_____

Date Restraint Applied: _____ **Time:** _____

Date Restraint ☐ **Ended /** ☐ **Renewed:** _____ **Time:** _____

Date: Time:am/pm	12	2	4	6	8	10	12	2	4	6	8	10
1. Hydration/Nutrition/Elimination												
2. Skin condition												
3. Range of motion/turn & position												
4. Communication (call light in reach)												
5. Circulation/Neurovascular Changes												
6. Assess chg. in clinical condition/behavior												
7. Assess for early release												
8. Restraint reduced/removed*												
9. Behavioral/Safety Check done q15"												
10. Vital Signs (if applicable)**												
Initials of assessor:												

Initials/Signature: _____   Initials/Signature: _____   Initials/Signature: _____

Comments: _____

_____

_____

_____

_____

* New order required when restraint removed or reduced. | ** Temperature not required unless indicated.

KEY: ✓ = Observation / Intervention; NN = Nurses' Notes; O = Patient Off Unit; R = Restraint Removed

Note: It is not necessary to document the Behavioral/Safety Check every 15 minute but nurse must note every 2 hours in the assessment documentation #7 that the observation was performed. *Any changes in behavior require an assessment.*

Caritas Christi · A Catholic Health Care System · Member

Written: 7/95; Revised: 29 January 1999

Figure 5-4 Behavioral restraint flow sheet. *Courtesy Holy Family Hospital and Medical Center, Methuen, Mass.*

Skill 5.4

SEIZURE PRECAUTIONS

A seizure involves sudden, violent, involuntary muscle contractions that occur rhythmically, such as during acute or chronic seizure disorders, febrile episodes (especially in children), and after a head injury. Seizure precautions include nursing interventions to protect the client from traumatic injury, positioning for adequate ventilation and drainage of secretions, providing privacy, and support after the seizure. It is important for the nurse to observe and accurately document the sequence of events before, during, and after the seizure, including the duration of the seizure.

Equipment
        Padded side rails and headboard
        Suction machine and oral catheter
        Clean, disposable gloves

ASSESSMENT

1. Assess whether the client experiences a visual, auditory, or other type of aura before a seizure.

PLANNING

Expected outcomes should focus on safety, prevention of airway obstruction and aspiration, and maintenance of self-esteem.

Expected Outcomes
1. Client does not suffer traumatic physical injury during a seizure episode.
2. Client's airway is maintained, and secretions are not aspirated during a seizure episode.
3. Client verbalizes positive self-feelings after a seizure episode.

DELEGATION CONSIDERATIONS

Setting up seizure precautions and protection for clients at risk for seizures may be delegated to AP. Stress the importance of protection from falls, avoiding attempts to restrain, and not placing anything in the client's mouth.

IMPLEMENTATION

Steps	Rationale

1. See Standard Protocol (inside front cover).
2. Prepare bed with padded side rails and headboard and bed in lowest position. Provide equipment for oral suction (see illustration).
3. Provide or encourage use of bracelet or identification card noting seizure disorder and medications taken.

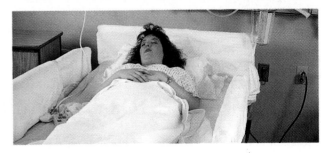

Step 2

4. If a seizure occurs:
    a. Stay with the client. Protect head from injury. Observe the sequence and timing of seizure activity, client's skin color and respirations.

NURSE ALERT

Injury may result from forcible insertion of a hard object. Soft objects may break or come apart and be aspirated. Do not place fingers near or in the client's mouth, because this could result in a bite injury. If   *the client has dentures, do not try to remove them during the seizure. If loosened, remove after the seizure (Lannon, 1995).*

Steps	Rationale

b. After the seizure, assess airway status, identify possible precipitating factors, assess for bruising or injury, and offer comfort and support. Remove gloves.

Client may be confused or drowsy.

c. Provide a quiet, nonstimulating environment.

5. See Completion Protocol (inside front cover).

• • •

EVALUATION

1. Assess client for traumatic injury during and after the seizure episode.
2. Observe client's color and respiratory rate and pattern during the seizure.
3. Ask client to verbalize feelings after the seizure.

Unexpected Outcomes and Related Interventions

1. Client suffers traumatic injury.
   a. Continue to protect client from further injury.
   b. Notify the physician.
2. Client verbalizes feelings of embarrassment and humiliation.
   a. Allow client to verbalize feelings.
   b. Encourage client and family to participate in decision making and planning care.

Recording and Reporting

Document events before, during, and after the seizure, including the following:

- Presence/absence of aura
- Level of consciousness

- Posture
- Color
- Sequence and movements of extremities
- Presence/absence of incontinence
- Objective and subjective data immediately afterward

Sample Documentation

1000 *Observed client sitting in chair in room. Cry heard, client observed sliding to floor, not responding to verbal stimuli. Client assisted to floor with head supported. Pillow placed under head. Tonic and clonic movements of all four extremities noted, lasting 2 minutes. Color remained good, respiratory pattern slightly irregular. No incontinence noted. At conclusion of tonic and clonic movements, client slept for 20 minutes, during which time respirations were 16 per minute and regular.*

1020 *Client awake and alert. Requested nurse to describe sequence of events. Stated that this was his "usual type of seizure."*

Skill 5.5

SAFETY MEASURES FOR RADIOACTIVE MATERIALS

Radiation and radioactive materials are used in the diagnosis and treatment of clients. Nurses may be exposed to radiation when assisting clients who are undergoing x-rays. Clients with some forms of cancer may be treated with radioactive implants placed in a body cavity, using sealed tubes, ribbons, wires, seeds, capsules, or needles. Nurses need to be familiar with agency policies for the care of clients who are receiving radiation and radioactive materials. Nurses who are or may be pregnant are not to be involved in the care of clients with radiation therapy. Nurses need to reduce the exposure to radiation by applying the principles of time, distance, and shielding. The time near the source is limited (a dosimeter badge may be worn to measure exposure), distance from the source is maximized,

and shielding devices (e.g., lead aprons) are used. Lead-shielded containers are used for storage of radioactive materials. Nurses need specific information about safe times and distances to ensure that their occupational exposure is as low as reasonably achievable.

Equipment

Protective lead shields (for x-rays)
Dosimeter badge
Sign for door: "Caution–Radioactive Material" (Figure 5-5)
Bright-colored tape for floor
Lead or disposable rubber gloves

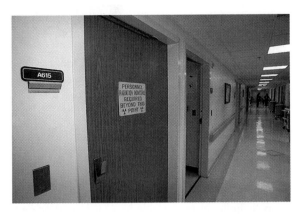

Figure 5-5 Signage indicates radioactive materials are in room.

ASSESSMENT

1. Consult with radiation safety officer to identify the type and amount of radiation to be used and its side effects and hazards.
2. Identify the restrictions related to time and distance.

PLANNING

Expected outcome focuses on minimizing exposure to radiation.

Expected Outcome

1. The client will be diagnosed or treated using radiation with the least exposure possible for client, visitors, and staff.

IMPLEMENTATION

Steps	Rationale

1. Explain the treatment plan to the client and family, including activity limitations and expected side effects.
2. Prepare the room with a sign on the door and yellow tape on the floor to mark the distance from the bed required for safety. A private room is required.
3. Explain safety regulations, time limits, and distance limits to client and visitors.
4. Wear a badge or dosimeter which indicates extent of radiation exposure.
5. Wear appropriate shield (e.g., lead apron or gloves, rubber gloves) when providing care. Wash gloves before removal, and dispose of in designated waste container. Wash hands thoroughly after removing gloves.
6. Wrap all nondisposable items that have come in contact with radiation source, and send to nuclear medicine department for decontamination.
7. Identify special requirements relating to laboratory specimens, dietary tray, secretions and excretions, dressings, linens, and trash.
8. Request a discharge survey by radiation safety officer to ensure that all sources of radiation have been removed at the completion of treatment.
9. See Completion Protocol (inside front cover).

NURSE ALERT

Rotate care providers to provide the nursing care needed while keeping exposure to radiation within safe limits. Avoid exposure to persons in early pregnancy to prevent risks related to fetal development.

• • • •

EVALUATION

1. Determine the amount of radiation exposure to client, visitors, and staff.

Unexpected Outcomes and Related Interventions

1. Questions arise about radiation exposure, spillage, dislodged implant, or systemic treatment.
   a. Notify radiation safety officer immediately.
   b. Avoid direct contact with source of radiation.
   c. Wash with soap and water if skin becomes contaminated.

Recording and Reporting

Document radiation therapy and related safety measures used, including the following:

- Length of exposure
- Apparent side effects if noted
- Teaching provided to client and family

Sample Documentation

1300　Admitted for radiation treatments. Client and family instructed on expectations relating to side effects of therapy and routines for minimizing unnecessary exposure by limiting time, maintaining appropriate distance, and use of protective equipment.

CRITICAL THINKING EXERCISES

1. A 88-year-old woman is admitted to a long-term care facility after having had several falls resulting from weakness and loss of balance. The most recent fall resulted in a fractured hip, which was surgically treated. She is being given Tylenol with codeine every 4 hours as needed for pain. She tells you she is accustomed to being very independent, having lived alone for several years since her husband died. She appears alert and oriented on arrival at the facility. However, during the first night she is found wandering in the hall, looking for the bathroom. What can be done to avoid restraining this client?

2. A client is admitted for surgery. She has a history of grand mal seizures for which she is taking medication. She has been ill for several days and has been unable to take the medication. When delegating the care of the client to AP, what information should you communicate about initiating seizure precautions and caring for the client if a seizure occurs?

3. As you are walking down the hall, you hear a client calling out for help. You assess the situation and realize that the client does not remember how to use the call light. What factors could contribute to the client's inability to remember, and how would you teach the client to use the call bell?

REFERENCES

Brady R et al: Geriatric falls: prevention strategies for the staff, *J Gerontol Nurs* 19(9):26, 1993.

Brians LK et al: Development of the RISK tool for fall prevention, *Rehabil Nurs* 16(2):67, 1991.

Chaff, 1994.

Ebersole P, Hess P: *Toward healthy aging: human needs and nursing process*, ed 4, St Louis, 1994, Mosby.

Ellis C: Nursing assessment and intervention for the patient experiencing seizures: a structured approach, *Clin Nurs Pract Epilepsy* 1(2):4, 1993.

Gordon M: *Manual of nursing diagnosis 1997-1998*, St Louis, 1997, Mosby.

Lannon S: Epilepsy in the elderly, *Clin Nurs Pract Epilepsy*, 2(2):5, 1995.

Miles SH, Irvine P: Deaths caused by physical restraints, *Gerontologist* 32, 1992.

Potter P, Perry A: *Fundamentals of nursing: concepts and practice*, ed 4, St Louis, 1997, Mosby.

Sorrentino SA: *Assisting with patient care*, St Louis, 1999, Mosby.

Stolley JM: Freeing your patients from restraints, *Am J Nurs* 95(2):27, 1995.

Tideiksaar R: Home safe home: practical tips for fall-proofing, *Geriatr Nurs* 11(6):284, 1989.

Weick M: Physical restraints: an FDA update, *Am J Nurs* 92(11): 1992.

UNIT THREE

Activities of Daily Living

Chapter 6
Promoting Activity and Mobility

Chapter 7
Promoting Hygiene

Chapter 8
Promoting Nutrition

Chapter 9
Assisting With Elimination

Chapter 10
Promoting Comfort, Sleep, and Relaxation

Chapter 11
Basic Infant Care

CHAPTER 6

Promoting Activity and Mobility

Skill 6.1
Assisting with Moving and Positioning Clients in Bed, 97

Skill 6.2
Minimizing Orthostatic Hypotension, 106

Skill 6.3
Transferring from Bed to Chair, 107

Skill 6.4
Using a Mechanical (Hoyer) Lift for Transfer from Bed to Chair, 112

Skill 6.5
Transferring from Bed to Stretcher, 115

Skill 6.6
Assisting Ambulation, 117

Activity is a basic human need that contributes to both physical and emotional well-being (McFarland and McFarlane, 1996). The benefits of physical activity include increased energy, improved sleep, better appetite, less pain, and improved self-esteem. It is useful to incorporate active exercises into activities of daily living (ADLs) (Box 6-1). Every effort must be made to promote functional mobility. Physical activities that clients are able to perform indicate their physical capacity and functional ability and desires.

Three elements are essential for mobility: (1) ability to move based on adequate muscle strength, control, and co-ordination and range of joint motion (ROJM); (2) motivation to move; and (3) absence of restriction in the environment. To prevent injury, use of good body mechanics is essential (Table 6-1).

Immobilized older adults with chronic illnesses are at a greater risk of developing complications that affect all body systems very quickly (Hogstel, 1992). These complications include muscle atrophy, loss of bone mass, contractures of joints, pressure ulcers, cardiovascular and respiratory problems, constipation, urinary stasis, and mental confusion.

Bed rest is a medical intervention in which the client is restricted to bed for one of the following purposes: (1) decreasing oxygen requirements of the body, (2) reducing pain, and (3) allowing rest and recovery.

For information about range of motion, see Chapter 26.

◢▶ NURSING DIAGNOSES

Activity Intolerance is a situation in which clients experience altered vital signs (pulse, respiration, or blood pressure) in response to activity. **Impaired Physical Mobility** is associated with pain or discomfort resulting from trauma or surgery, decreased strength and endurance, prolonged bed rest, or restrictive external devices such as casts, splints, braces, or drainage and intravenous (IV) tubing. Psychological factors such as **Fear** relating to a history of falling also result in a client's refusal to ambulate. **Risk for Disuse Syndrome** is a diagnosis that applies when inac-

Box 6-1 Examples of Incorporating Exercise into Activities of Daily Living

Upper Body

Nodding head "yes": neck flexion

Shaking head "no": neck rotation

Reaching to bedside stand for book: shoulder extension

Scratching back: shoulder hyperextension

Brushing or combing hair: shoulder hyperextension

Eating, bathing, and shaving: elbow flexion and extension

Writing and eating: fingers and thumb flexion, extension, and opposition

Lower Body

Walking: hip flexion, extension, and hyperextension; knee flexion and extension; ankle dorsiflexion; plantar flexion

Moving to side-lying position: hip flexion, extension, and abduction; knee flexion and extension

Moving from side-lying position: hip extension and adduction; knee flexion and extension

While sitting, lifting knees up and straightening legs: strengthens muscles used for walking

Table 6-1

Body Mechanics for Health Care Workers

Action	Rationale
1. When planning to move a client, arrange for adequate help. Use mechanical aids if help is unavailable.	Two workers lifting together divide the workload by 50%.
2. Encourage client to assist as much as possible.	This promotes client's abilities and strength while minimizing workload.
3. Keep back, neck, pelvis, and feet aligned. Avoid twisting.	Twisting increases risk of injury.
4. Flex knees, keep feet wide apart.	A broad base of support increases stability.
5. Position self close to client (or object being lifted).	The force is minimized. Ten pounds at waist height close to body is equal to 100 pounds at arms' length (Patterson, 1993).
6. Use arms and legs (not back).	The leg muscles are stronger, larger muscles capable of greater work without injury.
7. Slide client toward yourself using a pull sheet.	Sliding requires less effort than lifting. Pull sheet minimizes shearing forces, which can damage client's skin.
8. Set (tighten) abdominal and gluteal muscles in preparation for move.	Preparing muscles for the load minimizes strain.
9. Person with the heaviest load coordinates efforts of team involved by counting to three.	Simultaneous lifting minimizes the load for any one lifter.

tivity is desired or unavoidable, increasing the risk for deterioration of cardiovascular, respiratory, musculoskeletal, and psychosocial body systems (McFarland and McFarlane, 1996). In this case, maintenance of the client's present abilities is the primary focus. When a client has mental confusion, weakness, or orthostatic hypotension, **Risk for Injury** should be considered. Finally, a client with a nursing diagnosis of **Pain** is susceptible to developing impaired mobility resulting from the nature and extent of discomfort.

Skill 6.1

ASSISTING WITH MOVING AND POSITIONING CLIENTS IN BED

This skill includes moving dependent clients up in bed with one or two nurses and with or without a pull sheet and positioning clients in the Fowler's, supine, lateral, and semiprone (Sims') positions. The prone position is not included because it is uncomfortable, contraindicated for clients with respiratory problems, and rarely used (Bronstein, Popovich, and Stewart-Amidei, 1991). Each position offers advantages and limitations. It is important to be aware of potential pressure points (Figure 6-1). Mov-

ing a client even slightly changes the pressure points significantly.

Correct body alignment involves positioning so that no excessive strain is put on joints, tendons, ligaments, and muscles. Clients unable to move independently need to be repositioned according to activity level, perceptual ability, and daily routines (Bergstrom et al 1987a, 1987b). A standard turning interval of $1\frac{1}{2}$ to 2 hours may not prevent pressure sores. Clients need a regular program of as-

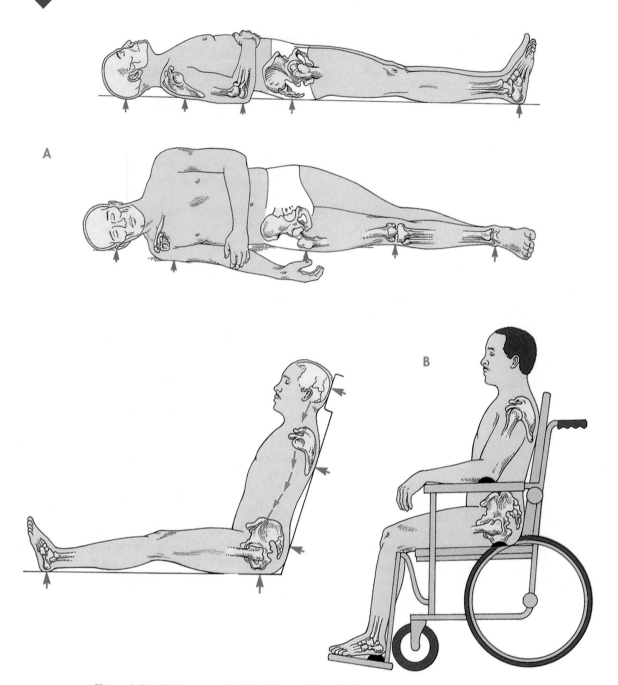

Figure 6-1   **A,** Pressure points in lying position. **B,** Pressure points in sitting position.

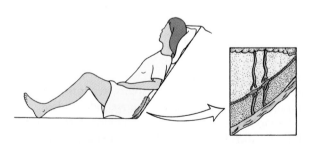

Figure 6-2   Shearing forces against sacrum cause tissue damage.

sisted range-of-motion (ROM) exercises. Care must be taken to protect the skin from damage caused by "shearing forces" resulting from sliding rather than lifting the client (Figure 6-2). Shear injury occurs when the skin remains stationary and the underlying tissue shifts, resulting in tissue damage. Friction injuries may be reduced by the use of lubricants (cornstarch or creams), protective films or dressings, and protective padding (AHCPR, 1992). This is especially important when the older client is thin, has fragile skin, is nutritionally compromised, or is unable to move independently.

For immobilized clients, pillows or foam wedges should be used to keep bony prominences such as heels and ankles from excessive or extended pressure. The use of air or water mattresses is also recommended (see Chapter 25).

Equipment

Pillows	Pull sheet
Hand rolls	Trapeze (optional)

ASSESSMENT

1. Assess client's weight, age, level of consciousness, and ability to cooperate. **Rationale: This information determines how much assistance will be needed.**
2. Assess strength of muscles and mobility of joints to be used by observing client movement in bed and by applying gradual pressure to a muscle group (e.g., attempting to extend client's elbow). Have client resist pressure by moving against the pressure (flex elbow). Compare strength in muscle groups, including arms and legs.
3. Assess willingness to cooperate.
4. Assess need for analgesic medication 30 to 60 minutes before position changes. **Rationale: Analgesics enhance client's ability to tolerate movement. Peak levels vary according to the specific analgesic and route of administration.**

PLANNING

Expected outcomes focus on mobility, self-care, interaction, and prevention of complications within the confines of the prescribed activity.

Expected Outcomes

1. Client's skin remains intact without redness.
2. Client verbalizes a sense of comfort after each repositioning.
3. Client maintains assisted changes in position in bed for at least 1 hour.
4. Client lists two benefits of position changes and good body alignment.
   a. Improved circulation
   b. Reduced skin breakdown

DELEGATION CONSIDERATIONS

The skills of moving and positioning clients in bed can be delegated to unlicensed assistive personnel. When delegating these skills, it is important for caregivers to know how to protect themselves from injury and to report changes in the client condition that indicate problems requiring the assessment and intervention of the professional nurse.

- Identify ability to maintain personal safety by use of good body mechanics, including height of bed, broad base of support, use of large muscles, and coordinated team effort.
- Encourage caregivers to have the client participate as much as possible in the process.
- Evaluate the client's comfort and alignment after repositioning, and assess pressure points for skin integrity.

Clients with acute spinal cord trauma usually require moving and positioning by professional nurses.

IMPLEMENTATION

Steps	Rationale

1. See Standard Protocol (inside front cover)
   Review principles of body mechanics (see Table 6-1).

NURSE ALERT

This move requires that the client can assist by pushing with feet and/or lifting with trapeze.

COMMUNICATION TIP

- *Encourage clients to assist as much as possible, discuss steps involved, and determine ways clients can assist while being moved.*
- *Review each step again as the move is about to be made.*
- *Include family in explanations.*

Steps	Rationale

2. **Moving a dependent client up in bed with one nurse and client assistance**
   a. Adjust position of IV pole, tubes, and catheters.
   b. Provide client with hearing aid and glasses if used.

   c. Lower the head of the bed to the lowest position. Place the pillow near the headboard.
   d. Assist client to flex knees so that soles of one or both feet are flat on the bed.
   e. If there is no trapeze, slide arm nearest the head of the bed under client's shoulders, reaching under and supporting client's opposite shoulder. Place other arm under client's upper back (see illustration). Have client push with feet as you lift on the count of three.
   f. If there is a trapeze, assist client to grasp it. Slide one arm under thighs and one arm under trunk. (see illustration).
   g. Have client lift with trapeze and/or push with feet on the count of three. Repeat if needed to move up farther in the bed.
   h. Ask what is needed to position client comfortably and adjust as necessary.

Facilitates movement without tension and disruption.
Promoting client involvement motivates and speeds progress toward independence and provides a sense of control and security.
Minimizes effort required to move client and minimizes potential trauma from head contacting headboard.
Positions client to exert effort when moving up in bed.

Coordinates client's movement with nurse's lifting action.

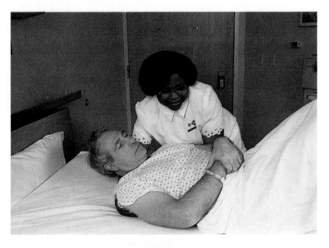

Step 2e

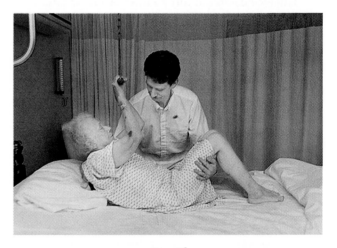

Step 2f

3. **Assisting client to move up in bed when client cannot assist**
   a. Lower the head of bed to the lowest position client can tolerate and lower side rails.
   b. Roll client side to side, placing a pull sheet that extends from shoulders to thighs. A pull sheet can be made using a small sheet folded in half.
   c. With one nurse on each side of client, grasp pull sheet firmly with hands near client's upper arms and hips, rolling sheet material until hands are close to client.

Clients with hypoxia may not tolerate lying flat.

The closer nurses are to client, the less height of lifting is required to clear the bed during the move.

Steps	Rationale

d. Nurses' knees are flexed with body facing the direction of the move. The foot away from the bed faces forward for a broader base of support (see illustration).

e. Instruct client to rest arms on body and to lift head on the count of three.

f. Lift client toward the head of the bed on the count of three. Repeat the move if necessary.

g. Assist client as needed to shift in order to attain position of comfort.

NURSE ALERT

Review principles of body mechanics (see Table 6-1). This move requires at least two nurses and pull sheet when client is unable to assist. If the client is very heavy, consider the need for more assistance.

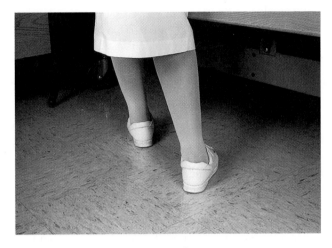

Step 3d

4. **Positioning in semi-Fowler's and Fowler's position**
   For the semi-Fowler's position the head of the bed is raised 45 to 60 degrees. The high Fowler's position, with the head of the bed raised 90 degrees, is recommended for eating. Both positions improve breathing by decreasing pressure on the diaphragm as gravity pulls abdominal contents downward. These positions also facilitate visiting and diversional activities. In this position clients tend to slide toward the foot of the bed.

   a. Raise the head of the bed to the appropriate level (45 to 90 degrees) (see illustrations).

   b. Use pillows to support client's arms and hands if upper body is immobilized.

   c. Position a pillow under the client's head if desired, and raise the knee break of the bed slightly. Avoid pressure under the popliteal space (back of the knee).

   d. Change the degree of elevation of the head of bed 5 to 10 degrees frequently.

   e. Identify potential pressure points, including scapulae, elbows, sacrum or coccyx, and heels (see Figure 6-1, p. 98) (see discussion of pressure ulcer prevention, Chapter 24).

Minimizes development of dependent edema and prevents shoulder dislocation if client has upper extremity impairment.

Pressure can interfere with circulation and contribute to thromboemboli (blood clots).

Alters the pressure points slightly and promotes comfort.

45°

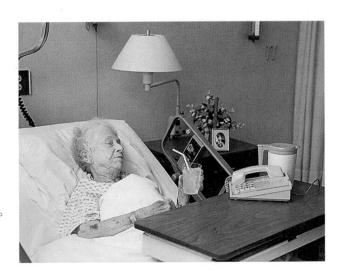

Step 4a

Steps	Rationale
5. Moving dependent client to 30-degree lateral (side-lying) position This move removes pressure from bony prominences of entire back.	If client can move freely, a side-lying position with upper and lower shoulders aligned is acceptable.
a. Lower the head of bed as much as client can tolerate keeping head of bed below 30-degree angle. Lower side rail.	Reduces shear. Avoids working against gravity.
b. Using a pull sheet, move client to the side of the bed opposite to the one toward which the client will be turned. Raise side rail. Go to opposite side of the bed and lower side rail.	Ensures that client will be in center of the bed when turned.
c. Assist client to raise arm nearest you above head, adjusting pillow if needed.	
d. Grasp client's shoulder and hip, and assist client to roll toward you onto side.	Turning client toward you promotes client's sense of security.
e. Flex both client's knees after the turn and support upper leg from knee to foot using a pillow or folded blanket.	Keep spine in good alignment.
f. Ease lower shoulder forward and bring upper shoulder back slightly. Check client's comfort.	Prevents excessive pressure directly on shoulder.
g. Support upper arm with pillows so that arm is level with shoulder.	Improves ventilation by minimizing pressure on chest.
h. Optional: Place pillow behind client's back and under so that it is tucked smoothly against back (see illustration).	Provides support and prevents client from rolling onto back.
i. Make sure client's back is straight without evidence of twisting. Adjust as needed for comfort.	
j. Pressure points to check include the ear, shoulder, anterior iliac spine, trochanter, lateral side of the knee, malleolus, and foot.	

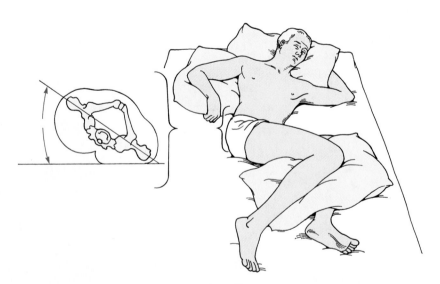

Step 5h

Steps	Rationale

6. **Logrolling to maintain neck and spinal alignment following injury or surgery.**

   a. Enlist the help of at least one additional person.

   b. Lower the head of the bed as much as the client can tolerate.

   Maintains alignment of the spinal column.

   c. Place a pillow between the legs. Use of a pull sheet placed between shoulders and knees can facilitate turning.

   Maintains position of the lower extremities.

   d. Extend the client's arm over the client's head unless shoulder movement is restricted.

   Prevents rolling over it during the turn. If shoulder movement is restricted, keep the arm in extension next to the body.

   e. With both caregivers on the same side of the bed, one places one hand on the client's shoulder and the other on the hip while the other places one hand to support the back and the other behind the knee. If a pull sheet is used, hands are placed alternately to provide even support for the length of the rolled sheet and to distribute weight evenly (see illustrations).

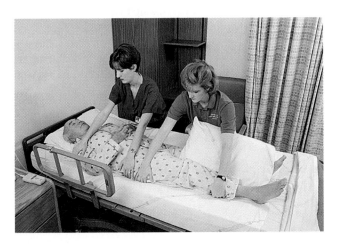 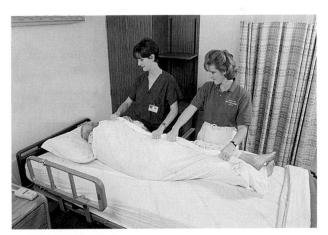

Step 6e *From Sorrentino SA: Assisting with patient care, St Louis, 1999, Mosby.*

   f. Using the count of three, turn the client with a continuous, smooth, and coordinated effort.

   Maintains body in alignment, preventing stress on any part of the body.

   g. Support the client with pillows as shown for the lateral position (Step 5h).

7. **Moving dependent client to Sims' (semiprone) position**

   For this alternative to the lateral position, client lies somewhat forward onto abdomen. This move is useful to discourage clients from rolling back to the supine position. It also minimizes pressure on the hip and shoulder.

Steps	Rationale

a. With client in the lateral position, arm against mattress is externally rotated with elbow extended. Prevent internal rotation of hip and adduction of leg by extending the lowermost leg and supporting the other leg level with the hip (see illustration).

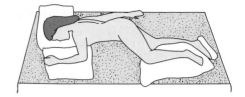

Step 7a

b. Support client's uppermost arm in flexed position level with shoulder.

Decreases internal rotation and adduction of shoulder and protects joint. Allows better chest expansion and improves ventilation.

c. Pressure points include ear, front of shoulder, iliac crest, lateral knee, malleolus, and side of foot of lower leg, as well as medial knee and malleolus of upper leg.

8. **Positioning dependent client in supine position**
This alternative to the Fowler's or semi-Fowler's position decreases pressure on buttocks and minimizes client's tendency to slide to the foot of the bed.
   a. Place client on back with head of bed flat.
   b. Place pillow under upper shoulders, neck, and head (see illustration).

Supports normal curvature of lumbar spine. Prevents excessive flexion of cervical spine.

   c. To position trochanter roll at client's hips, place a folded bath blanket under hips and roll ends under until toes point directly up (see illustration).

Prevents external rotation of hips and may be bilateral or unilateral depending on extent and location of muscle weakness.

   d. Place small support under ankles to minimize pressure on heels. High-top tennis shoes or a footboard may be used to prevent footdrop.

Shoes should be removed at least 3 times a day for range-of-motion exercises to prevent contractures.

   e. Place small supports under forearms with hand-wrist splints or small rolls to support fingers and thumb in a functional position.

A functional position allows the fingers to be flexed and the thumb to touch the fingertips.

   f. Pressure areas to check include the back of the head, scapulae, posterior iliac spine, sacrum or coccyx, ischium, Achilles tendons, and heels (see Figure 6-1, p. 98).
9. See Completion Protocol (inside front cover).

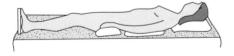

Step 8b

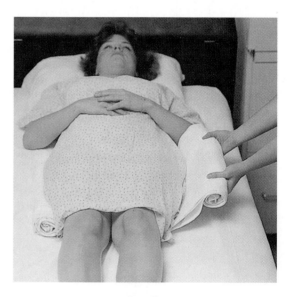

Step 8c

EVALUATION

1. Inspect skin overlying pressure areas for erythema (redness) and blanching. Observe again in 60 minutes.
2. Ask client if position is comfortable.
3. Observe client's body alignment and position.
4. Ask client to identify three benefits of position changes and correct body alignment.

Unexpected Outcomes and Related Interventions

1. Client develops areas of abnormal reactive hyperemia, blistering, or skin irritation.
   a. Change client's position more frequently.
   b. Avoid prolonged pressure on any one pressure area.
2. Client complains of discomfort from stretching because of altered alignment.
   a. Readjust position according to client's comfort level.
   b. Readjust supportive pillows to maintain alignment.
3. Client turns back to same position frequently and expresses discomfort with alternate positions.
   a. Reinforce the rationale for position changes.
   b. Provide diversional activities in various positions.
   c. Identify client's perception of position preference and attempt to create incentive for compliance with alternate positions.

Recording and Reporting

- Position client was moved from
- Position client was moved to
- Supportive devices used
- Condition of skin on pressure points
- Instructions given to client and/or family

Sample Documentation

0800 Turned from back to left lateral position. Area of erythema approximately 3 cm in diameter noted over coccyx. Blanches easily. Urged client not to lie on back.

1000 Found client lying on back. Turned to right side and supported with pillows. Coccyx remains reddened, blanches to fingertip pressure.

Geriatric Considerations

- Immobilized older adult clients are at higher risk of developing complications that affect all body systems. These complications include muscle atrophy, contractures, pressure ulcers, blood clots, pneumonia, constipation, urinary stasis, and mental confusion.
- Provide support to avoid strain on joints, tendons, ligaments, and muscles.
- Repositioning every 2 hours and a regular program of ROJM motion exercises are essential.
- Physical therapy or occupational therapy consultation is appropriate.
- In the presence of thin, fragile skin and/or nutritionally compromised state, lubricants or protective films or padding can reduce friction injury (see Chapter 24).
- Use a pull sheet to avoid shearing forces that damage client tissues.

Home Care and Long-Term Care Considerations

- Teach family members body mechanics
- In the absence of a hospital bed and equipment, creative adaptation will be required.
- Consider the need for a bed that places the bedridden client at caregiver's waist level.
- Teach caregivers to change client's position every 1-2 hours if possible, to maintain musculoskeletal alignment and reduce pressure on bony prominences. Develop a realistic turning schedule that is posted.
- Teach the dangers of immobility for all body systems (see Geriatric Considerations).

Skill 6.2

MINIMIZING ORTHOSTATIC HYPOTENSION

Orthostatic or postural hypotension involves a rapid drop in blood pressure of 25 mm Hg or more when changing from the supine to the sitting or standing position (Canobbio, 1990). The decreased blood pressure results in dizziness or sometimes fainting. Orthostatic hypotension may be related to bed rest, hypovolemia (decreased circulating blood volume), hypokalemia (low serum potassium level), and certain medications, including sedatives, hypnotics, analgesics, antihypertensives, antiemetics, antihistamines, diuretics, and antianxiety agents (McFarland and McFarlane, 1996).

Equipment

Blood pressure equipment
Stethoscope

ASSESSMENT

1. Check previous blood pressure and pulse readings and assess client's activity level. **Rationale: This establishes baseline criteria.**
2. Identify factors that may precipitate orthostatic hypotension, including decreased intravascular volume, hypokalemia, prolonged immobility, and medications.

PLANNING

Expected outcomes focus on preventing hypotension and increasing tolerance of activity with minimal risk of falls.

Expected Outcomes

1. Client demonstrates no evidence of weakness or dizziness in response to position changes.
2. Client states factors that influence incidents of orthostatic hypotension.
3. Client ambulates 10 feet while maintaining blood pressure within 25 mm Hg of systolic baseline.

DELEGATION CONSIDERATIONS

The following information is needed when delegating the skill of position changes to minimize orthostatic hypotension to nursing staff or family members:

- Have client wear shoes with a nonslip surface during transfer or ambulation.
- Make slow, gradual position changes.
- Observe for nausea, pallor, and dizziness.
- Have client sit in chair or return to bed if client has symptoms of orthostatic hypotension.

When assisting with ambulation:

- Do not try to hold clients if they become dizzy or faint. Ease them into a sitting position in a chair or on the floor.
- Be sure the area is free of clutter, wet areas, and rugs that may slide.

IMPLEMENTATION

Steps	Rationale
1. See Standard Protocol (inside front cover).	
2. Explain reason for gradual position change.	
3. Raise head of bed slowly to semi-Fowler's and then to high Fowler's position and reassess blood pressure, pulse, and respirations. Instruct client to report any dizziness or light-headedness during position change.	Raising slowly allows body to adjust to change in position. If client has a drop in blood pressure of 25 mm Hg (systolic) when upright, orthostatic hypotension is evident and risk of falls significant.
4. If no evidence of hypotension occurs, proceed to dangle (allow feet to hang over the side of the bed). Encourage client to move shoulders in circles and flex and extend ankles and knees. Reassess blood pressure.	Movement of muscles increases venous return and stimulates circulation.
5. Proceed with planned activity.	
6. See Completion Protocol (inside front cover).	

NURSE ALERT

DO NOT attempt to ambulate if client reports dizziness or pulse falls more than 10% of resting value. Lower head and allow client to rest for a few minutes and try again more gradually.

COMMUNICATION TIP

- *Include family in explanation.*
- *Explain to client the importance of slow, gradual position change to minimize dizziness, lightheadedness.*

EVALUATION

1. Observe client for signs of weakness or dizziness.
2. Assess blood pressure, pulse, and respirations if client experiences weakness or dizziness at any point and on completion of activity. Normally, blood pressure, pulse, and respirations increase slightly in response to exercise and return to baseline within 5 minutes of resting.
3. Ask client to describe three factors pertinent to the clinical condition that may cause orthostatic hypotension.

Unexpected Outcomes and Related Interventions

1. Client becomes light-headed and dizzy when upright.
   a. Return client to supine position.
   b. Take blood pressure immediately.
   c. After 3 to 5 minutes, attempt the same procedure. If unsuccessful, wait 1 to 2 hours before attempting again.

Recording and Reporting

- Resting pulse and blood pressure
- Type of exercise/exertion
- Repeated pulse and blood pressure after activity
- Subjective response (dizziness, weakness)

Sample Documentation

0900   BP with client lying down was 110/70, pulse 86, respirations 18. Was assisted to sitting position over 1 minute. Complained of dizziness. BP was 90/50, pulse 94, respirations 22. After resting in supine position for 5 minutes was assisted to upright position more slowly (over 3 minutes) without dizziness. BP 104/72, pulse 90, respirations 20. Ambulated to bathroom slowly with steady gait. Stated, "I feel weak, but not dizzy."

Geriatric Considerations

- Older adults who have volume losses or have undergone prolonged bed rest have greater risk for hypotension with postural change.
- Clients using medications to reduce blood pressure are at greater risk for orthostatic hypotension.

Home Care and Long-Term Care Considerations

Instruct family or caregiver in the rationale for slow gradual position change.

Skill 6.3

TRANSFERRING FROM BED TO CHAIR

This transfer technique can be done by one nurse. Moving clients to a chair after bed rest stimulates them physically and mentally and promotes involvement in self-care activities. It is important to allow clients to proceed at their own pace, encouraging as much independence as possible. Transfers may be from bed to chair, wheelchair, or bedside commode.

Equipment

     Transfer belt
     Sling
     Nonskid footwear
     Bath blanket
     Pillows
     Wheelchair: position chair close to bed, lock brakes, and remove or fold footrests out of the way.
     Bedside commode or supportive chair

NURSE ALERT

In general, nurses should not attempt to lift more than 35% of their own body weight. When in doubt about their ability to transfer a client safely, nurses should request assistance. It is advisable to use a transfer belt when clients have severe weakness, impaired balance, hemiparesis, or difficulty cooperating because of an altered mental state.

ASSESSMENT

1. Assess muscle strength of legs and upper arms, comparing right with left. **Rationale: Clients with hemiplegia have weakness on one side. Clients with paraplegia may have spastic or flaccid paralysis.**
2. Assess joint mobility and limitations caused by contractures or discomfort. Assess for history of osteoporosis, which may increase risk of pathological fractures with minimal stress.
3. Assess vision, hearing, and altered sensation. **Rationale: The presence of numbness or tingling of the feet or legs alters function.**
4. Assess ability to follow verbal instructions and appropriateness of response to simple commands.
5. Assess client's level of motivation. **Rationale: Clients who fear falling may avoid activity or make excuses.**
6. Determine the position and functioning of IV tubing and poles, need for oxygen therapy, Foley catheter, surgical drains, and other drains or tubes.
7. Assess the need for prescribed analgesic medication before transfer. Plan activity for the period in which adequate pain relief is apparent without dizziness or excessive sedation. **Rationale: Analgesics enhance client's ability to tolerate movement. Peak levels vary according to the specific analgesic and route of administration.**

PLANNING

Expected outcomes focus on improving the client's functional abilities and strength. It is also essential to promote body alignment and safety.

Expected Outcomes

1. Client assists with transfer to chair by standing erect, pivoting, and grasping arm of chair to sit.
2. Client tolerates sitting in chair 30 to 40 minutes and is able to shift weight independently, at least every 15 minutes.
3. Client benefits from change of environment while in the chair.

DELEGATION CONSIDERATIONS

The skills of safe and effective transfer techniques and moving and positioning clients in bed can be delegated to assistive personnel (AP) who have successfully demonstrated good body mechanics and safe transfer techniques for clients involved.

IMPLEMENTATION

Steps	Rationale

1. See Standard Protocol (inside front cover).
2. Position the chair or wheelchair so that the move will be *toward the client's stronger side.* Chair should be at an appropriate distance to allow client participation and safety. The stronger the client, the greater should be the distance.

    Facilitates balance and movement.

3. Lower bed to lowest position. Lower side rails and turn client to one side with knees flexed (see illustration).

NURSE ALERT

Check the equipment to be used and familiarize yourself with safety factors involved, such as wheelchair brakes, removable arm, adjustable footrest or leg rest, and reclining features.

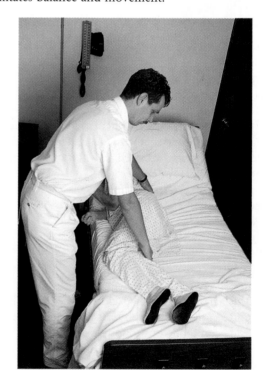

Step 3

Steps	**Rationale**

4. Raise the head of the bed to the highest position.

5. Face the client with feet comfortably apart and a broad base of support.

6. Assist client to the sitting position by lifting upper body as the legs swing over edge of the bed (see illustrations).

7. Encourage client to assist as much as possible as legs and feet are assisted over side of bed and client's shoulders are raised.

8. Instruct client to take a deep breath and sit for 1 to 2 minutes. Encourage movement of shoulders, legs, feet, and toes (see illustration).

9. Assist client to put on nonskid slippers or shoes and place feet flat on the floor.

10. Apply transfer belt if needed for stability.

Minimizes orthostatic hypotension (see Skill 6.2).

Maximizes nurse's stability and balance and prevents twisting that could result in muscle strain.

Client should be able to place feet flat on floor for balance and stability.

Muscle activity promotes venous circulation and allows adjustment to the sitting position.

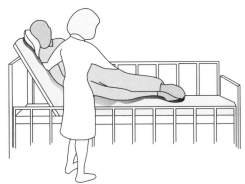

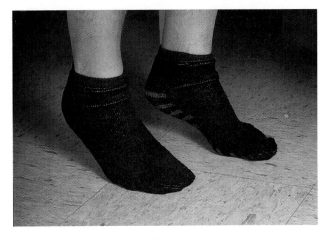

Step 6

COMMUNICATION TIP

Psychological support and encouragement during transfer is important.

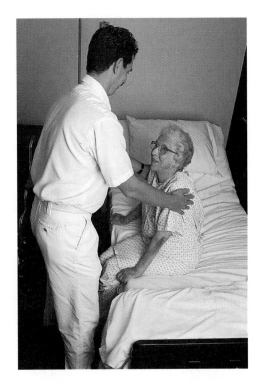

Step 8

Steps	Rationale
11. Apply a sling if client has flaccid arm.	Supports arm and prevents stress or injury.
12. Review the steps of the transfer procedure and ways client will assist with the move.	Encourages client to participate in transfer and increases muscle strength and a sense of control.
13. Facing the client, reach through client's axillae and place hands on client's scapulae or grasp the transfer belt with both hands toward the side of the client's back. Keep back straight, knees flexed with a wide base of support (see illustration). Client may place hands on your shoulders (not around neck).	Arms around neck could result in neck injury to nurse.
14. Instruct client to rock forward with each count and to stand erect on the count of three (see illustration). If needed, stabilize client's affected side with caregiver's knee against client's knee, placing foot in front of client's foot to prevent slipping.	Rocking motion gives client's body momentum and reduces the effort required to lift to standing position.
15. Once standing, pivot client toward seat of chair. Client should then reach for arm of the chair and assist to ease self into chair (see illustration).	
16. Observe client for proper alignment for sitting. Provide pillows to support affected (paralyzed) extremities (see illustration).	
17. See Completion Protocol (inside front cover).	

• • •

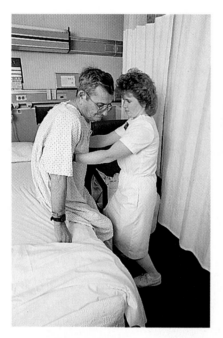

Step 13

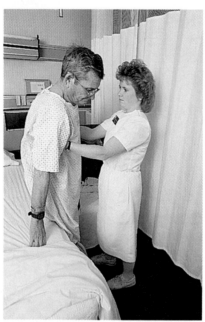

Step 14

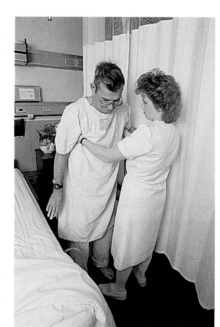

Step 15

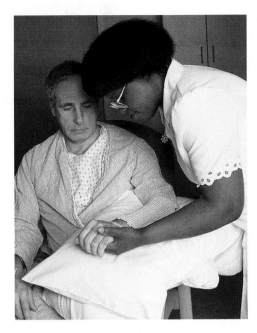

Step 16

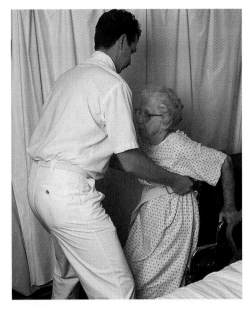

Figure 6-3   Gait belt facilitates balance and control.

EVALUATION

1. Observe client's ability to bear weight (or avoid bearing weight if prescribed), ability to pivot, and number of personnel needed. Ask client to describe level of strength and control.
2. Monitor length of time client sits in chair and ability to shift weight every 15 minutes.
3. Observe response to environment changes.

Unexpected Outcomes and Related Interventions

1. Client does not follow directions for transfer.
   a. Identify interfering factors (e.g., anxiety) and provide positive reinforcement for effort and achievement.
   b. Demonstrate the procedure for the client in a step-by-step manner.
2. Client's weakness of lower extremities does not permit active transfer. Consider physical therapy consultation.
   a. Develop a plan for isotonic or isometric leg-strengthening exercises to be done while lying in bed or sitting in chair.
   b. Use a gait belt for balance and support.
3. Client tends to bear weight on non–weight-bearing leg.
   a. Have another caregiver support affected leg as a reminder.
   b. Use a gait belt to facilitate balance and control (Figure 6-3).

Recording and Reporting

- Ability to bear weight and pivot
- Length of time
- Subjective response

Sample Documentation

0800   Transferred client from bed to chair with gait belt and assistance of one. Cooperative and able to stand erect with encouragement. Smiled when able to assist with self-feeding.

0815   Requested to return to bed. Stated, "I'm so tired, I just can't sit up any longer." Needed assistance of two with transfer back to bed. Knees buckled and legs were shaking during attempt to stand.

Geriatric Considerations

- Older persons who fear falling may be reluctant to move from bed to chair.
- Elderly clients who are depressed often prefer to stay in bed, especially when accustomed to being very independent and active and now need assistance.

Home Care and Long-Term Care Considerations

- Transfer ability at home is greatly enhanced by prior teaching of family, assessment of home for safety risks and functionality, and provision of applicable aids.
- Family should practice transfer in hospital to achieve success before taking client home.
- Alternatively, client (if living alone) should practice activities as they will be used at home, commode,

and shower. Clients should be taught to transfer to armchairs for ease of rising and sitting.
- Home should be free of risks (i.e., throw rugs, electric cords, slippery floors). If wheelchair is used, access must be possible through all doors, and space for transfer must be available in bedroom and bathroom.

Skill 6.4

USING A MECHANICAL (HOYER) LIFT FOR TRANSFER FROM BED TO CHAIR

Mechanical lifts are used for large, dependent clients who do not have spinal cord injury. Use of a lift does not require assistance from the client and should be used only when required (Baas and Ross, 1990).

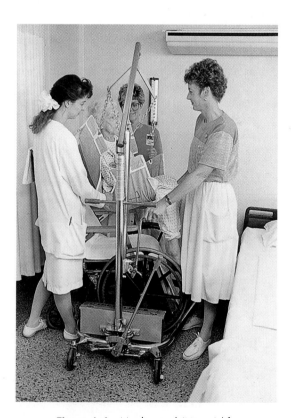

Figure 6-4   Mechanical (Hoyer) lift.

Equipment

Mechanical (Hoyer) lift: hydraulic lift frame with supporting boom and attached chains, canvas sling (Figure 6-4).
Pillow

NURSE ALERT

Before using the device, practice using controls that spread the base to provide stability, the lever that raises the sling, and the release that lowers the sling.

ASSESSMENT

1. Compare the weight limit for the lift with the client's current weight.
2. Assess muscle strength of legs and upper arms, joint mobility, and limitations from contractures or discomfort.
3. Assess vision, hearing, and altered sensation. **Rationale: Decreased vision or hearing influences ability to follow verbal instructions. The presence of numbness or tingling of the feet or legs alters function.**
4. Assess client's level of motivation. **Rationale: Clients who fear falling may avoid activity or make excuses.**

PLANNING

Expected outcomes focus on promoting safety and comfort during the transfer.

Expected Outcomes

1. Client verbalizes feeling secure and comfortable during transfer.
2. Client transfers safely.
3. Client maintains correct body alignment after transfer.
4. Client maintains heart rate and systolic blood pressure within 10% of resting baseline during transfer.

DELEGATION CONSIDERATIONS

The skills of safe and effective transfer techniques and moving and positioning clients in bed can be delegated to AP who have demonstrated ability to use good body mechanics and safe transfer techniques as well as equipment (Hoyer lift).

IMPLEMENTATION

Steps	Rationale

1. See Standard Protocol (inside front cover).
2. Ask another caregiver to assist. Move the lift to the bedside. Place a comfortable chair with supportive arms in a convenient location.
3. Raise the bed to a comfortable height. Turn client to side, and place the canvas sling under the client, extending from popliteal space of the knees to beneath the head. The hole of the canvas is placed under the buttocks.
4. With the client lying supine and arms crossed over the body, position the lift with the base under the bed and spread the base of the lift.
5. Attach the shorter chains to the section of the sling (may be narrower) that supports the upper body.
6. Raise the boom slightly and attach the longer chains to the (wider) sling that supports the hips and thighs.
7. Adjust the sling as necessary so that the client's weight is evenly distributed.
8. Pump the lift to elevate it just enough to clear the bed, and guide client's legs over the side (see illustration).

COMMUNICATION TIP

A mechanical lift may frighten the client. Reassurance and ability to convey knowledge of procedure by caregivers will decrease anxiety.

A broad base of support enhances stability and prevents tipping.

It may help if one caregiver supports and flexes the client's knees as another attaches the chains to the sling.

Promotes stability and security during the move.

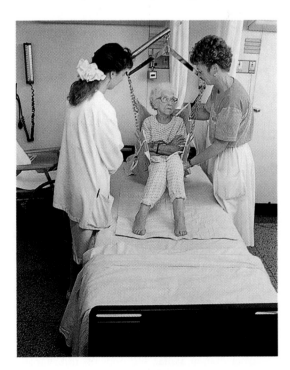

Step 8

Steps	Rationale
9. Instruct the client to keep arms folded during the transfer.	Keeps the device balanced and prevents injury from bumping against objects.
10. Check the chair's position and stability before the move. While supporting the client, guide the lift toward the chair, commode, or wheelchair so that when the boom is lowered, client will be centered in the chair.	
11. Release valve slowly and lower client into the chair. Protect client's head from striking the equipment. Once client is securely seated, remove the chains and store the lift nearby (see illustration).	Leaving the sling under client facilitates transfer back to bed.
12. See Completion Protocol (inside front cover).	

COMMUNICATION TIP

Psychological support and encouragement during transfer is important.

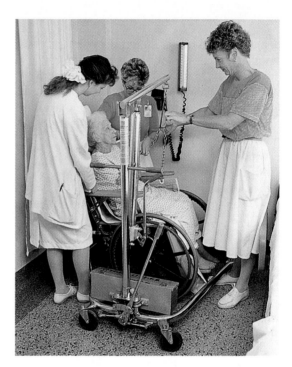

Step 11

• • •

EVALUATION

1. Ask client if the transfer felt safe, smooth, and comfortable.
2. Observe for correct body alignment.
3. Take blood pressure and compare with baseline.

Unexpected Outcomes and Related Interventions

1. Client's buttocks are too far forward in the chair seat, resulting in a slouched position.
   a. Have one caregiver stand in front of client to push the pelvis back into the chair.
   b. A second caregiver stands behind client, placing arms under client's axillae and grasping client's wrists, which places the force on client's arms rather than at axillae and prevents injury from pressure on axillae.

   c. As caregiver behind client lifts upward, second caregiver pushes the knees toward back of the chair, sliding the buttocks into alignment. Avoid shearing forces.
2. Blood pressure drops more than 10% of resting pressure.
   a. Have client extend and flex knees and ankles to encourage venous blood flow.
   b. If dizziness increases, have client lower head and close eyes and encourage deep breaths.
   c. Reassess blood pressure in 5 minutes.

Recording and Reporting

* Type of equipment and number of caregivers
* Subjective response
* Teaching done

Sample Documentation

0900 Transferred from bed to chair using Hoyer lift. Co-operative with move. Stated "I felt very secure with that." Noted a tendency to slide down in the chair while sitting. Propped with pillows and encouraged to call for assistance if uncomfortable. Call light is within reach.

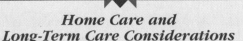

Home Care and Long-Term Care Considerations

- Transfer ability at home is greatly enhanced by prior teaching of family and support persons, assessment of home for safety risks and functionality, and provision of applicable aids.
- Family or support person should practice transfer in hospital to achieve success before taking client home. Arrangements must be made for home health nurse to continue to assist family or support person at home.

Geriatric Considerations

- Older clients may have fragile skin that tears easily and tissues that bruise easily. Take care to provide padding and prevent pinching of tissues during the transfer.
- Explain each step in simple language and avoid jerky and sudden movements

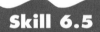

TRANSFERRING FROM BED TO STRETCHER

This transfer involves movement from the bed to a stretcher for client transport from one department to another, to surgery, or for diagnostic tests when the client is too ill to tolerate sitting, client is sedated, or equipment requires a supine position.

Equipment

Stretcher with side rails or safety straps and brake locks
IV pole (if needed and not attached to stretcher)
Roller device or plastic slider board (heavy plastic to minimize shearing forces while sliding client)
Bath blanket or sheet
Pillow

NURSE ALERT

As many as five caregivers may be required for a safe transfer of a heavy client who cannot assist.

ASSESSMENT

1. Assess client's level of consciousness and ability to cooperate with the move.
2. Assess client's joint mobility and limitations.

3. Assess client's pain, including location and severity. When appropriate, offer prescribed analgesic medication before transfer. **Rationale: Analgesics enhance client's ability to tolerate movement. Peak levels vary according to the specific analgesic and route of administration.**

PLANNING

Expected outcomes focus on comfort and safety.

Expected Outcomes

1. Client follows instructions for transfer to stretcher.
2. Client is transferred safely.
3. Client verbalizes feeling comfortable and secure during transfer.

DELEGATION CONSIDERATIONS

The skills of safe and effective transfer techniques and moving and positioning clients in bed can be delegated to assistive personnel (AP) who have successfully demonstrated good body mechanics and safe transfer techniques for clients involved. Clients who have acute spinal trauma or multiple acute injuries may require transfer and moving by professional nurses.

IMPLEMENTATION

Steps	Rationale

1. See Standard Protocol (inside front cover).
2. Position the bed flat and raise to the same height as the stretcher. Lower side rails.
3. Cover client with a sheet or bath blanket, and remove top covers of the bed without exposing client.
4. Check for IV line, Foley catheter, tubes, or surgical drains and position them to avoid tension during the move.
5. Position the stretcher as close to the bed as possible and lock the wheels of the bed and stretcher. Side rails should be lowered (see illustration).
6. **Transfer when client can assist**
   a. Stand near the side of the stretcher and instruct client to move feet, then buttocks, and finally upper body to the stretcher, bringing cover along.
   b. After moving, check to be sure client's body is centered on the stretcher.
7. **Client is unable to assist**
   a. Place a folded sheet or bath blanket so that it supports client's head and extends to midthighs.
   b. Roll the sheet or bath blanket close to client's body. Assist client to cross arms over chest.

> ### COMMUNICATION TIP
>
> - *Caution client not to move until all caregivers are in position. Explain to client to fold arms over chest to facilitate transfer.*
> - *Reassure client that move will be made slowly and gently according to client's level of tolerance.*

Promotes safety and security.

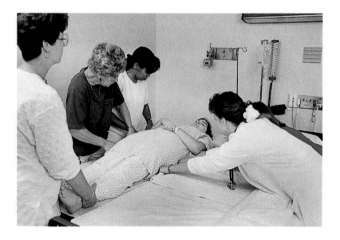

Step 5

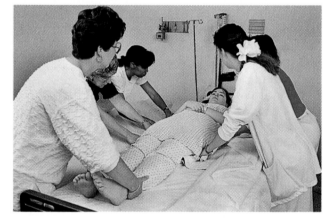

Step 7c

c. Two caregivers reach over the bed to client, and two caregivers stand as close as possible to the stretcher. A fifth caregiver stands at the foot of the bed to lift the feet (see illustration).
d. Using a coordinating count of three, all five caregivers simultaneously lift client to edge of the bed.
e. With another coordinated lift, move client from edge of the bed to the stretcher.

Being closer to weight being lifted reduces risk of back injury to caregiver.

Steps	Rationale

8. Raise both side rails and head of the stretcher if desired.
9. Instruct client to keep hands inside while moving and to avoid grasping side rail, which could bump against door frames during transport.

Improves breathing and comfort.

10. See Completion Protocol (inside front cover).

• • • •

EVALUATION

1. Observe client's ability to follow instructions and assist with transfer.
2. Ask client if the transfer felt safe, smooth, and comfortable.
3. Ask client if change in environment was positive.

Unexpected Outcomes and Related Interventions

1. Client resists transfer and interferes with move by grasping bed or caregivers.
   a. Explain reason for transfer to encourage client's cooperation.
   b. Identify client's reasons for resisting transfer.
   c. Assess for the possibility of premedication for pain before transfer.

Recording and Reporting

- Equipment used and number of caregivers
- Subjective response of client
- Destination for transport

Sample Documentation

1030   Transferred to stretcher with assistance of staff. Client unable to assist. Reports comfortable transfer. Transported to P.T.

Skill 6-6

ASSISTING AMBULATION

In the normal walking posture, the head is erect; the cervical, thoracic, and lumbar vertebrae are aligned; the hips and knees have slight flexion; and the arms swing freely. Illness, surgery, injury, and prolonged bed rest can reduce activity tolerance so that assistance is required. Clients with hemiparesis (one-sided weakness) have difficulty with balance. Temporary or permanent damage to the musculoskeletal or nervous system may necessitate use of an assistive device such as a cane, crutches, or walker (see Chapter 29). Clients with altered cardiovascular or respiratory function may experience difficulty with ambulation, evidenced by chest pain, altered vital signs, dyspnea, or fatigue.

NURSE ALERT

Check the availability of handrails on the walls. Consider whether the assistance of one or two caregivers is required, and determine the need for an assistive device.

Equipment
Robe
Nonskid footwear
Portable IV pole
Gait belt (required for clients with unsteady gait or balance)

ASSESSMENT

1. Assess client's most recent activity experience, including distance ambulated and tolerance of activity (see Skill 6.2). **Rationale: This facilitates realistic planning and identifies degree of assistance needed.**
2. Assess the best time to ambulate, considering other scheduled activities such as bathing and physical therapy. **Rationale: Rest is needed after activities requiring exertion and after meals. Energy is needed to digest food.**
3. Assess the environment and remove obstacles such as chairs, tables, and equipment. If client has an IV line, a rolling IV pole is needed.

4. Assess client's motivation and ability to cooperate. **Rationale: Comparing this activity with client plans for the home environment often enhances motivation.**

5. Assess for medications that may alter stability, including antihypertensive or narcotic medications. **Rationale: These drugs may cause hypotension, dizziness, or instability.**

6. Consider the need for a place where client can sit and rest during the ambulation.

7. Before beginning ambulation assess baseline vital signs.

PLANNING

Expected outcomes focus on developing activity and rest patterns that support increased tolerance of activity. It is essential that this is tailored to each client's needs and abilities (McFarland and McFarlane, 1996).

Expected Outcomes

1. Client ambulates to the end of the hall with assistance, stopping to rest fewer than 3 times.

2. Client maintains respirations, pulse, and blood pressure within 10% of resting values.

3. Client maintains erect posture while standing and walking.

DELEGATION CONSIDERATIONS

The skill of assisting the client with ambulation may be delegated to unlicensed personnel. The following information is needed when delegating this skill to nursing staff or family members:

- Have client wear shoes with a nonskid surface during ambulation.
- Do not try to hold clients if they become dizzy or faint. Ease them into a sitting position in a chair or on the floor.
- Be sure the area is free of clutter, wet areas, and rugs that may slide or buckle.

IMPLEMENTATION

Steps	Rationale
1. See Standard Protocol (inside front cover)	
2. Assist the client to put on shoes or slippers with nonslip soles.	Provides stable walking support.
3. Assist client to stand at the bedside. Encourage to stand fully erect with shoulders back and looking ahead (not at the floor).	
4. If client is unstable, seat client and apply safety belt before proceeding. Consider need for additional help.	If client is very heavy, unstable, or fearful, a second person is needed.
5. If client has an IV line, place the IV pole on the same side as the site of infusion, and instruct client to hold and push the pole while ambulating (see illustration).	
6. If a Foley catheter is present, client or caregiver carries the bag below the level of the bladder and prevents tension on the tubing.	Prevents reflux of urine from the bag back into bladder.
7. Take a few steps supporting client with one arm around the waist and the other under the elbow of the flexed arm. Grasp safety belt in the middle of client's waist.	This provides balance and facilitates lowering client to the floor if client is unable to continue because of weakness or dizziness.
8. When ambulating in a hallway, position client between yourself and the wall. Encourage client to use handrails if available.	The wall provides stable support for clients who start to fall away from nurse.
9. See Completion Protocol (inside front cover).	

COMMUNICATION TIP

Explain importance of nonskid shoes or slippers.

- ***Encourage client to move slowly at own pace.***

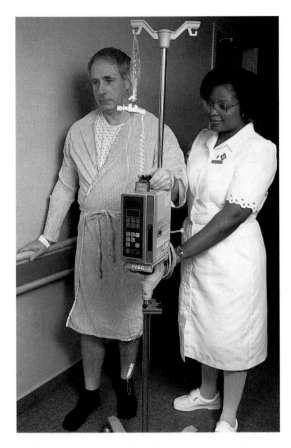

Step 5

EVALUATION

1. Observe tolerance of the activity by noting the frequency of rest periods.
2. Compare client's heart rate, respiratory rate, and blood pressure with baseline values immediately after ambulation and again after 5 minutes of rest.
3. Observe client's body alignment and balance while standing and walking.

Unexpected Outcomes and Related Interventions

1. Vital signs are altered: pulse more than 10% over resting rate or greater than 120 beats/min, systolic blood pressure increased or decreased more than 10% of resting value, or dyspnea, labored breathing, and wheezing present. Client reports feelings of excessive fatigue or weakness.
   a. Plan activity after adequate rest period.
   b. Pace activity to proceed more slowly, and allow time to stop and rest at regular intervals. Sitting periodically may be helpful.
   c. Provide a wheelchair to be pushed by the client to provide balance and support.
   d. Assistive devices such as a cane or walker may decrease energy required (see Chapter 29).

2. Client starts to fall.
   a. Call for help.
   b. Put both arms around client's waist from behind and spread feet apart for a broad base of support.
   c. If necessary, ease client slowly to the floor, bending knees to prevent strain on back muscles.
   d. Stay with client until assistance arrives to help lift client to wheelchair.

Recording and Reporting

- Distance ambulated
- Subjective response
- Changes in vital signs

Sample Documentation

1300   Ambulated client 100 feet in hall with assistance of one. Vital signs stable. States, "I am not as tired as yesterday." Gait steady. Systolic blood pressure increased by 15 mm Hg, and pulse increased 15 beats/min and returned to baseline within 5 minutes.

Geriatric Considerations

Older clients are often fearful of falling when ambulatory. Encouragement, reassurance, and assistance from family or caregiver decreases anxiety.

Home Care and Long-Term Care Considerations

- Client should be instructed on how to use the ambulation aid on various terrains (e.g., carpet, stairs, rough ground, inclines). Client should also be instructed on how to maneuver around obstacles such as doors and how to use the aid when transferring such as to and from a chair, toilet, tub, and car (Borgman-Gainer, 1996).
- Assess whether client is using the ordered ambulation aid correctly. If client is noncompliant, try to determine cause. Potential reasons for noncompliance are:
  - Lack of perception of reason and benefits of the aid
  - Time lapse between onset of disability and training with equipment
  - Lack of proper training
  - Decreased ability to attend to tasks

CRITICAL THINKING EXERCISES

1. Mrs. Smith has had a cerebral infarct (stroke), and her left side is paralyzed. She is on the unit with a plan to be discharged in 1 week. Her twin daughters, age 24, are anxious to care for her at home. Mrs. Smith lives with her 64-year-old husband in a one-story town house in a senior community. Her daughters live together 1 mile from their parents. Coordinate plan of home care for this family related to her activity, mobility, and normal daily routines.

2. Mrs. George is on bed rest at home. Develop a plan of care for the family to prevent pressure sores.

3. Safety is an important issue for all hospitalized clients. What important safety measure(s) was (were) overlooked in each of the following situations, and what consequence could have occurred to the clients as a result of the oversight?
   a. Sarah was transferring Martha from her bed to a stretcher. Sarah positioned the bed flat and placed a bath blanket beneath Martha from her shoulders to her hips. Sarah then moved the stretcher as close to the bed as possible and locked the wheels of the stretcher in place.
   b. Jim is in the process of transferring Mr. Blue from his bed to a chair using a mechanical lift. Jim has prepared the chair and placed it near the bed. Jim turns Mr. Blue to his side, places the sling under Mr. Blue to ensure adequate support of Mr. Blue's head, returns Mr. Blue to his back, and slowly begins to lift Mr. Blue from his bed.
   c. Tom has an order to ambulate Mrs. Rucker twice daily in her room. On entering Mrs. Rucker's room, Tom notes that she is lying in bed. He explains that she needs to take a short walk, assists her to a standing position, and encourages her to walk toward the door. Mrs. Rucker states that she is dizzy.

REFERENCES

Baas L, Ross D: Caring for patients on prolonged bedrest. In Swearingingen P: *Manual of nursing therapeutics: applying nursing diagnosis to nursing disorders,* St Louis, 1990, Mosby.

Bergstrom N et al: A clinical trial of the Braden Scale for predicting pressure sore risk, *Nurs Clin North Am* 23(2):417, 1987a.

Bergstrom N et al: The Braden Scale for predicting pressure sore risk, *Nurs Res* 36:205, 1987b.

Blue DL: Preventing back injury among nurses, *Orthop Nurs* 15(6):9, 1996.

Bronstein K, Popovich J, Stewart-Amidei C: *Promoting stroke recovery: a research based approach for nurses,* St Louis, 1991, Mosby.

Canobbio MM: *Cardiovascular disorders, Mosby's clinical nursing series,* St Louis, 1990, Mosby.

Hogstel MO: *Clinical manual of gerontological nursing,* St Louis, 1992, Mosby.

Kemp MG, Kroushap TA: Pressure ulcers: reducing incidence and severity by managing pressure, *J Gerontol Nurs* 20(9): 27, 1994.

Lane LD et al: Dangling practices of 51 nurses: a pilot project, *Am J Crit Care* 6(3): 177, 1997.

Logan P: Moving and handling: protecting yourself, *Community Nurse* 2(3): 22, 1996.

Mantee F: Moving experiences . . . complementary therapies . . . improving patients mobility, *Nurs Times* 92(14): 96, 1996.

McConnell EA: Clinical do's and don't's. Transferring a patient from bed to chair, *Nursing* 25(1): 30, 1995.

McFarland G, McFarlane E: *Nursing diagnosis and intervention,* ed 4, St Louis, 1996, Mosby.

Metzler DJ, Harr J: Positioning your patient properly, *Am J Nurs* 96(3): 33, 1996.

Neal C: The assessment of knowledge and application of proper body mechanics in the workplace, *Orthop Nurs* 16(1): 66, 1997.

Patterson DC: Minimizing back injuries in nursing home staff, *Nurs Homes* 42(4): 33, 1993.

Perry AG, Potter PA: *Clinical nursing skills and techniques,* St Louis, 1998, Mosby.

Agency for Health Care Policy and Research: *Pressure ulcers in adults: prediction and prevention,* pub no. 92-0047, Rockville, Md, 1992, US Department of Health and Human Services, Public Health Service, Agency for Health Care Policy.

CHAPTER 7

Promoting Hygiene

Skill 7.1
Complete Bathing,   123

Skill 7.2
Oral Care,   130

Skill 7.3
Hair Care,   135

Skill 7.4
Foot and Nail Care,   140

Skill 7.5
Bedmaking,   147

Personal hygiene is essential to maintain skin integrity by promoting adequate circulation and hydration. Intact skin functions include (1) defense against infection; (2) awareness of touch, pain, heat, cold, and pressure; and (3) control of body temperature. Bathing should be done when any body part becomes soiled. Linen changes usually are required as well. Problems such as incontinence, wound drainage, or diaphoresis may require frequent bathing. In addition to cleansing the skin, bathing a client has several benefits (Box 7-1).

Age influences the skin's condition. Normally the skin is elastic, well hydrated, firm, and smooth. With age the skin becomes thinner, dry, less vascular, more fragile, and prone to bruising and tears. Bathing is an excellent opportunity to assess the skin for common skin problems that may require special interventions (Table 7-1). Bathing older clients too frequently may contribute to dry skin and should be avoided. Three times a week may be adequate for many older clients; however, optimal frequency depends on individual needs.

Many clients require assistance with personal hygiene during illness or recovery. Maintenance of personal hygiene is necessary for comfort and a sense of well-being. Because personal hygiene requires close contact with the client, it provides an opportunity for interactions that focus on immediate and future emotional, social, and health-related concerns.

The nurse needs to convey sensitivity and respect for personal beliefs and habits and to ensure as much privacy as possible. Bathing should be done according to the client's usual routines and preferences. Some clients need encouragement to be independent and to participate in self-care. If the client cannot participate, the family or significant other may be encouraged to assist when possible. Some clients lack the physical energy to perform self-care and need to be temporarily dependent on others in order to enhance the healing and recovery process.

Box 7-1 Benefits of Bathing

Cleansing the skin: removal of perspiration, some bacteria, sebum, and dead skin cells minimizes skin irritation and reduces the chance of infection.

Stimulating circulation: muscle activity, warm water, and stroking extremities enhance circulation.

Promoting range of motion (ROM): movement of extremities maintains joint function.

Reducing body odors: secretions and excretions from axillae and perineal areas result in body odors that are eliminated by bathing.

Improving self-image: promotes relaxation and feeling clean and comfortable. Care of hair and teeth enhances appearance and sense of well-being.

NURSING DIAGNOSES

Bathing/Hygiene Self-Care Deficit is appropriate when the focus of care is helping the client move toward independence in bathing. The client may be unable to wash body parts, to obtain or have access to a water source, or to regulate water temperature or flow (Kim, McFarland, and McLane, 1997). Contributing factors may include impaired physical mobility in which range of motion (ROM) or muscle strength is limited or an alteration in mental state. Shortness of breath with activity or excessive fatigue when bathing may also be contributing factors. **Risk for Impaired Skin Integrity** should be considered when the client has reduced sensation, immobility, impaired circulation, incontinence, inadequate nutrition, or fragile skin associated with advancing age.

Altered Oral Mucous Membrane is appropriate when mucous membranes are damaged, such as by ulcerations, erythema, and irritation. Contributing factors may include sensory changes (pain, burning, numbness), decreased level of consciousness, and altered oral intake for any reason. **Dressing/Grooming Self-Care Deficit** is appropriate when the focus is to improve a client's ability to provide self-care with oral hygiene or hair care.

Body Image Disturbance is often appropriate when the client loses interest in grooming or experiences hair loss. This should also be considered when the client displays a lack of interest in appearance, especially when medical treatment alters body appearance or function.

Altered Health Maintenance is appropriate when client teaching related to foot care is the focus of care. **Impaired Skin Integrity** is an appropriate diagnosis for the client who has actually experienced a loss in skin integrity. Pressure ulcers, vascular ulcerations, and ecchymosis are examples of impaired skin integrity.

Table 7-1

Common Skin Problems and Related Interventions

Problem	Interventions
Dry skin: flaky, rough texture to skin, which may crack and become infected.	Bathe less frequently; rinse away all soap or use a waterless cleanser rather than soap; increase fluid intake; use moisturizing lotion.
Acne: inflammatory papulopustular skin eruption, usually involving bacterial breakdown of sebum, typically on face, neck, shoulders, and back.	Wash hair daily. Wash skin twice daily with warm water and soap to remove oils and cosmetics (if used); cosmetics that can accumulate in pores should be used sparingly. Topical antibiotics, if prescribed, may minimize problems.
Hirsutism: excessive growth of body and facial hair, especially in women; may cause negative body image by giving women a male appearance.	Shaving is safest method; electrolysis permanently removes hair by destroying hair follicles; tweezing and bleaching are temporary measures; depilatories may remove unwanted hair but may cause infection, rashes, or dermatitis.
Skin rashes: skin eruption from overexposure to sun or moisture or from allergic reaction; may be flat, raised, localized, or systemic; may be associated with pruritus (itching).	Wash thoroughly; apply antiseptic spray or lotion to prevent further itching and aid in healing process; warm or cold soaks relieve inflammation.
Contact dermatitis: inflammation of skin characterized by abrupt onset with erythema, pruritus, pain, and scaly, oozing lesions; usually results from contact with substance difficult to identify and eliminate.	Identify and avoid contributing agents; provide linens rinsed and sterilized to minimize irritation.
Abrasion: scraping or rubbing away of epidermis that results in localized bleeding and later weeping of serous fluid; easily infected.	Wash with mild soap and water; observe dressings for retained moisture, which can increase risk of infection.

COMPLETE BATHING

The extent of the bath and the methods used depend on the client's ability to participate and the skin's condition. A partial bath consists of bathing only body parts that would cause discomfort or odor if left unbathed, such as hands, face, breasts, perineal area, and axillae. Clients who cannot tolerate a complete bath and self-sufficient clients unable to reach all body parts may be given a partial bed bath. A tub bath or shower can be used to give a more thorough bath. In the tub or shower, washing and rinsing all body parts is easier; however, safety is of primary concern, and clients must have adequate strength, mobility, and mental capacity.

Equipment

Washcloths and towels
Bath blanket
Soap and soap dish
Warm water
Toiletry items (deodorant, powder, lotion)
Clean hospital gown or client's own pajamas
Laundry bag
Disposable gloves (when body secretions are present)

ASSESSMENT

1. Assess degree of assistance needed for bathing. Factors may include vision, ability to sit without support, hand grasp, ROM of extremities, and cognitive ability.
2. Assess client's tolerance of activity, level of discomfort with movement, and presence of shortness of breath or chest pain with exertion. **Rationale: This determines what type of cleansing bath is appropriate for the client.**
3. Assess client's preferences for time of day, products used, and frequency of bathing.
4. Identify any problems related to condition of the skin:
   a. Excessive moisture from secretions (diaphoresis) or incontinence
   b. Drainage or excretions from lesions or body cavities
   c. External devices (catheters, drains, dressings, restraints)
   d. Rashes or skin damage related to pruritus and scratching **Rationale: This determines what toiletry items and/or other equipment to have available for the client.**
5. Identify any prescribed limitations of activity or positioning required by client's illness or treatment plan. This information is available from the primary caregiver's report or information from a Kardex or nursing care plan. **Rationale: This determines safety need of the client to prevent injury.**

PLANNING

Expected outcomes focus on promoting comfort, mobility, and self-care abilities.

Expected Outcomes

1. Client's skin is clean and free of excretions, drainage, or odor.
2. Client demonstrates functional ROM of hands and shoulders.
3. Client demonstrates ability to wash face, hands, and chest independently.
4. Client expresses comfort and relaxation.

NOTE: This procedure assumes client is totally dependent. When client is able to assist, encourage and allow as much involvement as possible.

DELEGATION CONSIDERATIONS

Skills of bathing are often delegated to AP; however, assessment is not. The nurse should:

- Instruct care provider on what type of bath (complete, partial assist, tub, or shower) is appropriate to the client's diagnosis and needs.
- Remind the care provider to notify the nurse of any skin integrity problems so the nurse can inspect areas of breakdown.
- Tell care provider to allow the client to perform as much self-care as appropriate to encourage independence.

COMMUNICATION TIP

- *Use an organized approach and reassuring tone of voice so the client feels safe and comfortable during bathing.*
- *Encourage the client to report any concerns or discomfort during the bath.*
- *Encourage as much independence in the client's self-care skills as appropriate. Provide positive feedback.*

IMPLEMENTATION

Steps	Rationale
1. See Standard Protocol (inside front cover).	
2. Promote independence and participation as much as possible during bath. If appropriate, involve the family or significant other.	Increases client's cooperation and comfort.
3. Provide privacy. Close the door and/or pull the curtains around the area. Expose only the areas being bathed.	Promotes client's emotional and physical comfort.
4. Provide safety. If it is necessary to leave the room, be sure the call light is within reach. Provide assistance according to client's needs.	
5. The room should be comfortably warm. Protect the client from injury by assessing and controlling bath water temperature.	Avoids chilling the client and promotes safety.
6. Consider the client's cultural preferences in regard to grooming techniques and products. However, the nurse may have opportunities to caution against the use of products that can damage or injure skin, hair, or nails.	
7. With client supine, place bath blanket over client and remove top covers without exposing client. Place soiled linen in laundry bag.	Prevents chilling and provides privacy.

8. ![icon] Remove client's gown or pajamas.
   a. If an extremity is injured or has limited mobility, begin removal from unaffected side first.
   b. If client has IV line, remove gown from arm without IV first, then slide IV container and tubing through sleeve and rehang. Check flow rate and regulate if necessary (see illustration).

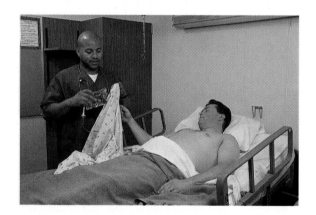

Step 8b

Steps	Rationale
c. If IV pump is in use, turn pump off, clamp tubing, remove tubing from pump, and proceed as in Step b. Unclamp tubing, insert into pump, and turn pump on at correct rate.	Sterility and patency of IV infusion must be maintained.
9. Remove pillow. Place one bath towel under client's head and another over chest.	Removing pillow facilitates bathing ears and neck. Towels absorb moisture.
10. Wash face. a. Form mitt with washcloth (see illustration) and wash client's eyes with plain warm water using a clean area of cloth for each eye, bathing from inner to outer canthus (see illustration). Dry eyes gently and thoroughly.	Mitt prevents loose ends from dripping or annoying client. Soap irritates eyes. Use of separate sections of cloth reduces transmission of microorganisms. Bathing inner to outer canthus prevents secretions from entering nasolacrimal duct.
b. Wash, rinse, and dry forehead, cheeks, nose, neck, and ears without using soap. Men may want to be shaved (see Skill 7.3).	Soap tends to dry face, which is exposed to air more than other body parts. If client has a preferred face wash, it should be used.

Steps

Rationale

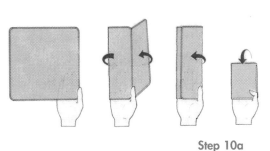

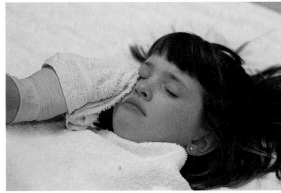

Step 10a

11. Eye care for the unconscious client.
  a. Cleanse the eyelids from the inner to outer canthus using gauze moistened with water or normal saline.

  b. Instill prescribed eyedrops or ointment as per physician's order or agency policy Reassess eyes every 2 to 4 hours or as ordered for dryness.
  c. In the absence of a blink reflex the eyelids should be kept closed and covered with an eye patch or shield. Avoid taping the eyelid.
12. Wash upper body.
  a. Remove bath blanket from over client's arm. Place bath towel lengthwise under arm. Bathe with minimal soap and water using long, firm strokes from distal to proximal (fingers to axilla).
  b. Raise and support arm above head (if possible) to wash, rinse, and dry axilla thoroughly.
  c. Repeat Steps a and b with other arm (see illustration). Apply deodorant or powder to underarms if appropriate.

Clients that are unconscious have lost the normal protective actions of the eye, which increases their risk for corneal drying, corneal abrasions, and eye infections.

Lubricants will help keep the client's eyes moist in the absence of tearing and/or blinking.

Eyelids should be kept closed to keep eyes moist and prevent injury. Taping can injure the eyelid.

Promotes circulatory return to heart.

Raising arm promotes ROM and facilitates thorough cleansing.

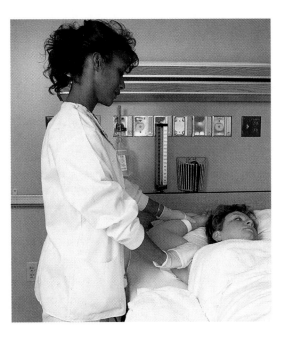

Step 12c

Steps	Rationale

   d. Cover client's chest with bath towel, and fold bath blanket down to umbilicus. Bathe chest using long, firm strokes. Take special care with skin under female clients' breasts, lifting breast upward if necessary. Rinse and dry well.

Skin under breasts is vulnerable to excoriation if not kept clean and dry.

13. Wash lower body.

   a. Place bath towel over chest and abdomen, and fold bath blanket down to just above pubic region. Bathe, rinse, and dry abdomen with special attention to umbilicus and skinfolds of abdomen and groin.

Keeping skinfolds clean and dry helps prevent odor and skin irritation.

   b. Expose client's leg nearest to you, leaving perineum covered. Place bath towel under leg, supporting leg at knee and with foot flat on bed. If desired, place client's foot in a basin to soak while washing and rinsing. If client is unable to support leg, assistance will be needed or soaking omitted. Wash and dry leg using long, firm strokes from ankle to knee, then knee to thigh (see illustration). Wash foot between toes. Rinse and dry thoroughly.

Soaking softens calluses and rough skin.

   c. Raise side rail, move to opposite side, and repeat Step b with other leg and foot. If skin is dry, apply lotion.

Promotes good body mechanics for the nurse.

   d. Cover with bath blanket, and raise side rail. Change bath water. Remove gloves.

Provides client warmth and safety.

14. Wash perineum.

   a. Assist client in assuming side-lying position, placing towel lengthwise along client's side and keeping client covered with bath blanket as much as possible.

If client is totally dependent, assistance is necessary to support client in side-lying position and to raise leg as perineum is bathed.

NURSE ALERT

It is not recommended to soak the feet of clients with diabetes mellitus or peripheral vascular disease. This may lead to maceration (excessive softening of the skin) and infection.

Avoid leg message especially when client is at risk of deep vein thrombosis (blood clots) or emboli.

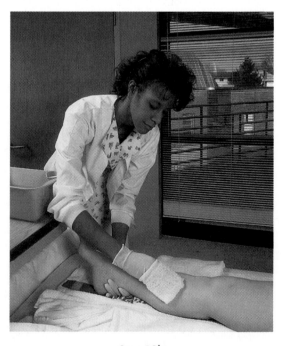

Step 13b

Steps	Rationale

b. If fecal material is present, enclose it in a fold of underpad and remove as much as possible with disposable wipes first. Cleanse buttocks and anus, washing from front to back or side to side. Cleanse anal area from front to back with special attention to folds of buttocks (see illustration). Use as many washcloths as necessary to cleanse and rinse thoroughly. Dry area completely. Remove and discard underpad and replace with a clean one.

Washing from front to back or side to side prevents transmission of microorganisms from anus to urethra or genitalia.

15. Provide female perineal care if applicable.
   a. Position waterproof pad under client's buttocks with client supine. Drape client with bath blanket placed in the shape of a diamond. Lift lower edge of bath blanket to expose perineum (see illustration). Wash labia majora using washcloth, soap, and warm water. Then gently retract labia from thigh and wash groin from perineum toward rectum.

   Washing from front to back prevents contamination of urethral meatus with fecal matter.

   b. Gently separate labia and expose urethra and vagina. Wash from pubic area toward rectum, cleansing thoroughly. Avoid tension on indwelling catheter if present and clean area around it thoroughly.

   Minimizes risk for developing infection because of presence of indwelling catheter or fecal incontinence.

   c. Rinse and dry area thoroughly. Assess for redness, swelling, discharge, irritation, or skin breakdown. Make sure catheter is secured with tape to upper thigh and positioned over (not under) the thigh.

   Prevents pulling of catheter on urethral canal and promotes urinary drainage.

16. Provide male perineal care if applicable.
   a. Gently grasp shaft of penis, and if client is not circumcised, retract foreskin.

   Gentle handling reduces risk of having an erection. Secretions and microorganisms tend to collect under foreskin.

   b. Wash tip of penis at urethral meatus first. Using circular motion, cleanse away from meatus (see illustration). Replace foreskin to its natural position.

   Discharge may indicate presence of infection or inflammation. Replacing foreskin prevents constriction of the penis, which may result in edema.

   c. Gently cleanse shaft of penis, and scrotum, washing underlying skinfolds. Rinse and dry.

17. Cover client with bath blanket, change bath water, and remove and discard gloves.

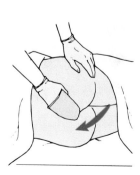

Step 14b

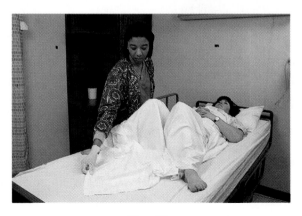

Step 15a

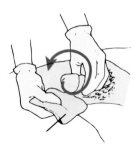

Step 16b

Steps	**Rationale**

18. Wash back.
   a. Assist client to side-lying position, and place towel lengthwise along the back. Wash, rinse, and dry back from neck to buttocks using long, firm strokes.
   b. Remove gloves and dispose of them properly.

19. Apply body lotion to skin as needed and topical moisturizing agents to dry, flaky, or scaling areas. Replace gown.

Dry skin results in reduced pliability and cracking. Moisturizers may help prevent skin breakdown (AHCPR, 1992).

20. Massage back.
   a. Position client prone (on abdomen) if possible. Side-lying position is also frequently used.
   b. Provide back massage using lotion to stimulate circulation (see illustration). Begin at sacral area. Massaging in circular motion, stroke upward from buttocks to shoulders and upper arms and over scapulas with smooth, firm strokes (see illustration). Keep hands on skin and continue massage pattern for 3 to 4 minutes.

NURSE ALERT

Massaging over bony prominences is no longer recommended. Evidence suggests that massage may result in decreased blood flow and tissue damage in some clients (AHCPR, 1992).

   c. Knead skin by grasping tissue between thumb and fingers. Knead upward along each side of spine and around muscles of neck, avoiding bony prominences.
   d. End massage with long stroking movements, and tell client you are ending massage.

Long strokes promote comfort and relaxation.

   e. Observe skin for redness and skin breakdown. Remove excess lotion from back with bath towel.

Excess lotion could promote maceration of skin.

   f. Apply clean gown or pajamas, dressing affected side first.

Allows easier manipulation of gown over restricted body part.

21. See Completion Protocol (inside front cover).

• • •

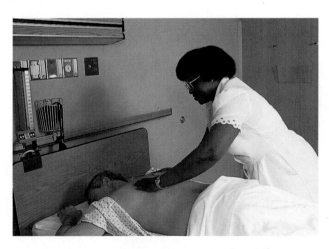 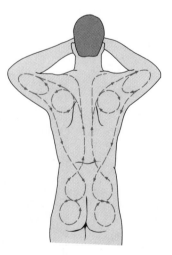

Step 20b

EVALUATION

1. Observe areas on skin for erythema, exudate, drainage, or breakdown.
2. Measure ROM in hands, arms, and shoulders, and compare with baseline. Assess vital signs if client is experiencing distress or restlessness.
3. Observe for improved ability to assist with self-bathing and hygiene to determine progress.
4. Ask client to view self in mirror and comment on appearance and comfort.

Unexpected Outcomes and Related Interventions

1. Client's skin on lower extremities is dry and flaky and itches.
   a. Limit the frequency of baths to every other day or less.
   b. Use a mild soap sparingly. Change cleansing agent.
   c. Blot skin dry after bathing, and apply lotion to skin.
   d. Increase hydration status.
   e. Administer antipruritics as ordered to control itching.
   f. Use distraction techniques to remove focus from itching.
2. The client has evidence of rashes, redness, scaling, or cracking.
   a. Evaluate the need for a change in frequency of bathing and soap product used.
   b. Collaborate with the physician regarding application of ointments or creams to provide a protective barrier and help maintain moisture within the skin.
3. The rectum, perineum, or genital region is inflamed, is swollen, or has foul-smelling discharge.

   a. Bathe area frequently enough to keep clean and dry.
   b. Apply protective barrier or antiinflammatory cream.

Recording and Reporting

Routine documentation may include check marks on a flow sheet. Observations made during the bath that should be charted may include:

- Type of bath given
- Client's ability to assist or cooperate
- Condition of client's skin and any nursing interventions related to skin integrity
- Client's response to bathing and any concerns voiced by client regarding self-care needs

Sample Documentation

0900   Complete bath given. Unable to assist but cooperative with turning. Skin on both legs dry and flaking, complains of severe itching. Bath oil added to bath water. Emollient lotion applied after bath. States itching is less now.

Home Care and Long-Term Care Considerations

- Type of bath chosen depends on assessment of the home, availability of running water, and condition of bathing facilities.
- In home setting, set up equipment according to established routines. Client is best resource for what works in terms of convenience and saving time.
- The three types of bath for the homebound client are the complete bed bath; the abbreviated bed bath, during which only parts of the body are washed that, if neglected, might cause illness, odor, or discomfort; and the partial bath, which may take place at the sink, in the tub, or in the shower.
- Never leave bathing client unattended. Adhesive strips on bottom of tub or shower, handrails, chairs, or stools in tub or shower will further protect client.
- Clients at risk for falls may wish to have grab bars installed around tub and have bathroom floor carpeted. Client also may use portable shower seat.
- If beds do not have side rails, positioning may be accomplished with pillows or by placing bed against wall.

Geriatric Considerations

- Consider conditions of older adult's skin when planning hygiene routine. Because of the aging process more moisture is needed; client's skin can be rehydrated with lotions and fluids.
- Older adults may chill easily.
- Older adults with limited mobility need assistance in perineal care. Using a side-lying position increases client's comfort and provides nurse with opportunity to provide perineal care and inspect surrounding skin as well.
- Older adults with urinary incontinence need meticulous skin care to reduce skin irritation from urine and feces.
- Older adults may require less frequent baths, more frequent application of skin lotion.

Skill 7.2

ORAL CARE

Oral hygiene helps maintain healthy structures of the oral cavity and comfort of the mouth, teeth, gums, and lips. Brushing cleanses the teeth of food particles, plaque, and bacteria; massages the gums; and relieves discomfort resulting from unpleasant odors and tastes. Flossing helps remove plaque and tartar between teeth to reduce gum inflammation and infection. Many factors can influence oral hygiene (Box 7-2). Inadequate oral hygiene can create a general sense of discomfort and also diminish appetite.

Clients may experience altered oral mucous membranes when they are dehydrated; have inadequate nutrition, particularly vitamin B deficiency; or are unable to take food or fluids orally (NPO). Mouth breathing may result in dry mucous membranes. Trauma to oral mucous membranes may also occur from oral tubes, oxygen therapy, suctioning, hot foods, or trauma from broken teeth or ill-fitting dentures. Chemical injury may result from irritating substances such as alcohol, tobacco, acidic foods, or side effects of medications, including chemotherapy, antibiotics, steroids, and antidepressants. Chronic inflammatory disease may be caused by bacteria, viral or fungal infections, or ineffective oral hygiene.

Dentures should be cleaned as regularly as natural teeth to prevent gingival infection and irritation. Loose dentures can cause discomfort and make it difficult for clients to chew food and speak clearly. Loose dentures may result from weight loss.

Box 7-2 Factors Influencing Oral Hygiene

Client lacks upper-extremity strength or dexterity to perform oral hygiene (e.g., is paralyzed or has limited ROM).

Client unable or unwilling to attend to personal hygiene needs (e.g., is unconscious, depressed, or confused).

Client is diabetic and prone to dryness of mouth, gingivitis, periodontal disease, and loss of teeth.

Client is prone to dehydration or has a fever. Thick secretions develop on tongue and gums. Lips become cracked and reddened.

Radiation therapy causes soreness, mild erythema, swollen mucosa, dysphagia, dryness, taste changes, and possible oral infection.

Chemotherapy causes ulcerations and inflammation of mucosa and possible oral infection.

Tissues in oral cavity become traumatized with swelling, ulcerations, inflammation, and possible bleeding.

Dentures can be easily lost or broken. They should be stored in an enclosed, labeled cup or should be soaking when not worn (e.g., during surgery or a diagnostic procedure), and they should be reinserted as soon as possible. The change in appearance when they are not worn may be of major concern to the client.

NURSING DIAGNOSES

Altered Oral Mucous Membrane is a nursing diagnosis for clients who have damage to oral mucous membranes. This may include mild generalized erythema, small ulcerations or white patches, or hemorrhagic ulcerations. Contributing factors could include sensory changes such as numbness, chronic irritation, or decreased level of consciousness and altered oral intake. **Altered Nutrition: Less Than Body Requirements** should be considered when a client's appetite and intake are diminished because of altered mucous membranes, and the aim is to increase oral intake by improving oral hygiene. **Bathing/Hygiene Self-Care Deficit** is appropriate when the focus is to promote independence in oral hygiene and teach the use of adaptive devices. **Risk for Infection** can apply in presence of trauma or lesions in the oral cavity. **Body Image Disturbance** may be appropriate when clients are unable to wear dentures for any reason.

Equipment (Figure 7-1)
Soft-bristled toothbrush or 4 × 4 gauze (if toothbrush is contraindicated)
Antiinfective solution or normal saline to loosen crusts (check agency policy)
Sponge toothette
Glass of water
Padded tongue blade
Emesis basin
Face towel
Suction equipment (optional)
Disposable gloves
Water-soluble lubricant

ASSESSMENT

1. Determine presence or absence of gag reflex by placing tongue blade or suction tip on back of tongue. **Rationale: Clients with no gag reflex are at risk for aspiration. Suction equipment must be available.**

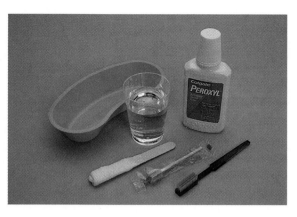

Figure 7-1 Oral hygiene equipment. *Clockwise from left;* emesis basin, water, mouthwash, toothbrush, sponge toothette, and padded tongue blade.

2. Inspect lips, teeth, gums, buccal mucosa, palate, and tongue, using tongue depressor and penlight if necessary (see Chapter 14). Observe for color, texture, moisture, lesions or ulcers, and condition of teeth (or dentures). Ask if areas of tenderness exist. **Rationale: Every effort should be made to prevent or minimize oral problems.**

3. Identify presence of oral problems and remove gloves.
   a. Dental caries: discoloration of tooth enamel
   b. Gingivitis: inflammation of gums
   c. Periodontitis: receding gum lines, inflammation, gaps between teeth, rough or jagged teeth
   d. Halitosis: bad breath
   e. Cracked lips
   f. Dry, cracked, coated tongue
      Rationale: Any oral problems put clients at risk for infection or nutritional deficiencies.

For Denture Care

1. Ask client if dentures fit and if there is any gum or mucous membrane tenderness or irritation.

2. ▧ Ask client to remove dentures and place them in basin or denture cup. Inspect oral cavity and denture surface after dentures are removed. **Rationale: If client is unable to remove dentures, grasp upper plate at front with gauze to prevent slipping. Use steady, downward pull and rotate sideways to reduce tension on lips. Gently lift lower denture from jaw and rotate to remove from mouth.**

3. Ask client about preferences for denture care and products used and remove gloves.

PLANNING

Expected outcomes focus on promoting comfort, preventing aspiration, and promoting integrity of oral mucous membranes.

Expected Outcomes

1. Client's oral mucous membranes are smooth, moist, pink, and without lesions.
2. Client maintains clean dental surfaces.
3. Client verbalizes comfort and displays no restlessness or grimace during oral care.
4. The client, spouse, or significant other demonstrates oral hygiene regimen.

DELEGATION CONSIDERATIONS

Skills of oral care, toothbrushing, and denture care can be delegated to AP. The nurse should:

- Instruct the care provider in what type of oral care is appropriate to the individual client and the amount of assistance and supervision the client may need.
- Remind the care provider to report any changes in oral mucosa.
- Review the use of oral suction with the care provider if the client may require it.
- Inform the care provider that many clients may be self-conscious about removing their dentures and privacy should be provided.

COMMUNICATION TIP

Use time assisting clients with oral care to teach proper oral hygiene practices, including flossing, and/or to provide reinforcement for the client's appropriate practices.

IMPLEMENTATION

Steps	Rationale

1. See Standard Protocol (inside front cover).
2. Position unconscious client in side-lying position with bed flat and towel placed under chin. Have emesis basin available.

   Side-lying position minimizes risk of aspiration. Debilitated client may be positioned with head of bed elevated if not in danger of aspirating.

3. [icon] Separate upper and lower teeth gently with padded tongue blade between back molars (see illustration). Client needs to be relaxed. Wait until client is relaxed with mouth open, then insert blade with smooth, quick motion and without using force.

   Some clients tend to bite on any object placed in mouth.

4. Oral suction should be on and ready for use if gag reflex is absent (see Chapter 31).

   Some clients who are unconscious do not have a gag reflex.

5. Clean mouth using brush or 4 × 4 gauze moistened with normal saline or water. Clean tooth surfaces, roof of mouth, inside cheeks, and tongue. Rinse with clean toothette and water. Avoid stimulating gag reflex (if present) and use as little fluid as possible to prevent aspiration.

6. If client cannot expectorate secretions, provide suction of oral cavity as they accumulate.

   Prevents aspiration.

7. Apply water-soluble jelly to lips (see illustration).

   Prevents drying and cracking.

8. For client with decreased level of consciousness or confusion, indicate that you are finished.

   Provides meaningful stimulation and reality orientation.

9. Provide oral care to prevent or minimize mucositis.
   a. Provide mouth care at least 4 times per day and often enough to keep the mouth clean and moist.

   Mucositis (inflammation of the mucous membranes in the mouth) is a common complication in hospitalized clients, especially those receiving radiation or chemotherapy.

   b. Clean the mouth by brushing the teeth with a soft-bristled toothbrush angled at 45 degrees or a sponge toothette and rinsing well with normal saline. Avoid the use of lemon and glycerine swabs.

   Angling the toothbrush or using the toothette avoids injury to the oral mucosa (Moore, 1995). Lemon and glycerine swabs are very drying to the oral mucosa.

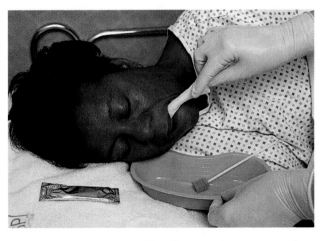

Step 3

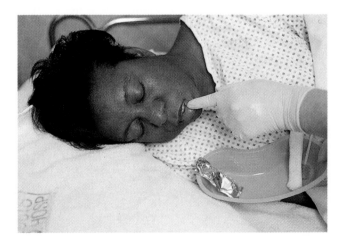

Step 7

Steps	Rationale
c. Rinse the mouth by teaching the client to carefully swish then spit the prescribed mouth rinse and remove gloves. (Check agency policy or specific order.)	Agencies and physicians have different protocols for oral rinses. These mouth rinse mixtures will generally include some combination of alcohol-free antifungals, a commercial oral rinse or very diluted hydrogen peroxide for cleaning, a topical anesthetic like lidocaine for pain, diphenhydramine hydrochloride, and a coating agent such as an antacid (Focazio, 1997).
d. Teach the client to keep lips well lubricated with water-soluble jelly or lip balm. Sucking on ice and drinking liquids will also help keep the mouth moist.	A moist mouth is less prone to break down and heals faster.
e. Remove and discard gloves.	
10. Provide care of dentures.	
a. Place washcloth in sink and fill with small amount of warm water.	Cloth protects dentures from breakage. Hot water could damage dentures. Dentures become very slippery when wet.
b. ![] Apply cleaning agent to brush, and cleanse biting surfaces of teeth. Use short strokes from top of denture to biting surfaces to clean outer and inner tooth surfaces (see illustration).	
c. Clean remaining surfaces of dentures with brush, then rinse thoroughly in tepid water.	
d. Apply toothpaste to soft toothbrush, and gently brush gums, palate, and tongue. Rinse mouth thoroughly.	Helps stimulate circulation to gums and removes residual film of debris on gums and mucosa.
e. Some clients use an adhesive to seal dentures in place. Apply a thin layer to undersurface before inserting.	
f. If client needs assistance with insertion of dentures, moisten upper denture and press firmly to seal it in place. Then insert moistened lower denture. Ask if dentures feel comfortable.	
11. Store dentures.	
a. Some clients prefer to remove and store dentures in a denture cup.	Removal gives the gums a rest and prevents bacterial buildup.
b. Label denture cup with the client's name and room number, and place in a secure place and remove gloves.	Keeping dentures moist prevents warping and facilitates easier insertion. Dentures are expensive to replace and can be easily misplaced.

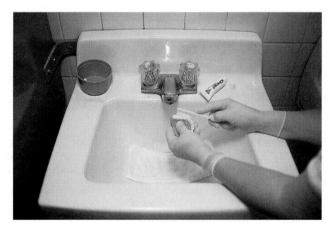

Step 10b

Steps	Rationale

12. Assist with flossing the teeth. (If the nurse is flossing the teeth of a dependent client, apply gloves.)

a. Once a day provide client with an 18-inch piece of dental floss before or after teeth are brushed (client's preference).

b. The client should wrap the floss around both index fingers. Assist the client as necessary but avoid injury if the client is confused or might bite.

c. Using a 1-inch piece of floss, the client should gently glide the floss between each tooth. The floss should be curved against each side of every tooth and gently scraped up and down between the teeth.

d. The floss should be rewrapped around the fingers so that a new section is used on the next tooth.

e. Continue until all the teeth are flossed. The client will probably want to rinse after flossing.

13. See Completion Protocol (inside front cover).

Toothbrushing alone does not reach the spaces between the teeth where the bacteria that cause gum disease are located.

Each side of every tooth and the back side of the rear tooth should all be flossed. Gentle motions should be used to avoid injury to the gums.

Advances to a clean piece of floss.

> ### NURSE ALERT
> *Clients who have coagulation abnormalities should avoid flossing because of the possibility of bleeding.*

• • • •

EVALUATION

1. Inspect oral mucous membranes for moistness, color, smoothness, and intact appearance.
2. Inspect dental surfaces for cleanliness.
3. Observe for restlessness or grimace during care. Ask client if mouth feels more comfortable.
4. Observe client, spouse, or significant other providing oral hygiene regimen.

Unexpected Outcomes and Related Interventions

1. Mucosa, tongue, or gums remain coated with thick secretions.
   a. Provide mouth care more frequently.
   b. To loosen and remove thick mucus, use toothette or soft toothbrush for cleaning and rinse with normal saline with sodium bicarbonate at least every 4 hours. Rinse more often if oral ulcers are present (Focazio, 1997).
2. Lips are cracked or inflamed.
   a. Lubricate lips more frequently.
3. Client has gurgles in back of throat from accumulation of liquid and is unable to clear throat or cough.
   a. Suction back of throat to clear airway and prevent aspiration.

Recording and Reporting

Routine documentation may include check marks on a flow sheet. Observations made during oral care that should be charted include:

• Condition of mucous membranes and lips

• Client's level of consciousness and ability to cooperate and/or swallow.
• Whether suction is necessary for oral care and if the client's gag reflex is present
• How the client tolerated the procedure

Sample Documentation

0800   Mouth care given. Mucous membranes and lips are moist, pink, and intact. Client unresponsive. No gag reflex elicited. Oral pharynx suctioned. No grimacing or evidence of bleeding noted.

> ### *Geriatric Considerations*
>
> • Older adults are more prone to oral injury and periodontal disease. Good oral hygiene practices can help older adults preserve their ability to eat.
> • Clients unable to grasp a toothbrush can have an enlarged handle placed on toothbrush (e.g., push handle through center of a plastic ball).
> • Clients with diabetes will require visits to the dentist at least every 6 months.
> • Older adults, especially those at risk for oral problems, should avoid spicy, course, acidic, and sugary foods, which can irritate the mouth and cause dental caries (Kim, McFarland, and McLane, 1997).

◆◆◆

Home Care and Long-Term Care Considerations

- During the initial admission visit, document the condition of the client's mouth, teeth, and gums, thus providing a baseline for assessment of the client's ability to comply with special diets and fluid intake and to carry out oral hygiene practices.
- Assess the state of dental health of family members and attitudes toward oral hygiene.

- On regular visits, assess for signs and symptoms of infection or irritation, including reddened, bleeding lesions.
- Provide special care to clients undergoing head and neck radiation, because gums may be dry and swollen and may interfere with proper denture fit.

Skill 7.3

HAIR CARE

A person's appearance and feeling of well-being are influenced by how the hair looks and feels. Brushing, combing, and shampooing are basic measures for all clients unable to provide self-care. Male clients should be offered the opportunity to shave or be shaved when their condition allows. Some hospitals have a beauty shop where clients can go for professional hair care.

Fever, malnutrition, emotional stress, and depression affect the condition of hair. Diaphoresis leaves hair oily and unmanageable. Excessively dry or oily hair may be associated with hormone changes. Dry, brittle hair occurs with aging and excessive use of shampoo.

Certain chemotherapy agents and radiation therapy may cause alopecia (hair loss). Many clients choose to wear a wig; however, some choose to wear head scarves or turbans (Figure 7-2). The average growth of healthy hair is $\frac{1}{2}$ inch per month. Table 7-2 describes common hair and scalp problems and nursing interventions.

When caring for clients from different cultures, it is important to learn as much as possible about the client's cultural customs and beliefs and be sensitive to the uniqueness of each client. Ask the client about preferred hair care methods or any cultural restrictions. For example, African Americans' hair is quite dry. Special lanolin conditioners may be used to maintain conditioning. The neglect of hair care may be interpreted by the client or family as rejection.

Frequency of shampooing depends on the hair's condition and the person's personal preferences. Dry hair, which often results from aging and protein deficiency, requires less frequent shampooing than oily hair or hair of people who exercise actively. Hospitalized clients who have excess perspiration or treatments that leave blood or solutions in the hair may need a shampoo.

Some clients are able to sit in a chair in front of a sink, positioned facing away from the sink with the head and neck hyperextended over the sink's edge. This is contraindicated for clients who have had neck injuries or back pain.

Some clients may be placed on a stretcher with head extended over a sink. A plastic shampoo trough or board facilitates a shampoo in bed. Water is poured over the client's head and allowed to drain into a container on the side of the bed.

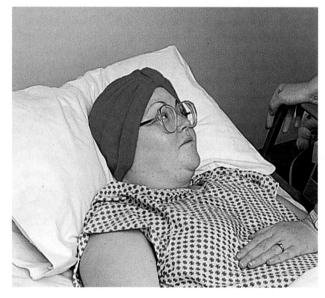

Figure 7-2   Clients may choose to wear a turban because of hair loss.

Table 7-2

Common Hair and Scalp Problems and Related Interventions

Problem	Interventions
Dandruff: scaling of scalp accompanied by itching; if severe, may involve eyebrows.	Shampoo regularly with medicated shampoo.
Pediculosis	
Head lice: parasites attached to hair strands. Eggs look like oval particles. Bites or pustules may be found behind ears and at hairline. May spread to furniture and other people.	Shampoo with a medicated shampoo or conditioner for lice and repeat 12 to 24 hours later. Change bed linens and follow isolation precautions for pediculosis according to agency policy.
Body lice: parasites tend to cling to clothing. Client itches. Hemorrhagic spots may appear on skin where lice are sucking blood. Lice may lay eggs on clothing and furniture.	For body lice, apply a medicated lotion for lice and repeat according to instructions on product. Follow appropriate agency isolation precautions.
Crab lice: found in pubic hair, are grayish white with red legs, and may spread via sexual contact.	For pubic lice, shave hair off affected area, use medicated product for lice, and notify sexual partner of proper treatment.
Alopecia (hair loss): chemotherapeutic agents kill cells that rapidly multiply, including both tumor and normal cells.	Some clients wear scarves. Some clients prefer hairpieces. Referral may be needed for professional consultation for long-term interventions.

NURSE ALERT

Caution is needed if clients have neck pain, neck or back injury.

Dependent clients with beards or mustaches need to have assistance keeping the facial hair clean, especially after eating. A brush or comb may be used. Shaving of facial hair is a task most men prefer to do for themselves. Men without beards usually shave daily. A beard or mustache should be combed or washed as needed. Food particles easily collect in the hair. Some religions and cultures forbid cutting or shaving any body hair (Galanti, 1991); therefore, nurses should not shave a client without consent.

Equipment

Brush
Comb
Shampoo board
Shampoo
Conditioner (optional)
Towels (two or more)
Razor
Shaving cream
Basin of very warm water

ASSESSMENT

1. Determine any restrictions that may be necessary. Often a physician's order is required. If exposure to moisture is contraindicated, dry shampoo may be used. **Rationale: Shampoo may be contraindicated if client has increased intracranial pressure; cerebrospinal fluid leaks; open incisions of face, head, or neck; cervical neck injuries; tracheostomy; facial edema; or respiratory distress.**

2. Assess condition of hair and scalp. Note distribution of hair, oiliness, and texture. Inspect scalp for abrasions, lacerations, lesions, inflammation, and infestation. **Rationale: This determines the need for further interventions, such as conditioner or medicated shampoo.**

3. Before shaving client, assess for bleeding tendency. Review medical history and check laboratory values, including platelet count, prothrombin time (PT), and activated partial thromboplastin time (aPTT). **Rationale: Clients with leukemia, hemophilia, or disseminated intravascular coagulation and clients receiving anticoagulant therapy (heparin or coumadin) or taking high doses of aspirin may have abnormally long clotting times. An electric razor is generally recommended for these clients. Electric razors may be a safety hazard in the presence of oxygen therapy.**

4. If client wants to shave himself, assess ability to manipulate razor to determine how much assistance will be needed.

PLANNING

Expected outcomes should focus on comfort and promoting self-concept.

Expected Outcomes

1. Client expresses increased sense of comfort.
2. Client verbalizes improved self-image.
3. Skin remains free of cuts.

DELEGATION CONSIDERATIONS

The skills of shampooing and shaving can be delegated to AP unless the client has a trauma or injury of the cervical spine. The nurse should:

- Instruct the care provider how to properly position individual clients and any special products indicated.
- Make sure the care provider knows how to correctly use medicated shampoos for lice or other conditions and the appropriate steps to prevent transmission to other clients.
- Remind the care provider to report how the client tolerated the procedure and any changes that may indicate inflammation, or injury.

IMPLEMENTATION

Steps	Rationale

1. See Standard Protocol (inside front cover).
2. **Shampoo for client confined to bed**
   a. Place a towel under head. Brush and comb client's hair by separating hair into small sections, releasing tangles with fingers.

   Moistening with water or mineral oil may help free tangles. Anchoring tangled hair at scalp prevents painful pulling of scalp.

   b. Place a waterproof pad under client's shoulders, neck, and head. Position client supine with plastic trough under head and spout extending beyond edge of mattress. Position container under spout to collect water (see illustration).
   c. Pour warm water over hair until it is completely wet (see illustration). The client or another caregiver can protect client's face with towel or washcloth over eyes, as needed.

   d. ⚡ If hair is matted with blood, apply hydrogen peroxide to dissolve it and rinse with saline.

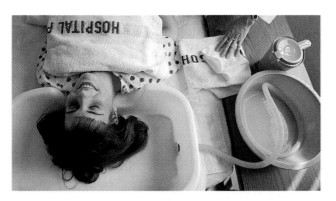

Step 2b

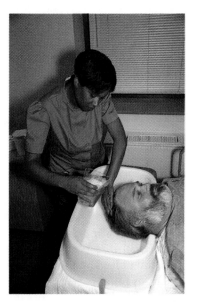

Step 2c

Steps	Rationale

e. Apply small amount of shampoo and work up a lather with both hands. Start at hairline and work toward back of neck. Lift head slightly to wash back of head. Massage scalp gently. Rinse thoroughly and repeat if necessary. Dry using a second towel if needed.

f. Assist client to a comfortable position and complete styling of hair. Braids may be helpful for clients with very long hair.

g. Remove gloves

3. **Braiding hair**

a. Comb or brush hair to remove tangles. Section the hair by parting it into the number of braids intended.

For clients on bed rest or those with long hair, braiding may help keep hair neat and comfortable.

b. Divide each section of hair to be braided into three equal strands. For a bedridden client avoid placing braid over the occipital area at the back of the head.

Pressure on the back of the head from the braid could cause discomfort.

c. Start the braid by crossing the hair strand on the left over the strand in the middle. Then cross the hair strand on the right over the strand in the middle. After each cross over pull the strands tight. Do not let go of the three hair strands. Braiding continues by alternately placing the left strand over the middle strand and then the right strand over the middle strand for the length of the client's hair (see illustration).

d. Finish the braid by fastening the end with a ribbon, barrette, or hair band.

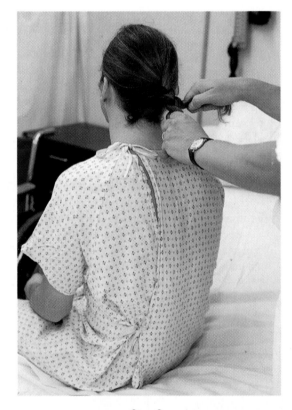

Step 3c

4. **Caring for coarse, curly hair**

a. Shampooing of coarse, curly hair is identical to shampooing wavy or straight hair, but the hair should be conditioned after washing. Ask clients if they use a particular product.

Coarse, curly hair, seen, for example, in African-American clients, does not retain moisture as other types of hair do.

b. To untangle wet coarse, curly hair use the wide teeth of a comb. Beginning at the nape of the neck, comb small subsections of the hair starting at the hair ends. Continue to work through small sections until hair is free of tangles.

Working on small sections of the hair keeps fragile hair from becoming entangled.

Steps	Rationale

c. To comb through dry hair it is best to lubricate the hair by applying a conditioner and loosening any tangles with your fingers. Then using a wide tooth comb, start on either side of the head, insert the comb with the teeth upward to the hair near the scalp. Comb through the hair in a circular motion by turning the wrist while lifting up and out. Continue until the hair is combed through and then comb into place using hands to shape.

Coarse, curly hair can be very dry and fragile and will be damaged if not combed carefully. Dry areas of the hair may require further lubrication with a leave-in conditioner and/or styling lotion.

5. **Shave beard**

a. Assist client to sitting position if possible, and place towel over chest and shoulders.

b. Place a warm, moist washcloth over client's face for several seconds. Apply shaving cream, using product client prefers.

Softens beard. Skin sensitivity can occur with some products.

c. ▨ With the razor at a 45-degree angle, shave in direction of hair growth using short strokes. Hold skin taut to avoid pulling. Ask client to direct you with his usual technique and tell you if it becomes uncomfortable (see illustration).

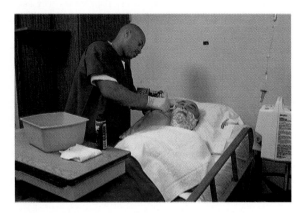

Step 5c

d. Rinse and dry face. Remove gloves. Apply aftershave if desired.

6. See Completion Protocol (inside front cover).

Provides a positive effect for comfort and self-esteem.

• • •

EVALUATION
1. Ask if client feels more comfortable.
2. Offer a mirror and ask how client feels and looks.
3. Inspect condition of shaved area of skin for nicks.

Unexpected Outcome and Related Intervention
1. Client has small nicks or cuts on skin.
   a. Apply pressure and if necessary a small dressing or Band-Aid.

Recording and Reporting
Routine documentation may include check marks on a flow sheet. Observations made during hair care that should be charted may include:

- Type of shampoo provided, for example, dry shampoo, shampoo in bed, shampoo with shower.
- Any special products used for shampoo.
- Condition of client's hair and scalp.
- Whether client was shaved, including whether a blade or electric razor was used.
- Client's response to shampoo or shave and any concerns voiced by client regarding hair care needs.

Sample Documentation
1000 Shampoo and shave completed by client with shower. Minimal assistance needed. Verbalized increased comfort and expressed satisfaction with appearance.

Geriatric Considerations

- Hair growth declines sharply between 50 and 60 years.
- Hair thinning and baldness accompany aging. Although hairline recession may begin during adolescence, it more commonly begins during the forties. Coarse hair becomes finer as hair follicles decrease in size. Some hair loss is usually common in both men and women after age 60. Common baldness (not hereditary baldness) is caused by a progressive decrease in the deep dermal blood vessels of the scalp (Gallagher, Kreidler, 1987).
- Graying of the hair may begin in the thirties. Graying before this time is considered "premature" (Gallagher and Kreidler, 1987). Graying is caused by decreased melanin production in the hair follicle.
- Usually the facial hair of older clients does not grow quickly, and thus a shave might not be necessary each day.

Home Care and Long-Term Care Considerations

- Assess room temperature, availability of water, and most satisfactory position for the client.
- Provide extra protection from wetness for clients with casts.
- Obtain dry shampoo preparations when a wet shampoo is contraindicated.
- Construct a trough by arranging a plastic shower curtain or tablecloth under the client's head and then tapering the cloth to form a narrow end that can drain into a bucket or basin next to the client's bed.
- In the home setting, one of the nurse's greatest challenges is to find ways the client can shampoo the hair without causing injury. For example, a client with a long leg cast may need to wash the hair at a sink until it is safe to shower or until the cast is removed and tub baths can be resumed.
- Caution clients about using chemicals and hot combs for straightening hair. Such practices can cause considerable damage to the hair. Misuse can result in scalp burns, hair loss, and allergic reactions that can cause severe skin rashes, urticaria, and conjunctivitis (Sawaya et al, 1992).

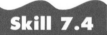

Skill 7.4

FOOT AND NAIL CARE

Most people are required to walk or stand to perform their jobs, and foot pain can cause strain on muscle groups. Often, people are unaware of foot or nail problems until pain occurs. Various skin problems involving the feet are the result of improperly fitted shoes. Tight shoes, socks, garters, or knee-high hose may interfere with circulation. Foot pain may cause a person to change gait, resulting in strain on different muscle groups. If job performance requires a person to walk or stand comfortably, a foot disorder can become a serious problem.

Nail and foot care should be included in a client's daily hygiene; the best time is during the client's bath. Feet and nails often require special care to prevent infection, odors, and injury to soft tissues. Problems often result from abuse or poor care of the feet and hands, such as biting nails or trimming them improperly, exposure to harsh chemicals, or wearing poorly fitting shoes. Changes also

occur in the shape, color, and texture of nails that may result from various nutritional, infectious, and circulatory disorders (Table 7-3, p. 142).

Many older clients may have poor vision, hand tremors, obesity, or limited joint mobility that contribute to difficulties with foot and nail care. Older clients may also have excessive dryness of the skin and poor circulation.

Circulation is assessed by palpation of the pedal and posterior tibial pulses. The nurse also palpates the skin for edema, texture, and coolness. Changes in skin color may be noted. Clients with peripheral vascular disease, such as diabetes, may have inadequate arterial or venous circulation or both. These clients are at high risk for neuropathy, a degeneration of peripheral nerves with loss of sensation. Sensation can be checked by light touch, use of a pinprick, or asking client to discriminate hot and cold temperatures.

These clients need to inspect their feet daily, because injuries may not be felt. These injuries are easily infected and heal slowly because of inadequate circulation.

Equipment

    Basin (appropriate size for soaking)
    Washcloth
    Bath or face towel
    Nail clippers
    Orange stick (optional)
    Emery board or nail file

ASSESSMENT

1. Identify client's risk for foot or nail problems.
   a. Poor vision, lack of coordination, and inability to bend over contribute to older adults' difficulty in performing foot and nail care. **Rationale: Normal physiological changes of aging also result in nail and foot problems.**
   b. Vascular changes associated with diabetes reduce blood flow to peripheral tissues. **Rationale: Break in skin integrity places diabetic clients at high risk for skin infection.**
   c. Edema associated with cardiac or renal conditions can have symptoms of increased tissue edema, particularly in dependent areas (e.g., feet). **Rationale: Edema reduces blood flow to neighboring tissues.**
   d. Presence of muscle weakness or paralysis of one lower extremity after a stroke. **Rationale: May result in altered walking patterns, which increase friction and pressure on feet.**
2. Inspect all surfaces of toes, feet, and nails. Pay particular attention to areas of dryness, inflammation, or cracking. Also inspect areas between toes, heels, and soles of feet. **Rationale: Changes in skin associated with aging include thinning of epidermis and dryness. The nails may become opaque, tough, scaly, brittle, and hypertrophied.**
3. Assess color and warmth of toes and feet. Assess capillary refill of nails. Palpate the dorsalis pedis pulse of both feet simultaneously, comparing the strength of pulses. **Rationale: Circulatory alterations may change integrity of nails and increase client's chance of localized infection when a break in skin integrity occurs.**

NURSE ALERT

Some agencies require a physician's order for trimming nails when circulatory compromise is apparent.

4. Determine client's ability to perform self-care. **Rationale: Limited vision, lack of coordination, and inability to reach feet influence degree of assistance required.**
5. Assess client's knowledge of foot and nail care practices and type of home remedies client uses for existing foot problems. **Rationale: Over-the-counter liquid preparations to remove corns may cause burns and ulcerations.**
   a. Cutting of corns or calluses with razor blade or scissors may result in infections. **Rationale: Proper foot care is essential if the client is to avoid foot ulcers, infections, and complications.**
   c. Use of oval corn pads may exert pressure on toes, thereby decreasing circulation to surrounding tissues.
   d. Application of adhesive tape may tear thin and delicate skin of older adults when removed.
6. Assess type of footwear worn by clients.
   a. Type and cleanliness of socks worn?
   b. Type and fit of shoes?
   c. Restrictive garters or knee-high nylons worn? **Rationale: Improper footwear and constrictive clothing contribute to foot problems.**

PLANNING

Expected outcomes focus on self-care practices that maintain healthy nails and feet and promote circulation and comfort.

Expected Outcomes

1. Client maintains nail integrity and cleanliness.
2. Client correctly demonstrates nail care.
3. Client walks steadily in appropriate footwear.
4. Client identifies ways to minimize sources of pressure or irritation when walking.

DELEGATION CONSIDERATIONS

The skill of care of the fingernails and foot care for the *nondiabetic* client can be delegated to the unlicensed assistive personnel. The nurse should:

- Instruct care provider in the proper way to use nail files and clippers. (Check agency policy on whether unlicensed assistive personnel may use nail clipper on clients).
- Caution care provider to use warm water.
- Remind care provider to report any changes that may indicate inflammation or injury.

Table 7-3

Common Foot and Nail Problems and Related Interventions

Problem	Prevention	Interventions
Callus: thickened epidermis, usually flat, painless, and on underside of foot or palm; caused by friction or pressure.	Wear gloves when working with hands. Wear proper footwear and always wear clean socks/stockings. Orthotic devices (insoles, pads) may help redistribute weight away from callus area.	Soak callus in warm water and Epsom salts to soften; use pumice stone to remove while soft. Creams or lotions can help prevent reformation. Refer diabetic client to a podiatrist.
Corns: caused by friction and pressure from shoes, mainly on toes, over bony prominence; usually cone shaped, round, raised, and tender; may affect gait (Figure 7-3).	Wear proper footwear and always wear clean socks or stockings. Avoid corn pads, which increase pressure and reduce circulation.	Surgical removal may be necessary.
Plantar warts: lesions on sole of foot caused by virus; may be contagious, are painful, and make walking difficult (Figure 7-4).	Avoid going barefoot, especially in public facilities.	Treatment ordered by physician may include applications of acid, burning, or freezing for removal.
Athlete's foot: fungal infection of foot; scaling and cracking of skin occur between toes and on soles of feet; may have small blisters containing fluid. Apparently induced by tight footwear. May spread to other body parts, especially hands; is contagious; and frequently recurs (Figure 7-5).	Feet should be well ventilated. Dry well after bathing; apply powder. Wear clean socks.	May be treated with medicated power or cream. Refer to physician if condition does not improve with medicated products.
Ingrown nails: toenail or fingernail grows inward into soft tissue around nail, often from improper nail trimming; may be painful with pressure (Figure 7-6).	Cut with a nail clipper and file toenails straight across after bathing when they are soft. If nails are thick or vision is poor, have toenails trimmed by a podiatrist.	Frequent warm soaks in antiseptic solution and surgical removal of portion of nail that has grown into skin. Diabetic clients should not soak feet and need to be referred to a podiatrist.
Ram's horn nails: long curved nails; attempts to cut may damage nail bed and risk infection.	Do not attempt to cut own nails.	Refer to podiatrist.
Fungus infection: thick, discolored nails with yellow streaks.	Keep feet and nails clean and dry. Check feet and nails daily.	Refer to podiatrist.

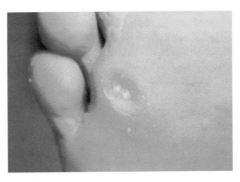

Figure 7-3   Corn.   *From Weston WL, Lane AT:* Color textbook of pediatric dermatology, *ed 2, St Louis, 1996, Mosby.*

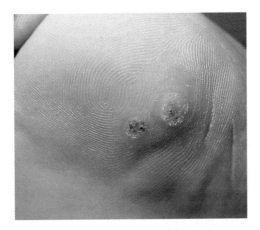

Figure 7-4   Plantar warts.   *From Zitelli BJ, Davis HW:* Atlas of pediatric physical diagnosis, *ed 3, St Louis, 1997, Mosby.*

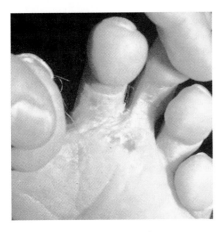

Figure 7-5   Athlete's foot, *tinea pedis.   From Greenberger NJ, Hinthorn DR:* History taking and physical examination: essentials and clinical correlates, *St Louis, 1993, Mosby.*

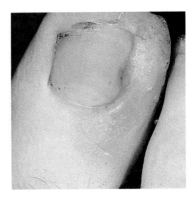

Figure 7-6   Ingrown toenail.   *From Habif TP:* Clinical dermatology: a color guide to diagnosis and therapy, *ed 1, St Louis, 1994, Mosby.*

IMPLEMENTATION

Steps	Rationale

1. See Standard Protocol (inside front cover).
2. **Soak feet**
   a. Explain that soaking requires 10 to 20 minutes.
   b. Assist ambulatory client to sit in chair with disposable bath mat under feet. If confined to bed, assist to a semi-Fowler's position with a waterproof pad and bath towel under feet.

COMMUNICATION TIP

Now is the time to stress to the client the importance of foot care routine. Nurse may say "Now let's look at your foot together to see any problem areas."

NURSE ALERT

It is not recommended to soak the feet of clients with diabetes mellitus or peripheral vascular disease. Soaking may lead to maceration (excessive softening of the skin), ulceration, or infection (Levin, 1995).

c. Fill wash basin with warm water. Test temperature of water with back of hand.

Warm water softens nails and thickened epidermal cells, reduces inflammation of skin, and promotes local circulation. Clients with decreased sensation to feet are unable to detect temperature of hot water.

d. Place basin on bath mat or towel and help client place one foot in basin. Place call light within client's reach and position overbed table in front of client. Offer diversional activity.

Clients with muscular weakness or tremors may have difficulty positioning feet.

e. If desired, allow client to soak fingers in a small basin on overbed table with arms in a comfortable position (see illustration).

Prolonged positioning can cause discomfort unless alignment is maintained.

f. Allow client's feet and nails to soak for 10 to 20 minutes. If necessary, rewarm water after 10 minutes. Begin care on foot that has soaked and place other foot in basin.

Softening of corns, calluses, and cuticles ensures easy removal of dead cells and easy manipulation of cuticle.

g. Using an orange stick, clean gently under nails while they are immersed in water. Remove from basin and dry thoroughly.

Thorough drying slows fungal growth and prevents maceration of tissues. Friction removes dead skin layers.

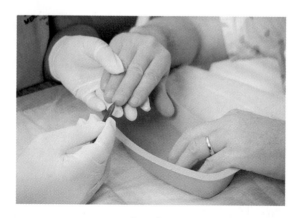

Step 2e

Steps	**Rationale**

3. **Trim nails**

a. With nail clippers, clip nails straight across and even with ends of digits. Shape nails with emery board or file (see illustration).

Cutting straight across prevents splitting of nail margins and formation of sharp nail spikes that can irritate lateral nail margins.

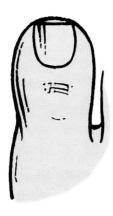

Step 3a

NURSE ALERT

Clients with severe hypertrophy of nails or diabetes should be referred to podiatrist for care to avoid risk of additional tissue injury.

b. If client has circulatory problems, file the nails.

Filing prevents cutting soft tissues, which could become infected and heal slowly.

c. Push cuticle back gently with orange stick and apply lotion to hands and feet and remove gloves.

Reduces incidence of inflamed cuticles. Lotion lubricates dry skin by helping to retain moisture.

4. **Teach foot care**

a. Instruct client to inspect feet daily: tops and soles, heels, and area between toes. Use a mirror to check soles and heels.

Irritated areas may not be painful initially, so are noted only by observation.

b. Instruct to wash and soak feet daily using lukewarm water and to dry thoroughly, especially between the toes.

c. Instruct to consult a physician or podiatrist rather than cutting corns or calluses or using commercial removers.

(1) Apply moleskin to areas of feet that are under friction.

Less likely to cause local pressure than corn pads.

(2) Spot adhesive bandages can guard corns against friction but do not have padding to protect against pressure.

(3) Wrap small pieces of lamb's wool around toes.

Reduces irritation of soft corns between toes.

d. If feet tend to perspire, instruct client to use a mild foot powder.

e. Instruct client to wear clean socks or stockings daily (change twice a day if feet perspire heavily). Check for holes or roughness that might cause pressure. Wearing absorbent liners also helps reduce perspiration and foot odors.

Light-colored or white cotton socks do not contain dyes and are more absorbent (Evanski, Reinherz, 1991).

f. If dryness is noted along the feet or between the toes, instruct client to apply lanolin, baby oil, or even corn oil and rub gently into skin.

g. Instruct client to avoid wearing elastic stockings, knee-high hose, or constricting garters and avoid crossing legs.

Impairs circulation to the lower extremities.

Steps	Rationale

h. Instruct client with impaired sensation to wear protective footwear at all times and check inside of shoes daily for pebbles, foreign objects, and roughness or tears in the inner liners.

i. Instruct client to wear shoes with flexible nonslip soles, sturdy porous uppers, and closed-in toes. Fit should not be restrictive to the feet.

j. Any minor cuts should be washed immediately and dried thoroughly. Only mild antiseptics (e.g., Neosporin ointment) should be applied to the skin. Avoid iodine or merbromin. Notify a physician.

5. See Completion Protocol (inside front cover).

Reduced circulation is often accompanied by reduced sensation, allowing injuries to go untreated unless detected by inspection. Foreign objects may cause sores that go unnoticed (Osterman, Stuck, 1990).

With reduced circulation, infections are more likely and heal more slowly.

EVALUATION

1. Inspect nails and surrounding skin surfaces after soaking and nail trimming. Note any remaining rough areas.
2. Ask client to explain and demonstrate nail care.
3. Observe client's walk using appropriate footwear.
4. Ask client to list ways to reduce irritation and pressure to feet when walking.

Unexpected Outcomes and Related Interventions

1. Nails are discolored, rough, and concave or irregular in shape. Cuticles and surrounding tissues may be inflamed and tender to touch. Localized areas of tenderness are present on feet, with calluses or corns at points of friction.
   a. Repeated soakings are necessary to help relieve inflammation and remove layers of cells from calluses or corns.
   b. Change in footwear or corrective foot surgery may be needed for permanent improvement in corns or calluses.
2. Client unable to explain or perform foot care.
   a. Provide repeated opportunities for practice in controlled setting.
   b. Refer to podiatrist for regular follow-up care.
3. Client complains of pain while walking and has unsteady gait.
   a. House slippers or special footwear may be required.
   b. Muscle-strengthening exercises may promote greater stability.
   c. Clients with chronic foot pain should be seen by physician.

Recording and Reporting

Foot care and condition of the feet and nails should be documented, including:

- Condition of feet and nails.
- Clients' ability to care for their own feet.
- Any apparent area of inflammation, infection, ulceration, or injury with any interventions provided.
- All teaching given to clients about foot care and their comprehension of information.

Sample Documentation

0900 Right great toe red, inflamed, and tender. Client states this was first noted before admission 1 week ago. Feet soaked for 10 minutes in warm water and dried thoroughly. Lotion applied. Client instructed on necessity of cutting nails straight across to avoid this problem. Stated, "This is so sore, I'll be careful how I trim my nails now."

Geriatric Considerations

- Changes in aging skin include thinning of epidermis and subcutaneous fat and dryness because of decreased activity of oil and sweat glands. These changes can be seen in the feet. In addition, nails become opaque, tough, scaly, brittle, and hypertrophied.
- A lifetime of limited exercise can result in laxity of foot ligaments and musculature and lead to instability and impaired mobility.
- Common foot problems of older adults include heel pain caused by tearing of plantar fascia and foot musculature, metatarsalgia (pain beneath metatarsal head), hammer toes and claw toes, corns and calluses, pathological nail conditions (e.g., ingrown toenails, fungal infections), arthritis, and neuropathies that cause diminished sensation in foot (Osterman, Stuck, 1990).
- Older persons are also more vulnerable to bunions because feet tend to spread with aging.

Home Care and Long-Term Care Considerations

- Alternative therapies: moleskin applied to areas of feet that are under friction is less likely to cause local pressure than corn pads; spot adhesive bandages can guard corns against friction, but do not have padding to protect against pressure; wrapping small pieces of lamb's wool around toes reduces irritation of soft corns between toes.

- Assess use of bathroom sink for soaking client's hands and tub for soaking feet.
- Financial constraints may contribute to clients' wearing poorly fitted shoes, which can cause foot problems.

Skill 7.5

BEDMAKING

The nurse makes a client's bed with safety and comfort in mind. The sheets must always be clean, dry, and wrinkle free. Whenever a client's bed is soiled, it must be changed. The sheets should be straightened out and tightened periodically throughout the day to keep them wrinkle free.

Within Skill 7.1 there are three bedmaking procedures:

1. Unoccupied bed, utilized when the client is able to get out of bed, is left open with the top sheets folded down.
2. Postoperative (postop) or surgical bed, utilized when clients have left for the operating room or procedural area, is left with the top sheets fanfolded lengthwise and not tucked in to facilitate the client's return to bed.
3. Occupied bed, utilized when the client is not allowed out of bed.

When a client is discharged and housekeeping cleans the unit, the bed is made with the top sheets left up. This is known as a *closed bed.*

Equipment
Linen bag or hamper
Bath blanket (if available)
Bottom sheet (flat or fitted)
Drawsheet (optional)
Waterproof pads (optional)
Top sheet

Blanket
Mattress pad (needs to be changed only when soiled)
Spread
Pillowcase
Disposable gloves

ASSESSMENT
1. Check the activity order and assess the client's ability to get out of bed. **Rationale: This determines whether an unoccupied or occupied bed should be made.**
2. Assess the client's self-toileting ability; note the presence of any wounds, drainage tubes, and so on. **Rationale: This determines if waterproof pads should be placed on the bed.**

PLANNING
Expected outcomes focus on the client's safety and comfort.

Expected Outcomes
1. Client has a clean, safe environment throughout hospitalization.
2. Client verbalizes a sense of comfort while in bed.
3. Client's skin remains free of irritation throughout hospitalization.

DELEGATION CONSIDERATIONS

Bedmaking is usually delegated to assistive personnel (AP). The nurse should:

- Instruct care provider on whether an unoccupied or occupied bed is to be made.
- Review safety precautions or activity restrictions for client with care provider. Stress the use of side rails and the call system in the event that staff assistance is needed.
- Tell care provider what to do if wound drainage, dressing material, drainage tubes, or intravenous (IV) tubing becomes dislodged or is found in the linen.
- Instruct care provider on what to do if the client becomes fatigued.

COMMUNICATION TIP

- *Use an organized approach and reassuring tone of voice so the client feels safe and comfortable during bedmaking.*
- *Encourage the client to report any discomfort or special requests while the bed is being made.*
- *When making an occupied bed, ask the client to assist as able and to report any discomfort or the need to rest.*
- *Interact throughout the entire procedure, even if client is not responsive.*

IMPLEMENTATION

Steps	Rationale
1. See Standard Protocol (inside front cover).	
2. **Unoccupied bed**	
a. Place linen on clean overbed table or chair near bed.	Organization facilitates efficiency.
b. Raise bed to comfortable working height and lower side rail.	
c. Remove spread and blanket, fold in quarters, and place over bottom of bed or on back of chair if they are clean and to be reused.	Gloves are worn to remove linen only if soiled with body secretions.
d. Disconnect call bell, and check for personal items in the bed. Loosen linen from top to bottom on one side. Go to opposite side, lower rail, and loosen linen.	Personal items may be lost in the linen.
e. Remove soiled pillowcase by grasping center of closed end with one hand and removing pillow with the other. Place pillow on client's chair or overbed table.	
f. Roll all soiled linen together, hold away from uniform, and place in linen hamper. Do not place on floor (see illustration).	Reduces transmission of organisms.
g. Slide mattress, using handles on sides, to head of bed frame if necessary.	
h. Clean mattress and dry, if necessary. Change mattress pad if soiled. Remove gloves, if worn, and dispose of them properly.	
i. Place clean bottom sheet on bed with seam side down.	
(1) Most bottom sheets are fitted.	

Steps	Rationale

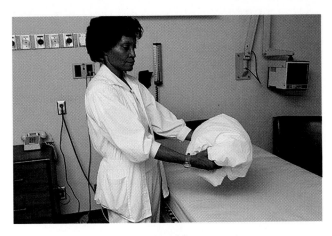

Step 2f

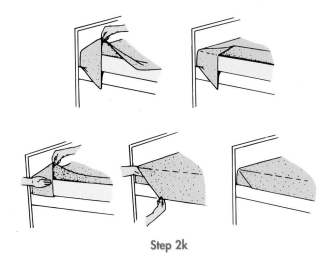

Step 2k

    (2) If flat, center sheet on bed and pull bottom
       hem to foot end of mattress. Fanfold sheet
       toward far side of bed.

j. Tuck top of sheet under head end of mattress.

k. Miter top corner of a flat bottom sheet, and tuck
   in side of sheet under mattress. To miter a corner:
   tuck sheet tightly under end of mattress, grasp
   edge of sheet, and bring it onto mattress at a right
   angle; tuck lower edge under mattress, then bring
   triangle fold down and tuck under mattress (see
   illustration).

l. Place folded drawsheet and/or waterproof pads (if
   necessary) on center of bed with seam side down.
   Fanfold toward far side of bed. Tuck drawsheet (if
   used) under mattress.

m. Place waterproof pads with absorbent side up and
    plastic side down. Some pads go under cloth
    drawsheet. Newer, larger absorbent pads go on
    top of drawsheet or replace it. (Check agency
    policy.)

n. Move to opposite side of bed. Tuck top of
   bottom sheet under mattress. Miter top corner
   (see Step k).

o. Grasp side of flat bottom sheet tightly. Keeping it
   taut, place it under mattress. Proceed from head
   to foot of bed.

p. Grasp drawsheet tightly at an angle. Keeping it
   taut, place it under mattress. Proceed from middle
   to top and then to bottom of bed.

q. Straighten out any waterproof pads that are on
   top of drawsheet.

Mitered corners do not loosen easily.

Waterproof absorbent pads protect bedding and keep
moisture away from client's skin.

Steps	Rationale

r. Place top sheet over bed, with vertical fold lengthwise. Open sheet from head to foot, leave excess sheet at bottom of bed. Make a horizontal toe pleat by fanfolding sheet 4 inches across near bottom of bed (see illustration).

A toe pleat allows for movement of client's feet, prevents top linen from forcing feet into plantar flexion, and prevents pressure ulcers from developing.

s. Place blanket and spread over top sheet in same manner. Cuff top edge of top sheet over blanket and spread.

Gives a neat appearance to bed and keeps client's face off blanket and spread.

t. Make a modified mitered corner with top linens at foot of bed. Miter corner, but do not tuck in lower edge of triangle (see illustration).

u. Go to other side of bed. Cuff sheet over blanket and spread. Make a modified miter corner.

v. Place clean pillowcase on pillow. Grasp center of closed end of pillowcase, and fold pillowcase inside out over closed end. Pick up pillow with same hand that is holding the pillowcase, grasping pillowcase and pulling it over pillow. Adjust corners of pillow in case. Place pillow at head of bed.

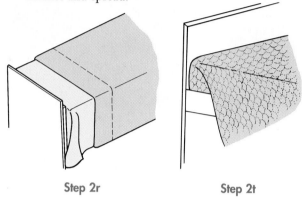

Step 2r   **Step 2t**

w. Fanfold top linen down to bottom third of bed for an open bed. For a closed bed, leave top linens up.

Closed bed is used when no client occupies room.

3. **Postoperative (postop) or surgical bed**

Facilitates transfer of postoperative client from stretcher to bed.

a. Fold all top linen from foot of bed toward center of mattress. Linen fold should be flush with bottom edge of mattress.

b. Fold top linen that is hanging down over sides of bed toward center of mattress. Face one side of bed and fold nearest bottom corner back and over toward opposite side of bed, forming a triangle. Repeat for top corner (see illustration).

c. Grasp apex of triangle and fanfold top linen over to far side of bed (see illustration).

d. Leave bed in high position with side rails down.

Matches height of stretcher and facilitates client transfer.

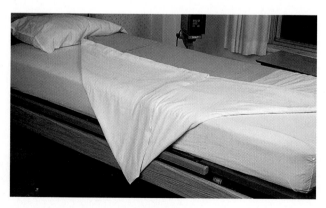

Step 3b

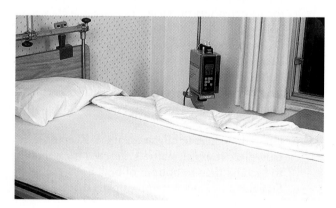

Step 3c

Steps	Rationale

4. Occupied bed

a. Raise entire bed to comfortable working height. Lower head of bed, if tolerated by client. Lower side rail on nurse's side, leave far side rail up.

b. ❖ Loosen all top linens. Remove spread and blanket, leaving client covered with top sheet or bath blanket. Fold spread and blanket in quarters and place over bottom of bed or on back of chair if they are clean and are to be reused.

c. Assist client to a side-lying position on far side of bed. Slide pillow over so it remains under client's head. Check that any tubing is not being pulled.

d. Roll bottom sheet, drawsheet, and any pads as far as possible toward client. Clean and dry mattress if necessary.

e. Place clean bottom sheet on bed with seam side down.
   (1) Bottom sheets may be fitted.
   (2) If flat, center sheet on bed and pull bottom hem to foot end of mattress. Open sheet toward client (see illustration).

f. Unfold flat bottom sheet lengthwise to cover mattress. Tuck top of sheet under head end of mattress.

g. Miter top corner of a flat bottom sheet, and tuck in side of sheet under mattress (see illustration).

h. Place folded drawsheet and/or waterproof pads on center of bed with seam side down. Fanfold toward client.

i. Cover unoccupied portion of bed with half the material, tucking drawsheet under mattress. Place remaining materials as close to client as possible.

It is easier to apply wrinkle-free, tight linens if bed is in the flat position.

Gloves are worn to remove linen only if it is soiled with body secretions.
Provides privacy and warmth.

Reduces transmission of organisms and keeps new linen dry.

Mitered corners do not loosen easily.

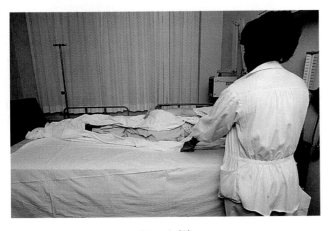

Step 4e(2)

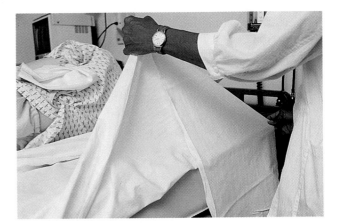

Step 4g

Steps	Rationale
j. Place waterproof pads with absorbent side up and plastic side down. Some pads go under cloth drawsheet. Newer, larger absorbent pads go on top of drawsheet or replace it. (Check agency policy.)	Waterproof absorbent pads protect bedding and keep moisture away from client's skin.
k. Assist client to log-roll over all linen and face you. Keep client covered with top sheet or bath blanket. Raise side rail on the side client is facing. Go to other side of bed and lower side rail.	
l. Remove soiled linens. Hold them away from uniform. Place on chair seat or in disposable bag or hamper if it is close by. Do not leave client alone with side rail down, even for a moment. Remove gloves if worn, and dispose of them properly.	Reduces transmission of microorganisms.
m. Gently slide clean linen toward you, and straighten the clean linen out.	Avoids friction of linen being pulled across skin.
n. Miter the top corner of bottom sheet as before.	
o. Grasp side of flat bottom sheet tightly. Keeping it taut, tuck it under mattress. Proceed from head to foot.	
p. Repeat by tucking drawsheet, proceeding from middle to top to bottom.	
q. Straighten out waterproof pads that are on top of drawsheet.	
r. Assist client into a supine position; place a clean top sheet, blanket, and spread over client, leaving several inches of sheet at top to be folded down.	
s. With client grasping clean top linens, slide out used top sheet or bath blanket (see illustration). Cuff top sheet over blanket and spread.	Prevents exposure of client. Gives a neat appearance to bed and keeps client's face off blanket.
t. Make a modified miter corner with top linens at foot of bed. Miter the corner as before, but do not tuck in lower edge of triangle (see illustration).	

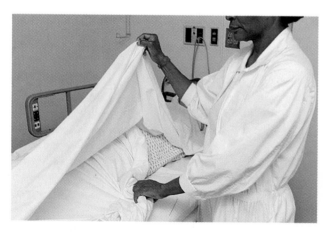

Step 4s

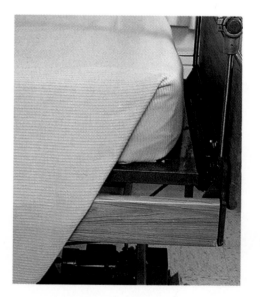

Step 4t

Steps	Rationale

u. Loosen linen at client's feet to client's comfort.

Allows for movement of client's feet, prevents top linen from forcing feet into plantar flexion, and prevents pressure ulcers from developing.

v. Supporting client's head, remove pillow and change pillowcase.

5. See Completion Protocol (inside front cover).

• • •

EVALUATION
1. Observe client's linens for cleanliness and tightness.
2. Ask if client is comfortable after bed is made.
3. Observe client's skin for signs of irritation.

Unexpected Outcomes and Related Interventions
1. Client is not comfortable in bed.
   a. Check that linens are clean and dry. Tighten them.
   b. Assist client to change position in bed.
2. Client's skin appears red and irritated.
   a. Reposition client frequently. Consider use of pressure-relieving mattress (see Chapter 25).
   b. Keep client's bedding clean and dry.

Recording and Reporting
Bedmaking is usually not documented. Some agencies require the nurse to check off this activity on a flow sheet.

Geriatric Considerations

- Older adults have fragile skin and require more protection. Be sure bed linens are clean, dry, and free of wrinkles.
- Encourage older adults to spend as much time out of bed as possible.
- Use drawsheets and waterproof pads with caution. Accumulation of moisture creates a risk for skin maceration and breakdown.

*Home Care and
Long-Term Care Considerations*

- Assess the primary caregiver's ability and willingness to maintain a clean environment for the client.
- Assess home laundry facilities to plan with the primary caregiver the frequency with which linens could reasonably be laundered.
- Assess the amount of linen in the home to establish with the primary caregiver the number of changes of sheets that could be reserved for the client's use.

CRITICAL THINKING EXERCISES

1. You are delegating morning care of Mr. Ray to the AP working with you. Mr. Ray is 78 years old, he has a history of diabetes mellitus, and he was recently admitted following a fall at home. The physician who saw him in the emergency room has ruled out any head injury or fractures. Mr. Ray has been living alone since his wife died 6 months ago. He is visibly dirty with body odor. Mr. Ray will need a full assessment, including his overall state of hygiene. He will also need a complete bath, shampoo, and shave.
   a. How should the you proceed with this client's care?
   b. Name particular hygiene concerns of your assessment.
   c. Which, if any, of these hygiene tasks could you appropriately delegate to AP?
   d. What special instructions could you give to the AP?

2. Mrs. Ryan is a 42-year-old client with liver failure due to chronic hepatitis B. She is admitted for ascites (fluid in the peritoneal cavity), which is causing increasing discomfort and shortness of breath. She is unable to walk without assistance and oxygen. Mrs. Ryan is jaundiced with 3 + pitting edema of both legs. She also has stress incontinence due to the ascites when she gets up or coughs.
   a. Identify factors that place Mrs. Ryan at risk for Impaired Skin Integrity.

3. Mrs. Otis is a 70-year-old client with a history of lung cancer. She is visiting the clinic for her third course of chemotherapy. Mrs. Otis is complaining of sore areas in her mouth, a decreased appetite, and decreased sensation of taste. She has lost 6 pounds since her treatment began 1 month ago. Mrs. Otis is able to perform her own hygiene care.
   a. Identify two priority nursing diagnoses for Mrs. Otis.
   b. Discuss proper oral hygiene for Mrs. Otis.

REFERENCES

Adams R et al: Answering patient's skin care questions, *Patient Care* 26(15):133, 1992.

AHCPR: *Pressure ulcers in adults: prediction and prevention* (clinical practice guidelines), Rockville, Md, 1992, US Dept of Health and Human Services.

American Diabetes Association: Footcare in patients with diabetes mellitus, *Diabetes Care* 20(Suppl 1):S31, 1997.

Avalon Industries: Personal communication, Antoinette Taylor, Education Coordinator, PO Box 388080, Chicago, 63063, 1994.

Colletti A: *Competency in cosmetology: a professional text*, ed 2, New York, 1988, Keystone Publications.

Crute S, editor: *Health and healing for African-Americans*, Emmaus, Pa, 1997, Rodale Press, Inc.

Evanski PM, Reinherz RP: Easing the pain of common foot problems, *Patient Care* 25:38, 1991.

Focazio B: Clinical snapshot of mucositis, *A J Nurs* 97(12):48, 1997.

Galanti G: *Caring for patients from different cultures*, Philadelphia, 1991, University of Pennsylvania Press.

Greifzu S, Radjeski D, Winnick B: Oral care is part of cancer care, *RN* 53:43, 1990.

Healy M, ed: *Standard textbook of cosmetology*, Bronx, NY, 1987, Milady Publishing Corp.

Kim MJ, McFarland GK, McLane AM: *Pocket guide to nursing diagnoses*, ed 7, St Louis, 1997, Mosby.

Laight S: The efficacy of eye care for ventilated patients: outline of an experimental comparative research pilot study, *Intensive Crit Care Nurs* 12(1):16, 1996.

Levin M: Preventing amputation in the patient with diabetes, *Diabetes Care* 18(10):1383, 1995.

Moore J: Assessment of nurse-administered oral hygiene, *Nurs Times* 91(9):40, 1995.

Mueller B et al: Mucositis management practices for hospitalized patients: national survey results, *J Pain Symptom Manage* 10(7):510, 1995.

Osterman HM, Stuck RM: The aging foot, *Orthop Nurs* 9:43, 1990.

Robertson C: Diabetes 2000: chronic complications, *RN* 58(9):34, 1995.

Sawaya M et al: Untangling misconceptions about hair, *Patient Care* 26(9):193, 1992.

Swearingen P, ed: *Manual of critical care nursing: nursing interventions and collaborative management* ed 3, St Louis, 1995, Mosby.

Wong D et al: *Nursing care of infants and children*, ed. 6, St Louis, 1999, Mosby.

CHAPTER 8

Promoting Nutrition

Skill 8.1
Feeding Dependent Clients, 156

Skill 8.2
Assisting Clients with Impaired Swallowing, 160

Skill 8.3
Obtaining Body Weights, 163

Nutrition is considered one of the foundations for life and health. It involves the process of ingesting food and using it to maintain body tissue and provide energy. The basic energy sources include carbohydrates, fats, and proteins. Other nutrients include vitamins, minerals, trace elements, and water. The body needs these sources in various combinations to continue daily activities, provide energy, heal, resist infection, grow, and survive. The U.S. Department of Agriculture has recommended the Food Guide Pyramid (Figure 8-1, p. 156) to emphasize the grain and cereal group as the basic food in the diet, with intake of foods in smaller quantities at the top.

Assessment of a client's nutritional status is essential for determining what dietary needs are present. Nurses are in an ideal position to perform this because of their frequent observation of the client. Registered dietitians possess primary expertise in assessing client's nutritional needs. Nurses and dietitians working together are able to develop a detailed plan of care to meet nutritional needs based on a sound nutritional assessment, the client's food preferences, and any cultural or religious requirements.

A nutritional assessment has four components: (1) a medical history, (2) physical assessment, (3) biochemical parameters (laboratory data), and (4) dietary history (Box 8-1). This can be performed by a dietitian or nurse.

Clients at risk for malnutrition include those with conditions that increase metabolism (e.g., hyperthyroidism, trauma, head injury, pregnancy, burns, sepsis)

diseases that impair absorption (e.g., diabetes, pancreatitis, liver disease, gastric surgery, Crohn's disease, diverticulosis); medical procedures (e.g., abdominal surgery, mouth/neck/jaw surgery, medications, radiation therapy); mechanical problems (e.g., difficulty chewing, paraplegia, quadriplegia, cerebrovascular accident [CVA], upper extremity injury, neuromuscular diseases such as poliomyelitis or muscular distrophy); and psychosocial problems (e.g., altered level of consciousness, alcoholism, depression, anorexia, loneliness, fear of choking, stress).

Box 8-1 Components of a Nutritional Assessment

History
- Swallowing, gastrointestinal, and elimination symptoms
- Functional status
- Social support
- Psychological status
- Ability to purchase food

Physical Assessment
- Height
- Weight
- Usual weight
- Ideal body weight
- Frame size
- Anthropometrics, such as triceps skinfold, midarm circumference, and midarm muscle circumference

Biochemical Parameters
- Serum proteins, such as albumin, prealbumin, transferrin, retinol binding protein
- Nitrogen balance
- Delayed cutaneous hypersensitivity (skin tests)
- Resting energy expenditure

Dietary History
- 24-hour food recall
- Food frequency questionnaire

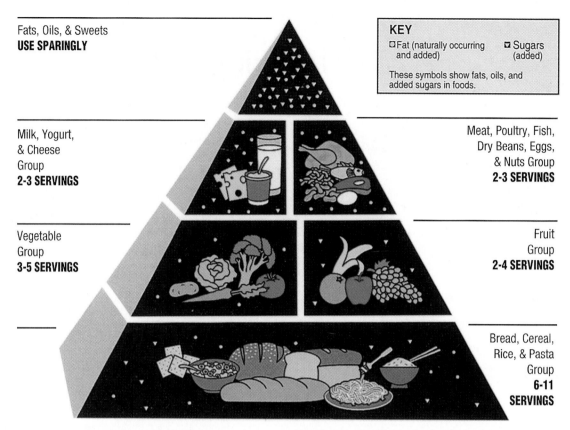

Figure 8-1 Food Guide Pyramid. *From US Department of Agriculture:* USDA's food guide pyramid, *USDA Human Nutrition Information Pub No 249, Washington, DC, 1992, US Government Printing Office.*

NURSING DIAGNOSES

Altered Nutrition, Less Than Body Requirements is the general nursing diagnosis for clients when the focus is increasing the quantity or quality of nutritional intake. **Feeding Self-Care Deficit** is more appropriate when clients are unable to prepare food or feed themselves because of mobility or coordination problems, such as with paralysis, casts, or missing limbs; visual problems, such as blindness or altered depth perception; or mental problems, such as confusion or dementia. **Impaired Swallowing** is appropriate if clients have an altered gag reflex or inability to cough, weakened muscles of chewing, or mechanical alterations such as cancer of the upper airway, an obstructing tumor, or a fistula (abnormal opening between the esophagus and adjacent body cavity). **Risk for Aspiration** may also be appropriate for clients who need assistance because of inability to position themselves or who are learning to swallow after neurological damage or surgery. **Altered Nutrition, More Than Body Requirements** is appropriate when clients are more than 10% to 20% over the desired weight range for their height.

Skill 8.1

FEEDING DEPENDENT CLIENTS

Many hospitalized clients are unable to feed themselves adequately because of the severity of their illness or the fatigue and debilitation associated with their disease. Others are limited by loss of arm or hand movement, by impaired vision, by brain injury, or by the need to remain in a flat or prone position. When assisting the client with feeding, the nurse must ensure the client ingests an adequate volume of food. It is important to facilitate independence when possible with the use of adaptive devices or finger foods and with comfortable and safe positioning for swal-

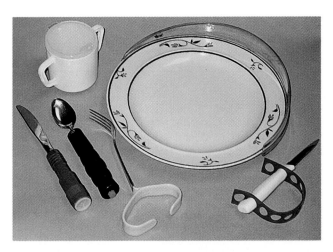

Figure 8-2 *Mealtime equipment. Clockwise from upper left:* two-handled cup with lid, plate with plate guard, utensils with splints, and utensils with enlarged handles.

lowing. Because mealtime is often viewed as a social time for clients, sitting and talking during mealtime is important.

Equipment
  Meal tray
  Overbed table
  Adaptive utensils if appropriate (Figure 8-2)
    Cups with lids and/or handles
    Plate guard to fit around plate
    Suction device to hold plate to tray
    Hand splints to help hold utensil in hand
    Utensils with padded or enlarged handles
  Damp washcloth (optional)
  Oral hygiene supplies (optional)

ASSESSMENT
1. Assess client's level of consciousness, ability to cooperate, mobility/activity orders, and physical limitations to determine appropriate positioning for meals.
2. Assess client's need for toileting, handwashing, and oral care before feeding. **Rationale: This reduces interruptions and improves appetite during the meal.**
3. Assess client's food tolerance, cultural and religious preferences, and food likes and dislikes to determine if special foods will improve appetite and desire to feed independently.

4. Assess gastrointestinal function, and determine whether the client requires a diet that has been altered in nutrients (low protein, low fat), flavoring (low salt, nonspicy), or consistency (pureed, liquid). Routine diets used in the hospital and sometimes in the home care or long-term care setting are shown in Table 8-1 on p. 158. **Rationale: Clients with chronic diseases, such as cardiac or renal disease, may need alterations in nutrient content or flavoring. After surgical procedures the client may progress from a clear liquid diet to a regular diet as the client's ability to digest or tolerance of more complex nutrients returns. The nurse should be aware of the client's prescribed diet.**

PLANNING
Expected outcomes focus on increased independence with eating, improved nutritional intake, and safe intake of food.

Expected Outcomes
1. Client's body weight remains stable or trends toward the normal level.
2. Client's nutrition-related laboratory values trend toward normal. (Note serum protein, albumin, and hemoglobin.)
3. Client demonstrates increased ability to feed self or open items on tray.
4. Client coughs appropriately when eating with no new signs of respiratory compromise.
5. Client demonstrates use of adaptive utensils as appropriate.
6. Client's intake improves in the quality of nutrients ingested.

DELEGATION CONSIDERATIONS

The skill of assisting the client with oral nutrition can be delegated to assistive personnel (AP) who have demonstrated ability to feed clients safely.

• Instruct care provider to observe for any swallowing problems and to notify nurse immediately. Clients with swallowing problems require the assistance of licensed personnel.

Table 8-1

Hospital Therapeutic Diets

Diet	Description
Regular	Is ordered for patients requiring no specific modifications. Generally, allows patients to select their food choices based on normal nutritional requirments for patient's age, sex, and activity level.
Clear-liquid	Allows clear, bland liquids, such as chicken broth, gelatin, and apple juice, that leave little residue and are easily absorbed. Is commonly ordered for short-term use (24 to 48 hours) after episodes of vomiting, diarrhea, or surgery.
Full-liquid	Consists of foods that liquefy at room or body temperature and are easily digested and absorbed. Includes foods allowed on clear-liquid diet plus milk and some milk-containing foods, such as creamed, strained soups. Is commonly ordered before or after surgery for patients who are acutely ill from infection or for patients who cannot chew or tolerate solid foods.
Pureed	Includes easily swallowed foods that do not require chewing. May be ordered for patients with head and neck abnormalities or who have had surgery.
Mechanical or dental-soft	Consists of foods that do not need chewing, such as chopped or ground foods. Avoids tough meats, nuts, bacon, and fruits with tough skins or membranes. May be ordered for patients who have chewing problems caused by lack of teeth or sore gums.
Soft	Includes foods that are low in fiber, easily digested, easy to chew, and simply cooked. Does not permit fatty, rich, and fried foods. Is sometimes referred to as *low-fiber diet*.
High-fiber	Includes sufficient amounts of indigestible carbohydrate to relieve constipation, increase gastrointestinal motility, and increase stool weight. May be ordered for patients with diverticulosis or irritable bowel syndrome.
Sodium-restricted	Allows low levels of sodium and may include a 4-g (no added salt), 2-g (moderate), 1-g (strict), or 500-mg (very strict) diet. May be ordered for patients with congestive heart failure, renal failure, cirrhosis, or hypertension.
Prudent (low cholesterol)	Is ordered to reduce high serum lipid levels. Reduces cholesterol intake to 300 mg daily and fat intake to 30% to 35% by eliminating or reducing fatty foods.
Diabetic	Is ordered as essential treatment for patients with diabetes mellitus. Provides patients with exchange list of foods recommended by American Diabetes Association, which allows for patients to select set amount of food from basic food groups.

From Cole G: *Foundations of nursing*, ed 2, St Louis, 1996, Mosby.

IMPLEMENTATION

Steps	Rationale
1. See Standard Protocol (inside front cover).	
2. Offer toileting and handwashing before meal.	
3. Offer toothbrush or mouthwash before meal.	May improve appetite in client with stomatitis or other oral hygiene problems.
4. Position client appropriately for safe eating within limitations of ability.	Positioning helps to improve swallowing and digestion and to avoid aspiration.
a. Up in chair	
b. High Fowler's position in bed (see illustration).	
c. Side-lying position if flat in bed	

Steps	Rationale

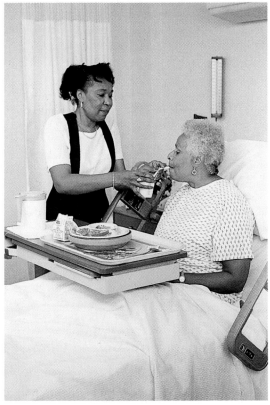

Step 4b

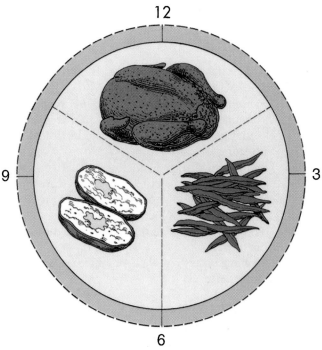

Step 7   For the visually impaired client: "The potatoes are at 9 o'clock."

5. Assist client with setting up meal tray if he or she is able: open packages, cut up food, apply seasonings/condiments, butter bread, place napkin.

6. Place adaptive utensils on tray if indicated, and instruct in their use.

7. If client is visually impaired, identify food location on plate as if it were a clock (i.e., the chicken is at 12 o'clock) (see illustration).

Visually impaired client may feed self if given adequate information about tray.

8. Pace feeding to avoid client fatigue. Ask client the order in which he or she wishes to eat food. Interact with client during mealtime.

Gives client some control of situation and avoids embarrassment of limitations. Social interaction may improve appetite.

9. Assist client with washing hands and repositioning as desired.

10. Monitor intake and output and calorie count.

These values help measure improvement in nutrition.

11. See Completion Protocol (inside front cover).

COMMUNICATION TIP

- *Check the environment for distractions. Reduce the noise level if possible.*
- *Use simple verbal prompts or touch to encourage self-feeding. For example, "Here is your bread" (place bread in the client's hand).*
- *Pantomime desired behaviors, such as drinking a beverage.*
- *Reinforce self-feeding attempts.*

EVALUATION

1. Monitor body weight and laboratory values.
2. Observe amount of food on tray after meal.
3. Observe client's technique for self-feeding: certain items, part or all of meal.
4. Observe client during eating for choking, coughing, gagging, or food left in the mouth.
5. Observe use of adaptive utensils.

Unexpected Outcomes and Related Interventions

1. Client refuses to eat food offered.
   a. Determine if client has other food preferences.
   b. Determine if different times of the day are better.
   c. Determine if pain or anxiety should be treated before eating.
   d. Determine if client is mentally incapable of cooperating.
2. Client chokes on food or does not choke but food sits on side or back of mouth (see Skill 8.2).
   a. Use suction equipment if necessary to clear food from airway.
   b. If choking occurs repeatedly, stop feeding and notify physician.

Reporting and Recording

- Position while eating
- Degree of participation/independence
- Client response
- Description of the presence/absence of suspected aspiration

Sample Documentation

0800   *Assisted client to high Fowler's position. Client able to feed self 5 bites with padded spoon and plate guard. Became fatigued, rest of breakfast fed to client. No coughing or aspiration noted.*

Geriatric Considerations

Changes in taste perception, oral mucus production, and dentition with aging may affect the client's food choices and ability to chew or swallow. The nurse needs to assess the client's food patterns for nutrient, calorie, and fluid adequacy.

Home Care and Long-Term Care Considerations

The nurse may suggest to caregivers of clients who are unable to feed themselves independently that the client join other family members for mealtimes to avoid social isolation.

Skill 8.2

ASSISTING CLIENTS WITH IMPAIRED SWALLOWING

Impaired swallowing is a decreased ability to voluntarily pass fluids and/or solids voluntarily from the mouth to the stomach (Kim et al, 1997). Swallowing is a complex event, requiring both voluntary and involuntary movements. It requires the coordination of cranial nerves V, VII, IX, X, and XII, as well as the muscles of the tongue, pharynx, larynx, and jaw. Clients with neuromuscular diseases involving the brain, brainstem, cranial nerves, myoneural junction, or muscles of swallowing should be assessed for swallowing difficulties before feeding (Baker, 1993).

Maintaining an upright position to enhance the effects of gravity is important. When feeding the client, the nurse should place food on the **unaffected** side of the mouth (as in clients with hemiparesis) and observe the swallowing event closely for delays. Reducing distractions in the room and providing verbal coaching throughout the swallowing process can also greatly help the client swallow more effectively. Food that is the consistency of mashed potatoes is easiest for dysphagic clients to swallow. Liquids and solids are more likely to pose a threat. In some cases, thickeners may be added to food or fluids to increase the consistency and thus allow the client more control of the volume in the mouth.

Equipment

    Meal tray
    Thickener (if ordered)
    Suction equipment
    Oxygen

ASSESSMENT

1. Assess client's level of alertness; drooling; problems with speech; and wet, gurgly voice. **Rationale: These factors indicate poor oral control and may put the client at risk for aspiration.**
2. Assess client's ability to cough on request, as well as the presence of gagging or involuntary coughing when back of the throat is tickled with a tongue depressor or wet cotton swab. **Rationale: Absence of these functions indicates that client is at high risk for aspiration with swallowing.**
3. Assess client's swallowing reflex before feeding by placing fingers on client's throat at level of the larynx, then asking client to swallow saliva. Movement of the larynx should be palpated.

PLANNING

Expected outcomes focus on adequate food and fluid intake to prevent malnutrition and dehydration while avoiding aspiration.

Expected Outcomes

1. Client swallows without retaining food in mouth.
2. Client demonstrates a complete effective swallowing event.
3. Client exhibits no symptoms of aspiration or respiratory distress after meals.
4. Client's body weight, thirst, skin turgor, and nutrition-related laboratory values all trend toward normal.

DELEGATION CONSIDERATIONS

The skill of assisting clients with impaired swallowing requires problem solving and knowledge application unique to a professional nurse.

IMPLEMENTATION

Steps	Rationale
1. See Standard Protocol (inside front cover).	
2. Position client upright in bed or chair with head slightly flexed forward.	This position reduces risk of aspiration.
3. Reduce distractions in the room to keep client focused on swallowing.	
4. Add thickener to thin liquids to the consistency of mashed potatoes or begin serving client pureed foods.	Thin liquids such as water and fruit juice are difficult to control in the mouth and are easily aspirated.
5. Place ½ to 1 tsp of food on unaffected side of the mouth, allowing utensil to touch the mouth or tongue.	
6. Place hand on throat as shown to gently palpate swallowing event as it occurs (see illustration). Swallowing twice is often necessary to clear the pharynx.	

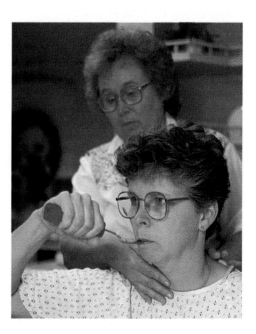

Step 6

Steps	Rationale

7. Provide verbal coaching while feeding client.
   a. Open your mouth.
   b. Feel the food in your mouth.
   c. Chew and taste the food.
   d. Raise your tongue to roof of your mouth.
   e. Think about swallowing.
   f. Close your mouth and swallow.
   g. Swallow again.
   h. Cough to clear airway.
	Verbal cueing keeps client focused on swallowing.

8. Provide positive reinforcement to client.	Enhances client's confidence in skill.
9. Observe for coughing, choking, gagging, and drooling of food; suction airway as necessary.	
10. Provide rest periods as necessary during meal to avoid fatigue.	
11. Maintain upright position for 15 to 30 minutes after eating.	Helps avoid aspiration or regurgitation.
12. Provide mouth care after meals.	This dislodges any food or fluids that may have accumulated inside client's cheeks.
13. Advance diet to thicker foods that require more chewing and finally to thin liquids as tolerated.	Dietitian and/or speech pathologist can direct safest advancement of diet.
14. See Completion Protocol (inside front cover).	

• • •

EVALUATION
1. Observe contents of client's mouth during meal for food pocketing.
2. Observe client for a continuous (not prolonged or delayed) swallowing event.
3. Observe client for coughing or choking during meal.
4. Monitor intake and output (Skill 9.1), calorie count, food eaten from tray, weight (Skill 8.3), and nutrition-related laboratory values.

Unexpected Outcomes and Related Interventions
1. Client begins coughing, choking, or turning blue.
   a. Stop feeding client.
   b. Position client in high Fowler's position or, if unable, position on side.
   c. Suction airway until clear.
   d. Provide oxygen if color has not returned to normal.
2. Food and/or fluids drain out of client's nose during the meal.
   a. Stop feeding client.
   b. Suction nasopharyngeal area.
   c. Resume feeding with increased head flexion.
3. On inspection, food is found pocketed in client's cheeks.
   a. Teach client to use the tongue or to massage the cheek externally to move food to a more functional area of the mouth.

4. A registered dietitian may calculate calorie count, which requires an accurate recording of the amount or percentage of food eaten in 24 hours.

Recording and Reporting
- Time of meal
- Amount of food and fluid ingested
- Any symptoms of intolerance to foods or fluids or symptoms of difficulty chewing, swallowing, or ingesting

Sample Documentation
1200   Client fed ½ of pureed diet and 4 oz juice with 1 tsp of thickener added. Stopped meal due to fatigue. No coughing or aspiration noted.

◆◆◆

Home Care and Long-Term Care Considerations

The nurse may suggest consultation with a speech therapist for recommendations about how to assist the client with impaired swallowing.

Skill 8.3

OBTAINING BODY WEIGHTS

This skill involves obtaining an accurate body weight for the client. Care must be taken in using the same scale at or near the same time of the day, weighing the same amount of clothing or linen, and avoiding weighing client drainage bags (e.g., full colostomy or catheter bag). The client's safety is extremely important, so a bed scale or chair scale may be used if the client is unable to safely stand independently.

Some of the newer models of beds have scales built into their structures. Obtaining a client's weight on this type of scale requires following the manufacturer's instructions.

Although obtaining a body weight is a fairly simple task, it must be done accurately because it is one of the more important parameters used to evaluate and treat many diseases, including congestive heart failure, fluid overload, and renal failure. The Joint Commission for the Accreditation of Healthcare Organizations (JCAHO) requires all hospitalized and home care clients to have height-weight measurement. Height is measured using a device attached to the standing scale (Figure 8-3). A height and weight chart is used to identify the appropriate weight.

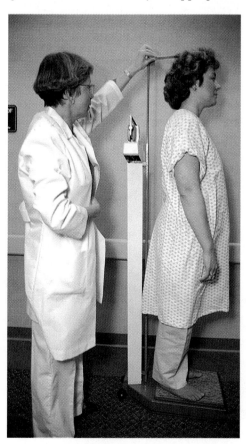

Figure 8-3 Measuring client's height.

Equipment

Standing platform scale
or
Stretcher scale or bed scale
or
Seated chair scale

ASSESSMENT

1. Assess client's weight-bearing status by asking client or by reviewing client's record to determine ability to stand independently and the previously recorded weight.
2. Assess client's level of consciousness. Alert, stable clients who have been on bed rest may require the assistance of two personnel to stand and be weighed safely or be transferred to a chair scale. If the client is not alert or is critically ill, a bed scale is the safest means to obtain a weight.

PLANNING

Expected outcomes focus on accuracy of the weight obtained and client's safety during the process.

Expected Outcomes

1. Client's correct weight is determined.
2. Client does not slip or fall during the weighing process.

DELEGATION CONSIDERATIONS

The skill of obtaining body weights can be delegated to unlicensed assistive personnel.

- Instruct care provider to obtain assistance for weights by floor scale or chair scale when the client is unable to stand alone.
- Instruct care provider to empty and record drainage containers, using Standard Precautions, prior to obtaining the client's weight.
- Instruct care provider to record the weight and to inform the nurse if the client's weight is greater or less than 5 pounds from the most recent weight.
- Instruct care provider to assist the client to a comfortable and safe position following the weight measurement.

IMPLEMENTATION

Steps	Rationale

1. See Standard Protocol (inside front cover).
2. Empty any pouches attached to client that contain drainage.

   Weight of drainage alters body weight. (500 mL = 1 lb)

3. Place appropriate scale at client's bedside.

   Chair scale should be used if client cannot stand independently. Bed scale should be used if client is non–weight bearing.

4. **Weigh client on platform scale.**
   Used when clients can bear weight.
   a. Balance and calibrate scale to "0" pounds (or kilograms). Balance beam should be in middle of mark; digital scale should read "0."
   b. Ask client to step up onto platform scale and stand still (see illustration).
   c. Adjust balance on scale until it is in middle of mark or until digital scale displays a reading (see illustration).
5. **Weigh client on chair scale.**

   Used when clients may be out of bed but are unable to stand independently.

   a. Balance and calibrate scale to "0" pounds (or kilograms). Balance beam should be in middle of mark; digital scale should read "0."

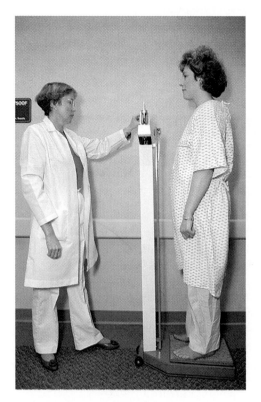

Step 4b

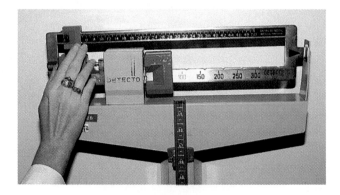

Step 4c

Steps	Rationale

b. Assist client onto chair scale.

c. Adjust balance on scale until it is in middle of mark or until digital scale displays a reading.

6. Weigh client on bed scale.   Used when clients are unable to bear weight.

  a. Place sling with same type and amount of linen and a client gown on arms of scale.

  b. Calibrate scale to "0" with linens and gown.   Calibrating with linen and gown allows these to be kept on client but not included in weight.

  c. With nurse on side of bed, roll client onto side. Place sling under client (see illustration) using good body mechanics (see Chapter 6). Two nurses may be required for clients who are unable to assist with procedure.

     Using two nurses protects client from rolling out of bed.

  d. Attach scale and elevate until clear of bed (see illustration).

  e. Instruct client to remain still, if possible.   Movement can cause inaccurate readings.

  f. Obtain weight from scale (see illustration).

  g. Lower client onto bed, roll over stretcher, then remove stretcher and scale from client's bed.

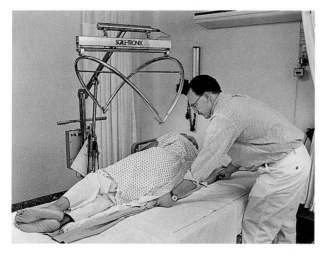

Step 6c

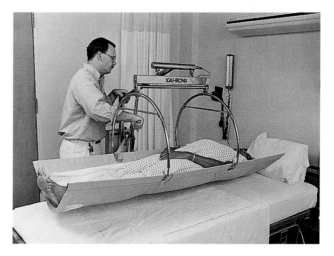

Step 6d

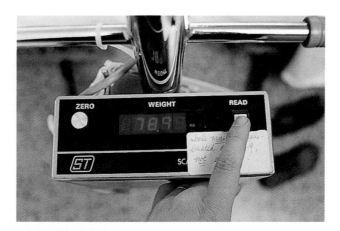

Step 6f

| Steps | Rationale |

7. Infants may be weighed on a calibrated beam balance scale or electronic scale. (see illustration). The infant can be unclothed or weighed with a dry disposable diaper. The weight of the diaper should be subtracted from the infant's weight if the diaper is on.
8. Discard gloves, if worn.
9. See Completion Protocol (inside front cover).

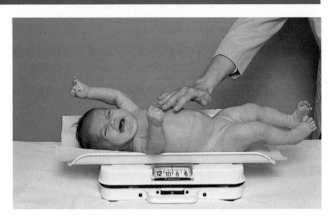

Step 7　*From Wong DL:* Whaley & Wong's Nursing Care of Infants and Children, *ed 5, St Louis, 1995, Mosby.*

• • •

EVALUATION
1. Determine how weight obtained compares with last weight obtained and current plan of treatment (e.g., fluid retention, diuretics, fluid bolus).
2. Observe for instability with type of scale used.

Unexpected Outcomes and Related Interventions
1. Weight obtained varies by greater than 5 pounds from previous reading.
   a. Recheck weight with another scale.
   b. Be sure that client is not touching scale and that no one is supporting him or her during procedure.
   c. Recalibrate scale to be certain it is balanced at "0."
2. Client falls during transfer or is injured during bed scale weighing (see Skill 8.3).
   a. Assist client immediately back to bed or out of injured position.
   b. Assess for physical injury.
   c. Contact physician as agency protocol dictates.

Recording and Reporting
- Weight changes +/− 2%
- Weight in kg or lbs according to agency policy

Sample Documentation
Usual documentation is simply the weight obtained recorded in the appropriate box on a flow sheet, for example, "72 kg/bed scale."

◀▶◀
Home Care and
Long-Term Care Considerations

Weights for ambulatory home care clients may be obtained using a good-quality standard bathroom scale; however, the scale should be tested periodically for accuracy with a known weight. The scale should be disinfected if it is taken from one client to another.

CRITICAL THINKING EXERCISES

1. Mr. Littlefeather has amyotrophic lateral sclerosis, a progressive neuromuscular disease, that affects his speech and throat muscles. What precautions should the nurse take in assisting this client with meals?

2. Identify the type of scale that is appropriate and precautions that should be taken for each of the following clients in order to obtain a weight safely and accurately:
   a. A 25-year-old client who has an ileostomy and is able to stand without assistance.
   b. A 75-year-old client who has had a recent amputation of his left leg, but is able to get up in a chair.
   c. A 15-year-old client with cerebral palsy who needs the assistance of two people to get out of bed.

REFERENCES
American Society for Parenteral and Enteral Nutrition (ASPEN): The 1995 ASPEN standards for nutrition support: hospitalized patients, *Nutr Clin Pract* 10(6):206, 1995.
Baker DM: Assessment and management of impairments in swallowing, *Nurs Clin North Am* 28(4):793, 1993.

Kim MJ, McFarland GK, McLane AM: *Pocket guide to nursing diagnosis,* ed 7, St Louis, 1997, Mosby.
Osborn CL, Marshall MJ: Self-feeding performance in nursing home residents, *J Gerontol Nurs* 19(3):7, 1993.
Van Ort S, Phillips LR: Nursing intervention to promote functional feeding, *J Gerontol Nurs* 21(10):6, 1995.

CHAPTER 9

Assisting with Elimination

Skill 9.1
Monitoring Intake and Output, 168

Skill 9.2
Providing a Bedpan and Urinal, 173

Skill 9.3
Caring for Incontinent Clients, 177

Skill 9.4
Applying an External Catheter, 181

Skill 9.5
Administering an Enema, 185

To promote normal elimination, nurses determine a client's normal pattern of elimination and attempt to accommodate that pattern. Client's elimination patterns are often disturbed by physiological and psychological factors during illness. Most people have been culturally indoctrinated to believe elimination is a very private activity. In a hospital or long-term care setting, bathroom facilities may be shared with a roommate. The sights, sounds, and odors associated with elimination may be embarrassing, which may prompt the client to decrease fluid intake to minimize the need to void or to ignore the urge to defecate for as long as possible. Clients who have difficulty lowering to and rising from a sitting position may need assistance with an elevated toilet seat. Those having difficulty ambulating may need assistance using a bedside commode, bedpan, or urinal. A young child recently toilet trained may have difficulty in unfamiliar circumstances.

Emotional factors often affect elimination. Anxiety may result in urinary frequency and urgency or urinary retention. Anxiety, fear, and anger may also accelerate peri-

stalsis, resulting in diarrhea and gaseous distention. Depressed persons may have decreased peristalsis resulting in reabsorption of water from the stool and constipation.

Urinary incontinence, the loss of control over voiding with continuous or intermittent leakage of urine, is a common problem among older clients; however, many could be helped. The U.S. Public Health Service's Agency for Health Care Policy and Research has concluded that approximately 80% of clients with urinary incontinence can be treated or cured (AHCPR, 1992). Most can be helped by bladder training and pelvic muscles exercises. Others can benefit from medication, electrostimulation, or surgery (Lewis, Collier, and Heitkemper, 1996).

Fecal incontinence, the involuntary passage of stool, may result from the stressors of illness and decreased mobility. Fecal incontinence in the elderly client and others is associated with a loss of sphincter control and impaired cognition (Anderson, Anderson, Glanze, 1998).

During illness fluid and electrolyte balance is often altered, therefore intake and output (I&O) are monitored. Intake to be measured and recorded includes liquids taken orally, intravenous (IV) solutions (see Skill 30.2), and tube feedings (see Skill 32.1). Output to be measured and recorded includes urine, vomitus, liquid stool, nasogastric drainage, and wound drainage (see Skill 21.4). Excessive fluid losses resulting from diarrhea, which also results in losses of sodium, potassium, chloride, and bicarbonate, contribute to fluid and electrolyte imbalance (see Chapter 37).

NURSING DIAGNOSES

Many different nursing diagnoses pertain to clients with altered elimination. **Self-Care Deficit: Toileting** is appropriate for clients when the focus is to promote independence with toileting activities. **Urinary Retention, Acute or Chronic** is inability to empty the bladder and may be associated with overflow incontinence. There are five nursing diagnoses related to urinary incontinence. **Functional Incontinence** refers to nonurinary problems, such as immobility. **Stress Incontinence** refers to loss of less than 50 ml of urine with increased abdominal pressure, as with coughing or sneezing. **Reflex Incontinence** occurs when there is no awareness of bladder fullness. **Urge Incontinence** is related to urgency with bladder spasms, decreased bladder capacity, increased fluid intake, or concentrated urine.

Colonic Constipation refers to decreased frequency of stool passage and/or passage of hard, dry stool resulting from inadequate dietary fiber, limited physical activity, altered routines, or chronic use of laxatives. **Perceived Constipation** results when a client expects a daily bowel movement at the same time and uses laxatives, enemas, or suppositories to achieve this.

Diarrhea is characterized by frequent loose, liquid, and unformed stools associated with abdominal pain, cramping, and urgency or loss of control. **Bowel Incontinence** involves weakness of the rectal sphincter or inability to know when a bowel movement occurs, which may be related to anal surgery, cerebrovascular accident (CVA), dementia, spinal cord injury, or ulcerative colitis.

Skill 9.1

MONITORING INTAKE AND OUTPUT

Measuring and recording I&O may be an independent or a dependent nursing intervention. The measuring and recording of I&O is appropriate if a client has a fever, has edema, is receiving IV or diuretic therapy, or is placed on restricted fluids. It is also important when a client has excessive fluid or electrolyte loss, as associated with vomiting, diarrhea, gastrointestinal drainage, or extensive open wounds. At specified times, usually every 8 hours, I&O is totaled and evaluated. Significant alterations are apparent by comparing 24-hour totals over several days.

Liquid intake includes all liquids taken orally, by feeding tube, and parenterally. Liquids include any substance that becomes liquid at room temperature, such as gelatin and ice cream, and liquid medications. Liquid output includes urine, diarrhea, vomitus, gastric suction, and contents of drainage devices. When possible, assistance from the alert client or family facilitates accuracy, independence, and a sense of accomplishment.

Equipment
Graduated measuring containers (Figure 9-1):
    180- to 240-cc container for intake
    1000-cc container for output
Bedpan, urinal, or bedside commode
Specipan or "hat" (a receptacle that fits inside the
    commode)
Disposable gloves

ASSESSMENT
1. Identify medications that may alter urine output. **Rationale: Diuretics cause water, sodium, and potassium excretion, resulting in an increased output** (Anderson, Anderson, and Glanze, 1998); **steroids (e.g., prednisone, cortisone) cause sodium and water retention and potassium excretion, resulting in a decreased output** (Lewis, Collier, Heitkemper, 1996).

2. Monitor hematocrit (Hct); **Rationale: increased Hct value suggests fluid volume deficit (FVD); decreased Hct value suggests fluid volume excess (FVE).** (Lewis, Collier, Heitkemper, 1996).

3. Weigh the client daily at the same time, on the same scale, in the same clothes. Weight loss greater than 2% suggests FVD, whereas sudden weight gain greater than 2% may indicate FVE (see Skill 8.3). **Rationale: Fluid retention or depletion is demonstrated by differences in weight before changes in edema appear** (Potter, Perry, 1998).

4. Assess signs and symptoms of dehydration and fluid overload (see Chapter 37).

5. Assess the client's and family's knowledge of the purpose of I&O measurement and ability to participate actively in measurement. **Rationale: Effective teaching and learning begins with the client's willingness and ability to learn** (Schrefer, 1995).

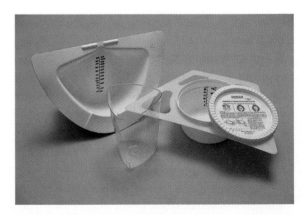

Figure 9-1 Graduated measuring containers. *Clockwise from left to right:* "hat" receptacle, specipan, and graduated measuring container.

PLANNING

Expected outcomes focus on maintaining fluid balance, encouraging adequate fluid intake, and achieving normal laboratory values and body weight.

Expected Outcomes

1. Client's urine is neither concentrated nor dilute, with specific gravity WNL (1.010 to 1.025).
2. Client maintains fluid balance, as evidenced by intake approximately 600 ml greater than output, with total 24-hour output at least 1500 ml.
3. Client's hematocrit level is within a range of 40% to 54% for males or 38% to 47% for females.
4. Client's weight remains within 2% of normal.

DELEGATION CONSIDERATIONS

The skill of measuring and recording I&O can be delegated to assistive personnel (AP).

- Stress the importance of accuracy in measuring and recording I&O.
- Ensure that the care provider uses Standard Precautions relating to body fluids.
- Verify that care provider is able to use the metric system to measure with standard containers.
- Have staff report changes in color, amount, and odor of stool and urine and presence of incontinence.

IMPLEMENTATION

Steps	Rationale
1. See Standard Protocol (inside front cover).	
2. Explain to client and family that accurate I&O measurements are important to identify potential fluid overload or excessive losses.	Alert, active clients and family members who understand the procedure can facilitate the recording and measuring of I&O (Schrefer, 1995).

3. Measure and record all fluid intake.
  a. Liquids with meals may include gelatin, custards, ice cream, popsicles, and sherbets. Ice chips are recorded as 50% of measured volume (e.g., 100 ml ice equals 50 ml water).
  b. Liquid medicines such as antacids are counted as fluid intake, as are liquids taken with medicines.
  c. Enteral nutrition (tube feedings) (see Chapter 33).
  d. IV fluids (see Chapter 30).
	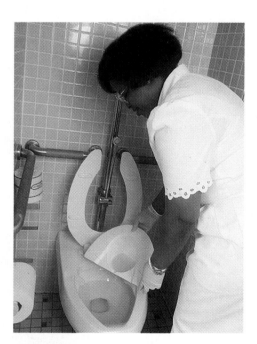
	Step 4

4. Instruct client and family to call nurse to empty urinal, drainage bag, bedpan, commode, or "hat" each time it is used (see illustration). Alert, cooperative clients may keep own tally using scratch paper or a copy of facility's I&O chart.	Promotes accurate method for recording output. Report any urine output less than 30 ml/hr, which may indicate decreased renal perfusion (Lewis, Collier, Heitkemper, 1996).

Steps	Rationale

5.   Empty and record urine output from Foley catheter into clean, graduated container at end of each shift (see illustration). Cleanse the drainage port before draining and before recapping.

6. Observe color and characteristics of urine in Foley tubing. Some clients may have a special device that is emptied into the larger container hourly. Urine output less than 30 ml/hr can indicate decreased renal perfusion and should be reported.

        Dark, concentrated urine suggests dehydration.

7. Measure and record all output from all other sources, including emesis, nasogastric suction, (see Chapter 32) and all measurable wound drainage (see illustration, *A*), or measure chest tube drainage by marking and recording the time on the collection chamber (see illustration, *B*) (see Chapter 21).

8. Remove gloves.

9. See Completion Protocol (inside front cover).

COMMUNICATION TIP

- *Tell client or family exactly what is to be measured and where to record it.*
- *Have client or family demonstrate ability to measure and record accurately.*

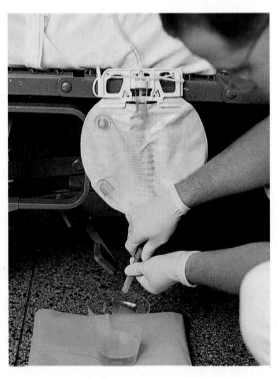

Step 5

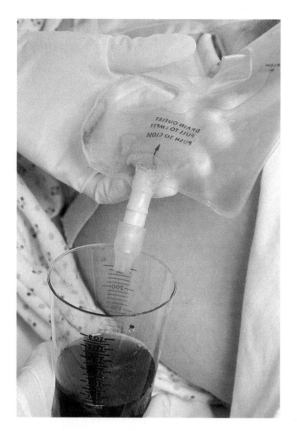

Step 7a

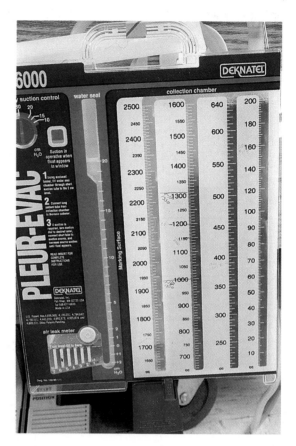

Step 7b

EVALUATION

1. Observe amount and characteristics of urine, including color and specific gravity (normal, 1.010 to 1.025). Specific gravity can be measured using a reagent test strip with a color chart. **Diluted watery urine indicates low specific gravity readings, and dark-yellow, concentrated urine indicates high specific gravity readings.**
2. Calculate total I&O at the end of each shift and for 24 hours.
3. Monitor serum Hct values.
4. Compare daily weights, noting increase or decrease greater than 2% within 48 hours.

Unexpected Outcomes and Related Interventions

1. Client develops fluid volume excess or fluid overload (see Chapter 37), as evidenced by intake greater than output and weight gain greater than 2% over 24 to 48 hours and a low Hct value.
   a. Assess other signs and symptoms of fluid excess.
   b. In collaboration with other health team members, administer diuretics and carefully regulate IV and oral intake.
   c. Reeducate client and family regarding fluid intake and medications.

2. Client develops FVD (see Chapter 37), as evidenced by output greater than intake, weight loss greater than 2% in 24 to 48 hours, and a high Hct value.
   a. Assess other signs and symptoms for FVD.
   b. In collaboration with other health team members, administer oral and IV fluids consistently (see Chapter 37).
   c. Reeducate client and family regarding fluid intake.

Recording and Reporting

- Collect I&O data from client's bedside at specified time, usually every 8 hours, and document it on the specified Intake and Output Summary in the client's chart (Figure 9-2, p. 172).
- Document any changes or clinical signs in nursing note.

Sample Documentation

1500   States will not eat or drink anything. 300 ml PO fluid intake in 8 hours, temperature 38.5° C; 350 ml dark, concentrated urine per Foley. Physician notified.

1515   1000 ml lactated Ringer's solution started IV in back of right hand with #18 angiocath and infusing per pump at 125 cc/hour without difficulty.

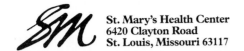

St. Mary's Health Center
6420 Clayton Road
St. Louis, Missouri 63117

PATIENT LABEL

INTAKE AND OUTPUT SUMMARY

	DATE 6-10-XX	2200 – 0600	0600 – 1400	1400 – 2200	24 Hr.	
INTAKE	P.O. Intake	120	800	650	1570	TOTAL INTAKE
	Tube Feedings					
	Hyperalimentation					
	I.V. Primary					
	I.V.P.B.	50		50	100	1670
	Blood/Blood Products					
OUTPUT	Urine	325	700	500	1525	TOTAL OUTPUT
	Emesis					
	G.I. Suction					1855
	Drainage	50	75	30	155	
	Chest tube	75	50	50	175	

	DATE	2200 – 0600	0600 – 1400	1400 – 2200	24 Hr.	
INTAKE	P.O. Intake					TOTAL INTAKE
	Tube Feedings					
	Hyperalimentation					
	I.V. Primary					
	I.V.P.B.					
	Blood/Blood Products					
OUTPUT	Urine					TOTAL OUTPUT
	Emesis					
	G.I. Suction					
	Drainage					

	DATE	2200 – 0600	0600 – 1400	1400 – 2200	24 Hr.	
INTAKE	P.O. Intake					TOTAL INTAKE
	Tube Feedings					
	Hyperalimentation					
	I.V. Primary					
	I.V.P.B.					
	Blood/Blood Products					
OUTPUT	Urine					TOTAL OUTPUT
	Emesis					
	G.I. Suction					
	Drainage					

	DATE	2200 – 0600	0600 – 1400	1400 – 2200	24 Hr.	
INTAKE	P.O. Intake					TOTAL INTAKE
	Tube Feedings					
	Hyperalimentation					
	I.V. Primary					
	I.V.P.B.					
	Blood/Blood Products					
OUTPUT	Urine					TOTAL OUTPUT
	Emesis					
	G.I. Suction					
	Drainage					

Figure 9-2 Intake and output summary. *Courtesy St Mary's Health Center, St Louis, Mo.*

Geriatric Considerations

- Older adults are more susceptible to fluid imbalances with fever, chronic illness, gasentroenteritis, or trauma.
- Incontinence may be discovered when I&O is monitored (though age is not the cause of incontinence).

Home Care and Long-Term Care Considerations

- Assess client's or primary caregiver's ability to maintain accurate I&O at home.
- Demonstrate measuring, recording, and weighing, and request return demonstration from client or home caregiver.
- Promote continuity between acute care and long-term care facilities.
- Client's in long-term care facilities can be an active part of their care if they are taught to measure and record I&O.

Skill 9.2

PROVIDING A BEDPAN AND URINAL

In many cultures squatting is the usual position for defecation and urination for females. For males squatting is the usual position during defecation and standing is the custom for voiding. For the client confined to bed, it is impossible to assume the customary positions, and the upright position needs to be facilitated to the extent possible. Adults may resist using a bedpan or urinal because of the emphasis on privacy. Children may find the equipment unfamiliar and threatening.

NURSE ALERT

Check physicians' orders for prescribed bed rest. When determining the need for a bedpan or urinal, consider factors that limit mobility (e.g., fractures, pain, surgery, postcardiac catheterization, arteriogram with potential for bleeding). Unless contraindicated, it is generally beneficial for clients to get up from bed to use the bathroom.

Equipment

Bedpan (regular or fracture) (Figure 9-3)
Urinal (male and female)
Specipan
Toilet paper
Underpads
Disposable gloves

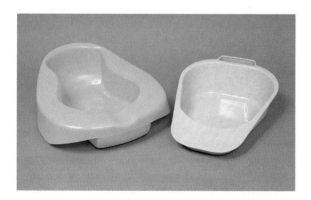

Figure 9-3 Types of bedpans. *Left,* regular bedpan; *right,* fracture bedpan. *From Sorrentino SA: Assisting with patient care, St Louis, 1999, Mosby.*

ASSESSMENT

1. Discuss client's elimination needs in a professional, open manner using common language familiar to client. **Rationale: Language and facial expressions that indicate disapproval or revulsion contribute to embarrassment and create communication barriers.**
2. Assess elimination pattern. When does client normally defecate (e.g., after breakfast)? Are laxatives or stool softeners routinely used? **Rationale: The normal patterns of elimination establishes a baseline for comparison.**
3. Assess the length and extent of immobility. **Rationale: Decreased mobility slows peristalsis of intestines and ureters.**
4. Assess client's ability to assist, including ability to lift hips or turn. **Rationale: Determines the type of assistance needed to assist client on and off bedpan.**
5. Determine if a urine or stool specimen is to be collected.

6. Assess patterns of fluid intake. Adequate hydration (1200 to 1500 ml water daily) facilitates normal bowel elimination by keeping stools soft. Hot fluids are especially effective in softening stool and increasing peristalsis. **Rationale: Decreased fluid intake slows the passage of food through the intestines, peristalsis slows, and there is increased absorption of fluid and hardening of feces.**

7. Assess dietary intake, including high-fiber foods such as raw fruit, whole grains, bran, and green leafy vegetables. **Rationale: High-fiber foods increase bulk, which helps increase fluid content in stool, normalize consistency, and decrease transit time in the colon.**

8. Assess extent and location of pain that may influence ability to void, defecate, or position on a bedpan. It may be advisable to administer a prescribed analgesic about a half hour before the normal time of elimination.

9. Assess bowel sounds and palpate abdomen and bladder for distention. Ask client if flatus is being passed. **Rationale: Abnormal bowel sounds or a distended bladder are indicative of urinary or bowel elimination problems.**

PLANNING

Expected outcomes focus on the management of bowel and urinary elimination.

Expected Outcomes

1. Client assists with movement onto bedpan and self-cleaning.
2. Client successfully defecates soft stool on the bedpan.
3. Client uses the bedpan or urinal to void more than 300 ml 2 times within an 8-hour period.
4. Client's skin remains intact without redness or irritation.

DELEGATION CONSIDERATIONS

The skill of assisting a client to use a bedpan or urinal can be delegated to AP.

- Ensure that personnel are aware of Standard Precautions guidelines relating to body fluids.
- Inform personnel about positioning needs of clients with specific limitations or therapeutic equipment, such as drains, casts, or traction.
- Clarify information that personnel are to report to the nurse about color, odor, amount, or incontinence of feces or urine.
- Verify that personnel are aware of proper hygiene, such as cleaning the perineal area front to back for the female.

IMPLEMENTATION

Steps	Rationale

1. See Standard Protocol (inside front cover).

Providing a Bedpan

2. Lower head of the bed so that it is nearly flat, and assist client to roll toward you.

3. Raise side rail and have client grasp it if necessary to maintain the side-lying position.

Facilitates placement of the bedpan.

4. Go to opposite side of the bed and place the powdered and warmed bedpan under the buttocks with the lower end just under the upper thighs.

Powder keeps pan from sticking to the skin. Many agencies have plastic bedpans. Warming a metal pan under running water promotes comfort and the relaxation necessary for elimination.

5. Press the bedpan firmly down into the mattress and against the buttocks. Keeping one hand against the bedpan, place the other on client's hip and assist client to roll back onto the pan (see illustration).

6. If client is able to lift buttocks, place the pan under the buttocks as they are lifted. Use of a fracture pan requires less lifting (see illustration). Check position of the pan by looking between client's legs. Front of the pan should be centered and visible.

COMMUNICATION TIP

- *Be matter-of-fact in your approach and tone of voice.*
- *Maintain a pleasant facial expression.*
- *Use terms the client will understand.*

Steps	**Rationale**

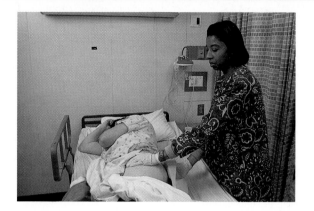

Step 5

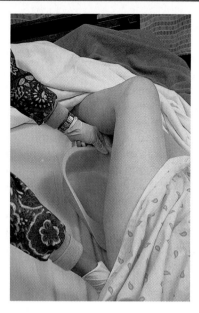

Step 6

7. If not contraindicated, raise head of the bed at least 30 to 45 degrees. Have client bend knees to assume a squatting position.

8. Raise the side rail and place the call light and toilet paper within easy reach. Discard gloves. Provide privacy.

9. ▨ When client is finished, lower head of bed and side rail and assist client to roll away from you onto one side as you hold the bedpan securely in place.

10. Assist client with wiping as needed; discard tissue in trash if on I&O. If necessary, clean perineum from front to back using a washcloth and warm soapy water.

11. Provide opportunity for client to wash hands.

12. Empty the contents into the toilet and rinse thoroughly with spray faucet attached to the toilet (see illustration).

This approximates the normal position for defecation as much as possible.

Privacy is essential for some clients to empty bowel and bladder successfully.

Prevents spilling contents on the bedding.

Cleaning front to back prevents transmission of microorganisms from anus to urethra, which may contribute to a urinary tract infection.

NURSE ALERT

Before emptying the bedpan, note the color and appearance of urine and stool. Measure the amount if I&O is being recorded, and check for whether a specimen is needed (see Skill 9.1)

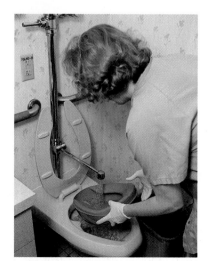

Step 12

Steps	Rationale

13. Store bedpan and urinal in appropriate location, normally in the bathroom. Some clients need or want to have the bedpan within easy reach. If so, bedpan may be placed on a chair seat and covered with a disposable cover.

Promotes rapid accessibility when there is urgency or frequency of bowel or bladder elimination.

14. Discard gloves.

Providing a urinal for a male client

15. Position client on side, back, or sitting with head of the bed elevated, or assist to a standing position.

Men find it easier to void and empty the bladder while standing.

16. ▨ If lying in bed, client should hold urinal with base flat on the bed between the thighs, and if possible, client places penis into neck of the urinal. Assist as needed and discard gloves.

Minimizes spilling.

17. Instruct client to notify caregiver so that the urinal can be emptied each time it is used. If needed, measure and record urine output.

Avoids overfilling; minimizes odors and growth of microorganisms. Provides accuracy in recording amount of each voiding.

18. Urinals may be attached to the side rail for easy access (see illustration).

19. Remove and discard gloves.

20. See Completion Protocol (inside front cover).

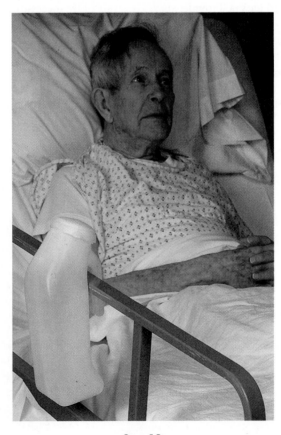

Step 18

EVALUATION

1. Observe client's ability to assist with movement onto and off the bedpan and participate in self-cleaning.
2. Observe and record the appearance and characteristics of stool, including color, odor, consistency, frequency, amount, shape, and constituents. Observe and record the appearance, odor, and amount of urine.
3. Observe skin integrity in the perineal area.

Unexpected Outcomes and Related Interventions

1. Client is unable to void using a bedpan or urinal.
   a. Provide sensory stimulation that promotes voiding, such as running water in the sink or pouring warm water over perineum, stroking the inner thigh, placing hand in warm water, or providing a drink (if not contraindicated).
   b. Male clients may need to stand in order to void. Obtain adequate assistance if client is at risk of falling.
2. Client is unable to defecate using a bedpan.
   a. Assist to as normal a position as possible. Encourage client to massage upper abdomen from right to left to promote peristalsis.
   b. Provide reading materials and allow ample time and privacy for the process.
   c. Consider use of a bedside commode rather than the bedpan if client is able to be up in a chair.
   d. Consider collaborating with the physician for stool softener or laxative orders.
3. Client is incontinent (see Skill 9.3).
   a. Identify detailed information about episodes of incontinence, including how often, amount, and circumstances involved.
   b. Offer bedpan or urinal more frequently (e.g., every 2 hours).
   c. If client experiences the urge but cannot wait, place urinal within client's reach.
   d. Male clients may benefit from an external catheter (see Skill 9.4).

Recording and Reporting

- Document client signs and symptoms.
- Describe feces and urine, including odor, consistency, amount, and any other pertinent characteristics.

Sample Documentation

0800   C/O abdominal cramping. Large, loose, light brown stool on bedpan.

Geriatric Considerations

- The aging process alters defecation and micturition. The older client may require the bedpan or urinal more frequently and more quickly, or may not perceive the need to void or defecate.
- The older client may have a greater need for the "normal" position to empty the bowel or bladder because of long-ingrained cultural practices.
- The nurse may need to teach the older client the importance of diet and exercise in elimination.

Home Care and Long-Term Care Considerations

- Assess client and caregiver for ability to carry out bowel and bladder care.
- Assess environment for accessibility of facilities and safety features such as elevated toilet seat.
- Personnel in long-term care facilities can better facilitate bowel and bladder care for the client when provided with a history of the client's elimination patterns.

Skill 9.3

CARING FOR INCONTINENT CLIENTS

Incontinence is a very common problem, especially among older adults. Regardless of the cause, incontinence is a psychologically distressing and socially disruptive problem.

Urinary incontinence occurs because pressure in the bladder is too great or because the sphincters are too weak. The nurse can collaborate with other members of the health care team to assess the cause and extent of incontinence and to assist in the management of the problem. The physical therapist, for example, can assess the extent of musculoskeletal involvement and determine methods of treatment (Frahm 1997.)

Incontinence may involve a small leakage of urine when the person laughs, coughs, or lifts something heavy.

The client can be taught exercises to strengthen muscles around the external sphincters to help manage this type of incontinence. Pelvic floor exercises (Kegel's exercises) involve tightening of the ring of muscle around the vagina and anus and holding them for several seconds. This is done at least 10 times, 3 times a day.

Alert clients need an incontinence product that is discreet and promotes self-care. Some incontinence products are designed for small amounts of leakage. Persistent urge, stress, or overflow incontinence may need referral for urological evaluation (Lewis, Collier, Heitkemper, 1996).

When urinary incontinence results from decreased perception of bladder fullness or impaired voluntary motor control, bladder training can be helpful. Bladder training provides cooperative clients with opportunity to void at regular intervals (every $1\frac{1}{2}$ to 2 hours) to achieve continence. On such a schedule, clients need to be asked if they are wet or dry, checked for wetness, reminded or assisted to the toilet, and praised for appropriate toileting. Limiting fluids after the evening meal minimizes the need for voiding during the night.

When paralyzed clients have overflow incontinence, Crede's method may be used. This involves manual pressure over the lower abdomen to express urine from the bladder at regular intervals. Crede's method requires a measure of expertise to prevent injury to the bladder (Lewis, Collier, Heitkemper, 1996).

The first step in care of the client with fecal incontinence is to assess if fecal impaction is the cause and to remove the impaction (see Skill 34.1). Management of fecal incontinence includes educating the client about dietary measures, abdominal exercises, and physical activity (Lewis, Collier, and Heitkemper, 1996).

Incontinence characterized by urine or fecal flow at unpredictable times requires the use of disposable adult undergarments or underpads as the primary means of management. Urine and feces are very irritating to the skin. Skin that is continuously exposed quickly becomes inflamed and irritated. Cleansing the skin thoroughly after each episode of incontinence with warm soapy water and drying it thoroughly help prevent skin breakdown.

ASSESSMENT

1. Assess the frequency of episodes of incontinence. Determine if there is a pattern.
2. Assess the amount of leakage experienced. Determine if it is frequent dribbling of small amounts or unpredictable loss of large amounts of urine and stool. **Rationale: Helps determine type of incontinence and appropriate choice of therapies.**
3. Assess episodes related to specific events such as coughing, sneezing, or exercise.
4. Assess the condition of client's skin in the perineal area. **Rationale: Identifies the need for special skin care products, barrier films, or creams.**
5. Assess fluid intake and the color, odor, and appearance of urine. **Rationale: Some clients drink less to minimize incontinence, resulting in dark, concentrated urine and increased risk for infection.**

PLANNING

The expected outcomes focus on promoting continence.

Expected Outcomes
1. Client achieves continence 75% of the time.
2. Client remains clean and dry 90% of the time.
3. Client maintains skin integrity without redness or irritation of the perineum.

DELEGATION CONSIDERATIONS

The skill of providing care for incontinent clients can be delegated to AP.

- Caution personnel to be aware of the client's dignity and self-esteem needs and to take measures to avoid violating these needs.
- Ensure personnel know Standard Precautions guidelines related to body fluids.
- Be sure personnel report information to the nurse such as abdominal pain, increased episodes of incontinence, changes in appearance of urine or stool, and evidence of skin breakdown.
- Crede's maneuver is to be done by the nurse.

IMPLEMENTATION

Steps	Rationale
1. See Standard Protocol (inside front cover).	
2. Provide client with opportunity to use the bathroom, bedpan, or commode to void and defecate at appropriate regular times.	Promotes episodes of continence.
3. Keep a record of episodes of continence and incontinence for 48 hours.	Record allows identification of patterns of elimination.

Steps	Rationale

4. Turn client to the supine position with legs abducted (see Skill 6.1).

   a. **Female.** Wash labia using a washcloth, soap, and warm water. Then gently retract labia from thigh and wash groin from perineum toward rectum (front to back).

Cleansing from front to back prevents transmission of microorganisms from anus to urethra.

   b. **Male.** Wash the penis beginning with the urinary meatus, retracting the foreskin if client is uncircumcised. Gently cleanse shaft of penis and scrotum, taking care to thoroughly reach all skinfolds. Return foreskin to its natural position.

COMMUNICATION TIP

Avoid all negative verbal and nonverbal expressions. Cleanse the perineum in a professional, caring, and matter-of-fact manner. Under no circumstances should client be reprimanded or humiliated for having "accidents."

5. Turn client to side and continue cleansing, using as many washcloths as necessary and drying thoroughly.

6. Place absorbent underpad from waist to knees with absorbent side toward client; or use other appropriate incontinent product if absolutely necessary.

Use of these products emphasizes the incontinence and affects the client's dignity and self-esteem.

7. If skin is red or irritated, exposure to air whenever possible is beneficial. A vitamin-enriched cream may promote healing. Apply a skin barrier or sealant to protect the skin from moisture (see Chapter 24).

8. Ambulatory clients may wear briefs with pads to absorb urine (Box 9-1, p. 180).

Sanitary pads can hold small amounts of urinary leakage but are not intended for this purpose.

9. Discard gloves.

10. See Completion Protocol (inside front cover).

• • •

EVALUATION

1. Determine percentage of continent episodes in relation to total number of events of elimination in specified time.
2. Observe effectiveness of absorbent pads or garments used to contain incontinent episodes.
3. Observe the perineum for evidence of redness or irritation.

Unexpected Outcomes and Related Interventions

1. Client describes episodes of incontinence as urgency, associated with frequency and burning with voiding.
   a. Increase fluid intake and encourage cranberry juice.
   b. Consider the possibility of urinary tract infection. Report to physician for evaluation and treatment.
2. Client experiences overflow incontinence associated with urinary retention and bladder distention.
   a. Teach and encourage voiding according to a planned schedule.
   b. Notify physician if prescribed drugs may be contributing to urinary retention (e.g., anticholiner-gics, antispasmodics, antidepressants, seizure medications). Dosage or schedule of administration may be adjusted.
   c. Consult with physician regarding catheterization for residual urine (see Chapter 35).

Recording and Reporting

- Document each episode of incontinence.
- Include appearance and amount of stool or urine.
- Include appearance of skin.
- Document interventions that are carried out.

Sample Documentation

0800 C/O urgency and frequency of urination that started 24 hours ago, C/O burning with some pain when urinating. Voided 50 ml concentrated urine every 1 to 2 hours in the last 24 hours. Reddened area around urinary meatus and labia. Perineal area cleansed with warm soapy water and dried thoroughly. Increased fluid intake encouraged, 200 cc of water intake now. Physician notified. Culture sent to lab as ordered.

Box 9-1 Containment Devices

Diapers can hold large amounts of urinary leakage. They are large and bulky and best used for clients with total incontinence and confined to bed or wheelchair.

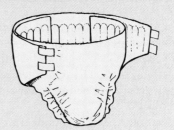

Adult undergarments can hold relatively large amounts of urinary leakage and are best for ambulatory clients.

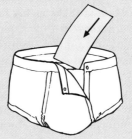

Underpants with absorbent pads can hold relatively large amounts of urinary leakage.

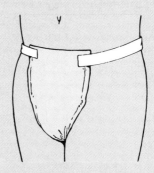

Sanitary pads can hold small amounts of urinary leakage. They are constructed for menstrual flow and are not as absorbent as incontinent pads.

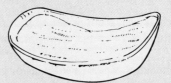

Male drip collectors can absorb small amounts of urine and fit comfortably over the penis.

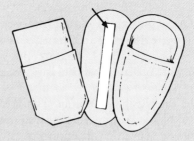

Modified from Gray M: *Genitourinary disorders,* Mosby's Clinical Nursing Series, St Louis, 1992, Mosby.

Geriatric Considerations

- The aging process contributes to changes in voiding and defecating. The aging client may require immediate response to a request for the bedpan or urinal or a trip to the toilet.
- Incontinence of urine or stool is NOT an expected result of the aging process.

Home Care and Long-Term Care Considerations

- Assess the client before determining a treatment program; include health history, voiding diary, cognitive ability, physical functions, urinalysis, and environment (Colling, 1996).
- Teach the primary home caregiver methods of assisting the client to manage incontinence, such as prompted voiding or a voiding schedule.
- Personnel in long-term care facilities need to emphasize methods to manage incontinence, instead of emphasizing custodial care.
- Long-term use of incontinence products can lead to skin breakdown, although this can be minimized with conscientious care.
- Personnel in long-term care facilities must maintain professional, respectful attitudes toward both cognitively impaired and alert clients experiencing repeated, continuing problems with incontinence

Skill 9.4

APPLYING AN EXTERNAL CATHETER

The external application of a urinary drainage device is a convenient, safe method of draining urine in male clients. There does not seem to be an effective external catheter for women. (Pieper, Cleland, 1993). The external catheter is suitable for incontinent or comatose clients who have complete and spontaneous bladder emptying. The external catheter is a soft, pliable rubber sheath that slips over the penis. External catheters have elastic adhesive provided to secure them in place. The catheter may be attached to a leg drainage bag or a standard urinary drainage bag.

An external catheter should be assessed at least every 4 hours to detect potential problems and changed once every 24 hours for aseptic purposes. With each catheter change, the urethral meatus and penis are cleansed thoroughly and inspected for signs of skin irritation.

A new external catheter has been developed that is held by a sheath attached to a brieflike man's undergarment. A clinical trial demonstrated ease of use by the client, increased dryness, decreased odor, and decreased skin irritation or breakdown (Peifer, Hanover, 1997).

Equipment

Urinary external catheter (appropriate size) with elastic or Velcro adhesive (if not using self-adhesive device)
Urinary collection bag with drainage tubing or leg bag and straps
Skin preparation (tincture of benzoin)
Towels and washcloths
Bath blanket
Clean disposable gloves
Scissors

ASSESSMENT

1. Assess urinary elimination patterns, ability to urinate voluntarily, and continence. **Rationale: External catheter is suitable for incontinent or comatose male clients with complete and spontaneous bladder emptying, who are at risk for skin breakdown.**
2. Assess mental status of client so appropriate teaching related to external catheter can be implemented. Teaching can include self-application. Assess client's knowledge of the purpose of an external catheter.
3. Assess condition of penis. **Rationale: Provides a baseline to compare changes in condition of skin after application of the external catheter.**

PLANNING

Expected outcomes focus on promoting dryness and preventing continual exposure of skin to urine.

Expected Outcomes

1. Client voids 5 or more times daily.
2. Client's penis remains free from skin irritation or breakdown.
3. Client remains dry with catheter secure and adequate circulation to the penis.

IMPLEMENTATION

Steps	Rationale
1. See Standard Protocol (inside front cover).	
2. Assist client into supine position with a bath blanket over upper torso and lower extremities covered; only genitalia should be exposed.	Promotes comfort and prevents unnecessary exposure of body parts.
3. Prepare urinary drainage collection bag and tubing. Clamp off drainage exit ports. Secure collection bag to bed frame; bring drainage tubing up between side rails and bed frame. Be sure tubing is not pulled when side rails are raised. Prepare leg bag for connection to external catheter, if necessary.	Provides easy access to drainage equipment.
4. ✋ Using warm soapy water remove all secretions from the penis and dry thoroughly.	Prevents skin breakdown from exposure to secretions. Rubber sheath rolls onto clean, dry skin more easily.
5. Clip hair at base of penis if necessary.	Hair adheres to adhesive and pulls during external catheter removal.
6. Apply skin preparation to penis and allow to dry. A thin layer of plasticized skin spray protects skin from irritation. If client is uncircumcised, return foreskin to normal position.	Skin preparation has an alcohol base. Evaporation prevents irritation. Returning foreskin prevents foreskin from tightening around penile shaft, which impedes circulation to penis, and causes trauma to tissue.
7. **With self-adhesive external catheter** Application: a. A plastic collar positions the inner flap for application (see illustration).	

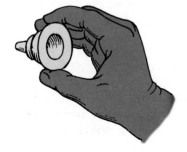

Step 7a

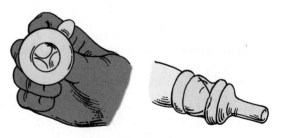

Step 7b

Steps	Rationale

b. Pinch catheter closed (see illustration). Place against glans as shown so tip, not entire glans, protrudes approximately 0.6 cm (¼ inch) into opening (see illustration). Foreskin should remain in natural position so tip of glans and foreskin protrude 0.6 cm (¼ inch) into opening.

Allows free flow of urine into collecting tubing when client voids.

c. With nondominant hand, grasp penis along shaft. With the other hand, unroll catheter up the shaft of the penis with as little wrinkling as possible. Discard plastic collar.

Plastic collar is for application of external catheter. *Do not push it onto the penis.*

d. Gently squeeze catheter to adhere sheath to skin. Once applied, do not attempt to reposition catheter. Pinch wrinkles to seal openings.

Catheter must be snug, but not tight enough to cause constriction of blood flow.

8. For external catheter without adhesive (see illustration)

Application:

a. Apply sheath to penis as in Step 7c.

Allows free passage of urine into collecting tubing when client voids.

b. Allow 2.5 to 5 cm (1 to 2 inches) of space between tip of glans penis and end of external catheter.

c. Encircle penile shaft with strip of elastic adhesive kept only in contact with sheath. Apply snugly, but not tightly.

Constriction of blood flow may occur if applied too tightly.

NURSE ALERT

Do not apply standard adhesive tape around the penis; this could interfere with circulation and cause necrosis of the skin and penis.

9. Connect drainage tubing to the end of the external catheter. A urine drainage bag is used at night (see illustration *A*), and a leg bag attached above or below the knee may be used for ambulation (see illustration *B*).

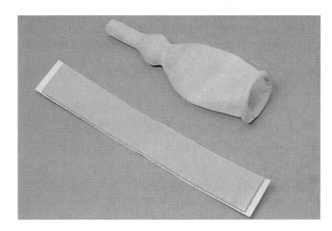

Step 8

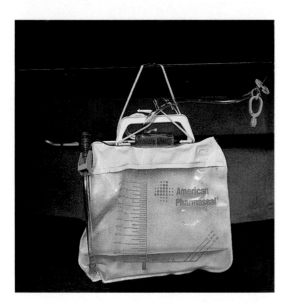

Step 9a

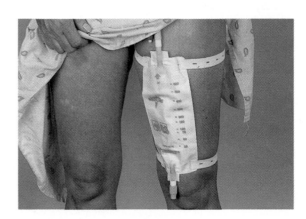

Step 9b

Steps	Rationale

10. Secure so that the tubing is not looped and the sheath is not twisted. Discard gloves.

Promotes free drainage of urine.

11. Remove sheath for 30 minutes every 24 hours to allow assessment and cleansing of skin. Remove and discard gloves and wash hands.

12. See Completion Protocol (inside front cover).

• • • •

EVALUATION

1. Observe frequency and amount of urine output in drainage container every 4 hours.
2. Remove sheath and inspect skin on penile shaft for signs of breakdown or irritation at least daily during hygiene and when external catheter is reapplied.
3. Observe circulation of glans penis 1 hour after application and every 4 hours thereafter to determine that sheath has not been applied too tightly.

Unexpected Outcomes and Related Interventions

1. Urination is reduced or infrequent, indicating possible urinary retention.
   a. Check for urinary retention and bladder distention.
   b. Monitor urine output.
2. Skin irritation occurs. Client may have allergy to adhesive product or irritation from contact with urine.
   a. Increase frequency of skin cleansing, and remove external catheter for 30 minutes each shift to promote healing.
   b. Make sure urine drains readily rather than sitting in contact with penis.
   c. Investigate the possibility of the new product with a sheath instead of adhesive.
3. Urine leaks from tubing. Remove catheter and reapply more snugly.
4. Penile swelling occurs.
   a. Remove catheter and allow swelling to decrease.
   b. Reapply more loosely.

Recording and Reporting

- Client responses, signs, symptoms (such as condition of the penis, scrotum) are included. Documentation must indicate justification for use of the external catheter.
- Description of product is included.

Sample Documentation

0900　Urinary dribbling has been constant for 1 week. Perineal area reddened, even with frequent washing, drying, and application of barrier lubricant. Skin of penis intact without edema. Self-adhesive external catheter applied, connected to leg drainage bag.

1000　Voided 200 cc in leg bag without discomfort. Circulation to penis intact. No skin irritation on penis.

Geriatric Considerations

- External catheters are contraindicated in clients with prostatic obstruction.
- Catheters are contraindicated in clients with prostatic obstruction.
- Clients with neuropathy must be carefully evaluated before application of an external catheter and at more frequent intervals, at least twice daily.
- The skin on the penis will be very delicate on the older person and prone to tearing; extreme caution is needed with the adhesives.

Home Care and Long-Term Care Considerations

- External catheters may contribute to urinary tract infections; therefore teach the caregiver signs and symptoms of infection and emphasize medical asepsis.
- Encourage use of a leg bag during the day and a bedside drainage bag at night.
- Loose fitting clothing may be needed to promote adequate drainage.
- Long-term use of external catheters is discouraged as skin breakdown becomes a major problem.

Skill 9.5

ADMINISTERING AN ENEMA

The primary reason for an enema is promotion of defecation. The volume and type of fluid instilled can lubricate or break up the fecal mass, stretch the rectal wall, and initiate the defecation reflex. Clients should not rely on enemas to maintain bowel regularity because they do not treat the cause of irregularity or constipation. Frequent enemas disrupt normal defecation reflexes, resulting in dependence on enemas for elimination. Fluid and electrolyte imbalances can occur with frequent enemas.

An enema is the instillation of a solution into the rectum and sigmoid colon. Cleansing enemas promote complete evacuation of feces from the colon by stimulating peristalsis through infusion of large volumes of solution.

An impaction involves presence of a fecal mass too large or hard to be passed voluntarily. Either constipation or diarrhea can suggest the presence of an impaction. An oil-retention enema lubricates the rectum and colon, softens the feces, and facilitates defecation. An oil-retention enema can be used alone or as adjunct therapy to manual removal of a fecal impaction.

Medicated enemas contain pharmacological therapeutic agents and are used to reduce dangerously high serum potassium levels, as with a sodium polystyrene sulfonate (Kayexalate) enema, or to reduce bacteria in the colon before bowel surgery, as with a neomycin enema.

Enema administration may be considered an evil practice in some cultures, thus introducing a conflict when the client is in need of an enema. A young child may be frightened by administration of an enema.

Equipment

Enema bag (disposable or reusable) (Figure 9-4)
Disposable gloves
Waterproof absorbent underpads
Adult: 750 to 1000 ml warm water or prepackaged disposable enema with prelubricated tip (Figure 9-5)
Water-soluble lubricant
Bath blanket
Toilet tissue
Bedpan, bedside commode, or access to toilet
Wash basin, washcloths, towel, and soap
IV pole

ASSESSMENT

1. Assess last bowel movement and presence or absence of bowel sounds. **Rationale: Reduced bowel motility may indicate need for enema.**
2. Assess ability to control external sphincter. **Rationale: Client with paralysis and no sphincter control must be placed on bedpan because enema solution cannot be retained.**
3. Assess presence or absence of hemorrhoids, which may obscure the rectal opening and cause discomfort or bleeding with evacuation.
4. Assess for abdominal pain. **Rationale: Indicates an enema is contraindicated until further assessment rules out danger of bowel perforation.**
5. Determine client's level of understanding and previous experience with enemas in order to provide appropriate teaching measures.
6. Assess limitations of mobility.

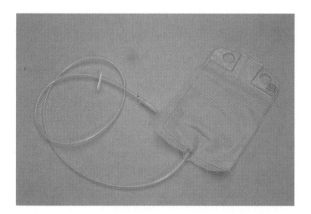

Figure 9-4   High-volume enema bag with tubing.

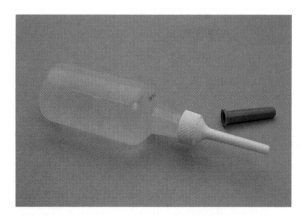

Figure 9-5   Prepackaged enema container with rectal tip(s).

PLANNING

Expected outcomes focus on establishing a normal pattern of bowel elimination and normal consistency of stools.

Expected Outcomes

1. Client verbalizes relief of abdominal discomfort.
2. Client expels gas and feces from the colon.
3. Client empties rectum and lower colon of stool.

DELEGATION CONSIDERATIONS

The skill of administering an enema can be delegated to AP.

- Stress importance of Standard Precautions for body fluids.
- Instruct care provider to use alternative positioning if there are mobility restrictions.
- Instruct care provider to stop and report inability to hold enema solution, severe cramping, bleeding, or severe abdominal pain.

IMPLEMENTATION

Steps	Rationale
1. See Standard Protocol (inside front cover).	
2. If using an enema bag, fill it with 750 to 1000 ml warm tap water as it flows from faucet. Check temperature of water by pouring small amount over inner wrist. Remove air from tubing by allowing solution to fill tubing. Clamp tubing.	Hot water can burn intestinal mucosa. Cold water can cause abdominal cramping and is difficult to retain.
3. Add castile soap if ordered.	Causes mild level of bowel irritation, facilitating mucus secretion
4. Assist client into left side-lying (Sims') position with right knee flexed.	Allows enema solution to flow downward by gravity along natural curve of sigmoid colon and rectum, thus improving retention of solution (Lewis, Collier, and Heitkemper, 1996).

COMMUNICATION TIPS

- *Adapt terms to developmental level of client.*
- *Ask a parent to assist if a child is to receive the enema.*

NURSE ALERT

Clients with minimal sphincter control may not be able to retain all of enema solution and will require placement of a bedpan under the buttocks. Administering enema with client sitting on toilet is ineffective because solution will not effectively infuse against gravity into bowel.

5. Place waterproof pad absorbent side up under hips and buttocks to prevent soiling of linen.	
6. Cover client with bath blanket, exposing only rectal area, and clearly visualize anus.	Provides warmth, reduces exposure of body parts, allows client to feel more relaxed and comfortable. Presence of hemorrhoids obscures anal opening and increases discomfort with bowel elimination.
7. If client will be expelling contents in toilet, ensure that toilet is available and place client's slippers and bathrobe in easily accessible location. If client is unable to get out of bed, place bedpan in easily accessible position. Place client in as private and comfortable an environment as possible.	
8. **Prepackaged disposable container**	
a. Remove plastic cap from rectal tip. Tip may be already lubricated. More lubricant can be applied if needed.	Lubrication provides for smooth insertion of rectal tube without rectal irritation or trauma.

Steps	**Rationale**

b. 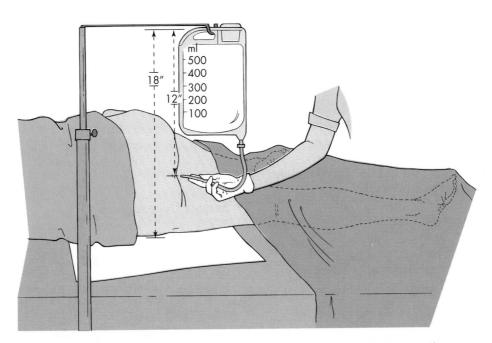 Gently separate buttocks and locate anus. Instruct client to relax by breathing out slowly through mouth.

> Breathing out promotes relaxation of external rectal sphincter. Presence of hemorrhoids obscures location of anus. Probe gently with gloved finger to locate rectal opening if necessary.

c. Insert lubricated tip of bottle gently into rectum approximately 7.5 to 10 cm (3 to 4 inches) for an adult.

d. Squeeze bottle continuously until all of solution has entered rectum and colon. (Most bottles contain approximately 250 ml solution.)

> Hypertonic solutions require only small volumes to stimulate defecation. Intermittent squeezing results in return of solution to the bottle.

9. **Enema bag**

   a. Lubricate 7.5 to 10 cm (3 to 4 inches) of tip of rectal tube with lubricating jelly.

   b. Gently separate buttocks and locate anus. Instruct client to relax by breathing out slowly through mouth.

   > Breathing out promotes relaxation of external anal sphincter.

   c. Insert tip of rectal tube slowly by pointing tip in direction of client's umbilicus. *Adult:* 7.5 to 10 cm (3 to 4 inches) past the internal sphincter.

   > Careful insertion prevents trauma to rectal mucosa from accidental lodging of tube against rectal wall. Forceful insertion beyond 10 cm (4 inches) could cause bowel perforation.

   d. Hold tubing in rectum constantly until end of fluid instillation.

   > Bowel contraction can cause expulsion of rectal tube.

   e. With container at client's hip level, open regulating clamp and allow solution to enter slowly.

   > Rapid infusion can stimulate evacuation and cause cramping.

   f. Raise height of enema container slowly to 30 to 45 cm (12 to 18 inches) above the anus. Infusion time varies with volume of solution administered (e.g., 1 L may take 7 to 10 minutes). Hang container on IV pole (see illustration).

   > Raising container too high causes rapid infusion and possible painful distention of colon.

Step 9f   *From Sorrentino SA: Assisting with patient care, St Louis, 1999, Mosby.*

Steps	Rationale

g. Lower container or clamp tubing if client complains of cramping or if fluid escapes around rectal tube.

Temporary cessation of infusion minimizes cramping and promotes ability to retain all the solution.

h. Clamp tubing after all the solution is infused. Tell client that the procedure is completed and that you will be removing rectal tube. Then gently withdraw tube.

Clients may misinterpret the sensation of removing the tube as loss of control.

10. Explain to client that feeling of distention is normal. Ask client to retain solution as long as possible (5 to 10 minutes) while lying quietly in bed.

Solution distends bowel. Length of retention varies with type of enema and client's ability to contract rectal sphincter. Longer retention promotes more effective stimulation of peristalsis and defecation.

11. Discard enema container and tubing in proper receptacle, or rinse out thoroughly with warm soap and water if container is to be reused.

12. Assist client to bathroom or commode if possible. If necessary to use the bedpan, assist to as near the normal position for evacuation as possible.

Normal squatting position promotes defecation.

13. Instruct clients with a history of cardiovascular disease to exhale while expelling enema to avoid the Valsalva maneuver (forced effort against a closed airway), especially if client is dehydrated.

The Valsalva maneuver in strenuously trying to move a constipated stool may result in cardiac arrest (Anderson, Anderson, and Glanze, 1998).

14. Instruct client to call for nurse to inspect results before flushing the toilet. Observe character of feces and solution.

When enemas are ordered "until clear," enemas are repeated until client passes fluid that is clear and contains no formed fecal matter. Usually three consecutive enemas are adequate.

15. Assist client as needed to wash anal area with warm soap and water.

Fecal contents can irritate skin. Hygiene promotes client's comfort.

16. Discard gloves.

17. See Completion Protocol (inside front cover).

• • •

EVALUATION

1. Ask client if abdominal discomfort has been relieved. Palpate abdomen to determine if distention is relieved.
2. Inspect color, consistency, and amount of stool and fluid passed. Observe abnormalities such as presence of blood or mucus.
3. When "enemas until clear" is ordered in preparation for surgery or diagnostic testing, the water expelled should be colorless and contain no particles of feces.

Unexpected Outcomes and Related Interventions

1. Client is unable to hold enema solution.
   a. Pinch the buttocks together to assist retention.
   b. Position on bedpan while administering the solution.
2. Severe cramping, bleeding, or sudden severe abdominal pain occurs and is unrelieved by temporarily stopping or slowing flow of solution.
   a. Stop enema.
   b. Notify physician.

3. With an order for "enemas until clear," after three enemas the water is highly colored or contains solid fecal material.
   a. Notify the physician before continuing.
   b. Excessive loss of electrolytes is a dangerous possibility.

Recording and Reporting

- Client signs and symptoms and responses
- Type of enema given
- Results, including color, amount, and appearance of stool

Sample Documentation

2000   Last BM 5 days ago. C/O abdominal fullness and rectal pressure. Abdomen distended, firm. Rectum free of fecal material on palpation. 900 ml tap water enema given with "mild" abdominal cramping during administration. Solution returned with large amount of dark brown, soft-formed stool.

2100   States is comfortable with no fullness in abdomen. Abdomen soft, nondistended.

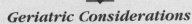

Geriatric Considerations

- Older adults may become fatigued more quickly and are at greater risk for fluid and electrolyte imbalances; therefore caution is needed when administering enemas "until clear."
- Teach older adults and their caregivers dietary and activity measures to avoid constipation.

Home Care and Long-Term Care Considerations

- Assess client's and primary caregiver's ability and motivation to administer enema and provide instruction as needed.
- Assess client's ability to administer enema if enema ordered is self-administrative type.
- Assess client's environment to identify location where enema may be administered with privacy.
- Teach skill; observe to determine level of understanding. Review possible complications and what action to take.
- Teach long-term care assistive personnel signs and symptoms (diaphoresis, pallor, shortness of breath, palpitations) that require stopping enema administration and to report immediately to the nurse.

CRITICAL THINKING EXERCISES

1. Mrs. Thorne had extensive abdominal surgery 3 days ago. She has a T-tube, nasogastric tube, and IV. Based on the following information, calculate Mrs. Thorne's I&O from 6 A.M. to 2 P.M.
   - Wound drainage in the T-tube: 35 ml emptied at 1:45 P.M.; 10 ml of this had been marked at 5:30 A.M., left in the bag and included in the 10 P.M. to 6 A.M. I&O calculation.
   - Enteral feedings: continuously at 50 ml per hour through a nasogastric tube.
   - Water: 30 ml instilled through the nasogastric tube every 2 hours on the even hour.
   - 1000 ml lactated Ringer's was started at 8 A.M. and will infuse by 4 P.M.
   - Urination for the day was 200 ml at 7 A.M., 150 ml at 10 A.M., and 300 ml at 1:00 P.M.

2. The home health aid tells the nurse that Mr. Ralph Smith, 76, has been incontinent of urine for 2 weeks.
   a. What further information does the nurse need to gather to assist in determining the most effective treatment plan?
   b. What do Mr. Smith and his primary caregiver need to be taught about his incontinent care?
   c. The nurse decides an external catheter will be helpful. Discuss measures the nurse needs to teach the home health aid, Mr. Smith, and his primary caregiver.

3. Mrs. Pradil, 90, is from India and has been in the nursing home 3 years. Although she has been in the United States 15 years, she does not speak English. She has had small amounts of fecal incontinence intermittently for 2 days. She has not had a bowel movement for 1 week
   a. What further assessment will the nurse do?
   b. Mrs. Pradil will receive a soap solution enema. Discuss how the nurse can explain each step to Mrs. Pradil.

REFERENCES

Anderson KN, Anderson LE, Glanze WD: *Mosby's medical, nursing, and allied health dictionary,* ed 5, St Louis, 1998, Mosby.

Colling J: Noninvasive techniques to manage urinary incontinence among care-dependent persons, *Journal of WOCN* 23(6):302, 1996.

Frahm J: The role of the PT in incontinence innovation and communication to improve patient care, *Ostomy/Wound Manage* 43(1):42, 1997.

Lewis SM, Collier IC, Heitkemper MM: *Medical surgical nursing: assessment and management of clinical problems,* ed 4, St Louis, 1996, Mosby.

Peifer DJ, Hanover RY: Clinical evaluation of the Easy-Flow Catheter, *J Rehabil Res Dev* 34(20):215, 1997.

Peiper B, Cleland V: An external urine-collection device for women: a clinical trial, *J ET Nurs* 20(2):51, 1993.

Potter PA, Perry AG: *Fundamentals of nursing: concepts, process, and practice,* ed 4, St Louis, 1998, Mosby.

Schrefer S: *Mosby's patient teaching tips,* St Louis, 1995, Mosby.

Urinary Incontinence Guideline Panel: Urinary incontinence in adults: clinical practice guidelines, AHCPR Publication no 92-0038, Rockville, Md, March 1992, Public Health Services U.S. Department of Health and Human Services, Agency for Health Care Policy and Research.

CHAPTER 10

Promoting Comfort, Sleep, and Relaxation

Skill 10.1
Comfort Measures that Promote Sleep, 191

Skill 10.2
Relaxation Techniques, 195

The theory that sleep is associated with healing suggests that achieving optimum sleep quality is important for the recovery of health care clients. Identifying sleep disturbances and promoting sleep, comfort, and relaxation are basic aspects of the nursing role.

The major problem in sleep disturbances is insufficient quantity and quality of sleep and is usually associated with some underlying physical (e.g., pain) or psychological (e.g., anxiety) disorder. The benefits of sleep often go unnoticed until a person develops problems resulting from sleep deprivation, which lead to changes in reflexes, memory, equilibrium, pain tolerance, and attention span. Severity of symptoms is highly variable and relates to the duration of the sleep deprivation (Box 10-1). Research has shown that older adults tend to experience changes in sleep patterns that can result in impaired judgment and concentration. The use of sedatives or hypnotics tends to create troublesome side effects (Johnson, 1993).

Sleep studies have revealed the phases and stages of sleep. Sleep involves two phases: non-rapid eye movement (NREM) and rapid eye movement (REM) sleep. During NREM a sleeper progresses through four stages in a typical sleep cycle. The cycles do not occur once but cycle back and forth several times during the course of sleep. At the end of each NREM phase, REM sleep occurs. REM sleep is the deepest level of sleep and is associated with changes in cerebral blood flow and vivid dreams. REM sleep assists learning, emotional adaptation, and problem

solving. People progress in various ways through cycles depending on the amount of time spent sleeping. The 24-hour sleep-wake cycle is a circadian rhythm that influences physiological function and behavior.

Pain and discomfort are subjective and highly individualized sensations and are greatly influenced by psychosocial and cultural factors. The gate control theory suggests that pain impulses can be regulated or blocked by "closing gates" that transmit pain sensations to the spinal cord. A bombardment of sensory impulses, such as from a backrub, closes the gates to pain stimuli. This theory also suggests that gating mechanisms can be altered by thoughts, feelings, and memories. (For additional information on pain management, refer to Chapter 22.) The focus of this chapter is the nurse's role in providing basic comfort measures.

Box 10-1 Sleep Deprivation Symptoms

Physiological
Hand tremors
Decreased reflexes
Slowed response time
Reduction in word memory
Decreased reasoning and judgment abilities
Cardiac irregularities Decreased alertness

Psychological
Moods
Disorientation
Irritability
Decreased motivation
Fatigue and sleepiness
Hyperactivity
Agitation

Pain has been shown to stimulate the autonomic nervous system as part of the stress response. This response involves physiological changes, including increased heart rate, respirations, blood pressure, oxygen consumption, metabolism, and muscle tension. Nurses must be able to use and teach stress management techniques and comfort measures that can promote falling and remaining asleep.

Life-threatening illness, changes in family structure, job stress, depression, and grief increase the anxiety of clients and their families. Anxiety can increase a client's level of pain and discomfort, interfere with learning, lower resistance to disease, and delay the recovery process (McFarland, McFarlane, 1993). Stress-related conditions frequently bring clients into the health care system. Recent studies support the effectiveness of progressive relaxation and guided imagery in managing pain and stress-related conditions. Although these techniques alone will not cure a disease, they do have a positive effect on stress-related symptoms, pain, and disease processes accelerated by stress, when used in addition to prescribed medical treatment (Benson, McKee, 1993).

NURSING DIAGNOSES

Sleep pattern disturbance is the state in which disruption of sleep causes discomfort or interferes with desired lifestyle (Kim et al, 1997). Related factors may include physical discomfort, personal or family stress, depression, environmental or habit changes, inactivity, or fear. The focus of care involves reducing factors that interfere with sleep. **Fatigue** is an overwhelming sense of exhaustion and decreased capacity for physical and mental work, even after sleeping. The focus for clients with fatigue becomes conservation of energy and the provision of rest periods. **Anxiety** is a vague, uneasy feeling of apprehension and tension with a nonspecific or unknown cause and frequently is associated with insomnia and depression. The nursing focus with anxiety is promoting relaxation and stress management.

Powerlessness is a perception that one's own action will not significantly affect an outcome, or a perceived lack of control over a current situation or immediate happening (Kim et al, 1997). Related factors include the health care environment, interpersonal interaction, and illness-related regimen. The focus of care includes activities that empower the client by allowing the experiencing of an increased sense of control over life situations and personal activities.

Skill 10.1

COMFORT MEASURES THAT PROMOTE SLEEP

The hospital environment is likely to influence clients' ability to fall and remain asleep. Acutely ill clients require frequent assessment and are exposed to unavoidable environmental stimulation to the point of having difficulty differentiating night and day. Disruptive sounds include paging systems, alarms, monitors, telephones, flushing toilets, suctioning equipment, and nursing activities. This is especially problematic for clients in intensive care units (ICUs). In this environment, normal sleep-wake cycles are frequently disrupted.

In addition, any illness that causes pain, difficulty breathing or swallowing, itching, nausea, or nocturia (urination at night) results in discomfort. Discomfort, emotional stress, anxiety, and depression may interfere with falling asleep or may cause frequent awakening or early awakening.

When comfort measures are inadequate, the short-term use of prescribed sedatives or hypnotics may be necessary. A sedative is medication that relaxes the client and promotes rest. A hypnotic actually produces sleep.

Equipment
Night light
Side rails
Alarm system (optional) for clients at risk for falls
Television monitoring system (optional) for clients at risk for falls

ASSESSMENT
1. Ask client to describe location of any discomfort, as well as onset, precipitating factors, quality, duration, and severity.
2. To identify client's normal sleep pattern, ask:
    a. What time do you usually go to sleep?
    b. How quickly do you fall asleep?
    c. What is the average number of hours you sleep?
    d. How many times do you awaken during that time?
    e. When do you typically awaken?
    f. Do you rise once you awaken, or do you stay in bed?

3. When a problem is identified, use open questions to help the client describe the problem more fully.
   a. What interferes with your sleep?
   b. What type of sleep problem do you experience?
   c. When did you notice the problem? How long has it lasted?
   d. How often do you have trouble sleeping?
   e. Compare your sleep now with your normal sleep.
   f. What do you do just before going to bed?
   g. What do you think about as you fall asleep?
   h. Have you had any recent changes at work or at home?
   i. How has the loss of sleep affected you?
   j. Have you or your partner noted any changes in behavior since the sleep problem started? Irritability, fatigue, trouble concentrating, others?
4. Identify medications that may influence sleep patterns (Table 10-1).
5. Identify indications of sleep apnea. **Rationale: Sleep apnea is the temporary cessation of airflow through the nose and mouth for 10 seconds or more during sleep** (Barkauskas et al, 1998). The sleeping partner may be a better source of information than the client.
   a. Snores loudly and irregularly?
   b. Stops breathing for a while and then starts up again?
   c. Has headaches after awakening?
   d. Awakens coughing or choking?
   e. Makes grunting or gurgling noises during sleep?

COMMUNICATION TIP

Before discussing specific sleep problems with the client, use this time to inform the client and family about factors, such as diet and exercise, that could impact positively or negatively on sleep patterns.

PLANNING

Expected outcomes focus on providing comfort and assisting the client to identify and adopt sleep-promoting measures.

Expected outcomes
1. Client is relaxed and comfortable after technique as evidenced by: slow, deep respirations, calm facial expressions, calm tone of voice, relaxed muscles, and relaxed posture.
2. Client demonstrates and describes sleep-promoting measures.
3. Client verbalizes restful sleep.

Table 10-1

Effects of Some Medications on Sleep

Drug Class	Effects
Hypnotics	Interfere with reaching deeper sleep stages
	Provide only temporary (1 week) increase in quantity of sleep
	Eventually cause "hangover" during day: excess drowsiness, confusion, decreased energy
	May worsen sleep apnea in adults
Beta blockers	Cause nightmares, insomnia, awakening from sleep
Antianxiety agent (Valium)	Decreases stage 2, stage 4, and REM sleep; decreases awakenings
Narcotic analgesics (morphine, meperidine [Demerol])	Suppress REM sleep
	If discontinued quickly, can increase risk of cardiac dysrhythmias because of rebound
	Cause increased awakenings and drowsiness
Antidepressants and stimulants	Suppress REM sleep

DELEGATION CONSIDERATIONS

The nurse, in collaboration with the client, is responsible for the assessment, planning, initial implementation, and evaluation of needed comfort and sleep-enhancing measures. The following information is necessary when delegating skills to assistive personnel (AP) or family members:

- Have staff report changes in client's condition.
- Identify and eliminate environmental conditions that might inhibit sleep.
- Plan comfort measures to provide maximum rest periods.
- Be aware that turning, positioning, and reducing environmental stimuli are important for comfort, pain control, and promotion of sleep.

IMPLEMENTATION

Steps	Rationale

1. See Standard Protocol (inside front cover).
2. Promote usual bedtime routines (reading, eating a snack, watching television). Encourage client to empty bladder. Provide opportunity to wash face and hands, brush teeth or dentures, and cleanse mouth.
3. Suggest avoiding caffeine at bedtime. Schedule diuretics early in the day to minimize nocturia. Teach client to eliminate/reduce physical activities 1 hour before bedtime. Decrease fluid intake before bedtime.

   Caffeine in coffee, tea, colas, and chocolate is a stimulant and can interfere with sleep. It also acts as a diuretic and may cause the need to void during the night.

4. Make sure client gown and linens are clean and dry. Tighten and smooth wrinkled bed linen. Provide adequate warmth, especially for feet and shoulders.
5. Provide cutaneous stimulation such as a massage (see Skill 10.2). A warm bath or a warm or cold compress may promote comfort.

   Massage promotes muscle relaxation. The gate control theory suggests that stimulation of certain nerve fibers closes gates to transmission of discomfort.

6. Assist client to a comfortable position, providing support to body parts to minimize muscle tension. Place a pillow at the client's back to support in lateral position (see illustration).

   This position is good for relaxation in general.

7. Raise side rails and place call light within reach. Remind client to call for help if getting up for any reason is necessary. Assure client you will respond to calls as quickly as possible.

   Clients who have urinary urgency may attempt to go to the bathroom alone rather than experience soiling the bed.

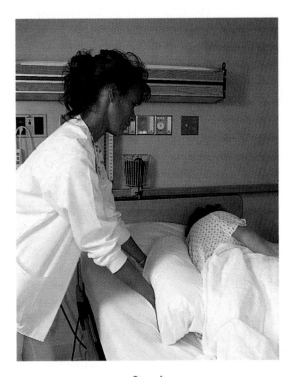

Step 6

Steps	Rationale

8. Identify need for safety system. Some beds have alarm systems that alert nurses to client getting out of bed. Some rooms can be monitored by a television screen for safety (see illustration).

9. Eliminate environmental noise as much as possible. Closing door to the hallway may minimize disturbing sounds. Some clients are accustomed to music or the sound of radio or television (Box 10-2).

Many clients become disoriented when in an unfamiliar environment, which increases risk for falls (see agency policy).

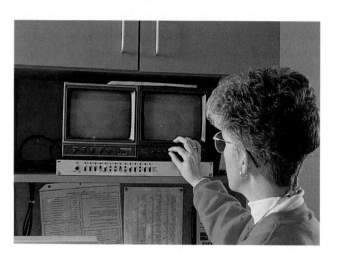

Step 8

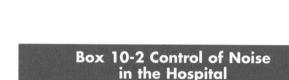

Box 10-2 Control of Noise in the Hospital

Close doors to client's room.
Provide a sign on the door requesting avoidance of interruptions.
Reduce volume of nearby telephone and paging equipment.
Wear rubber-soled shoes.
Turn off equipment if possible (e.g., oxygen, suction).
Drain humidified oxygen tubing of water accumulation periodically.
Avoid flushing a toilet or moving beds if possible.
Keep talking at low levels, especially at night.
Conduct nursing reports and discussions in areas away from client rooms.
Turn off television or radio or provide soft music.

10. Provide an acceptable level of indirect light. Use of a night light may be beneficial.

11. Schedule necessary assessments, medications, and treatments to minimize the number of times client must be awakened and assure client of this plan.

12. See Completion Protocol (inside front cover).

May reduce confusion if client awakens at night.

Increases the opportunity for quality sleep and REM/NREM sleep cycling.

• • •

EVALUATION

1. Ask client to rate discomfort level on a scale of 0 to 10 (10 is the worst).

2. Observe client for evidence of sleep 30 minutes after preparing for sleep and every hour thereafter.

3. Ask client to describe methods used to promote sleep and discuss their effectiveness.

4. Assess client's perception of feeling rested on awakening.

Unexpected Outcome and Related Interventions

Client reports frequent awakenings during the night or not feeling rested on awakening.

1. Have client keep a sleep-wake log. Each morning, record evening and bedtime rituals, the time attempting to begin sleep, number and length of awakenings, and time of morning awakening.

2. Monitor for signs of sleep deprivation.

3. Offer hypnotics or antianxiety agents (if ordered) 30 to 40 minutes before usual bedtime. Sedative-hypnotics should be used short-term only (less than 1 week).

4. Clients should avoid alcohol, smoking, and drinking caffeine while taking hypnotics. **Alcohol can increase the sedation produced by these drugs and can dangerously depress brain function. Smoking and drinking caffeine interfere with effectiveness.**

Recording and Reporting

- Report continued sleep pattern disturbance to charge nurse or physician.
- Record findings of ongoing assessment, interventions completed, and client's response to interventions.
- Report client's response to techniques to nurse in charge and to staff at change of shift.

Sample Documentation

0700   States awakened frequently when turning, on care-givers' entering room, and with roommate movement. Lethargic with flat affect. Closes eyes repeatedly during interaction with nurse. Expresses desire for uninterrupted sleep. Discussed using soft music or a fan for distraction and obtaining pillow from home.

Geriatric Considerations

Visual, hearing, cognitive, and motor impairments may make it difficult for older adults to sleep and may contribute to sleeplessness.

Home Care and Long-Term Care Considerations

- Use same noise control strategies as in the hospital environment (see Box 10-2 on p. 194).
- Inform friends and relatives about the best time to phone or visit the client.
- Turn off ringer on phone when client is trying to sleep during the day. Be sure to instruct client to turn the phone ringer back on.

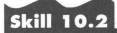

Skill 10.2

RELAXATION TECHNIQUES

Clients can alter the ability to relax physically and mentally, resulting in many physical and psychological benefits. Relaxation can promote rest and sleep as well as significantly relieve tension headaches and acute and chronic pain.

For effective relaxation, the client's participation and cooperation are needed. The technique requires practice and is best taught when the client is not experiencing acute pain. The nurse guides the client slowly through the steps of the exercise. Relaxation training may take 5 to 10 training sessions before clients can use it effectively. It can be practiced indefinitely and usually has no side effects.

PROGRESSIVE RELAXATION

By teaching clients the use of progressive relaxation techniques, the nurse offers the client a sense of self-control when pain occurs. Progressive relaxation may be used independently or with other pain-relief measures. This technique eases muscle tension and reduces anxiety associated with pain (Jurf, Nirschl, 1993). Relaxation techniques may require a physician's order if the stability of a client's condition is in question. The nurse should be available to assist the client in performing relaxation techniques, as well as in timing procedures (such as dressing changes) so that the technique can be most beneficial. The client's full participation and cooperation are necessary for progressive relaxation to be effective (Perry, Potter, 1998).

GUIDED IMAGERY

Guided imagery is a creative sensory experience that can effectively reduce pain perception and minimize reaction to pain. The goal of imagery is to have the client use one or several of the senses to create an image of the desired result. This image creates a positive psychophysiological response (Dossey, 1992; Stephens, 1993). Pain relief associated with imagery may be related to the release of endorphins (Tiernan, 1994).

Choosing images that clients find pleasant requires a careful assessment by the nurse. For example, a scene of rolling waves at the seashore may be restful to one client but desolate or frightening to another. Imagery may be used with progressive relaxation, massage or as a distraction (Perry, Potter, 1998).

MASSAGE

A gentle massage is a form of cutaneous stimulation that activates large-diameter sensory nerve fibers in the skin to prevent painful stimuli from reaching the brain's conscious awareness (Jurf, Nirschl, 1993). A proper massage not only blocks the perception of pain impulses but also helps relax muscle tension and spasm that otherwise might increase pain (Ferrell-Torry, Glick, 1993). The high state of relaxation often achieved with massage adds to the effects of other pain-relief measures (Ferrell-Torry, Glick, 1993; Meintz, 1995). A massage of the back, shoulders, and lower part of the neck is sometimes referred to as a *backrub*. A nurse should offer a backrub after a bath or before a client prepares for sleep to promote relaxation and comfort, relieve muscle tension, and stimulate circulation. An effective backrub takes 3 to 5 minutes and is an important intervention for decreasing pain and improving the sense of well-being (Perry, Potter, 1998).

Equipment
Progressive muscle relaxation: cassette tape player, taped instructions for relaxation, nature sounds, or music
Massage: lotion or oil, folded sheet, bath towel

ASSESSMENT
1. Assess facial expressions and verbal indications of discomfort. Clients may cry, moan, grimace, clench jaws, or tightly close or widely open mouth or eyes.
2. Observe body movement indicating physical or psychological distress. This may include restlessness, muscle tension, hand and finger movements, pacing, rhythmical or rubbing motions, or immobilization.
3. Observe social interactions that suggest physical or psychological distress. Clients may avoid conversation, have reduced attention span, avoid eye contact, or display irritability, anger, or withdrawal.
4. Assess for physiological signs of anxiety or stress, which may include tachycardia (increased heart rate), increased respirations or hyperventilation, elevated blood pressure, sweaty palms, trembling, and dry mouth.

PLANNING
Expected outcomes focus on alleviating or reducing discomfort, increasing client's sense of control, and providing client empowerment through education.

Expected Outcomes
1. Client verbalizes feelings of well-being and relaxation.
2. Client verbalizes an increased sense of control over life situations as evidenced by integration of relaxation techniques into activities of daily living.
3. Client increases knowledge and skill of basic relaxation techniques as evidenced by ability to use and demonstrate techniques correctly.

DELEGATION CONSIDERATIONS

The nurse, in collaboration with the client, is responsible for the assessment, planning, initial implementation, and evaluation of needed comfort measures. The following information is necessary when delegating skills to unlicensed assistive personnel or family members:

- Instruct staff to alert nurse if signs of discomfort increase.
- Emphasize importance of controlling environment to ensure quiet and privacy.

IMPLEMENTATION

Steps	Rationale

A. Progressive muscle relaxation:
  1. See Standard Protocol (inside front cover).
  2. Begin relaxation technique
    a. Assist client to assume position of comfort with entire body well supported. Encourage to settle in comfortably. Instruct client to notice areas of tension.
      (1) Sitting: entire back rests against back of chair and head supported in line with spine, feet flat on floor, legs apart, and arms resting comfortably on arms of chair or lap (see illustration).
      (2) Lying: keep head aligned with spine, with a thin small pillow under head, arms resting at sides without touching sides of body, legs separated, and toes slightly outward (see illustration).
	Adequate support enhances relaxation.

Steps	Rationale

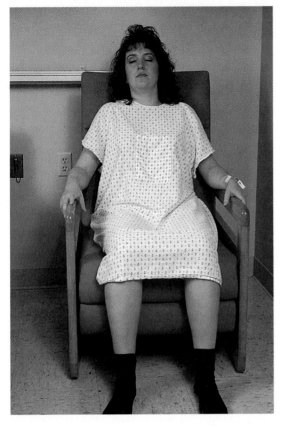

Step 2a(1)

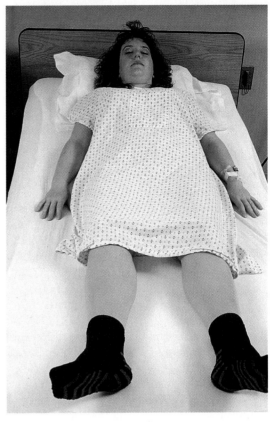

Step 2a(2)

b. Tell client to close eyes, relax, and breathe slowly and deeply, allowing the abdomen to rise and fall with each breath.

3. Instruct client to follow verbal cues for relaxation; use calm, soft voice.

a. Begin series of alternating tightening and relaxing muscle groups: (1) clench right fist, relax; (2) clench left fist, relax; (3) clench both fists, relax; (4) tighten right biceps, relax; (5) tighten left biceps, relax.

Deep, regular breathing pattern creates a sensation of removing all discomfort and stress.

Relaxation is guided verbally or by tape until individual is comfortable with sequence and no longer needs verbal guidance.

Alternating tension and relaxation in muscle groups allows client to feel difference.

NURSE ALERT

Tension of each muscle group is maintained for 5 to 7 seconds except for the feet. Allows time to focus on the muscle group; cramps can easily occur in the feet.

b. As each muscle group is completed, ask client to enjoy relaxed feeling and allow mind to drift and think how nice it is to be relaxed; ask client to breathe deeply.

Distracts client from perceiving pain. Enhances the relaxation response.

Breathing deeply prevents Valsalva response, which can increase intrathoracic pressure and compromise cardiac function.

Steps	Rationale
c. Instruct client to repeat each step 2 times: (1) reach with right arm, relax; (2) reach with left arm, relax; (3) reach with both arms, relax; (4) wrinkle forehead, relax; (5) squint eyes, relax; (6) tighten jaw muscles, relax; (7) press head into pillow, relax; (8) bring right shoulder to earlobe, relax; (9) bring left shoulder to earlobe, relax; (10) bring both shoulders to earlobe, relax; (11) tighten abdominal muscles, relax; (12) tighten hips and buttocks, relax; (13) press right leg into mattress, relax; (14) press left leg into mattress, relax; (15) point right toes and stretch, relax; (16) point left toes and stretch, relax; (17) stretch right leg, relax; (18) stretch left leg, relax; (19) stretch both legs, relax; (20) flex right foot, relax; (21) flex left foot, relax; (22) flex both feet, relax; (23) tense right leg, relax; (24) tense left leg, relax; (25) tense both legs, relax; (26) tense entire body, relax.	Relaxation is integrated response associated with diminished sympathetic nervous system arousal; decreased muscle tension is desired outcome. Relaxation decreases pulse rate, respiration rate, and blood pressure and reduces anxiety.

NURSE ALERT

If muscle group tightens after relaxation has proceeded to other muscles, return to that group and repeat tension-relaxation until relaxation is achieved.

Steps	Rationale
d. Calmly explain during exercise that client may feel sensations of tingling, heaviness, floating, or warmth as relaxation occurs.	Prevents anxiety should sensation occur without warning.
e. Ask client to continue slow, deep breaths.	Allows opportunity to enjoy feelings of relaxation.
4. When exercise is complete, instruct client to inhale deeply, exhale, and then initially move about slowly after resting a few minutes.	Returns client to more awake and alert state. When deeply relaxed, client may experience dizziness on arising too rapidly.
B. Guided imagery	
1. Assist client to assume position of comfort with entire body well supported (see Skill 10.2, Step 2).	The ability to relax physically promotes mental relaxation.
2. Sit close to client and speak in a soft, calm voice.	The experience of discomfort can be altered by concentrating on a serene, tranquil voice.
3. Begin by helping client breathe in a slow, rhythmical fashion as you count, and suggest inhaling on 1 and 2, exhaling on 3 and 4.	
4. Suggest relaxation with a phrase such as "Your body is beginning to relax . . . think relax . . . continue to breathe slowly and relax."	Focusing on the sensation of relaxation enhances the ability to relax.
5. Direct client through guided imagery exercise: a. Instruct client to imagine that inhaled air is ball of healing energy.	Development of specific images assists in removal of pain perception.
b. Imagine inhaled air travels to area of pain.	Client's ability to concentrate decreases pain perception.
6. Alternatively, nurse may direct imagery: a. Suggest client think about going to pleasant place such as beach or mountains.	Directs imagery after selection of restful place by nurse and client.
b. Direct client to experience all sensory aspects of restful place (e.g., for beach: warm breeze, warm sand between toes, warmth of sunshine, rhythmic sound of waves, smell of salt air, gulls gliding and swooping in air).	Helps client concentrate and relax.

Steps	Rationale

    c. Describe the scene identified by client as pleasurable and relaxing; for example, "Imagine yourself lying on a cool bed of grass with the sounds of rushing water from a nearby stream. It's a sunny day, and there is a gentle cool breeze." Have client travel mentally to the scene.

    d. Ask questions to help client experience the scene: "How does this look? Sound? Smell? Feel? Taste?"

7. Encourage client to practice the imagery. It may be helpful to tape-record the imagined experience for repeated practice opportunities.

8. Continue deep, slow rhythmic breathing.

9. End the experience: "Experience the comfort and relaxation. When you open your eyes, you will feel alert and renewed. Breathe deeply. Be aware of where you are now, stretch gently, and when you are ready, open your eyes."

C. Massage

    1. Adjust bed to high, comfortable position and lower side rail.

    2. Place client in comfortable position such as prone or side-lying position.

    3. Drape client to expose only area to be massaged.

    4. Warm lotion in hands.

    5. Choose stroke technique based on desired effect:

      a. Effleurage (see illustration)

Rationale (for Massage section):

Ensures proper body mechanics and prevents strain on nurse's back muscles.

Enhances relaxation and exposes area to be massaged.

Maintains client's privacy and warmth.

Warm lotion is soothing, and warmth helps to produce local muscle relaxation (Meintz, 1995).

Gliding stroke, used without manipulating deep muscles, smooths and extends muscles, increases nutrient absorption, and improves lymphatic and venous circulation (Meintz, 1995).

NURSE ALERT

Clients with respiratory difficulties may lie on side with head of bed elevated.

NURSE ALERT

Do not use lotion or oils before massaging head and scalp.

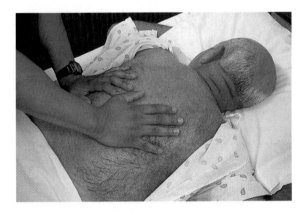

Step 5a

Steps	Rationale
b. Pétrissage (see illustration)	Use on tense muscle groups to "knead" muscles, promote relaxation, and stimulate local circulation.
c. Friction	Strong circular strokes bring blood to surface of skin, thereby increasing local circulation and loosening tight muscle groups (Meintz, 1995).

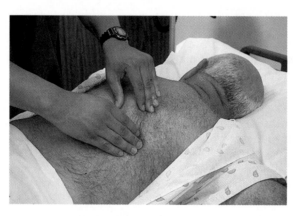

Step 5b

6. Encourage client to breathe deeply and relax during massage.	
7. Massage head and scalp.	Strong circular strokes (friction) stimulate local circulation and relaxation.
8. Standing behind client, stimulate scalp and temples.	
9. Supporting client's head, rub muscles at base of head.	
10. Massage hands and arms:	Releases tension in hands and arms. Studies indicate that anxious behaviors may be significantly reduced with hand massage (Snyder et al, 1995).
a. Support hand and apply friction to palm using both thumbs.	Encourages relaxation; enhances circulation and venous return.
b. Support base of finger and work each finger in corkscrewlike motion.	
c. Complete hand massage using effleurage strokes from fingertips to wrist.	
d. Knead muscles of forearm and upper arm between thumb and forefinger.	
11. Massage neck:	
a. Place client in prone position unless contraindicated.	Reduces tension that often localizes in neck muscles.
b. Knead each neck muscle between thumb and forefinger.	Helps relax muscle body.
c. Gently stretch neck by placing one hand on top of shoulders and other at base of head and gently move hands away from each other.	

Steps	**Rationale**

12. Massage back:
    a. Place client in prone or side-lying position.

    b. Do not allow hands to leave client's skin.

    c. Apply hands first to sacral area, and massage in circular motion (see illustration). Stroke upward from buttocks to shoulders. Massage over scapulas with smooth, firm stroke. Continue in one smooth stroke to upper arms and laterally along sides of back down to iliac crests. Continue massage pattern for 3 minutes.

Side-lying position is indicated for clients unable to lie prone.

Continuous contact with skin's surface is soothing and stimulates circulation to tissues. Breaking contact with skin can startle client.

Gentle firm pressure applied to all muscle groups promotes relaxation.

NURSE ALERT

Be certain to massage muscular region, not bruised, swollen, or inflamed areas or bones of the spine (Meintz, 1995).

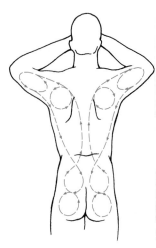

Step 12c

d. Use long, gliding strokes along muscles of spine in upward and outward motion.
e. Knead muscles of each shoulder toward front of client.
f. Use palms in upward and outward circular motion from lower buttocks to neck.
g. Knead muscles of upper back and shoulder between thumb and forefinger.
h. Use both hands to knead muscles up one side of back, then other.
i. End massage with long stroking movements.

13. Massage feet:
    a. Place client in supine position.
    b. Hold foot firmly. Support ankle with one hand or support sides of foot with each hand while performing massage.
    c. Make circular motions with thumb and fingers around bones of ankle and top of foot.
    d. Trace space between tendons with firm finger pressure, moving from toe to ankle.
    e. Massage sides and top of each toe.
    f. Use top of fist to make circular motions on bottom of foot.

14. See Completion Protocol (inside front cover).

Massage follows distribution of major muscle groups.

Area often tightens because of tension.

These muscles are thick and can be vigorously massaged.

Most soothing of massage movements.

EVALUATION

1. Inspect client's physiological (e.g., vital sign changes, posture) and behavioral (facial expressions, tone of voice, affect) responses to technique.
2. Ask client to rate level of comfort using a scale of 0 to 10.
3. Observe client performing relaxation technique.

Unexpected Outcomes and Related Nursing Interventions

1. Client's level of comfort declines.
   a. Assist client with relaxation technique.
   b. Consider analgesic.
2. Client is unable to perform relaxation technique.
   a. Reinstruct client and demonstrate procedure.
   b. Coach client through relaxation procedure.

Recording and Reporting

- Record client's level of comfort before and after procedure, document relaxation technique used, client vital signs, and overall client response.
- Report client's response to relaxation technique and any unusual responses to technique to charge nurse or physician.

Sample Documentation

2000 Client reported restlessness and severe headache (10 on scale 1 to 10). States cannot sleep. Participated in progressive relaxation exercise. States headache is relieved (3 on scale 1 to 10). Resting in bed with eyes closed.

2200 Guided imagery practiced for 5 minutes in preparation for sleep. States feeling "much more relaxed and comfortable now." Verbalizes plans to practice this regularly using "favorite fishing spot" as setting.

2330 Reports "dull ache in neck and shoulders" (8 on scale 1 to 10). Massage given to shoulder, neck, and back regions. Verbalizes pain decreasing (5 on 1 to 10 scale). Resting with eyes closed.

◆ Geriatric Considerations

- Visual, hearing, cognitive, and motor impairments may make it difficult for client to effectively use procedure.

►◄ Home Care and Long-Term Care Considerations

- Teach family member how to perform relaxation technique.
- Teach family how to reduce home environmental noises.

CRITICAL THINKING EXERCISES

1. Mrs. Jones is scheduled for an open laparotomy in the morning. She verbalizes at 2100 that she feels quite anxious and cannot sleep. Discuss the nursing interventions you will use to promote relaxation and sleep.

2. Discuss the outcome criteria you will use in evaluating the effectiveness of the relaxation techniques performed with Mrs. Jones in the above situation.

3. Mr. Williams, a 70-year-old male, has COPD. He states he feels "tense in my shoulders and neck" and would like a massage. He exhibits mild dyspnea. Discuss adaptations you would make in the massage technique to accommodate his respiratory problem.

REFERENCES

Barkauskas VH et al: *Health and physical assessment,* ed 5, St Louis, 1998, Mosby.

Benson H, McKee MG: Relaxation and other alternative therapies, *Patient Care* 27(20):65, 1993.

Dossey B: Psychophysiologic self-regulation. In Dossey B, Guzzetta C, eds: *Cardiovascular nursing: holistic practice,* St Louis, 1992, Mosby.

Ferrell-Torry A, Glick O: The use of therapeutic massage as a nursing intervention to modify anxiety and the perception of cancer pain, *Cancer Nurs* (1692):93, 1993.

Johnson JE: Progressive relaxation and the sleep of older men and women, *J Community Health Nurs* 12(10):31, 1993.

Jurf J, Nirshl A: Acute postoperative pain management: a comprehensive review and update, *Crit Care Nurs Q* 16(1):8, 1993.

Kim, M et al: *Pocket guide to nursing diagnosis,* ed 7, St Louis, 1997, Mosby.

McFarland G, McFarlane E: *Nursing diagnosis and intervention,* ed 4, St Louis, 1996, Mosby.

Meintz S: Whatever became of the back rub? *RN* 58(4):49, 1995.

Perry AG, Potter, PA: *Clinical nursing skills and techniques,* ed 4, St Louis, 1998, Mosby.

Snyder M, Egan EL, Burns KR: Efficacy of hard massage in decreasing agitation behavior associated with care activities in persons with dementia. *Geriatric Nursing–American Journal of Care for the Aging* 16(2):60, 1995.

Stephens R: Imagery: a strategic intervention to empower clients. II. A practical guide, *Clin Nurse Specialist* (795):235, 1993.

Tiernan P: Independent nursing interventions: relaxation and guided imagery in critical care, *Crit Care Nurse* (1495):47, 1994.

CHAPTER 11

Basic Infant Care

Skill 11.1
Thermoregulation Using a Radiant Warmer, 204

Skill 11.2
Infant Feeding, 206

Skill 11.3
Infant Bathing, 212

Skill 11.4
Changing a Diaper, 215

Skill 11.5
Swaddling and Use of a Mummy Restraint, 218

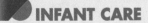

INFANT CARE

Nursing care of infants is concerned with providing for the infant's basic needs, as well as incorporating parent teaching. Newborn infants experience intense changes as they make the transition from intrauterine life into the world. Immediate nursing care is directed toward maintaining an open airway, stabilizing body temperature, and protecting from infection.

The first priority after birth is maintaining an open airway, which routinely involves suction with a bulb syringe. The newborn is immediately placed under a radiant warmer and dried thoroughly. Next to establishing respiration, heat regulation is most critical to the newborn's survival (Wong and Perry, 1998). Several factors predispose the infant to heat loss, including the large body surface area and the thin layer of subcutaneous fat. Radiant warmers regulate the temperature of the environment, which will help maintain an appropriate body temperature for the newborn.

As soon as physiological stability is achieved and identification bracelets are in place, it is important to respond to the needs related to close parent-infant contact. Most healthy newborns are alert for the first 30 minutes after birth, and, if the parents are receptive, this is an excellent time to promote the bonding process.

Infants depend on caregivers for all of their basic needs, including nutrition, cleanliness, and safety. Breast-feeding is recommended because it is uniquely suited to the infant's needs. Breast milk provides antibacterial and antiviral properties, immunoglobulins, and anti-allergic factors to protect the infant. The decision to feed a baby infant formula may result from the mother's or partner's personal preference, the influence of significant family members, or a lack of information about the benefits and techniques of breast-feeding. Inexperienced mothers need to learn how to successfully feed their infants whether they are breast-feeding or bottle feeding.

Infant bathing provides the opportunity to inspect the infant from head to toe, provide socialization, and cleanse the skin. The initial bath is given after the infant's body temperature has stabilized, and gloves are worn for all contact with the infant before this bath. A bath demonstration is routinely provided for new parents and it provides an excellent opportunity to demonstrate normal characteristics of the newborn, umbilical cord care, how to change the diaper, and how to hold and dress the infant.

Box 11-1 Traditional Cultural Beliefs Relating to Infant Care

Hispanic

Breast-feeding begins after the third day, with colostrum considered "spoiled."

Males are not circumcised; females' ears are pierced.

The infant is protected from the "evil eye."

African-American

Feeding is very important; a "good baby" eats well; solid foods are introduced very early.

Parents fear "spoiling" the baby.

There are strong family, community, and religious influences.

Asian-American

The father heads the household, and the wife plays a subordinate role.

Boy babies are preferred.

Parents may delay naming the child.

European-American

Breast-feeding begins as soon after birth as possible.

There is an emphasis on the bonding process.

Native American

The infant is not fed colostrum.

Herbs are used to increase milk flow.

Babies are not handled often; cradle boards may be used.

Data from Wong DL, and Perry SE: *Maternal child nursing care*, St. Louis, Mosby 1998.

Many cultural beliefs and practices surround pregnancy, childbirth, and infant care (see Box 11-1). Women from cultural-ethnic groups may adhere to some, all, or none of the practices typical of that culture. It is important for nurses to become familiar with each family and validate their cultural beliefs. However, if certain beliefs are identified as harmful, they need to be carefully explored and modified for the benefit of the infant (Wong and Perry, 1998).

Risk for Ineffective Airway Clearance may be related to excessive secretions. **Risk for Ineffective Thermoregulation** may be related to environmental factors and evaporation of moisture on the skin. **Risk for Infection** is related to immature immunological defenses and/or environmental exposure. **Effective Breast-feeding** is appropriate for a mother who was well prepared to begin breast-feeding and for whom the emphasis is promoting continued success. **Ineffective Breast-feeding** is the appropriate term when factors interfere with success, such as temporary separation because of illness of either the mother or the newborn or problems such as difficulty with latching on or sore nipples. **Ineffective Infant Feeding** is appropriate when the infant has impaired ability to suck or coordinate the suck-and-swallow response. **Health-seeking Behaviors** is the appropriate diagnosis when inexperienced parents are eager to learn as much as possible about infant care and feeding. **Risk for Altered Parent-Infant Attachment** is applied appropriately when circumstances alter the opportunity or ability for parents to participate in the normal bonding process.

Skill 11.1

THERMOREGULATION USING A RADIANT WARMER

If thermoregulation is not adequately maintained, the newborn may suffer from cold stress, which can impact oxygenation and result in hypoxia, respiratory distress, hypoglycemia, and metabolic acidosis. In some settings the baby is held by the mother immediately after birth in a "skin-to-skin" fashion with warm blankets used to protect the newborn from lower room temperatures. This maintains optimal body temperature and promotes parental bonding (Vaughns, 1990). Radiant warmers may be used to prevent heat loss while performing assessments and procedures; they can also be used therapeutically if the infant's body temperature has dropped. An isolette can also be helpful in this situation. Newborns are also at risk for hyperthermia because of their ability to perspire. Signs of hyperthermia include flushed or hot skin, lethargy, and poor feeding.

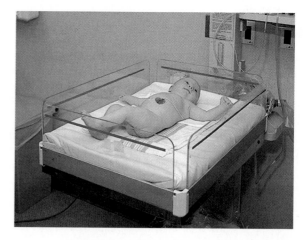

Figure 11-1   Thermal skin sensor.

Equipment

Radiant warmer
Thermal skin sensor (see Figure 11-1)
Aluminum heat deflector patch
Blankets and clothing
Thermometer

ASSESSMENT

1. Assess infant's body temperature. **Rationale: If a newborn's temperature falls below 36.4° C (97.5° F), there is an increased oxygen consumption and use of calories. This may lead to cold stress.**
2. Assess skin integrity. **Rationale: Taping the thermal skin sensor to the infant's skin may cause damage to the tissue.**

PLANNING

Expected outcomes focus on preventing complications.

Expected Outcomes

1. Infant's temperature will stabilize between 36.4° and 37.2° C (97.5° and 99° F).
2. Infant's skin integrity will remain intact.

DELEGATION CONSIDERATIONS

The skill of using a radiant heater requires problem solving and application unique to a professional nurse. For this skill, delegation is inappropriate.

IMPLEMENTATION

Steps	Rationale
1. See Standard Protocol (inside front cover).	
2. Prewarm the radiant warmer to between 36° and 37° C (96.8° and 98.6° F).	
3. Remove shirt from infant, leaving a diaper on.	
4. Place infant under the heater.	
5. Place thermal skin probe on the abdomen and attach by an aluminum heat deflector patch.	The aluminum heat deflector will prevent heating the probe and causing a false reading.
6. Set the radiant warmer controls according to agency protocol.	This will prevent hyperthermia and too rapid increase of body temperature. Rapid warming can cause apneic spells; therefore warming over a period of 2 to 4 hours is recommended.
7. Assess infant's body temperature every 30 minutes or according to agency protocol (see Skill 12.1).	Monitors temperature stability.
8. As the infant's temperature stabilizes, prewarm blankets.	Use of prewarmed blankets prevents heat loss from the infant to the cool blankets by conduction.
9. When the infant's temperature reaches 37° C (98° F), dress the infant, wrap in prewarmed blankets, and place a dry cap on the infant's head.	
10. Place infant in an open crib.	
11. Recheck axillary temperature in 1 hour.	
12. See Completion Protocol (inside front cover).	

• • •

EVALUATION

1. Assess body temperature to verify stability between 36.4° and 37.2° C (97.5° and 99° F).
2. Inspect infant's skin for absence of redness and irritation.

Unexpected Outcomes and Nursing Implications

1. Infant's body temperature is greater than 37.2° C (99° F).
   a. Remove infant from radiant warmer.
   b. Dress in T-shirt and wrap in one blanket.
   c. Retake axillary temperature in 1 hour.
2. Infant's temperature does not stabilize and stays below 36.4° C (97.5° F).
   a. Continue to use radiant warmer to reheat.
   b. Prevent drops in temperature when not under warmer by:
      (1) Keeping clothing and bedding dry.

(2) Double wrapping the infant and putting a cap on the head.

(3) Using the radiant warmer during procedures and when bathing.

(4) Warming objects that come in contact with the infant.

(5) Preventing exposure to drafts.

  c. Assess for complications that may be producing fluctuations in temperature.

  d. Assess temperature every hour until stabilized.

Recording and Reporting

- Temperature of infant before and after warming
- Length of time under the warmer
- Temperature of infant 1 hour after removing from the warmer
- Condition of skin after warming process

Sample Documentation

0915 Axillary temperature 96° F. Placed under radiant warmer, skin probe applied to abdomen.

1025 Skin temperature 98° F. Dressed, wrapped in two warmed blankets, and placed in an open crib. Skin area under probe pink, intact.

1125 Axillary temperature 97.2° F.

Skill 11.2

INFANT FEEDING

Good nutrition in infancy fosters optimal growth and development. Selection of a method of feeding is a major decision new parents face. To make an informed decision about feeding, parents must be given facts about the nutritional and immunological needs of the newborn that are met with human milk, the potential benefits to the mother's health, and the facts related to the use of infant formula. There is a special closeness that usually develops quickly between a mother who is breast-feeding and her baby. The nurse's attitude and choice of words are extremely important. Nurses should realize that when they convey positive expectations about a mother's ability to feed her baby effectively, they strongly influence the mother's sense of competence and success.

Once the choice is made, the nurse must provide support and teaching that promote success. Effective breast-feeding patterns must be learned, and several weeks may be required for both the mother and the baby to settle into a comfortable routine. The infant who is obtaining the necessary nutrients will exhibit a steady increase in weight, a regular elimination pattern, good skin and muscle tone, a vigorous feeding behavior, and a regular sleep pattern.

Mothers who are formula-feeding also need teaching and support. Emphasis on the beneficial use of feeding times for close contact and socializing with the infant is appropriate and helpful. When an infant's needs are met, a sense of trust develops between the baby and the parent. It is also important for new parents to realize that babies cry not only to communicate hunger or thirst, but also to communicate pain, boredom, and the need for human contact. Babies may act hungry and suck vigorously when they have gas pains, in which case feeding does not relieve the problem.

Many types of formulas are available, including ready-to-use, concentrate, and powder. Ready-to-use formula is used in the hospital setting, but at home many parents choose a concentrate or powder, because these are less expensive options. The amount of water used to dilute the formula must be carefully measured. If too much water is added, the infant will not get the nutrients needed for proper growth. If too little water is added, the formula will be too concentrated. Resulting in serious illness.

The schedule for introducing solid foods and the types of foods to offer are topics generally discussed at the well-baby check-ups at ages 4 and 6 months. New foods should be offered one at a time so that any reaction (gas, colic, diarrhea, vomiting, diaper rash, or other skin rashes) can be related to the suspected food and eliminated. Common allergens to be avoided for small babies include cow's milk, egg whites, oranges, and strawberries. These foods should not be offered until the infant is a year old (Wong and Perry, 1998).

Equipment

  Breast-feeding requires no special equipment.

  Bottle-feeding: A sterile nipple/bottle unit

  Infant formula: According to parent or physician preference

  Water (if concentrated formula or powdered formula is used)

ASSESSMENT

1. Assess for feeding readiness cues, which may be present even during sleep. These cues include bringing the fist to the mouth, rooting, and sucking motions.

Rationale: The optimal time to begin a feeding is when the baby exhibits these cues rather than waiting until the baby is crying and distraught.

2. Determine when the infant was last fed and the quality of that feeding time. **Rationale: Infants develop a pattern of feeding every 3 to 4 hours. If much less time has elapsed, the infant's cries may be related to some need other than feeding, such as gas, a wet or soiled diaper, or the need for human contact.**

3. Assess physical development of infant and suck reflex. **Rationale: Different positions and techniques are used depending on the developmental stage of the infant.**

4. Assess for tolerance of last feeding of formula. **Rationale: Some infants develop allergic reactions or sensitivities to a particular prepared formula.**

PLANNING

Expected outcomes focus on adequate nutritional intake and successful parent-infant bonding.

Expected Outcomes

1. Infant will consume an appropriate amount of formula (see Box 11-2) or, if breast-feeding, nurses up to 30 to 40 minutes and softens at least one breast each feeding.

2. Infant will be content for at least 2 to 2½ hours between feedings.

3. Infant will have at least six wet diapers and two bowel movements each 24 hours by 4 days of age.

4. Infant will regain birth weight in 7 to 10 days and double birth weight in 6 months.

Box 11-2 Feeding Patterns

Newborns
Typically 10 to 15 ml, gradually increasing during the first week. Most babies take 3 to 5 oz at a feeding by the end of the second week or sooner.

After 2 Weeks
Under 10 lb (4.5 kg): approximately 840 ml per 24 hours
More than 10 lb: 960 ml in 24 hours

Growth Spurts
Increased appetite occurs periodically between 10 days and 2 weeks, 6 and 9 weeks, and 3 and 6 months to correspond with growth spurts. The amount of formula placed in the bottle should be increased by ¹/₂ to 1 ounce to meet the baby's needs.

Feeding Times
During the day, newborns should be fed at least every 3 hours, even if that requires waking the baby for feedings. If the baby is fussy earlier and other comfort measures do not help, the baby may be hungry and should be fed. At night the infant with adequate weight gain can be allowed to sleep and be fed only on awakening.

Data from Wong DL, and Perry SE: *Maternal child nursing care*, St Louis, Mosby 1998.

DELEGATION CONSIDERATIONS

The skill of assisting and/or teaching a new postpartum mother with breast-feeding or bottle feeding requires the problem solving unique to a professional nurse. The skill of feeding an infant without eating or swallowing problems can be delegated to assistive personnel (AP), with instructions on the following:

- Check with the nurse for proper formula to be fed to the infant.
- Proper methods to position the infant during feeding and burping.
- Signs of choking and vomiting and how to suction the infant.
- Report signs of formula intolerance to the nurse.

IMPLEMENTATION

Steps	Rationale

1. See Standard Protocol (inside front cover).
2. Encourage thorough handwashing before infant feeding.

Assisting with Breast-Feeding
3. Assist the mother to a comfortable position.
   a. In bed with the head of the bed elevated and pillows to provide support as needed or side lying.
   b. In a chair with arms on pillows to provide additional support as needed (see illustration).

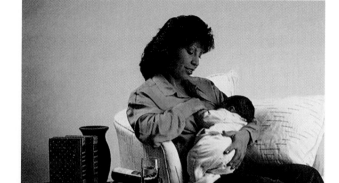

Step 3b   *Courtesy Ross Laboratories, Columbus, Ohio.*

4. Assist the mother to position the infant in one of four positions and to use a variety of positions.
   a. The football hold: tuck the baby's hips and legs under the mother's arm and support the baby's back and head with the mother's hand (see illustration).
   b. The cradle hold: cradle the baby with the baby's head in the crook of the arm nearest the breast in use. Have the baby's body facing the mother (see illustration) tummy to tummy.

Using a variety of positions minimizes pressure on the same spot of the mother's nipple and reduces the development of nipple soreness.

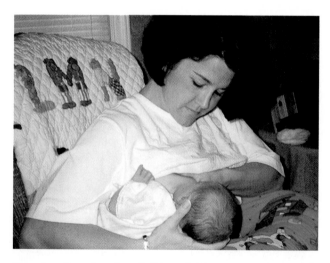

Step 4a   *From Lowdermilk DL et al: Maternity nursing, ed 5, St Louis, 1999, Mosby.*

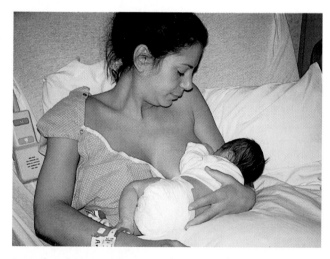

Step 4b   *Courtesy Marjorie Pyle, RNC, Lifecircle, Costa Mesa, California.*

Steps	Rationale

c. Across the lap: lay the baby on firm pillows across the mother's lap with the baby facing the mother. Support the baby's neck and shoulders within the palm of the mother's hand (see illustration).

d. Lying down: have mother lie on her side with a pillow at her back with the baby facing her. To start, have the mother prop herself up on her elbow and support her breast with that hand. Once the baby is feeding, lie down (see illustration).

5. Assist the baby to latch on to the mother's breast effectively.

a. Have the mother support the breast in one hand with the fingers underneath and the thumb on top (see illustration).

b. Have the mother lightly touch the baby's lower lip and the tip of the tongue with her nipple, which tends to encourage the baby to open the mouth.

c. When the mouth is open wide and the tongue is down, have the mother pull the baby quickly to the breast. It is important to bring the baby to the breast and not the breast to the baby.

6. Evaluate for a proper latch on.

a. The mother feels a firm tug on her nipple and no pinching or sliding sensation.

b. Ask if nursing hurts after the first 10-12 sucks. If there is pain, have the mother release the suction by placing a finger in the corner of the infant's mouth (see illustration), remove the infant from the breast, and start over.

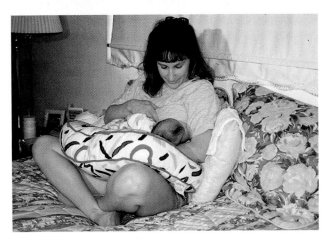

Step 4c   *Courtesy Marjorie Pyle, RNC, Lifecircle, Costa Mesa, California.*

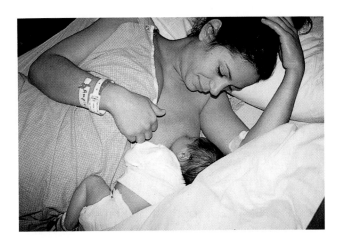

Step 4d   *Courtesy Marjorie Pyle, RNC, Lifecircle, Costa Mesa, California.*

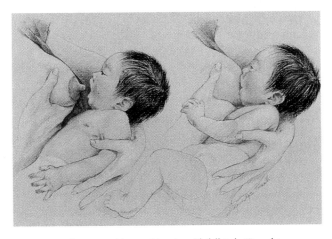

Step 5a   *Courtesy Karen Martin, Childbirth Graphics, Waco, Texas.*

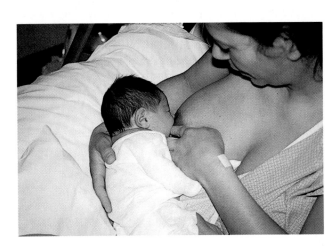

Step 6b   *Courtesy Marjorie Pyle, RNC, Lifecircle, Costa Mesa, California.*

| **Steps** | **Rationale** |

7. Assess for the following evidence of success:
   a. After the milk comes in, at least one breast softens with each feeding.
   b. The baby has bursts of 10 or more sucks and swallows at the beginning and slows down to 2 to 3 suck/swallows as the breast softens. The swallowing can be heard.
   c. As the let-down reflex occurs, there may be leaking from the other breast.
8. After the breast has softened, encourage the mother to burp the infant and, if possible or desired, continue nursing on the opposite breast. Encourage the mother to begin feedings on the opposite breast each time.

Formula Feeding

9. Identify and prepare the appropriate type and amount of formula. Room temperature formula is usually not heated.
10. Identify the infant using identification bracelet.
11. Prepare the infant by providing a clean diaper and clothing and wrap snugly.
12. Position the infant: cradle head in one hand or on one arm, support body on the lap (see illustration).
13. Place bib or small cloth under the infant's chin.
14. Touch the corner of the infant's mouth with nipple.

15. Insert nipple into mouth, holding bottle so that nipple is completely filled with formula.

16. Allow infant to suck, and observe for suck-swallow-breathe reflex.

17. Observe for choking, gagging, or regurgitation during feeding.
18. Burp infant about halfway through feeding. Place infant in a sitting position and gently rub the back in an upward direction (see illustration). Observe the infant's face for signs of choking or regurgitation. The infant may also be placed prone on the lap of the caregiver or on the shoulder.

19. Continue to feed remainder of formula.
20. Burp infant at the end of the feeding.
21. Check diaper and change if needed. Place infant in bed on right side or back.

22. Observe for choking, gagging, or regurgitation after feeding.
23. Dispose of bottle and unused formula in an appropriate container.
24. See Completion Protocol (inside front cover).

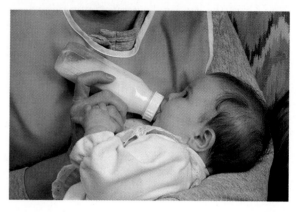

Step 12   *From Sorrentino SA: Assisting with patient care, St Louis, 1998, Mosby.*

By decreasing other discomforts, the infant will be more relaxed and able to concentrate on feeding.
Holding the head in a slightly elevated position will facilitate swallowing.

This will elicit the rooting reflex in infants under 4 to 7 months of age. The infant's mouth will open for ease of insertion of the nipple.
Allowing air into the nipple area will increase the amount of air swallowed. This may lead to abdominal distention, discomfort, and sometimes regurgitation.
The suck-swallow-breathe reflex must be present for proper feeding. Special feeding precautions should be implemented if it is absent.
The nurse must be alert to regurgitation during feeding to prevent aspiration.
By gently patting or rubbing the back, the cardiac sphincter will relax and allow the release of air that rises to the top of the stomach. When the air is removed, overdistention of the stomach is prevented.

NURSE ALERT

It is unsafe to leave an infant unattended while positioned on abdomen.

This position will prevent possible aspiration if the infant spits up. Also, because the sphincter is on the left side of the stomach, placing the infant on the right side will help prevent regurgitation of formula.

Warm formula is a source of bacterial growth. Unused formula should not be saved for later use.

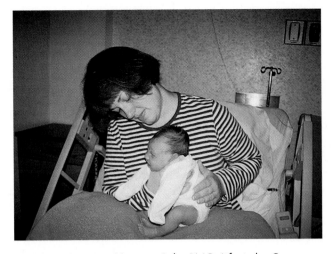

Step 18   *Courtesy Marjorie Pyle, RNC, Lifecircle, Costa Mesa, Calif.*

• • •

EVALUATION

1. Infant consumes an appropriate amount of formula (see box) or, if breast-feeding, nurses up to 30 to 40 minutes and softens at least one breast each feeding.
2. Infant is content for at least 2 to 2 ½ hours between feedings.
3. Infant has at least six wet diapers and two bowel movements each 24 hours by 4 days of age.
4. Infant regains birth weight in 7 to 10 days and doubles birth weight in 6 months.

Unexpected Outcomes and Nursing Interventions

1. Infant vomits repeatedly or develops diarrhea.
   a. Report to primary health care provider. Further assessment is necessary to determine the cause of the problem. If it is formula related, a change in the type of formula may be needed. If the care giver is using a concentrate or powder formula, the preparation technique may need to be assessed. The problem may also be related to amount of formula given, feeding techniques, or physical problems.
   b. Assess infant for dehydration:
      (1) Decreased urinary output (less than 1 ml/kg/hour)
      (2) Weight loss
      (3) Dry mucous membranes
      (4) Sunken fontanels
      (5) Poor skin turgor
      (6) Hematocrit increased by 10% or more
   c. Treat diaper area to prevent irritation.

Recording and Reporting

- Amount of formula infant drank or if breastfed, length of feeding
- Length of feeding
- How infant sucked
- Infant's tolerance of feedings
- Positive/negative bonding response of parents

Sample Documentation

0800   Took 2 ounces of Similac with Iron in 20 minutes. Infant demonstrated suck-swallow-breath reflex. No regurgitation. Observed mother calling infant by given name, talking to infant in eye-to-eye position. Mother able to properly hold infant while feeding and burping.

◤◢◤◢

Home Care and Long-Term Care Considerations

If formula is prepared with a water source in the home, checking on the safety of the water supply is important. If there is a doubt about the purity of the water supply it should be tested for safety before use. Assessing for proper refrigeration of formula is important if it is prepared ahead of time. Caregivers should be warned that formula heated in the microwave may produce hot spots that can burn the infant's mucous membranes.

Skill 11.3

INFANT BATHING

Bathing an infant is an excellent time for the nurse to assess the child and to do parent teaching. Bathing cleanses the skin and provides both sensory and social stimulation. Because of the risk for hypothermia, the infant must be kept covered to the extent possible and the bath should be completed quickly. A sponge bath is recommended until after the umbilical cord separates, usually within 10 to 14 days. After the site is completely healed, a tub bath can be given. It is adequate to bathe the infant once or twice a week and as needed when the skin is soiled with body secretions.

Equipment

Washbasin or small tub
Mild soap (type according to agency protocol)
Clean gloves
Three soft washcloths
Towel or cloth diapers
Blanket
Soft-bristled brush or fine-toothed comb
Clothing (shirt, cap, sleeper), as needed
Diaper (disposable or plain cloth and safety pins)
Cord care product as needed (according to agency
    protocol)

ASSESSMENT

1. Inspect the infant's skin for dryness, peeling, or signs of infection. **Rationale: Care of the skin during and after the bath may need to be altered to prevent infection or the spread of infections.**
2. Assess the site of the umbilical cord for redness, drainage, drying, and intactness. **Rationale: If the umbilical cord is still intact, then a sponge bath is indicated. Redness or drainage at the umbilical site may indicate irritation and/or infection.**
3. Assess the infant's temperature if at high risk for hypothermia. **Rationale: Newborns with a rectal temperature greater than 36.8° C (98° F) can be bathed at any time (Penny-MacGillivray, 1996).**
4. Assess parents' knowledge of how to give a bath and any cultural deviations that may alter the care of the infant. **Rationale: This determines the parent teaching needed and how care may need to be altered to respect the parents' cultural diversity.**

PLANNING

Expected outcomes focus on maintaining the infant's safety, maintaining skin integrity, thermoregulation, and parent teaching.

Expected Outcomes

1. Parents will demonstrate ability to safely bathe, handle, and dress the infant while maintaining body temperature.
2. Parents will identify ways to provide sensory and social stimulation while bathing the infant.

DELEGATION CONSIDERATIONS

The skill of teaching basic infant care, including bathing, handling, and dressing the infant and the initial newborn bath, requires the problem solving and professional knowledge unique to the professional nurse. The skill of bathing an infant after the initial bath can be delegated to AP, with instructions as to the following:

*   Inform care provider about early signs of impaired skin integrity and infection at the cord site. Tell provider to have nurse assess the skin if changes are noted.
*   Test the bath water for proper warmth before the bath by placing drops of water on the inside surface of the forearm. The water temperature can then be adjusted if too hot or too cold.
*   Report a pre-/post-bath axillary temperature of less than 36.8° C (98° F) to the nurse.

IMPLEMENTATION

Steps	Rationale

COMMUNICATION TIP

Talk to the infant throughout the bath to demonstrate how to provide appropriate social stimulation for the infant. Ask the parents if any specific bathing techniques or methods are important to their family or culture. Assess these techniques for safety, and, if feasible, try to incorporate them into the infant care.

1. See Standard Protocol (inside front cover).
2. Prepare washbasin with warm water at about 36.6° to 37.8° C (98° to 100° F). Nurse tests water temperature by placing drops on inside surface of forearm. Water should feel comfortably warm.

   This temperature will prevent skin burns or chilling.

3. Place infant in crib or bassinet with sides and have all supplies within reach.

   This will prevent infant falls.

   Clean gloves are to be worn if this is the first newborn bath or if the nurse is to come in contact with body secretions during any bath.

4. Keep infant covered with a blanket to maintain warmth.

   Infants are prone to hypothermia, which can be produced by evaporation during the bathing process.

5. Cleanse the eyes with plain water. Wash each eye from the inner to the outer canthus, using a clean portion of the washcloth with each swipe. If crusts are present on eyelid margins, apply a moistened washcloth for 1 to 2 minutes before cleansing.

   This prevents transferring microorganisms from one eye to the other.

6. Cleanse the external ears with plain water and a twisted end of the washcloth.

NURSE ALERT

Teach parents not to attempt to clean the internal ear with cotton-tipped applicators because of the risk of injury.

7. Cleanse the face and neck with plain water. Give special attention to areas behind the ears and creases in the neck. A very small amount of soap may be used for soiled creases, rinsing well after washing.
8. Dry face and neck with a towel using a gentle patting motion.

   Excessive rubbing may cause skin breakdown.

9. With fresh washcloth dampened with plain water, cleanse the infant's mouth. Wash inside the lips, cheeks, dorsal surface of the tongue, the roof of the mouth, and all along the upper and lower gum pads.

   Good oral hygiene removes excess breast milk or formula that stays on the infant's gums and may encourage bacteria and plaque and lead to tooth decay (Van Burg et al, 1995).

10. Cover infant's lower body with a blanket.
11. Cleanse infant's upper body with warm water and washcloth. Quickly rinse soap, if used, from the infant's hands.

    Infants frequently put a fist in the mouth, which may lead to soap ingestion if the fists are not rinsed.

12. Thoroughly rinse the rest of the upper body and dry completely by using a patting motion.
13. Cleanse the abdomen around the umbilicus with warm water, keeping the cord dry. Dry the area. Apply cord care product according to agency protocol until area is healed.

    This prevents infection.

14. Cover the upper body with a dry towel or blanket.
15. Cleanse the legs and outer buttocks with warm water. Dry thoroughly.

Steps	Rationale

16. With a fresh washcloth, cleanse the genitalia with plain water.
   a. For a female infant:
      (1) Gently retract labia and wash from front to back toward the anus. Use separate portions of the washcloth for each swipe.
      (2) Wash the other portions of the labia and the folds in the groin.
   b. For an uncircumcised male infant:
      (1) Wash from the urethra outward and down toward the scrotum.
      (2) Wash scrotum and folds of the groin.
      (3) In uncircumcised newborns the foreskin may adhere to the glans and should not be retracted.
      (4) In older children, gently retract the foreskin only as far as it will go; do not force the foreskin. Cleanse around the glans penis in circular motion, moving from the urethra outward. Dry and return the foreskin to its normal position.
   c. In a circumcised newborn, circumcision care is done.
      (1) Assess area for bleeding.
      (2) Cleanse the area gently with warm tap water and cotton gauze or cotton balls.
      (3) Sterile gauze dressing with sterile petroleum jelly added is placed between the penis and diaper. This dressing should be changed with each diaper change after the first 12-24 hours.
      (4) If a Plastibell was used in the circumcision process, the gauze and petroleum jelly may not be needed.
17. Cleanse anal area with soap, rinse and dry.
18. Apply clean diaper and remove gloves (see Skill 11.4).
19. **Shampooing infant's hair**
   a. Wrap the infant in the blanket using a swaddling technique (see Skill 11.5).
   b. Hold the infant in a "football" hold over the washbasin (see illustration) or leave infant in crib and gently pick up head, supporting it in one hand.
   c. Lather scalp with a small amount of mild soap. A soft washcloth may be used to wash the scalp if there is excess soiling.
   d. Rinse the scalp thoroughly by pouring water from a small cup over the infant's scalp into the washbasin.
   e. Dry thoroughly with a towel.
20. Comb or brush infant's hair gently.
21. Dress infant in regular clothing or sleeper if desired by parents.
22. Replace the damp sheets and blankets. Remove and discard gloves and wash hands.
23. See Completion Protocol (inside front cover).

This will prevent contamination of the urinary and vaginal areas by anal secretions.

Forcing the foreskin into a retracted position may constrict the blood vessels and cause trauma and edema. Full sparation of the foreskin may not occur for several years.

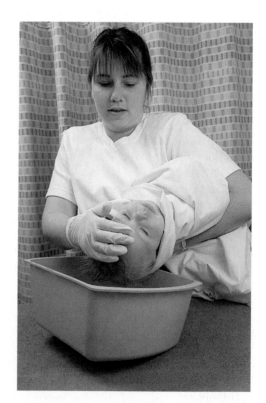

Step 19b

EVALUATION

1. Observe parents' ability to bathe, handle, and dress the infant during a return demonstration.
2. Observe parents' interactions with infant in relation to sensory and social stimulation.

Unexpected Outcomes and Nursing Interventions

1. Diaper rash develops.
   a. Immediately cleanse and thoroughly dry area after each voiding and stooling.
   b. Expose area to warm air and filtered sunlight.
2. Skin becomes very dry, cracked, and peeling
   a. Limit bathing to 2 to 3 times per week and use plain water.
   b. Avoid the use of lotions and products with perfumes or chemicals.
3. Infant experiences cradle cap.
   a. Shampoo head daily, allowing shampoo or mineral oil to remain on scalp until crusts are softened.
   b. Thoroughly rinse scalp of all soap.
   c. Use a fine-toothed comb or soft brush to gently remove loosened crusts from the strands of hair.
4. Redness and/or drainage is present around the umbilical site.
   a. Keep area clean and dry.
   b. Keep diaper folded below umbilical site to prevent irritation and to expose area to the air.
   c. Report to health care provider for additional treatment.

5. Infant's temperature falls below 36.8° C (98° F).
   a. Wrap infant in extra blanket and place cap on head.
   b. Reassess temperature in 1 hour.
6. Parents are unable to explain and demonstrate proper bath procedure.
   a. Establish rapport and allow parents to verbalize concerns.
   b. Reassess teaching techniques and learning levels.
   c. Assess for unmet needs the parents have that may prevent learning.
   d. Assess for cultural differences. Build on parent's cultural practices by reinforcing the positive and promoting change only if a practice is harmful.

Recording and Reporting

- Record temperature on the graphic sheet.
- Describe skin condition.
- Record parent teaching and response.

Sample Documentation

1030 Baby bath demonstration given. Infant's mother, father, and maternal grandmother present. Mother did return demonstration with few verbal cues and asked appropriate questions.

Skill 11.4

CHANGING A DIAPER

Hospitals have used disposable diapers for many years because of the decreased cross-contamination and reduced laundry costs. Some hospitals are now beginning to use cloth diapers in response to environmental issues. The parent's preference for cloth or disposable diapers should be supported. If an infant is readmitted to the hospital for any reason, the same type of diaper should be used if possible.

Diapers are available in a wide variety of sizes and shapes. The appropriate size is determined as that which allows the diaper to fit securely around the infant's waist and legs. If the umbilical cord is still intact, the diaper must be folded so that the umbilical cord is exposed to the air to promote drying and prevent irritation.

To fold a cloth diaper, place the cloth on a flat surface and fold the long sides toward the middle. The width can be changed as the infant grows by folding less material into the center. Folding one end can also alter the length

of the diaper. For optimal absorption of urine, the thickest area is placed toward the front for a male infant and toward the back for a female infant (see Figure 11-2, p. 216).

Equipment

Diaper (cloth or disposable)
Washcloth
Pins (if cloth diaper used)
Clean gloves

ASSESSMENT

1. Assess the infant's diaper for wetness.
2. Determine the infant's physical developmental stage. **Rationale: This will help the nurse to know the child's ability to assist by lying still or rolling over if necessary. Also, the nurse should assess for safety problems.**

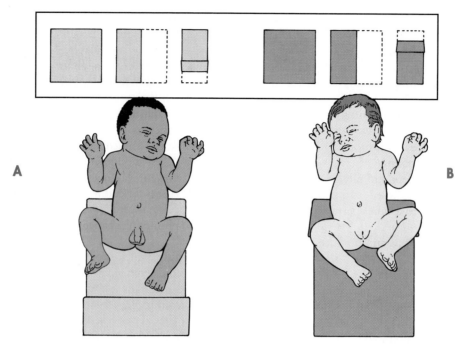

Figure 11-2 Changing a diaper. **A,** Fold cloth diaper in front for boys. **B,** The diaper has a fold in the back for girls.   *From Sorrentino SA: Assisting with patient care, St Louis, 1998, Mosby.*

3. Assess the type and size of diaper to be used. **Rationale: This should be parent choice or agency procedure.**
4. Assess for skin integrity. **Rationale: The use of diapers puts the infant at high risk for skin disorders because of prolonged contact with urine, reaction to the ammonia formation, localized irritation from the chemicals in the diaper, and/or irritation from the cleansing agents used during diaper changes.**

PLANNING

Expected outcomes focus on maintaining skin integrity and promoting comfort.

Expected Outcomes
1. Infant will be clean and dry without skin rash, irritation, or injury.
2. Diaper will fit securely and comfortably.

DELEGATION CONSIDERATIONS

The skills of diapering may be delegated to AP, with instructions to inform the nurse regarding the following:

*   Early signs of impaired skin integrity and tell provider to have nurse assess the skin when changes are noted.
*   Diaper contents (urine, meconium, diarrhea, etc.).

IMPLEMENTATION

Steps	Rationale

1. See Standard Protocol (inside front cover).
2. If using cloth diaper, fold the diaper as necessary (see Figure 11-2).

    Clean gloves should be worn when in contact with body substances.
3. Place the infant on a flat surface, keeping one hand in contact with the infant at all times.

NURSE ALERT

Do not leave infant with sides of the crib down or on changing table.

Steps	Rationale

4. Remove soiled diaper and assess the amount, color, and consistency of the contents. Roll soiled diaper so that the cleanest area is toward the outside, and place it out of the infant's reach. If diaper pins are used, close them and place out of reach of the infant. If diaper pins become dull, stick them into a bar of soap.

Diaper pins are a choking hazard. Open diaper pins can cause injury or be swallowed. Use of soap allows pins to penetrate the diaper more easily.

5. Cleanse the diaper area with damp washcloth. Clean from the front toward the anus for a female and from the tip of the penis toward the scrotum for a male. Cleanse all folds of the groin area.

Cleansing the skin removes residual urine or feces that may cause skin irritation. Cleansing from the meatus to the anus keeps from spreading microorganisms.

6. Lift the infant's buttocks with one hand and place clean diaper under the infant (see illustration).

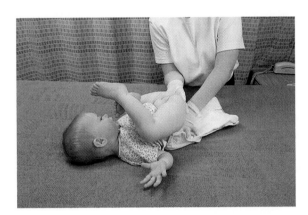

Step 6

7. Pull the diaper toward the anterior section through the legs. Fit the diaper snugly around the legs to prevent leaks. Fit the diaper around the waist and fold the diaper below the umbilical cord if it is still healing.

This promotes exposure to air, which facilitates the drying and healing process.

NURSE ALERT

When using pins, your fingers should be placed between the diaper and the infant's skin while pinning the diaper. Also, insert the pin from front to back so that the sharp point is away from the infant, thus preventing injury with the sharp point if it should come unhooked.

8. Change other clothing and/or blanket if soiled or wet.
9. Place infant in a secure crib with side rails up.
10. Dispose of the soiled diaper and gloves in the appropriate container.
11. See Completion Protocol (inside front cover).

• • •

EVALUATION
1. Diaper area is free of any skin irritation.
2. Diaper is secure. Diaper pins are securely closed.

Unexpected Outcomes and Nursing Interventions
1. Infant's skin around the perineum is red and may have macular eruptions.

   a. Change diapers more frequently.
   b. Cleanse the diaper area thoroughly with each change; if soap is used, rinse thoroughly.
   c. Following agency protocol, use a protective ointment on the skin after cleansing and drying.
   d. You may leave the area open to room air several times a day.

Recording and Reporting
- Note the number of diaper changes.
- Note the characteristics of stool and any unusual color or odor of urine.
- If infant is on intake and output monitoring, the diapers may need to be weighed before applying to infant and on removal. By subtracting the weight of the unused diaper from the weight of a used diaper, urinary output can be estimated. Record this difference on the flow sheet as output.

Sample Documentation
1100   Since 0700 small meconium stool × 1 and 3 small voids with dark yellow urine.

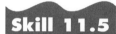

SWADDLING AND USE OF A MUMMY RESTRAINT

Parents may be taught how to swaddle their newborns as a comfort measure. Wrapping snugly often provides security, because the newborn has been accustomed to the uterine confinement. Some nurses suggest leaving the hands exposed to allow the infant to begin exploring the environment. Certain procedures and diagnostic tests require the use of a mummy restraint to keep the infant from moving and disrupting the procedure. Such restraint should be used only for short periods.

Equipment
Blanket or sheet of sufficient size to wrap infant's limbs

ASSESSMENT
1. Observe for fussiness and crying. **Rationale: If all other physical causes for crying have been eliminated, then swaddling may provide security to the infant.**
2. Identify infant's need for restraint (i.e., procedures that require the infant to be held securely). **Rationale: Restraints should be used only to maintain the safety of the infant and only for a short-term period.**

Planning
Expected outcomes focus on infant safety and security.

Expected Outcomes
1. Infant is content.
2. Infant is held securely without movement during procedure.

DELEGATION CONSIDERATIONS

The skill of swaddling for comfort may be delegated to AP. Use of a mummy restraint for a procedure may be delegated to the AP under the direct supervision of a professional nurse or physician. Restraints should be used only for a short period of time and only to maintain safety.

IMPLEMENTATION

Steps	Rationale
1. See Standard Protocol (inside front cover).	
2. Place blanket or sheet on a flat surface.	
3. Fold one corner of the sheet down toward the center.	
4. Place the infant on the sheet with shoulders toward the folded corner and feet toward the opposite corner (see illustration).	
5. Align the infant's arm toward the body, and bring the corner closest to the left arm over top of the body, tucking it under the body on the opposite side (see illustration).	By properly aligning arms before restraining them, possible injury may be avoided.

Steps	Rationale

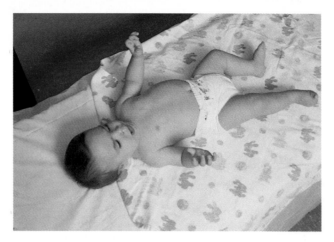

Step 4   *From Wong DL:* Whaley & Wong's nursing care of infants and children, *ed 5, St Louis, 1995, Mosby.*

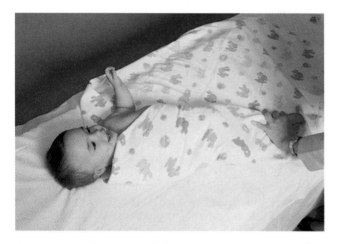

Step 5   *From Wong DL:* Whaley & Wong's nursing care of infants and children, *ed 5, St Louis, 1995, Mosby.*

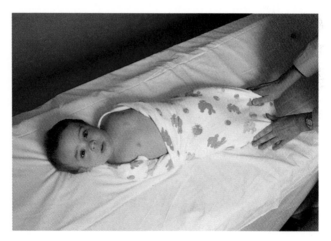

Variation for procedure involving right chest or neck.

6. Align the infant's other arm toward the body, and bring the corner closest to that arm over top of the body, tucking it under the infant's body on the opposite side (see illustration).
7. Align the infant's legs, and pull the corner of the sheet near the feet up toward the body and tuck snugly in place.

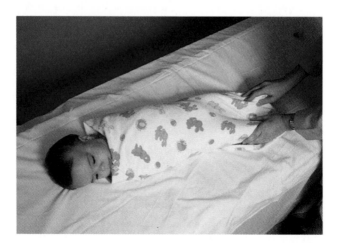

Step 6   *From Wong DL:* Whaley & Wong's nursing care of infants and children, *ed 5, St Louis, 1995, Mosby.*

Steps	Rationale

8. If a blanket is used as a restraint, remain with the infant. Remove the restraint immediately after treatment is complete. If restraint is required for an extended time, remove it at least every 2 hours and perform range of motion exercises on all extremities.

9. See Completion Protocol (inside front cover).

Restricted movement may cause circulatory problems. A restraint too tightly wrapped around the chest may cause restricted breathing.

EVALUATION

1. Infant is held securely for required procedure.
2. Inspect for evidence of altered circulation.

Unexpected Outcomes and Nursing Interventions

1. Infant's circulation is impaired.
    a. Remove restraints.
    b. Promote warmth and activity to improve circulation.

Recording and Reporting

- Reason for restraints
- Length of time in restraints
- Type of restraint used
- Assessment of circulation before and after restraining

Sample Documentation

1230   Mummy restraint used for venipuncture for 15 minutes. No evidence of circulatory compromise after restraints removed. Moves all extremities without difficulty.

REFERENCES

Association of Women's Health Nurses and Neonatal Nurses: Guideline for the care of the healthy newborn. In *Standards and guidelines for professional nursing practice in the care of women and newborns,* ed 5, Washington D.C. 1998.

Committee on Injury and Poison Prevention: Selecting and using the most appropriate car safety seats for growing children: guidelines for counseling parents, *Pediatrics* 97(5):761-763, May 1996.

Dickason E, Silverman B, Kaplan J: *Maternal-infant nursing care,* St Louis, 1998, Mosby.

Guntheroth W, Spiers P: Sleeping prone and the risk of sudden infant death syndrome, *JAMA* 267(17): 2359, 1992.

Lowdermilk D, Perry S, Bobak I: *Maternity & women's health care,* ed 6, St Louis, 1997, Mosby.

Penny-MacGillivray T: Newborn's first bath: when? *JOGNN* 25(6):481-487, 1996.

Sigman-Grant M, Bush G, Anantheswaran R: Microwave heating of infant formula: a dilemma resolved, *Pediatrics* 90(3):412-415, Sept 1992.

Van Burg MM, Sanders BJ, Weddell JA: Baby bottle tooth decay: a concern for all mothers, *Pediatr Nurs* 21(6):515-521, 1995.

Vaughns B: Early maternal-infant contact and neonatal thermoregulation, *Neonate Netw* 8(5):19, 1990.

Ventura M: Air bag safety alert, *RN* 60(4):43-44, April 1997.

Wong D: *Whaley & Wong's nursing care of infants and children,* ed 5, St Louis, 1995, Mosby.

Wong D, Perry S: *Maternal-child nursing care,* St Louis, 1998, Mosby.

CRITICAL THINKING EXERCISES

1. A teenage mother is considering breastfeeding. What information about benefits of breastfeeding is most likely to be effective in encouraging her to do it?

2. During an infant bath demonstration with the mother, father, and grandmother present, the grandmother keeps interrupting and correcting the nurse with comments such as "the baby needs to be bathed every day with plenty of soap and water" and "always use baby powder (that keeps them smelling sweet.")

3. The nurse assesses the bonding process of a newborn boy and the 17-year-old mother during feeding time. The mother lays the infant on the bed and holds the bottle in his mouth. She then turns the television on and watches a soap opera. The mother feeds the infant 2 oz without burping and then asks the nurse to take him back to the nursery.

UNIT FOUR

Assessment Skills

Chapter 12
Vital Signs

Chapter 13
Shift Assessment

Chapter 14
Comprehensive Health Assessment

Chapter 15
Laboratory and Diagnostic Tests

CHAPTER 12

Vital Signs

Skill 12.1
Assessing Temperature, Pulse, Respirations, and Blood Pressure, 231

Skill 12.2
Tympanic Temperature, 243

Skill 12.3
Electronic Blood Pressure Measurement, 245

Skill 12.4
Measuring Oxygen Saturation with Pulse Oximetry, 249

Temperature, pulse, respirations, and blood pressure (BP) are the vital signs, which indicate the body's ability to regulate body temperature, maintain blood flow, and oxygenate body tissues. Vital signs indicate clients' responses to physical, environmental, and psychological stressors. Vital signs may reveal sudden changes in a client's condition.

A change in one vital sign (e.g., pulse) can reflect changes in the other vital signs (temperature, respirations, BP). The nurse's findings aid in determining whether it is necessary to assess specific body systems more thoroughly. The nurse must be able to measure vital signs correctly, understand and interpret the values, begin interventions as needed, and report findings appropriately. Part of the nurse's clinical judgment involves deciding which vital signs to measure, when measurements should be made (Box 12-1), and when measurements can be safely delegated to assistive personnel. For example, after assessing an abnormal respiratory rate, the nurse also auscultates lung sounds. In certain situations, vital sign assessment may be limited to measurement of a single vital sign for the purpose of reviewing a specific aspect of a client's condition. For example, after administering an antihypertensive medication, the nurse measures the client's BP to evaluate the drug's effect.

Keeping clients informed of their vital signs promotes understanding of their health status.

 TEMPERATURE

Body tissues and cell processes function best within a relatively narrow temperature range between 36° and 38° C (96.8° and 100.4° F), but no single temperature is normal for all people. The temperature range of a normal adult depends on age, physical activity, status of hydration, and state of health, including the presence of infection (Table 12-1). Temperature fluctuates in a 24-hour cycle, being lowest between 1 and 4 AM, rising steadily throughout the day, and peaking at about 6 PM. Body temperature is physiologically regulated by vasodilatation, vasoconstriction,

Box 12-1 When to Take Vital Signs

1. On client's admission to a health care facility.
2. In a hospital or care facility on a routine schedule according to a physician's order or institution's standards of practice.
3. When assessing client during home health visits.
4. Before and after a surgical or invasive diagnostic procedure.
5. Before and after the administration of medications or application of therapies that affect cardiovascular, respiratory, and temperature control functions.
6. When the client's general physical condition changes (e.g., loss of consciousness or increased severity of pain).
7. Before and after nursing interventions influencing a vital sign (e.g., before and after a client previously on bed rest ambulates or before and after client performs range of motion exercises).
8. When the client reports specific symptoms of physical distress (e.g., feeling "funny" or "different").

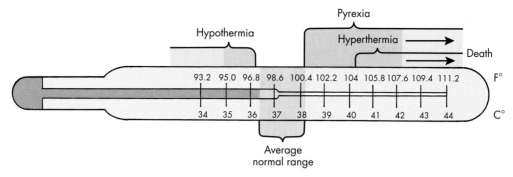

Figure 12-1 Celsius and Fahrenheit temperatures related to temperature ranges.

shivering, and sweating. Behaviorally, body temperature is adjusted by the avoidance of temperature extremes, adding or removing external clothing or coverings, and the ingestion of fluids and drugs. Average body temperature varies depending on the measurement site used; each site has advantages and disadvantages (Table 12-2). Three types of thermometers measure body temperature: mercury-in-glass, electronic, and disposable. To ensure accuracy and client safety, each type of thermometer must be used correctly and appropriately.

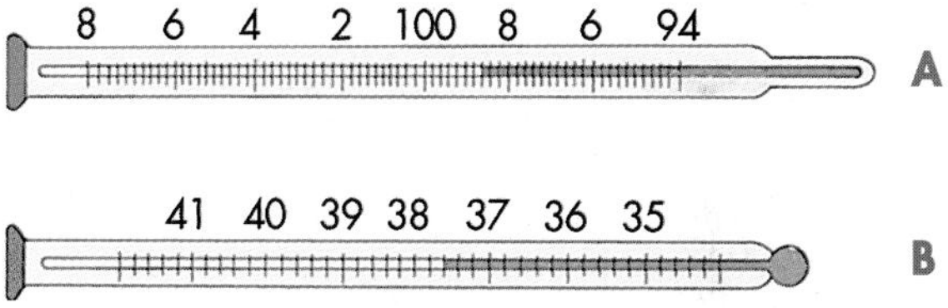

Figure 12-2 **A,** Oral or axillary thermometer. **B,** Stubby thermometer.

Types of Thermometers

Mercury-in-glass thermometers consist of a glass tube sealed at one end and a mercury-filled bulb at the other. Exposure of the bulb to heat causes the mercury to expand and rise in the tube. Glass thermometers may have either a Celsius or a Fahrenheit scale (Figure 12-1). Conversion charts are available to convert from one system to the other. Glass thermometers are available with a slim-tipped bulb for oral use, a pear-shaped bulb for rectal use, and a stubby-tipped bulb for use orally or rectally (Figure 12-2). The slim-tipped or stubby-tipped glass thermometer can be used for axillary temperatures. To reduce the risk of cross-contamination, a glass thermometer is stored at the client's bedside and sent home when the client is discharged. If a mercury-in-glass thermometer is broken, the nurse must take immediate action to protect the client and the environment (Box 12-2, p. 225). Special procedures are implemented for decontaminating a mercury spill area.

Electronic thermometers consist of a rechargeable battery-powered display unit, a thin wire cord, and a temperature-processing probe covered by a disposable cover (Figure 12-3, p. 225). Separate probes are available for oral temperature measurement (blue tip) and rectal temperature measurement (red tip). A special form of electronic thermometer is used exclusively for tympanic temperature. An otoscope-like speculum with an infrared sen-

Table 12-1

Vital Signs: Normal Ranges for Adults

Vital Sign	Normal Ranges
TEMPERATURE	
Oral/tympanic	37.0° C; 98.6° F (range, ± 1° F)
Rectal	37.6° C; 99.6° F (range, ± 1 − F)
Axillary	36.4° C; 97.6° F (range, ± 1 − F)
PULSE	60-100 beats/min, strong and regular
RESPIRATIONS	12-20 breaths/min, deep and regular
BP*	Systolic: 90-140 mm Hg (average, 120) Diastolic: less than 90 mm Hg
PULSE PRESSURE	30–50 mm Hg

*In some clients, BP is consecutively measured lying, sitting, and standing or in both arms. In normal individuals the change from lying to standing causes a decrease in systolic BP of less than 15 mm Hg (Barkauskas et al, 1994). Record the position and extremity, and compare the measurements for significant differences.

Table 12-2

Advantages and Disadvantages of Frequently Selected Temperature Measurements Sites and Methods

Advantages	Disadvantages
TYMPANIC MEMBRANE SENSOR	
Easily accessible site	Hearing aids must be removed before measurement
Minimal client repositioning required	Should not be used with clients who have had surgery of the ear or tympanic membrane
Provides accurate core reading	Does not accurately measure core temperature changes during and after exercise (Yeo and Scarbough, 1996)
Very rapid measurement (2–5 sec)	
Can be obtained without disturbing or waking client	Should not be used in newborns because of weak correlation with rectal and axillary temperatures (Bliss-Holtz, 1995)
Eardrum close to hypothalamus; sensitive to core temperature changes	Requires disposable probe cover
	Expensive
ELECTRONIC THERMOMETER	
Plastic sheath unbreakable; ideal for children	May be less accurate by axillary route
Quick readings	
RECTAL SITE	
Contended to be more reliable when oral temperature cannot be obtained	May lag behind core temperature during rapid temperature changes
	Should not be used with clients who have had rectal surgery, a rectal disorder, or bleeding tendencies
	Should not be used for routine vital signs in newborns
	Requires positioning and may be a source of client embarrassment and anxiety
	Risk of body fluid exposure
	Requires lubrication
ORAL SITE	
Accessible–requires no position change	Affected by ingestion of fluids or foods, smoke, and oxygen delivery (Neff J, et al, 1992)
Comfortable for client	Should not be used with clients who have had oral surgery, trauma, history of epilepsy, or shaking chills
Provides accurate surface temperature reading	
Indicates rapid change in core temperature	Should not be used with infants, small children, or confused, unconscious, or uncooperative clients
	Risk of body fluid exposure
AXILLARY SITE	
Safe and noninvasive	Not recommended to detect fever in infants and young children (Haddock, Merrow, and Swanson, 1996).
Can be used with newborns and uncooperative clients	Long measurement time
	Requires continuous positioning by nurse
	Measurement lag behind core temperature during rapid temperature changes
	Requires exposure of thorax
SKIN	
Inexpensive	Lags behind other sites during temperature changes, especially during hyperthermia
Provides continuous reading	Diaphoresis or sweat can impair adhesion
Safe and noninvasive	

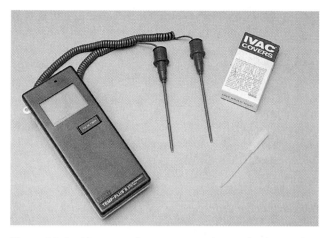

Figure 12-3   Electronic thermometer. *Blue probe* for oral or axillary use. *Red probe* for rectal use.

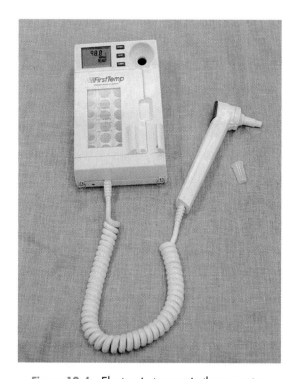

Figure 12-4   Electronic tympanic thermometer.

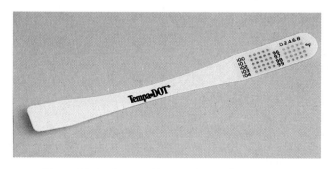

Figure 12-5   Disposable, single-use thermometer.

Box 12-2 Steps to Take in the Event of a Mercury Spill

1. Do NOT touch spilled mercury droplets. If skin contact has occurred, immediately flush area with water for 15 minutes.
2. If possible, remove client from immediate contaminated environment.
3. Change any clothing or linen that has been contaminated with mercury. Wash hands thoroughly after changing. Wash clothing before reuse.
4. Notify the Environmental Services Department or obtain a mercury spill kit if available.
5. Follow procedures for mercury removal as directed by Material Safety Data Sheet (MSDS). Spills are removed using special absorbent materials, filtered vacuum equipment, and protective clothing.
6. Promote exhaust ventilation to reduce concentration of mercury vapors.
7. Complete occurrence report as directed by institution procedure.

sor tip detects heat radiated from the tympanic membrane of the ear (Figure 12-4). Electronic thermometers display digital readings in Celsius or Fahrenheit in less than a minute.

Disposable, single-use thermometers are thin strips of plastic with chemically impregnated paper (Figure 12-5). Temperature changes the chemical dots on the paper to reflect a skin temperature, usually within 45 seconds. One type of chemical strip adheres to the skin. Disposable temperature strips are used to screen clients for altered temperature and are not appropriate for monitoring temperature therapies.

PULSE

The pulse is a palpable bounding of blood flow caused by pressure wave transmission from the left ventricle to the aorta, large arteries, and peripheral arteries. Assessing the pulse provides indications of heart function and tissue perfusion (circulation). In adults the radial pulse is the site for routine pulse assessment (Figure 12-6, p. 226). The brachial or apical pulse is the site for routine pulse assessment in infants. The pulse should be easily palpable, regular in rhythm, and range between 60 and 100 beats/min in adults. When palpated, a normal pulse does not fade in and out and is not easily obliterated by pressure. If abnormalities are identified, such as an irregular rhythm or an inability to access or palpate the radial pulse, an apical pulse must be obtained (Figure 12-7, p. 226). The apical pulse, the most accurate measure of heart rate and rhythm, is obtained us-

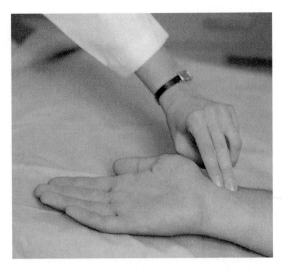

Figure 12-6 Palpating the right radial pulse.

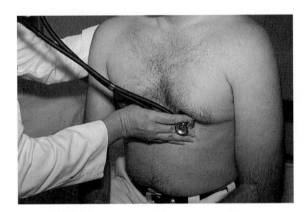

Figure 12-7 Assessing apical pulse.

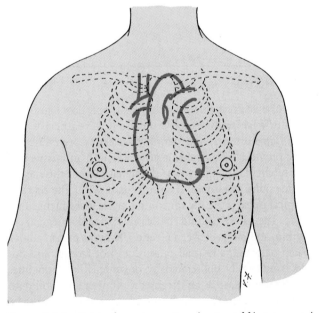

Figure 12-8 Point of maximum impulse is at fifth intercostal space.

ing a stethoscope. The stethoscope magnifies the sounds as they are transmitted from the chest wall, through the tubing, to the listener. The apical pulse is auscultated (heard with a stethoscope) by placing the diaphragm over the point of maximum impulse at the fifth intercostal space on the left midclavicular line (Figure 12-8).

Familiarity and practice using a stethoscope improve assessment skills (Box 12-3). Pulse abnormalities include bradycardia (pulse less than 60 beats/min), tachycardia (pulse greater than 100 beats/min), and dysrhythmia (irregular pulse). *Weak, feeble,* and *thready* are descriptive words for a pulse of low volume that is difficult to palpate. *Bounding* is the term used to describe a pulse that is easy to palpate. Strength (amplitude) of pulses may be rated by the following scale: 4+ bounding, 3+ full, 2+ normal, 1+ weak, 0+ absent. Changes in the pulse can reflect the client's metabolic rate and physiological responses to stress, exercise, blood loss, and pain.

RESPIRATIONS

Movement of air between the environment and the lungs involves three interrelated processes: *ventilation,* which is mechanical movement of air in and out of the lungs; *diffusion,* which involves movement of respiratory gases (oxygen and carbon dioxide) between the alveoli and red blood cells (RBCs); and *perfusion,* which involves distribution of blood through the pulmonary capillaries.

These processes are evaluated by observing the rate, depth, and rhythm of respiratory movements. *Rate* refers to the number of times the person breathes in and out in 1 minute. *Depth* of respirations is estimated by observing the movement of the chest during inspiration and can be described as deep or shallow. *Rhythm* of respirations is normally regular; however, irregular respiration patterns may occur (Table 12-3, p. 228).

Breathing patterns can be determined by observing the chest or the abdomen. Diaphragmatic breathing results from the contraction and relaxation of the diaphragm and is most visible in the abdomen. Healthy men and children usually demonstrate diaphragmatic breathing, whereas women breathe more with the thorax, most apparent in the upper chest (Figure 12-9, p. 228). Labored respirations usually involve the accessory muscles of respiration in the neck. When something such as a foreign body interferes with the movement of air into the lungs, the intercostal spaces retract during inspiration. A longer expiration phase is evident when the outward flow of air is obstructed (e.g., asthma). If a client is experiencing *dyspnea,* a subjective experience of inadequate or difficult breathing, lung sounds should be assessed with a stethoscope. In some clients, abnormal sounds, such as wheezing, can be heard even without a stethoscope. Dyspnea may be associated with increased effort to inhale and exhale and active use of

Box 12-3 Learning to Use a Stethoscope

1. Place earpieces in both ears with tips of earpieces turned toward the face. *Lightly* blow against the diaphragm (flat side of chestpiece). Now place the earpieces in both ears with the tips turned toward the back of the head and again blow against the diaphragm. Compare comfort in the ears and amplification of sounds with earpieces in both directions. Most people find pointing earpieces toward the face more comfortable and effective.

2. If the stethoscope has both a diaphragm (flat side) and a bell (bowl shaped with a rubber ring) (see illustration below) put earpieces in ears and lightly blow against the diaphragm. If sound is faint, lightly blow into the bell. Then turn the chestpiece and blow again against both the diaphragm and the bell. NOTE: The chestpiece can be turned to allow sound to be carried through either side (bell or diaphragm) of the chestpiece. The diaphragm is used for higher-pitched heart sounds, bowel sounds, and lung sounds. The bell is used for lower-pitched heart sounds and vascular sounds (see illustration below).

3. With earpieces in place and amplification set for the diaphragm, move the diaphragm lightly over the hair on your arm. The bristling sound mimics a sound heard in the lungs. When listening for significant sounds, the diaphragm should be held firmly and still eliminating extraneous sounds.

4. Place the diaphragm over the front of your chest and listen to your own breathing, comparing the bell and the diaphragm. Repeat the process while listening to your heart beat. Ask someone to speak in a conversational tone and note how the speech detracts from hearing clearly. When using a stethoscope, both the client and the examiner should remain quiet.

5. With the earpieces in your ears, gently tap tubing. Note that this also generates extraneous sounds. When listening to a client, maintain a position that allows tubing to extend straight and hang free. Movement may allow tubing to rub or bump objects, creating extraneous sounds. Kinked tubing muffles sounds.

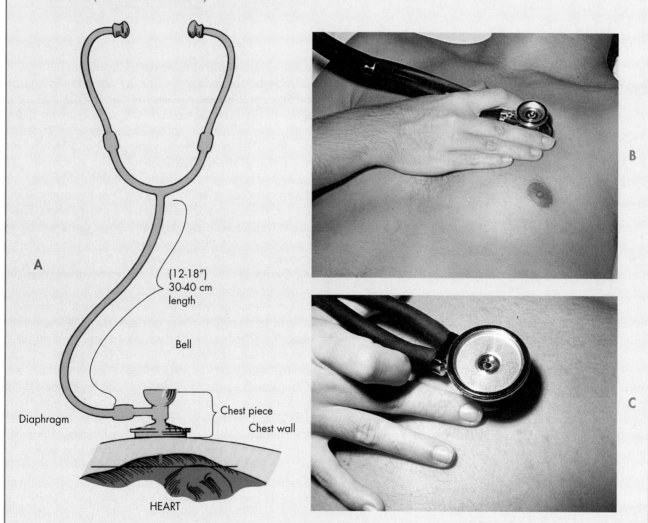

A, Parts of a stethoscope. **B,** The diaphragm is placed firmly and securely when auscultating high-pitched lung and bowel sounds. **C,** The bell must be placed lightly on the skin to hear low-pitched vascular and heart sounds.

Table 12-3

Alterations in Breathing Pattern

Alteration	Description	Alteration	Description
Bradypnea	Rate of breathing is regular but abnormally slow (less than 12 breaths/min).	Cheyne-Stokes respiration	Respiratory rate and depth are irregular, characterized by alternating periods of apnea and hyperventilation. Respiratory cycle begins with slow, shallow breaths that gradually increase to abnormal rate and depth. The pattern reverses, and breathing slows and becomes shallow, climaxing in apnea before respiration resumes.
Tachypnea	Rate of breathing is regular but abnormally rapid (greater than 20 breaths/min).		
Hyperpnea	Respirations are increased in depth. Hyperpnea occurs normally during exercise.		
Apnea	Respirations cease for several seconds. Persistent cessation results in respiratory arrest.		
		Kussmaul respiration	Respirations are abnormally deep but regular.
Hyperventilation	Rate and depth of respirations increase. Hypocarbia may occur	Biot's respiration	Respirations are abnormally shallow for 2 to 3 breaths followed by irregular period of apnea.
Hypoventilation	Respiratory rate is abnormally low, and depth of ventilation may be depressed. Hypercarbia may occur.		

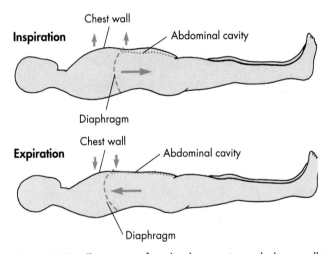

Figure 12-9 Illustration of a diaphragmatic and chest wall movement during inspiration and expiration.

intercostal and accessory muscles. *Orthopnea* is difficulty breathing while lying flat and is relieved by sitting or standing. Lung sounds should also be assessed if the client has excessive secretions, complains of chest pain, or has sustained trauma to the chest (see Chapter 14).

BLOOD PRESSURE

Blood pressure (BP) is the force exerted by the blood against the vessel walls. The systolic pressure is the peak pressure occurring during the heart's contraction as blood is forced under high pressure into the aorta. The level of pressure before the next ventricular compression and the minimal pressure exerted against the arterial wall at all times is the diastolic pressure. BP reflects many factors within the circulatory system including: cardiac output, peripheral resistance, blood volume, blood viscosity, and vessel wall elasticity. When the heart fails to contract adequately (e.g., congestive heart failure), the decreased cardiac output can result in a low BP. Peripheral resistance is increased when peripheral vessels constrict, such as during stress, which results in a high BP. Drugs can affect BP by changing one or all the factors regulating the circulatory system.

Normally, the volume of blood circulating remains constant: approximately 5000 ml in an adult. If circulating blood volume increases, such as after a rapid intravenous (IV) infusion, BP may temporarily rise. During hemorrhage or dehydration, BP falls. Vessel wall elasticity is affected by arteriosclerosis when the fibrous tissue in the arterial walls does not stretch easily. Arteriosclerosis contributes to a sustained elevated BP, or hypertension. Hypertension is a major contributing factor for death, heart attack, and cerebrovascular accident (CVA, stroke) in the United States and Canada. Factors that increase the risk of arteriosclerosis and hypertension include obesity, increased sodium intake, smoking, and lack of exercise. The diagnosis of hypertension in nonpregnant adults is made when an average of two or more diastolic readings on at least two subsequent visits is 90 mm Hg or higher or when the average of multiple systolic BP on two or more subsequent visits is consistently higher than 140 mm Hg. One BP recording does not qualify as a diagnosis of hypertension.

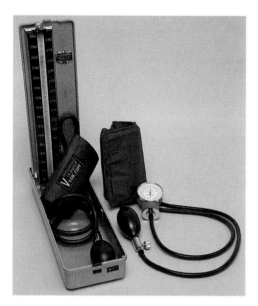

Figure 12-10   *Right,* Mercury and, *left,* aneroid sphygmomanometers.

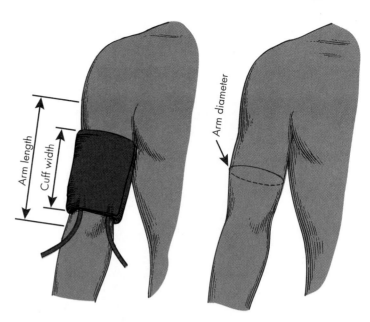

Figure 12-11   Guidelines for proper cuff size. Current width 20% more than upper arm diameter, or 40% of circumference and two-thirds of arm length.

Measurement of BP requires the use of a sphygmomanometer and a stethoscope. A sphygmomanometer includes a pressure manometer, an occlusive cloth cuff that encloses an inflatable rubber bladder, and a pressure bulb with a release valve that inflates the bladder. There are two types of manometers: mercury and aneroid (Figure 12-10). Both types can be wall-mounted or portable units. The mercury manometer is an upright tube containing mercury. Pressure created by inflation of the bladder moves the column of mercury upward against the force of gravity. Millimeter calibrations mark the height of the mercury column. When using a mercury manometer, care must be taken to protect the device from damage, because mercury is a potentially toxic substance. The mercury column must be at zero when the cuff is deflated. When reading BP values, the mercury column must be at eye level and fall freely when the cuff pressure is released. The aneroid manometer has a glass-enclosed circular gauge containing a needle that registers millimeter calibrations. The metal parts of an aneroid manometer are subject to temperature expansion and contraction; routine maintenance for calibration is required. The needle of the aneroid manometer should move freely when the cuff pressure is released. Although the circular gauge of the aneroid manometer is easy to read when measuring BP, the mercury manometer is the most accurate of the sphygmomanometers.

The cuff of the sphygmomanometer contains an inflatable bladder that is placed around the arm. Results will not be accurate unless the correct-sized BP cuff is used (Figure 12-11). The cuff is quickly inflated until blood flow ceases. The cuff is slowly deflated while the mercury column falls gradually (mercury manometer) or the aneroid

needle begins to fall. Korotkoff sounds are auscultated with the stethoscope (Figure 12-12, p. 230). Korotkoff sounds are auscultated over the artery distal to the BP cuff. In some clients the sounds are clear and distinct, whereas in others, only the beginning and ending sounds are heard. The BP is recorded with the systolic and diastolic numbers written as a fraction. The systolic pressure is the first sound heart. Before the sounds cease, they may become distinctly muffled (second sound). The diastolic pressure is the third and last sound heard. The American Heart Association (AHA, 1993) recommends that in adults the systolic and diastolic BP readings are identified and recorded by the pressures corresponding to the first of two consecutive sounds heard and the disappearance of sounds (not muffling) respectively. Confirm the last sounds by continuing to listen for 10-20 mmHg below the last sound heard.

The nurse promotes accuracy in measurement by being aware of the various factors that influence accurate BP values when a stethoscope and sphygmomanometer are used (Table 12-4, p. 230). The importance of accuracy in BP measurement cannot be overemphasized.

NURSING DIAGNOSES

When a client's body temperature is above the upper range of normal (over 38° C or 100.4° F), the nursing diagnosis is **hyperthermia.** Conversely, a body temperature below the lower value of 36° C (96.8° F) is **hypothermia. Risk for Altered Body Temperature** is an appropriate nursing di-

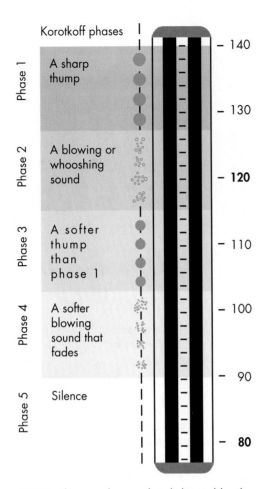

Korotkoff phases

Phase 1 — A sharp thump
Phase 2 — A blowing or whooshing sound
Phase 3 — A softer thump than phase 1
Phase 4 — A softer blowing sound that fades
Phase 5 — Silence

— 140
— 130
— **120**
— 110
— 100
— 90
— **80**

Figure 12-12 The sounds ausculated during blood pressure measurement can be differentiated into five Korotoff phases. In this example the blood pressure is 140/90.

Table 12-4	
Common Mistakes in BP Assessment	
Error Causing False Low	Errors Causing False High

Bladder or cuff too wide
Cuff wrapped too loosely
Deflating cuff too quickly
  (false low systolic)
Inflation level too low
Arm placed above level
  of heart
	Bladder cuff too narrow
	Deflating cuff too slowly
	Deflating cuff too quickly
	  (false high diastolic)
	Stopping during deflation
	  and reinflating to recheck
	Failure to wait 30 seconds
	  before repeating BP
	Arm placed lower than level
	  of heart

NOTE: Multiple examiners using different Korotkoff sounds for diastolic readings results in inaccurate records. Inflating cuff too slowly results in decreased quality of Korotkoff sounds.

agnosis for a client who demonstrates risk factors for hypothermia because the client is unable to maintain a body temperature within a normal range. Clients at risk include those at the extremes of age (elderly and the young), the extremes in weight (obese and malnourished), and exposure to environmental extremes. Altered health status, including dehydration, infection, surgery, compromised neurological status, medication use, and alcohol consumption can affect body temperature. **Ineffective Thermoregulation** is an appropriate nursing diagnosis when an individual's body temperature fluctuates between hyperthermia and hypothermia. This may be related to ineffective temperature-regulating mechanisms.

Decreased Cardiac Output is manifested by decreased BP, decreased or irregular peripheral pulses, and/or difficulty breathing. Decreased cardiac output to meet body demands increases the risk of **Activity Intolerance** (Kim, McFarland, & McLane, 1997). Activity Intolerance should be considered when an individual has insufficient energy to endure or complete required or desired daily activities.

Ineffective Airway Clearance is appropriate for clients who are unable to clear secretions or obstructions and maintain airway patency. **Ineffective Breathing Pattern** is appropriate when the client's rate, depth, and rhythm of respirations or chest and abdominal movements are not adequate for gas exchange to occur. Decreased energy, pain, musculoskeletal disease, or neurological dysfunction can contribute to ineffective breathing patterns. **Impaired Gas Exchange** refers to altered oxygen or carbon dioxide exchange in the lungs or at the cellular level. The lowered oxygen level can be assessed by noting circumoral, nailbed, or mucous membrane cyanosis, tachycardia, dizziness, and mental confusion.

Altered Tissue Perfusion (Cardiopulmonary, Peripheral) should be considered when a client exhibits decreased pulses, cold extremities, and BP changes. A decreased BP, increased pulse rate, and increased body temperature can characterize a state of **Fluid Volume Deficit.** In this condition, clients have decreased body fluids from hemorrhage or failure of body regulatory mechanisms (e.g., diabetes insipidus). **Fluid Volume Excess** is noted by altered respirations, BP changes, and abnormal breath sounds (see Chapter 13), (Kim et al, 1997).

Skill 12.1

ASSESSING TEMPERATURE, PULSE, RESPIRATIONS, AND BLOOD PRESSURE

The nurse routinely obtains a baseline measurement of vital signs at initial contact with a client to provide a means for comparison with subsequent vital sign values. This skill includes temperature measurement with an electronic thermometer using the oral, rectal, and axillary sites, palpating the radial pulse, and auscultating an upper extremity BP.

Equipment

Electronic thermometer
Oral and rectal probes
Disposable probe covers
Water-soluble lubricant (for rectal measurements only)
Stethoscope
Sphygmomanometer
BP cuff of appropriate size
Alcohol swab
Watch that displays seconds
Vital signs flow sheet

ASSESSMENT

1. Consider normal daily fluctuations in vital signs. **Rationale: BP and body temperature tend to be lowest in early morning, peak in late afternoon, and gradually decline during the night. When temperatures are taken between 5 pm and 7 pm, fever is more accurately assessed** (Beaudry et al, 1996).

2. Identify medications or treatments that may influence vital signs. **Rationale: Antiarrhythmics, cardiotonics, antihypertensives, vasodilators, and constrictors affect BP and pulse rate. Antiinflammatory drugs, steroids, warming or cooling blankets, and fans affect temperature. Oxygen and bronchodilators affect respiratory assessment.**

3. Identify factors that influence vital signs. **Rationale: Exercise increases metabolism and heat production, resulting in increased temperature, pulse, respirations, and BP. Anxiety and pain also tend to increase vital signs through hormonal and neural stimulation.**

4. Identify factors likely to interfere with accuracy of temperature reading or blood pressure. **Rationale: Temperature can be altered by intake of hot or cold food and fluids, and smoking. Blood pressure and pulse can be altered by caffeine and nicotine. Wait 30 minutes after ingestion/use of substances before measuring vital signs.**

5. Identify conditions that influence blood pressure. **Rationale: High BP is associated with pain, rapid IV infusion of fluids or blood products, increased intracranial pressure, cardiovascular disease, and renal disease. Low BP is associated with rapid vasodilation, shock, hemorrhage, and dehydration.**

6. Assess pertinent laboratory values, including complete blood count (CBC) and arterial blood gases (ABGs). **Rationale: A low hemoglobin, hematocrit, and RBC count are associated with decreased oxygen transport to tissues and hypoxia. ABGs reflects adequacy of oxygenation and ventilation (see Appendix D). Low hemoglobin levels, decreased oxygenation, and decreased ventilation can increase pulse rate, BP readings, and respiratory rate. A WBC count greater than 12,000 in a nonpregnant adult suggests the presence of infection, which can lead to hyperthermia; a WBC count less than 5000 suggests that the body's ability to fight infection is compromised, which can lead to ineffective thermoregulation.**

7. Determine previous baseline vital signs from client's record. **Rationale: This allows the nurse to assess for change in condition by comparing future temperature measurements.**

8. Determine appropriate temperature site for client, considering advantages and disadvantages of each site (see Table 12-2).

9. Determine device most appropriate for client. **Rationale: Mercury-in-glass thermometer is used for client who is on isolation precautions (Box 12-4, p. 240). Electronic BP device can be used when frequent measurements are required.**

PLANNING

Expected outcomes focus on identifying abnormalities and restoring homeostasis.

Expected Outcomes

1. Client's vital signs are within normal range for client's age group.
2. Client identifies factors that influence vital signs.
3. Baseline is established for clients with chronic diseases such as arteriosclerosis, that alter vital signs.
4. Client states strategies to reduce personal risk factors for hypertension.

DELEGATION CONSIDERATIONS

The skill of vital sign measurements can be delegated to assistive personnel (AP). After staff have shown competency delegate to trained assistive personnel by clarifying:

- Appropriate route and device for assigned client to measure temperature.

- Any special considerations for positioning a client for vital signs.
- Client history of, or risk for abnormal vital signs.
- Appropriate limb for BP measurement.
- Appropriate-size BP cuff for designated extremity.
- Frequency of specific vital sign measurements.
- Need to report any abnormalities to the nurse.

IMPLEMENTATION

Steps	Rationale

1. See Standard Protocol (inside front cover).
2. Assist client to comfortable position either lying or sitting. Avoid injured arm or one with IV infusion, previous breast or axilla surgery, cast, or arteriovenous shunt for renal dialysis.

Good circulation facilitates accuracy in BP measurement. BP measurement temporarily disrupts circulation.

3. **Oral temperature**
   a. Remove thermometer pack from charging unit; attach oral (blue tip) probe to thermometer unit. Grasp top of probe stem, being careful not to apply pressure on the ejection button. Slide disposable plastic probe cover over thermometer probe until cover locks in place (see illustration).

   b. Ask client to open mouth, and gently place probe under tongue in posterior sublingual pocket lateral to center of lower jaw (see illustration). Ask client to hold thermometer with lips closed.

Heat from superficial blood vessels in sublingual pocket produces temperature reading. With electronic thermometer, temperatures in right and left posterior sublingual pockets are significantly higher than in area under front of tongue.

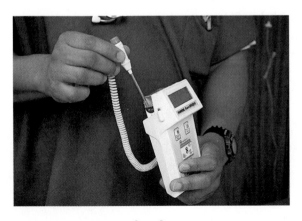

Step 3a

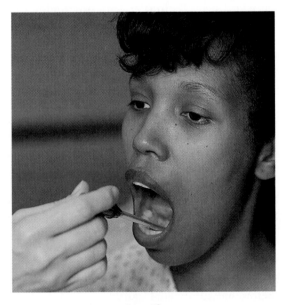

Step 3b

Steps	Rationale
c. When audible signal indicates completion, note reading and remove probe from under tongue. Inform client of temperature reading and record measurement.	Probe must stay in place until signal occurs to ensure accurate reading.
d. Push ejection button on thermometer stem to discard plastic probe cover into an appropriate receptacle. Return probe to storage position of thermometer unit. Return thermometer to charger.	Returning probe automatically causes digital reading to disappear.

NURSE ALERT

If temperature is abnormal, repeat measurement. If indicated, select an alternative site or instrument.

4. Rectal temperature

a. Draw curtain around bed and/or close room door. Assist client to Sims' position with upper leg flexed. Move aside bed linen to expose only anal area. Keep client's upper body and lower extremities covered with sheet or blanket.

Maintains client's privacy, minimizes embarrassment and promotes comfort.

NURSE ALERT

Use of rectal thermometer is not recommended following anal surgery, in client with history of decreased platelets, and children with diarrhea (Haddock, 1996). Use of rectal temperatures in neonates is controversial because of the danger of rectal perforation. Recent information indicates rectal measurement is more accurate for detection of high fevers and the risk of perforation is less than one in two million measurements (Morley et al, 1992).

b. Remove thermometer pack from charging unit, and attach rectal (red tip) probe to thermometer unit. Grasp top of probe stem, being careful not to apply pressure on the ejection button. Slide disposable plastic probe cover over thermometer probe until cover locks in place.

c. Squeeze liberal portion of lubricant on tissue. Dip thermometer's blunt end into lubricant, covering 2.5 to 3.5 cm (1 to 1½ inches) for adult.

Lubrication minimizes trauma to rectal mucosa during insertion. Tissue avoids contamination of remaining lubricant in container.

d. With nondominant hand, separate client's buttocks to expose anus. Ask client to breathe slowly and relax.

Relaxes anal sphincter for easier thermometer insertion.

e. Gently insert thermometer into anus in direction of umbilicus. 3.5 cm (1½ inches) for adult. Do not force thermometer. If resistance is felt during insertion, withdraw thermometer immediately.

Steps	Rationale
f. Hold thermometer probe in place until audible signal indicates completion, remove thermometer from anus, and note reading.	Probe must stay in place until signal occurs to ensure accurate reading.
g. Push ejection button on thermometer stem to discard plastic probe cover into appropriate receptacle. Return probe to storage position of thermometer unit.	Returning probe automatically causes digital reading to disappear.
h. Wipe client's anal area with soft tissue to remove lubricant or feces. Discard tissue and remove gloves.	
i. Inform client of temperature reading and record measurement. Return thermometer to charger.	

5. Axillary temperature

Steps	Rationale
a. Draw curtain around bed and/or close room door. Assist client to supine or sitting position and move clothing or gown away from shoulder and arm.	Maintains client's privacy, minimizes embarrassment, and promotes comfort. Exposes axilla for correct thermometer probe placement.

NURSE ALERT
In an infant or young child it may be necessary to hold the arm against the child's side when using the axillary method. If infant is in a side-lying position, the lower axilla will record the higher temperature.

Steps	Rationale
b. Remove thermometer pack from charging unit; attach oral (blue tip) probe to thermometer unit. Grasp top of probe stem, being careful not to apply pressure on the ejection button. Slide disposable plastic probe cover over thermometer probe until cover locks in place.	
c. Insert thermometer probe into center of axilla, lower arm over thermometer, and place arm across client's chest.	Maintains proper placement of thermometer against blood vessels in axilla.
d. Hold thermometer in place until audible signal indicates completion, remove thermometer from axilla, and note reading. Inform client of temperature reading and record measurement.	Probe must stay in place until signal occurs to ensure accurate reading.
e. Push ejection button on thermometer stem to discard plastic probe cover into appropriate receptacle. Return probe to storage position of thermometer unit. Return thermometer to charger.	Returning probe automatically causes digital reading to disappear.

6. Pulse

Steps	Rationale
a. If client is supine, place client's forearm straight alongside or across lower chest or upper abdomen with wrist extended straight (see illustration). If client is sitting, bend client's elbow 90 degrees and support lower arm on chair or on nurse's arm. Slightly flex the wrist with palm down.	Relaxed position of lower arm and extension of wrist permits full exposure of artery to palpation.
b. Place tips of first two fingers of hand over groove along the radial or thumb side of the client's inner wrist (see illustration).	Fingertips are most sensitive parts of hand to palpate arterial pulsation. Nurse's thumb has pulsation that may interfere with accuracy.
c. Lightly compress against radius, obliterate pulse initially, and then relax pressure so pulse becomes easily palpable.	
d. Determine strength of pulse. Note whether thrust of vessel against fingertips is bounding, strong, weak, or thready.	

Steps	Rationale

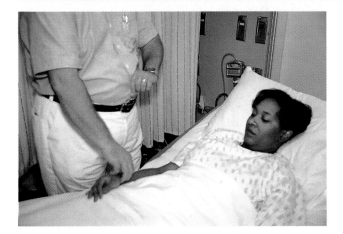

Step 6a

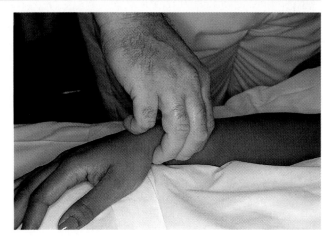

Step 6b

e. After pulse can be felt regularly, look at watch's second hand and begin to count rate: when sweep hand hits number on dial, start counting with zero, then one, two, and so on.

If pulse is regular, count rate for 30 seconds and multiply total by 2.

If pulse is irregular, count rate for 60 seconds. Assess frequency and pattern of irregularity.

7. **Respirations**

a. Without changing the position of your hand on the pulse, observe one complete respiratory cycle (one inspiration and one expiration) (see illustration).

Rate is determined accurately only after nurse is assured pulse can be palpated. Timing begins with zero. Count of one is first beat palpated after timing

A 30-second count is accurate for regular pulse rates.

Inefficient contraction of heart fails to transmit pulse wave, interfering with cardiac output, resulting in irregular pulse. Longer time period ensures accurate count.

Maintaining the same position keeps client from being aware that you are counting respirations. Inconspicuous assessment prevents client from consciously or unintentionally altering rate and depth of breathing. Viewing an entire respiratory cycle promotes accurate measurement.

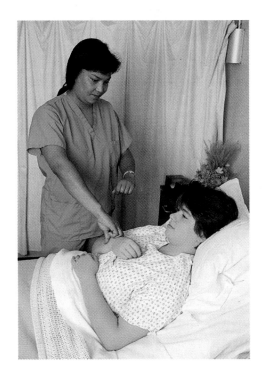

Step 7a

NURSE ALERT

If pulse is irregular, assess for a pulse deficit, which may indicate alteration in cardiac output. Count apical pulse (Chapter 13) while colleague counts radial pulse. Begin apical pulse, counting out loud to simultaneously assess pulses. If pulse count differs by more than 2, a pulse deficit exists.

Steps	Rationale

b. After cycle is observed, look at watch's second hand and begin to count rate: when sweep hand hits number on dial, begin time frame, counting one with first full respiratory cycle.

Timing begins with count of one. Respirations occur more slowly than pulse; thus timing does not begin with zero.

c. If rhythm is regular, count number of respirations in 30 seconds and multiply by 2. If rhythm is irregular, less than 12, or greater than 20, count for 1 full minute.

Respiratory rate is equivalent to number of respirations per minute. Suspected irregularities require assessment for at least 1 minute (see Table 12-3 p. 228).

d. Note depth of respirations, subjectively assessed by observing degree of chest wall movement while counting rate. Nurse can also objectively assess depth by palpating chest wall or auscultating the posterior chest during respiratory excursion (Chapter 13) after rate has been counted. Depth is shallow, normal, or deep.

Character of ventilatory movement may reveal specific disease state, restricting volume of air from moving into and out of the lungs.

e. Note rhythm of ventilatory cycle. Normal breathing is regular and uninterrupted. Sighing should not be confused with abnormal rhythm. Periodically people unconsciously take single deep breaths or sighs to expand small airways prone to collapse.

NURSE ALERT

Position of discomfort may cause client to breathe more rapidly.

Respiratory rate less than 12 or greater than 20 breaths/min and shallow and slow respirations (hypoventilation) may require immediate intervention.

f. Observe for evidence of dyspnea (increased effort to inhale and exhale). Ask client to describe subjective experience of shortness of breath compared with usual breathing pattern.

Clients with chronic lung disease may experience difficulty breathing all the time and can best describe their own discomfort from shortness of breath.

NURSE ALERT

Occasional periods of apnea is a symptom of underlying disease in the adult and must be reported to the physician or nurse in charge. Irregular respirations and short apneic spells are normal in a newborn.

8. **Upper extremity BP**

a. Determine the best site for BP assessment. Avoid applying cuff to extremity when intravenous fluids are being infused; when an arteriovenous shunt or fistula is present; when breast or axillary surgery has been performed on that side; or when extremity has been traumatized, diseased, or requires a cast or bulky bandage. The lower extremities may be used when the brachial arteries are inaccessible (Box 12-5, p. 241).

Inappropriate site selection may result in poor amplification of sounds, causing inaccurate readings. Application of pressure from inflated bladder temporarily impairs blood flow and can further compromise circulation in extremity that already has impaired blood flow.

NURSE ALERT

Client should be seated or lying in a quiet environment, free from temperature extremes, for at least 5 minutes before BP is obtained.

COMMUNICATION TIP

This is a good time to discuss with client the benefits of exercise and weight control in reducing the risks for hypertension and coronary artery disease or lowering an existing BP elevation.

Steps	**Rationale**
b. Select appropriate cuff size (see Figure 12-11, p. 229).	Improper cuff size results in inaccurate readings (see Table 12-4, p. 230). If cuff is too small, it tends to come loose as it is inflated or results in false-high readings. If the cuff is too large, false-high readings may be recorded.
c. Expose upper arm by removing restrictive clothing.	Ensures proper cuff application. Tight clothing causes congestion of blood and can falsely elevate BP readings.
d. With client sitting or lying, position client's forearm, supported if needed, with palm turned up at level of the heart.	If arm is unsupported, client may perform isometric exercise that can increase diastolic pressure 10%. Placement of arm above the level of the heart causes false-low reading. Placement of arm lower than the level of the heart causes false-high readings.
e. Palpate brachial artery (see illustrations). Position cuff 2.5 cm (1 inch) above site of brachial pulsation (antecubital space). Center bladder of cuff above artery (see illustration). With cuff fully deflated, wrap cuff evenly and snugly around upper arm (see illustration).	Inflating bladder directly over brachial artery ensures proper pressure is applied during inflation. Loose-fitting cuff causes false-high readings.

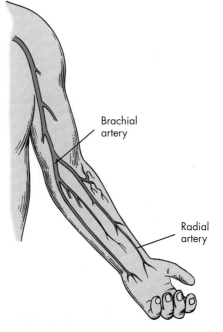

Brachial artery

Radial artery

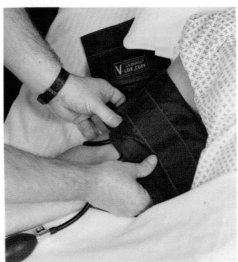

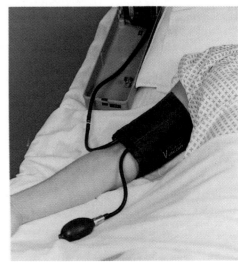

Step 8e

Steps	Rationale

f. Position manometer vertically at eye level. Observer should be no farther than 1 m (approximately 1 yard) away.

Accurate readings are obtained by looking at the meniscus of the mercury at eye level. The meniscus is the point where the crescent-shaped top of the mercury column aligns with the manometer scale. Looking up or down at the mercury results in distorted readings.

g. If you do not know client's baseline BP, estimate systolic pressure by palpating the brachial or radial artery with fingertips of one hand while inflating cuff rapidly to pressure 30 mm Hg above point at which pulse disappears. Slowly deflate cuff and note point when pulse reappears.

Estimating prevents false-low readings, which may result from the presence of an auscultatory gap (inaudible sounds below the actual systolic pressure). This phenomenon occurs in about 5% of adults and is prevalent in individuals with hypertension (Barkauskas et al, 1994).

NURSE ALERT

Eliminate extraneous noise, such as television and conversation. Noise interferes with accuracy. Falsely elevated readings will be obtained if client moves, talks, or coughs during BP measurement.

h. Deflate cuff fully and wait 30 seconds.
i. Place stethoscope earpieces in ears.
j. Relocate brachial artery and place bell or diaphragm chestpiece of stethoscope lightly over it. Do not allow chestpiece to touch cuff or clothing (see illustration).

Excess pressure results in falsely low diastolic BP readings.

k. Close valve of pressure bulb clockwise until tight.
l. Rapidly inflate cuff to 30 mm Hg above palpated systolic pressure.
m. Slowly release pressure bulb valve and allow mercury (or needle of aneroid manometer gauge) to fall at rate of 2 to 3 mm Hg/sec. Make sure there are no extraneous sounds at this point.

Too rapid or slow a decline in mercury level or aneroid pressure can cause inaccurate readings. Noise interferes with precise hearing of Korotkoff sounds.

NURSE ALERT

If you hear sounds immediately, release the pressure, wait 60 seconds, and estimate systolic pressure at higher reading. Reinflate cuff 30 mm Hg above the sound first heard. Reinflation of a partially deflated cuff is uncomfortable for client and may render an inaccurate reading.

n. Note point on manometer when first clear sound is heard (first Korotkoff sound reflects systolic BP). The sounds will slowly increase in intensity.

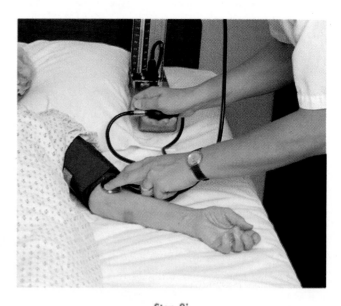

Step 8j

Steps	Rationale
o. Continue to deflate cuff gradually, noting point at which sound disappears in adults. Note pressure to nearest 2 mm Hg. Listen for 10 to 20 mm Hg after the last sound, and then allow remaining air to escape quickly.	Beginning of the fifth Korotkoff sound is recommended by American Heart Association as indication of diastolic pressure in adults. Fourth Korotkoff sound involves distinct muffling of sounds and is recommended by the American Heart Association as indication of diastolic pressure *in children*.
p. If this is first assessment of client, repeat procedure on other arm.	Comparison of BP in both arms detects circulatory problems. (Normal difference of 5 to 10 mm Hg exists between arms.)
q. Remove cuff from client's arm unless measurement must be repeated.	Continuous cuff inflation causes arterial occlusion, resulting in numbness and tingling of client's arm.
r. Record readings from both arms. Use arm with highest BP measurement for all subsequent BP recordings.	
s. Inform client of the BP. If possible, discuss risk factors for high BP. If BP is elevated, inquire as to any factors that may have affected BP, including general health, life stress or diet changes. If client takes blood pressure medication, determine if anything has interferred with prescribed regimen.	
9. See Completion Protocol (inside front cover).	

• • •

EVALUATION

1. Compare vital signs with client's baseline and normal expected ranges.
2. Ask client to identify factors that influence vital signs.
3. Identify a baseline for clients with chronic diseases that alter vital signs.
4. Ask client to describe changes in vital signs related to therapies (e.g., ambulation, medications).

Unexpected Outcomes and Related Interventions

1. Client has a temperature 1° C or more above normal range.
   a. Assess for additional related data suggesting systemic infection, including loss of appetite, headache, hot, dry skin, flushed face, thirst, general malaise, or chills.
   b. Further assess for possible site of localized infection, including pain or tenderness, purulent drainage, redness, or area of unusual warmth.
   c. Increase fluid intake to at least 3 L daily (unless contraindicated by client's condition).
   d. Control environmental temperature at 21° to 27° C (70° to 80° F).
   e. Reduce external covering on client's body to promote heat loss. Do not induce shivering.
   f. Keep clothing and bed linen dry.
   g. Limit physical activity and sources of emotional stress.
   h. Initiate measures to stimulate appetite and provide nutrients to meet increased energy needs (Chapter 8).
   i. Encourage oral hygiene because oral mucous membranes dry easily from dehydration (Chapter 7).
   j. Implement measures to determine etiology of fever, for example, obtain necessary culture specimens for lab analysis (e.g., urine, blood, sputum, and wound sites) (Chapter 15).
   k. Implement measures to prevent or control spread of infection; for example, pulmonary hygiene and postural drainage (Chapter 31), wound care (Chapter 24), and adequate urinary elimination (Chapter 9).
   l. If fever persists or reaches unacceptable level as defined by physician, administer antipyretics and antibiotics as ordered, and apply hypothermia blanket.
2. Client has a temperature 1° C or more below normal range.
   a. Cover client with warm blankets.
   b. Close room doors or windows to eliminate drafts.
   c. Encourage warm liquids.
   d. Apply hyperthermia blankets as indicated.
   e. Remove wet clothes and replace with dry garments.
   f. Monitor apical pulse rate and rhythm (Chapter 13), because hypothermia may cause bradycardia, cardiac dysrhythmias, and electrolyte imbalances.

3. Client has a weak or difficult-to-palpate radial pulse.
   a. Assess both radial pulses and compare findings. Local obstruction to peripheral blood flow (e.g., clot or edema of hand and wrist) may cause pulse to be difficult to palpate.
   b. Have another nurse assess pulse.
   c. Perform complete assessment of all peripheral pulses (see Chapter 13)
   d. Observe for symptoms associated with altered peripheral tissue perfusion, including pallor or cyanosis of tissue distal to pulse and cold extremities.
   e. Auscultate the apical pulse to determine a pulse deficit.

   f. Observe for factors associated with a decrease in cardiac output that result in diminished peripheral pulses, such as hemorrhage, hypothermia, or heart muscle damage.

4. Client has pulse greater than 100 beats/min (tachycardia).
   a. Identify related data, including pain, fear or anxiety, recent exercise, low BP, blood loss, elevated temperature, or inadequate oxygenation.
   b. Observe for symptoms associated with abnormal cardiac function, including dyspnea, fatigue, chest pain, orthopnea, syncope, palpitations (unpleasant awareness of pulse), jugular vein distention, edema of dependent body parts, cyanosis, or pallor of skin.

Box 12-4 Using a Mercury-in-Glass Thermometer

Equipment

Mercury-in-glass thermometer (Glass thermometers should not be shared between clients unless terminal disinfection is performed between each measurement).
Disposable plastic thermometer sleeve
Soft tissue
Lubricant (rectal measurements only)

Preparing the Thermometer

1. 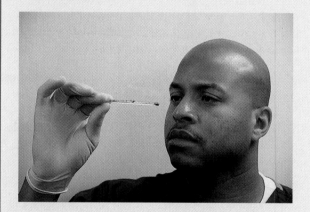 Hold end of glass thermometer with fingertips (if color coded, thermometer end will be blue for oral and axillary use, red for rectal use).
2. Read mercury level while gently rotating thermometer at eye level (see illustration). If mercury indicates a temperature above 35.5° C (96° F), grasp thermometer securely, stand away from solid objects, and sharply flick wrist downward. Continue brisk shaking until reading is below 35.5° C (96° F).

Nurse reading mercury thermometer at eye level.

3. Insert thermometer into plastic sleeve cover to protect from contact with feces and body secretions.
4. If obtaining rectal temperature, squeeze liberal portion of lubricant onto tissue and dip thermometer's blunt end into lubricant, covering 2.5 to 3.5 cm (1 to 1½ inches).

Obtaining Temperature

5. Insert thermometer using steps similar to those for electronic thermometer probe.
6. Oral temperature
   a. Ask client to hold thermometer under side of tongue toward back of mouth, lips closed to maintain proper position of thermometer while recording. Caution client against biting down on thermometer.
   b. Leave thermometer in place for 3 minutes (Holtzclaw, 1992) or according to agency policy.
7. Rectal temperature
   a. Hold thermometer in place for 2 minutes (Holtzclaw, 1992) or according to agency policy.
8. Axillary temperature
   a. Hold thermometer in place for at least 3 minutes for adults (Stephen & Sexton, 1987) and at least 5 minutes for children (Eoff & Joyce, 1981).
9. Carefully remove thermometer, then remove and discard plastic sleeve in appropriate receptacle. Wipe off any remaining secretions with clean tissue, wiping in a rotating fashion from fingers toward bulb.
10. Read thermometer at eye level. Gently rotate until scale appears. Store thermometer in appropriate protective storage container to prevent breakage and reduce risk of mercury spill.
11. Remove gloves and wash hands.

5. Client has pulse less than 60 beats/min (bradycardia).
   a. Auscultate the apical pulse (Chapter 13).
   b. Observe for factors that may alter heart rate and regularity, including medications such as digoxin and antiarrhythmics; it may be necessary to withhold prescribed medications until the physician can evaluate the need to alter the dosage.
6. Client has irregular rhythm.
   a. Auscultate the apical pulse (Chapter 13) and identify the pattern of irregularity. Assess for the presence of a pulse deficit.
   b. Clients with an irregular rhythm may require an electrocardiogram (ECG) or 24-hour heart monitor per physician's order to detect heart abnormalities.
7. Client has abnormal respiratory rate, depth, or pattern of dyspnea with complaints of feeling short of breath.
   a. Observe for related factors, including obstructed airway; noisy respirations; cyanosis of nail beds, lips, mucous membranes, and skin; restlessness; irritability; confusion; dyspnea (labored breathing); shortness of breath; productive cough; and abnormal breath sounds.
   b. Consider possible effects of anesthesia or medications such as narcotic analgesics (pain relievers).
   c. Assist client to a supported sitting position (semi-Fowler's or high Fowler's unless contraindicated), which improves ability to take a deep breath.
   d. Provide oxygen as ordered by physician (Skill 31.1) if client exhibits signs or symptoms of respiratory distress.
8. Client has elevated BP, as evidenced by pressure greater than 140 mm Hg systolic or 90 mm Hg diastolic.
   NOTE: A diagnosis of hypertension involves two or more elevated readings on separate occasions.
   a. Assess BP in other arm and compare findings. Recheck or have another nurse recheck readings.
   b. Observe for related symptoms. Often symptoms are not apparent unless BP is extremely high. Client may have a headache (usually occipital), flushing of face, or nosebleed; older adult client may notice fatigue.
   c. Be certain size of cuff is appropriate. A cuff that is too small gives false-high readings. Recheck or have another nurse recheck readings.
   d. Administer antihypertensive medication as ordered. If none is ordered, report BP to initiate appropriate evaluation and treatment.
9. Client is hypotensive when BP is not sufficient for adequate perfusion and oxygenation of tissues.
   a. Compare to baseline. A systolic reading of 90 may be normal for some persons and cause no ill effects.
   b. Observe for symptoms associated with hypotension related to decreased cardiac output, which include tachycardia; weak, thready pulse; weakness, dizziness, or confusion; pale, dusky, or cyanotic skin; or cool, mottled skin over extremities.
   c. Position client in supine position to enhance circulation and restrict activity that may drop BP further.
   d. Increase rate of IV infusion or administer vasoconstricting drugs if ordered.
   e. Observe for factors that would contribute to a low BP such as hemorrhage, dilation of blood vessels resulting from hyperthermia or anesthesia, and medication side effects.

Box 12-5 Obtaining BP from Lower Extremity by Auscultation

Equipment
Stethoscope
Sphygmomanometer
Large-leg BP cuff, wide and long enough to allow for larger girth of thigh

1. Assist client to prone position that provides the best access to the popliteal artery. If client is unable to assume prone position, assist client to supine position with knee slightly flexed.
2. Move aside bed linen and any constrictive clothing to ensure proper cuff application.
3. Locate and palpate the popliteal artery just below the thigh in the back of the knee in the popliteal space.
4. Apply BP cuff 2.5 cm (1 inch) above popliteal artery around middle thigh, centering arrows marked on BP cuff over the artery (see illustration). If there are no center arrows on the BP cuff, estimate the center of the cuff bladder and place this center over the artery.
5. Obtain BP using auscultatory method. Systolic pressure in the legs is usually 10 to 40 mm Hg higher than the brachial artery, but the diastolic pressure is the same.

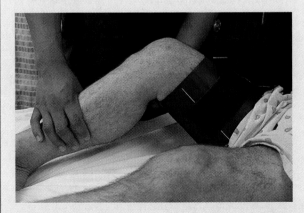

Lower extremity BP cuff positioned above popliteal artery at mid-thigh.

Box 12-6 Palpating the Systolic BP

1. Apply BP cuff to the upper arm in the same manner as the auscultation method.
2. Palpate the radial artery.
3. Inflate BP cuff 30 mm Hg above the point at which the radial pulse can no longer be palpated.
4. Release valve and allow mercury to fall 2 mm Hg per second.
5. As soon as the radial pulse is palpable, note the manometer reading.

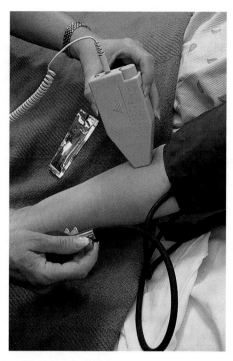

Figure 12-13 Doppler stethoscope over brachial artery to measure BP.

10. Client BP is inaudible or difficult to obtain.
    a. Determine that no immediate crisis is present by obtaining respiratory rate and pulse rate.
    b. Implement palpation method to obtain systolic BP (Box 12-6).
    c. Use an ultrasonic Doppler instrument to obtain BP (Figure 12-13).
    d. Auscultate BP in lower extremity (see Box 12-5, p. 241)

Recording and Reporting

- Record vital signs promptly on vital sign flow sheet (Appendix A), computer database, or nurse's notes. Record associated findings and related factors in narrative from nurse's notes.
- Record site of BP and position of client, pulse, and temperature measurement.
- Report abnormal findings to nurse in charge or physician.

Sample Documentation

2300   Client vomited 50 ml clear green fluid. NPO maintained. BP 104/56 RA, supine. L radial pulse 112, regular but weak. Respirations 24 and regular. Temperature 36.8° C tympanic. Client denies dyspnea, nausea, or pain. Physician notified.

Geriatric Considerations

- Temperatures considered within normal range may reflect a fever in an older adult.
- Older adults are very sensitive to slight changes in temperature.
- Adults who wear dentures and who do not have them in place or older adults with muscle weakness may be unable to close their mouth tightly enough to obtain accurate oral temperature readings.
- A decrease in sweat gland reactivity in the older adult results in higher threshold for sweating at high temperatures, which can lead to hyperthermia.
- Older adults are at high risk for hypothermia because of diminished sensation to cold, abnormal vasoconstrictor responses, and impaired shivering.
- With aging, a loss of subcutaneous fat reduces the insulating capacity of the skin.
- Older adults, especially the frail elderly, have lost

upper arm mass, requiring special attention to selection of smaller BP cuff.
- Older adults have an increase in systolic pressure related to decreased vessel elasticity.
- Older adults often experience a fall in BP after eating.
- Older adults are instructed to change position slowly and wait after each change to avoid postural hypotension and to prevent injuries.
- It is often difficult to palpate the pulse of an older adult or obese client. A Doppler device provides a more accurate reading.
- The arteries of an older adult may feel stiff and knotty because of atherosclerosis and decreased elasticity.
- Once elevated, the pulse rate of an older adult takes longer to return to normal resting rate (Wold, 1993).

Home Care and Long-Term Care Considerations

- Assess temperature and ventilation of environment to determine existence of any conditions that may influence client's temperature.
- Assess safe storage of mercury-in-glass thermometers to protect from breakage and mercury spills.
- Assess home noise level to determine the room that will provide the quietest environment for assessing BP.

- Assess family's financial ability to afford a sphygmomanometer for performing BP evaluations on a regular basis.
- Consider an electronic BP cuff for home if client or caregiver has hearing difficulties.

Skill 12.2

TYMPANIC TEMPERATURE

The measurement of body temperature is aimed at obtaining a representative average of temperature of the core body tissues. Sites reflecting core temperatures are more reliable indicators of body temperatures than sites reflecting surface temperatures (Box 12-7). The tympanic membrane reflects core body temperature because it shares its blood supply with the hypothalamus, the body's temperature control center in the brain. The tympanic thermometer detects heat radiated from the tympanic membrane of the ear and is used exclusively for measuring tympanic temperature. This skill involves obtaining an accurate core temperature measurement with a tympanic thermometer (Figure 12-14).

Equipment

Electronic tympanic thermometer
Disposable speculum covers specified by the manufacturer

ASSESSMENT

1. Consider normal daily fluctuations in temperature. **Rationale: Body temperature tends to be lowest in** **early morning, peak in late afternoon, and gradually decline during the night. When temperatures are taken between 5 pm and 7 pm fever is more accurately assessed (Beaudry et al, 1996).**

2. Identify medications or treatments that may influence temperature. **Rationale: Temperature is affected by anti-inflammatory drugs, steroids, warming or cooling blankets, and fans.**

3. Identify factors that influence temperature. **Rationale: Age, exercise, hormonal variations, stress, and environmental temperature can affect the body temperature.**

4. Identify factors likely to interfere with accuracy of tympanic temperature reading, including recent facial or aural surgery, presence of cerumen (ear wax), or the presence of a hearing aid. An ear infection

Box 12-7 Core and Surface Temperature Measurement Sites

Core	Surface
Rectal	Skin
Tympanic membrane	Oral
Esophageal	Axillary
Pulmonary artery	
Urinary bladder	

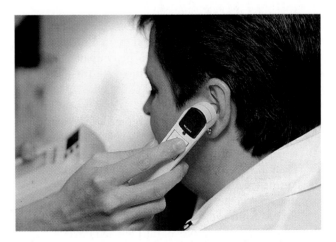

Figure 12-14 Tympanic membrane thermometer with probe cover being placed in client's ear.

(otitis) of the middle or external ear will cause the ear canal to be sensitive and painful to touch and should be avoided. **Rationale: Conditions that alter regional blood flow or obstruct tympanic membrane cause inaccurate temperature measurement.**

5. Determine previous baseline vital signs from client's record. **Rationale: Baseline information provides basis for comparison and assists in assessment of current status. Temperature should be assessed at same site for accurate comparison.**

PLANNING

Expected outcomes focus on monitoring and restoring body temperature to within normal ranges.

Expected Outcomes

1. Client's temperature is within normal range for client's age-group.

2. Client describes environmental factors that increase risk of altered body temperature.
3. Client's body temperature returns to normal or baseline range after nursing interventions and medical therapies for altered temperature.

DELEGATION CONSIDERATIONS

The skill of tympanic temperature measurement can be delegated to AP. Be sure to inform AP of:

- Factors that can falsely raise or lower temperature
- Frequency of temperature measurement
- Need to report any abnormalities to the nurse

IMPLEMENTATION

Steps	Rationale
1. See Standard Protocol (inside front cover).	
2. Assist client in assuming a comfortable position with head turned toward side, away from nurse, so that ear canal is easily viewed.	
3. Remove thermometer handheld unit from charging base, being careful not to apply pressure to the ejection button. Slide disposable speculum cover over otoscope-like tip until it locks in place.	
4. For an adult, pull ear pinna back, up, and out; insert speculum into ear canal snugly to make a seal, pointing toward the nose. Some manufacturers recommend moving the speculum in a rocking or figure-of-eight pattern to scan the tympanic membrane. Refer to manufacturer's instructions for each instrument.	The ear tug straightens the external auditory canal, allowing maximum exposure of the tympanic membrane. Some manufacturers recommend movement of the speculum tip in a figure-of-eight pattern that allows the sensor to detect maximum tympanic membrane heat radiation. Gentle pressure seals the ear canal from ambient air temperature.
5. As soon as the probe is in place, depress scan button on handheld unit. Leave thermometer probe in place until audible signal occurs and client's temperature appears on digital display.	Depression of scan button causes infrared energy to be detected from tympanic membrane. Otoscope tip must stay in place until signal occurs to ensure accurate reading.
6. Carefully remove speculum from auditory meatus. Push ejection button on thermometer stem to discard speculum cover into appropriate receptacle. Return handheld unit to charging base.	Returning handheld unit automatically causes digital reading to disappear and protects sensor tip from damage.
7. See Completion Protocol (inside front cover).	

• • • •

EVALUATION

1. Compare tympanic temperature with client's baseline and normal expected ranges.
2. Ask client to identify factors that influence temperature.
3. Monitor changes in temperature related to therapies (e.g., removal of excess clothing, cool sponge bath).

Unexpected Outcomes and Related Interventions

1. Client has a tympanic temperature 1° C or more below normal range.
   a. Repeat measurement in other ear. A scarred eardrum may have a lower temperature than an unscarred one. Temperature variations exist from ear to ear.
   b. Assess ear canal for cerumen, obtain physician order, and remove if needed. Cerumen is a poor conductor of heat and can lower tympanic measurements in large amounts (Hasel and Erickson, 1995).
   c. Remove wet clothes and cover client with warm blankets.
   d. Close room doors or windows to eliminate drafts.

For further Outcomes and Related Interventions see Skill 12.1.

Recording and Reporting

- Record temperature promptly on vital sign flow sheet (Appendix A) or nurse's notes. Record associated findings and related factors in narrative form in nurses' notes.
- Record site of temperature measurement.
- Report abnormal findings to nurse in charge or physician.

Sample Documentation

12/7/98, 11 AM   Client excused from class by teacher complaining of feeling warm. Tympanic temperature 37° C; skin pink, warm, and dry. Returned to class.

Geriatric Considerations

- With aging, cerumen is drier and cilia become coarse and stiff, contributing to the buildup of cerumen. It is estimated that one third or more of older adults may have occlusive amounts of cerumen in one or both ear canals (Hasel and Erickson, 1995).

Skill 12.3

ELECTRONIC BLOOD PRESSURE MEASUREMENT

Many electronic devices are available to determine BP automatically (Figure 12-15). These devices are applied when frequent BP assessment is required, such as in the critically ill or potentially unstable clients, during or after invasive procedures, or when therapies require frequent monitoring (e.g., trials of new drugs). Electronic BP devices can be found in public areas such as shopping malls or in clients' homes. While the sphygmomanometer-stethoscope technique of measuring BP relies on auscultation of Korotkoff sounds, electronic devices rely on the principle of oscillometry. A pressure sensor located in the BP cuff responds to the rush of blood into the vessel when the cuff is deflated. The released blood causes the vessel wall to oscillate or vibrate. The sensor determines the initial burst of oscillations and translates the information into a systolic pressure reading. The diastolic pressure is measured when the oscillations are lowest, just before they stop (Bridges and Middleton, 1997). Anatomical and physiological factors specific to each client can affect the accuracy of oscillometric pressure measurements (Box 12-8, p. 246). The nurse must know the appropriate applications, advantages, and limitations of these devices to ensure accurate measurements (Box 12-9, p. 246).

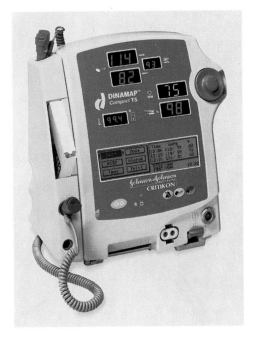

Figure 12-15 Automatic BP monitor. *DINAMAP® Compact Monitor is a trademark of Critikon. Photo Courtesy Critikon, Tampa, Fla.*

Equipment

Electronic BP machine

Cloth or disposable vinyl pressure cuff of appropriate size for client's extremity and recommended by machine manufacturer (Table 12-5).

Box 12-8 Client Conditions that are not Appropriate for Electronic BP Measurement

Irregular heart rate

Peripheral vascular obstruction (e.g., clots, narrowed vessels)

Shivering

Seizures

Excessive tremors

Unable to cooperate to minimize arm motions

Box 12-9 Advantages and Disadvantages of Electronic BP Measurement

Advantages

Ease of use

Efficient when repeated measurements are indicated

Ability to use a stethoscope not required

Not sensitive to outside noise

Disadvantages

Expensive

Sensitive to outside motion interference

Requires source of electricity

Requires space to position machine

ASSESSMENT

1. Determine appropriateness of using electronic BP machine for measurement of BP. **Rationale: Accuracy of oscillometric method is decreased for clients with certain conditions (see Box 12-8). The expense of electronic BP machines requires they be used for frequent pressure monitoring. The BP cuff remains in place, which may be inappropriate for active or uncooperative clients.**

2. Determine client baseline BP using auscultatory method **Rationale: The oscillometric method is not accurate for monitoring hypotension (BP less than 90 mm Hg systolic) or conditions where there is reduced blood flow, as in shock. Baseline information provides bases of comparing auscultatory and oscillometric methods and assists in the assessment of current status.**

3. Identify factors that influence BP. **Rationale: High BP is associated with pain, rapid IV infusion of fluids or blood products, increased intracranial pressure, cardiovascular disease, and renal disease. Low BP is associated with rapid vasodilation, shock, hemorrhage, and dehydration.**

Table 12-5

Proper Cuff Size for Electronic Monitor*

Cuff Type	Limb Circumference (cm)
Small adult	17–25
Adult	23–33
Large adult	31–40
Thigh	38–50

*It is mandatory for the 12- to 24-foot cord to be used for adult monitoring.

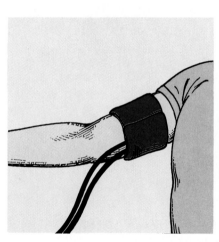
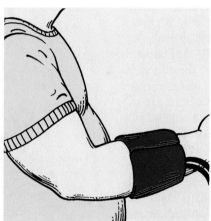
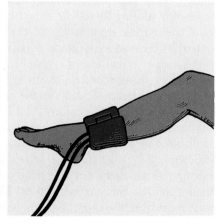

Figure 12-16 Placement of BP cuff for electronic monitoring.

4. Assess pertinent laboratory values, including platelet count and coagulation studies (e.g., PT, PTT) if client receiving anticoagulant therapy. **Rational: Repeated inflations of BP cuff can result in microvascular rupture, which can lead to abnormal bleeding in a client who has poor ability to clot.**

5. Determine best site for BP assessment. Avoid applying cuff to extremity when intravenous fluids are being infused; when an arteriovenous shunt or fistula is present; when breast or axillary surgery has been performed on that side; or if extremity has been traumatized, is diseased, or requires a cast or bulky bandage. Upper arm, forearm, or lower leg is appropriate as long as circulation is adequate and cuff is correct size (Figure 12-16).

PLANNING

Expected outcomes focus on identifying abnormalities and restoring homeostasis.

Expected Outcomes

1. Auscultatory BP reading is equivalent to oscillometric BP recorded by electronic device.
2. Client's BP is within normal range for client's age-group.

DELEGATION CONSIDERATIONS

The skill of BP measurement using an electronic BP machine can be delegated to AP. Be sure to inform AP of:

- Appropriate limb for BP measurement
- Appropriately sized BP cuff for designated extremity
- Appropriate alarm limit settings for client condition
- Frequency of BP measurements
- Need to report any abnormalities to the nurse

IMPLEMENTATION

Steps	Rationale

COMMUNICATION TIP

Because BP measurement can frighten children, this is a good time to prepare the child for the squeezing feeling of the inflated BP cuff by saying "This will feel like a tight hug for a minute" or "This will feel like rubberband on your finger."

If using an electronic BP machine, tell the client and family that these machines have audible alarm systems. Explain and allow the client to hear sound. Inform client that "the alarms do not always mean you have a problem, but also show that the machine needs attention."

1. See Standard Protocol (inside front cover).
2. Assist client to comfortable position, either lying or sitting. Place electronic BP machine near client and plug in machine to source of electricity.

3. Locate on/off switch and turn machine on.

4. Select appropriate cuff size for client extremity and appropriate cuff for machine. Note that the inner surface of the cuff has marked placement ranges. When wrapped around the extremity, an appropriately sized and placed cuff will end within the noted placement range. If an ideal cuff size is not available, a larger cuff will result in the smallest measurement error (Bridges and Middleton, 1997).

5. Expose extremity by removing restrictive clothing.

Length of connector hose between cuff and machine requires planning appropriate placement of electronic BP machine between client and electricity source.

Machine will self-test computer systems when power is activated.

NURSE ALERT

Electronic BP cuff and machine must be matched by the manufacturer. Do not interchange BP cuffs from machines of different manufacturers.

Oscillometric vibrations can be affected by tight clothing, which causes congestion of blood and distention of vessel walls.

Steps	Rationale

6. Prepare BP cuff by manually squeezing all the air out of the cuff and connecting cuff to connector hose.

7. Wrap cuff snugly around extremity, verifying that only one finger can fit between cuff and client's skin. Make sure the "artery" arrow marked on the outside of the cuff is correctly placed.   Correct sensing of vibrations depends on consistent contact between cuff sensor and limb.

8. Verify that connector hose between cuff and machine is not kinked.

9. Following manufacturer's directions, set the frequency control for automatic or manual, then press the start button. The first BP measurement sequence will pump the cuff to a peak pressure of about 180 mm Hg. After this pressure is reached, the machine begins a deflation sequence that determines the BP. The first reading determines the peak pressure inflation for additional measurements.

10. Follow manufacturer's directions to set frequency of BP measurements and upper and lower alarm limits for systolic, diastolic, and mean BP readings. Additional readings can be determined at any time by pressing the "start" button. Pressing the "cancel" button immediately deflates the cuff. Intervals between BP measurements may be set from 1 to 90 minutes. The monitor displays the most recent reading and flashes the time in minutes that has elapsed since that measurement occurred.   The frequency of BP measurement is determined by physician order or nursing clinical judgment. Alarms are determined for each client based on initial BP measurement and therapy goals.

11. When BP determinations are frequent, the cuff may be left in place. Remove cuff at least every 2 hours to assess underlying skin, and if possible alternate sites.

12. See Completion Protocol (inside front cover).

• • •

EVALUATION
1. Compare electronic BP reading with BP obtained by sphygmomanometer-stethoscope.
2. Review readings at specific intervals for trends outside normal range for client's age.

Unexpected Outcomes and Related Interventions
1. Client has elevated BP.
   a. Assess BP in other arm and compare findings. Recheck cuff size and position or have another nurse recheck. A difference of more than 10 mm Hg between BP measurements on upper extremities indicates potential alteration in vascular anatomy and signals need for further medical assessment.
   b. Observe for related symptoms. Often symptoms are not apparent unless BP is extremely high. (See Skill 12.1.)

   c. Administer antihypertensive medication as ordered. If none is ordered, report BP to initiate appropriate evaluation and treatment.
2. Client is hypotensive when BP is not sufficient for adequate perfusion and oxygenation of tissues.
   a. Obtain BP with sphygmomanometer and compare with electronic BP readings. Electronic BP measurements are less accurate in low blood flow conditions.
   b. Position client in supine position to enhance circulation and restrict activity that may cause BP to continue to drop.
   c. Administer vasoconstrictor medications and IV solutions as ordered. If none are ordered, report BP to initiate appropriate evaluation and treatment.

Recording and Reporting

- Record vital signs promptly on vital sign flow sheet (Appendix A) or nurse's notes. Record associated findings and related factors in narrative form in nurse's notes.
- Record site of BP and use of electronic BP machine.
- Report abnormal findings to nurse in charge or physician.
- If reading abnormal, record action taken in narrative form in nurse's notes.

Sample Documentation

1430   Client returned from esophageal dilation procedure. Vital signs on admission: HR 82, regular; BP right arm 128/84, RR 14; temp 98.02 tympanic, R ear; automatic BP machine placed on right arm; see vital signs flow sheet.

Geriatric Considerations

- Skin of older adults is more fragile and susceptible to cuff pressure when BP measurements are frequent. More frequent assessment of skin under cuff or rotation of BP sites is recommended.

Home Care and Long-Term Care Considerations

- Consider an electronic BP cuff for home if client or caregiver has hearing difficulties.

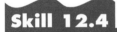

Skill 12.4

MEASURING OXYGEN SATURATION WITH PULSE OXIMETRY

Pulse oximetry is a noninvasive measurement of arterial oxygen saturation (SaO_2) that assesses the level of oxygen in the blood available to the body tissues. SaO_2 reflects the percent of hemoglobin that is bound with oxygen in the arteries and is expressed as a percentage; for example, an SaO_2 of 96% indicates that 96% of the hemoglobin molecules are carrying oxygen molecules. The more the hemoglobin is saturated with oxygen, the higher the SaO_2. SaO_2 is normally over 90% and can be measured with an arterial blood gas (ABG) sample, an invasive procedure. The pulse oximeter is a device that measures pulse saturation (SpO_2), a reliable estimate of SaO_2. For an SaO_2 over 70% the SpO_2 is accurate to ± 2% (Tittle and Flynn, 1997). The measurement of SpO_2 is simple, is painless, and has fewer risks than obtaining an ABG to measure SaO_2.

A pulse oximeter includes a probe with a light-emitting diode (LED) connected by cable to an oximeter (Figure 12-17). Light waves emitted by the LED are absorbed and then reflected back by oxygenated and deoxygenated hemoglobin molecules. The reflected light is processed by the oximeter, which calculates SpO_2. In adults the oximeter sensor probe is applied to the finger, toe, earlobe, or bridge of the nose. In addition, sensors for infants and children can be applied to the palm or sole of the foot. The nurse selects the appropriate sensor probe for the client's condition (Box 12-10, p. 250). SpO_2 can be assessed continuously, intermittently, or with spot checks, depending on the client's condition. Pulse oximetry is indicated in clients who have an unstable oxygen status or in those who are at risk for alterations in oxygenation (Box, 12-11 p. 250).

Equipment

Oximeter
Oximeter probe appropriate for client and
    recommended by the manufacturer
    (see Box 12-11, p. 250)
Acetone or nail polish remover

ASSESSMENT

1. Identify clients at risk for unstable oxygen status (see Box 12-11, p. 250).
2. Identify medications or treatments that may influence oxygen saturation. **Rationale: Oxygen therapy, respiratory therapy such as postural drainage and**

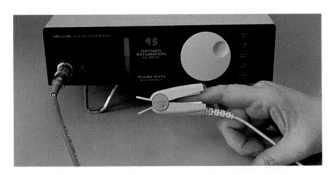

Figure 12-17   Pulse oximeter.

Box 12-10 Characteristics of Pulse Oximeter Sensor Probes and Sites

Reusable Probe

Digit probe
Easy to apply, conforms to various sizes
Yields strong correlation with SaO_2
Earlobe
Clip-on is smaller and lighter, although more positional than digit probe
Research suggests greater accuracy at lower saturations (Tittle and Flynn, 1996)
Yields strong correlation with SaO_2
Good when uncontrollable movements are a problem, such as hand tremors seen with Parkinson's disease
Ear site is least affected by decreased blood flow (Carroll, 1997)

Disposable Sensor Pad

Can be applied to variety of sites: earlobe of adult or nose bridge, palm, or sole of infant
Less restrictive for continuous SpO_2 monitoring
Expensive
Contains latex
Skin under adhesive may become moist and harbor pathogens
Available in variety of sizes, pad can be matched with infant weight (Hanna, 1995)

Box 12-11 Conditions that can Require SpO₂ Monitoring

Acute respiratory disease (e.g., pneumonia or asthma)
Chronic respiratory disease (e.g., emphysema)
Ventilator dependence
Chest pain
Activity intolerance
Recovery from general anesthesia after surgery
Recovery from conscious sedation after procedures such as endoscopy, bronchoscopy, or cardiac catheterization.
Traumatic injury to chest wall
Changes in supplemental oxygen therapy

Box 12-12 Factors Affecting Determination of Pulse Oxygen Saturation

Interference with Light Transmission

Outside light sources can interfere with the oximeter's ability to process reflected light
Carbon monoxide (caused by smoke inhalation or poisoning) artificially elevates SpO_2 by absorbing light similar to oxygen
Client motion can interfere with the oximeter's ability to process reflected light
Jaundice may interfere with the oximeter's ability to process reflected light
Intravascular dyes (methylene blue) absorb light similar to deoxyhemoglobin and artificially lower saturation

Reduction of Arterial Pulsations

Peripheral vascular disease (Raynaud's, atherosclerosis) can reduce pulse volume
Hypothermia at assessment site decreases peripheral blood flow
Pharmacological vasoconstrictors (epinephrine, neosynephrine, dopamine) will decrease peripheral pulse volume
Low cardiac output and hypotension decrease blood flow to peripheral arteries
Peripheral edema can obscure arterial pulsation

percussion, and bronchodilators will affect client's ability to ventilate and perfuse lung tissue.

3. Identify factors that influence oxygen saturation: **Rationale: Any abnormalities in the type or amount of hemoglobin affect the ability of oxygen to be carried to the tissues (Box 12-12).**

4. Identify factors likely to interfere with accuracy of pulse oximeter. **Rationale: Skin pigmentation affects the ability of SpO2 to predict SaO2. Darker pigments can result in false-high readings (Tittle and Flynn, 1997).**

5. Assess pertinent laboratory values, including hemoglobin and ABGs if available. **Rationale: Anemia affects the ability of oxygen to attach to the hemoglobin molecule. ABGs measure SaO2, which serves as a standard and provides a basis for comparison to assist in the assessment of respiratory status.**

6. Determine client-specific site appropriate to place pulse oximeter probe by measuring capillary refill (see Chapter 13), if less than 3 seconds select alternative site, note presence of moisture or nail polish. **Rationale: Site must have adequate local circulation for sensor to detect hemoglobin molecules that absorb emitted light. Changes in SpO2 are reflected in the circulation of finger capillary bed within 30 seconds and earlobe capillary bed within 5 to 10 seconds. Moisture, dark nail polish, and acrylic nails impede sensor detection of emitted light and produce falsely elevated SpO2 levels (Tittle and Flynn, 1997).**

7. Determine previous baseline SpO$_2$ from client's record. **Rationale: Baseline information provides basis for comparison and assists in assessment of current status and evaluation of interventions.**

PLANNING

Expected outcomes focus on monitoring and maintaining adequate oxygenation when client is at risk for hypoxemia.

Expected Outcomes

1. SaO$_2$ level greater than 90% is maintained, with or without oxygen therapy, during sleep, after removal of secretions with suctioning, and with exertion of ambulating in the hall for 5 minutes. (NOTE: Acceptable level must be individualized for each client.)
2. Client maintains skin integrity beneath pulse oximeter probe.

DELEGATION CONSIDERATIONS

The skill of measuring oxygen saturation with a pulse oximeter can be delegated to AP. Be sure to inform AP of:

- Appropriate sensor probe and site for client
- Factors that can falsely lower SpO$_2$
- Appropriate client position when obtaining SpO$_2$
- Frequency of SpO$_2$ measurement
- Need to report any measurement lower than 90% to nurse

IMPLEMENTATION

Steps	Rationale
1. See Standard Protocol (inside front cover).	
2. Select site, which may include ear, nailbed, or bridge of nose. Disposable adhesive sensor pads are available to conform to digits, palm of hand, or sole of foot for infants and toddlers. If finger is selected, remove fingernail polish and acrylic nail (if worn) with acetone or polish remover.	Opaque coatings decrease light transmission, and nail polish containing blue pigments can absorb light emissions and falsely alter saturation.

NURSE ALERT

Mixing probes from different manufacturers can result in burn injury to the client.

Adhesive probe contains latex and should not be used if client has a latex allergy or latex sensitivity.

Steps	Rationale
3. Determine capillary refill at site. If less than 3 seconds, select alternative site.	Cold temperature with vasoconstriction or vascular disease may decrease circulation, impair refill, and prevent sensor probe from measuring SpO$_2$.
4. Position client comfortably. If finger is chosen as monitoring site, support lower arm. Instruct client to keep sensor probe site still.	Movement interferes with SpO$_2$ determination.
5. Attach sensor probe to selected site (see illustration), making sure photodetectors of light sensors are aligned opposite each other.	
6. Turn on oximeter by activating power. Observe pulse waveform/intensity display and audible beep. Compare oximeter pulse rate with client's radial pulse.	Pitch of audible beep is proportional to SpO$_2$ value. Double-check pulse rate to ensure oximeter accuracy.

Steps	Rationale

COMMUNICATION TIP

1. *The pressure of the sensor probe's spring tension on a peripheral digit or earlobe may be unexpected. Inform client that clip on probe "feels like a clothespin on your finger but will not hurt."*
2. *Inform client that oximeter alarm will sound if the probe falls off or if he or she moves the probe.*

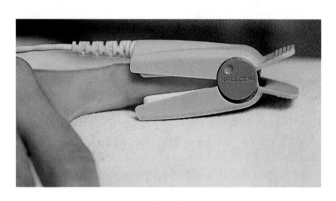

Step 5

NURSE ALERT

Oximeter pulse rate, client's radial pulse rate, and apical pulse rate should be the same. Any differences require reevaluation of oximeter sensor probe placement and reassessment of pulse rates.

7. Leave sensor probe in place until oximeter reaches constant value and pulse display reaches full strength during each cardiac cycle. Read SpO$_2$ on digital display.

Reading may take 10 to 30 seconds, depending on site selected.

8. If continuous SpO$_2$ monitoring is planned, check SpO$_2$ alarm limits, which are preset by the manufacturer at a low of 85% and a high of 100%. Limits for SpO$_2$ and pulse rate should be determined as indicated by client's condition. Verify that alarms are on. Relocate sensor probe at least every 4 hours.

Spring tension of sensor probe or sensitivity to disposable sensor probe adhesive can cause skin irritation and lead to disruption of skin integrity.

9. If intermittent or spot-checking SpO$_2$ measurements are planned, remove probe and turn oximeter power off. Store probe in appropriate location.

Sensor probes are expensive and vulnerable to damage.

10. See Completion Protocol (inside front cover).

• • •

EVALUATION

1. Compare SpO$_2$ levels whenever oxygen therapy is initiated or discontinued, before and during sleep, before and after removal of secretions with suctioning and during activity.
2. Assess skin integrity under probe every 2 hours.

Unexpected Outcomes and Related Interventions

1. Client's SpO_2 is less than 90%.
   a. Observe for indications of hypoxemia, which include the presence of cyanosis, restlessness, altered respiratory patterns, and tachycardia. Skin beneath oximeter probe is intact without irritation.
   b. Compare SpO_2 with SaO_2 on ABG. A SpO_2 of 85% to 89% may be acceptable for certain chronic disease conditions and reflects the client's baseline oxygen saturation. An SpO_2 less than 85% is abnormal and is often accompanied by changes in respiratory rate, depth, and rhythm. Immediate medical intervention is required.
   c. Observe for and minimize factors that decrease SpO_2, such as lung secretions, increased activity, altered neurological status, and hyperthermia.
   d. Assist client to a position that maximizes ventilatory effort, for example, placing an obese client in a high Fowler's position.
   e. Verify appropriate oxygen delivery system and liter flow; administer oxygen according to physician's orders.
   f. Implement measures to reduce client's energy consumption by avoiding unnecessary activity, anxiety, or emotional stress.

2. Pulse rate indicated on oximeter is less than radial or apical pulse rate.
   a. Change sensor probe site. Clients who have cold hands or peripheral vascular disease may have decreased blood flow to extremity.
   b. Check sensor probe for excessive spring pressure, which can constrict blood flow.
   c. Assess apical and radial pulse along with other signs and symptoms, which would indicate compromised cardiac status or decreased peripheral blood flow.

3. Pulse rate intensity display indicated on oximeter is dampened or irregular.
   a. Request that client not move extremity or area with sensor probe because movement interferes with measurements. Motion artifact is most common cause of inaccurate readings (Carroll, 1997).
   b. Reposition sensor probe for better contact with underlying skin.
   c. Protect sensor from room light by covering sensor probe site with opaque covering or washcloth.

Sample Documentation

1715   Continuous pulse ox on R index finger relocated to L index finger. Good capillary refill R = L, 2 seconds. Skin intact, no redness noted. SpO_2 93% with 3 L O_2 via nasal cannula. RR 24, client denies dyspnea, remains in semi-Fowler's position.

Geriatric Considerations

- Identifying an acceptable sensor probe site may be difficult on older adults because of the likelihood of peripheral vascular disease, cold-induced vasoconstriction, and anemia.
- Older adults require more frequent assessment of sensor probe site because of tissue fragility and poor elasticity caused by aging.

Home Care and Long-Term Care Considerations

- Pulse oximetry is used in home care to spot-check the effectiveness of oxygen therapy or need for therapy changes.

CRITICAL THINKING EXERCISES

1. During afternoon report, an AP reports to you that Mrs. Coburn, a client with insulin-dependent diabetes who resides in the assistive living area of your long-term care facility, was "breathing funny" during her bath.
   a. How should you proceed?
   b. What instructions you should give the AP?
   c. After determining Mrs. Coburn's respiratory rate is 16 and irregular, what additional information should you obtain?

2. A 72-year-old gentleman arrives back on the medical unit after a diagnostic endoscopy. An IV is running in the right antecubital space, and the left arm is in a cast from a previous fall and fracture.
   a. What instructions should you give the AP regarding post-procedure vital signs?
   b. You are told by the AP that the tympanic temperature is 35.8° C (96.4° F) in the right ear. How should you proceed?

3. A 35-year-old African-American man arrives at the cardiac clinic for follow-up of suspected hypertension. He is 5'6", weighs 285 pounds, and has chewing tobacco in his mouth. He is a long-distance truck driver and is determined to get his truck unloaded this morning. The clinic appointments are backed up by 45 minutes.
   a. What factors should you consider when obtaining this client's BP?
   b. What factors can influence this client's BP reading?
   c. The client tells you that he stopped at the mall yesterday during lunch and took his own BP at "one of those instant machines." He reported it said he was "OK," and he doesn't understand what all the fuss is about. What is your reply?

REFERENCES

American Heart Association: *Recommendations for human blood pressure determination by sphygmomanometers,* Dallas, 1993, The Association.

American Heart Association National Committee on Detection, Evaluation and Treatment of High Blood Pressure: Report, *Arch Intern Med* 153:154–183, Jan 1993.

Anderson DA, Cunningham SG, Maloney JP: Indirect blood pressure measurement: a need to reassess, *Am J Crit Care* 4(2):269, 1993.

Barkauskas VH et al: *Health and physical assessment,* ed 4, St Louis, 1994, Mosby.

Beaudry M et al: Research utilization: once-a-day temperatures of afebrile patients, *Clin Nurse Specialist* 10(1):21, 1996.

Bliss-Holtz, J: Methods of newborn infant temperature monitoring: a research review, *Issues Comp Pediatr Nurs* 18:287, 1995.

Bridges EJ, Middleton R: Direct arterial oscillometric monitoring of blood pressure: stop comparing and pick one, *Crit Care Nurse* 17(3):58, 1997.

Carroll P: Using pulse oximetry in the home, *Home Healthcare Nurse* 15(2):89, 1997. axillary temperatures, *Pediatr Nurs* 22(2):121, 1997.

Cusson RA et al: The effect of environment on body site temperatures in full-term neonates, *Nurs Res* 46(4):202, 1997.

Eoff M, Joyce B: Temperature measurements in children, *Am J Nurs* 81(12):1010, 1981.

Haddock BJ et al: The falling grace of axillary temperatures, *Pediatr Nurs* 22(2):121, 1996.

Hanna D: Equipment guidelines for pulse oximetry use in pediatrics, *J Pediatr Nurs* 10(2):124, 1995.

Hasel KL, Erickson RS: Effect of cerumen on infrared ear temperature measurement, *J Gernontol Nurs* 21(2):6, 1995.

Holtzclaw B: The febrile response in critical care: state of the science, *Heart Lung* 21(5):482, 1992.

Kim MJ, McFarland GK, McLane AM: *Pocket guide to nursing diagnoses,* ed 7, St Louis, 1997, Mosby.

Morley CJ, Hewson PH, Thornton AJ, Cole TJ: Axillary and rectal temperature measurements in infants, *Arch Dis Child,* Jan, 67(1): 1992.

Stephen SB, Sexton Pr: Neonatal axillary temperatures: increases in readings over time, *Neonat Netw* 5(6):25, 1987.

Tittle M, Flynn MB: Correlation of pulse oximetry and co-oximetry, *Dimen Crit Care Nurs* 16(2):88, 1997.

Wold G: *Basic geriatric nursing,* St Louis, 1998, Mosby.

Yeo S, Scarbough M: Exercise-induced hyperthermia may prevent accurate core temperature measurement by tympanic membrane thermometer, *West J Nurs Res* 24(3):82, 1996.

CHAPTER 13

Shift Assessment

Skill 13.1
General Survey and Inspection of Integument, 257

Skill 13.2
Auscultating Lung Sounds, 262

Skill 13.3
Auscultating Apical Pulse, 266

Skill 13.4
Assessing the Abdomen, 269

Skill 13.5
Assessing Extremities and Peripheral Circulation, 274

In many situations nurses are the first to detect changes in a client's condition. The skills of physical assessment are important for the detection of significant changes in the client's health. Hospitalized clients are likely to be acutely ill, and changes may occur rapidly. In acute care settings a brief systematic assessment is done at the beginning of each shift to identify changes in the client's status compared with the previous assessment. This routine brief assessment takes 10 to 15 minutes and reveals information that supplements the database for the client.

Once data are gathered, the nurse groups significant findings into patterns of data that confirm or reveal actual or high-risk nursing diagnoses. Information gathered provides the information about a client's functional abilities and serves as a comparison for future assessment findings. Each abnormal finding directs the nurse to gather additional data and helps to select appropriate nursing measures.

A shift assessment is performed using a consistent, organized sequence that improves accuracy of findings. Priorities for assessment are based on a client's presenting signs and symptoms or health care needs. For example, a client who develops sudden shortness of breath should first undergo an assessment of the lungs.

Clients are often knowledgeable about their physical condition. Many can verify whether certain findings are normal for them, as well as noting whether actual changes have occurred. A client's sensory or physical limitations can affect how quickly the nurse is able to complete the assessment. For example, if the nurse realizes that the client has short-term memory loss, communication will be limited, or if a client becomes fatigued, a brief rest period may be necessary.

Inspection, palpation, auscultation, olfaction (smell), and percussion are techniques used in physical examination. All, except percussion, are used for a shift assessment. *Percussion* is a more advanced technique used in comprehensive examinations (see Chapter 14).

Inspection involves visual examination of body parts (see Chapter 14).

Palpation involves use of the sense of touch to detect characteristics of body parts such as texture, temperature, perception of vibration or movement, and consistency (see Chapter 14). Cultural factors also need to be acknowledged (Box 13-1). Brief explanations during the examination will reduce stress.

Auscultation is listening with a stethoscope for sounds created in body organs to detect variations from normal (see Chapter 14). To auscultate, the nurse needs to hear well, have a good stethoscope, and know how to use the stethoscope properly (see Chapter 12).

The final skill a nurse may use during assessment is *olfaction* (smell). Certain changes in body functions create characteristic body odors (Table 13-1, p. 256). The sense of smell can detect abnormalities that go unrecognized by any other means.

Performing a shift assessment efficiently requires skill and practice. The nurse may need to integrate additional assessment into routine nursing care, such as bathing, administration of medications, or other therapies, or while conversing with a client. In addition, health education can be integrated with assessment activities. The nurse also can teach clients about their health problems during assessments. This is a good time to discuss changes in symp-

Box 13-1 Cultural Considerations

- Consider the need for an interpreter when language barriers exist.
- Physical contact is perceived differently by clients with various cultural backgrounds. Individual differences must be identified and respected.
  - Hispanics are very modest and prefer a health care provider of the same gender.
  - Asians avoid touch as much as possible. Patting the head is taboo.
  - African Americans and Native Americans prefer not to be touched without having given permission. Some individuals may have a high level of fear. Nonverbal communication is considered very important.

toms, the implications for changes, and approaches the client may use for self-assessment. More comprehensive assessment skills are described in Chapter 14.

 NURSING DIAGNOSES

Shift assessment involves gathering data about the client's status and changes in comparison to the previous shift. It is important to be aware of nursing diagnoses previously established. The client may present any nursing diagnosis. However the following are easily screened for during shift assessment.

Impaired Skin Integrity or **Risk for Impaired Skin Integrity** is appropriate when the client is at risk for or has experienced skin breakdown. Influencing factors may include immobility, moisture from incontinence, or circulatory alterations..

Ineffective Airway Clearance is appropriate when the client is unable to clear secretions or obstructions from the respiratory tract. **Ineffective Breathing Pattern** involves altered inhalation or exhalation and may include either hypoventilation or hyperventilation. Influencing factors may include decreased muscle strength or energy, pain, and anxiety.

Activity Intolerance applies when physiological energy is inadequate for the completion of desired activities because of altered cardiac function. Activity intolerance may also be related to prolonged immobility, weakness, and muscle atrophy. **Decreased Cardiac Output** is appropriate when there is a need to reduce cardiac workload or improve cardiac performance.

Pain related to unknown etiology may be appropriate when the focus of nursing care involves identifying factors that contribute to pain. Such as when the client presents signs and symptoms of discomfort and/or suffers a condition that may cause pain. Abdominal pain is one of the most common symptoms clients present.

Constipation or **Diarrhea** may be associated with abdominal pain or cramping and altered peristalsis resulting in either infrequent hard stools or frequent unformed stools and fluid loss.

Altered Peripheral Tissue Perfusion involves a chronic deficit in blood supply to the extremities and is appropriate when findings reveal alteration in arterial or venous circulation.

Table 13-1

Assessment of Characteristic Odors

Odor	Site or Source	Potential Causes
Alcohol	Oral cavity	Ingestion of alcohol
Ammonia	Urine	Urinary tract infection
Body odor	Skin, particularly in areas where body parts rub together (e.g., under arms, beneath breasts)	Poor hygiene, excess perspiration (hyperhidrosis), foul-smelling perspiration (bromhidrosis)
Feces	Wound site	Wound abscess
	Vomitus	Bowel obstruction
	Rectal area	Fecal incontinence
Foul-smelling stools in infant	Stool	Malabsorption syndrome
Halitosis	Oral cavity	Poor dental and oral hygiene, gum disease
Sweet, fruity ketones	Oral cavity	Diabetes acidosis
Stale urine	Skin	Uremic acidosis
Sweet, heavy, thick odor	Draining wound	*Pseudomonas* (bacterial) infection
Musty odor	Casted body part	Infection inside cast
Fetid, sweet odor	Tracheostomy or mucous secretions	Infection of bronchial tree (*Pseudomonas* bacteria)

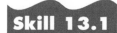

GENERAL SURVEY AND INSPECTION OF INTEGUMENT

The general survey is the preliminary portion of the assessment during which the client's vital signs, general behavior, and appearance are identified. If abnormalities or signs of problems are revealed during the assessment, the nurse can direct attention to specific concerns. This information influences how the nurse communicates instructions to the client and conducts remaining portions of the assessment.

Clients develop skin lesions from trauma to the skin, exposure to pressure while immobilized, continued exposure to moisture and irritating fluids, or reaction to medications used in therapy. This is a particular concern for debilitated or older adults. Nurses routinely assess the skin each shift using inspection, palpation, and olfaction.

Equipment

Stethoscope
Sphygmomanometer and cuff
Wristwatch with second hand
Tape measure (optional)
Penlight
Thermometer

ASSESSMENT

1. Obtain previous vital signs from client records. Often this information is kept on a clipboard just outside the door. **Rationale: Previous data provide a means to compare nurse's assessment findings to detect change. Compare current data with previous data to detect alterations.**
2. Consider factors or conditions that may normally alter vital sign readings (see Chapter 12).
3. Review client's recent fluid intake and output (I & O) records. Intake includes all liquids taken orally, by feeding tube, and parenterally. Liquid output includes urine, diarrhea, vomitus, gastric suction, and drainage from postsurgical tubes, such as chest tubes or Jackson-Pratt drains. **Rationale: Provides data regarding client's risk for fluid imbalance which can be detected through behavioral changes, vital sign changes, and skin integrity.**
4. Assess client's general perceptions about personal health. **Rationale: Nurse's assessment of client's general appearance coupled with client's own perceptions may reveal problem areas.**

PLANNING

Expected outcomes focus on accuracy in collection of assessment data.

Expected Outcomes

1. Client demonstrates alert, cooperative behaviors without evidence of physical or emotional distress during assessment.
2. Client's skin is smooth, soft, dry, and warm.
3. Client provides appropriate subjective data related to physical condition.

DELEGATION CONSIDERATIONS

Shift assessment requires problem solving and knowledge unique to the professional nurse. Assistive personnel (AP) may measure daily weight, I&O, and vital signs. The professional nurse must clarify expected findings and provide parameters for what is to be reported. Acute distress, difficulty breathing, pain, and anxiety must be promptly reported to the professional nurse.

IMPLEMENTATION

Steps	Rationale
1. See Standard Protocol (inside front cover).	
2. Take temperature, pulse, respiration, and blood pressure (BP) unless gathered within last 3 hours (see Chapter 10). Inform client of vital signs.	Data used to compare with client's baseline.
3. Assess the following aspects of behavior and appearance.	
a. Signs of distress (e.g., shortness of breath, acute pain, anxiety).	Such distress requires immediate attention and helps establish priorities.
b. Race, gender, and age.	These are important variables that influence assessment findings and techniques to use.

Steps	Rationale

NURSE ALERT

If pulses were previously palpable and cannot be located, ask another nurse to assess client's pulses. Loss of peripheral pulse must be reported to the physician immediately for appropriate medical intervention.

COMMUNICATION TIP

Tell clients you are going to check them over to get a clear picture of how they are progressing. Ask "What is your greatest concern at this time?," which helps with setting priorities as you proceed with the assessment.

4. Determine the level of consciousness and orientation by talking to client.
   a. Is client alert, confused, or lethargic?
   b. Eyes open spontaneously, to speech, to pain, or not at all.
   c. Verbal response may be oriented, confused, inappropriate, or incomprehensible.
   d. Motor response may be appropriate in relation to commands, withdraw in response to pain only, or no response apparent.

May reveal subtle or obvious change in client's condition. Level of consciousness influences ability to cooperate. Timing of recent medications, especially pain medication and sedatives, may also alter assessment data.

5. Assess affect and mood: note if verbal expressions match nonverbal behavior. Note appropriateness to situation.

Reflects client's feelings and emotional status.

6. Assess if speech is understandable and properly paced. Is there an association with client's behavior?

Alterations reflect neurological impairment, injury or impairment of mouth, or differences in dialect and language.

7. Note body type (trim and muscular, obese, excessively thin).

Reflects level of health, risk factors, and lifestyle.

8. Assess position and posture: note alignment of shoulders and hips (see illustration). Reposition for comfort if needed.

9. Assess body movements: are they purposeful? Are there tremors of the extremities?

Indicates neurological problem or emotional stress.

10. Assess hygiene and grooming: observe for presence or absence of makeup, type of clothes (hospital or personal), and general state of cleanliness.

May reflect client's mood, sociocultural preferences, economic status, self-care habits, culture, and life-style.

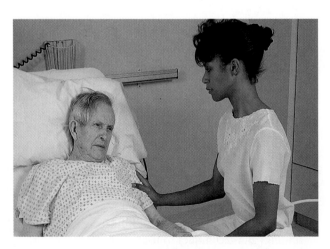

Step 8

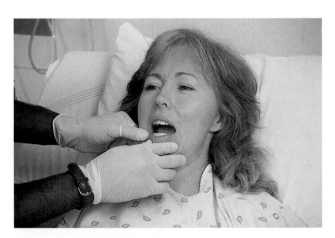

Step 13

Table 13-2

Pathological Color Changes

Color Changes	Light Skin	Dark Skin
Cyanosis: related to hypoxia (late sign of decreased oxygen) heart or lung disease, cold environment	Blue tinge, especially in conjunctivae, nailbeds earlobes, oral membranes, soles, and palms	Ashen-gray lips and tongue
Pallor: related to decreased perfusion (blood flow, anemia, shock)	Loss of rosy glow in skin, especially face	Ashen-gray appearance in black skin
Erythema: related to increased blood flow (fever, irritation)	Redness easily seen anywhere on body	Difficult to assess; rely on palpation for warmth or edema
Jaundice: related to deposits of bilirubin in tissue, liver disease	Yellow staining in sclerae of eyes, skin, fingernails, soles, palms, and oral mucosa	Most reliably assessed in sclerae, hard palate, palms, and soles
Ecchymoses: related to bleeding into skin, often trauma	Purple to yellowish green areas resulting from bleeding into skin, usually related to trauma	Difficult to see except in mouth or conjunctivae
Petechiae: minute hemorrhages into skin	Purple pinpoints most easily seen on buttocks, abdomen, and inner surfaces of arms or legs	Usually invisible except in oral mucosa, conjunctivae, or eyelids and covering eyeballs

Modified from Whaley LF, Wong DL: *Nursing care of infants and children*, ed 5, St Louis, 1995, Mosby.

Steps	Rationale
11. Assess for presence or absence of body odor.	Results from physical exercise, inadequate hygiene, or certain conditions, including infections or tissue necrosis.
12. Inspect color of skin surfaces. Compare color of symmetrical body parts, including areas unexposed to sun.	Changes in color can indicate pathological alterations (Table 13-2).
13. Inspect oral mucosa, tongue, teeth, and gums of oral cavity for hydration and obvious lesions (see illustration).	Reveals need for oral hygiene. Identifies sources of irritation that can affect ability to chew or swallow.
14. Inspect color of oral mucosa, nailbeds, lips, palms of hands, sclerae, and conjunctivae.	Nurse can more readily identify abnormalities in areas of body where melanin production is least. Pallor or cyanosis suggests compromised oxygenation or circulation.
15. Palpate texture, smoothness, and moisture of the skin using fingertips.	Changes in skin texture may be the first indication of skin rashes in dark-skinned clients. Skin moisture is affected by environment and body temperature.
a. If lesions, secretions, or drainage is noted, note color, odor, amount, consistency (e.g., thin and watery or thick and oily), and exact location.	Description of secretions helps to identify type of lesion.
b. Remove gloves. Use dorsum (back) of hand to palpate temperature of skin. Compare symmetrical body parts and upper to lower body parts. Note distinct temperature differences and localized areas of warm or cool skin.	Cool skin temperature often indicates decreased blood flow. A stage 1 pressure ulcer may cause warmth and erythema (redness) of an area (see Chapter 24).
c. Palpate for presence of edema (swelling), and note location and extent.	Localized edema associated with redness and tenderness suggests inflammation. Peripheral edema suggests circulatory problems. Dependent edema gravitates according to position to lowermost part of the body (e.g., in feet and ankles when client is sitting).

Steps	Rationale

d. Assess skin turgor by first grasping fold of skin over client's sternum, forearm, or abdomen. Release skinfold, and note ease and speed with which skin returns to place (see illustration).

Turgor is measure of skin's elasticity and hydration status. Skin may remain suspended or "tented" for a few seconds before slowly returning to place, indicating dehydration, inadequate nutrition, and effects of aging. Do not test over back of hand because of looseness of skin (Seidel, 1995).

16. Inspect condition of skin. If areas of redness are noted, place fingertip over area and apply gentle pressure, then release.

Normal reactive hyperemia (redness) is visible effect of localized vasodilation, the body's normal response to lack of blood flow to underlying tissue. Affected area of skin will blanch with fingertip pressure.

a. Assess for redness with particular attention to areas of pressure (e.g., sacrum, greater trochanter, heels, and clavicles).

If pressure is not relieved, tissue damage can occur in as little as 90 minutes from tissue hypoxia.

b. If lesions are detected, inspect color, location, size, type, grouping (e.g., clustered or linear), and distribution (localized or generalized). Be sure skin is well illuminated.

Certain skin lesions can be identified by a characteristic pattern of features (Box 13-2).

c. Gently palpate any lesion to determine mobility, shape, contour (flat, raised, or depressed), and consistency (soft or hard). Open lesions require use of gloves

Gentle palpation prevents accidental rupture of underlying cysts.

d. Ask if client has tenderness during palpation.

Tenderness may be indicative of inflammation or pressure on body part.

e. Palpate any intravenous (IV) site (see illustration) for evidence of inflammation (redness, heat, swelling, or tenderness) or infiltration (puffiness, pallor and coolness). Note when site is due to be changed (see Chapter 30).

Report or correct identified problems with infusion immediately. Presence of phlebitis or infiltration requires relocation of IV catheter or needle.

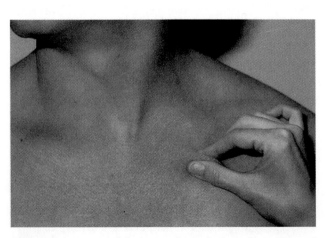

Step 15d *From Seidel HM et al: Mosby's guide to physical examination, ed 3, St Louis, 1995, Mosby.*

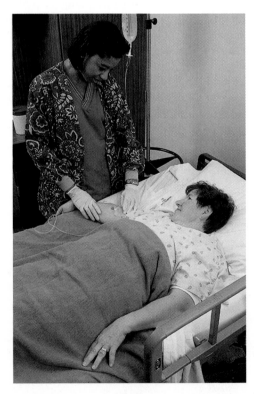

Step 16e

Steps	Rationale
17. Check intravenous fluids and medications, including type of fluids and rate of infusion. Note expiration date of fluids and tubing.	Infusion rate that is too rapid may result in fluid volume excess; a rate too slow can result in inadequate fluid replacement.
18. If client has dressings, cast, restraints, or other constricting devices, compare right and left body parts for impaired circulation, sensation, and motion (CSM). Inspect distal areas for pallor. Palpate for decreased capillary refill and coolness. Ask if client has numbness or tingling, and have client move body part (see Chapters 27 and 28).	Altered CSM may indicate circulatory compromise or pressure on a nerve.

Box 13-2 Types of Skin Lesions

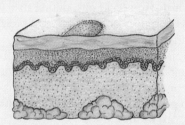

Macule: flat, nonpalpable, change in skin color, smaller than 1 cm (e.g., freckle or petechia)

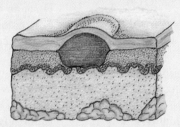

Papule: palpable, circumscribed, solid elevation in skin, smaller than 0.5 cm (e.g., elevated nevus)

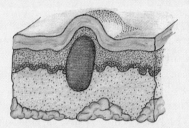

Nodule: elevated solid mass, deeper and firmer than papule, 0.5 to 2.0 cm (e.g., wart)

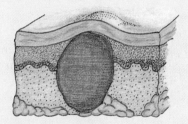

Tumor: solid mass that may extend deep through subcutaneous tissue, larger than 1 to 2 cm (e.g., epithelioma)

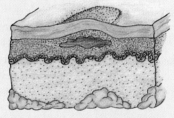

Wheal: irregularly shaped, elevated area or superficial localized edema, varies in size (e.g., hive or mosquito bite)

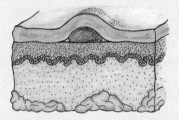

Vesicle: circumscribed elevation of skin filled with serous fluid, smaller than 0.5 cm (e.g., herpes simplex or chickenpox)

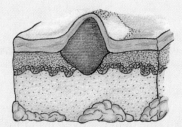

Pustule: circumscribed elevation of skin similar to vesicle but filled with pus, varies in size (e.g., acne or staphylococcal infection)

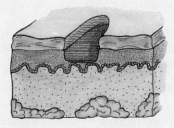

Ulcer: deep loss of skin surface that may extend to dermis and frequently bleeds and scars, varies in size (e.g., venous stasis ulcer)

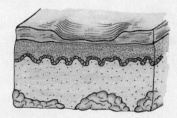

Atrophy: thinning of skin with loss of normal skin furrow with skin appearing shiny and translucent, varies in size (e.g., arterial insufficiency)

Steps	Rationale
19. Observe drainage (color, amount, consistency) and function of any drainage systems (see Skill 21.4).	Character and amount of drainage to expect will vary with type of drainage system.
20. Inspect dressings to determine if they are clean, dry, and intact. If the dressing is loose or drainage is visible, change the whole dressing.	A dressing that is loose or has drainage provides a potential for infection.
21. Remove gloves.	
22. See Completion Protocol (inside front cover).	

• • •

EVALUATION

1. Observe throughout the assessment for evidence of physical or emotional distress.
2. Compare assessment findings with previous observations of skin.
3. Ask the client if there is information about physical condition that has not been discussed.

Unexpected Outcomes and Related Interventions

1. Client displays signs of distress, such as shortness of breath, acute pain, or anxiety.
   a. Respond immediately to identified need (reposition, administer oxygen or medication as appropriate).
   b. Notify charge nurse or physician if orders are needed for relief of acute symptoms.
2. Client's skin has abnormal coloring, dry texture, reduced turgor, lesion, or erythema.
   a. Identify contributing factors (see Chapter 24).
   b. Prevent continued irritation and damage as appropriate (e.g., loosen constricting or pressure-causing devices, turn, provide hygiene).
3. Client is unwilling or unable to provide subjective information relating to identified concerns.
   a. Seek information from family members if present.
   b. Review client's record for baseline data.

Recording and Reporting

- Document vital signs if taken on graphic flow sheet. Compare to previous data for significant changes (see Chapter 12 and Skill 14.6).
- Document significant changes in level of consciousness, mood, speech, and body movements on neurological flow sheet (see Skills 14.1, 14.9, and 14.10).
- Describe abnormal skin conditions, noting size, location, color, whether raised or indented, and presence or absence of drainage.
- Describe abnormal sensations such as pruritus, pain, burning, or numbness, including specific location and bilateral comparison as subjective data using quotes. Determine if sequential changes are related to therapy (i.e., cast or dressings).
- Report skin breakdown and draining lesions to physician and/or clinical specialist.
- Record condition of IV site on IV flow sheet including presence/absence of redness, tenderness, swelling, or leaking.

Sample Documentation

Documentation routinely involves use of an assessment flow sheet (see Appendix A). Changes in condition need a description in nurse's notes.

Skill 13.2

AUSCULTATING LUNG SOUNDS

Assessment of respiratory function is one of the most critical assessment skills, because alterations can be life-threatening. Routine shift assessment is essential because changes in respirations can occur quickly as a result of a variety of factors, including immobility, infection, and fluid overload. Shift assessment includes auscultation, which assesses the movement of air through the tracheo-bronchial tree. Normally, air flows through the airways unobstructed. Recognizing the sounds created by normal airflow allows the nurse to detect sounds caused by obstruction of the airways. Auscultation of the lungs requires familiarity with landmarks of the chest. During the assessment, the nurse should keep a mental image of the location of the lung lobes. To locate the position of each rib,

Table 13-3

Adventitious Sounds

Sound	Site Auscultated	Cause	Character
Crackles (also called *rales*)	Are most commonly heard in dependent lobes: right and left lung bases	Random, sudden reinflation of groups of alveoli*	Are fine, short, interrupted crackling sounds heard during inspiration, expiration, or both; vary in pitch: high or low; may or may not change with coughing*; sound like crushing cellophane
Gurgles (also called *rhonchi*)	Are primarily heard over trachea and bronchi; if loud enough, can be heard over most lung fields	Fluid or mucus in larger airways, causing turbulence	Are low-pitched, continuous sounds heard more during expiration; may be cleared by coughing; sounds like blowing air through milk with a straw
Wheezes	Can be heard over all lung fields	Severely narrowed bronchus	Are high-pitched, musical sounds heard during inspiration or expiration; do not clear with coughing†
Pleural friction rub	Is heard best over anterior lateral lung field (if client is sitting upright)	Inflamed pleura, parietal pleura rubbing against visceral pleura	Has grating quality heard best during inspiration; does not clear with coughing

*Data from Forgacs P: *Chest* 73:399, 1978.
†Modified from Wilkins RL, Hodgkin JE, Lopez B: *Lung sounds: a practical guide,* St Louis, 1988, Mosby.

the nurse locates the angle of Louis by palpating the "speed bump" on the sternum where the second rib articulates with the sternum. The ribs and intercostal spaces are counted from this point. Auscultation involves listening to breath sounds using a stethoscope and are best heard when the person breathes deeply through the mouth.

Adventitious sounds are abnormal sounds resulting from air passing through moisture, mucus, or narrowed airways; alveoli suddenly reinflating; or an inflammation between the pleural linings. The four types of adventitious sounds include *crackles* (also referred to as *rales*), *gurgles* (also referred to as *rhonchi*), *wheezes*, and *pleural friction rub* (Table 13-3). The location and characteristics of the sounds should be noted, as well as diminished breath sounds or the absence of breath sounds (found with collapsed or surgically removed lobes). Because deep palpation and percussion are not included in a routine shift assessment, they are not described in this skill.

Equipment
Stethoscope
Watch with second hand

ASSESSMENT

1. Check client record to determine if client has smoking history: length of time client has smoked, number of cigarettes per day, cigar or pipe smoking, or length of time since smoking stopped. To calculate pack years, multiply the number of packs smoked per day times the number of years a smoker; for example, ½ pack per day times 4 years equals 2 pack years. **Rationale: Determine the age smoking started and, if applicable, describe efforts that have been made to quit. Smoking predisposes client to lung disease and affects secretion of mucus in airways.**
2. Ask if client is experiencing any of the following: persistent cough (productive or nonproductive), sputum production, shortness of breath with exertion, chest pain, or orthopnea, or dyspnea. If cough is productive, obtain a description of sputum. **Rationale: Warning signs of lung cancer include persistent cough, bloody sputum, and recurrent lung infections.**
3. Check for history of allergies to pollens, dust, or other airborne irritants, as well as to any foods, drugs, or chemical substances. **Rationale: Allergies are associated with wheezes on auscultation, dyspnea, cyanosis, and diaphoresis.**
4. Determine the rate, rhythm, and depth of breathing (see Chapter 10). **Rationale: Used to compare with baseline to assess change in client condition.**

PLANNING

Expected outcomes focus on identifying alterations in respiratory function.

Expected Outcome

Client's breath sounds are clear to auscultation in all lung fields.

DELEGATION CONSIDERATIONS

Lung auscultation requires the knowledge and problem-solving skills unique to a professional nurse. Delegation is inappropriate. For clients with abnormal lung sounds, AP must be instructed to observe client's respirations and report changes in rate and depth as well as the need to keep head of bed elevated in order to breathe.

IMPLEMENTATION

Steps	Rationale

1. See Standard Protocol (inside front cover).
2. Position for auscultation of lungs.
   a. Have client sit upright, or elevate head of bed 45 to 90 degrees for bedridden client.   Promotes full lung expansion during examination.
   b. If client cannot tolerate sitting, supine position is allowed for anterior chest and side-lying position is used for posterior chest.

COMMUNICATION TIP

Tell client to relax and breathe deeply and normally through the mouth. If sounds are faint, ask client to temporarily breathe deeper.

3. Remove or raise gown, avoiding unnecessary exposure and providing full visibility of thorax (see illustration).
4. Auscultate breath sounds. For adult, place diaphragm of stethoscope on chest wall over intercostal spaces. Move stethoscope systematically from apex of lung down to lower lobes. Ask client to take slow, deep breaths through the mouth each time you place the stethoscope on the chest.   Easy, passive movement indicates no respiratory distress.
5. Listen to entire inspiration and expiration at each stethoscope position. Systematically compare breath sounds over right and left sides (see illustrations for posterior and anterior stethoscope placement).
6. Assess client's respiratory character, observing symmetry and degree of chest wall and abdominal movement.   Assesses client's effort to ventilate.

Steps	Rationale

7. If adventitious sounds are auscultated, have client cough. Listen again with stethoscope to determine if sound has cleared with coughing (see Table 13-3).

8. If client has a productive cough, and mucus is purulent, obtaining a specimen may be indicated (see Chapter 15).

9. See Completion Protocol (inside front cover).

Gurgles caused by fluid or mucus in larger airways can be diminished or eliminated by effective coughing. Crackles may or may not change with coughing.

• • •

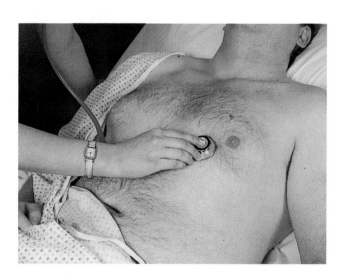

Step 3

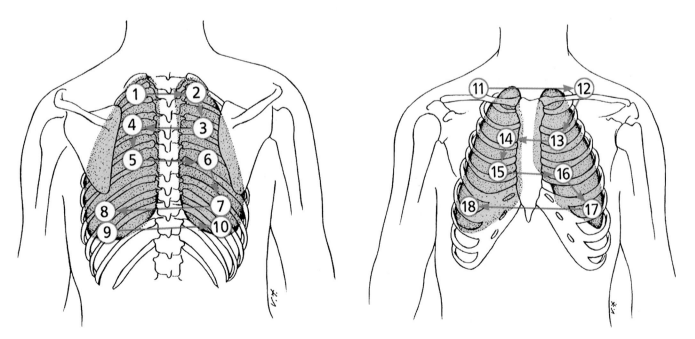

Step 5

EVALUATION

Compare respirations (depth, regularity, rate) and breath sounds with findings of previous shift.

Unexpected Outcomes and Related Interventions

Client is unable to clear secretions from airway, and adventitious sounds are auscultated over one or both lungs.

    a. Encourage increased fluid intake if not contraindicated, to liquefy secretions for the ease of expectoration.

    b. Position with head of bed elevated, turning side-to-side every 2 hours.

    c. If client is experiencing respiratory distress, suction and/or oxygen administration may be indicated (see Chapter 31).

Recording and Reporting

- Record adventitious breath sounds, including type; location; presence on inspiration, expiration, or both; and changes noted after coughing.
- Record ability/inability to clear airways by effective coughing and, if cough is productive, the amount, color, odor, and consistency of sputum.
- Report increased dyspnea and acute respiratory distress immediately.

Sample Documentation

0730   *Wheezes noted over anterior upper lobes bilaterally. Respiratory rate 26. C/O shortness of breath even at rest. M.D. notified. HOB raised to 90 degrees.*

Skill 13.3

AUSCULTATING APICAL PULSE

The apical pulse provides information about the heart rate and rhythm. Changes in the client's pulse may result from responses to many factors, including stress, exercise, fatigue, blood loss, and pain. Responses to medications and medical treatment can also be monitored by changes in the pulse.

    Auscultation of the apical pulse is done as part of the routine shift assessment after auscultation of the lungs, because the client is already in a suitable position with the chest exposed. The nurse forms a mental image of the heart's location in the center of the chest to the left of the sternum. The apex of the heart is the bottom tip (Fig. 13-1) and actually touches the anterior chest wall at approximately the fourth to fifth intercostal space along the midclavicular line (MCL), known as the *point of maximal impulse (PMI)*. In children under 7 years of age the PMI is located just lateral to the MCL at the fourth intercostal space (Fig. 13-2).

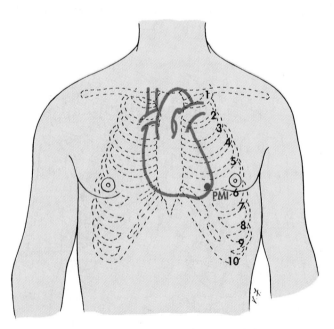

Figure 13-1 Location of PMI in adult.

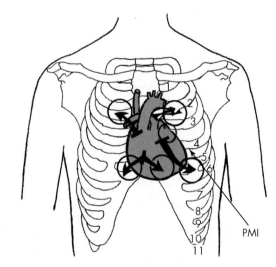

Figure 13-2 Location of PMI in child under 7 years of age. *From Wong DL:* Whaley & Wong's nursing care of infants and children, *ed 5, St Louis, 1995, Mosby.*

ASSESSMENT

1. Review records for history of smoking family history of heart disease, alcohol ingestion, cocaine use, absent or reduced regular exercise, and intake of foods high in carbohydrates and cholesterol. **Rationale: These are important risk factors for cardiovascular disease.**

2. Determine medications the client is taking related to cardiovascular function (e.g., digoxin, antidysrhythmics, antihypertensives). Determine if client knows their purpose, dosage, and side effects.

3. Review the history for evidence of dyspnea, chest pain, fatigue, edema of feet and ankles, and orthopnea. **Rationale: Clinical signs of heart failure.**

4. If chest pain is present, determine onset (sudden or gradual), precipitating factors, quality, region, severity, and timing (how long it lasts). **Rationale: Symptoms may reveal coronary artery disease.**

5. Ask if client has had congestive heart failure, congenital heart disease, coronary artery disease, a pacemaker, or an irregular heart rate.

PLANNING
Expected Outcome

Client's heart rhythm is regular and at a rate appropriate for age:

Adults and adolescents:	60 to 100 beats/min
Children 2 to 10 years old:	70 to 110 beats/min
Infants (1 month to 2 years):	80 to 150 beats/min
Neonates (up to 1 month):	100 to 180 beats/min

DELEGATION CONSIDERATIONS

AP can be trained to count the apical pulse rate. Cardiac assessment requires the problem-solving ability and knowledge unique to a professional nurse.

IMPLEMENTATION

Steps	Rationale
1. See Standard Protocol (inside front cover).	
2. Prepare client: have client assume semi-Fowler's or supine position.	Provides adequate visibility and access to left thorax and mediastinum. Client with heart disease may experience shortness of breath while lying flat.
3. Explain procedure and be sure client is relaxed and comfortable.	Client with previously normal cardiac history may become anxious if nurse shows concern.
4. Locate anatomical landmarks used to assess cardiac function including angle of Louis, sternum, intercostal spaces, and midclavicular line.	Familiarity with landmarks allows nurse to describe findings more clearly and ultimately may improve assessment.
5. Locate PMI by palpating with fingertips along fifth intercostal space in midclavicular line (see illustration). Note a light tap in an area 1 to 2 cm (½ to 1 inch) in diameter at the apex.	NOTE: In the presence of cardiac enlargement associated with left-sided heart disease, PMI is located to the left of the midclavicular line. If associated with right-sided heart failure, PMI is moved toward the sternum.

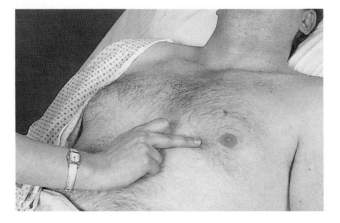

Step 5

Steps	Rationale

6. If palpating PMI is difficult, turn client onto left side (see illustration).

Maneuver moves the heart closer to the chest wall.

7. Ask client not to speak. Place the diaphragm of the stethoscope lightly against the chest wall over the PMI (see illustration).

Pressing too firmly may decrease transmission of sounds. Cardiovascular sounds may be difficult to hear, so a quiet room and focused attention are essential (Barkauskas et al, 1998).

   a. Listen for "lub-dub" sounds (S_1 and S_2).
   b. After both sounds are heard clearly as "lub-dub," count each combination of S_1 and S_2 as one heart beat. Count the number of beats for 1 minute to determine the apical pulse rate.
   c. Determine if heart sounds are clear, strong, and regular.

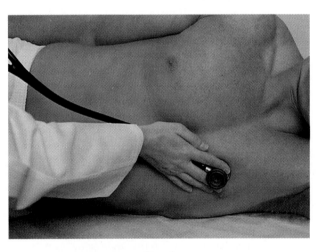

Step 6

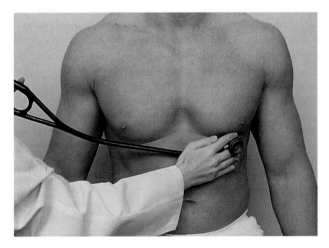

Step 7

8. Identify if the rhythm is regular or irregular. This may be further identified as regularly irregular or irregularly irregular.

An irregular heart beat is a dysrhythmia, which interferes with heart's ability to pump effectively and may result in decreased cardiac output.

9. When heart rate is irregular, compare apical and radial pulses. This is best done with a colleague, who can count the radial pulse simultaneously while the apical pulse rate is counted (see Chapter 14). NOTE: Additional information about cardiac assessment is included in Skill 14.6.

If a pulse deficit exists (radial pulse is slower than apical), this indicates that ineffective contractions of the heart fail to send pulse waves to the periphery.

10. See Completion Protocol (inside front cover).

• • •

EVALUATION

Compare heart rate and rhythm with previous shift assessment.

Unexpected Outcome and Related Interventions

Client's heart rate is irregular; rate is less than 60 or greater than 100 beats/min.

a. Respond immediately to acute distress (oxygen or medication if ordered).
b. Identify and alleviate contributing factors if possible.
c. Notify charge nurse or physician if orders are needed for relief of acute symptoms.

Recording and Reporting

- Document quality (clear or muffled), intensity (weak or pounding), rate, and rhythm (regular, regularly irregular, or irregularly irregular).
- Document activity level and subjective data related to fatigue, shortness of breath, and chest pain.
- Document preferred position, medications and/or treatments used, and client's response.

Sample Documentation

0730   Pulse rate 104 and irregularly irregular. Blood pressure 120/70. Client denies discomfort. Resting quietly in bed without complaints of distress. (See Routine Nursing Assessment: Cardiovascular, Appendix A.)

Skill 13.4

ASSESSING THE ABDOMEN

Routine abdominal assessment may identify changes resulting from dietary changes, procedures that interfere with peristalsis, or prolonged bed rest. Abdominal pain can be caused by many different problems relating not only to the gastrointestinal (GI) system but also to the urinary system, reproductive system, or spinal or muscular injury. When performing abdominal assessment, the nurse should maintain a mental image of the anatomical location of each of the organs, including the kidneys, which are toward the back.

Abdominal shift assessment includes inspection, auscultation, and palpation. The order of an abdominal assessment differs from previous assessments in that auscultation precedes palpation. Otherwise, palpation may alter the frequency and character of bowel sounds.

Equipment

Stethoscope
Tape measure

ASSESSMENT

1. If client has abdominal or low back pain, assess the character of pain in detail (location, onset, frequency, precipitating factors, aggravating or relieving factors, type of pain, severity). Compare findings with baseline. **Rationale: Knowing characteristics of pain helps determine its source.**
2. Carefully observe client's movement and position.
   a. Lying still with knees drawn up.
   b. Moving restlessly to find a comfortable position.
   c. Lying on one side or sitting with knees drawn up to chest.

Rationale: Positions assumed by the client may reveal nature and source of pain (e.g., peritonitis, renal [kidney] stone, pancreatitis).
3. Assess when client last had a stool, character of stool, and any recent changes in character of stools.
4. Identify measures usually used to promote elimination (e.g., laxatives, enemas, dietary intake, eating and drinking habits). **Rationale: This may help to identify cause and nature of elimination problems.**
5. Determine if client has had abdominal surgery or trauma. **Rationale: Surgery or trauma influences approach to assessment of the abdomen and can be associated with pain.**
6. Assess if client has had any recent changes in weight or intolerance to diet (e.g., nausea, vomiting, cramping), especially in last 24 hours. **Rationale: Changes may indicate stomach, gallbladder, or lower intestinal tract alterations.**
7. Assess for difficulty in swallowing, belching, flatulence, bloody emesis (hematemesis), black or tarry stools (melena), heartburn, diarrhea, or constipation.
8. Ask if client takes antibiotics or antiinflammatory medications (e.g., aspirin, steroids, or non-steroidal antiinflammatory drugs [NSAIDs]). **Rationale: These drugs may cause gastric irritation with bleeding or gastrointestinal upset.**

PLANNING

Expected outcomes should focus on identifying alterations in function relating to organs located within the abdomen (stomach, gallbladder, intestines, kidneys).

Expected Outcomes

1. Abdomen is soft and symmetrical with even contour. No mass, distention, or tenderness when palpated. No rebound tenderness on quick release of finger pressure.
2. Bowel sounds are active and audible in all four quadrants.

DELEGATION CONSIDERATIONS

This skill requires problem solving and knowledge unique to a professional nurse. Delegation is not appropriate. AP should report any problems related to bowel habits or dietary intake, the presence of abdominal pain, and changes in the size or shape of the abdomen.

IMPLEMENTATION

Steps	Rationale
1. See Standard Protocol (inside front cover).	
2. Prepare client.	
a. Ask if client needs to empty bladder.	Palpation of full bladder can cause discomfort and feeling of urgency and can make it difficult for client to relax.
b. Keep upper chest and legs covered.	Maintains client's warmth during examination, promoting relaxation.
c. Have client lie supine with arms down at sides and knees flexed.	Position promotes optimal relaxation of abdominal muscles. Tightening of muscles prevents adequate palpation of underlying muscles.

COMMUNICATION TIP

Maintain general conversation during assessment (except when auscultating). Carefully observe non-verbal response to palpation and further assess for subjective information relating to severity and location of discomfort.

Steps	Rationale
d. Ask client to locate tender areas, and assess painful areas last.	Manipulation of body part can increase pain and client's anxiety and make remainder of assessment difficult to complete.
3. Describe observations or findings in relation to quadrants. A line extending from tip of xiphoid process to symphysis pubis crossed by a line intersecting umbilicus divides abdomen into four equal sections (see illustration).	Provides consistent reference points.
4. Inspect skin of abdomen's surface for scars, venous patterns, rashes, lesions, silvery white striae (stretch marks), and stomas or ostomies.	Scars reveal evidence client has had past trauma or surgery. Striae indicate stretching of tissue by growth, obesity, pregnancy, ascites, or edema. Venous patterns may reflect liver disease (portal hypertension). Artificial openings indicate bowel or urinary diversion (see Chapters 33 and 34).
5. Observe for visible pulsations and movement as client inhales and exhales.	Normal ventilation involves rhythmical movement of abdomen as diaphragm descends and rises. Normally, the aorta pulsates slightly with each beat of systole.
6. To assess bowel sounds, provide a quiet environment. Ask client not to talk. If nasogastric (NG) or intestinal tube is connected to suction, turn off momentarily.	Sound obscures bowel sounds.

Steps	Rationale

7. Place the stethoscope's diaphragm lightly over each of the four abdominal quadrants. Listen until repeated gurgling or bubbling sounds are heard at each location (see illustration).

8. Describe sounds as normal or audible, absent, and hyperactive or hypoactive.

Normal bowel sounds occur irregularly every 5 to 15 seconds. Hyperactive sounds occur almost continuously. This is normal after meals. Hypoactive bowel sounds occur less than once every 15 to 20 seconds.

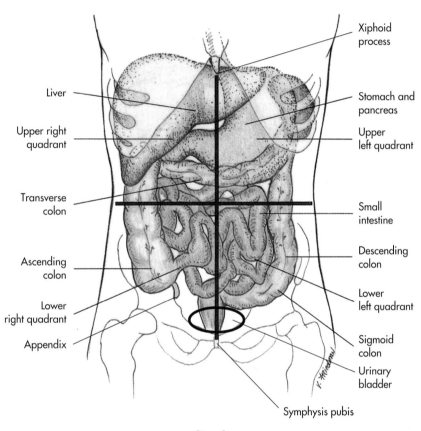

Labels: Xiphoid process; Liver; Upper right quadrant; Transverse colon; Ascending colon; Lower right quadrant; Appendix; Stomach and pancreas; Upper left quadrant; Small intestine; Descending colon; Lower left quadrant; Sigmoid colon; Urinary bladder; Symphysis pubis

Step 3

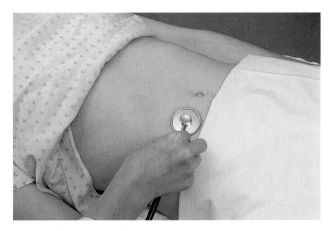

Step 7   *From Doughty DB, Jackson DB:* Gastrointestinal disorders, *Mosby's clinical nursing series, St Louis, 1993, Mosby.*

Steps	Rationale
9. Listen 3 to 5 minutes before reporting bowel sounds are absent.	Absence of peristalsis, may require surgical intervention.
10. Ask client if abdomen feels unusually tight. Observe skin for a taut, stretched, shiny appearance.	Continued sensation of fullness helps to detect distention. Feeling of fullness after a heavy meal causes only temporary distention. Tightness is not felt with obesity.
11. If distention is suspected, place tape measure around abdomen at level of umbilicus and note measurement. Compare with previous measurements if available (see illustration).	Assesses changes in abdominal size. All measurements of abdominal girth should be done at the umbilicus.
12. Have client roll onto side. If distention is present, entire abdomen protrudes.	Distention may result from a variety of sources easily remembered as the "6 F's"—fat, fetus, flatus, fluid, feces, foreign growth (i.e., tumor). If gas causes distention, flanks do not bulge. If fluid is source of distention, flanks bulge and protuberance forms on dependent side.
13. Lightly palpate over each abdominal quadrant, using palm and pads of fingertips in smooth, coordinated movement. Depress skin approximately 1 cm ($\frac{1}{2}$ inch) (see illustration). Note if abdomen is firm or soft to touch. Palpate painful areas last, avoiding quick jabs.	Detects areas of localized tenderness, degree of tenderness, and presence and character of underlying masses. Palpation of sensitive areas last minimizes guarding, which is voluntary tightening of underlying abdominal muscles.

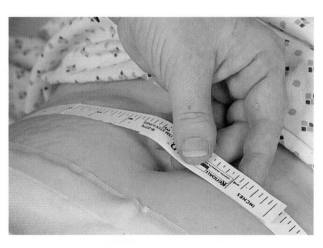

Step 11

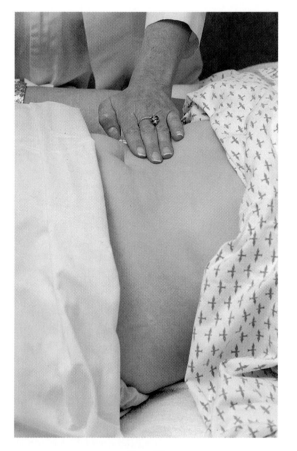

Step 13

Steps	Rationale

14. Observe client's verbal and nonverbal cues, which may indicate discomfort from tenderness. Firm abdomen may indicate accumulation of fluid or gas.

15. Palpate for a full bladder just above symphysis pubis, felt as a smooth, rounded mass.

Detects presence of a distended bladder.

16. If masses are palpated, note size, location, shape, consistency, tenderness, mobility, and texture.

Characteristics help to reveal type of mass.

17. If tenderness is present, press one hand slowly and deeply into the involved area and then let go quickly. Note if pain is aggravated.

Tests for rebound tenderness. Results are positive if pain increases. Additional assessment may include increased pain with coughing or dropping onto heels from a tiptoe position. Rebound abdominal tenderness, if found, can result from peritoneal irritation (e.g., appendicitis, pancreatitis).

18. See Completion Protocol (inside front cover).

• • •

EVALUATION

1. Observe throughout the assessment for evidence of discomfort.
2. Compare assessment findings with previous shift assessment.

Unexpected Outcomes and Related Interventions

1. Client has a firm, protruding, symmetrical abdomen with taut skin. Client complains of tightness and is not passing flatus, resulting in gaseous distention.
   a. Encourage ambulation (if permitted).
   b. Encourage hot liquids (if permitted).
   c. Nasogastric (NG) intubation may be required if bowel sounds are absent and client has nausea and vomiting (see Chapter 32).
2. Client has an increased abdominal girth with ascites (a buildup of fluid within peritoneal cavity).
   a. Determine the extent of the pressure, which can press against the diaphragm, causing difficulty breathing.
   b. Position with head of bed elevated to minimize discomfort and knee gatch slightly elevated to decrease pull on abdominal muscles.
3. Client has a distended urinary bladder palpable over the symphysis pubis.
   a. If a Foley catheter is in place, check that it is properly secured and that tubing and bag are positioned to promote drainage.
   b. Ask if there has been a change in voiding pattern (ability to urinate) or pain when urinating.
   c. If client is unable to urinate, see Chapter 35.

4. Hyperactive bowel sounds are evident, which results from an increase in GI motility.
   a. Assess for anxiety, diarrhea, and use of laxatives, which stimulate peristalsis.
   b. Caution clients about dangers of excessive regular use of laxatives or enemas, which can result in dependence.
   c. Bowel sounds normally tend to be increased after meals.
5. Absence of bowel sounds when assessed for 3 to 5 minutes in each quadrant.
   a. Instruct client to remain NPO.
   b. Report to physician for evaluation for paralytic ileus.
   c. Expected finding in early postoperative period.

Recording and Reporting

• Record abnormalities, such as absent bowel sounds, hyperactive or hypoactive bowel sounds, nausea and vomiting, or acute pain, including onset, precipitating factors, quality, region, severity, and timing (OPQRST)
• Record presence of masses, bulging (hernias), or distention. If distended, note if soft or firm, measure abdominal girth, and note whether or not client is passing flatus.

Sample Documentation

1030   Client complains of feeling "bloated." Denies nausea. Abdomen firm and nontender. Abdominal girth increased from 38″ to 41″ since yesterday. Bowel sounds hypoactive. Denies passing flatus. Encouraged to drink hot tea and ambulate more frequently. (See Routine Nursing Assessment: Gastrointestinal and Abdomen, Appendix A.)

Skill 13.5

ASSESSING EXTREMITIES AND PERIPHERAL CIRCULATION

Prolonged illness or immobility may result in muscle weakness and atrophy. Hospitalized clients may experience altered peripheral circulation as a result of high or low BP, immobility, prolonged bed rest, altered fluid balance, or pressure and constriction of the extremities with dressings or a cast.

Inadequate tissue perfusion results in an inadequate delivery of oxygen and nutrients to cells, a condition called *ischemia*. This can be caused by constriction of the vessels or by occlusion (blockage) from clot formation. The effects of the ischemia depend on the duration of the problem and the metabolic needs of the tissues. Ischemia results in pain. If lack of oxygen to tissues is unrelieved, tissue necrosis (death) occurs. An embolus is a blood clot that breaks loose and travels through the circulation. If the clot obstructs circulation to the lungs or the brain, it can be life-threatening.

Assessment of extremities and circulation routinely includes inspection and palpation.

Equipment
Stethoscope

ASSESSMENT

1. Determine if client is taking medications for cardiovascular function (e.g., antidysrhythmics, antihypertensives) and if client knows their purpose, dosage, and side effects. **Rationale: This allows nurse to assess client's compliance with and understanding of drug therapies. Medications for cardiovascular function cannot be taken intermittently.**

2. Ask if client experiences dyspnea, chest pain or discomfort, palpitations, excess fatigue, fainting, cyanosis, orthopnea, or edema of the feet. Ask if symptoms occur at rest or during exercise. **Rationale: These are the cardinal symptoms of heart disease. Cardiovascular function may be adequate during rest but not during exercise.**

3. Ask if client experiences leg cramps, numbness or tingling in extremities, or sensation of cold appendages. Also determine if client has noted swelling of feet, ankles, or hands. **Rationale: These are common signs and symptoms of peripheral vascular disease.**

4. If client experiences pain or cramping in the lower extremities, ask if it is relieved or aggravated by walking. Assess the distance walked and degree, location, and characteristics of pain before, during, and after activity. **Rationale: Pain caused by certain vascular conditions tends to increase with activity.**

PLANNING

Expected outcomes focus on identifying alterations in muscle strength and altered peripheral circulation.

Expected Outcomes

1. Client demonstrates strong grasp and leg strength that is equal bilaterally.

2. Client's peripheral pulses are normal (3+) and equal; extremities are warm and pink, with capillary refill less than 3 seconds.

3. Client has no dependent edema.

DELEGATION CONSIDERATIONS

AP can be trained to palpate peripheral pulses, and this skill can be delegated. Evaluation of diminished or absent pulses requires the problem-solving ability unique to a professional nurse. Instruct AP to assess and report altered or absent pulses, especially if noted after orthopedic interventions (i.e., casts, traction), vascular surgery, and cardiac catheterization. Also instruct AP to recognize and report temperature and color changes associated with altered arterial blood flow.

IMPLEMENTATION

Steps	Rationale

1. See Standard Protocol (inside front cover).
2. Observe ability to use arms and hands for grasping objects (see illustration).

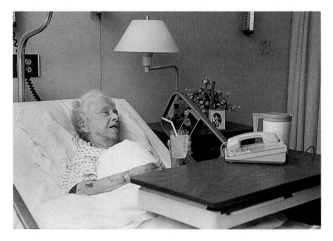

Step 2

Table 13-4

Comparison of Venous and Arterial Insufficiency

Assessment	Arterial	Venous
Pain	Burning, throbbing, cramping, increases with exercise	Aching, increases in evening and with dependent position
Paresthesia	Numbness, tingling, decreased sensation	None
Temperature/ color	Cool to touch, pale when elevated	Warm, flushed, cyanotic, brown discolorations on ankles
Capillary refill	>3 seconds	Not applicable
Pulses	Diminished or absent	Present
Ulcerations	Deep, well defined at site of trauma or tips of toes	Shallow ulcers around ankles (chronic venous stasis); edema apparent

3. Assess muscle strength of upper extremities by asking client to grasp your hands and squeeze as hard as possible. Note weakness, and compare right with left.
4. Inspect the knees, ankles, and feet for redness or swelling. Note abnormal positioning or alignment.

Muscle weakness may be generalized or confined to certain muscle groups. Dominant side is often slightly stronger.

COMMUNICATION TIP

Some clients need instructions repeated or a visual example to understand how to do strength assessments.

5. Assess strength of lower extremities by having client move legs. Then ask client to push and pull feet against your hands. Note weakness, and compare right with left.
6. Inspect lower extremities for changes in color and condition of the skin (Table 13-4). Note skin and nail texture, hair distribution, venous patterns, edema, and scars or ulcers. Compare skin color lying and standing.

Determines if venous or arterial insufficiency is present. Changes in circulation may be related to gravitational pull.

7. Inspect areas of skin for edema, paying particular attention to dependent body parts such as feet and ankles, sacrum, and scapular areas. Note color, location, and shape of area.
   a. Palpate edematous areas, noting mobility, consistency, and tenderness.

Edema results from fluid in tissues. Inadequate venous return causes edema in the sacrum if client is confined to bed, in the feet and ankles if sitting. Direct trauma causes localized edema.
Assists in determining extent of edema.

Steps	Rationale

b. Assess for pitting edema by pressing area firmly for 5 seconds, then releasing. Depth of edema determines severity (see illustration).

2 mm indentation: ⁺1 edema

4 mm indentation: ⁺2 edema

6 mm indentation: ⁺3 edema

8 mm indentation: ⁺4 edema

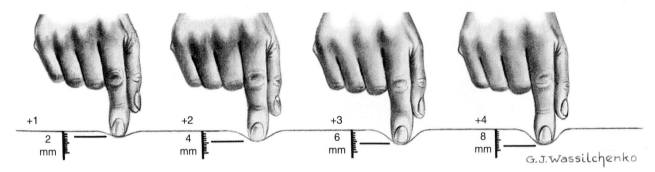

+1   2 mm   +2   4 mm   +3   6 mm   +4   8 mm

G.J.Wassilchenko

Step 7b *From Cannobbio MM: Cardiovascular disorders,* Mosby's Clinical Nursing Series, *St Louis, 1990, Mosby.*

8. Check capillary refill by grasping client's fingernail, and note color of nailbed. Next, apply gentle, firm pressure with the thumb to the nailbed. Release thumb quickly. Watch for color change. On release of pressure, circulation is restored and normally returns to pink color in less than 3 seconds.

Cold temperature with vasoconstriction and vascular disease may impair refill. Local pressure from cast or bandage may also impair refill.

9. If client complains of tenderness or pain in legs, test for Homans' sign.

A positive Homan's sign suggests the possibility of thrombophlebitis (inflammation of the vein) and (deep venous thrombosis) (DVT).

a. Support the leg while flexing the foot in dorsiflexion.

b. Note if client complains of pain.

10. Note tenderness or firmness of leg muscle and gently palpate calf muscles.

Signs of phlebitis include inflammation of veins and reddened or swollen areas over vein sites.

11. Palpate temperature of extremities with dorsum (back) of hand.

Temperature measures degree of blood flow to body part.

12. Assess each peripheral artery for following characteristics.

Palpation of peripheral arteries determines adequacy of blood flow to extremities.

a. Elasticity of vessel wall: depress and release artery, noting ease with which it springs back to shape.

Determines integrity of vessel. Artery should be easily palpable and should return to shape after pressure is released.

b. Rate and rhythm of pulse.

Radial pulse is chosen to assess heart rate. Other peripheral pulses are assessed only to determine condition of local blood flow.

c. Strength of pulse (force of blood against arterial wall).

Radial pulse is chosen to assess heart rate. Other peripheral pulses are assessed only to determine condition of local blood flow

Steps	Rationale

Rating scale for strength (Seidel, 1995):

    0: No pulse is palpable.

    1+: Pulse is difficult to palpate, weak and thready in character, and easy to obliterate.

    2+: Pulse located with light pressure, and touch senses it is stronger than 1+.

    3+: Normal pulse, easy to palpate, and not easily obliterated.

    4+: Strong pulse, easily palpated, bounds against fingertips, and cannot be obliterated.

d. Equality of pulses: comparison of both sites allows nurse to determine any localized obstruction or disturbance in blood flow.

13. Palpate dorsalis pedis (pedal pulses). Have client lie supine with feet relaxed. Gently place fingertips between great and first toe and slowly move along groove between extensor tendons of great and first toe until pulse is palpable (see illustration).

       Artery lies superficially and does not require deep palpation. Too much pressure can obliterate pulse. Pulse is absent from birth in some healthy individuals.

14. If pedal pulses are not palpable, palpate posterior tibial pulse. Have client relax and slightly extend feet. Place fingertips behind and below medial malleolus (ankle bone) (see illustration).

       Posterior tibial pulses are more easily palpated in some individuals.

15. If it is difficult to palpate a pulse or the pulse is not palpable, use a Doppler instrument over the pulse site (see Chapter 14).

       Doppler amplifies sounds, allowing nurse to hear low-velocity blood flow through peripheral arteries.

16. See Completion Protocol (inside front cover).

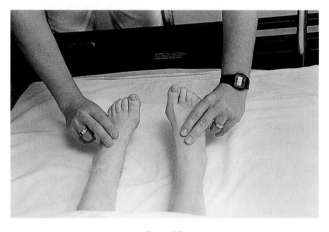

Step 13

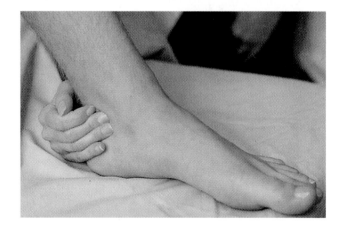

Step 14

• • •

EVALUATION

1. Compare muscle strength and range of motion with previous shift assessment.
2. Compare pulses and capillary refill bilaterally with previous shift assessment.
3. Compare absence or presence and extent of edema with previous shift assessment.

Unexpected Outcomes and Related Interventions

1. Previously palpable pedal pulses are diminished or absent.
2. Client's lower extremities have pale, cool, thin, and shiny skin, with reduced hair growth and nail thickening, indicating chronic arterial insufficiency.
   a. Client may benefit from having legs in dependent position (hanging down) to promote circulation.

b. Assess strength of pedal pulses. Absent pulses or pulses less than 2+ help to determine the extent of the problem.

3. Client has warm but cyanotic skin with dependent edema present in ankles; brown pigmentation is noted, indicating venous stasis (decreased venous circulation).

   a. Keep legs elevated to promote venous circulation.

4. Client demonstrates a positive Homans' sign, which indicates risk for clot in client's deep leg veins.

   a. Assess for redness, tenderness, and warmth.

   b. Measure circumference of both legs at the same distance from the knee to determine presence of swelling.

   c. Do not massage extremity, which could dislodge clot, resulting in an embolus.

   d. Report condition promptly to nurse in charge or physician.

Recording and Reporting

- Report the absence of any peripheral pulses, including position of extremity and possible contributing factors immediately. Absence of pulses can result in tissue damage. A Doppler instrument can detect pulses that are not palpable (see Chapter 12).
- Record elasticity of vessel wall (ease of compression and ability to spring back) and strength of pulse (scale 1 to 4), comparing right and left.
- Note position for maximizing blood flow, along with color changes accompanying with position changes.
- Record teaching done and client response.

Sample Documentation

1530 Client's right lower leg red, warm, and tender to touch. Circumference of right leg 16" and left leg 14". Client instructed to remain in bed. Findings reported to Dr. H. (See Routine Nursing Assessment: Cardiovascular, Appendix A.)

Home Care and Long-Term Care Considerations

- In the client's home the nurse must be aware of being on the client's own turf. The assessments are done periodically, perhaps weekly, and it is important to make plans with the realization that care can be safely continued in the absence of health care professionals. Clients and family members must be very aware of what changes to watch for and how to determine when to call the physician (Burke and Walsh, 1997).
- In long-term care settings, residents are often in a very stable condition and head-to-toe assessments are done less frequently, for example, monthly or as client condition dictates. The professional nurse is responsible for identifying acute conditions that may arise, as well as serious gradual or sudden deterioration that can develop. As condition changes are identified by assessment data, it is important to plan and implement accordingly. The acuity of care in this setting is increasing, as state and federal regulations have influenced eligibility requirements.

Pediatric Considerations

- Allow significant other to hold and assist during assessment.
- Keep all strange and potentially threatening equipment out of sight to minimize child's anxiety.
- Allow children to use equipment (i.e., stethoscope) on a doll, family member, or nurse to facilitate cooperation.
- Use language appropriate for age when explaining what you will do.
- Perform more invasive techniques, for example, rectal temperature, last. Auscultation is most easily accomplished when the child/infant is asleep. To encourage deep breaths, ask the child to blow out the light on your penlight or blow a cotton ball off your palm. Note changes related to crying and physical resistance.
- Keep infants covered as much as possible to prevent chilling.
- Commonly, skin rashes occur from contact and food allergies.
- Adolescents have the right to confidentiality and respond better when treated as adults and individuals. Provide opportunity to talk with them without parents present.

CRITICAL THINKING EXERCISES

1. Jessica is a 3-year-old who has had minor surgery requiring an overnight stay. As you prepare to do your shift assessment, she clings to her mother and screams. What approaches might be the most helpful in this situation? What terminology could you use to explain vital signs and lung assessment?

2. When caring for a 73-year-old man with severe respiratory distress you determine that he has a frequent, nonproductive cough, diminished lung sounds in lower lobes bilaterally, and shallow respirations. He complains of a sharp pain when he coughs. When delegating vital signs to the AP, what parameters would be appropriate in clarifying what is significant to report?

3. You are preparing to do a shift assessment for a 66-year-old African-American man whose wife and four children are visiting. During the report you were told that the client has been complaining of severe right lower quadrant abdominal pain, for which he was given a narcotic by injection. What should you consider when approaching this situation? What should be included in the abdominal assessment, and in what sequence should you proceed?

REFERENCES

Barkauskas VH et al: *Health and physical assessment,* ed 4, St Louis, 1998, Mosby.

Burke MM, Walsh MB: *Gerontologic nursing: wholistic care of the older adult,* ed 2, St Louis, 1997, Mosby.

Canobbio MM: *Cardiovascular disorders,* Mosby's Clinical Nursing Series, St Louis, 1996, Mosby.

Doughty DB, Jackson DB: *Gastrointestinal disorders,* Mosby's Clinical Nursing Series, St Louis, 1993, Mosby.

Gordon M: *Manual of nursing diagnosis, 1997–1998,* St Louis, 1997, Mosby.

McFarland GK, McFarlane EA: *Nursing diagnosis and intervention: planning for patient care,* ed 3, St Louis, 1997, Mosby.

Seidel HM et al: *Mosby's guide to physical examination,* ed 3, St Louis, 1995, Mosby.

Wong DL, Perry SE: *Maternal child nursing care,* St Louis, 1998, Mosby.

CHAPTER 14

Comprehensive Health Assessment

Skill 14.1
Assessing the Head, Face, and Neck,   283

Skill 14.2
Assessing the Nose, Sinuses, and Mouth,   288

Skill 14.3
Assessing the Eyes and Ears,   293

Skill 14.4
Assessing the Thorax, Lungs, and Breasts,   299

Skill 14.5
Assessing the Heart and Circulation,   309

Skill 14.6
Assessing the Abdomen,   317

Skill 14.7
Assessing the Genitalia and Rectum,   322

Skill 14.8
Assessing Neurological Function,   327

Skill 14.9
Assessing Musculoskeletal Function,   339

A comprehensive health assessment includes a detailed review of the client's reason for seeking health care, history of present illness, if applicable (the client may be healthy and establishing a primary care relationship), past medical history, hospitalizations, and surgeries. It also includes a family history; social history, including use of alcohol, street drugs, and smoking history; allergies; review of body systems; functional status related to activities of daily living (ADLs); and the physical examination. The physical examination reveals information that refutes, confirms, or supplements the database for the client. The nurse groups significant history and physical examination findings into patterns that reveal nursing diagnoses. Identification of abnormal findings requires that additional data be gathered.

Results of a health assessment and physical examination allow the nurse and the physician to collaborate on an appropriate plan of care. The information provides a baseline for the client's functional abilities and helps the nurse select nursing interventions to facilitate management of the client's health problems or health promotion.

For priorities for health assessment and techniques used in a shift assessment, refer to Chapter 13.

GENERAL SURVEY

The nurse begins the health assessment process with a general survey of the client by observing the client's behavior, mannerisms, appearance, posture, body structure and size, hygiene, dress, and positioning (see Chapter 13). The nurse observes how the client walks, stands, and sits. The overall mood and general mental status of the client is noted. Does the client make eye contact; is he or she crying, angry, withdrawn, or cheerful? Note if the client has good hygiene, appears the stated age, and is able to answer questions appropriately, follow the conversation, and respond appropriately. During the neurological examination, the mental status will be assessed.

PHYSICAL EXAMINATION SKILLS

Inspection, palpation, percussion, and auscultation are examination techniques that enable the nurse to collect a broad range of physical data about clients. Inspection, palpation, percussion, and auscultation are skills used in the shift assessment (see Chapter 13) as well as in a comprehensive examination.

Inspection is the process of observation, a visual examination of the client's body parts to detect normal characteristics or significant physical signs. It is important to recognize normal physical characteristics of clients of all ages before trying to distinguish abnormal findings. An examiner methodically takes the time necessary to carefully inspect body parts. If an examiner becomes hurried, significant signs may be overlooked and incorrect conclusions may be made about a client's condition. *Do not hurry. Pay attention to details.* Experience is needed to recognize normal variations among clients, as well as ranges of normal in an individual. An experienced nurse learns to make several observations, almost simultaneously, while becoming very perceptive of early warnings of abnormalities.

Good lighting and full exposure of the body parts being inspected are essential. Each area is inspected for size, shape, color, symmetry, position, and the presence of abnormalities. Compare each area inspected with the same area on the opposite side of the body. Use additional light, such as a penlight, to inspect body cavities such as the mouth and throat.

Palpation involves the use of the sense of touch. Through palpation the hands can make delicate and sensitive measurements of specific physical signs, including resistance, resilience, roughness, texture, temperature, and mobility. Palpation is often used with or after inspection. The nurse uses different parts of the hand to detect specific characteristics. For example, the dorsum (back) of the hand is sensitive to temperature variations. The pads of the fingertips detect subtle changes in texture, shape, size, consistency, and pulsation, of body parts. The palm of the hand is especially sensitive to vibration. The nurse measures position, consistency, and turgor by lightly grasping the body part with the fingertips.

The client should be relaxed and positioned comfortably because muscle tension during palpation impairs the ability to correctly palpate. Asking the client to take slow, deep breaths may enhance muscle relaxation. Tender areas are palpated last. The nurse asks the client to point out sensitive areas and notes any nonverbal signs of discomfort. Clients appreciate warm hands, short fingernails, and a gentle approach. Palpation may be either light or deep and is controlled by the amount of pressure applied with the fingers or hand (Figure 14-1). The nurse must not palpate without considering the client's condition, the area being palpated, and the reason for using palpation. For example, a client admitted to the emergency department following an automobile accident will be examined for obvi-

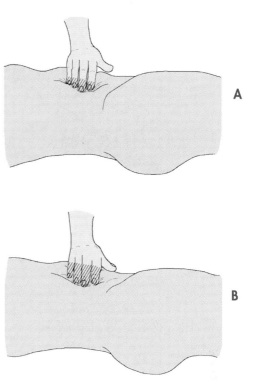

Figure 14-1 A, During light palpation, gentle pressure against underlying skin and tissues can be used to detect areas of irregularity and tenderness. **B,** During deep palpation, depress tissue to assess condition of underlying organs.

ous external as well as potential internal injury. The nurse should consider factors surrounding the client's injury and inspect the chest wall carefully before performing any palpation around the area of the ribs.

Light palpation always precedes deep palpation. The nurse applies tactile pressure, slowly, gently, and deliberately; depressing the area examined about 1 cm (½ inch). Deeper palpation is used to examine the condition of the organs. The area being examined is depressed approximately 2 cm (1 inch). Caution is the rule. A student nurse should not attempt deep palpation without the assistance of a qualified instructor to ensure the client does not suffer internal injury.

Percussion involves tapping the body with the fingertips to evaluate the size, borders, and consistency of body organs and to discover fluids in body cavities. When the body's surface is struck with a finger, a vibration travels through the body tissues. The sound from the vibration depends on the density of the underlying tissues. Direct percussion involves striking the body surface directly with one or two fingers. Indirect percussion involves placing the middle finger of the examiner's nondominant hand firmly against the body surface. With palm and fingers remaining off the skin, the tip of the middle finger of the dominant hand strikes the other, using a quick, sharp stroke (Figure 14-2, p. 282). The wrist must remain relaxed

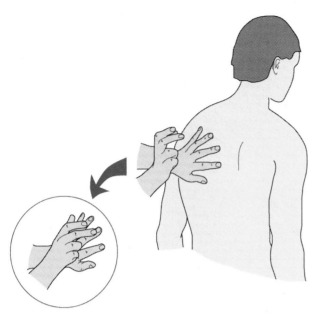

Figure 14-2 Percussing the chest.

to deliver the proper blow. Accurate use of percussion takes time and practice.

There are five different percussion sounds. Tympany is a drumlike sound that indicates an air-containing space such as a gastric air bubble or a puffed-out cheek. Resonance is a hollow sound heard over a normal lung. Hyperresonance is a louder booming sound heard over a hyperinflated lung, as with emphysema. Dullness is a soft or moderate thud, as heard over the liver. Flatness is a soft sound heard over muscle. Each sound allows an examiner to locate anatomical landmarks as well as underlying abnormalities.

Auscultation is listening to sounds produced by the body. Some sounds can be heard with the unaided ear, although most sounds are heard only with a stethoscope. To auscultate correctly, listen in a quiet environment. Listen for the presence of the sound, as well as its characteristics. It is important for a student to recognize normal sounds, such as the passage of blood through an artery, heart sounds, and movement of air through the lungs, to detect abnormal sounds. The nurse is more successful in auscultation after knowing what type of sounds arise from each body structure and the location in which they can most easily be heard. Likewise, the nurse becomes familiar with areas that normally do not emit sounds.

Various instruments are used for physical examination. Instruments should be clean or sterile and in good working order. An ophthalmoscope has a light and system

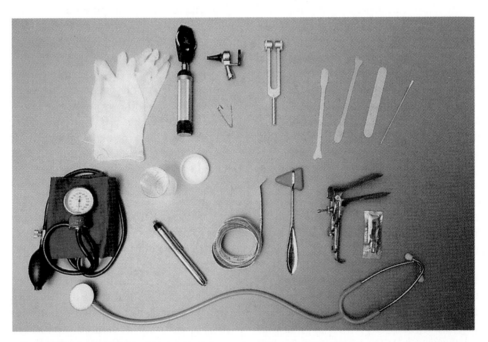

Figure 14-3 Standard equipment for physical assessment. Equipment shown includes: *(top, left to right)* disposable gloves, ophthalmoscope with battery handle, otoscope attachment, safety pin, tuning fork, cervical spatulas, tongue depressor, cotton-tipped swab; *(middle, left to right)* sphygmomanometer, specimen cup, penlight, tape measure, reflex hammer, vaginal speculum, lubricant *(bottom)* stethoscope.

of lenses and mirrors and is used to examine the interior structures of the eyes. An otoscope illuminates the ear canal and tympanic membrane (eardrum) and can be used for examination of the nose. A percussion (reflex) hammer is used to test deep tendon reflexes. A vaginal speculum is used to examine the vaginal canal and cervix. A tuning fork is used to test hearing and vibratory percep- tion (Figure 14-3). Other pieces of equipment needed for the physical examination include a tape measure, scale for height and weight, blood pressure manometer, thermometer, and stethoscope. All equipment should be ready for use when the examination begins, preventing delays and facilitating a smooth, organized approach to the physical examination.

Skill 14.1

ASSESSING THE HEAD, FACE, AND NECK

Although many structures are located in the head, neck, and face, this skill focuses on the skull, face, thyroid gland, trachea, and lymph node chains. Assessment of the carotid and jugular veins is usually deferred until the cardiovascular assessment (Skill 14.5). Facial muscles are innervated by cranial nerve (CN) V (trigeminal) and CN VII (facial). The function of these nerves is also tested as part of the neurological examination (Skill 14.8) but is usually carried out at this time. The assessment techniques are normally painless and involve inspection, palpation, and auscultation.

NURSING DIAGNOSES

Risk for Infection is appropriate when the assessment findings reveal enlarged lymph nodes with accompanying signs and symptoms, such as fever, chills, and grayish-white plaques on the tonsils. An enlarged lymph node alone does not indicate infection. **Impaired Skin Integrity** is appropriate when lesions are found on the scalp, face, or neck. **Impaired Swallowing** is appropriate for the client who has a decreased ability to pass fluids or solids from the mouth to the stomach (Kim, McFarland, and McLane, 1997) (see Chapter 8).

Equipment

    Stethoscope
    Transparent pocket ruler
    Cup of water

ASSESSMENT

1. Assess client for a history of recent cold or infection. **Rationale: Potential cause for lymph node enlargement.**
2. Determine if client has history of thyroid problem or takes thyroid medicine.

3. Ask if client has history of neck pain or has noted any enlargements or nodules.
4. Determine if medical condition indicates pneumothorax, hemothorax, pleural effusion, or bronchial tumor.

PLANNING

Expected outcomes focus on health teaching and identification of alterations of the head, face, and neck.

Exected Outcomes

1. Client has no deviation from normal:
   a. Lymph nodes are nonpalpable or small, mobile, and nontender.
   b. Cervical nodes may be palpable in a healthy person and would be soft, discrete, nontender, and moveable.
   c. Trachea is at midline.
   d. Facial nerves are intact.
   e. Scalp is clean and intact.
2. Client able to recall or demonstrate instructions.

DELEGATION CONSIDERATIONS

The skill of assessing the head, face, and neck requires problem solving and knowledge application unique to a professional nurse. Delegation is inappropriate. AP provide routine hygiene to a client and must know what changes in the client's hair and scalp are indicative of problems. All findings should be reported to the registered nurse (RN) for assessment.

IMPLEMENTATION

Steps	Rationale

COMMUNICATION TIP

- *During the examination of head and neck, instruct client about lymph nodes and how infection can commonly cause node tenderness.*
- *Inform client that certain hair care products or lubricants can clog sebaceous glands and promote scalp infection.*

1. See Standard Protocol (inside front cover)
2. Have client sit upright. Ask client to remove wigs, hairpieces, or toupees. Nurse examines posterior, lateral, and anterior skull and scalp.

   Provides easy access. Client may choose to defer this part of the examination.

3. Inspect and palpate the following:
   a. Skull for size, shape, contour, and position.

   Note size in proportion to overall body size; ovoid shape; long diameter on anteroposterior axis; symmetrical and smooth with prominent occipital and frontal areas. Assess lesions in same manner as for skin lesions (see Skill 13.1).

   b. Scalp for color, texture, lesions, hygiene, and tenderness. Part hair in several areas to inspect fully.

   Head and crab lice attach their eggs to the hair shaft.

   c. Face for color, proportions, expressions, and movement.
4. Assess trigeminal and facial nerves.

   May reveal facial nerve involvement.

   a. CN V: Instruct client to clench teeth while examiner palpates muscles over jaw (see illustration).

   Determines presence of bilateral equal muscle strength.

   b. CN VII: Instruct client to raise eyebrows, close eyes tightly, frown, smile, show teeth, and puff out cheeks (see illustration).

   Reveals symmetrical facial movement.

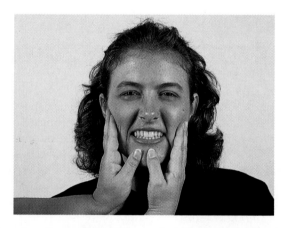

Step 4a *From Chipps E et al: Neurological disorders, Mosby's Clinical Nursing Series, St Louis, 1992, Mosby.*

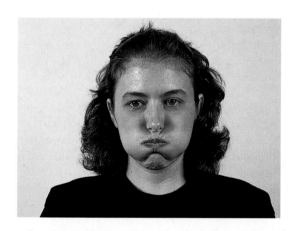

Step 4b *From Chipps E et al: Neurological disorders, Mosby's Clinical Nursing Series, St Louis, 1992, Mosby.*

Steps	Rationale

5. Palpate temporal artery bilaterally for rhythm and tenderness.

6. Assess temporomandibular joint (TMJ) just in front of each ear for crepitation, range of motion (ROM), and tenderness on palpation.

7. Assess CN XI (spinal accessory). Instruct client to shrug shoulders against resistance of examiner's hands and then to turn head to one side against resistance of examiner's hand.

    Maneuver shows ability to oppose resistance or presence of pain, weakness, or discomfort.

8. Inspect neck for symmetry, masses, scars, movement, and ROM.

    When evaluating ROM, proceed slowly and judge each movement separately.

  a. Have client flex neck with chin toward sternum.

    Observe for reduced flexion less than 70 degrees.

  b. Have client extend neck with chin pointing toward the ceiling without tensing neck muscles. Palpate any apparent masses to determine size, shape, tenderness, consistency, and mobility. Use pads of fingers.

    Neck extension provides for exposure of underlying structures. Observe for reduced extension less than 30 degrees. Tensing muscles prevents access to lymph nodes for palpation.

  c. Have client bend neck laterally with ear toward shoulder, then rotate neck, with chin toward shoulder, right and left.

    Observe for reduced lateral bending less than 35 degrees from midline and rotation with chin less than 70 degrees.

9. Inspect and palpate trachea for location. Place the thumbs on each side of the trachea, just above the suprasternal notch (see illustration). Note space between thumb and sternocleidomastoid muscle. Trachea is normally in midline above suprasternal notch. Avoid forceful pressure.

    Gentle palpation prevents eliciting cough reflex.

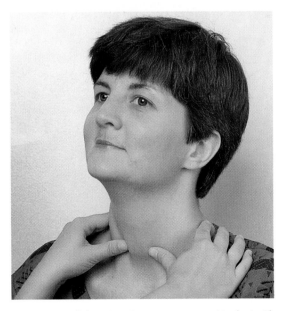

Step 9   *From Belcher AE: Cancer nursing, Mosby's Clinical Nursing Series, St Louis, 1992, Mosby.*

Steps	Rationale
10. Assess lymph nodes.	Allows for clear view of all lymph node chains.
a. Inspect both sides of neck as client relaxes with neck slightly flexed forward.	
b. Stand either in front of or to the side of client and palpate each lymph node chain systematically (see illustration). Use pads of fingers and gently palpate in rotary fashion over region where nodes are normally found. Be sure to press underlying tissue. Note size, shape, location, mobility, symmetry, and surface characteristics.	Improves access for node palpation. Methodical palpation over each lymph chain prevents omission of any nodes. Vigorous palpation may obliterate small nodes and cause stimulation of carotid sinus with a slowing of the heart rate.
c. Ask client to bend head forward and relax shoulders. Palpate supraclavicular nodes. It may be necessary to hook the index and third fingers over the clavicle, lateral to the sternocleidomastoid muscle, to palpate these nodes.	Position relaxes the muscles to ease palpation of nodes.
11. Assess the thyroid.	
a. Stand in front of client and inspect the lower neck overlying the thyroid gland for symmetry, visible masses, and any subtle fullness at the base of the neck.	Gross inspection may reveal gland enlargement.

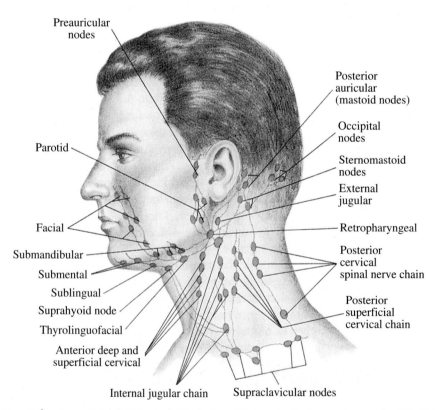

Step 10b *From Seidel HM et al: Mosby's guide to physical examination, ed 3, St Louis, 1995, Mosby.*

Steps	Rationale

b. Provide client with a glass of water. Ask client to extend neck and take a sip of water; note any bulging of the thyroid gland.

c. To palpate the thyroid gland use light, gentle palpation, allowing fingers to drift over the gland. Palpate for size, shape, configuration, consistency, tenderness, and presence of nodules.

d. Posterior approach (see illustration)
   (1) Place both hands around client's neck, with two fingers of each hand on the sides of the trachea just beneath the cricoid cartilage.
   (2) As client swallows, feel for movement of the thyroid isthmus, noting any enlargement.

e. Anterior approach (see illustration)
   (1) Stand at client's side. Palpate the left lobe with the pads of the index and middle fingers of the right hand and the right lobe with the pads of the index and middle fingers of the left hand as the client swallows.
   (2) Move the skin medially over the sternocleidomastoid muscle, and reach under its anterior borders while the fingers stay beneath the cricoid cartilage.

12. See Completion Protocol (inside front cover).

Hyperextension helps to tighten the skin for better visualization. Swallowing causes an enlarged gland to bulge.

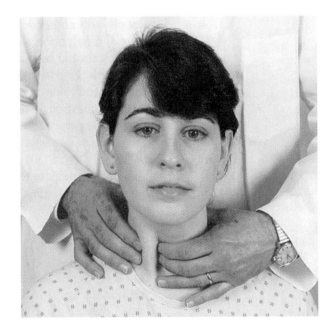

Step 11d *From Seidel HM et al: Mosby's guide to physical examination, ed 4, St Louis, 1999, Mosby.*

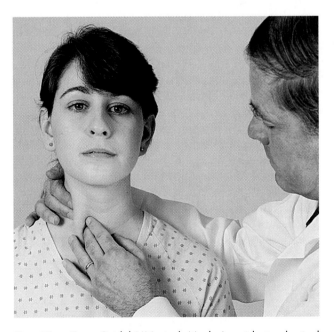

Step 11e *From Seidel HM et al: Mosby's guide to physical examination, ed 4, St Louis, 1999, Mosby.*

EVALUATION

1. Compare findings with client's baseline and normal expected findings.
2. Ask for feedback on whatever instruction was given to the client.

Unexpected Outcomes and Related Interventions

1. Lymph nodes are palpable, nontender, fixed, and hard. **Refer to physician; fixed, hard, nontender nodule may indicate malignant lesion.**
2. Lymph nodes are large, tender, and mobile.
   a. Ask more questions about infection, because findings indicate inflammation or infection.
   b. Check temperature.
3. Trachea is deviated to right or left. **Assess for lung problems, including degree of respiratory distress (Skill 14.4).**

Recording and Reporting

- Note any unexpected findings.
- Describe what is assessed as completely as possible.
- Report findings of concern to the physician, including any pertinent history and vital signs.

Sample Documentation

Head, face, and neck negative for any lesions. No lymphadenopathy or thyroid enlargement noted.

Geriatric Considerations

- The thyroid gland may move to a lower position in relation to the clavicles and becomes more flexible and nodular on palpation.
- The neck may curve backward as a result of changes in the vertebral column.
- The older client has more wrinkles around the eyes, less orbital fat, and a relaxation of the tissues of the face.

Skill 14.2

ASSESSING THE NOSE, SINUSES, AND MOUTH

Assessment of the client's nose and sinuses takes little time, and procedures are relatively simple, using inspection and palpation. If clients have nasogastric (NG) or nasotracheal (NT) tubes inserted, however, the nurse should take care to inspect the nasal mucosa thoroughly. Presence of tubes can cause mucosal irritation, necrosis, and even erosion. Nasal flaring, especially in children, may indicate respiratory difficulty. Discharge and foul odor from only one nostril may indicate a foreign body in the naris (nostril).

Condition of the oral cavity can reveal significant information about a client's health, such as state of hydration, nutritional status, hygiene practices, and specific pathological conditions. The procedure is to be done thoroughly so as not to miss a lesion or local area of inflammation under or around the tongue and along the mucosal surfaces. A convenient time to perform this assessment is during administration of oral hygiene.

NURSING DIAGNOSES

Ineffective Breathing Pattern is appropriate when a client's inhalation or exhalation pattern is inadequate. **Pain** is appropriate when open lesions or inflammation occur. **Altered Oral Mucous Membrane** is appropriate when observation reveals a break in the oral mucosa. **Bathing/Hygiene Self-Care Deficit** is appropriate if the client exhibits inability to use upper extremities.

Equipment

   Tongue depressor
   Penlight
   Disposable gloves
   Gauze square

ASSESSMENT

1. Determine if client has experienced any trauma to the nose or mouth.
2. Assess if client has history of allergies, nasal discharge, epistaxis, postnasal drip, smoking, chewing tobacco, alcohol consumption, recent change in appetite, dentures (comfort and fit). Assess dental hygiene practices.
3. Ask if client uses nasal sprays or drops, or sniffs toxic substances.
4. Ask if client snores at night or has difficulty breathing through the nose.

PLANNING

Expected outcomes focus on health teaching and identification of alterations of the nose, sinuses, and mouth.

Expected Outcomes

1. Client has no deviations from normal:
   a. Nose is aligned, symmetrical, without obvious lesions, and nontender.
   b. Nasal mucosa is pink, clear, and dry; septum is midline.
   c. Sinuses are nontender and glow when illuminated.
   d. Mouth mucosa is glistening pink or red, soft, moist, and smooth.
   e. Teeth, if present, are white, smooth, and shiny.
   f. Gums are pink, moist, smooth, and firm.
   g. Tongue is midline, moist, and mobile, with smooth lateral margins.
2. Client is able to describe appropriate hygiene measures, use of nasal spray, and signs of oral cancer.

IMPLEMENTATION

Steps	Rationale

COMMUNICATION TIP

Use this time to review use of OTC nasal decongestants and nasal sprays, proper oral hygiene, and discuss early warning signs of oral cancer: a sore that bleeds easily and does not heal, a lump or thickening, a persistent red or white patch on mucosa, or difficulty chewing or swallowing.

Steps	Rationale
1. See Standard Protocol (inside front cover).	
2. Examine nose and sinuses.	
a. Inspect nose externally for placement, alignment, and symmetry. If swelling or deformities exist, palpate more gently for tenderness, swelling, or deviations.	Asymmetry may indicate trauma and may affect patency.
b. Place a finger on the side of the client's nose and occlude one naris (nostril) while client breathes with mouth closed. Repeat with other nostril.	Assesses patency of nares.
c. Use penlight to illuminate anterior nares and inspect nasal mucosa and position of septum at anterior end of nose. If nasal tubes are present, inspect for excoriation, inflammation, or sloughing of skin.	Reveals any nasal obstruction interfering with breathing. Character of discharge and inflammation reveals allergy (clear or whitish color) or infection (yellowish color). Swallowing or coughing reflex causes movement of tubes against nares. Failure to anchor tube properly results in pressure against mucosa.
d. Ask client to tip head back slightly. Inspect septum for alignment, perforation, or bleeding.	Position provides clear view of septum and turbinate.
e. Percuss and palpate frontal sinus over ridge and upper orbit of each eye.	Pressure elicits tenderness if sinus is swollen or inflamed.

Steps	**Rationale**

f. Percuss and palpate maxillary sinuses just to each side of nose, (see illustration).

g. If sinus tenderness is present or infection is suspected, transillumination should be performed:

   (1) Darken room.

   (2) View maxillary sinus by placing the transilluminator light lateral to the client's nose, just beneath the medial aspect of the eye.

   (3) Have client open mouth and check to see if hard palate is illuminated.

   (4) View frontal sinus by placing the light against the medial aspect of each supraorbital rim. A dim red glow of light should be seen just above the eyebrow.

Elicits tenderness in presence of inflammation.

Light passes through bone to illuminate frontal sinuses. Normally the light outlines the sinuses.

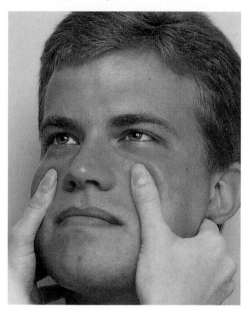

Step 2f Palpation of maxillary sinuses. *From Potter P, Perry A: Basic nursing, St Louis, 1999, Mosby.*

3. **Examine mouth.**

   a. Have client open mouth halfway and inspect lips for color, texture, hydration, contour symmetry, and lesions.

   b. Inspect inner mucosa by gently pulling lower then upper lip from teeth (see illustration). Note color, texture, hydration, and any ulcers, abrasions, or cysts.

   c. If lesions present, palpate with fingers for tenderness, size, and consistency.

   d. Ask client to open mouth; inspect lining of cheeks by gently retracting lips and cheeks with tongue depressor. View surface of mucosa right to left and top to bottom (see illustration).

Allows discrimination between cancerous lesion, ulceration, and cyst.

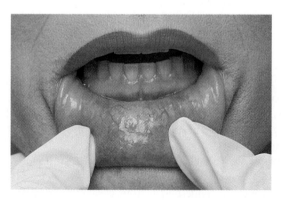

Step 3b

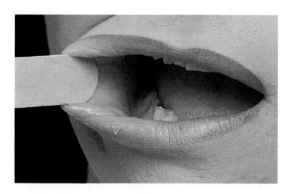

Step 3d

Steps	**Rationale**

 e. Palpate cheek with one finger along the inner mucosa and the thumb along the outside cheek.

 f. While retracting cheeks, inspect gums for color, edema, retraction, bleeding, and lesions. Ask if client has any tenderness. If client wears dentures, be sure they are removed.

 g. Palpate gums gently with tongue blade and note resistance.   Determines firmness.

 h. To examine teeth, ask client to open lips and clench teeth. Note position of teeth. Ask to open mouth wide and note caries or missing teeth. May reveal hygiene or chewing problems.

 i. To assess tongue, ask client to relax mouth and protrude tongue halfway. Note color, size, position, and texture. Ask client to elevate it, then move it side to side. Illuminate with penlight. Tongue should move freely. Tongue positions test for hypoglossal nerve function.

 j. Inspect undersurface of tongue by asking client to lift tongue toward roof of mouth (see illustration). Undersurface of tongue and floor of mouth are common sites for cancerous lesions.

 k. To palpate tongue, first explain procedure. Then, as client protrudes tongue, grab tip with gauze and gently retract to side. Palpate full length of tongue, base, and any lesions of floor of the mouth. Release tongue. Client may fear sensation of not being able to swallow. Detects areas of hardness.

 l. With client extending head backward and holding mouth open, inspect hard and soft palates using penlight for illumination. Hard palate is anterior; soft palate extends toward pharynx.

 m. Ask client to say "ah." Place tongue blade on middle third of tongue (see illustration). Tongue depressor placed anteriorly may cause posterior tongue to mound up and obstruct view; placed posteriorly may elicit gag reflex. Assesses CN X (vagus). Uvula and soft palate should rise without deviation to either side.

 n. With penlight, inspect posterior pharynx, including anterior and posterior tonsillar pillars. Observe color, exudate, and any lesions. Note the tonsils in cavity between the pillars. Tonsils are graded as visible 1+, enlarged 2+ to 4+. Common sites for infection.

4. Remove and discard gloves.

5. See Completion Protocol (inside front cover).

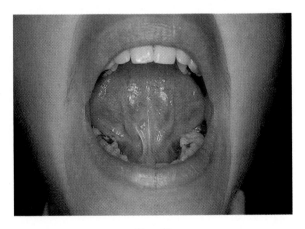

Step 3j

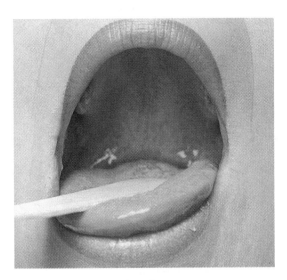

Step 3m

EVALUATION

1. Compare findings with client's baseline and normal expected findings.
2. Ask client to describe recommended hygiene schedule, indications for use of nasal spray, or signs of oral cancer.

Unexpected Outcomes and Related Interventions

1. Client has evidence of asymmetry, inflammation, drainage, lesions, tenderness, dry mucosa, or inadequate oral hygiene. Tongue is edematous and coated. Sinuses are tender or obstructed. Illuminated areas are dark in color.
   a. Increase frequency of oral hygiene and increase hydration (as appropriate).
   b. Report any lesions to M.D.
2. Tonsils are enlarged, red, with exudate or plaques. Obstructed nares, deviated septum, rhinitis, nasal polyps, deviation of tongue or uvula.
   a. Ask client more details about history as related to findings.
   b. Consult with physician for treatment options.

Recording and Reporting

- Report any abnormal findings to the physician and any associated information, (e.g., duration of finding, intensity, associated vital signs).
- Record abnormal findings.

Sample Documentation

2300   Nasal passages patent without deviation, lesions, or abnormal drainage. Oral mucous membranes and palates clear and moist. No lesions, redness, or tenderness. Full dentition without apparent dental caries. Intact cranial nerve X. Tonsils present.

Geriatric Considerations

- Older adults may report problems with sense of smell during examination. Instruct them in importance of installing smoke detectors throughout home and to always check dated food labels for possible spoilage.
- In older adults, gum recession occurs from loss of tissue elasticity or periodontal tissue.
- Loose or missing teeth are common because bone resorption increases.
- Yellow or darkened teeth are also common in the older adult because of the general wear and tear that exposes the darker underlying dentin.
- An older adult's teeth often feel rough when tooth enamel calcifies.
- The mucosa is normally dry because of reduced salivation.
- Varicosities (swollen veins) under the tongue are common in the older adult.
- Older adults may need to eat soft foods and cut food into small pieces because of difficulty in chewing and changes in the teeth.
- Taste perception is altered due to changes in the number of taste buds.
- The tissue of the oral cavity is more friable due to decreased hydration, thinning of the epithelial layer and reduced resistance to injury and infection (Lueckenotte, 1996).

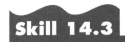

Skill 14.3

ASSESSING THE EYES AND EARS

Vision is vital to performing ADLs, communicating effectively with others, and analyzing and learning about events. Clients often have preexisting visual alterations or may be undergoing diagnostic or therapeutic procedures that can impair vision.

A hearing disorder is caused by one of four types of problems: (1) mechanical dysfunction–blockage of external ear by cerumen or a foreign body; (2) trauma impact from blows, falls, motor vehicle accidents or foreign bodies or excess noise exposure; (3) neurological disorders–auditory nerve damage (e.g., after use of medications); and (4) acute illnesses after inner ear infection. Conduction deafness results from sound waves failing to pass through external or middle ear structures; it is often treatable. Nerve deafness, which involves the internal ear, is more serious.

Examination of the eyes include skills for assessing visual acuity, visual fields, extraocular movements, and external eye structures. Assessment of the ear includes inspection of the external ear and the test for gross hearing.

NURSING DIAGNOSES

Risk for Injury is appropriate when the deficit impairs the client's ability to be functional or perform ADLs. **Sensory/Perceptual Alterations: Visual or Auditory** is appropriate when the client has a deficit in vision or hearing. **Pain** is appropriate for clients with eye or ear discomfort.

Equipment

　　Newspaper or magazine
　　Penlight
　　Cotton-tipped applicator

ASSESSMENT

1. Question if client has history of eye disease, trauma, itching, discharge, diabetes, or hypertension; also ask about blurred vision, diplopia, spotters, floaters, flashes of light, or halos around lights. **Rationale: These warning signs may indicate visual problems.**

2. Question if client has history of ear disease or trauma; ask if there is itching, discharge, or tinnitus (ringing) of the ears.
3. Determine occupational history and use of glasses, contacts, hearing aid, and medications (e.g., antibiotics, large doses of aspirin).

PLANNING

Expected outcomes focus on health teaching and identification of alterations of the eyes and ears.

Expected Outcomes

1. Client has no deviations from normal:
   a. Normal visual acuity with or without correction.
   b. Full visual fields and parallel eye movement in each cardinal gaze.
   c. Normal position of eyes, lids, and eyebrows; clarity of sclera with clear conjunctivae; equal, round, briskly reactive pupils; and equal corneal light reflexes.
   d. Clear and smooth ear canal, cerumen and hair present; tympanic membrane pearly gray color, with cone of light reflex visualized; normal hearing acuity.
2. Client is able to list early signs and symptoms of visual and hearing loss.

DELEGATION CONSIDERATIONS

The skill of assessment of the eyes and ears requires problem solving and knowledge application unique to a professional nurse. Delegation is inappropriate. AP may be able to determine a problem with a client's visual acuity while the client reads a menu, newspaper, or other printed material. AP should know how to recognize clients with obvious hearing impairments. Review for the staff member how to communicate most effectively with the client. Findings should be reported to the RN for assessment.

IMPLEMENTATION

Steps	Rationale

1. See Standard Protocol (inside front cover).
2. Test visual acuity: CN II.
   a. If client wears glasses or contact lenses, ask to read print from newspaper while wearing glasses. Note distance from the eyes that client holds the newspaper (see illustration).

       Be sure client is able to read and can read English. It may help to have client read aloud if illiteracy is suspected.

   b. If client is unable to see print clearly, test each eye separately by placing index card over one eye at a time. (A more detailed examination involves use of a Snellen eye chart.)

       Determines extent of involvement of each eye.

3. Test visual fields.
   a. Have client sit or stand 60 cm (2 feet) away and face you. Your eyes should be at eye level of client (see illustration).

       Allows for standardization of findings.

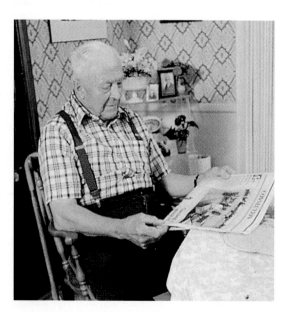

Step 2a *From Barkauskas VH et al: Health and physical assessment, St Louis, 1994, Mosby.*

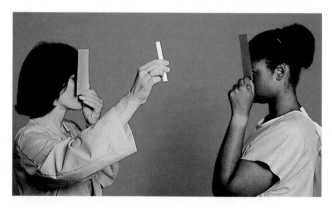

Step 3a *From Barkauskas VH et al: Health and physical assessment, St Louis, 1994, Mosby.*

Steps	**Rationale**

b. Ask client to gently close or cover one eye and to look at your eye directly opposite. Close or cover other eye on side of client's closed eye.

Nurse's field of vision is superimposed on client's.

c. Fully extend arm midway between client and yourself, then move it centrally with fingers moving.

d. Move finger or object equidistant from you and client outside of own field of vision. Slowly bring it back into field, asking client to state when it is first seen. Repeat procedure for all visual fields and for both eyes.

The point at which finger can first be viewed indicates farthest limit of visual field for that direction.

4. Test extraocular movements: CNs III, IV, and VI.

a. Instruct client to look straight ahead toward nurse, keeping head motionless throughout examination.

Tests for parallel eye movement.

b. Hold finger 15 to 30 cm (6 to 12 inches) in front of client's eyes.

Comfortable distance prevents nystagmus.

c. Ask client to follow movement of finger with eyes, keeping head still. Move finger slowly through each of the six cardinal gazes (see illustration).

The point at which finger can first be viewed indicates farthest limit of visual field for that direction.

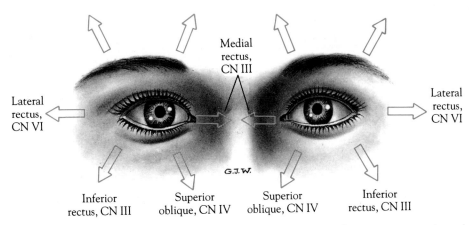

Step 4c Six dimensions of gaze. Nurse directs client to follow finger movement through each gaze. *From Potter P, Perry A: Basic nursing, ed 4, St Louis, 1999, Mosby.*

d. Nurse keeps finger within normal field of vision.

Forcing client to look beyond visual field may cause nystagmus.

e. Nurse observes parallel eye movement, position of upper lid in relation to iris, and presence of nystagmus (rhythmical oscillation of eyes).

Eyes move together in parallel. Upper eyelid should cover iris only slightly. Eyelid does not cover pupil.

5. Test pupillary reflexes: CN III.

a. Dim room lights to test reaction to light.

Darkened room normally ensures brisk response of pupils to light. Pupil that is illuminated constricts; pupil in other eye should constrict equally (consensual light reaction).

Steps	**Rationale**

b. As client looks straight ahead, move light source from side of client's face and direct light onto pupil (see illustration).

c. Observe pupillary response of both eyes (see illustration). Normal pupils are round and equal in size with a brisk response.

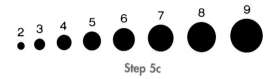

Step 5c

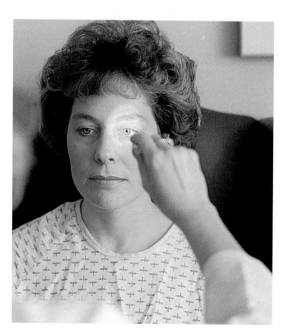

Step 5b

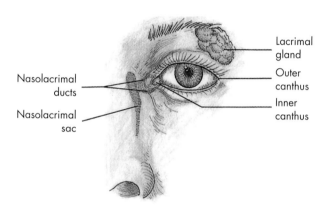

Step 7c

d. Note corneal light reflex. Normal is bright orange glow (red reflex).

e. Defects along inner margins of the iris may be from surgical correction for glaucoma.

6. Test accommodation.

a. Ask client to look at wall in distance. Quickly bring finger within 10 to 15 cm (4 to 6 inches) of client's nose and ask client to look at finger.

b. Move finger smoothly toward nasal bridge; watch for pupil constriction and convergence.

7. Assess external eye.

a. Inspect eye position with eyes open. Note if any portion of lower conjunctiva is visible.

b. Ask client to close both eyes; inspect lid position. Raise eyebrows and inspect upper eyelids for color, edema, and presence of lesions. Have client open eyes, and note blink reflex.

c. Inspect lacrimal apparatus (see illustration) and note edema or inflammation. Palpate gently to detect tenderness.

d. Inspect condition of nasolacrimal ducts, noting edema or excess tearing. Gentle palpation of duct may cause regurgitation of tears.

When focusing on near object, pupils in both eyes should constrict when gaze comes in from a distance. Pupils normally converge.

Normally, eyelids do not cover pupil, and sclera cannot be seen above iris.

Eyelids should close completely. Persons blink as many as 20 times per minute.

Normally, lacrimal gland cannot be seen or palpated.

NURSE ALERT

A pair of new gloves should be worn to examine each eye to prevent cross-contamination.

Steps	Rationale

e. 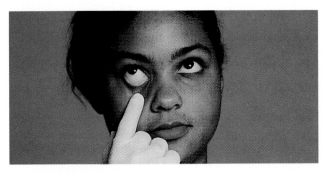 Inspect conjunctivae for color, edema, or lesions by gently depressing lower lid against bony orbit. Ask client to look up (see illustration). Dispose of gloves and wash hands.

Prevents pressure from being exerted on eye.

f. Inspect cornea for opacities by shining light at an angle toward the cornea. Check pupils for size, shape, and equality. Inspect iris for symmetry.

Illumination should show a clear and transparent cornea. Normal pupils are round, clear, and equal in size. Defects along inner margins of iris may be from surgical correction for glaucoma.

Step 7e   *From Barkauskas VH et al: Health and physical assessment, ed 2, St Louis, 1998, Mosby.*

8. Examine external ear.
   a. Inspect auricle for placement, size, symmetry, and color.

Normally, ears are level with each other, and upper point of attachment to head is in straight line with lateral outer canthus or corner of eye.

   b. Palpate auricle for texture, tenderness, and presence of lesions. If client complains of pain, gently pull auricle and press on tragus and behind ear over mastoid bone.

If palpation of external ear increases the pain, external ear infection is likely. If palpation does not increase pain, infection may involve middle ear. Palpate any lesions gently.

   c. Observe opening of ear canal for lesions, discharge, swelling, foreign bodies, or inflammation. Illumination should show a clear and translucent tympanic membrane.
   d. Inspect canal for buildup of cerumen. If canal is clear, ask how often client usually cleans ears.

Small amounts of cerumen normally should be in ears. Cerumen can cause conduction deafness. Cotton-tipped swabs or other objects should not be used to clean ear canals.

9. Assess hearing acuity.
   a. Ask client to remove hearing aid and close eyes.
   b. Test one ear at a time.
   c. Stand 15 to 60 cm (6 inches to 2 feet) away, exhale fully, and softly whisper a sequence of numbers with two equally accented syllables, e.g., nine four.
   d. Ask client to repeat. Repeat in conversational or loud tones if needed.

Determines if client can hear voice tones. Reflects hearing deficit.

10. If hearing loss if suspected, perform a tuning fork test.

Checks for lateralization of sound. Sound is transmitted through bone directly to the inner ear structures, bypassing external and middle ear.

Steps	Rationale

a. Weber's test
   (1) Hold fork at its base and tap lightly against heel of palm. Place base of vibrating fork on midline vertex of client's head or middle of forehead (see illustration).
   (2) Ask client if sound is heard equally in both ears or better in one ear.

Client with normal hearing hears sound equally in both ears or in midline of head. In conduction deafness, sound is heard in impaired ear. In unilateral sensorineural hearing loss, sound is heard only in normal ear.

b. Rinne test
   (1) Place stem of vibrating tuning fork against client's mastoid process (see illustration).
   (2) Ask client to tell you when sound is no longer heard. The nurse observes the length of time in seconds.
   (3) Quickly place the still-vibrating tines 1 to 2 cm (½ to 1 inch) from ear canal (see illustration).
   (4) Ask client to tell you when sound is no longer heard. Again, time with a watch.
   (5) Compare the number of seconds for bone conduction vs. air conduction.

Air-conducted sound should be heard twice as long as bone-conducted sound.

In sensorineural loss, sound is not as loud and is heard longer through air and leads to distortion of sounds and misinterpretation of speech. Conductive hearing loss results when sound transmission is impaired through external or middle ear.

11. See Completion Protocol (inside front cover).

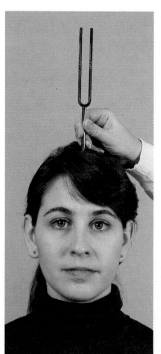

Step 10a(1) *From Seidel HM et al: Mosby's guide to physical examination, ed 4, St Louis, 1999, Mosby.*

Step 10b(1) & (3) *From Seidel HM et al: Mosby's guide to physical examination, ed 4, St Louis, 1999, Mosby.*

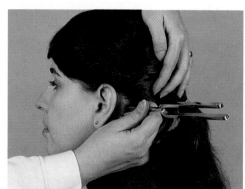

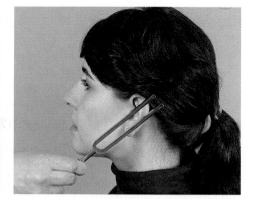

Step 10a(1)   Step 10b(1)   Step 10b(3)

EVALUATION

1. Compare findings with client's baseline and normal expected findings.
2. Ask client to describe early symptoms of visual deficits and hearing loss.

Unexpected Outcomes and Related Interventions

1. Client has evidence of decreased visual acuity or visual fields, inflammation, change in color of sclerae from white, ptosis of eyelids, or crusty yellow or white drainage on lid margins.
   a. Gently cleanse eyes, taking care not to facilitate transmission of microorganisms (see Skill 7.2).
   b. Consider need for referal to ophthalmologist.
2. Nurse detects auricle or ear canal that is swollen, inflamed, or tender to palpation; drainage or lesions; or decreased hearing acuity.
   a. Gently cleanse auricle.

Recording and Reporting

- Record observations made.
- Note all abnormal findings.
- Report abnormal findings to physician.

Sample Documentation

0730 Client exhibits no dysfunction in accommodation, visual fields, hearing, and visual acuity. Extraocular muscle function intact without nystagmus. Pupils equal, react briskly to light bilaterally, and constrict from 4 to 2 mm.

Geriatric Considerations

- Instruct older adult client to take the following precautions because of normal visual changes: avoid driving at night, increase lighting in home to reduce risk of falls, paint first and last steps of a staircase and edge of each step in between a bright color to aid depth perception.
- Common visual changes with aging include reduced acuity (presbyopia), loss of or reduction in peripheral vision, reduced tearing, sensitivity to glare or bright lights, fading of iris, and loss of outer third of eyebrows.
- Arcus senilis, a halo around cornea, is common in older adults but is abnormal in anyone younger than age 40.
- Older adults experience an inability to hear high-frequency sounds and consonants (e.g., s, z, t, and g). Deterioration of cochlea and thickening of tympanic membrane cause older adults to gradually lose hearing acuity.

Skill 14.4

ASSESSING THE THORAX, LUNGS, AND BREASTS

Any alteration in pulmonary function usually affects other body systems. Care must be taken to assess findings from all body systems when determining the nature of pulmonary problems. For example, if a client's ventilation is impaired, the nurse should also assess the client's level of consciousness, skin color, and capillary refill to assess the adequacy of blood flow and oxygen to the tissues.

The optimal time to complete the thorax and chest assessment is when the client is dangling or sitting in a chair. To perform an assessment accurately, the nurse should be familiar with the anatomical landmarks of the chest (Figure 14-4, p. 300).

Assessment of the male and female breast is similar, with a more detailed female examination. Breast cancer affects one of every eight women in the United States (American Cancer Society, 1998) and is the second leading cause of death in women with cancer. Early detection is essential to survival and cure.

NURSING DIAGNOSES

Anxiety is appropriate when a client has a history of air hunger, cancer, or high-risk factors related to cancer. **Ineffective Airway Clearance** might be indicated with reduced chest excursion or inability to elicit a cough. **Impaired Gas Exchange** might occur when trauma, congestion, or infection is present in the lungs unilaterally or bilaterally. **Ineffective Breathing Pattern** is appropriate when the client's rate, depth, timing, rhythm, and chest wall movement do not maintain optimal ventilation. **Knowledge Deficit** regarding breast self-examination (BSE) is appropriate for clients who are inexperienced or not using the proper technique. (Kim, McFarland, and McLane, 1997).

Equipment

Gloves
Stethoscope

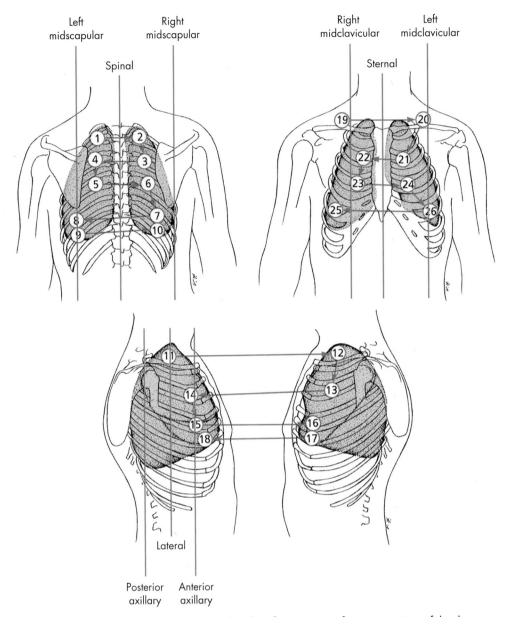

Figure 14-4 Anatomical landmarks and order of progression for examination of the thorax.

ASSESSMENT

1. Review family history for cancer, tuberculosis, allergies, asthma, and chronic obstructive pulmonary disease (COPD).
2. Ask if client experiences any of the following: persistent cough (productive or nonproductive), shortness of breath at rest or with activity, chest pain, orthopnea, frequent respiratory infections, or hemoptysis.
3. **Assess Risk Factors for Lung Cancer.**
   a. Determine if client works in environment or participates in hobbies that contain pollutants (e.g., asbestos, coal dust, chemical irritants).
   b. Ask if client has smoking history or exposure to smoke: length of time; number of cigarettes per day, cigar, pipe, or marijuana smoking; or length of time since exposure or smoking stopped.
4. **Assess Risk Factors for Breast Cancer.**
   a. Determine if female client has family history of breast cancer, previous breast cancer, history of fibrocystic disease, never had children or had first child after age 30, or did not breast-feed. Determine if client is taking oral contraceptives, digitalis, diuretics, steroids, or estrogen hormones.
   b. Ask if client (either sex), has noticed pain, lump, thickening, or tenderness in breast; discharge, dis-

tortion, retraction, or scaling of nipple; or changes in size of breast. Have client point out any lumps.
5. Determine if female client performs monthly BSEs and when in relation to menstrual cycle. Have client demonstrate or describe method.

PLANNING
Expected outcomes focus on health teaching and identification of alterations of the thorax, lungs, and breasts.

Expected Outcomes
1. Client has no deviations from normal:
   a. Symmetrical chest excursion, regular nonlabored respirations, and clear breath sounds bilaterally.
   b. Breasts of young or middle age women smooth, symmetrical without retraction or flattening; firm, elastic tissue with presence of soft lobular underlying tissue; smooth, symmetrical nipples and areolas; no nipple drainage.
   c. Breasts of older women smaller, shrunken, wrinkled, and sagging; stringy, nodular tissue; nipples may point downward.
   d. Nonpalpable lymph nodes.

2. Client is able to list the risk factors for and signs of lung disease.
3. Client is able to demonstrate BSE and state when to perform in relation to menses (woman only).

DELEGATION CONSIDERATIONS

The skill of assessment of the lungs and thorax requires problem solving and knowledge application unique to a professional nurse. AP should learn to monitor the client's respirations and report changes in rate, depth, and positioning to the RN.

The skill of breast assessment and client education requires problem solving and knowledge application unique to the professional nurse. The RN is responsible for providing the health education necessary for the client to understand fully the personal risks for breast cancer and how to perform the examination correctly. AP can be taught to reinforce the importance of BSE with clients.

IMPLEMENTATION

Steps	Rationale

1. See Standard Protocol (inside front cover).
2. Sequence of assessment moves from posterior to lateral, then to anterior thorax, and then to breast assessment. Describe findings made during the examination in relation to the imaginary lines formed from anatomical landmarks: sternum, intercostal spaces, clavicle, spine, scapulae, and axilla (see Figure 14-4).

COMMUNICATION TIPS

This examination provides an opportune time to discuss smoking cessation with clients who smoke and avoidance of environmental and occupational exposure for clients with chronic lung disease and lung cancer; to review energy-conserving techniques for clients with COPD: pacing activities, limiting activity in the morning, pursed-lip and diaphragmatic breathing exercises, and upper body strengthening exercises; and to discuss the warning signs of lung cancer: persistent cough, sputum streaked with blood, chest pain, and recurrent pneumonia or bronchitis.

3. Assess posterior thorax.
   a. Standing at midline position behind the client, inspect thorax for shape, deformities, retractions, or bulging of intercostal spaces, slope of ribs, and alignment of scapulae. Note client's posture.
   b. Determine rate, depth, and rhythm of breathing (see Skill 12.1).

Allows for identification of factors that may impair chest expansion. Normal anterior/posterior ratio of the adult thorax is 1:2 or 5:7. COPD results in a 1:1 chest ratio. A client with breathlessness often leans forward with hands on knees for support (orthopneic position).

Steps	Rationale

c. Palpate posterior chest wall and costal and intercostal spaces for localized areas of tenderness or masses. If swollen area or suspicious mass is detected, palpate for size, shape, and qualities of lesion. Do not palpate deeply in the presence of pain.

Fractured ribs can be painful and should not have unnecessary pressure applied. Localized tenderness or swelling may indicate trauma to the thorax and possibly the underlying lung tissue.

d. Palpate for chest expansion. Place hand on lower third of each rib cage, with hands parallel and thumbs approximately 5 cm (2 inches) apart, pointing to spine. Fingers point out laterally. Press hands toward client's spine to form small skinfolds between thumbs (see illustration *A*). After exhalation, client takes deep breath. Note movement of thumbs, which normally separate 3 to 5 cm (1½ to 2 inches) during chest excursion (see illustration *B*).

Assesses client's ability to breathe deeply.

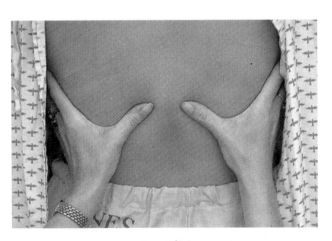

Step 3d(A)

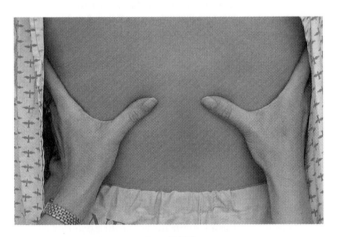

Step 3d(B)

e. Palpate for vocal or tactile fremitus by first placing ball or lower palm of hands on area of thorax over intercostal space. Then ask client to say "99" in voice of uniform intensity. Place hands over symmetrical areas of thorax (see illustration). Feel faint vibration.

Vibration created by movement of vocal cords travels through lung tissue to chest wall. Failure to palpate vibration indicates airway obstruction. Palm of hand is most sensitive to vibrations.

f. Ask client to fold arms forward across chest. Follow same pattern as with palpation; using indirect percussion, percuss intercostal spaces (see illustration) for comparison of posterior lobes.

g. Auscultate lung sounds (see Skill 13.2).

h. If any abnormalities, place stethoscope over intercostal spaces systematically. Ask client to say "e" and "99" in a normal tone of voice.

Position separates scapulae to expose more lung tissue. Percussion determines underlying lung tissue density. Normal is resonant. Dull or flat sounds reflect fluid-filled tissue. Tests for spoken voice sounds. Normally, expect "e" to sound like "e" and "99" to sound muffled. Abnormal if "e" sounds like "a" and "99" is clear and distinct, reflecting fluid or consolidation of lung tissue.

| Steps | Rationale |

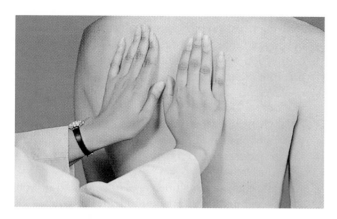

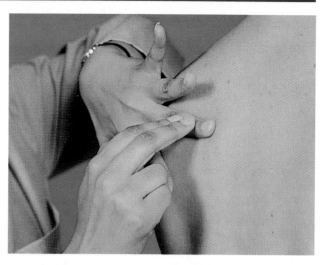

Step 3e *From Barkauskas VH et al: Health and physical assessment, ed 2, St Louis, 1998, Mosby.*

Step 3f *From Barkauskas VH et al: Health and physical assessment, ed 2, St Louis, 1998, Mosby.*

4. Assess lateral thorax.
   a. Instruct client to raise arms straight into air and inspect, palpate, percuss, and auscultate chest wall. Omit excursion maneuver.
   b. Give particular attention during auscultation to the right lateral wall at the fourth to fifth intercostal spaces, because this is the location of the right middle lobe.

   The right middle lobe is the most common site for aspiration.

5. Assess anterior thorax.
   a. Inspect the width or spread of angle made by costal margins and tip of sternum; it is usually greater than 90 degrees between margins.

   Indicates congenital, acquired, or traumatic alterations.

   b. Measure client's respiratory character, observing for symmetry and degree of chest wall and abdominal movement.

   Assesses client's effort to ventilate.

   c. Palpate for areas of swelling, tenderness, and tactile fremitus. In female, retract breast tissue and lift breasts gently for chest wall palpation.
   d. Percuss thorax between intercostal spaces by using same sequence as in palpation.

   Percussion over anterior thorax enables nurse to locate position of the heart, liver, and stomach. Location of findings by common reference points helps successive examiners to confirm findings and locate abnormalities.

   e. For auscultation, see Skill 13.2.
6. Inspect breasts.
   a. Describe findings made during examination in relation to imaginary lines that divide breasts into four quadrants and tail (see illustration).

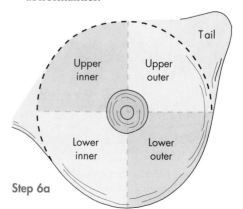

Step 6a

Steps	**Rationale**

b. Inspect both breasts for size, symmetry, position of breasts, and position of the nipples in relation to underlying intercostal space.

Changes in size or shape may indicate underlying mass or presence of inflammation.

c. Observe contour or shape of breast and note any masses, retraction of tissue, or flattening. If retraction is suspected, ask client to raise arms above head or press hand against hips (see illustration). If the client has large or pendulous breasts, ask client to lean forward.

Underlying mass, swelling, or inflammation may cause bulging or retraction of breast tissue. Maneuver causes contraction of pectoral muscles, which accentuates presence of retraction.

d. Inspect overlying skin for color and venous pattern. If breasts are large, carefully lift breasts to inspect underlying surfaces. Normal breasts are the same color as surrounding skin surfaces.

Vascular changes, edema, and inflammation may cause skin color changes. Breast undersurface is a common site for redness and excoriation caused by rubbing against chest wall.

e. Inspect areolas and nipples for color, size, and shape. Note direction in which nipples point and presence of rashes or ulcerations. If nipple discharge present, apply gloves. Note color and amount of discharge.

Hormonal changes cause differences in color and size of areolas and nipples throughout the life span.

f. Remove gloves when examination of the nipple is complete.

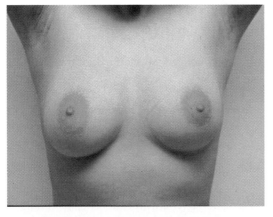
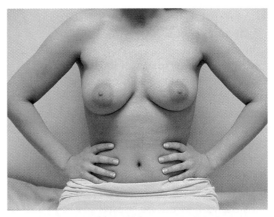
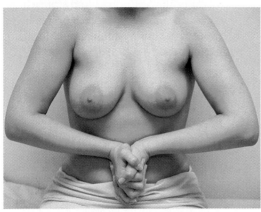
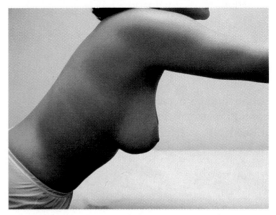

Step 6c *From Seidel HM et al: Mosby's guide to physical examination, ed 4, St Louis, 1999, Mosby.*

Steps	**Rationale**

7. Palpate lymph nodes.
   a. Client position: arms at side and muscles relaxed. Face client, stand on the side being examined, and support this arm while abducting arm from chest wall.

   Position allows for easy palpation of axillary nodes.

   b. Place hand against client's chest wall and high in the axilla. Palpate axillary nodes with fingertips, pressing gently down over the surface of the ribs and muscles (see illustration).

   c. Palpate the following areas: edge of the pectoralis major muscle along anterior axillary line; chest wall in midaxilla; upper part of humerus; and anterior edge of latissimus dorsi muscle along posterior axillary line (see illustration).

   Breast cancer can metastasize to lymph nodes.

   d. Palpate along upper and lower clavicular ridges.

   e. Note number, location, consistency, mobility, and size of nodes. If enlarged node is present, ask if tender.

   Location of supraclavicular and infraclavicular nodes. Characteristics of node help to determine cause of enlargement.

   f. Repeat on other side.

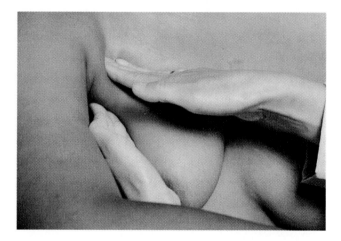

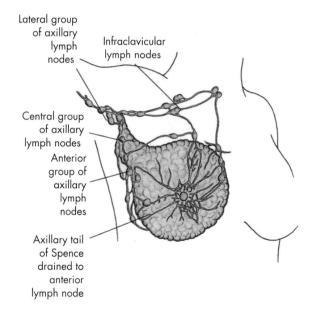

Lateral group of axillary lymph nodes

Infraclavicular lymph nodes

Central group of axillary lymph nodes

Anterior group of axillary lymph nodes

Axillary tail of Spence drained to anterior lymph node

Step 7b   *From Barkauskas VH et al: Health and physical assessment, St Louis, 1994, Mosby.*

Step 7c

8. Palpate breasts.
   a. If client has lump or mass, examine opposite breast first.

   Ensures objective comparison between normal and abnormal tissue.

   b. Client position: lying with right arm abducted and hand placed above head. A small towel can be placed under right shoulder blade. During this portion, nurse can ask client to demonstrate BSE, or nurse can perform and teach to client (Box 14-1, p. 306).

   Position allows breast tissue to flatten evenly against client's chest wall.
   Allows client time to understand and feel maneuvers. Helps client develop comfort level with touching own breasts.

Box 14-1 Breast Self-Examination

Breast self-examination (BSE) should be done once a month so that you become familiar with the usual appearance and feel of your breasts. Familiarity makes it easier to notice any changes in the breast from one month to another. Early discovery of a change from what is "normal" is the main idea behind BSE.

If you menstruate, the best time to do BSE is 2 or 3 days after your period ends, when your breasts are least likely to be tender or swollen. If you no longer menstruate, pick a day, such as the first day of the month, to remind yourself it is time to do BSE.

Here is how to do BSE:

1. Stand before a mirror. Inspect both breasts for anything unusual, such as any discharge from the nipples, puckering, dimpling, or scaling of the skin.

   The next two steps are designed to emphasize any changes in the shape or contour of your breasts. As you do them, you should be able to feel your chest muscles tighten.

2. Watching closely in the mirror, clasp hands behind your head and press hands forward.

3. Next, press hands firmly on hips and bow slightly toward your mirror as you pull your shoulders and elbows forward.

Some women do the next part of the examination in the shower. Fingers glide over soapy skin, making it easy to appreciate the texture underneath.

4. Raise your left arm. Use three or four fingers of your right hand to explore your left breast firmly, carefully, and thoroughly. Beginning at the outer edge, press the flat part of your fingers in small circles, moving the circles slowly around the breast. Gradually work toward the nipple. Be sure to cover the entire breast. Pay special attention to the area between the breast and the armpit, including the armpit itself. Feel for any unusual lump or mass under the skin.

5. Gently squeeze the nipple and look for a discharge. Do not squeeze too tightly, will cause bruising. Repeat the examination on your right breast.

6. Steps 4 and 5 should be repeated lying down. Lie flat on your back, right arm over your head and a pillow or folded towel under your right shoulder. This position flattens the breast and makes it easier to examine. Use the same circular motion described earlier.

Repeat on your left breast.

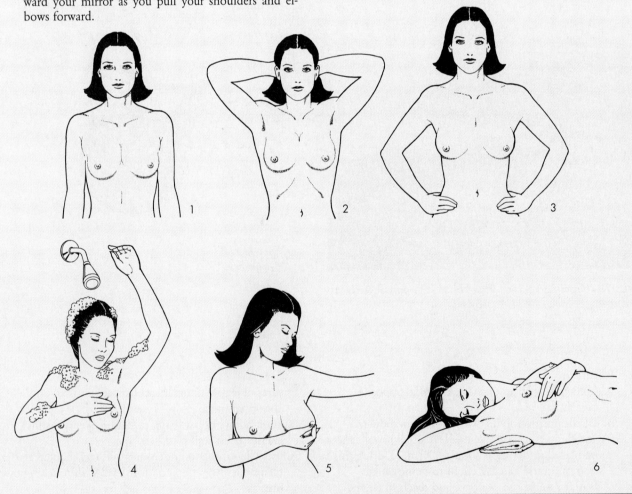

From Seidel HM et al: *Mosby's guide to physical examination*, ed 4, St Louis, 1999, Mosby.

Steps	Rationale

c. Stand at client's right side. Using systematic approach, gently palpate breast tissue with palmar surface of first three fingers of right hand moving in rotary fashion and compressing breast tissue against chest wall. Thoroughly examine all surfaces and tail. Each area may be examined by moving from nipple outward (see illustration).

Entire breast must be thoroughly palpated to rule out presence of a mass. Young women: breast normally firm and elastic; older women: normally often feels stringy and nodular. Note time of examination vs. time of menstrual cycle. If done during the week before or within the first few days of the menstrual cycle, examination may not reveal true findings. Menstrual cycle may cause breast to be tender and engorged.

d. Note consistency of breast tissue.

Consistency of underlying tissue changes with age, pathological conditions, and hormonal variations.

e. If mass is found, palpate for location in relation to quadrants, size in centimeters, shape (round or discoid), consistency (soft, firm, hard), tenderness, mobility, and discreteness (are boundaries of mass easily detected?).

Lower edge of breast, inframammary ridge, may normally feel firm and hard.

f. Use finger to compress areola gently. Then, with thumb and index finger, gently compress nipple while observing for a discharge (see illustration).

Involvement of glandular tissue may cause discharge from nipple. Signs of breast cancer are same as for female client.

g. Repeat procedure in opposite breast after repositioning client.

h. For large breasts, bimanual palpation may be needed; support inferior portion of breast in one hand while palpating breast tissue against supporting hand (see illustration).

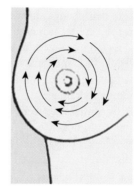

Step 8c *From Payne WA, Hahn DB:* Understanding your health, *ed 2, St Louis, 1989, Mosby.*

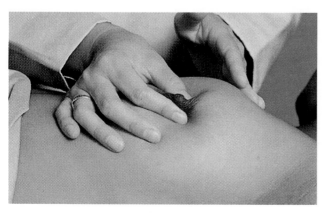

Step 8f *From Barkauskas VH et al:* Health and physical assessment, *ed 2, St Louis, 1998, Mosby.*

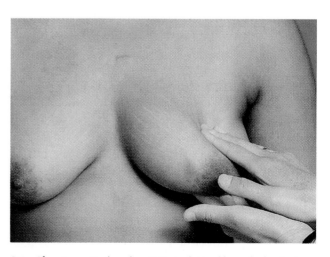

Step 8h *From Barkauskas VH et al:* Health and physical assessment, *ed 2, St Louis, 1998, Mosby.*

Steps	**Rationale**

i. In male clients, conduct same technique and note any breast swelling.

9. See Completion Protocol (inside front cover).

• • •

EVALUATION

1. Compare findings with client's baseline and normal expected findings.
2. Ask client to explain risk factors predisposing to lung disease.
3. Ask client to demonstrate BSE.

Unexpected Outcomes and Related Interventions

1. Client has evidence of anterior/posterior diameter in ratio of 1:1, limited chest excursion, and abnormal chest auscultation, percussion, and palpation.
   a. Compare to baseline for client, consider presence of pain, and consider recent use of medication (e.g., sedatives).
   b. Monitor frequently for changes back to normal or deterioration of respiratory condition.
   c. Communicate new changes in condition to appropriate health care team member.
2. Client has evidence of localized hard, fixed, nontender, and irregularly shaped mass; dimpling or retraction unilaterally; palpable lymph nodes; or serous, bloody nipple drainage.
   a. These are signs of breast cancer.
   b. Refer to client's physician.
3. Client has evidence of lumpy, painful breasts, occasional nipple discharge; and lumps that are soft, well differentiated, and movable.
   a. These are common signs of fibrocystic disease.
   b. Encourage client to become familiar with own breast tissue and to notify physician if abnormalities present.

Recording and Reporting

- Record assessment findings.
- Clearly describe any abnormal findings, including location.
- Record instructions given to client.
- Record client's understanding of information given and ability to return demonstrate BSE.

Sample Documentation

0800   Client in no acute respiratory distress. Lungs clear to auscultation and percussion. Breast exam negative for tenderness, masses, lesions, nipple drainage, or abnormal contour. Instructed in BSE. Able to return demonstrate independently and verbalize understanding of when to do BSE.

Geriatric Considerations

- Older adults have a costal angle (anteriorly) of slightly less than 90 degrees. The anteroposterior diameter may be increased from kyphosis.
- In older adults chest expansion is reduced because of calcification of rib cartilage and partial contraction of inspiratory muscles.
- In older adults ligaments supporting breast tissue weaken, causing breasts to sag and nipples to lower. Actual breast tissue feels stringy and nodular. Older women may ignore BSE, assuming that changes are a result of aging. These changes mimic breast cancer.
- Many older women fail to perform regular BSE or seek routine medical screening because of limited fixed income. The nurse should help find access to free screening programs.
- Musculoskeletal limitations, diminished peripheral sensation, reduced eyesight, and changes in joint range of motion can limit an older woman's ability to palpate and inspect the breasts. A friend or family member may need to learn how to perform a breast examination.

Skill 14.5

ASSESSING THE HEART AND CIRCULATION

Assessment of the heart and vascular system should be performed together, because alterations in either system may be manifested as changes in the other. A client who presents with findings of cardiac problems, such as chest pain, may have a life-threatening condition. The nurse therefore must be able to respond to the client's presenting symptoms and prioritize essential assessments.

Assessment of the heart includes inspection, palpation, and auscultation. Assessment of the vascular system includes measuring blood pressure (see Chapter 12) and assessing the integrity of accessible arteries and veins using inspection, palpation, and auscultation.

NURSING DIAGNOSES

Altered Peripheral Tissue Perfusion is appropriate when the client has cyanotic extremities, diminished peripheral pulses, cold clammy skin, and a change in level of consciousness (LOC). **Pain** is appropriate when diminished peripheral arterial flow or stagnant venous flow presents in acute or chronic fashion or when compromised cardiac circulation produces cardiac pain. **Decreased Cardiac Output** is indicated when the client has diminished cardiac contractility or a damaged heart. **Activity Intolerance** is appropriate when the client has insufficient physiological energy (e.g., from a low blood count) to endure or complete daily activities.

Equipment

    Stethoscope
    Doppler stethoscope with conducting gel (optional)
    Regular and centimeter rulers

ASSESSMENT

1. Assess client for risk factors for heart/vascular disease, including history of smoking; alcohol ingestion; high-fat, low-fiber diet; cocaine use; absent or irregular exercise; stressful life-style; diabetes; hypertension; family history of heart disease; obesity; excessive caffeine intake; history of phlebitis or varicose veins; or wearing tight-fitting clothing about the legs.
2. Ask if client has experienced leg cramps; edema of hands, ankles, or feet; numbness; or tingling in extremities or a sensation of cold extremities. **Rationale: Reveals circulatory alterations.**

3. If client experiences pain or cramping in the lower extremities, ask if it is relieved or aggravated by walking. **Rationale: Differentiates vascular from musculoskeletal pain.**

PLANNING

Expected outcomes focus on health teaching and identification of alterations of the heart and circulation.

Expected Outcomes

1. Client has no deviations from normal:
    a. Normal rhythm and heart rate, normal heart sounds, and a point of maximal impulse (PMI) at the fifth intercostal space, midclavicular line.
    b. Blood pressure (BP) within normal parameters for client; equal, strong, bilateral pulses; no jugular vein distention; and warm, pink extremities with normal hair growth and nails.
2. Client describes changes in own behavior that may improve cardiovascular function.
3. Client lists risks for heart disease.
4. Client describes purpose, schedule, and dosage of medications being taken for cardiovascular function.

DELEGATION CONSIDERATIONS

The skill of comprehensive heart and vascular assessment requires problem solving and knowledge application unique to a professional nurse. Delegation is inappropriate. AP can be trained to assess apical pulse and peripheral pulses correctly. Assessment of peripheral pulses is important, particularly in specialty areas such as vascular surgery and orthopedics, where the skill is performed frequently.

-   Familiarize the staff member with the importance of assessing peripheral pulses in specific clients.
-   Instruct the AP to recognize temperature and color changes along with changes in peripheral pulses.
-   Instruct AP to notify RN immediately of any abnormal findings.

IMPLEMENTATION

Steps	Rationale

COMMUNICATION TIP

- *Assessment of the heart and circulation is a good time to discuss risk factors for heart disease: high dietary intake of saturated fat or cholesterol, lack of regular aerobic exercise, smoking, obesity, stressful life-style, hypertension, and family history.*
- *Inform client of blood pressure reading.*

- *Inform clients of ways to reduce vascular insufficiency in the lower extremities: avoid tight clothing over lower body or legs, avoid standing or sitting for long periods of time, walk regularly, and elevate feet when sitting.*

1. See Standard Protocol (inside front cover).
2. **Heart assessment**
   a. With client in a semi-recumbent position stand on client's right side and view chest at an angle to the side. Locate anatomical landmarks used to assess cardiac function (see illustration). Inspect systematically over the six landmarks. Look for visible pulsations. Be sure your hands are warm.
   b. With client supine, systematically palpate over the six anatomical landmarks. Palpate each site with the proximal halves of the four fingers held gently together or with the whole hand (see illustration). Touch gently noting any pulsations and allow the movements to rise to your hand. Note any thrill—a fine, palpable rushing vibration—felt best over the base of the heart near the right or left second intercostal space.

Familiarity with landmarks allows nurse to describe findings more clearly and ultimately may improve assessment.

The fingertips best sense pulsations; the ball of the hand detects vibrations.

NURSE ALERT

Presence of a thrill is not normal and may indicate a disruption of blood flow caused by a defect in closure of a heart valve or atrial septal defect.

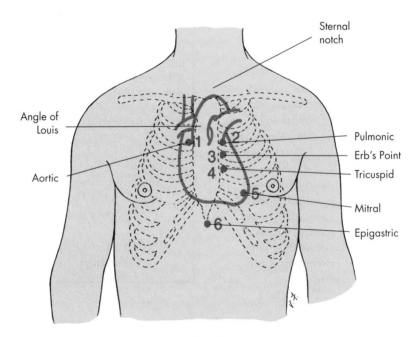

Step 2a

Steps	Rationale

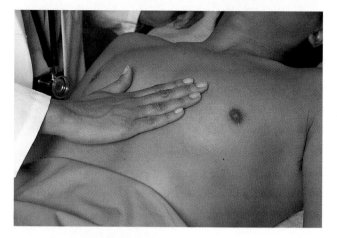

Step 2b *From Canobbio MM:* Cardiovascular disorders, *Mosby's Clinical Nursing Series, St Louis, 1990, Mosby.*

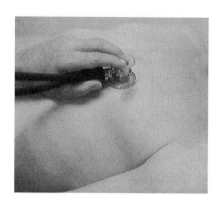

Step 2f(1) *From Seidel HM et al:* Mosby's guide to physical examination, *ed 2, St Louis, 1991, Mosby.*

c. If pulsations or vibrations are palpated, time their occurrence in relation to systole or diastole by feeling the carotid pulse simultaneously.

d. Locate the PMI by palpating with fingertips at apex at fifth intercostal space in an area 1 to 2 cm in diameter (about the size of a quarter). Normally at the PMI, the apical pulse is felt as a light tap. If locating PMI is difficult, turn client onto left side.

The PMI (apical impulse) may be located to the left of the midclavicular line in clients with enlarged hearts.

e. Inspect the epigastric area; palpate the abdominal aorta. Note a localized strong beat.

Rule out reduced blood flow or diffuse pulse.

f. Auscultate heart sounds (see illustration).

(1) With client supine and head of bed elevated 45 degrees, locate the anatomical sites for auscultation of cardiac function.

(a) Angle of Louis is felt as a ridge in the sternum approximately 5 cm (2 inches) below the sternal notch (see illustration Step 2a).

(b) Intercostal spaces are just below each rib. The second intercostal space on the right is the aortic area *(1)* and on the left is the pulmonic area *(2)* (see illustration Step 2a).

(c) Erb's point is at the third intercostal space *(3)* (see illustration Step 2a).

(d) Tricuspid area *(4)* is at the fourth intercostal space (see illustration Step 2a).

(e) Apical area is located at the fifth intercostal space at the left midclavicular line *(5)* (see illustration Step 2a).

NOTE: In clients with serious heart disease, the PMI is located to the left of the midclavicular line.

(f) Epigastric area is at tip of the sternum *(6)* (see illustration Step 2a).

Steps	**Rationale**

(2) If locating PMI is difficult turn client onto left side (see illustration).

Maneuver moves the heart closer to the chest.

(3) Ask client not to speak. Place stethoscope's diaphragm lightly against chest wall.

Pressing too firmly may decrease transmission of sounds.

(4) Listen at the apex. Normal first and second heart sounds (S_1, S_2) are high pitched, are best heard with diaphragm, and sound like "lub-dub."

(5) After both sounds are heard clearly as "lub-dub," count each combination of S_1 and S_2 as one heartbeat. Count the number of beats for 1 minute to determine the apical pulse rate.

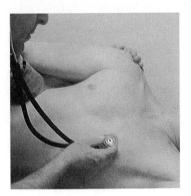

Step 2f(2)   *From Seidel HM et al: Mosby's guide to physical examination,* ed 2, St Louis, 1991, Mosby.

g. Identify if heart rhythm is regular or irregular. This may be further identified as regularly irregular or irregularly irregular.

An irregular heartbeat is a dysrhythmia, which interferes with the heart's ability to pump effectively.

h. When heart rate is irregular, compare apical and radial pulses. This is best done with a colleague, who can assess the radial pulse while the nurse simultaneously assesses the apical pulse.

If a pulse deficit exists (radial pulse slower than apical), ineffective heart contractions are failing to send pulse waves to the periphery.

i. Listen for clicks as short, high-pitched extra sounds.

Clicks are caused by abnormalities such as mitral valve prolapse or prosthetic valves.

j. Listen for pericardial friction rubs as "squeaky" or rubbing sounds.

Rubs result from inflamed visceral and parietal layers of the pericardium rubbing against one another.

k. Auscultate for heart murmurs using the bell of the stethoscope. Murmurs are swishing or blowing sounds caused by altered blood flow.

Sounds may be caused by increased flow through a normal valve, forward flow through a stenotic (narrowed) valve or into a dilated vessel or chamber, or backward flow through a valve that fails to close.

3. **Vascular assessment**

The sequence of vascular assessment is blood pressure, carotid arteries, jugular neck vein distention, and then peripheral pulses.

a. Compare lying and standing blood pressures.

Abnormalities may suggest atherosclerosis or diseases of aorta. Comparing pressure readings with client in different positions rules out orthostatic hypotension and volume depletion.

NURSE ALERT

A fall in the systolic blood pressure greater than 20 mm Hg and a fall in the diastolic blood pressure signify orthostatic hypotension. Client may become dizzy and light-headed.

b. Assess carotid arteries with client in sitting position. Inspect neck bilaterally for obvious pulsations, then palpate each artery separately (see illustration). Note if pulsation changes with inspiration or expiration.

Simultaneous occlusion of both arteries could cause loss of consciousness from inadequate circulation.

c. Place bell of stethoscope over each carotid artery, auscultating for blowing sound or bruit (see illustration).

Narrowing of lumen results in turbulence with a harsh blowing sound.

Steps	**Rationale**
d. Examine the right jugular vein to assess venous pressure (see illustration). First have client sit upright at a 45- to 90-degree angle. Have client slowly lean backward into supine position. Avoid neck hyperextension or flexion. Determine venous pressure by measuring the vertical distance between the angle of Louis and the level of the highest visible point of vein pulsation. Use both metric and regular rulers. Measure in centimeters.	Normal veins are flat when client in sitting position. Puslations become evident as client's head is lowered. Height of pulsation reflects venous pressure in right atrium. Higher than 2.5 indicates fluid overload.

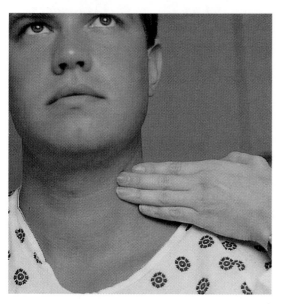

Step 3b

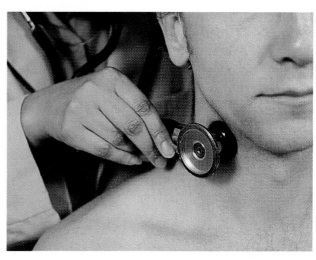

Step 3c *From Barkauskas VH et al: Health and physical assessment, ed 2, St Louis, 1998, Mosby.*

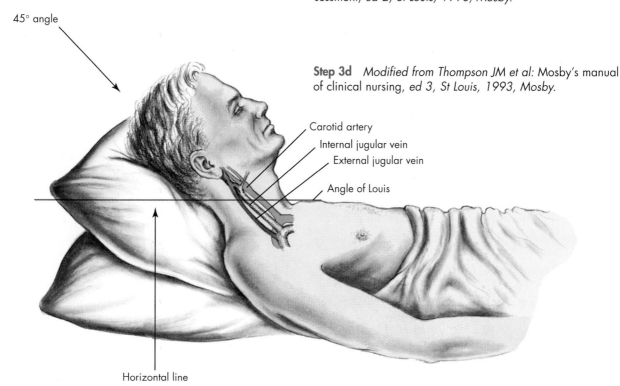

45° angle

Step 3d *Modified from Thompson JM et al: Mosby's manual of clinical nursing, ed 3, St Louis, 1993, Mosby.*

Carotid artery

Internal jugular vein

External jugular vein

Angle of Louis

Horizontal line

Steps	**Rationale**

e. Assess integrity of vascular system.

   (1) Inspect skin, mucous membranes, nailbeds (see illustration) and lower extremities for changes in color, texture, edema, ulcers, or hair distribution (see Table 13.2, p. 259). Normal nail angle is 160 degrees. Nail angles of 180 degrees are seen in late clubbing. The normal capillary refill is 2 seconds or less (Seidel et al, 1999).

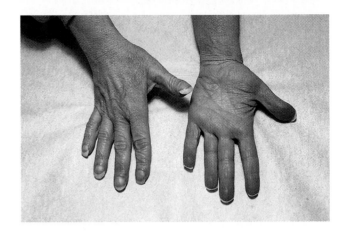

Step 3e *From Canobbio MM: Cardiovascular disorders, Mosby's Clinical Nursing Series, St Louis, 1990, Mosby.*

   (2) If veins in calves reddened or swollen, palpate gently for tenderness or firmness of muscle. With tenderness, support the leg while client dorsiflexes foot. Note if client complains of sharp pain.

Homans' test for thrombophlebitis.

   (3) If edema present, assess for pitting (see Skill 13.5). Palpate and note temperature.

The higher degree of pitting, the more severe the edema.

f. Palpate peripheral arteries. Assess each site for rate and rhythm, strength, and elasticity. (Depress and release artery, noting ease with which it springs back.)

Rating scale for strength of pulses:
   0,   No pulse, not palpable
   1+, Weak, thready, barely palpable
   2+, Normal pulse
   3+, Full, increased
   4+, Strong, bounds against fingertips

   (1) Radial (see illustration). Lightly place tips of first and second fingers in groove formed along radial side of forearm, lateral to flexor tendon of wrist.

   (2) Ulnar (see illustration). Place fingertips along ulnar side of forearm.

   (3) Brachial (see illustration). Locate groove between biceps and triceps muscles above elbow at antecubital fossa. Place tips of first three fingers in muscle groove.

   (4) Femoral (see illustration). With client supine, place first three fingers over inguinal area below inguinal ligament, midway between symphysis pubis and anterosuperior iliac spine.

   (5) Popliteal (see illustration). With client lying supine or prone, flex knee slightly. Palpate with fingers of both hands deep into popliteal fossa, just lateral to midline.

   (6) Dorsalis pedis (see illustration). With client supine and feet relaxed, gently place fingertips between great and first toe and slowly move along groove between extensor tendons of these toes until pulse is palpated.

   (7) Posterior tibial (see illustration). Have client relax and slightly extend feet. Place fingertips behind and below medial malleolus (ankle bone).

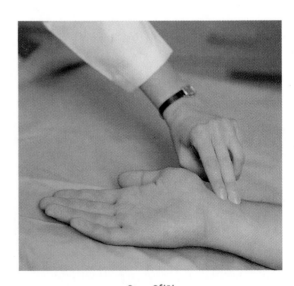

Step 3f(1)

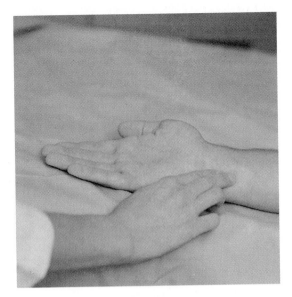

Step 3f(2)

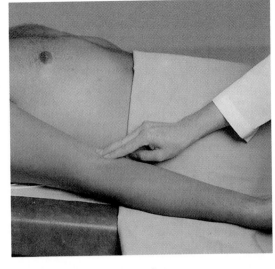

Step 3f(3)

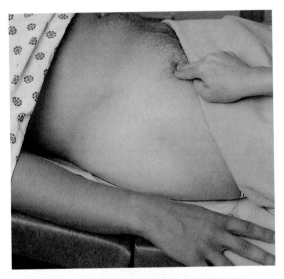

Step 3f(4)

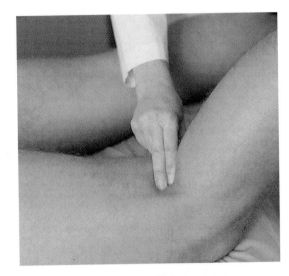

Step 3f(5)

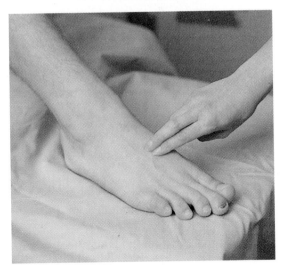

Step 3f(6)

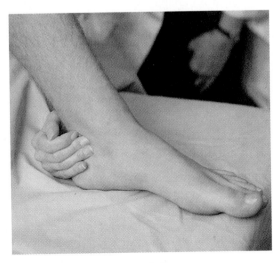

Step 3f(7)

Steps	Rationale

g. If pulses are difficult to palpate, use an ultrasound stethoscope over the pulse site. Apply conductance gel over site; then apply probe at a 45- to 90-degree angle on skin (see illustration). Turn up volume as needed.

4. See Completion Protocol (inside front cover).

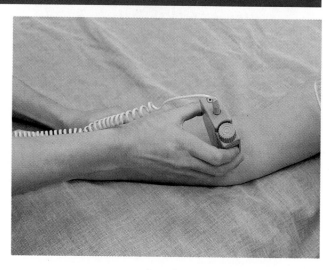

Step 3g

• • •

EVALUATION

1. Compare findings with client's baseline and normal expected findings.
2. Have client explain exercise routine to follow for improvement of cardiovascular function.
3. Ask client to describe risk factors of cardiovascular disease.
4. Ask client to describe purpose, schedule, and dosage of prescribed blood pressure medication.

Unexpected Outcomes and Related Interventions

1. Client has evidence of hypertension, hypotension, or elevated neck vein distention.
   a. Monitor closely for changes in vital signs.
   b. Notify physician of findings.
   c. If client is unstable, be sure resuscitation equipment is nearby (see Chapter 38).
2. Evidence of edema of extremities, diminished arterial circulation, or stasis of venous circulation.
   a. Instruct client on factors that can further impair circulation.
   b. Determine client's knowledge of foot care practices.
3. Positive Homans' sign is detected.
   a. Evaluate for additional evidence of thrombophlebitis (i.e., redness, swelling, and inflammation).
   b. Instruct client to remain in bed.
   c. Notify physician.
4. Heart sounds are abnormal with gallops or rubs.
   a. Refer to past history. Compare with previous findings.

b. If findings differ, refer client to physician for follow-up.
5. Client is unable to offer interventions to improve cardiovascular function.
   Review with client means to improve cardiovascular function, exercise, elimination of risk factors.

Recording and Reporting

- Record findings, describing exact location and abnormality.
- Record instructions given to client.
- Record client's ability to return demonstrate or describe instructions given.
- Report abnormal findings to physician, including relevant vital signs, past history, and history of present illness.

Sample Documentation

0930 Heart: regular rate and rhythm. S_1 and S_2 WNL. No murmurs, rubs, or gallops. Apical pulse present and equal to radial pulse. NVD at 30 degrees absent. Extremities: Pulses 3+; warm, dry, and pink. Adequate hair distribution to lower extremities. No edema present.

Geriatric Considerations

- PMI may be difficult to find in an older adult because anteroposterior diameter of the chest deepens.
- Accidental massage of the carotid sinus during palpation of the carotid artery can be a particular problem for older adults, causing a sudden drop in heart rate from vagus nerve stimulation.

- Varicosities are common in the older adult because the veins fibrose, dilate, and stretch.
- The older adult should be carefully assessed for carotid bruits.

Skill 14.6

ASSESSING THE ABDOMEN

Within the abdominal cavity are multiple organs: stomach, intestines, pancreas, gallbladder, liver, kidneys, and bladder. When performing the assessment, the nurse should maintain a mental image of the anatomical location of each organ (Table 14-1; Figure 14-5). Specific historical data are essential to pinpoint findings to localize organ involvement.

The abdominal assessment should be completed in depth for any client reporting gastrointestinal (GI) and urinary complaints. The sequence of the examination differs for the abdominal area in that inspection is followed by auscultation. Percussion and palpation are done last because these maneuvers stimulate an increase in bowel sounds.

Table 14-1

Location of Abdominal Organs

Right Upper Quadrant	Left Upper Quadrant
Liver and gallbladder	Left lobe of liver
Pylorus	Spleen
Duodenum	Stomach
Head of pancreas	Body of pancreas
Right adrenal gland	Left adrenal gland
Portion of right kidney	Portion of left kidney
Hepatic flexure of colon	Splenic flexure of colon
Portions of ascending and transverse colon	Portions of transverse and descending colon

Right Lower Quadrant	Left Lower Quadrant
Lower pole of right kidney	Lower pole of left kidney
Cecum and appendix	Sigmoid colon
Portion of ascending colon	Portion of descending colon
Bladder (if distended)	Bladder (if distended)
Ovary and salpinx	Ovary and salpinx
Uterus (if enlarged)	Uterus (if enlarged)
Right spermatic cord	Left spermatic cord
Right ureter	Left ureter

NURSING DIAGNOSES

Acute Pain is appropriate if the client reports discomfort of the anterior or posterior trunk. Altered elimination, such as **Diarrhea, Constipation,** or **Urinary Retention,** is indicated when assessment data confirm abnormal peristalsis of the intestines, resulting in loose or constipated stools or bladder dysfunction with inability to void. **Altered Nutrition: More** or **Less than Body Requirements** is appropriate if the client reports factors of indigestion, cramping, or emesis after eating and if the client's weight is 20% over or under ideal body weight.

Equipment
Stethoscope
Tape measure
Marking pen

ASSESSMENT

1. Elicit details of abdominal or low back pain: location, onset, frequency, precipitating factors, aggravating factors, type of pain, and severity. For female clients, determine if they are pregnant.
2. Note position and movement of client. Usually leans into, splints, or positions toward the pain? Moves more slowly? **Rationale: Positioning may reveal nature of pain.**

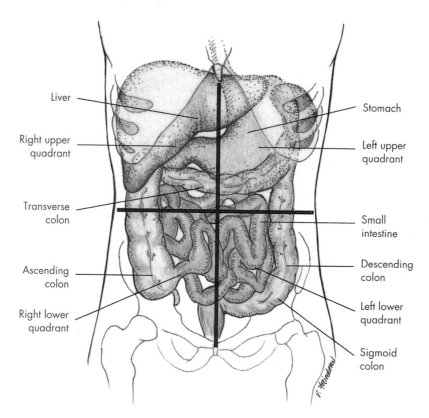

Figure 14-5 Abdominal quadrants.

3. Obtain detailed data about elimination patterns for bowel and bladder along with measures used to promote elimination: laxatives, enemas, and eating and drinking habits vs. patterns of weight gain or loss.
4. Inquire about history of surgeries of the trunk and family history of cancer, kidney disease, alcoholism, drug use, and hypertension.

PLANNING

Expected outcomes focus on health teaching and identification of alterations of the abdomen.

Expected Outcomes

1. Client has no deviations from normal:
   a. Soft, symmetrical abdomen with even contour and no masses or tenderness; active bowel sounds in all four quadrants; percussion reveals tympanic sounds.
   b. Normal borders of liver without any enlargement or tenderness.
   c. No costovertebral angle or suprapubic tenderness.
2. Client states warning signs of colon cancer.

DELEGATION CONSIDERATIONS

The skill of assessing the abdomen requires problem solving and knowledge application unique to a professional nurse. Delegation is inappropriate. AP should know to report to the RN any changes in the client's bowel habits or dietary intake and the development of abdominal pain.

IMPLEMENTATION

Steps	Rationale

1. See Standard Protocol (inside front cover).
2. After client empties bladder, have client assume a recumbent position with knees slightly flexed or a small pillow under knees. Ask client to point with one finger to any painful areas and to show how pain moves or radiates.

   Full bladder can cause discomfort and feeling of urgency, preventing ability to relax. Position promotes optimal relaxation of abdominal muscles.
   Painful areas are assessed last.

3. Inspect abdominal surface from the client's right side for:

   Position helps to detect shadows and movement.

   a. Skin alterations: scars, venous patterns, and openings.
   b. Contour and symmetry.
   c. Position, shape, and color of umbilicus and visible pulsations.

   An everted, pouched-out umbilicus usually indicates distention or hernia.

   d. Distention, ask client if abdomen feels tight. If distention suspected, measure size of abdominal girth by placing tape measure around abdomen at level of umbilicus and note measurement. Mark site with marker pen.

   Assesses increases in abdominal size caused by distention.

4. Repeat inspection with client taking a deep breath and holding it, then raising head up. At this time, observe for bulges.

   Position causes superficial abdominal wall masses and hernias to become apparent.

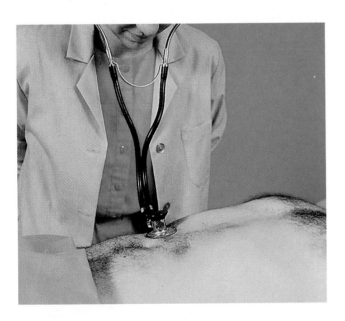

COMMUNICATION TIP

- *Use this time to discuss dangers of excessive use of laxatives or enemas.*
- *Explain that factors such as diet, regular exercise, limited use of OTC drugs causing constipation, establishment of regular elimination schedule, and good fluid intake promote normal bowel elimination.*

Step 5 *From Barkauskas VH et al:* Health and physical assessment, *ed 2, St Louis, 1998, Mosby.*

5. Auscultate bowel by placing diaphragm of stethoscope lightly over each of the four quadrants (see illustration). Ask client not to speak. If NG tube present, disconnect it from suction or turn suction off during auscultation. If client has no history of bowel problems, only the left lower quadrant needs to be auscultated for bowel sounds. Listen 2 to 5 minutes. If sounds are abnormal here, assess all quadrants.

   Determines presence or absence of peristalsis. Absent sounds indicate cessation of gastric motility in the large bowel.

Steps	Rationale
6. Listen 2 to 5 minutes for succession of clicks or gurgles in each quadrant before deciding bowel sounds are absent. Describe sounds as audible or normal, absent, hyperactive (prolonged, loud, multiple gurgles), hypoactive (paralytic ileus with absent or infrequent sounds), or borborygmi (exaggerated waves of peristalsis that indicate attempt to push fluid and air against an obstruction).	Normal sounds range from 8 to 20 per minute.
7. Percuss abdomen. Gently percuss each of the four quadrants systematically to note areas of tympany and dullness (see illustration).	Normal percussion sounds are tympanic sounds.
8. Palpate abdomen. Lightly palpate over abdominal quadrants by using palm and pads of fingertips in smooth, coordinated movement. Depress skin approximately 1.25 cm (½ inch) and note muscle tone, abdominal stiffness, presence of masses, and tenderness. Observe client's face for grimacing, which may indicate tenderness or pain. Note if abdomen is firm or soft to touch (see illustration). Remember to palpate painful areas last and to avoid quick jabs.	Detects areas of localized tenderness, degree of tenderness, and presence and character of underlying masses.
9. Just below umbilicus and above symphysis pubis, palpate for smooth, rounded mass.	Detects the top of a distended bladder.
10. If abdominal masses are palpated, note size, location, shape, consistency, tenderness, mobility, and texture.	
11. If tenderness is present, press one hand slowly and deeply into the involved area, then let go quickly.	Tests for rebound tenderness. Results are positive if pain increases with maneuver. Note if pain is aggravated.

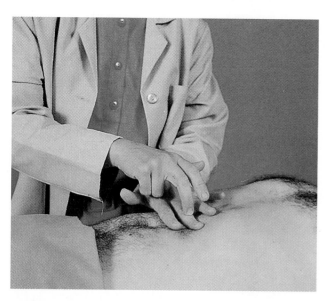

Step 7 *From Barkauskas VH et al: Health and physical assessment, ed 2, St Louis, 1998, Mosby.*

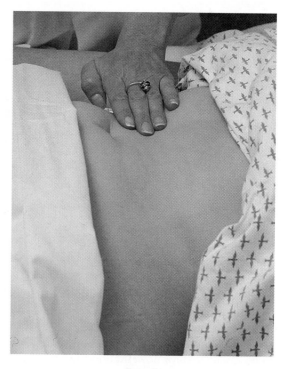

Step 8

Steps	Rationale

12. Assess liver. Locate the liver's lower border by placing left hand under client's right posterior thorax, just under small of the back. Apply gentle upward pressure with left hand. With fingers pointing toward right costal margin, place right hand on right upper quadrant below costal margin. Ask client to take a deep breath, and gently palpate right hand in and up. As client inhales, liver's edge may be felt (see illustration) as it descends.

Liver's edge cannot usually be palpated in normal adults. If liver is enlarged, pressure in this area causes pain; be sure to observe client's face during this maneuver.

13. Place bell of stethoscope over midline of abdomen and auscultate for vascular sounds. If aortic bruit is heard, stop assessment and notify physician.

Determines presence of turbulent blood flow (bruits) through thoracic or abdominal aorta.

14. Assess posterior trunk. Have client sit upright. Place bell of stethoscope posteriorly over costovertebral angle (CVA) (see illustration) and listen for bruits. If found, stop and notify physician. Next, firmly percuss over each CVA along scapular lines. Use ulnar surface of fist to percuss directly or indirectly. Note if client has pain.

Pain may indicate presence of kidney inflammation.

15. See Completion Protocol (inside front cover).

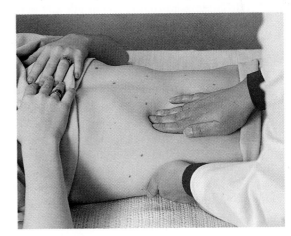

Step 12 *From Seidel HM et al: Mosby's guide to physical examination, ed 4, St Louis, 1999, Mosby.*

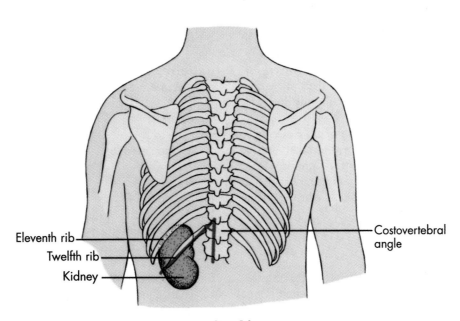

Eleventh rib

Twelfth rib

Kidney

Costovertebral angle

Step 14

EVALUATION

1. Compare findings with client's baseline and normal expected findings.
2. Ask client to describe signs of colon cancer.

Unexpected Outcomes and Related Interventions

1. Client has abnormal bowels sounds, abdominal pain; asymmetrical abdomen with palpable masses, dullness to percussion, rebound abdominal tenderness, or findings of enlarged liver.
   a. Compare established baseline with new findings.
   b. Report to physician any new findings.
   c. Position to reduce abdominal discomfort.
2. Client has bladder that is palpable over the symphysis pubis or has a tender kidney area.
   a. Report findings to appropriate health care personnel, charge nurse, or physician.
   b. Implement actions to facilitate bladder emptying, or insert urinary catheter as ordered (see Chapter 35).
3. Client is unable to describe signs of colon cancer. Review with client appropriate signs of colon cancer.

Recording and Reporting

- Record all abnormal findings, indicating the exact location on the abdomen.
- Report all abnormal findings to the physician; include all pertinent history and vital signs.

- Record instructions given to the client.
- Record the client's understanding of the instructions and any return demonstration.

Sample Documentation

0800   *Abdomen soft and nontender to palpation. Bowel sounds (BS) present in left lower quadrant (LLQ). No hepatomegaly noted. Bladder not palpable.*

Geriatric Considerations

- Older adult often lacks abdominal tone; underlying organs are more easily palpable.
- A weakened intestinal musculature and decreased peristalsis affect the large intestine. Constipation along with nausea, flatulence, and heartburn are common.
- Stress to older adults importance of adequate fluid intake, regular exercise, and a diet with at least 4 servings daily of fresh fruit and vegetables and high-fiber foods to promote normal defecation.

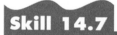

Skill 14.7

ASSESSING THE GENITALIA AND RECTUM

The nurse should complete the assessment of the external genitalia and rectum after obtaining a sexual activity health history. This is especially important to screen for sexually transmitted disease (STD). These data will guide the nurse in what to inspect in more detail or defer to another health care team member.

Typically, the client feels anxious during the examination. To avoid embarrassing the client, the nurse uses a calm, reassuring, and attentive approach. Comfort is established through correct positioning and draping. Each portion of the examination is explained so that the client can anticipate the nurse's action.

NURSING DIAGNOSES

Impaired Skin Integrity is appropriate when lesions, rashes, or drainage are evident. **Knowledge Deficit** is indicated if the client has inadequate perineal care or verbalizes minimal knowledge in the prevention of STDs or

cancer risk factors. **Risk for Infection** is appropriate if the client reports multiple sexual partners or unprotected sexual activity. **Sexual Dysfunction** or **Altered Sexuality Patterns** is indicated if reported by the client.

Equipment

Gloves
Examination light

ASSESSMENT

1. Assess client's sexual history for use of safe sex behaviors; reproductive history; pain during intercourse; and history of any lesions or drainage in the perineal area.
2. Assess client for elimination problems such as change in bowel habits; melena; hemorrhoids; use of laxatives, iron, or codeine; rectal pain; and history of genitourinary problems.

3. Determine if client has had previous illness or surgery involving reproductive organs or rectal area.
4. For males, determine if client has had prior feelings of heaviness or painless enlargement of the testes.
5. Assess dietary history for intake of fat and fiber.
6. Determine family history for cancer of the reproductive organs or colon.

PLANNING
Expected outcomes focus on health teaching and identification of alterations of the genitalia or rectum.

Expected Outcomes
1. Client exhibits normal genitalia.
   a. Female: symmetrical labia majora, triangular pattern of hair growth, pink clitoris and labia minora, symmetrical vaginal orifice without tissue prolapse, nonpalpable Bartholin's and Skene's glands, and absence of lesions, inflammation, edema, or foul-smelling drainage.
   b. Male: pink, smooth glans with meatus at tip; freely hanging scrotum with both testes descended; loose scrotal skin; smooth, ovoid, and nontender testes; shaft without swelling; and no bulging or protrusion in scrotal or inguinal area.
   c. Client exhibits anal area without redness, lesions, or hemorrhoids.

2. Client describes symptoms of STD.
3. Client describes the findings of reproductive organ cancers and methods for screening.

DELEGATION CONSIDERATIONS

The skill of physical examination of a client's genitalia requires problem solving and knowledge application unique to a professional nurse. Delegation is inappropriate. Assistive personnel are trained to perform routine hygiene for a client, including catheter care. This gives the staff member the opportunity to observe the condition of the client's genitalia frequently. The nurse should be sure that AP:

- Know to report any unusual discharge, client complaint of tenderness, or presence of any obvious lesions or masses.
- Explain thoroughly to a client the purpose of perineal hygiene and catheter care.
- Avoid any attempt to manipulate or inspect the client's genitalia other than that required for hygiene.

IMPLEMENTATION

Steps	Rationale

1. See Standard Protocol (inside front cover).
2. **For female client**
   a. After client empties bladder, position in lithotomy position: supine, knees flexed perpendicular to the bed, thighs relaxed with legs abducted to the side, and arms to the side or over chest.
   b. Place rectangular sheet with corner draping over sternum, adjacent corners falling over each knee, and fourth corner covering perineum (see illustration, p. 324). | Provides for privacy. |
   c. With perineum well illuminated, inspect quantity and distribution of hair growth, color of skin, and size and contour of labia. Note any areas of inflammation, edema, lacerations, lesions, or discharge. Inspect skin and hair of pubic area for lice. If structures appear distorted or if vaginal orifice is asymmetrical, palpate tissues later in examination.

Steps	Rationale

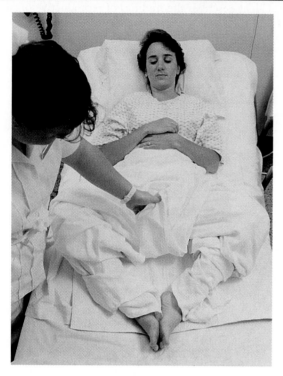

Step 2b

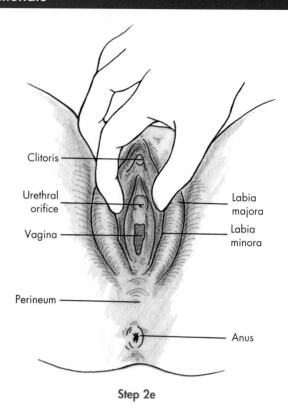

Clitoris

Urethral
orifice

Vagina

Labia
majora

Labia
minora

Perineum

Anus

Step 2e

d. Before touching perineum, touch neighboring thigh. Explain that it is necessary to inspect deeper perineal structures.

e. With nondominant hand, gently place thumb and index finger inside labia minora and retract tissues outward (see illustration). Be sure to have firm hold during retraction.

Ensures clear view for inspection.

f. Inspect clitoris, labia minora, vaginal opening, and urethral orifice (a small slit or pinhole opening just above vaginal canal) for size, color, drainage, edema, inflammation, or lesions.

g. Nurse may also examine rectal area at this time. Use nondominant hand and retract buttocks. Inspect condition of perianal tissues, noting color of skin, closure of anal sphincter, and presence of lesions, hemorrhoids, ulcers, inflammation, rashes, or discoloration.

Perianal area is more pigmented and more coarse than skin overlying buttocks.

h. Ask client to bear down as though having a bowel movement.

Maneuver causes any hemorrhoids or fissures within anal canal to appear.

i. Clean any moisture or drainage from perineal area. Assist client to sitting position while draping protects privacy.

Restores comfort.

j. Remove and discard gloves.

3. For male client

a. After client empties bladder, have him lie supine with chest, abdomen, and lower legs draped. Throughout the examination, manipulate genitalia gently.

Steps	Rationale

b. Expose genitalia, then observe size and shape of the penis and testes, color of the scrotal skin, and character and distribution of pubic hair.

Scrotal skin is darker than surrounding skin and is wrinkled. Adult client has pubic hair extending from base of penis over the symphysis pubis; hair is coarse and curly.

c. Inspect skin over genitalia for lice, rashes, excoriations, or lesions.

d. Inspect structures of penis.

   (1) In uncircumcised males, retract foreskin to reveal glans and urethral meatus. Note position of meatus and observe for discharge, edema, inflammation, and lesions of glans. Be sure to check entire circumference (see illustration).

   (2) Carefully inspect area between foreskin and glans.

Common site for venereal lesions. Small amount of thick, white secretion between glans and foreskin is normal. Be sure to replace foreskin over glans if it was retracted, because edema will result if it is not replaced properly.

   (3) Inspect scrotum's size, shape, and symmetry and for presence of lesions.

Normally, left testis is lower than right. Scrotum should hang freely from perineum behind penis.

   (4) Gently lift scrotal sac to view posterior surface. Gently palpate each testis and epididymis using thumb and first two fingers. Palpate for size, shape, and consistency. Ask if client has sensation of tenderness (see illustration).

Teach or reinforce principles and technique of testicular self-examination at this time.

e. Explain technique of testicular self-examination (to be performed monthly after age 15) (Box 14-2, p. 326). Have client perform exam after warm bath or shower, when scrotum is relaxed. Client should stand naked in front of mirror and look for swelling of or lumps in skin. Using both hands, he should place the index and middle fingers under testicles and place thumbs on top, then gently roll testicle, feeling for lumps, thickening, or hardening.

Testicular cancer is the most common solid tumor among young men age 18 to 34.

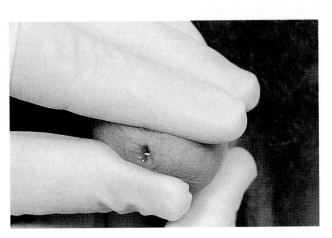

Step 3d(1) *From Barkauskas VH et al: Health and physical assessment, ed 2, St Louis, 1998, Mosby.*

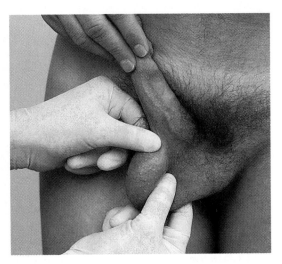

Step 3d(4) *From Seidel HM et al: Mosby's guide to physical examination, ed 4, St Louis, 1999, Mosby.*

Steps	Rationale

f. Ask client to assume a side-lying position.
   Examine the rectal area. Refer to Steps 2g and 2h
   to complete examination.
g. Remove and discard gloves.

4. See Completion Protocol (inside front cover).

Box 14-2 Genital Self-Examination for Men

Because testicular tumors are the most common cancer occurring in young men, all male clients should be instructed in the technique of genital self-examination (GSE). The client should obviously be made aware of the rationale. GSE is also recommended for anyone who is at risk for contracting a sexually transmitted disease STD. This includes sexually active persons who have had more than one sexual partner or whose partner has had other partners. In these cases the purpose of GSE is to detect any signs or symptoms that might indicate the presence of an STD. Many people who have an STD do not know they have one, and some STDs can remain undetected for years. GSE should become a regular part of routine self-health care practices.

You should explain and demonstrate the following procedure to your clients and give them the opportunity to perform a GSE with your guidance.

Instruct the client to hold the penis in his hand and examine the head. If not circumcised, he should pull back the foreskin to expose the head. Inspection and palpation of the entire head of the penis should be performed in a clockwise motion, while the client carefully looks for any bumps, sores, or blisters on the skin. Bumps and blisters may be red or light colored, or may resemble pimples. Have the client also look for genital warts, which may look sim-

ilar to warts on other parts of the body. At first they may be small bumpy spots. Left untreated, they could develop a fleshy cauliflower-like appearance. The urethral meatus should also be examined for any discharge.

Next the client will examine the entire shaft and look for the same signs and symptoms. Instruct him to separate the pubic hair at the base of the penis and carefully examine the skin underneath. Make sure he includes the underside of the shaft in the examination; a mirror may be helpful.

Instruct the patient to move on to the scrotum and examine it. He should hold each testicle gently and inspect and palpate the skin for the same signs, including the underneath of the scrotum. The client should also be alert to any lump, swelling, soreness, or irregularities in the testicle. (Suggest to the client that self-examination of the scrotum at home be performed while bathing, because the warmth is likely to make the scrotal skin less thick.)

Educate the patient about other symptoms associated with STDs, specifically, pain or burning on urination or discharge from the penis. The discharge may vary in color, consistency, and amount.

If the client has any of the above signs or symptoms, he should see a health care provider.

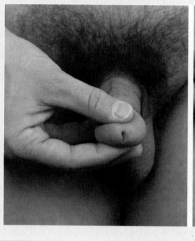 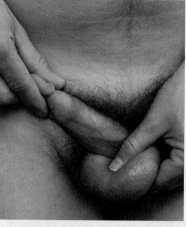

Modified from Burroughs Wellcome Co, 1989. (Instructional pamphlets available.) (From Seidel HM et al: *Mosby's guide to physical examination*, ed 4, St Louis, 1999, Mosby.)

EVALUATION

1. Compare findings with client's baseline and normal expected findings.
2. Ask client to describe the findings of STDs.
3. Ask client to demonstrate/describe screening for reproductive organ cancers.

Unexpected Outcomes and Related Interventions

1. Client has evidence of inflammation, foul-smelling discharge, lesions, or edema in genitalia area or tender, reddened anal area with or without hemorrhoids.
   a. Obtain further details of history as indicated.
   b. Obtain ordered culture of any vaginal or urethral discharge.
   c. Refer to appropriate agency for follow-up and treatment.
2. Client is unable to describe the risk factors for colorectal cancer or STDs or when to monitor for reproductive organ cancers.
   a. Review selected risks that are pertinent to client.
   b. Provide supplementary reading materials.

Recording and Reporting

- Record any abnormal findings, describing the location and appearance.
- Report abnormal findings to the physician, including appropriate history and vital sign information.
- Record client's instruction in relation to safe sexual activity and sexually transmitted diseases.
- Record client instruction about reproductive organ cancers.

Sample Documentation

0845 Genitalia development appropriate for age. No lesions, discharge, or vermin. Rectum without hemorrhoids, lesions, or discharge. Bowel patterns normal without use of laxatives or cathartics.

Geriatric Considerations

- External anal sphincter may be slightly lax.
- Constipation is common in older adults; fecal mass may be palpated.
- An older client may require more time and assistance to assume the lithotomy position.
- With menopause the labia majora become thin, and with advancing age they atrophy. The pubic hair thins and the vaginal introitus constricts.
- Because of hormonal and structural changes, the older woman is predisposed to vaginitis, painful intercourse (dyspareunia), bleeding, and uterine prolapse (Lueckenotte, 1996).
- Older women may have scarring of perineum caused by lacerations or episiotomies from childbirth.
- Older women may have malignant changes that result in dry, scaly nodular lesions of the clitoris.
- With aging the testes decrease in size and firmness.
- The scrotum becomes more pendulous.

Skill 14.8

ASSESSING NEUROLOGICAL FUNCTION

Neurological and mental status assessment may be conducted simultaneously. Information gathered from both examinations is valuable in determining a client's ability to make judgements, perform ADLs, or to tolerate exercise.

The extensiveness of the neurological assessment may be limited if the client's LOC is diminished. A client's chief complaint often determines whether a neurological assessment is necessary. For example, if a client has headaches, this assessment is mandatory. However, if a client complains of oral pain or skin rash, a neurological assessment is not as urgent.

Mental status has six components: orientation, attention and concentration, judgment, memory, thought content and processes, and mood and affect. The level of consciousness is a priority concern. The client's level of consciousness influences the ability to follow directions and participate in a complete health assessment and examination.

Nonverbal observation findings such as crying, frowning, or a masklike face give the nurse clues for further questioning of a client's mental health. Mental health status can be impacted by situational and maturational crises. The client's race, culture, gender, and age also need to be considered. These important variables influence assessment findings and techniques used.

NURSING DIAGNOSES

Altered Thought Processes is appropriate when the client lacks orientation to time, place, person, and/or event or demonstrates an abnormality in any of the six components of the mental health examination.

Acute confusion is appropriate when the client has an abrupt onset of global, transient changes and disturbances in attention, cognition, sleep-wake cycle, and psychomotor activity (Kim, McFarland, and McLane, 1997). **Impaired memory** is appropriate when the client experiences the inability to remember or recall information or behavioral skills (Kim, McFarland, and McLane, 1997).

Risk for Injury is appropriate when the client has muscle weakness or altered LOC. **Impaired Physical Mobility** may apply when clients have indications of cerebellar disease, parkinsons paresis, and any form of plegia (e.g. paraplegia or hemiplegia). **Risk for Impaired Skin Integrity** is appropriate if client is unconscious or has impaired voluntary movement. **Unilateral Neglect** applies when a client who has suffered a stroke is perceptually unaware of and inattentive to one side of the body.

Equipment

Two sterile safety pins
Cotton-tipped applicator or cotton ball
Wartenberg wheel
Two test tubes, one filled with hot water and one with cold water
Reflex hammer
Vials containing coffee or vanilla extract

ASSESSMENT

1. Determine if the client is taking medications, such as analgesics, sedatives, hypnotics, antipsychotics, antidepressants, or nerve stimulants. **Rationale: Medications can depress mental status or cause agitation.**
2. Screen client for headaches, seizures, dizziness, vertigo, numbness or tingling of body part, visual changes, weakness, pain, or changes in speech.
3. Discuss with significant other any recent changes in client's behavior, such as increased irritability, mood swings, or memory loss.
4. Assess client for history of changes in any of the senses: vision, hearing, smell, taste, or touch.
5. Assess if the client is pain free and comfortable without recent pain medication.
6. Assess if the client has a history of deviations in mental status and if these are recent or long-standing.

PLANNING

Expected outcomes focus on health teaching and identification of alterations related to neurological function.

Expected Outcomes

1. Client has no deviations from normal:
   a. Alert and oriented and carries on appropriate discussion.
   b. Intact pain, light touch, temperature, and position sensation.
   c. Cranial nerves intact.
   d. Normal and symmetrical muscle strength, even and balanced gait, reflexes symmetrical and 2+.
2. Client and family identify safety factors related to neurological deficits.
3. Client demonstrates immediate recall of recent and past events.
4. Client is able to interpret abstract ideas and make associations of related concepts.

DELEGATION CONSIDERATIONS

The physical examination of the neurological system requires problem solving and knowledge application unique to a professional nurse. Delegation is inappropriate. AP should know to inform the nurse of any changes in a client's behavior or level of consciousness. Some neurological conditions can be life threatening.

IMPLEMENTATION

Steps	Rationale

1. See Standard Protocol (inside front cover).
2. Assess mental status, behavior, appearance, language function, and intellectual function (See Skill 13.1.)
   a. Assess LOC, directing questions and giving instructions that require response. Be sure client is as fully awake as possible before testing alertness.

   Alteration in mental status may result from brain disorders, drug effects, or electrolyte and metabolic changes. Nurse can assess client's optimal level of alertness only by being assured client is fully responsive.

   b. Use Glasgow Coma Scale (GCS) to measure consciousness objectively (Table 14-2).

   GCS is used to evaluate neurological status over time. A score less than 15 is considered a decrease in LOC. A communication or language problem rather than deterioration of mental status may cause client's inappropriate response.

   c. Note appropriateness of emotions, responses, and ideas expressed.
   d. Rephrase or ask similar questions if it is uncertain whether client understands.
   e. If client has inappropriate responses, ask questions such as, "Tell me your name," "Tell me where you live," "Tell me what day this is," and "Tell me the name of this place."

   Measures client's orientation to person, place, and time within environment.

COMMUNICATION TIP

- *Be sensitive to cultural and educational background when asking questions.*
- *Discuss with family and friends the implications of any behavioral or mental impairment shown by client.*
- *Explain measures to ensure safety in clients with sensory or motor impairments.*

Table 14-2

Glasgow Coma Scale

Action	Response	Score
Eyes open	Spontaneously	(4)
	To speech	3
	To pain	2
	None	1
Best verbal response	Oriented	(5)
	Confused	4
	Inappropriate words	3
	Incomprehensible sounds	2
	None	1
Best motor response	Obeys commands	(6)
	Localized pain	5
	Flexion withdrawal	4
	Abnormal flexion	3
	Abnormal extension	2
	Flaccid	1
	Total Score	(15)

From Potter PA, Perry AG: *Basic nursing,* ed 4, St Louis, 1999, Mosby.

Steps	**Rationale**
f. If signs of early dementia are present (Box 14-3), conduct mental status examination.	Folstein's Mini-Mental State (MMS) is a tool that can be used if the client has positive findings in any of the six areas (Box 14-4). An MMS score of less than 21 indicates cognitive impairment.
g. If client is unable to respond to questions of orientation, offer simple commands: "Squeeze my fingers" or "Move your toes."	LOC exists along a continuum from fully alert and responsive, to inability to initiate meaningful behaviors consciously, to unresponsiveness to external stimuli.
h. When client fails to respond to verbal command, test painful stimuli response.	The more reduced the level of consciousness, the greater the impairment of cerebral function.
(1) Apply firm pressure with thumb on root of client's fingernail.	Client should withdraw from pain.
(2) DO NOT pinch the skin to elicit response to pain.	Causes bruising.
3. Assess behavior, appearance, mood, and affect.	Mood and behavioral responses may indicate a specific disease process. Client is normally concerned and anxious about findings. Euphoria or lack of concern is inappropriate.
a. Observe client's mannerisms and actions. Note response to directions and what mood client displays. Does client participate with examination?	
b. Observe manner of speech.	Tone, pitch of voice, and speed of spoken word may reveal mood and behavior status.
c. Observe appearance: hygiene, cleanliness, appropriateness of makeup, clothes (state of repair, appropriateness to weather and setting).	Appearance can reflect numerous conditions. An unkempt appearance may reflect poor self-image, inability to groom, an emergency, inability to keep clothing clean, or a lack of finances or resources.

Box 14-3 Symptoms That May Indicate Dementia

Learning and Retaining New Information
Trouble remembering recent conversations, events, and appointments
Frequently misplaces objects

Handling Complex Tasks
Difficulty following a complex train of thought
Difficulty performing tasks that require many steps

Reasoning Ability
Unable to develop plan to address problems at work or home
Displays uncharacteristic disregard for rules of social conduct

Spatial Ability and Orientation
Difficulty driving
Difficulty in organizing objects around the house
Difficulty finding way around familiar places

Language
Increasing difficulty with expressing self
Difficulty following conversations

Behavior
Appears more passive and less responsive
More irritable and suspicious than usual
Misinterprets visual and auditory stimuli

Data from Agency on Health Care Policy and Research: *Recognition and initial assessment of Alzheimer's disease and related dementias,* 1996, Agency on Health Care Policy and Research, Rockville, Maryland.

Box 14-4 Folstein's Mini-Mental State Examination

Maximum Score	Score	

Orientation

5　( )　What is the (year) (season) (date) (day) (month)?

5　( )　Where are we: (state) (county) (town) (hospital) (floor)?

Registration

3　( )　Name 3 objects: 1 second to say each. Then ask the patient all 3 after you have said them. Give 1 point for each correct answer. Then repeat them until all 3 are repeated correctly. Count trials and record.

Attention and Calculation

5　( )　Serial 7's. 1 point for each correct. Stop after 5 answers. Alternatively spell "world" backwards.

Recall

3　( )　Ask for the 3 objects repeated above. Give 1 point for each correct.

Language

9　( )　Name a pencil, and watch (2 points)
Repeat the following: "No ifs, ands or buts" (1 point)
Follow a 3-stage command:
"Take a paper in your right hand, fold it in half, and put it on the floor" (3 points)
Read and obey the following:

Close Your Eyes (1 point)

Write a sentence (1 point)
Copy design (1 point)
_____ Total score
ASSESS level of consciousness along a continuum

Alert	Drowsy	Stupor	Coma

Instructions for Administration of Mini-Mental State Examination

Orientation

(1) Ask for the date. Then ask specifically for parts omitted, e.g., "Can you also tell me what season it is?" One point for each correct.

(2) Ask in turn "Can you tell me the name of this hospital?" (town, county, etc.). One point for each correct.

Registration

Ask the patient if you may test his memory. Then say the names of 3 unrelated objects, clearly and slowly, about one second for each. After you have said all 3, ask him to repeat them. This first repetition determines his score (0–3) but keep saying them until he can repeat all 3, up to 6 trials. If he does not eventually learn all 3, recall cannot be meaningfully tested.

Attention and Calculation

Ask the patient to begin with 100 and count backwards by 7. Stop after 5 subtractions (93, 86, 79, 72, 65). Score the total number of correct answers.

If the patient cannot or will not perform this task, ask him to spell the word "world" backwards. The score is the number of letters in correct order, e.g., dlrow = 5, dlorw = 3

Recall

Ask the patient if he can recall the 3 words you previously asked him to remember. Score 0–3.

Language

Naming: Show the patient a wrist watch and ask him what it is. Repeat for pencil. Score 0–2.

Repetition: Ask the patient to repeat the sentence after you. Allow only one trial. Score 0 or 1.

3-Stage command: Give the patient a piece of plain blank paper and repeat the command. Score 1 point for each part correctly executed.

Reading: On a blank piece of paper print the sentence "Close your eyes" in letters large enough for the patient to see clearly. Ask him to read it and do what it says. Score 1 point only if he actually closes his eyes.

Writing: Give the patient a blank piece of paper and ask him to write a sentence for you. Do not dictate a sentence, it is to be written spontaneously. It must contain a subject and verb and be sensible. Correct grammar and punctuation are not necessary.

Copying: On a clean sheet of paper, draw intersecting pentagons, each side about 1 inch, and ask him to copy it exactly as it is. All 10 angles must be present and 2 must intersect to score 1 point. Tremor and rotation are ignored.

Estimate the patient's level of sensorium along a continuum, from alert on the left to coma on the right.

From Folstein and others: Mini-Mental State: a practical method for grading the cognitive state of patients for the clinician, *J Psychiatr Res* 12:189, 1975.

Steps	Rationale
4. Assess language function. If client's communication is unclear, assess the following, asking client to: a. Name a familiar object to which you point. b. Respond to a simple verbal or written command such as, "Sit up." c. Read simple sentences out loud.	Assesses client's ability to understand spoken or written English words.
5. Assess intellectual function (attention, concentration, memory, judgment, thought content and processes). a. Ask client to repeat a short series of numbers forward, then backward (e.g., 7, 3, 1, 4). Gradually increase number of digits until client fails to repeat digits correctly.	Assesses immediate recall. Normally a person can recite a series of five to eight digits forward and four to six backward.
b. Ask client to recall what was eaten for breakfast or the form of transportation used to arrive at the clinic or hospital. Validate accuracy with family member.	Assesses recent memory.
c. Ask client to recall birthday and previous medical history or family history.	Assesses past memory.
d. Ask what client knows about illness or reason for examination or hospitalization.	Assesses knowledge level and ability to learn.
e. Have client explain meaning of simple proverb such as, "Don't count your chickens before they hatch." Note if explanation is literal or abstract.	Determines ability for higher level of intellectual functioning for abstract thinking. Client with altered mentation interprets phrase literally or merely rephrases words.
f. Ask client to identify similarities or associations between terms or simple concepts, for example, "A dog is to a beagle as a cat is to a _____" or "What do a tree and a rose have in common?"	Association is a higher intellectual function.
6. Assess function of each cranial nerve if not completed in previous examinations (Table 14-3). a. CN I: Ask client to identify different aromas, such as coffee, vanilla, and alcohol swab (see illustration). (Have client close eyes if test aroma has labeled container.)	Detects presence of motor and sensory impairment of nerves extending from intracranial sites. Tests sensory and motor function.
b. CNs II, III, IV, and VI: Refer to Skill 14.3	Tests sensory and motor function.
c. CNs V and VII: Ask client to close eyes, and lightly measure sensation of soft touch across skin of face (see illustration). As client smiles, frowns, puffs out cheeks, and raises and lowers eyebrows, look for symmetry. Have client identify salty or sweet taste on front of tongue.	Tests sensory and motor function.
d. CN VII: Assess client's ability to hear the spoken word at normal and whispered levels of voice.	Tests auditory sensory function.
e. CNs IX, X, and XII: Ask client to identify sour, salty, or sweet taste on back of tongue. Use a tongue blade to elicit gag reflex. Ask client to say "ah" while you observe movement of palate, pharynx, signs of hoarseness, and ability to stick out tongue to midline and move side to side.	Tests sensory and motor function.
f. CN XI: Have client shrug shoulders and turn head against examiner's passive resistance. (See Skill 14.1.)	Tests motor function.

Table 14-3

Cranial Nerve Function and Assessment

Number	Name	Type	Function	Method
I	Olfactory	Sensory	Sense of smell	Ask client to identify different nonirritating aromas such as coffee and vanilla.
II	Optic	Sensory	Visual acuity	Use Snellen chart or ask client to read printed material while wearing glasses.
III	Oculomotor	Motor	Extraocular eye movement	Assess directions of gaze.
			Pupil constriction and dilation	Measure pupil reaction to light reflex and accommodation.
IV	Trochlear	Motor	Upward and downward movement of eyeball	Assess directions of gaze.
V	Trigeminal	Sensory and motor	Sensory nerve to skin of face	Lightly touch cornea with wisp of cotton. Assess corneal reflex. Measure sensation of light pain and touch across skin of face.
			Motor nerve to muscles of jaw	Palpate temples as client clenches teeth.
VI	Abducens	Motor	Lateral movement of eyeballs	Assess directions of gaze.
VII	Facial	Sensory and motor	Facial expression	As client smiles, frowns, puffs out cheeks, and raises and lowers eyebrows, look for symmetry.
			Taste	Have client identify salty or sweet taste on front of tongue.
VIII	Auditory	Sensory	Hearing	Assess ability to hear spoken word.
IX	Glossopharyngeal	Sensory and motor	Taste	Ask client to identify sour or sweet taste on back of tongue.
			Ability to swallow	Use tongue blade to elicit gag reflex.
X	Vagus	Sensory and motor	Sensation of pharynx	Ask client to say "ah." Observe palate and pharynx movement.
			Ability to swallow	Use tongue blade to elicit gag reflex.
			Movement of vocal cords	Assess speech for hoarseness.
XI	Spinal accessory	Motor	Movement of head and shoulders	Ask client to shrug shoulders and turn head against passive resistance.
XII	Hypoglossal	Motor	Position of tongue	Ask client to stick out tongue to midline and move it from side to side.

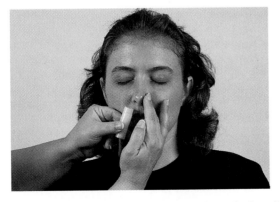

Step 6a *From Chipps E et al: Neurological disorders, Mosby's Clinical Nursing Series, St Louis, 1992, Mosby.*

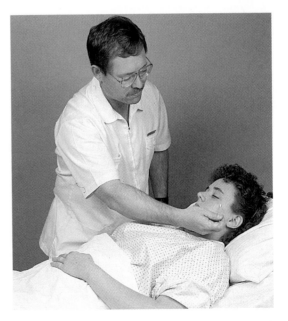

Step 6c

Table 14-4

Assessment of Sensory Nerve Function

Function	Equipment	Method	Precautions
Pain	Sterile safety pin or sharp end of broken sterile tongue blade.	Ask client to voice when dull or sharp sensation is felt. Alternately apply pointed and blunt ends of pin to skin's surface. Note areas of numbness or increased sensitivity.	Remember that areas where skin is thickened, such as heel or sole of foot, may be less sensitive to pain.
Temperature	Two test tubes, one filled with hot water and other with cold	Touch skin with tube. Ask client to identify hot or cold sensation.	Omit test if pain sensation is normal.
Light Touch	Cotton ball or cotton-tipped applicator	Apply light wisp of cotton to different points along skin's surface. Ask client to voice when sensation is felt.	Apply at areas where skin is thin or more sensitive (e.g., face, neck, inner aspect of arms, top of feet and hands).
Vibration	Tuning fork	Apply vibrating fork to distal interphalangeal joint of fingers and interphalangeal joint of great toe. Have client voice when the vibration stops.	Be sure client feels vibration and not merely pressure.
Position		Grasp finger, holding it by its sides with thumb and index finger. Alternate moving finger up and down. Ask client to state when finger is up or down. Repeat with toes.	Avoid rubbing adjacent appendages as finger or toe is moved.
Two-point discrimination	Two safety pins, Wartenberg wheel, or fingers	Lightly apply two points simultaneously to skin's surface. Ask client if one or two pinpricks are felt.	Apply to same anatomical site (e.g., fingertips, palm of hand, or upper arms). Minimum distance at which client can discriminate two points varies (2–3 mm on fingertips).

Steps	Rationale

7. Assess sensory function.
   a. Perform all sensory testing with client's eyes closed. Sensory can be integrated into site-specific assessments.
   b. Assess sensation to pain, temperature, light touch, vibration, position, and two-point discrimination (Table 14-4).
   c. Apply sensory stimuli in random, unpredictable order. Note anatomical area where sensation is reduced.
   d. Compare symmetrical areas of body while applying stimuli to face, arms, legs, and trunk.
   e. Ask client to say when particular stimulus is perceived.
8. Assess motor function.
   a. Assess gait, stance, and muscle strength and tone.

   b. Have client stand with feet close together and eyes closed (see illustration *A*). Then ask client to stand on one foot, then the other (see illustration *B*).
   c. Ask client to sit. Demonstrate method for rapidly striking thigh with palm of hand evenly and without hesitation. Have client repeat.

Client should not be able to see when or where stimulus strikes skin.

Changes may reflect lesions in peripheral nerves, spinal cord, or cerebral cortex.
Note swaying. Romberg's test assesses balance. Cerebellar disease causes imbalance even with eyes open.

Note smoothness of movement. Assesses upper extremity coordination.

A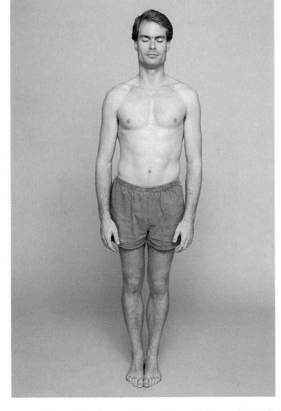

B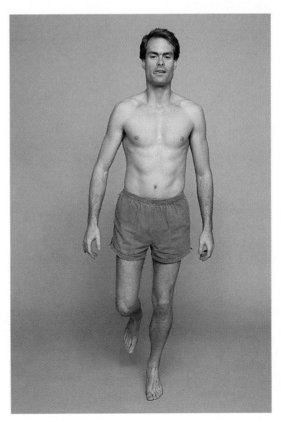

Step 8b   *From Chipps E et al:* Neurological disorders, *Mosby's Clinical Nursing Series, St Louis, 1992, Mosby.*

Steps	Rationale
d. Have client alternately strike thigh with hand supinated and then pronated.	Speed and symmetry of movement are disturbed in cerebellar dysfunction. Note tremors of hand or awkward movement.
e. Stand in front of client; hold index finger 60 cm (2 feet) stationary in front of client's face. Ask client to touch your index finger with his or her index finger and then to touch the nose alternately (see illustrations).	Point-to-point test assesses upper extremity coordination.
f. Ask client to close eyes and place heel of one foot just below knee of opposite leg and then slide heel down to shin toward foot. Repeat for other leg (see illustration).	Presence of involuntary movements or difficulty in controlling heel may indicate cerebellar problem.

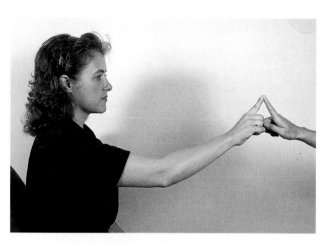 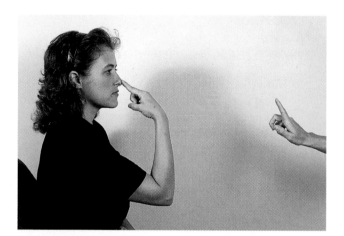

Step 8e   *From Chipps E et al: Neurological disorders, Mosby's Clinical Nursing Series, St Louis, 1992, Mosby.*

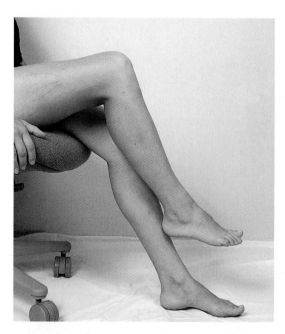 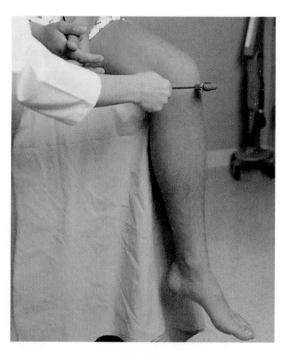

Step 8f *From Chipps E et al: Neurological disorders, Mosby's Clinical Nursing Series, St Louis, 1992, Mosby.*

Step 9e

Steps	Rationale

g. With client supine, place hand at ball of client's foot. Ask client to tap hand with foot as quickly as possible.

Note speed and smoothness of movement. Assesses lower extremity coordination.

9. Assess reflexes.
   a. Assess deep tendon reflexes (Table 14-5). Reflexes should be symmetrical on both sides of body.
   b. Ask client to relax extremity.
   c. Position limb to slightly stretch muscle being tested.
   d. Hold reflex hammer loosely between thumb and fingers.
   e. Tap tendon briskly (see illustration).

The more commonly tested reflexes are *plantar* and *patellar*. Reflexes are graded on scale:
   0, No response
   1+, Low-normal slight muscle contraction
   2+, Normal visible muscle twitch
   3+, Brisker than normal
   4+, Hyperactive, very brisk; spinal cord disorder suspected

   f. Compare symmetry of reflex from one side of body to the other.

Asymmetry of reflex response indicates alteration in reflex pathway.

10. See Completion Protocol (inside front cover).

• • •

Table 14-5

Assessment of Common Reflexes

Type	Procedure	Normal Reflex
DEEP TENDON REFLEXES		
Biceps	Flex client's arm at elbow with palms down. Place your thumb in antecubital fossa at base of biceps tendon. Strike thumb with reflex hammer.	Flexion of arm at elbow
Triceps	Flex client's elbow, holding arm across chest, or hold upper arm horizontally and allow lower arm to go limp. Strike triceps tendon just above elbow.	Extension at elbow
Patellar	Have client sit with legs hanging freely over side of bed or chair or have client lie supine and support knee in flexed position. Briskly tap patellar tendon just below patella.	Extension of lower leg at knee
Achilles	Have client assume same position as for patellar reflex. Slightly dorsiflex client's ankle by grasping toes in palm of your hand. Strike Achilles tendon just above heel.	Plantar flexion of foot
Plantar (Babinski's)	Have client lie supine with legs straight and feet relaxed. Take handle end of reflex hammer and stroke lateral aspect of sole from heel to ball of foot, curving across ball of foot toward big toe.	Bending of toes downward
CUTANEOUS REFLEXES		
Gluteal	Have client assume side-lying position. Spread buttocks apart and lightly stimulate perineal area with cotton applicator.	Contraction of anal sphincter
Abdominal	Have client stand or lie supine. Stroke abdominal skin with base of cotton applicator over lateral borders of rectus abdominis muscle toward midline. Repeat test in each abdominal quadrant.	Contraction of rectus abdominis muscle with pulling of umbilicus toward stimulated side

EVALUATION

1. Compare findings with client's baseline and normal expected findings:
   a. Observe ability to relate history in sequential and logical manner.
   b. Ask if client has altered sensations of pain, touch, temperature, or position sense.
   c. Observe status of cranial nerve function.
   d. Compare right to left in relation to muscle strength, gait, and reflexes.
2. Ask what safety measures are being taken to motor/sensory deficits.
3. Verify accuracy of history and recall of recent and past events.
4. Verify ability to interpret abstract ideas and associate related concepts.

Unexpected Outcomes and Related Interventions

1. Client is confused and at times difficult to arouse by verbal stimulus.
   a. Stop examination and investigate reasons for confusion or unresponsiveness.
2. Client is not consistently oriented to person, place, time, or events.
   a. Provide reorientation frequently.
   b. Have family provide items that help orient the client (e.g., photographs, familiar personal items).
3. Client demonstrates evidence of confusion; intact sensory and motor function but slow response to instructions; reduced sensation to temperature, touch, and painful stimuli; unsteady gait or dragging foot; reflexes of 0 to 1+ or 3+ to 4+; or abnormal cranial nerve function.
   a. Provide for client's safety (e.g., remove barriers to mobility in the home; provide appropriate assistive devices; supervise ambulation).
   b. Compare findings to prior history to identify if they are new.
   c. If new findings, refer client and significant other to appropriate health care professional or agency.
4. Speech is slow and slurred. Provide more time for examination. If this represents a change, notify physician.
5. Client is able to recall past events but unable to repeat a series of five numbers.
   Be sure to note age of client; older adults may normally have this problem.

6. Client is unable to interpret proverbs or associate related concepts.
   Reassess client's cultural and educational background. Nurse may need to rephrase concepts in terms with which client is familiar.

Recording and Reporting

- Record all abnormalities or changes in LOC and behavior, describing in specific detail.
- Report all mental status changes to physician immediately.
- Report abnormal findings to the physician, including pertinent history and vital sign information.

Sample Documentation

0645   Client carries on appropriate conversation. Oriented to person, place, and time. Past and recent memory intact. Able to recall 4/4 in 3 minutes. Higher level of intellect demonstrated by interpretation of proverb and association of related concepts. Responded to questions quickly and with cooperation. No deficits in mobility, coordination, or motor and sensory functioning of upper and lower extremities. Deep tendon reflexes 2+.

Geriatric Considerations

- Older adults have decreased ability to respond to multiple stimuli.
- Older adult has reduced number of taste buds and reduced ability to discriminate odors.
- Sense of touch and pain may be diminished.
- Deep tendon and superficial reflexes are present but may also be slightly decreased.
- Older adults are at risk for acute confusion, resulting from an adverse or unwanted effect of a diagnostic or therapeutic intervention.

Skill 14.9

ASSESSING MUSCULOSKELETAL FUNCTION

Musculoskeletal assessment includes a general inspection of gait, posture, and body position, as well as thorough assessment of specific muscle, bone, and joint groups. This assessment is easily integrated into routine activities of care or when assessing other body systems.

With aging, a person's ability to respond to multiple stimuli decreases, and ROM decreases in all joints because of reduction in muscle fiber size and tightening of joints. Allow more time for older adults because they are slower to complete tasks.

NURSING DIAGNOSES

Risk for Injury is appropriate when the client is not immobilized and has a deficit in musculoskeletal functioning. **Body Image Disturbance** is indicated when the client expresses concern or negative comments about lack of abilities for locomotion. **Impaired Physical Mobility** is appropriate when findings of muscle weakness, loss of strength, or skeletal abnormalities are present. **Pain** is indicated with a report of injury or misalignment of the skeletal frame accompanied by discomfort.

Equipment

Tape measure

ASSESSMENT

1. Ask client to describe history of problems in bone, muscle, or joint function (e.g., recent falls, trauma, lifting heavy objects) and history of bone or joint disease with sudden or gradual onset.
2. Assess nature and extent of client's pain: type, location, severity, predisposing and aggravating factors, and relieving factors.
3. Determine how alterations influence client's ability to perform ADLs, household chores, work, and social functions.

4. Assess height loss of women older than age 50 by subtracting current height from recall of maximum adult height. **Rationale: May be indicator for osteoporosis.**

PLANNING

Expected outcomes focus on health teaching and identification of alterations related to musculoskeletal function.

Expected Outcomes

Client has no deviations from normal:

a. Gait is even and balanced with arms swinging freely at side, and posture is erect.
b. Full active ROM in all joints, joints without deformities or crepitus, and normal thoracic and lumbar curves.
c. Strong muscle groups without deformity.

DELEGATION CONSIDERATIONS

The skill of assessment of musculoskeletal function requires problem solving and knowledge application unique to a professional nurse. Delegation is inappropriate. Assistive personnel will often assist clients with ambulation, transfer, and positioning. As a result, the staff member should be trained in recognizing problems with gait and ROM. The nurse should be responsible for informing AP about the following:

- Clients at risk for gait problems.
- Importance of never moving or forcing a joint beyond the client's current ROM.
- Clients with muscular weakness will require special assistance with transfer and ambulation.
- Need to report any problems noted in ROM, appearance of a joint, or muscle strength.

IMPLEMENTATION

Steps	Rationale
1. See Standard Protocol (inside front cover).	
2. Inspect gait as client walks into examination room and stands. Observe for foot dragging, shuffling, or limping; balance; and presence of obvious deformity in lower extremities.	Gait is more natural if client is unaware of observation. Nature of gait may indicate type of alteration. Ambulation can accentuate presence of deformity.

Steps	**Rationale**

COMMUNICATION TIP

- *Discuss benefits of correct postural alignment.*
- *Discuss benefit of proper weight-bearing exercise 3 times per week or more to promote bone health.*
- *Review proper lifting to avoid back injury.*

- *Review fall prevention techniques with older adults and clients with altered mobility.*
- *Discuss need to pace activities to compensate for loss in muscle strength in the older adult.*
- *Review energy-conserving techniques and self-care assistive devices, as indicated.*

3. Stand behind client and observe postural alignment: position of hips relative to shoulders. Look sideways at cervical, thoracic, and lumbar curves (see illustration). Note abnormalities.

4. Make a general observation of symmetry of joints, muscles, and extremity length. Look for obvious deformities.

General review helps to pinpoint areas requiring in-depth assessment.

5. Assist client in putting each joint through its full ROM (see illustration). Observe for equality of motion in same body parts.
   a. Active motion: Client needs no support or assistance and is able to move joint independently.
   b. Passive motion: Nurse supports extremity and moves joints through full ROM.

Assessment of client's normal ROM provides baseline for assessing later changes after surgery or procedures.

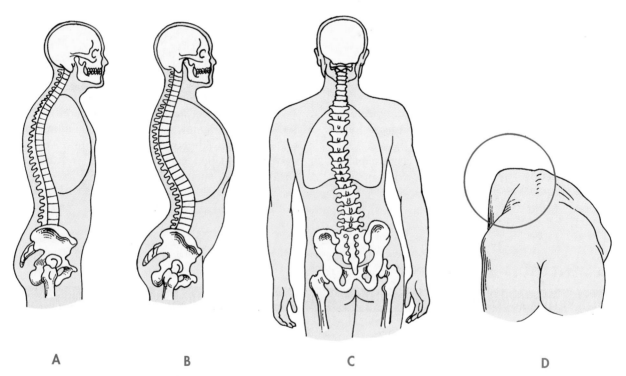

A   B   C   D

Step 3 *Spinal deformities:* **A,** *kyphosis;* **B,** *lordosis;* **C,** *scoliosis;* **D,** *scoliosis with client bending forward.*

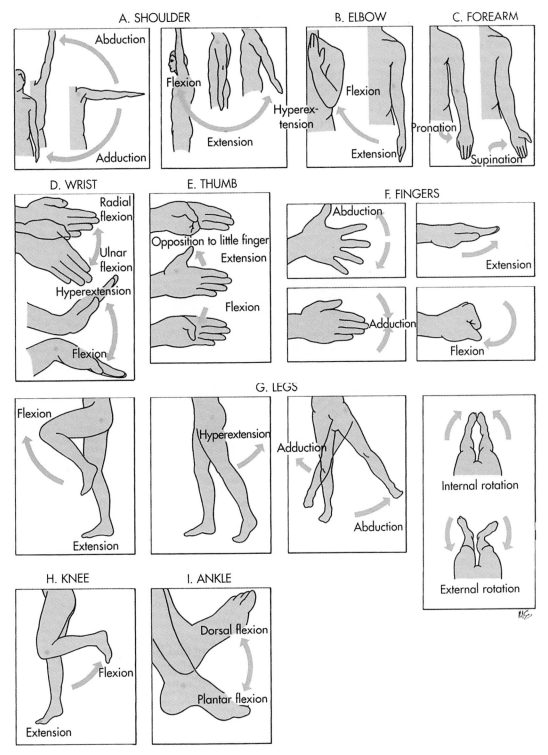

Step 5 *Modified from Beare PG, Myers JL:* Adult health nursing, *ed 3, St Louis, 1998, Mosby.*

Steps	Rationale

6. While observing ROM, note any instability of joint. Palpate for unusual movement of joint during its movement and for swelling, stiffness, tenderness, redness, and heat.

Crepitus is crunching or grating that occurs when joint is moved; it indicates a pathological condition.

7. While assessing ROM, ask client to allow extremity to relax or hang limp. Support extremity, move through full ROM to detect muscular resistance. Observe position changes (standing, sitting, lying) for coordination, strength, and flexibility.

Detects muscle tone in major muscle groups. Normal tone causes mild, even resistance to movement through ROM. If tone is increased (hypertonicity), any sudden movement of joint is met with considerable resistance.

8. Assess muscle strength by having client resist pressure applied to the muscle group by the nurse to move against resistance (e.g., push with foot) (see illustration). Have client hold resistance until told to stop. Compare symmetrical groups.

Hypotonic muscle moves without resistance and feels flabby.

9. If muscle weakness is identified, measure muscle size with tape measure placed around body of muscle (see illustration). Compare with same muscle on opposite side of body.

10. See Completion Protocol (inside front cover).

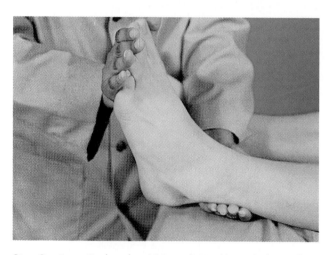

Step 8 *From Barkauskas VH et al: Health and physical assessment, ed 2, St Louis, 1998, Mosby.*

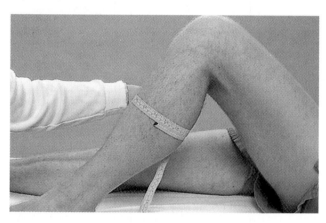

Step 9 *From Seidel HM et al: Mosby's guide to physical examination, ed 4, St Louis, 1999, Mosby.*

• • • •

EVALUATION
Compare findings with client's baseline and normal expected findings.

Unexpected Outcomes and Related Interventions
Client demonstrates evidence of reduced ROM in one or more major joints, weakness in one or more muscle groups, or postural abnormalities with poor balance and shuffling or stumbling feet.
a. Provide for client's safety.
b. Compare findings to prior history to identify if these are new findings.

c. Refer to the appropriate health care agency or physician.

Recording and Reporting
- Record all abnormal findings.
- Report acute pain or sudden muscle weakness to the physician.
- Report abnormal findings to the physician, including pertinent history and vital signs.

Sample Documentation
0900   ROM without restriction for all joints. Strength equal bilaterally. Gait steady and smooth.

Geriatric Considerations

- Older adult's gait normally has smaller steps and a wider base of support.
- Older adults tend to assume a stooped, forward-bent posture, with hips and knees somewhat flexed and arms bent at the elbows and the level of the arms raised (Ebersole and Hess, 1998).
- In older adults joints often become swollen and stiff, with reduced ROM resulting from cartilage erosion and fibrosis of synovial membranes.
- Older adults may develop kyphosis because of osteoporosis.

CRITICAL THINKING EXERCISES

1. Discuss the rationale for the order of progression for assessment of the lungs and thorax.

2. Ms. Emma Bradley, a 32-year-old married woman, presents to the medicine clinic to establish a primary care provider. Her health history and physical are significant for the following:
   a. Current medications: none
   b. Family history: paternal grandfather died at age 72 with an acute myocardial infarction, paternal grandmother alive at age 77 with coronary artery disease, maternal grandfather alive at age 71 with insulin-dependent diabetes mellitus and peripheral vascular disease, maternal grandmother alive at age 69 with non–insulin-dependent diabetes mellitus; father alive with at age 50 with coronary artery disease, and mother alive at age 49 with hypertension.
   c. Social history: married with three children, ages 8, 6, and 4. Cigarette smoker, 10 per day times 12 years. Social drinker, 1 to 3 glasses of wine per week. Den mother, room mother, and part-time secretary. No regular exercise program.
   d. Physical examination: Vital signs: BP 150/92; weight 15 lb over recommended weight; remainder of physical examination unremarkable. Identify three priorities for the nursing plan of care.

3. Discuss the rationale for completing the neurological and muscoskeletal examination together.

REFERENCES

Agency on Health Care Policy and Research (AHCPR): *Recognition and initial assessment of Alzheimer's disease and related dementias,* Clinical Practice Guideline no. 19, pub. no. N97-0702, 1996, Agency on Health Care Policy and Research, Rockville, Maryland.

American Cancer Society: *1998 Cancer facts and figures,* New York, 1998, The Society.

Barkauskas VH et al: *Health and physical assessment,* St Louis, 1994, Mosby.

Beare PG, Myers JL: *Principles and practices of adult health nursing,* ed 3, St Louis, 1998, Mosby.

Belcher AE: *Cancer nursing,* Mosby's Clinical Nursing Series, St Louis, 1992, Mosby.

Canobbio MM: *Cardiovascular disorders,* Mosby's Clinical Nursing Series, St Louis, 1990, Mosby.

Chipps E et al: *Neurological disorders,* Mosby's Clinical Nursing Series, St Louis, 1992, Mosby.

Ebersole P, Hess P: *Toward healthy aging,* ed 5, 1998, Mosby.

Folstein MF, Folstein S, McHugh PR: Mini-Mental State: a practical method for grading the cognitive state of patients for the clinician, *J Psychiatric Res* 12:189, 1975.

Kim MJ, McFarland GK, McLane AM: *Pocket guide to nursing diagnosis,* ed 7, St Louis, 1997, Mosby.

Lueckenotte AG: *Gerontologic nursing,* St Louis, 1996, Mosby.

Lueckenotte AG: *Pocket guide to gerontologic assessment,* ed 3, St Louis, 1998, Mosby.

Payne WA, Hahn DB: *Understanding your health,* ed 2, 1989, Mosby.

Potter PA, Perry AG: *Basic Nursing,* ed 4, St Louis, 1999, Mosby.

Seidel HM et al: *Mosby's guide to physical examination,* ed 4, St Louis, 1999, Mosby.

Thompson JM et al: *Mosby's clinical nursing,* ed 4, St Louis, 1997, Mosby.

Wilson SF, Thompson JM: *Respiratory disorders,* Mosby's Clinical Nursing Series, St Louis, 1990, Mosby.

CHAPTER 15

Laboratory and Diagnostic Tests

Skill 15.1

Specimen Collection (Urine, Stool, Sputum Cultures), 346

Skill 15.2

Blood Specimens (Venipuncture; Vacutainer; Blood Cultures), 360

Skill 15.3

Unit Specimen Testing (Glucose, Chemstrip/Multistix, Hemoccult, Gastroccult), 368

Skill 15.4

Contrast Media Studies (Arteriogram, Computed Tomography, Intravenous Pyelogram, 376

Skill 15.5

Nuclear Imaging Studies (Bone Scan, Brain Scan, Thyroid Scan), 380

Skill 15.6

Assisting with Diagnostic Studies (Aspirations [Bone Marrow, Lumbar Puncture, Paracentesis, Thoracentesis, Liver Biopsy], Bronchoscopy, Endoscopy, Magnetic Resonance Imaging), 383

Skill 15.7

Cardiac Studies (Electrocardiograms, Exercise Stress Test, Dobutamine Stress Echocardiography, Cardiac Nuclear Scanning, Cardiac Catheterization), 396

Proficiency in assisting with diagnostic procedures is more important than ever for the professional nurse. Skill and judgment in obtaining specimens and assisting with diagnostic procedures affect client safety and comfort and ensure the quality of diagnostic samples. Accountability is increasing, and there is more attention to monitoring outcomes. Additionally, current health care economics insist that laboratory and diagnostic procedures be performed accurately and timely.

Nurses often assume the responsibility for collecting specimens of body secretions and excretions (Table 15-1). Depending on the type of specimen needed and skill required, the nurse may be able to delegate this task to the assistive personnel (AP). Laboratory examination of specimens of urine, stool, sputum, blood, and wound drainage provides important information about body functioning and contributes to the assessment of health status. Laboratory test results can aid the diagnosis of health care problems, provide information about the stage and activity of a disease process, and measure the response to therapy.

Clients often experience embarrassment or discomfort when giving a sample of body excretions or secretions. It is important to handle excretions discreetly and to provide the client with as much comfort and privacy as possible. The nurse needs to be aware that sociocultural variations may impact the client's response and willingness to participate in various diagnostic procedures. Anxiety is also provoked by the invasive nature of some collection procedures or by fear of unknown test results. Clients who are given a clear explanation about the purpose of the specimen and how it is to be obtained will be more cooperative in its collection. With proper instruction many clients are able to obtain their own specimens of urine, stool, and sputum, thus avoiding embarrassment. Often the success of specimen collection depends on cooperation.

Laboratory tests are often expensive. The nurse can prevent unnecessary costs by using the correct procedure for obtaining and processing specimens. When there are questions about laboratory tests, the nurse should consult the institution's procedure manual or call the laboratory.

Normal values for laboratory tests can be found in reference books, but the nurse should know that each laboratory establishes its own values for each test. These values

Table 15-1

Specimen Collection

Source	Type of Specimen	Assessment
Urine	Routine urinalysis Culture/sensitivity Clean-voided (midstream) From indwelling catheter	Urinary tract infection: frequency, urgency, dysuria, hematuria, back pain, cloudy urine with sediment, foul odor, fever
	Twenty-four-hour timed collection	Renal function, amino acids, creatinine, hormones, glucose, adrenocorticosteroids
Stool	Hemoccult Culture	Possibility of blood in stool, visible or not visible (occult) Diarrhea
Nose and throat	Culture	Sore throat, upper respiratory or sinus infection
Sputum	Culture	Productive cough; if client is unable to cough productively, a suction trap may be used
Wound drainage	Culture	Fever; increased tenderness/deep pain at wound site; drainage, especially purulent, foul smelling, green, yellow, or brown

are usually readily available on the laboratory slips of the agency. Any major deviations should be discussed with the physician immediately.

Diagnostic tests are performed within the hospital at the client's bedside or in specifically equipped rooms for diagnostic or therapeutic purposes either within the hospital or in outpatient settings. Responsibilities of the nurse include assessing the client's knowledge of the procedure, preparing the client, maintaining a safe environment throughout the procedure, and providing postprocedure care. The nurse supervises care delegated to assistive personnel (AP). If testing was done on an outpatient basis, the nurse provides detailed, printed home care instructions. Knowledge of each test and application of the nursing process ensures safe performance of the procedure.

Certain diagnostic procedures require the client to receive IV conscious sedation (IVCS). IVCS is the administration of pharmacological agents to provide a minimally depressed level of consciousness. During IVCS the client independently and continuously maintains an airway and is responsive to physical stimulation and verbal commands. The use of IVCS provides client comfort along with safe and effective performance during the procedure. Although IVCS may be administered by a registered nurse with a physician in attendance, it is the responsibility of the physician to order the appropriate drugs and their dosages. Check agency policy for recommended and maximum doses of medications.

Client risks during IVCS include airway compromise, hemodynamic instability, and/or altered levels of consciousness. Emergency equipment (see Chapter 38) must be immediately accessible where IVCS is administered. After IVCS, clients need continuous monitoring of vital signs (i.e., pulse, blood pressure, respiration) and oxygen saturation by pulse oximetry. In addition, the client's level of sedation and level of consciousness must be assessed and documented according to agency policy by the registered nurse (RN) or delegated to an licensed practical nurse (LPN) or respiratory therapist. Check agency policies regarding specific monitoring parameters and frequency both during and after the procedure.

The nurse must know legal implications for diagnostic testing. Most invasive diagnostic tests require a signed informed consent. The physician is ultimately responsible for disclosure, but the nurse must be aware of institutional policies regarding consent forms and ensure that informed consent is obtained before the procedure (Cushing, 1991). The nurse must also record and report the client's status before, during, and after the procedure. The nurse assists the client throughout a procedure. Most of these procedures cause moderate discomfort, and the client may tolerate the procedure better if a well-informed nurse stays at the bedside and explains each step.

NURSING DIAGNOSES

Anxiety may result from the manner in which a specimen is obtained or a procedure is performed. **Fear** may result from the unknown test results. There may be a **knowledge deficit** regarding the way the specimen is to be collected or the test performed. **Risk for infection** exists when skin or tissue integrity is altered, and **Pain** is often associated with invasive diagnostic tests. Nursing diagnoses related to promoting optimum oxygenation during diagnostic procedures involving the airway include **Impaired Gas Exchange, Ineffective Breathing, Risk for Aspiration, and Ineffective Airway Clearance.**

Skill 15.1

SPECIMEN COLLECTION (URINE, STOOL, SPUTUM, CULTURES)

Laboratory examination of specimens provides valuable information about body system functions. A urinalysis can provide data about kidney or metabolic function, nutrition, and systemic diseases. A culture and sensitivity measurement of urine may be collected either as a clean-voided midstream specimen or under sterile conditions from an indwelling urinary catheter. Some tests of renal function and urine composition require urine to be collected over 2 to 72 hours. The 24-hour timed collection is most common and allows for measurement of elements such as amino acids, creatinine, hormones, glucose, and adrenocorticosteroid, the level of which changes over time.

Analysis of stool provides useful information about pathological conditions such as tumors, infection, and malabsorption problems. A nasal or throat culture specimen is a simple diagnostic tool for determining the nature of a client's problem when signs and symptoms of upper respiratory or sinus infections are present. Examination of sputum may aid in the diagnosis and treatment of several conditions, ranging from bronchitis to lung cancer. A specimen of wound drainage is analyzed to determine the type and number of pathogenic microorganisms present.

Clients can often assist the nurse or unlicensed care provider in obtaining specimens. Clients should receive careful instructions about the purpose and technique of urine and stool collection to ensure specimens are not accidentally contaminated. For cultures of the nose, throat, or wound, the specimen is collected by the nurse according to agency policy with the client's cooperation.

Equipment

All specimens

Completed specimen identification label

Completed laboratory requisition form (date, time, name of test, source of specimen/culture)

Small plastic bag for delivery of specimen to laboratory (or a container as specified by agency)

Random urine specimen

Disposable gloves

Washcloth, towel, soap, and water

Clean collection container (e.g., specimen "hat") to place under toilet seat (Figure 15-1), bedpan, or urinal

Wide-mouth specimen container with lid

Midstream (clean-voided) urine specimen

Disposable gloves

Commercial kit for clean-voided urine (Figure 15-2) containing:

Antiseptic towelettes

Sterile specimen container

Soap, water, washcloth, and towel

Bedpan (for nonambulatory client), specimen hat (for ambulatory client), or potty chair (for young child)

Sterile urine specimen from an indwelling catheter

Disposable gloves

3-ml syringe with 1-inch needle (21 to 25 gauge) for culture

or

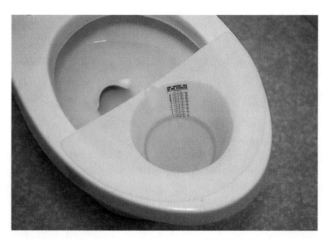

Figure 15-1 Specimen hat.

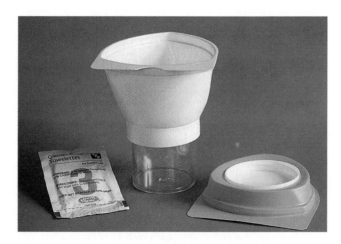

Figure 15-2 Clean voided urine kit.

20-ml syringe with 1-inch needle (21 to 25 gauge) for routine analysis

Metal clamp or rubber band

Alcohol, povidone-iodine, or other disinfectant swab

Specimen container (nonsterile for routine urinalysis, sterile for culture)

24-hour urine collection (timed urine collection)

Large collection bottle with cap that may contain a chemical for urine preservation (consultation with laboratory is usually necessary to obtain bottle and determine appropriate chemical additive [e.g., toluene or acetic acid])

Bedpan, urinal, specimen hat, or potty chair if client does not have indwelling catheter

Graduated measuring cup if intake and output (I&O) are to be measured

Basin large enough to hold collection bottle surrounded by ice if immediate refrigeration is required

Signs that remind client and staff of timed urine collection

Clean disposable gloves

Stool specimen

Disposable gloves

Plastic container with lid

Two tongue blades

Paper towel

Bedpan, specimen hat, or bedside commode

"Save Stool" signs

Completed specimen identification label

Completed laboratory requisition form

Nasal and throat specimen

Disposable gloves

Two sterile swabs in sterile culture tubes (Flexible wire swab with cotton tip may be used for nose cultures.)

Nasal speculum (optional)

Emesis basin or clean container (optional)

Tongue blades

Penlight

Facial tissues

Sputum specimen

Sterile specimen container with cover

Clean disposable gloves

Facial tissues

Emesis basin (optional)

Toothbrush (optional)

Suctioned sputum specimen

Suction device (wall or portable)

Sterile suction catheter (size 14, 16, or 18 Fr [not large enough to cause trauma to nasal mucosa])

Sterile gloves

Sterile saline in container

In-line specimen container (sputum trap)

Oxygen therapy equipment if indicated

Protective eyewear (if required)

Wound drainage specimen

Culture tube with swab and transport medium for aerobic culture

Anaerobic culture tube with swab (tubes contain carbon dioxide or nitrogen gas)

5- to 10-ml syringe and 21-gauge needle

Sterile gloves

Protective eyewear

Antiseptic swab

Sterile dressing materials (determined by type of dressing)

Paper or plastic disposable bag

ASSESSMENT

1. Assess client's ability to assist with urine and stool specimen collection: able to position self and hold container. **Rationale: This determines ability to cooperate and level of assistance required.**

2. Assess client's understanding of need for the specimen. **Rationale: This determines the need for health teaching. Client's understanding of purpose promotes cooperation.**

3. Determine if fluid, dietary requirements, or medications need to be administered in conjunction with test. **Rationale: Certain substances affect excretion and levels of urinary constituents. Specific amounts of fluid may be required for concentration/dilution tests.**

4. Assess for signs and symptoms of urinary tract infection (frequency, urgency, dysuria, hematuria, flank pain, cloudy urine with sediment, foul odor, fever), upper respiratory infection (increased cough, increased sputum production, changes in sputum color), sinus infection (sinus headache or tenderness, nasal congestion, sore throat, inflammation or purulent drainage of posterior pharynx), and wound infection (fever, increasing tenderness and deep pain at the wound site, change in color or amount of drainage, elevated white blood cell [WBC] count in conjunction with erythematous wound). Signs and symptoms help reveal nature of problem.

5. Assess stool or urinary elimination pattern to allow for more effective planning.

PLANNING

Expected outcomes focus on the collection of an uncontaminated specimen by nurse or client with client knowledgeable of the purpose of the specimen examination.

Expected Outcomes

All specimens

1. Client explains procedure for specimen collection before collection is attempted.

2. Client explains purpose of specimen analysis before collection is attempted.

24-hour urine collection

3. Client's specimen is free of contaminants, such as urine or toilet tissue in stool or stool or toilet tissue in urine.

Urine and stool specimens

4. All of client's urine voided during time period is saved.

Suction sputum specimen

5. Client maintains adequate oxygenation throughout procedure.

Wound drainage specimen

6. Specimen is free of contaminants from skin.

DELEGATION CONSIDERATIONS

The collection of a clean midstream urine specimen, a sterile specimen from an indwelling catheter, a timed urine specimen, a stool specimen, and a sputum specimen may be performed by assistive personnel (AP). For these specimen collections, determine that the AP understands the specific specimen collection procedure, which may include use of sterile technique. Inform AP of when to collect specimen and proper storage of specimen (if not to be sent to the laboratory immediately). Specific considerations and instructions are necessary for obtaining the following specimens:

- Clean midstream urine specimen: Inform AP how to cleanse urethra before obtaining specimen.
- Sputum specimens: Instruct AP to collect specimen before a meal and how to position client with impaired mobility.

The skills of obtaining throat, nasal, and nasal pharyngeal cultures and obtaining wound drainage specimens require problem solving and knowledge application unique to a professional nurse. Delegation of this skill is inappropriate.

IMPLEMENTATION

Steps	Rationale
1. See Standard Protocol (inside front cover).	
2. **Perform random urine collection.**	
a. Explain how to obtain specimen free of feces and tissue.	Promotes cooperation. Client may be able to obtain the specimen independently. Prevents accidental disposal of urine.
b. Give client or family member towel, washcloth, and soap to cleanse perineal area, or assist client to cleanse perineum.	Cleansing prevents contamination of specimen as urine passes from urethra.
c. Give male client specimen container and direct to bathroom; give female client specimen hat and direct to bathroom. Assist client as needed to void into bedpan or urinal.	Maintains as much independence in client as possible.
d. If client did not void directly into specimen container, transfer 4 oz of urine into it.	Avoids contamination of specimen and ensures collection of correct volume.
e. Place lid tightly on container without touching inside of lid.	Prevents contamination of specimen by other substances and loss from spillage.
f. If urine has been splashed on outside of container, wash it off. Remove and discard gloves.	Prevents spread of bacteria.
g. Follow Steps 9-13 on p. 358.	

Steps	Rationale

3. Collect midstream (clean-voided) urine specimen.

   a. Explain procedure to client and/or family member. Discuss reason midstream specimen is needed, how client/family member can assist, and how to obtain specimen free of feces and tissue.

       Promotes cooperation and participation. Client may be able to obtain specimen independently. Prevents accidental disposal of specimen. Feces and tissue alter chemical composition of specimen.

   b. Give client or family member towel, washcloth, and soap to cleanse perineum, or assist client to cleanse perineum.

       Prevents contamination of specimen after urine passes from urethra.

   c. Assist bedridden client onto bedpan.

       Provides easy access to perineal area to collect specimen.

   d. Using sterile technique, open commercial specimen kit (see Figure 15-2), maintaining sterility of inside of specimen container.

   e. Open specimen container, and place cap with sterile inside surface up. Do not touch inside of container.

       Contaminated specimen is most frequent reason for inaccurate reporting on urine cultures and sensitivities.

   f. Assist or allow client to cleanse perineum and collect specimen independently.

     (1) *Male:* Hold penis with one hand; using circular motion and antiseptic towelette, cleanse end, moving from center to outside (see illustration).

       Decreases bacterial levels at urinary meatus.

COMMUNICATION TIP

Be sensitive that diverse age and sociocultural groups may use different words to describe urine and stool.

COMMUNICATION TIP

Forewarn client that antiseptic solution may feel cold to touch.

In uncircumcised males, foreskin must be retracted for effective cleansing of meatus and during voiding.

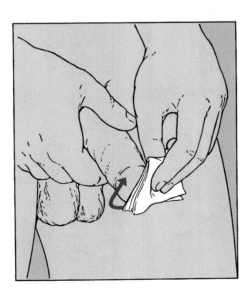

Step 3f(1) *Modified from Grimes D:* Infectious diseases, *Mosby's Clinical Nursing Series, St Louis, 1991, Mosby.*

Steps	Rationale

(2) *Female:* Spread labia minora with fingers of nondominant hand. Use dominant hand to cleanse area with antiseptic towelette, moving from front (above urethral orifice) to back (toward anus) (see illustration).

Provides access to urethral meatus.
Prevents contamination of urinary meatus with fecal material.

g. If agency procedure indicates, rinse area with sterile water and dry with cotton.

Prevents contamination of specimen with antiseptic solution.

h. While continuing to hold labia apart, or hold penis, client should initiate urine stream. After stream is achieved, pass specimen container into stream and collect 30 to 60 ml (see illustration).

Initial urine stream flushes out microorganisms that normally accumulate at urethral meatus.

i. Remove specimen container before flow of urine stops and before releasing labia or penis. Client finishes voiding into bedpan or toilet.

Prevents contamination of specimen with skin flora.

j. Replace cap securely on specimen container (touch only outside).

Maintains sterility of inside of container and prevents spillage of urine.

k. Cleanse urine from exterior surface of container.

Reduces transmission of microorganisms.

l. Follow Steps 9-13 on p. 358.

NURSE ALERT

Indicate on the laboratory slip if client is menstruating.

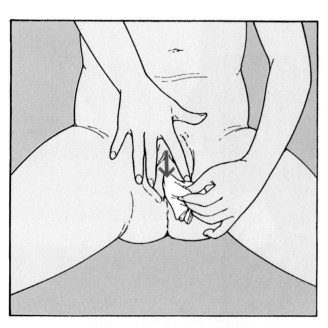

Step 3f(2) *Modified from Grimes D:* Infectious diseases, *Mosby's Clinical Nursing Series, St Louis, 1991, Mosby.*

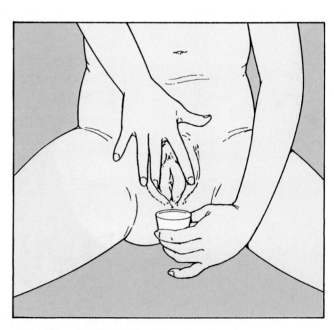

Step 3h *Modified from Grimes D:* Infectious diseases, *Mosby's Clinical Nursing Series, St Louis, 1991, Mosby.*

Pediatric Considerations

- It is not possible to obtain a midstream urine collection on a non–toilet-trained child; consequently, urine for culture should be obtained by use of a sterile plastic urine-collecting bag that adheres to the perineum (Figure 15-3). The same cleansing procedure should be followed as indicated in Step 3f of Implementation

Home Care and Long-Term Care Considerations

- Ideally, a specimen for culture should not be collected at home because the time delay before applying it to a culture medium in a laboratory setting would greatly enhance bacterial growth. If a specimen is collected, keep on ice until it reaches the laboratory.

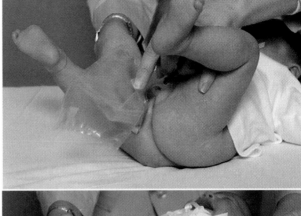

A

B

Figure 15-3   A and **B,** Application of pediatric urine collection bag. *From Wong DL:* Whaley and Wong's nursing care of infants and children, *ed 6, St Louis, 1999, Mosby.*

Steps	Rationale
4. Collect sterile urine specimen from an indwelling catheter.	
a. Emphasize that although a syringe with a needle is used to remove the urine from the catheter, client will not experience any discomfort.	Prevents anxiety when nurse manipulates catheter and aspirates urine with syringe and needle. Promotes client cooperation.
b. Explain why catheter will need to be clamped for 30 minutes before obtaining a urine specimen and why it is not obtained from drainage bag.	Prevents development of anxiety over clamping and promotes understanding of need for urine to collect within bladder.
c. Clamp drainage tubing with clamp or rubber band for up to 30 minutes (see illustration, p. 352) below the site chosen for withdrawal.	Permits collection of fresh, sterile urine in catheter tubing.
d. Return to room and inform client that the procedure to collect a specimen from a catheter will begin.	Allows client to anticipate manipulation of urinary catheter and cope more effectively with discomfort that may occur when catheter is moved.
e. Position client so catheter is easily accessible.	

Steps	Rationale

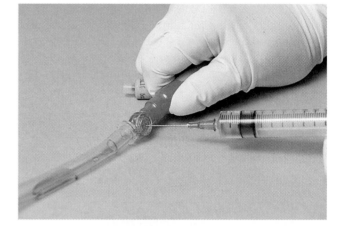

Step 4c   Step 4g

f. Cleanse entry port for needle with disinfectant swab.

Prevents entry of microorganisms into catheter.

g. Insert needle at 30-degree angle just above where catheter is attached to drainage tube or at 90-degree angle from a collection port in the drainage tube of an indwelling catheter (see illustration).

Ensures entrance of needle into catheter lumen and prevents accidental puncture of lumen leading to balloon that holds catheter in place in bladder. Aspiration of water from lumen can result in catheter falling out of bladder.

h. Draw urine into 3-ml syringe for culture, or draw urine into 20-ml syringe for routine urinalysis.

Allows collection of urine without contamination. Proper volume is needed to perform test.

i. Transfer urine from syringe into nonsterile urine container for routine urinalysis, or transfer urine from syringe into sterile urine container for culture.

Prevents contamination of urine during transfer procedure.

j. Do not recap needle. Dispose of uncapped contaminated needle in proper receptacle.

Reduces risk of needle stick injury.
Prevents contamination of specimen by air and loss by spillage.

k. Place lid tightly on container.

l. Unclamp catheter and allow urine to flow into drainage bag. Ensure flow.

Allows urine to drain by gravity and prevents stasis of urine in bladder.

m. Follow Steps 9-13 on p. 358.

5. Collect 24-hour timed urine specimen.

a. Discuss reason for specimen collection and how client can assist. Explain that urine must be free of feces and tissue.

Client who understands procedure is more likely to cooperate and may be able to obtain the specimen independently. Prevents accidental disposal and chemical changes resulting from feces and tissue.

b. Have client drink 2 to 4 glasses of water about 30 minutes before timed collection is to begin.

Enables client to void old urine (collected in bladder) at time test begins.

c. Provide privacy for and assist client in collecting specimen.

Clients prefer collecting specimens themselves. Timed specimens are not sterile.

Steps	Rationale

d. Discard this first specimen as test begins. Print time that test began on laboratory requisition.

Collection period begins with empty bladder.

e. When applicable, have client drink required amount of liquid or take ordered medication.

Required for specific types of tests to measure elimination of urine constituents.

f. Place signs indicating timed urine specimen collection on client's door and toileting area.

Prevents uninformed staff and relatives from accidentally discarding urine specimens.

g. Measure volume of each voiding if output is recorded.

Measures client's fluid balance.

h. Place all voided urine in labeled specimen bottle with appropriate additive.

Preserves urine specimen and prevents deterioration.

i. Unless instructed otherwise, keep specimen bottle in specimen refrigerator or in container of ice in bathroom.

Coldness prevents decomposition of urine.

j. Remove and discard gloves and wash hands after collection of each voiding.

Reduces transmission of microorganisms.

k. Encourage client to drink 2 glasses of water 1 hour before timed urine collection ends.

Facilitates client's ability to void at end of period.

l. Encourage client to empty bladder during last 15 minutes of urine collection period.

Ensures urine collected for precise amount of time.

m. Remove signs and remind client that specimen collection period is completed.

Allows client to resume usual voiding habits.

n. Follow Steps 9-13 on p. 358.

NURSE ALERT

If urine is accidentally discarded or contaminated or client is incontinent, restart timed period.

6. **Collect stool specimen.**

a. Discuss reason stool specimen is needed, how client/family member can assist, and how to obtain specimen free of urine and tissue.

Promotes cooperation.

b. Assist client as needed into bathroom or onto commode or bedpan.

Client's physical mobility and level of fatigue influence amount of assistance needed.

c. Instruct client to void into toilet before defecating (discard urine before collecting specimen in bedpan).

Feces should not be mixed with urine or toilet tissue. Urine inhibits fecal bacterial growth. Toilet tissue contains bismuth, which interferes with test results. Feces should not be mixed with urine or water.

d. Provide client with clean, dry bedpan and specimen hat in which to defecate.

e. If needed, assist client in washing after toileting and leave in safe, comfortable position after defecation.

Promotes comfort and sense of well-being.

f. Take covered bedpan or container with stool to bathroom or utility room.

Covering bedpan and removing it from client's room reduces odor and client's embarrassment.

g. Obtain specimen.

(1) *For culture.* Remove swab from sterile test tube, gather bean-sized piece of stool, and return swab to tube. If stool is liquid, soak cotton swab in it and return to tube.

Stool is touched only by sterile swab to prevent introduction of bacteria.

(2) *For other tests.* Obtain specimen by using tongue blades to transfer portion of stool to container (2.5 cm [1 inch] of formed stool or 15 ml of liquid stool).

Use of tongue blades prevents transfer of bacteria to hands or other objects.

Steps	Rationale
(3) *For timed stool specimen.* All of each stool is placed in waxed cardboard containers for specific time ordered and kept in specimen refrigerator.	Tests for dietary products and digestive enzymes such as fat content or bile require analysis of all feces over time.
h. For timed tests, place signs that read "Save all stool (with appropriate dates)" over client's bed, on bathroom door, and above toilet.	Helps prevent accidental disposal of stool.
i. Immediately place lid on container tightly.	Prevents spread of microorganisms by air or contact with other articles.
j. Follow Steps 9-13 on p. 358.	
7. Collect throat, nasal, nasopharyngeal, and sputum cultures.	
a. Explain that client may have tickling sensation or gag during swabbing of throat, urge to sneeze during nasal swabbing, and tickling or painful sensation during swabbing of wound. State that procedure takes only a few seconds.	Decreases anxiety and promotes cooperation. Clients who have been made aware of sensations to expect are able to cooperate with uncomfortable experiences.
b. Ask client to sit erect in bed or chair facing you for nose or throat culture. Acutely ill client may lie back against bed with head of bed raised to 45-degree angle.	Provides easy access to nasal or oral structures.
c. Have swab in tube ready for use. You may want to loosen top so swab can easily be removed.	Nurse should be able to grasp swab easily without danger of contaminating it. Most commercially prepared tubes have a top that fits securely over end of swab, which allows nurse to touch outer top without contaminating swab stick.
d. Collect throat culture.	
(1) Instruct client to tilt head backward. For clients in bed, place pillow behind shoulders.	Facilitates visualization of pharynx.
(2) Ask client to open mouth and say "ah."	Permits exposure of pharynx, relaxes throat muscles, and minimizes gag reflex.
(3) If pharynx is not visualized, depress tongue with tongue blade and note inflamed areas of pharynx or tonsils. Depress anterior third of tongue only. (Illuminate with penlight as needed.)	Area to be swabbed should be visualized. Placement of tongue blade along back of tongue more likely initiates gag reflex.
(4) Insert swab without touching lips, teeth, tongue, or cheeks (see illustration).	Touching lips or oral mucosal structures can contaminate swab with resident bacteria.
(5) Gently but quickly swab tonsillar area side to side, making contact with inflamed or purulent sites.	These areas contain the most microorganisms.
(6) Carefully withdraw swab without striking oral structures. Immediately place swab in culture tube, and crush ampule at bottom of tube. Push tip of swab into liquid medium.	Retains microorganisms within culture tube. Mixing swab tip with culture medium ensures life of bacteria for testing.
(7) Follow Steps on p. 358.	
e. **Collect nasal culture**	
(1) Encourage client to blow nose, and check nostrils for patency with penlight.	Clears nasal passage of mucus that contains resident bacteria.

Steps	Rationale
(2) Ask client to occlude each nostril alternately and exhale.	Determines nostril with greater patency, from which specimen will be collected.
(3) Ask client to tilt head back. Clients in bed should have pillow behind shoulders.	Facilitates visualization of nasal septum and sinuses.
(4) Gently insert nasal speculum in one nostril (optional). Carefully pass swab through center of speculum (if used) into nostril until it reaches that portion of mucosa that is inflamed or containing exudate.	Allows retraction of mucosa for easier swab insertion. Swab should remain sterile until it reaches area to be cultured.
(5) Rotate swab quickly.	Rotating swab covers all surfaces with exudate.
(6) Remove swab without touching sides of speculum.	Prevents contamination of swab by resident bacteria.
(7) Carefully remove nasal speculum (if used) and place in basin. Offer client facial tissue.	
(8) Insert swab into culture tube. Crush ampule at bottom of tube, and push tip of swab into liquid medium.	Retains microorganisms within culture tube. Mixing swab tip with culture medium ensures life of bacteria for testing.
(9) Follow Steps 9-13 on p. 358.	

f. **Collect nasopharyngeal cultures** Follow steps for nasal culture, *except* use a special swab on a flexible wire that can be flexed downward to reach the nasopharynx via the nose.

g. *Sputum culture collected by expectoration:*

Steps	Rationale
(1) Position client on side of bed or in high semi-Fowler's position.	
(2) Provide opportunity to cleanse or rinse mouth with water.	Reduces oral contamination that can alter results.
(3) Provide sputum cup and instruct client not to touch inside.	
(4) After client takes several deep breaths, tell client to inhale deeply and cough forcefully, expectorating sputum directly into specimen container (see illustration).	Full inhalation provides enough force to move sputum out of deeper airways.
(5) Repeat until 5 to 10 ml (1 to 2 tsp) of sputum (not saliva) has been collected.	

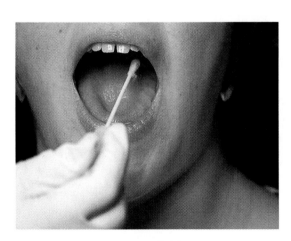

Step 7d(4)

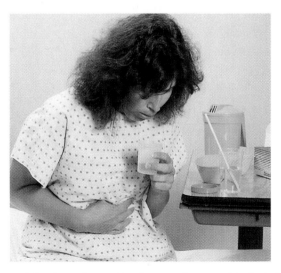

Step 7g(4)   *From Grimes D: Infectious diseases, Mosby's Clinical Nursing Series, St Louis, 1991, Mosby.*

Steps	Rationale

(6) Continue by following Steps 9-13 on p. 358.

(7) Remove and discard gloves.

h. *Sputum culture collected by suctioning:*

(1) 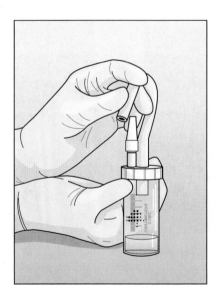 Prepare suction machine or device and determine if it functions properly.

Adequate amount of suction is necessary to aspirate sputum.

(2) Connect suction tube to adapter on sputum trap.

Establishes suction that passes through sputum trap to aspirate specimen.

(3) Apply sterile gloves (required only for dominant hand).

Tracheobronchial tree is sterile body cavity. Allows nurse to manipulate suction catheter without contamination.

(4) With gloved hand, connect sterile suction catheter to rubber tubing on sputum trap.

Aspirated sputum will go directly to trap instead of to suction tubing.

(5) Other hand should have glove on for application of suction. Thumb should be on trap to provide suction, and trap should be covered.

(6) Gently insert lubricated tip of suction catheter through nasopharynx, endotracheal tube, and tracheostomy without applying suction (see Chapter 30).

Minimizes trauma to airway as catheter is inserted. Lubrication allows for easier insertion.

(7) Advance catheter into trachea.

Entrance of catheter into larynx and trachea triggers cough reflex.

(8) As client coughs, apply suction for 5 to 10 seconds, collecting 2 to 10 ml of sputum.

Ensures collection of sputum from deep within tracheobronchial tree. Suctioning longer than 15 seconds can cause hypoxia.

(9) Remove catheter without applying suction, then turn off suction.

Suction can damage mucosa if applied during withdrawal.

(10) Detach catheter from specimen trap, and dispose of catheter into appropriate receptacle.

Decreases risk of spreading microorganisms.

(11) Secure top on specimen container tightly. For sputum trap, detach suction tubing and connect rubber tubing on sputum trap to plastic adapter (see illustration).

Contains microorganisms within container, preventing exposure to personnel handling specimen.

Step 7h(11)

Steps	Rationale
(12) If any sputum is present on outside of container, wash it off with disinfectant.	Prevents spread of infection to persons handling specimen.
(13) Offer client tissues after expectorating. Dispose of tissues in emesis basin or trash container.	
(14) Remove and dispose of glove(s).	
(15) Offer client mouth care, if desired.	
(16) Follow Steps 9-13 on p. 358.	

8. Wound drainage culture

a. Remove old dressing. Observe drainage. Fold soiled sides of dressing together and then dispose of in bag.

b. Cleanse area around wound edges with antiseptic swab. Remove old exudate.	Removes skin flora, preventing possible contamination of specimen.
c. Discard swab and dispose of soiled gloves in bag.	Reduces spread of infection.
d. Open package containing sterile culture tube and dressing supplies.	Provides sterile field from which nurse can pick up and handle sterile supplies.
e. Apply sterile gloves.	Allows nurse to maintain sterility of items while collecting specimen.

f. Obtain culture.

(1) Aerobic culture

Take swab from culture tube, insert tip into wound near area of drainage, and rotate swab gently. Remove swab and return to culture tube (see illustration). Crush ampule of medium and push swab into fluid (see illustration).	Swab should be coated with fresh secretions (not drainage) from within wound. Medium keeps bacteria alive until analysis is complete.

NURSE ALERT

Placing a gauze pad around ampule of medium before crushing it protects nurse's fingers from trauma.

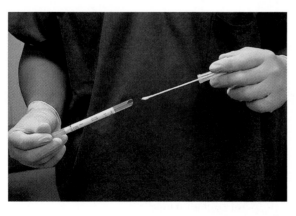
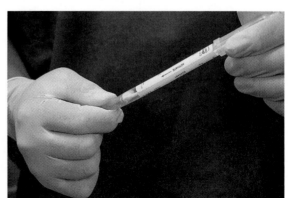

A   B

Step 8f(1)

Steps	Rationale

(2) Anaerobic culture

Take swab from special anaerobic culture tube, swab deeply into body cavity, and rotate gently. Remove swab and return to culture tube.

Specimen is taken from deep cavity where oxygen is not present. Carbon dioxide or nitrogen gas keeps organisms alive until analysis is complete.

or

Insert tip of syringe (without needle) into wound and aspirate 5 to 10 ml of exudate. Attach 21-gauge needle, expel all air, and inject drainage into special culture tube. Clean wound as ordered, and apply new sterile dressing. Place top on culture tube securely.

Air injected into tube would cause organisms to die.

Prevents contamination from microorganisms.

9. Securely attach properly completed identification label and laboratory requisition to side of specimen container (not lid).

Incorrect identification of specimen could result in diagnostic or therapeutic errors.

10. Enclose in a plastic bag (see illustration).

11. Send specimen immediately to laboratory, or refrigerate.

Specimen left at room temperature may increase bacterial content.

12. Remove and discard gloves.

13. See Completion Protocol (inside front cover).

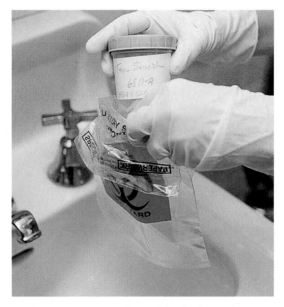

Step 10

• • •

EVALUATION

1. Ask client to identify steps in specimen collection procedure.
2. Ask client to state purposes of specimen collection.
3. Inspect specimen for contamination with toilet tissue or stool in urine/urine in stool.
4. Intermittently during collection period, observe/ask if all urine has been saved.
5. Observe client's respiratory status throughout procedure, especially during suctioning. Note anxiety or discomfort in client.
6. Inspect color and amount of wound drainage.

Unexpected Outcomes and Related Interventions

1. Client is unable to produce a urine or stool specimen.
   a. Offer fluids (if permitted) to enhance ability to void.
   b. Administer a suppository or enema as ordered to promote passage of stool.
2. Client's urine specimen is contaminated with stool and tissue.
   a. Reinforce importance of obtaining specimen free of contaminants.

b. Assist client with specimen collection: place specimen hat as close to front of commode as possible.

3. Client experiences minor nasal bleeding.
   a. Apply mild pressure over bridge of nose.
   b. Apply ice pack over bridge of nose.

4. Client becomes hypoxic; increased respiratory rate and effort are necessary; client feels short of breath.
   a. Discontinue procedure until stable; provide oxygen therapy as needed.
   b. Monitor vital signs and pulse oximetry.

5. Specimen contains saliva.
   a. Reattempt after several deep breaths and forceful coughs.

6. Wound cultures reveal heavy bacterial growth.
   a. Notify physician.
   b. Administer medications as ordered.

7. Wound culture is contaminated from superficial skin cells.
   a. Repeat specimen collection.

Recording and Reporting

- Record method used to obtain specimen, date and time collected, type of test ordered, and laboratory receiving specimen.
- Describe characteristics of specimen.
- Describe client's tolerance to procedure of specimen collection.
- When available, report abnormal findings.

Sample Documentation

1215 Voided 150 ml of dark amber urine at 1145. Urine discarded. 24-hour urine for protein started at 1200 noon. Client instructed to save all urine and place in container in bathroom. Verbalized understanding.

Geriatric Considerations

- Older adults may need assistance in positioning to obtain specimen. In confused clients, auxiliary personnel may be necessary to hold client's hands while sample is being obtained.
- The older client may need a reminder placed in the bathroom on the mirror for the ambulatory client. The verbal reminders will further enhance continuing the sample collection.

Pediatric Considerations

- If procedure is to be performed on a child and is anticipated to be painful, some agencies prefer performing procedure in area other than child's room, thus maintaining feeling that child's room is safe place.
- Ask parents if they wish to help hold child or if they prefer nurse to do so.
- Immobilization of child's head and arms is important when obtaining nose or throat culture and should be done in firm, gentle, kind manner. Ask another nurse to assist, if necessary. Ask parents to act as coach with their child.
- Showing tongue blade and penlight to child and demonstrating how to say "ah" helps to decrease anxiety.
- School-age child will be more cooperative if given opportunity to ask questions about procedure and results.
- Throat cultures should not be attempted if acute epiglottitis is suspected, because trauma from swab might cause increase in edema and resulting occlusion of airway (Wong, 1995).

Home Care and Long-Term Care Considerations

- If client is to produce sputum specimen at home, instruct client and/or family member regarding proper technique and importance of having specimen sent to laboratory in timely manner.
- Discuss ways to avoid contaminating specimen (e.g., handwashing, using clean equipment).

Skill 15.2

COLLECTING BLOOD SPECIMENS (VENIPUNCTURE; VACUUM TUBE; BLOOD CULTURES)

Blood tests, one of the most commonly used diagnostic aids in the care and evaluation of clients, can yield valuable information about nutritional, hematological, metabolic, immune, and biochemical status. Tests allow physicians and other healthcare providers to screen clients carefully for early signs of physical alterations, plot the course of existing disease, and monitor responses to therapies.

The nurse is often responsible for collecting blood specimens; however, many institutions have specially trained technicians whose sole responsibility is to draw blood. Nurses must be familiar with their institution's policies and procedures and their state's Nurse Practice Act regarding guidelines for drawing blood samples.

Venipuncture, the most common method, involves inserting a hollow-bore needle into the lumen of a large vein to obtain a specimen. The nurse may use a needle and syringe or a special vacuum tube that allows the drawing of multiple blood samples.

Blood cultures aid in detection of bacteria in the blood. Because bacteremia may be accompanied by fever and chills, blood cultures should be drawn at this time. It is important that at least two culture specimens be drawn from two different sites. If only one culture produces bacteria, the assumption is that the bacteria were contaminants rather than the infecting agent. Bacteremia exists when both cultures grow the infecting agent.

Because culture specimens obtained through an IV catheter are frequently contaminated, tests using them should not be performed unless catheter sepsis is suspected. Cultures should be drawn before antibiotic therapy is started, because the antibiotic may interrupt the organism's growth in the laboratory. If the client is receiving antibiotics, the laboratory needs to be notified and told what specific antibiotics the client is receiving. (Pagana and Pagana, 1997).

Because veins are major sources of blood for laboratory testing and routes for IV fluid or blood replacement, maintaining their integrity is essential. The nurse should be skilled in venipuncture to avoid unnecessary injury to veins.

Regardless of the method used to obtain a blood specimen, the nurse must anticipate the client's anxiety. The procedures can be painful, and often just the appearance of a needle is frightening, especially to children. The nurse's calm approach and skilled technique help to limit anxiety.

Equipment

Blood
- Alcohol or antiseptic swab (check agency policy for specific antiseptic solution)
- Disposable gloves
- Small pillow or folded towel
- Sterile gauze pads (2 × 2 inch)
- Rubber tourniquet
- Band-Aid or adhesive tape
- Appropriate blood tubes
- Completed identification labels according to agency policy
- Completed laboratory requisition (date, time, type of test)
- Plastic bag for delivery of specimen to laboratory (or container as specified by agency)

Syringe Method
- Sterile needles (20 to 21 gauge for adults, 23 to 25 gauge for children, 23 to 25 gauge butterfly for older adults)
- Sterile syringe of appropriate size

Vacuum Tube Method
- Vacuum tube with needle holder
- Sterile double-ended needles (20 to 21 gauge for adults, 23 to 25 gauge for children)

Blood Cultures
- Povidone-iodine (Betadine) (check agency policy for specific antiseptic solution)
- 70% alcohol (check agency policy)
- Two 20-ml syringes
- Sterile needles (20 to 21 gauge for adults, 23 to 25 gauge for children, 23 to 25 gauge butterfly for older adults)
- Anaerobic and aerobic culture bottles

ASSESSMENT

1. Assess if special conditions need to be met before specimen collection (e.g., client NPO, specific time for collection after medication or meal). **Rationale: Some tests require meeting specific conditions to obtain accurate measurement of blood elements (e.g., fasting blood sugar, drug peak and trough, timed endocrine hormone levels).**

2. Assess client for possible risks of venipuncture, which include anticoagulant therapy, low platelet count, bleeding disorder, presence of arteriovenous shunt or fistula, after breast or axillary surgery performed on that side. **Rationale: History may include abnormal**

clotting abilities caused by low platelet count, hemophilia, medications that increase risk for bleeding and hematoma formation, or compromised circulation in extremity that already has impaired blood flow.

3. Determine client's ability to cooperate with procedure. **Rationale: Some clients may need assistance of another member of the health care team. Procedure can appear threatening to client.**

4. Review physicians's orders for type of tests. **Rationale: Multiple samples may be needed; physician's order is required.**

PLANNING

Expected outcomes focus on the collection of an uncontaminated blood specimen by the nurse or trained technician.

Expected Outcomes

1. Client will discuss purpose and benefits of obtaining blood specimens.
2. Client's venipuncture site shows no evidence of continued bleeding or hematoma.
3. Client denies anxiety or discomfort.
4. Test results are within normal limits (see Appendix D).

DELEGATION CONSIDERATIONS

The phlebotomy trained staff are the personnel used to obtain venipuncture samples. They may be AP or licensed staff. Usually they are IV certified by the agency that employs them. However, check agency policy to determine who may perform blood drawing.

IMPLEMENTATION

Steps	Rationale
1. See Standard Protocol (inside front cover).	**COMMUNICATION TIP** *Explain procedure to client: describe purpose of tests; explain how sensation of tourniquet, alcohol swab, and needle stick will feel.*
2. Assist client to supine or semi-Fowler's position with arms extended to form straight line from shoulders to wrists. Place small pillow or towel under upper arm.	Helps to stabilize extremity because arms are most common sites of venipuncture. Supported position in bed reduces chance of injury to client if fainting occurs.
3. ⬛ Apply tourniquet 5 to 10 cm (3 to 4 inches) above venipuncture site selected (antecubital fossa site is most often used). Encircle extremity and pull one end of tourniquet tightly over other, looping one end under other. Apply tourniquet so it can be removed by pulling end with single motion.	Tourniquet blocks venous return to heart from extremity, causing veins to dilate for easier visibility.
4. Palpate distal pulse (e.g. radial) below tourniquet. If pulse is not palpable, reapply tourniquet more loosely.	If tourniquet is too tight, pressure will impede arterial blood flow.

NURSE ALERT

Some specimens have special collection requirements before or after collection:

• *Cryoglobulins need prewarmed test tubes.*
• *Ammonia levels require tube to be placed in ice for delivery to laboratory.*

• *Do not use tourniquet for lactic acid levels.*
• *Avoid exposure of test tube to light when measuring vitamin levels.*

Steps	Rationale

5. Keep tourniquet on client no longer than 1 to 2 minutes. If tourniquet is left on arm is too long, remove and assess other extremity, or wait 60 seconds before reapplying.

Prolonged time may alter test results and cause pain and venous stasis (e.g., falsely elevated serum potassium level). Minimizes effects of hemoconcentration.

6. Ask client to open and close fist several times, finally leaving fist clenched.

Facilitates distention of veins by forcing blood up from distal veins.

7. Quickly inspect extremity for best venipuncture site, looking for straight, prominent vein without swelling or hematoma.

Straight and intact veins are easiest to puncture.

8. Palpate selected vein with fingers. Note if vein is firm and rebounds when palpated or if vein feels rigid and cordlike and rolls when palpated (see illustration).

Patent, healthy vein is elastic and rebounds on palpation. Thrombosed vein is rigid, rolls easily, is difficult to puncture.

NURSE ALERT

Avoid vigorous opening and closing of fist, which may cause erroneous laboratory results of hemoconcentration.

NURSE ALERT

Inspect needle for defects, such as burrs, which can cause increased discomfort and damage to the client's vein.

9. Select venipuncture site.

Prevents discomfort to client and inaccurate test results.

10. Obtain blood sample:
    a. Syringe Method
    (1) Have syringe with appropriate needle securely attached.

Needle should not dislodge from syringe during venipuncture.

    (2) Cleanse venipuncture site with alcohol swab (70% isopropyl alcohol is recommended), moving in circular motion from site for approximately 5 cm (2 inches) (see illustration). Allow to dry.

Antimicrobial agent cleans skin surface of resident bacteria so organisms do not enter puncture site. Allowing alcohol to dry reduces "sting" of venipuncture. Alcohol left on skin can cause hemolysis of sample.

    (3) Remove needle cover and inform client that "stick" lasting only a few seconds will be felt.

Client has better control over anxiety when prepared for what to expect.

    (4) Place thumb or forefinger of nondominant hand 2.5 cm (1 inch) below site, and pull skin taut.

Stabilizes vein and prevents rolling during needle insertion.

    (5) Hold syringe and needle at 15- to 30-degree angle from client's arm with bevel up.

Reduces chance of penetrating both sides of vein during insertion. Keeping bevel up reduces vein trauma.

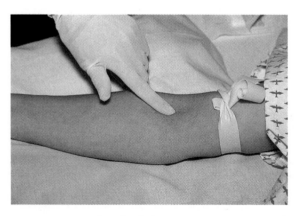

Step 8 Palpate vein.

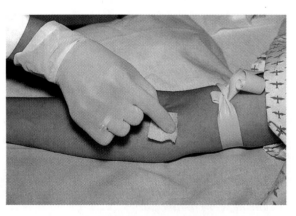

Step 10a(2) Cleanse site.

Steps	**Rationale**

(6) Slowly insert needle into vein (see illustration).

Prevents puncture on opposite side.

(7) Hold syringe securely and pull back gently on plunger (see illustration).

Syringe held securely prevents needle from advancing. Pulling on plunger creates vacuum needed to draw blood into syringe.

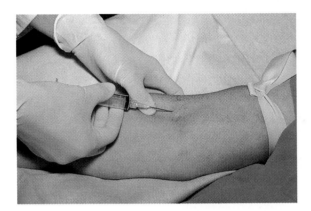

Step 10a(6)   Insert needle.

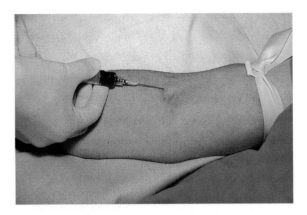

Step 10a(7)   Pull back on plunger.

(8) Look for blood return.
(9) Obtain desired amount of blood, keeping needle stabilized.

If blood flow fails to appear, needle is not in vein.
Test results are more accurate when required amount of blood is obtained. Some tests cannot be performed without minimal blood requirement. Movement of needle increases discomfort.

(10) After specimen is obtained, release tourniquet.

Reduces bleeding at site when needle is withdrawn.

(11) Apply 2- × 2-inch gauze pad or alcohol swab over puncture site without applying pressure, and quickly but carefully withdraw needle from vein and apply pressure following removal of needle (see illustrations).

Pressure over needle can cause discomfort. Careful removal of needle minimizes discomfort and vein trauma.

NURSE ALERT

When filling tubes with an anticoagulant additive, let tube fill until the vacuum is exhausted. Ratio of blood to additive is important.

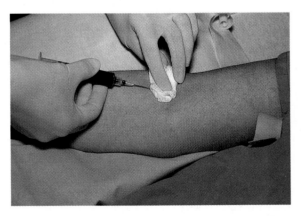

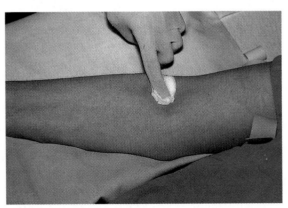

Step 10a(11)

Steps	Rationale
(12) Discard needle without recapping in proper receptacle.	Reduces risk of needle-stick injury.
(13) Remove and discard gloves.	

b. *Vacuum Tube Method*

Steps	Rationale
(1) 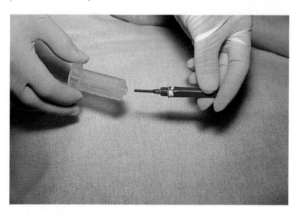 Attach double-ended needle to vacuum tube (see illustration).	Long end of needle is used to puncture vein. Short end fits into blood tubes.

Step 10b(1)

Steps	Rationale
(2) Have proper blood specimen tube resting inside vacuum tube, but do not puncture rubber stopper.	Causes loss of tube's vacuum.
(3) Cleanse venipuncture site with alcohol swab, moving in circular motion out from site for approximately 5 cm (2 inches).	Cleans skin surface of resident bacteria so that organisms do not enter puncture site.
(4) Remove needle cover and inform client that "stick" lasting only a few seconds will be felt.	Client has better control over anxiety when prepared for what to expect.
(5) Place thumb or forefinger of nondominant hand 2.5 cm (1 inch) above or below site and pull skin taut. Stretch skin down until vein is stabilized.	Helps to stabilize vein and prevent rolling during needle insertion.
(6) Hold vacuum tube at 15- to 30-degree angle from arm with bevel up.	Reduces chance of penetrating both sides of vein during insertion. Keeping bevel up causes less trauma to vein.
(7) Slowly insert needle into vein (see illustration).	Prevents puncture on opposite side.
(8) Grasp vacuum tube securely and advance specimen tube into needle of holder (do not advance needle in vein).	Pushing needle through stopper breaks vacuum and causes flow of blood into tube. If needle in vein advances, vein may become punctured on other side.
(9) Note flow of blood into tube (should be fairly rapid) (see illustration).	Failure of blood to appear indicates that vacuum in tube is lost or needle is not in vein.
(10) After specimen tube is filled, grasp vacuum tube firmly and remove tube (see illustration). Insert additional specimen tubes as needed.	Prevents needle from advancing or dislodging. Tube should fill completely because additives in certain tubes are measured in proportion to filled tube. Tubes with additives should be inverted as soon as possible.
(11) After last tube is filled, release tourniquet (see illustration).	Reduces bleeding at site when needle is withdrawn.
(12) Apply 2- × 2-inch gauze pad over puncture site without applying pressure, and quickly but carefully withdraw needle from vein (see illustration).	Pressure over needle can cause discomfort. Careful removal of needle minimizes discomfort and vein trauma.
(13) Remove and discard gloves.	

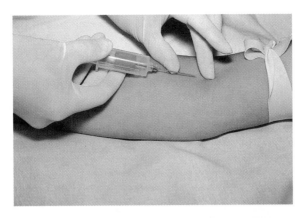

Step 10b(6)   Hold vacuum tube at 15°-30° angle.

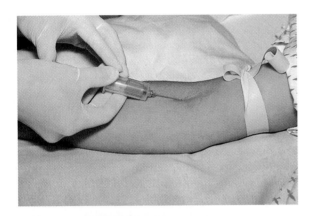

Step 10b(9)   Note flow of blood.

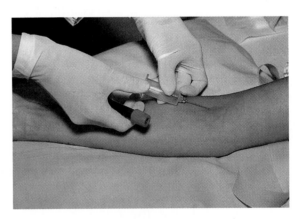

Step 10b(10)   Remove filled tube.

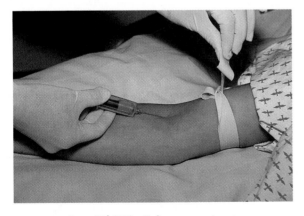

Step 10b(11)   Release tourniquet.

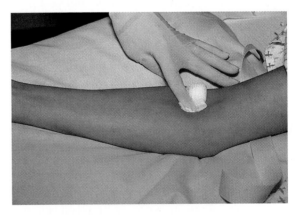

Step 10b(12)   Apply pressure.

Steps	Rationale

c. Blood Cultures

(1) Carefully prepare proposed site with povidone-iodine (Betadine). Allow skin to dry. Antimicrobial agent cleans skin surface so organisms do not enter puncture site or contaminate the culture.

(2) Clean tops of the vacuum tubes or culture bottles. Check agency policy regarding cleaning with 70% alcohol after cleaning with antiseptic solution and air drying.

Reduces transmission of organisms into bottle.

(3) Collect 10 to 15 ml of venous blood by venipuncture in a 20-ml syringe from each site.

(4) Discard needle on syringe; replace with second sterile needle before injecting blood sample into culture bottle.

(5) Inoculate anaerobic bottle first if both anaerobic and aerobic cultures are needed (Pagana and Pagana, 1997).

Anaerobic organisms may take longer to grow.

(6) Immediately apply pressure over venipuncture site with gauze or antiseptic pad for 2 to 3 minutes or until bleeding stops (see Step 10a[11]). Apply pressure over site, and tape gauze dressing securely.

Direct pressure minimizes bleeding and prevents hematoma formation. Pressure dressing controls bleeding.

11. For blood obtained by syringe, transfer specimen to tubes.

a. Using one-handed technique, insert needle through stopper of blood tube and allow vacuum to fill tube. Do not force blood into tube.

Blood should not be forced into tube; this prevents hemolysis of red blood cells or can invalidate test with tubes containing anticoagulants or additives. The Occupational Safety and Health Administration OSHA, recommends one-handed technique to avoid needle-stick injury.

b. Alternative method is to remove needle from syringe and stopper to each test tube. Gently inject required amount of blood into each tube. Reapply stopper.

Blood injected too quickly may cause frothing or hemolysis of red blood cells. Stopper maintains sterility of specimen.

12. For blood tubes containing additives, gently rotate back and forth 8 to 10 times. For blood obtained for blood cultures, gently mix each bottle after inoculation.

Additives should be mixed with blood to prevent clotting. Shaking can cause hemolysis of red blood cells, producing inaccurate test results.

13. Inspect puncture site for bleeding and apply adhesive tape with gauze.

Keeps puncture site clean and controls any final oozing.

14. Check tubes for any sign of external contamination with blood. Decontaminate with 70% alcohol if necessary. Remove and discard gloves.

Prevents cross-contamination. Reduces risk of exposure to pathogens present in blood.

15. Securely attach properly completed identification label to each tube and affix proper requisition.

Incorrect identification of specimen could result in diagnostic or therapeutic errors.

16. Additional information needed for blood culture requisitions includes time of collection and any medications that may affect blood culture results.

Steps	**Rationale**

17. Dispose of needles, syringe, vacutainer holder, and soiled equipment in proper container. Do not cap needles.

Prevents cross-contamination through needle sticks and contact with blood.

18. Place specimens in bag to be sent to laboratory.
19. Remove disposable gloves after specimen is obtained and any spillage is cleaned.

Reduces risk of exposure to HIV, hepatitis, and other blood-borne pathogens.

20. Wash hands after procedure.

Reduces transfer of microorganisms.

21. Send specimens immediately to laboratory.

Fresh specimen ensures accurate results.

22. See Completion Protocol (inside front cover).

• • •

EVALUATION
1. Ask client to explain purposes of tests.
2. Reinspect venipuncture site.
3. Determine if client remains anxious or fearful.
4. Check laboratory report for test results.

Unexpected Outcomes and Related Interventions
1. Client develops hematoma at venipuncture site.
   a. Apply pressure to site and document.
   b. Continue to observe site.
2. Client continues to have bleeding at site.
   a. Apply pressure and pressure dressing.
   b. Continue to observe site.
3. Laboratory tests reveal abnormal blood constituents.
   a. Report to physician.
   b. Institute medical regimen as ordered.

Recording and Reporting
• Record method used to obtain blood specimen, date and time collected, type of test ordered, and laboratory receiving specimen.
• Describe venipuncture site after specimen collection.
• Describe client's tolerance to procedure of specimen collection.
• Report any STAT results to physician or charge nurse.
• Report any abnormal results to physician or charge nurse.

Sample Documentation
1000 Left antecubital site used for venipuncture. Serum chemistry and complete blood count specimens obtained and sent to hematology laboratory. Client had no complaints. No hematoma present at venipuncture site. Bandage in place.

Geriatric Considerations

Older adults have fragile veins that are easily traumatized during venipuncture. Sometimes application of warm compresses may help in obtaining samples. Using a small-bore catheter also may be beneficial.

Pediatric Considerations

• Ask staff member to restrain child so venipuncture site is immobilized. Prevents sudden movement, which can cause serious injury to vessel wall or soft tissues.
• When performing venipuncture on children, the nurse needs to explore a variety of sources for vein access: scalp, antecubital fossa, saphenous, hand veins.
• Application of local anesthetic cream 30 minutes before procedure may be ordered to reduce pain in infants and young children.

Home Care and Long-Term Care Considerations

• In the home care setting a blood pressure cuff, rather than a tourniquet, can be used for venipuncture.
• Instruct client to notify nurse or physician if persistent or recurrent bleeding or expanding hematoma occurs at venipuncture site.

Skill 15.3

UNIT SPECIMEN TESTING (GLUCOSE, CHEMSTRIP/MULTISTIX, HEMOCCULT, GASTROCCULT)

This skill includes tests done on the nursing unit (Table 15-2). Assessing chemical properties of urine can be done by immersing a specially prepared strip of paper (Chemstrip) into clean urine specimen. When the screening test for the presence of substances in the urine is positive, other tests are used to determine the diagnosis or measure the effectiveness of treatment. The capillary blood glucose test is used to measure blood glucose for monitoring the control of diabetes mellitus. Test results are used to direct diet, amount and type of medication, and exercise prescription. The Hemoccult test measures microscopic amounts of blood in the stool. It is a useful diagnostic tool for conditions such as colon cancer, upper gastrointestinal (GI) ulcers, and localized gastric or intestinal irritation.

Measuring gastric occult blood via the Gastroccult test reveals bleeding in the esophagus, stomach, or duodenum and is similar to measuring stool for occult blood. The Gastroccult test also measures pH level of GI secretions.

The nurse can easily perform these tests at the bedside with minimal discomfort to the client. Clients should receive instructions about the purpose of the tests and whether any discomfort is to be anticipated, such as during skin puncture for a capillary blood sample for glucose measurement and during insertion of a nasogastric (NG) tube if needed for the Gastroccult test.

Equipment

Urine screening
Disposable gloves
Reagent test strip
Test strip color chart
Specimen hat, bedpan, urinal, or potty chair
Watch with second hand or digital counter
Clean disposable gloves (if person other than client tests urine)
Blood glucose monitoring (Figure 15-4)
Disposable gloves
Antiseptic swab
Cotton ball
Sterile blood-letting device
Paper towel
Glucose testing meter (Table 15-3)
Sharps box
Blood glucose reagent strips (brand determined by meter used)
Hemoccult
Disposable gloves
Paper towel
Wooden applicator
Hemoccult test (Figure 15-5)
    Cardboard Hemoccult slide
    Hemoccult developing solution
Gastroccult
Disposable gloves
Facial tissues
Emesis basin
Wooden applicator or 1-ml syringe
Gastroccult test (Figure 15-6, p. 370)
    Cardboard Gastroccult slide
    Gastroccult developing solution
60-ml bulb or catheter-tip syringe
NG tube and supplies for insertion (if indicated)

Table 15-2

Tests Done by Nurses on the Unit

Test	Assessment
Blood glucose monitoring (capillary glucose)	Hyperglycemia (high blood glucose): thirst, polyuria, polyphagia, weakness, fatigue, headache, blurred vision, nausea, vomiting, abdominal cramps Hypoglycemia (low blood glucose): sweating, tachycardia, palpitations, nervousness, tremors, weakness, headache, mental confusion, fatigue
Multistix (urine screening test for pH, protein, glucose, ketones, and/or blood)	Protein or blood: abnormal kidney function or urinary tract infection pH: concentration Glucose: inadequate glucose metabolism Ketones: abnormal metabolism of proteins associated with inadequate food intake or excessive vomiting
Hemoccult (stool) Gastroccult (gastric contents or drainage from NG tube)	Gastrointestinal alterations: abdominal cramping, pain, vomiting, diarrhea, appearance of blood or suspected presence of unseen (occult) blood in stool, vomitus, or gastric aspirate

ASSESSMENT

1. Assess client's understanding of need for the specimen. **Rationale: This provides nurse with a database on which to provide necessary teaching.**

2. Assess client for types of medications received and foods eaten. **Rationale: Drugs such as cortisone preparations, diuretics, and anesthetics increase** blood glucose levels. **Anticoagulants increase risk of bleeding in the GI tract, and long-term use of steroids and acetylsalicylic acid can irritate the gastric mucosa.**

3. Assess client for related signs and symptoms (see Table 15-2), which help reveal nature of the problem.

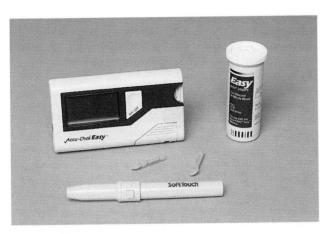

Figure 15-4 Blood glucose monitor test strips and blood-letting device.

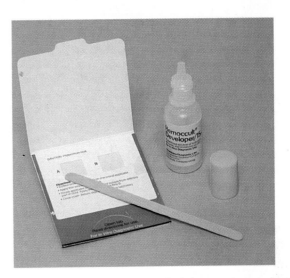

Figure 15-5 Cardboard Hemoccult slide, wooden applicator, and developing solution.

Table 15-3

Glucose Meters Currently Available

Meter	Glucose Range (mg/dL)	Test Strip Used	Test Time	Memory
Accu-Chek Advantage	10–600	Advantage	40 seconds	100 readings
Accu-Check Easy	20–500	Easy Test Strips	15–60 seconds	350 readings
Accu-Check Instant	20–500	Instant Glucose	12 seconds	9 readings
Accu-Check III	20–500	Chemstrip bG	2 minutes	20 readings
CheckMate Plus	25–500	CheckMate Plus	15–70 seconds	255 readings
Diascan-S	10–600	Diascan	90 seconds	10 readings
ExacTech	40–450	ExacTech	30 seconds	Last reading recall
ExacTech RSG	40–450	ExacTech RSG	30 seconds	–
Glucometer Elite	20–500	Glucometer Elite	30 seconds	Last reading recall
Glucometer Encore	10–600	Glucometer Encore	15–60 seconds	10 readings
MediSense 2 Card	20–600	MediSense 2 or Precision Q.I.D.	20 seconds	Extended memory
MediSense 2 Pen	20–600	MediSense 2 or Precision Q.I.D.	20 seconds	Extended memory
One Touch Basic	0–600	Genuine One Touch	45 seconds	Last reading recall
One Touch Profile	0–600	Genuine One Touch	45 seconds	250 readings
Precision Q.I.D.	20–600	Precision Q.I.D.	20 seconds	Extended memory
Prestige	25–600	Prestige	20–50 seconds	–
Select GT	30–600	Select GT	50 seconds	100 readings
Supreme II	30–600	Supreme	50 seconds	100 readings
SureStep	0–500	SureStep	15–30 seconds	10 readings
Ultra +	30–600	Ultra +	45 seconds	–

Data from American Diabetes Association: 1998 Buyer's Guide to Diabetes Products, *Diabetes Forecast* 50(10):68–71, 1997.

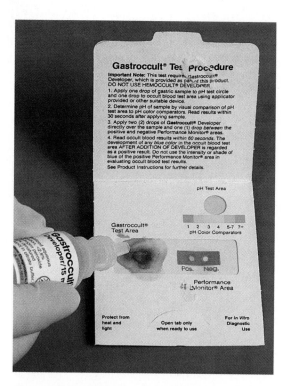

Figure 15-6 Apply developer to Gastroccult slide.

Expected Outcomes

1. Client explains purpose of the unit test ordered before specimen collection is attempted.
2. Client explains basic steps of the procedure for the unit test ordered before specimen collection is attempted.
3. Client's specimen is appropriate for the unit test analysis.
4. Client verbalizes lack of fear of specimen collection and unit test results after nurse reviews the procedure.
5. Client who requires daily or more frequent testing will be able to perform test independently.

DELEGATION CONSIDERATIONS

The screening of urine specimens for glucose, pH, protein, ketones, and blood and testing stool for occult blood may be performed by AP. For these specimen collections, determine that care provider understands the specific specimen collection procedure and reports the results of the test to the nurse. Inform AP to notify nurse immediately if blood is detected in stool and not to discard specimen, so the nurse may repeat the testing.

The skills of obtaining and testing blood glucose measurement and gastric secretion specimens require problem solving and knowledge application unique to a professional nurse. Delegation of these skills is inappropriate.

PLANNING

Expected outcomes focus on collecting an appropriate specimen, with client knowledgeable of the purpose of specimen examination, and decreasing client's anxiety when these types of specimens are collected. Institute dietary or medication restrictions as needed.

IMPLEMENTATION

Steps	Rationale
1. See Standard Protocol (inside front cover).	
2. Explain procedure to client and/or family member.	Promotes cooperation.
3. **Perform urine screening test for glucose, pH, protein, ketones, and blood.**	
a. Obtain double-voided specimen when testing urine for glucose.	
(1) Ask client to collect random urine specimen and discard.	Stagnant urine stored in bladder overnight or for long periods does not reveal amount of glucose excreted by kidney at time of testing.
(2) Have client drink at least 8 oz water or preferred liquid.	Facilitates ability to void again within short period.
(3) 30 to 45 minutes later, have client collect another random specimen.	Fresh specimen provides accurate test measurements. If client is catheterized, a single, fresh specimen from catheter is adequate.

Steps	Rationale

b. ▨ Use Multistix reagent test strip to assess for glucose, pH, protein, ketones, and/or blood simultaneously.

(1) Immerse end of chemically impregnated test strip into urine.

Exposes reagent to urine.

(2) Remove strip immediately from container and tap it gently against container's side.

Excess urine can dilute reagents.

(3) Hold strip in horizontal position.

(4) Time for number of seconds specified on container, and compare color of strip with color chart on container (see illustration).

Prevents possible mixing of chemical reagents.
Accurate interpretation of results depends on precise timing.

c. Remove and discard gloves.

d. Discuss test results with client.

Participation in care improves understanding and compliance.

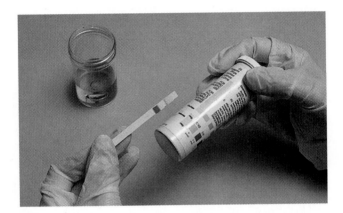

Step 3b(4)

4. **Perform blood glucose measurement (Accu-Chek used as example).**

a. Instruct client to wash hands with soap and warm water, if able.

Reduces presence of microorganisms. Promotes vasodilation at selected puncture site. Establishes practice for client when test is performed at home.

b. Position client comfortably in chair or semi-Fowler's position in bed.

Ensures easy accessibility to puncture site.

c. Remove reagent strip from container and tightly seal cap.

Protects strips from accidental discoloration.

d. Turn on glucose meter.

Activates meter.

e. Insert strip into glucose meter (see manufacturer's directions) and make necessary adjustments.

Some machines must be calibrated; others require zeroing of timer. Each meter is adjusted differently.

f. Remove unused reagent strip from meter and place on paper towel or clean, dry surface with test pad facing up.

Moisture on strip can change its color, altering reading of final test results.

g. ▨ Choose a vascular area as a puncture site.

Side of finger is less sensitive to pain.

h. Hold finger to be punctured in dependent position while gently massaging finger toward puncture site.

Increases blood flow to area before puncture.

i. Clean site with antiseptic swab and *allow to dry completely.*

Alcohol can alter accuracy of test.

j. Remove cover of blood-letting device.

Cover keeps tip of needle sterile.

Steps	**Rationale**
k. Place blood-letting device firmly against finger and push release button, causing needle to pierce skin (see illustration).	Pierces skin to appropriate depth, ensuring adequate blood flow.
l. Wipe away first droplet of blood with cotton ball. (See manufacturer's directions for meter used.)	First droplet of blood generally contains large portions of serous fluid, which can dilute specimen and cause false results.
m. Lightly squeeze (but do not touch) puncture site until large droplet of blood has formed.	Ensures proper coverage of test pad on reagent strip.
n. Hold reagent strip test pad close to drop of blood, and lightly transfer droplet to test pad (see illustration). Do not smear blood.	Ensures proper chemical reaction. Smearing causes inaccurate test results.
o. Immediately press timer on glucose meter, and place reagent strip on paper towel or on side of timer. (See manufacturer's directions for meter used.)	Accurate timing ensures correct results. Strip should lie flat so blood does not pool on only one part of pad. Some meters (e.g., One Touch) require blood sample to be applied to test strip already in meter.
p. Apply pressure to skin puncture site.	Promotes hemostasis.

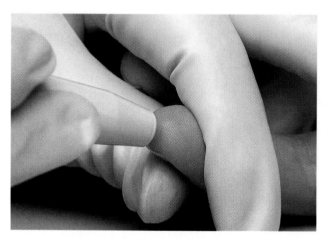

Step 4k

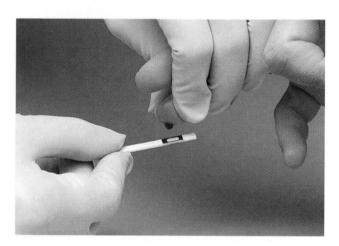

Step 4n

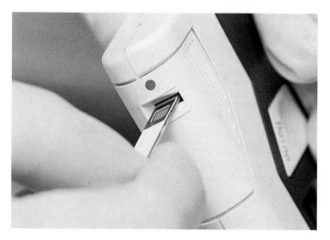

Step 4r

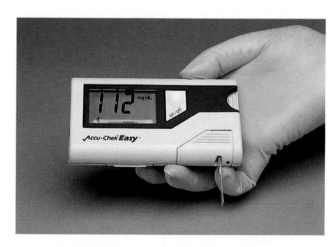

Step 4s

Steps	Rationale
q. When timer displays 60 seconds (for Accu-Chek III model), use moderate pressure to wipe blood from test pad with cotton ball. No blood should remain on test pad for some meters. (See manufacturer's directions for meter used.)	For meter to read glucose levels, some strips must be dry. Refer to product directions for timing used with each type of meter.
r. While timer continues to count, place reagent strip into meter (see illustration).	Strip must be inserted correctly to obtain accurate reading.
s. Read meter, noting reading on display (see illustration).	
t. Turn meter off. Dispose of test strip, cotton balls, and blood-letting device in proper receptacles.	Meter is battery powered. Proper disposal reduces spread of microorganisms.
u. Remove and discard gloves.	
v. Share results with client.	Promotes participation and compliance with therapy.

5. Perform Hemoccult test.

Steps	Rationale
a. Obtain uncontaminated stool specimen (see Skill 15.1) in clean, dry container. Avoid contamination with urine, water, or toilet tissue.	
b. Use tip of wooden applicator to obtain small portion of feces.	Small specimen is sufficient for measuring blood content.
c. Open flap of Hemoccult slide and apply thin smear of stool on paper in first box.	Guaiac paper inside box is sensitive to fecal blood content. Occult blood from upper GI tract is not always equally dispersed through stool.
d. Obtain second fecal specimen from different portion of stool and apply thinly to slide's second box (see illustration).	Findings of occult blood are more conclusive when entire specimen is found to contain blood.
e. Close slide cover and turn slide over to reverse side. Open cardboard flap and apply 2 drops of Hemoccult developing solution on each box of guaiac paper (see illustration).	Developing solution penetrates underlying fecal specimen. Blood is indicated by change in color of guaiac paper.
f. Read results of test after 30 to 60 seconds. Note color changes.	Bluish discoloration indicates occult blood (guaiac positive). No change in color of guaiac paper indicates negative results.
g. Remove and discard gloves.	

6. Perform Gastroccult test.

Steps	Rationale
a. To obtain specimen of gastric contents using NG tube, position client in high Fowler's position in bed or chair.	Minimizes aspiration of gastric contents. Position relieves pressure on abdominal organs. If client is nauseated, flat position in bed or one in which client cannot sit straight may cause abdominal discomfort.

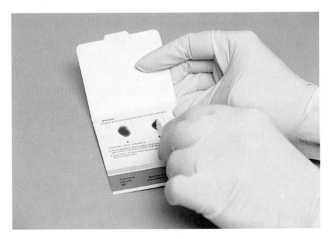

Step 5d

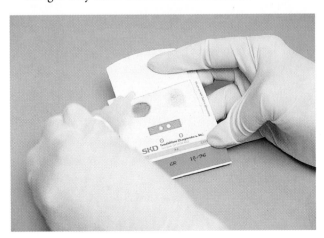

Step 5e

Steps	Rationale

b. Insert NG tube as indicated, if not already placed (see Skill 32.1).

Allows aspiration of gastric contents.

c. Obtain specimen of gastric contents by attaching bulb syringe to NG tube and aspirating 5 to 10 ml. Obtain sample of emesis with 1-ml syringe or wooden applicator.

Only small amount of specimen is needed for pH and occult blood testing.

d. Apply 1 drop of gastric sample to Gastroccult blood test paper.

Sample must cover guaiac paper for test reaction to occur.

e. Apply 2 drops of commercial developer solution over sample and 1 drop between positive and negative performance monitors (see illustration).

Developer initiates chemical reaction of solution with guaiac paper.

f. After 60 seconds, compare color of gastric sample with that of performance monitors.

Positive performance monitor turns blue in 30 seconds, and negative monitor remains white or beige. If sample turns blue, test is positive for occult blood. If sample turns green, test is negative.

g. Remove and discard gloves.
h. Explain results to client.

Immediate results are obtained. Allows client to participate in care.

7. See Completion Protocol (inside front cover).

• • •

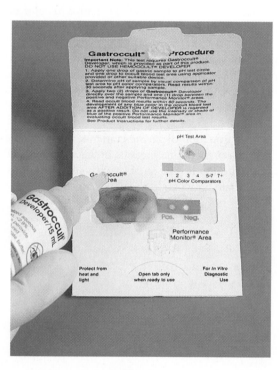

Step 6e

EVALUATION

1. Ask client to state purpose of the specific unit test ordered.
2. Ask client to state the specimen collection procedure required.
3. Inspect client's specimen for appropriateness.
4. Ask if client has questions or concerns about the unit test procedure before specimen collection and later about unit test results. Assess nonverbal behaviors of anxiety before, during, and after procedure.
5. Observe client's ability to perform test independently.

Unexpected Outcomes and Related Interventions

1. Puncture site from Accu-Chek is bruised or continues to bleed.
   a. Apply pressure to site for at least 1 minute.
   b. Apply pressure to site for at least 5 minutes if client is taking anticoagulants or acetylsalicylic acid.
2. Hemoccult test results are positive.
   a. Assess client for hemorrhoids that can cause bleeding. (Bleeding could be misinterpreted as upper GI bleeding.)
   b. Assess client for intake of medications that may increase risk of GI bleeding (e.g., anticoagulants, steroids, acetylsalicylic acid) (Pagana and Pagana, 1997).
   c. Repeat Hemoccult at least 3 times while client is on a meat-free, high-residue diet. (Red meats cause false-positive results.)

3. Glucose meter malfunctions.
   a. Repeat test, following directions.
   b. Follow company directions for malfunctions.
4. Client expresses misunderstanding of procedure and results.
   a. Reevaluate client knowledge base and explain steps again if needed.
   b. Provide printed information if necessary.

Recording and Reporting

- Record method used to obtain specimen, date and time collected, type of test ordered, and laboratory receiving specimen.
- Describe client's tolerance to procedure of specimen collection.
- Report any STAT results to physician or charge nurse.
- Report any abnormal results to physician or charge nurse.

Sample Documentation

0730   Blood glucose 110. No sliding-scale insulin administered.

1200   Blood glucose 240. Regular insulin (4u) administered SQ as ordered per sliding scale.

1000   Nasogastric tube draining 100 ml of light-brown fluid with dark flecks. Gastroccult test is positive for occult blood. Physician notified of results.

1030   Infusion of Zantac 250 mg in 250 ml 5% dextrose initiated via IV at 10 ml per hour.

Geriatric Considerations

- Older adults may have difficulty seeing color charts. Clients with visual impairments can still perform glucose testing independently because there are several audio blood glucose meters on the market that give verbal instructions to guide the client through the procedure.
- Older adults with musculoskeletal alterations may not have fine motor coordination necessary to obtain samples on reagent strips.
- Warming fingertips may facilitate obtaining blood specimen.
- If serial fecal specimens are required, older adult may need assistance from family member or friend.

Home Care and Long-Term Care Considerations

- Many clients are instructed to collect specimens at home and return them to clinic or physician's office.
- Clients who collect specimen at home are asked to prepare slide with feces, close cardboard slide, and return it to office or clinic.
- Most kits sold in drug stores contain all equipment necessary for testing urine except specimen container.
- Clients at home may prefer to use large clock with second hand for timing urine tests.
- Glucose meters may be used routinely by clients in their homes.
- Self-testing of blood glucose is performed by two methods. The first method involves visually reading a reagent strip by comparing it to the color chart on the strip container. The second type of self–blood-glucose monitoring is done by inserting a test strip into a reflectance meter. A variety of meters are on the market (Table 15-3).
- Blood glucose levels are usually assessed before meals, before taking medication, and at bedtime to determine required insulin or other hypoglycemic agents.
- In the home the client need not cleanse the finger with an antiseptic swab because this can aggravate callus formation. Washing hands with soap and warm water is sufficient before the procedure.

Pediatric Considerations

- Children of school age and older are often very curious and may ask many questions about specimen collection. Questions should be answered honestly and at the child's level of understanding. Allow child to watch, if desired, while test is performed.
- Heel and great toe are frequently used as puncture sites in infants.
- Heel warming can be used to facilitate obtaining blood specimen from neonate.

Skill 15.4

CONTRAST MEDIA STUDIES (ARTERIOGRAM, COMPUTED TOMOGRAPHY, INTRAVENOUS PYELOGRAM)

The diagnostic procedures addressed in this skill may be performed by a variety of health care personnel in radiology or a special procedures department. Roles of the nurse include assisting with the preparation of the client before the procedure, providing support during the procedure if indicated, and providing appropriate nursing care after the procedure (Table 15-4).

Equipment

Angiogram (arteriogram)
Special packs are usually available from central supply.
The packs contain various sizes and types of catheters for performing the procedures, as well as the necessary specialized equipment.
Sterile gown
Sterile gloves
Mask
Goggles
Computed tomography
CT scanning
None

Intravenous pyelogram
None
Oral cholecystogram
None

ASSESSMENT

1. Assess client's knowledge of the procedure to determine level of understanding and what education may be necessary.
2. Observe verbal and nonverbal behaviors to determine level of client's anxiety.
3. Assess if client is allergic to iodine dye or shellfish; if so, notify cardiologist or radiologist. **Rationale: In angiography and CT scanning, a hypoallergenic contrast medium can be used.**
4. Assess vital signs to provide baseline data for comparison with findings during and after procedure.
5. Assess peripheral pulses (for clients undergoing angiography) to provide baseline data for comparison with findings during and after procedure.
6. Assess hydration status of client. **Rationale: Severe dehydration can cause renal shutdown and failure** (Pagana and Pagana, 1997).

Table 15-4

Contrast Media Studies

Procedure	Description	Assessment Specific to Test
Angiography (arteriography)	Injection of radiopaque material through catheter threaded into femoral, brachial, or carotid artery and viewed with x-ray study to show vasculature of heart and arterial system	Assess peripheral pulses to establish baseline. Auscultate heart and lung sounds to establish baseline. Assess complete blood count, platelets, prothrombin time, electrolytes, blood urea nitrogen, and creatinine levels to evaluate possible contraindications (Schroeder et al., 1992).
Computed tomography (CT or CAT scan)	Multiple x-ray studies of specific body organs and tissues to provide three-dimensional view	Assess for claustrophobia, which indicates need for sedation or alternative diagnostic test.
Intravenous pyelogram (IVP)	IV injection of radiopaque material to visualize the kidneys or renal pelvis, ureters, and bladder	Assess for allergy to iodinated dye or shellfish, dehydration, renal insufficiency (Pagana and Pagana, 1997).
Oral cholecystogram	Radiological visualization of gallbladder following ingestion of radiopaque iodinated dye.	Assess for allergy to iodine dye or shellfish, pregnancy, or bilirubin greater than 2 mg/dL (Pagana and Pagana, 1997).

7. Auscultate heart and lung sounds (for clients undergoing angiography) to provide baseline data for comparison with findings during and after procedure.
8. Assess whether client has signed consent form (check institution policy). **Rationale: Angiography and CT (if dye used) require a signed consent form to reduce legal risk to institution.**
9. Assess time of last ingested fluid or food. **Rationale: Prevent possible aspiration if client is to receive IVP or must lie flat (CT or angiogram). Excessive hydration causes dilution of contrast medium, making structure more difficult to visualize. Iodine dye may cause nausea.**
10. Assess client's ability to remain still and cooperate throughout the procedure.
11. Assess according to procedure being performed (see Table 15-4).

5. Client does not experience postprocedural complications, such as the following:
   a. Flushing, itching, and urticaria, which signify possible allergic reaction to dye.
   b. Respiratory depression, decreased cardiovascular function, confusion, and diminished reflexes, which are side effects of drugs used for IV sedation.
   c. Diminished or absent peripheral pulses, which may signify thrombosis or embolism.
   d. Hypotension and tachycardia, which may signify hemorrhage or allergic reaction to dye.
   e. Decreased or absent urine output **related to renal failure.**

PLANNING

Expected outcomes focus on client's knowledge of the procedure, client's level of anxiety, prevention of complications, and control of discomfort during and after the procedure.

Expected Outcomes
1. Client explains the purpose and basic steps of the procedure before it is begun.
2. Client assumes the correct position and remains still throughout the entire procedure.
3. Client verbalizes fear of procedure and results, even after the procedure is reviewed by nurse.
4. Client has little pain, which requires no analgesia after the procedure.

DELEGATION CONSIDERATIONS

Diagnostic studies requiring the use of contrast medium are subject to potentially life-threatening complications. Monitoring vital signs following the procedures may be delegated to AP, but assessment can not. Inform AP to report immediately to the RN indications of allergic reactions and bleeding.

IMPLEMENTATION

Steps	Rationale
1. See Standard Protocol (inside front cover).	
2. Assist client to empty bladder before procedure.	Ensures that client will not need to void during procedure.
3. Assist with angiography (arteriography). (Illustration on p. 378 shows an example of abdominal angiography.)	
a. Establish IV access using large-bore cannula (see Chapter 30).	Provides access for delivery of IV fluids and/or drugs.
b. Assist client in assuming comfortable position on x-ray table.	Position may need to be maintained for 1 to 3 hours.
c. Structures can be visualized as dye circulates.	

NURSE ALERT

Consent form must be completed before administration of preprocedural sedation or IVCS.

| **Steps** | **Rationale** |

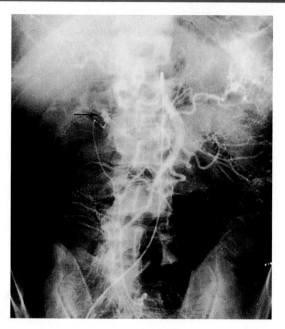

Step 3 *From Doughty DB, Jackson DB: Gastrointestinal disorders, Mosby's Clinical Nursing Series, St Louis, 1993, Mosby.*

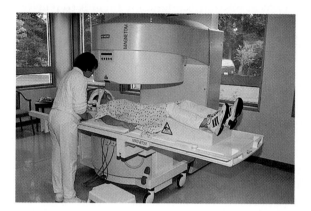

Step 4

4. **Assist with CT (see illustration).**
   a. Instruct client not to move, talk, or sigh during procedure once technician assists to desired position.
   b. Observe client for signs of anaphylaxis if iodinated dye administered.
5. **Assist with IVP.**
   a. Explain to client that skin testing for iodine allergy may be done.
   b. Instruct that a peripheral IV may be started and that a contrast dye will be administered.

Movement causes computer-generated artifacts on image produced.

Signs include respiratory distress, palpitations, itching, and diaphoresis.

Helps reduce anxiety by providing information.

COMMUNICATION TIP

Inform client that dye injection often causes a transitory flushing of the face, a feeling of warmth, a salty taste in the mouth, or even transient nausea (Pagana and Pagana, 1997).

   c. Following procedure, assess client's urinary output.
   d. Assess for delayed reaction (dyspnea, rash, tachycardia) to the dye, which may occur within the first 2 to 6 hours after the test (Pagana and Pagana, 1997).
6. Remove and discard gloves.
7. See Completion Protocol (inside front cover).

A decreased output may be an indication of renal failure.

Prevents dye-induced renal failure and promotes dye excretion.

• • • •

EVALUATION

1. Ask client to explain purpose and basic steps of the procedure.
2. Ask client to demonstrate body position required for procedure. Assess client's body position during procedure.
3. Ask if client has questions or concerns about the procedure before it begins and later about test results. Assess nonverbal behaviors of anxiety before, during, and after procedure.
4. Assess client's level of *comfort* during and after procedure.
5. Assess the client for postprocedural complications.
   a. Assess client for flushing, itching, and urticaria (could signify allergic reaction to dye).
   b. Assess client's respiratory status for sudden, severe shortness of breath, which could indicate allergic reaction to dye.
   c. Palpate for diminished or absent peripheral pulses, which may signify thrombosis or embolism.
   d. Assess client for hypotension, changes in heart rate and/or rhythm (usually bradycardia). (side effects of IVCS).
   e. Assess for decreased output, which may be an indication of renal failure.

Unexpected Outcomes and Related Interventions

1. Client's dorsalis pedis pulses are nonpalpable bilaterally 2 hours after an angiogram.
   a. Assess dorsalis pedis pulses with a Doppler scope.
   b. Notify physician immediately.
2. Hematoma or hemorrhage is present at catheter insertion site.
   a. Maintain adequate pressure over insertion site.
   b. Monitor catheter site every 30 minutes for 2 to 3 hours, then as ordered.
   c. Monitor client for complications.
   d. Notify physician.
3. Client experiences allergic reaction to dye.
   a. Assess client for anaphylaxis.
   b. Assess vital signs.
   c. Administer antihistamine if ordered.
   d. Notify physician.

Recording and Reporting

- Record preprocedure client preparation.
- Record client's condition on return to nursing unit: vital signs, status of pulses, urine output, client's level of responsiveness.
- Record type of dressing, type and amount of any drainage, and client's level of comfort.
- Report to physician or charge nurse immediately:
  - Changes in vital signs and/or oxygen saturation, urine output, and level of client responsiveness.
  - Excessive bleeding or increased in hematoma.
  - Decreased or absent peripheral pulses.

Sample Documentation

0800   Client returned from angiogram per stretcher. Dorsalis pedis and posterior tibial pulses are 12 bilaterally. No bleeding, swelling, or discoloration noted at catheter insertion site in left groin. Sandbag in place over left groin. Left leg extended. Complains of mild discomfort at left groin, but denies need for analgesics.

Geriatric Considerations

- In the older adult, slight alterations in vital signs or behavior may be precursors to impending problems; therefore skilled observations are critical.
- Older adult clients may have reduced drug clearance from decreased glomerular filtration rate (GFR) and nephron activity or decreased hepatic function. Therefore the nurse must monitor the effects of narcotics and hypnotics that may interfere with breathing.

Home Care and Long-Term Care Considerations

Upon discharge, client will be instructed to contact the physician (or affiliated emergency department) if the following occurs after cardiac catheterization:

- Bleeding from the catheterization puncture site; apply gentle pressure with a clean gauze or cloth
- Formation of a knot or lump under the skin that increases in size
- Worsening of a bruise or its movement down the extremity rather than disappearing
- Pain at puncture site or in the extremity used for the catheterization
- Extremity where arterial puncture is made becomes pale and cool to touch
- Appearance of redness, swelling, or warmth of the affected extremity

Although bathing or showering may be allowed the day after the catheterization, the client should be cautioned to avoid slipping, because the leg (if this extremity was used) may feel stiff.

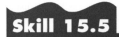

NUCLEAR IMAGING STUDIES (BONE SCAN, BRAIN SCAN, THYROID SCAN)

The diagnostic procedures addressed in this skill may be performed by a variety of health care personnel. Roles of the nurse include assisting with the preparation of the client before the procedure, providing support during the procedure if indicated, and providing appropriate nursing care after the procedure (Table 15-5).

Equipment

> *Bone scan*
> IV equipment
> Radionuclide material
> *Thyroid scan*
> IV equipment
> Radioactive iodine
> *Brain scan*
> IV equipment
> Radioisotope

ASSESSMENT

1. Assess client's knowledge of the procedure to determine level of understanding and what education may be necessary.
2. Observe verbal and nonverbal behaviors to determine level of client's anxiety.
3. Assess vital signs to provide baseline data for comparison with findings during and after procedure.

4. Assess for any allergies, particularly to iodine (brain scan and thyroid scans) or shellfish (thyroid scan).
5. Determine pregnancy status of client (for clients undergoing bone, brain, and thyroid scans). **Rationale: There is risk of fetal damage.**
6. Determine if client is lactating (for bone scan). **Rationale: There is risk of infant contamination.**
7. Assess for dietary intake of iodine, for administration of medications containing iodine, and for the use of antithyroid drugs before the test (for thyroid scan). **Rationale: Test results may be affected by the ingestion of any of these** (Thompson et al., 1997).
8. Check with laboratory regarding whether fasting is required (thyroid scan).
9. Assess client's ability to remain still and cooperate throughout the procedure.
10. Assess according to procedure being performed (see Table 15-5).

PLANNING

Expected outcomes focus on client's knowledge of the procedure, client's level of anxiety, prevention of complications, and control of discomfort during and after the procedure.

Table 15-5

Nuclear Imaging Studies

Procedure	Description	Assessment Specific to Test
Bone scan	Examination of the skeleton by a scanning camera following IV injection of a radionuclide material (Pagana and Pagana, 1997)	Assess for pregnancy or lactation.
Brain scan	Scanning used for detection of pathological cerebral conditions by counter scanning of client's brain following IV injection of a radioisotope (Pagana and Pagana, 1997)	Assess for pregnancy. Determine client's ability to cooperate during the test. Consider sedative order for agitated clients. Assess for allergy in case an iodinated solution will be used.
Thyroid scan	A determination of the size, shape, position, and physiological function of the thyroid gland with the use of radionuclear scanning	Assess for iodine or shellfish allergy. Assess for pregnancy. Assess for recent administration of x-ray contrast agents and medications that might affect results of tests, such as cough medicines, multiple vitamins, some oral contraceptives, and thyroid medications (Pagana and Pagana, 1997).

Expected Outcomes

1. Client explains the purpose and basic steps of the procedure before it is begun.
2. Client assumes the correct position and remains still throughout the entire procedure.
3. Client expresses fears and anxiety related to testing and test results.
4. Client does not experience postprocedural complications, such as hematoma, redness, or edema at site of injection.

IMPLEMENTATION

Steps	Rationale
1. See Standard Protocol (inside front cover).	
2. Explain purpose and steps of procedure.	Reduces anxiety and increases cooperation.
3. Assist client to empty bladder before procedure.	Ensures that client will not need to void during procedure.
4. Assist with bone scan.	
a. Client receives IV injection of an isotope (usually sodium pertechnetate–technetium-99m) in a peripheral vein.	
b. Encourage client to drink several glasses of water between injection of radioisotope and the scanning. Approximate waiting time before scanning is 1 to 3 hours.	Facilitates renal clearance of the circulating tracer not picked up by bone (Pagana and Pagana, 1997).
c. Instruct client to urinate.	
d. Explain to client that scanning table will feel hard and a radionuclide detector will be placed over client's body and will record radiation emitted by the skeleton.	Reduces anxiety and increses cooperation.
e. Explain that client will be repositioned in the prone and lateral positions during test.	
f. Explain to client that nuclear medicine technician performs scan in 30 to 60 minutes, and it is interpreted by physician trained in nuclear medicine imaging (Pagana and Pagana, 1997).	
g. Following procedure, encourage client to drink fluids.	Aids in excretion of radioactive substance, which usually takes 6 to 24 hours (Pagana and Pagana, 1997).
h. Inspect injection site for redness or swelling.	
5. Assist with brain scan.	
a. Explain to client that following IV administration of radioisotope, he or she will be placed in various positions while a counter is placed over the head.	

COMMUNICATION TIP

Assure clients that they won't be exposed to large amounts of radioactivity, because only trace doses of isotope are used and no precautions need to be taken to prevent radioactive exposure to others present (Pagana and Pagana, 1997).

Explain that a slight discomfort during the injection of radioisotope might be felt.

COMMUNICATION TIP

Explain to client that no discomfort other than the peripheral IV puncture needed for radioisotope injection will be felt during the study. Explain that a technician performs the study in the nuclear medicine department in approximately 35 to 45 minutes.

Explain to client the need to remain very still during the procedure. Explain that when cerebral flow studies are performed, the counter is immediately placed over the head (Pagana and Pagana, 1997).

Steps	Rationale

   b. Following procedure, explain to client that the radioactive material is usually excreted within 6 to 24 hours.

   c. Encourage client to drink fluids.

Aids in excretion of isotope.

   d. Assess injection site for redness and swelling.

6. Assist with thyroid scan.

   a. Tell client that an oral dose of radioactive technetium is given.

   b. Explain to client that at designated times during the scanning, client will be supine while a detector is passed over the thyroid area.

   c. After the procedure, explain that no special isolation or urine precautions are necessary.

COMMUNICATION TIP

Assure client the capsule is tasteless and that minute, harmless doses of radioactive technetium will be used (Pagana and Pagana, 1997).

Assure client there will be no discomfort associated with this study.

• • •

EVALUATION

1. Ask client to explain purpose and basic steps of the procedure.
2. Ask client to demonstrate body position required for procedure. Assess client's body position during procedure.
3. Ask if client has questions or concerns about the procedure before it begins and later about test results. Assess nonverbal behaviors of anxiety before, during, and after procedure.
4. Observe client's level of comfort during and after procedure. Inspect injection site for hematoma, redness, or edema.

Unexpected Outcomes and Related Interventions

1. Client's injection site becomes red and swollen.
   a. Monitor site until resolution of swelling.
   b. Instruct client to check site at home if procedure is performed on an outpatient basis.

Recording and Reporting

- Record preprocedure client preparation. Include the amount and type of contrast material injected.
- Record client's tolerance to procedure.

Sample Documentation

0820   Client transported to nuclear medicine for noncontrast bone scan. Client reports being "tired," but no other complaints. Client resting.

Geriatric Considerations

Because of the normal aging process, an older adult is at risk for skin breakdown and joint stiffness. The client may require assistance with frequent position changes.

   The older adult client may experience increased discomfort during the procedure because of lying motionless for an extended period of time.

   After the procedure, be aware of the need to change positions slowly in older adult clients to minimize safety risks and possible postural changes.

Skill 15.6

ASSISTING WITH DIAGNOSTIC STUDIES (ASPIRATIONS [BONE MARROW, LUMBAR PUNCTURE, PARACENTESIS, THORACENTESIS, LIVER BIOPSY], BRONCHOSCOPY, ENDOSCOPY MAGNETIC RESONANCE IMAGING).

Diagnostic studies are performed at the client's bedside or in a treatment room by a physician assisted by a nurse or other health care personnel. A consent form is signed by the client. Most of these procedures cause moderate discomfort, and the client may tolerate the procedure better if a well-informed nurse stays at the bedside and explains each step.

Equipment

Aspiration trays: Most institutions purchase trays with contents appropriate for the specific aspiration, or the trays are compiled by the institution's central supply department. Contents of trays may differ from one institution to another. Equipment needed but not found in aspiration trays includes:
Two pair sterile gloves of appropriate size for physician
Laboratory requisitions and labels
Mask, goggles, and gowns for physician and nurse
Standard aspiration trays may contain:
Antiseptic solution (e.g., povidone-iodine)
Gauze sponges (4 × 4)
Sterile towels
Anesthetic agent (e.g., lidocaine 1%)
Two 3-ml sterile syringes with 23- to 25-gauge needles
2-inch adhesive tape
Adhesive bandages
Box 15-1 lists equipment usually found in specific aspiration trays.
Bronchoscopy
Bronchoscopy tray, if available from central supply, may include:
Flexible fiberoptic bronchoscope
Gauze sponges (4 × 4)
Local anesthetic spray (lidocaine)
Sterile tracheal suction catheters
Sterile gloves
Sterile water-soluble lubricating jelly
Mask, goggles, and gown
Emesis basin
Oxygen equipment
Endoscopy
Endoscopy tray may include:
Fiberoptic endoscope
Camera

Box 15-1 Contents of Aspiration Trays

Bone Marrow Aspiration Tray
Sterile syringes: two 10 ml and two 50 ml for marrow aspiration
Two bone marrow needles with inner stylus
Test tubes and/or glass slides

Lumbar Puncture Tray
Three spinal needles (various sizes) with inner obturators (5 to 12.5 cm [2 to 5 inches] long)
Glass or plastic manometer with three-way stopcock
Four test tubes

Paracentesis Tray
Four 10- to 60-ml syringes with 19- to 20-gauge needles
Small, sterile knife blade
Two sterile cannula needles, sizes 10 or 12, with inner trochar or catheter
Sterile specimen cups and receptacle

(2 to 3 L IV fluids and macrodrip-size (10 gtt/ml) IV tubing [as ordered by physician] are not included in tray.)

Thoracentesis Tray
Two 50-ml syringes with 14- to 17-gauge needles, 5 to 7 cm (2 to 3 inches) long, for drainage of pleural fluid
Receptacle for fluid
Three-way stopcock
Two-way stopcock with extension tubing
Test tubes

Liver Biopsy Tray
Scalpel
Two True-Cut disposable needles (4½-inch straight and 6-inch straight)
One 30-ml bottle sterile 0.9% normal saline
Formalin solution

Solutions for biopsied specimens
Local anesthetic spray
Tracheal suction equipment
Blood pressure equipment
Sterile water-soluble jelly
Mask, goggles, and gown
Magnetic Resonance Imaging (*MRI*)
Contrast medium: gadolinium (Magnevist) (optional and must be ordered by physician)

ASSESSMENT

1. Assess client's knowledge of procedure to determine level of health teaching required.
2. Observe verbal and nonverbal behaviors to determine client's anxiety.
3. Assess client's ability to understand and follow directions. **Rationale: Procedure requires client to follow directions closely and assume proper position.**
4. Assess client's ability to assume position required for procedure and ability to remain still. **Rationale: Client must maintain position without moving, to avoid complications during needle or trochar insertion.**
5. Determine whether client is allergic to antiseptic or anesthetic solutions to decrease risk of complications. **Rationale: Common allergic reactions to**
anesthetic agents are central nervous system depression, respiratory difficulties, and hypotension. Allergic reactions to antiseptic solutions are usually skin irritations.
6. Assess whether client has signed consent form (check institution's policy). **Rationale: Bronchoscopy, MRI (if dye used), and endoscopy require a signed consent form to reduce legal risk to institution.**
7. Assess time of last ingested fluid or food (for clients undergoing, bronchoscopy , and upper GI endoscopy). Clients should receive nothing by mouth (NPO), 8 hours before endoscopy and bronchoscopy. **Rationale: Excessive hydration causes dilution of contrast medium, making structures more difficult to visualize. Iodine dye may cause nausea. NPO decreases chance of aspiration of stomach contents.**
8. Assess vital signs to provide baseline data for comparison with postprocedural vital signs.
9. Assess client's coagulation status (use of anticoagulants, platelet count, prothrombin time) to determine factors that can increase risk of bleeding.
10. Auscultate heart and lung sounds (for clients undergoing bronchoscopy) to provide baseline data for comparison with findings during and after procedure.

Table 15-6

Aspirations

Procedure	Description	Assessment Specific to Test
Bone marrow aspiration	Removal of cells from bone marrow for diagnosis of leukemias and other malignancies, anemias, and thrombocytopenia	Assess complete blood count for abnormalities.
Lumbar puncture	Aspiration of spinal fluid for testing and/or measurement of pressure for diagnosis of meningitis, encephalitis, brain or spinal cord tumors, and cerebral hemorrhage	Assess neurological status, including movement, sensation, and muscle strength of legs, to provide baseline for comparison after procedure.
Paracentesis	Removal of fluid from peritoneal cavity to determine presence of blood, bile, bacteria, or protein; also to decrease intraabdominal pressure in presence of ascites (accumulation of fluid in peritoneal cavity)	Assess bladder for distention and determine last voiding. Bladder should be empty to minimize risk of puncture. Weigh client, assess abdomen, and measure abdominal girth at largest point. Mark location.
Thoracentesis	Aspiration of fluid to evaluate cell types for the presence of a tumor. May also be used to remove excess fluid in pleural cavity to minimize difficulty breathing	Establish baseline by assessing respiratory rate and depth, symmetry of chest on inspiration and expiration, type of cough, and sputum.
Liver biopsy	Aspiration of cells from liver for diagnosis of cancer, effects of hepatotoxic drugs, or assessment of treatment for chronic liver disease such as hepatitis	Assess bladder for distention.

Table 15-7

Selected Diagnostic Procedures

Procedure	Description	Assessment Specific to Test
Bronchoscopy	Examination of tracheobronchial tree with flexible fiberoptic bronchoscope. Sputum or mucus plugs may be aspirated, or tissues can be examined or biopsied for abnormalities	Assess heart and lung sounds, type of cough, and sputum to establish baseline. Assess for allergy to local anesthetic used to spray throat, which could cause laryngeal edema or laryngospasm.
Endoscopy	Visualization of GI tract using a long, flexible fiberoptic scope with a light source attached	Assess for upper GI bleeding, which may obscure viewing lens with blood, preventing visualization.
Esophagogastroduoden-oscopy (EGD)	Visualize upper GI tract	
Proctoscopy, colonoscopy, or sigmoidoscopy	Visualize lower GI tract	
MRI	Noninvasive scanning to visualize internal organs and structures by use of magnetic forces rather than radiation	Assess for cardiac pacemaker, aneurysm clips, or history of valve replacement, which are contra-indications because magnet may move metal or electronic objects (Pagana and Pagana, 1997). Additional items that may interfere with MRI are found on the informational diagram. Assess client for claustrophobia.

11. Assess respiratory status–lung sounds, type of cough, and sputum produced (for clients undergoing bronchoscopy)–to provide baseline data for comparison with respiratory status during and after procedure.

12. Assess according to aspiration or diagnostic procedure being performed (Tables 15-6 and 15-7).

13. Assess need for preprocedural pain medication. **Rationale: Procedure may be painful, and client must remain still throughout procedure because of potential complications.**

PLANNING

Expected outcomes focus on client's knowledge of the procedure, including the need to remain still to prevent complications; client's anxiety regarding procedure and results; and control of discomfort during and after the procedure.

Expected Outcomes

1. Client explains purpose and basic steps of the procedure before it is begun.
2. Client does not verbalize fear of procedure and its results after nurse reviews procedure.
3. Client assumes the correct position and remains still throughout the entire procedure.
4. Client verbalizes minimal pain, which requires no analgesics after procedure.

5. Client has nonlabored respirations within normal range after abdominal paracentesis, thoracentesis, and bronchoscopy.
6. Client maintains heart rate and blood pressure within normal limits during and after aspiration.
7. Puncture site dressing remains clean, dry, and intact.
8. Client does not experience postprocedural complications, such as:
   a. Hypotension and tachycardia, which may signify hemorrhage or allergic reaction to dye.
   b. Flushing, itching, and urticaria, which signify possible allergic reaction to dye.
   c. Sudden, severe shortness of breath, which signifies laryngospasm and bronchospasm in response to irritation from bronchoscope or topical anesthetic.
   d. Abdominal pain, fever, and bleeding, which occur with perforation of abdominal structures.
   e. Respiratory depression, decreased cardiovascular function, confusion, and diminished reflexes, which are side effects of drugs used for IV sedation (client conscious).
9. Client is able to explain position and activity restrictions after aspirations.

DELEGATION CONSIDERATIONS

Diagnostic studies are invasive and can result in potentially life-threatening complications. Monitoring vital signs after the procedures may be delegated to assistive personnel, but assessment can not. Inform AP to report immediately to the professional nurse indications of allergic reactions, respiratory distress or bleeding.

IMPLEMENTATION

Steps	Rationale
1. See Standard Protocol (inside front cover).	
2. **Assist with bone marrow aspiration.**	
a. Explain steps of skin preparation, anesthetic injection, needle insertion, and position required.	Anticipation of expected sensation reduces anxiety.

> **NURSE ALERT**
>
> *Obtain a premedication order (i.e., sedative) if client is extremely anxious.*

b. Set up sterile tray or open supplies to make accessible for physician.	Reduces risk of contamination of sterile field and promotes prompt completion of procedure.
c. Assist client in maintaining correct position. (Position required depends on bone marrow aspiration site. Iliac crest is most common site, but sternum or tibia may also be used.) Reassure client while explaining procedure.	Decreases chance of complications during procedure. Explanations increase client comfort and relaxation.

> **NURSE ALERT**
>
> *This procedure may be contraindicated in clients who cannot cooperate or remain still during the procedure (Pagana and Pagana, 1997).*

d. Remove and discard gloves.	
e. Assess client's condition during procedure: comfort, respiratory status, and vital signs if indicated.	Identifies any changes that may indicate a complication.
f. Note characteristics of bone marrow aspirate (e.g., amount, color).	Characteristics are used for observation, reporting, and recording.

> **NURSE ALERT**
>
> *A pressure dressing may be in place. If so, do not remove.*

3. Assist with lumbar puncture.	
a. Explain steps of procedure, and assist client in assuming flexed side-lying position for entire procedure (see illustration).	Ensures no movement of spinal needle within spinal column and canal. Spinal needle is inserted into spinal canal anywhere between third lumbar (L3) and first sacral (S1) vertebrae (see illustration).

Steps	Rationale

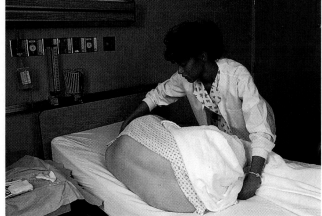

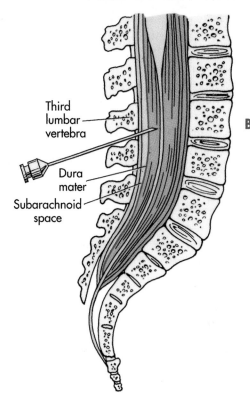

Third lumbar vertebra

Dura mater

Subarachnoid space

Step 3a

b. Set up sterile tray or open supplies to make accessible for physician.

c. Gently but firmly hold client's arms and legs in flexed position.

Prevents sudden movement by client.

d. Caution client not to cough and to breathe slowly and deeply.

Coughing or changes in breathing increase cerebrospinal fluid (CSF) pressure and give false reading.

e. Explain each step that may cause discomfort.

Client should know exactly what is occurring so that discomfort can be anticipated and surprises eliminated.

Pediatric Considerations

- Very young children may receive a general anesthetic for this procedure.
- Allow child to practice procedure beforehand, using doll as a model (Broome et al., 1992).

Geriatric Considerations

- Older adults with arthritis may have difficulty sustaining the position required for the procedure.

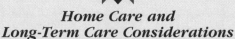

Home Care and Long-Term Care Considerations

- Instruct client that some clients experience tenderness at the puncture site for several days after this study and that mild analgesia may be ordered by the physician.

Steps	Rationale

f. Properly label tubes with client information and name of test desired.

Nurse is responsible for labeling tubes with client's name and tests desired. Test tubes are numbered in sequence of collection (e.g., 1 through 4).

g. Assist with placement of direct pressure and gauze dressing over puncture site.

Pressure helps minimize CSF loss and bleeding.

h. Ask client to maintain dorsal recumbent position (flat), usually for 4 to 12 hours after procedure. Client may turn from side to side.

Dorsal recumbent position reduces risk of spinal headache, which may result if client sits upright.

i. Provide for client's comfort with medication as ordered.

Procedure is usually described as painful by client. Postprocedural headache may require that client be medicated.

NURSE ALERT

If client has a central nervous system disorder a sedative or analgesic may be contraindicated so as not to further cloud client's consciousness.

j. Remove and discard gloves.
k. During and after procedure, observe client for:
   (1) Changes in level of consciousness (LOC) and pupil size/reaction.
   (2) Respiratory status and vital signs.
   (3) Numbness, tingling, or pain radiating down legs.

Changes in LOC, pupil size/reaction, respiratory status, and vital signs indicate increasing intracranial pressure.

May result from spinal nerve irritation.

l. Encourage client to force fluids by mouth if not contraindicated.

Needed to replace CSF lost and resume hemodynamics.

4. Assist with paracentesis.
a. Explain steps of procedure and position required (either semi-Fowler's in bed or sitting upright on side of bed or in chair with feet supported) (see illustration).
b. Set up sterile tray or open sterile supplies and make accessible for physician.

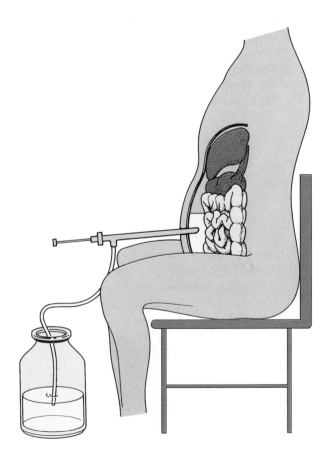

NURSE ALERT

Report any excessive drainage (e.g., saturation of gauze dressing) from the insertion site, which may predispose client to postpuncture headache and infection (moisture may function as growth medium for bacteria). If excessive drainage occurs, place pressure dressing on site.

Step 4a *Modified from Beare PG, Myers JL: Adult health nursing, ed 3, St Louis, 1998, Mosby.*

Steps	**Rationale**
c. Have client void before procedure.	Full or distended bladder increases possibility of puncturing bladder.

> **NURSE ALERT**
>
> *If unable to void and bladder is distended, obtain order to catheterize client.*

d. Describe steps of procedure as they are implemented by physician.	Allows client opportunity to ask questions and helps to decrease anxiety.
e. Assess vital signs every 15 minutes during procedure.	Identifies possible complications of procedure, such as shock.
f. Maximum amount of ascitic fluid usually allowed to drain is 4 L (Pagana and Pagana, 1997). Collect any necessary laboratory specimens in sterile containers.	Maximum of 4 L drainage prevents hypovolemic shock if ascites is rapidly accumulated (Pagana and Pagana, 1997).
g. Remove and discard gloves.	

◆ Geriatric Considerations

In older adults, skin is normally inelastic and thin; therefore special care should be used when removing adhesive bandages or tape at puncture site.

5. Assist with thoracentesis.
   a. Explain steps of procedure and position required.
   b. Set up sterile tray or open supplies to make them accessible to physician.
   c. Assist client in assuming correct position: leaning over a bedside table padded with pillows (see illustration).

◆◆ Home Care and Long-Term Care Considerations

If paracentesis is done on an outpatient basis, inform client to notify physician of fever or any swelling, pain, or drainage at puncture site. In males, scrotal edema should be reported to the physician (Society of Gastroenterology Nurses and Associates [SGNA], 1993).

Positions client appropriately for procedure and prevents sudden movement by client.

> **NURSE ALERT**
>
> *Client must remain immobile during the procedure to prevent trauma to visceral pleura.*

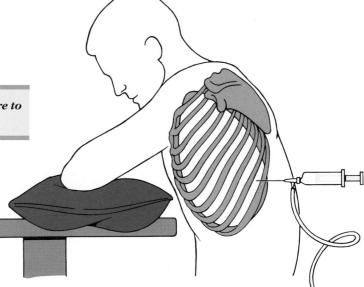

Step 5c *Modified from Beare PG, Myers JL: Adult health nursing, ed 3, St Louis, 1998, Mosby.*

Steps	Rationale
d. Assist client through procedure by holding shoulders or sides and reassuring in coaching manner.	Procedure is usually uncomfortable.
e. Assess client's respiratory status during procedure: rate, difficulty, and color of mucous membranes and nailbeds.	Enables nurse to detect tolerance to procedure and possible complications.
f. Assist client in assuming comfortable position in bed after procedure.	If leakage into pleural space is suspected, client is positioned recumbent with punctured chest side up.
g. Remove and discard gloves.	

NURSE ALERT

The complications of liver and spleen perforation are less common than lung perforation. Symptoms are subtle and may not be noted for several days. Symptoms include decreasing hemoglobin and hematocrit values and possibly abdominal pain.

NURSE ALERT

Obtain a premedication order (i.e., sedative) if client is extremely anxious.

This procedure is contraindicated in clients who are uncooperative or who cannot remain still and hold their breath during sustained exhalation.

Geriatric Considerations

During all aspects of this procedure, be aware of ineffective breathing patterns in the older adult because of age-related changes such as reduced elastic lung recoil, declining chest expansion, reduced cough efficiency, and weaker thoracic and diaphragmatic muscles (Stanley and Beare, 1995).

After the procedure, be aware of need to change positions in older adult clients slowly to minimize safety risks and possible postural changes.

6. **Assist with liver biopsy.**
   a. Explain steps of procedure and position required.
   b. Set up sterile tray or open sterile supplies and make them accessible for physician.
   c. Ask client to empty bladder.
   d. Assist client to correct position: supine at far right edge of bed with head turned left and right arm extended above head (see illustration).

Facilitates access to liver biopsy site. Needle is inserted through the lower chest, between the sixth and seventh ribs (see illustration).

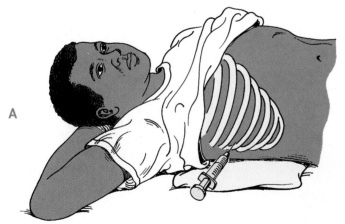
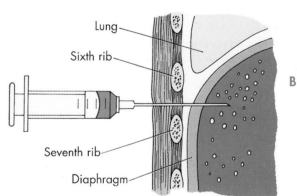

Lung

Sixth rib

Seventh rib

Diaphragm

A   B

Step 6d

Steps	Rationale

e. Teach client breathing used during procedure: take deep breath in, blow all air out, and hold breath. After physician removes needle, client can breathe normally.

This brings the liver and diaphragm to their uppermost position and immobilizes them (Wilkinson, 1990).

f. Assist client in changing position after the procedure: move to center of bed and roll onto right side. Instruct to maintain position for 2 hours.

Liver capsule is compressed against the chest wall at the site of needle insertion, which prevents blood from leaking (Wilkinson, 1990).

g. Advise client to remain in bed for 6 hours.

h. Remove and discard gloves.

i. Assess pulse, blood pressure, and respirations every 15 minutes for 1 hour, every 30 minutes for 2 hours, every 1 hour for 4 hours, then every 4 hours.

Enables nurse to identify possible complications of procedure, such as shock.

NURSE ALERT

Clients who have severe arthritic conditions or who are orthopneic may be unable to assume this position.

▶◆◀
Home Care and
Long-Term Care Considerations

- Teach client symptoms of complications related to liver and spleen perforation that may not present for several days after procedure.
- Encourage client to report any dyspnea, chest pain, or cough after procedure.
- Inform the client that no food or fluid restrictions are necessary before or after the test.

7. **Assist with bronchoscopy (see illustration).**
   a. Remove and safely store client's dentures and eyeglasses (if applicable).

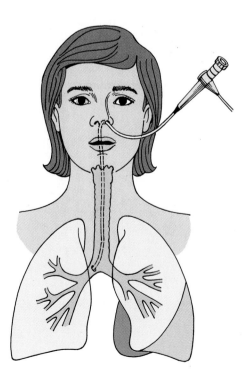

Step 7

Steps	Rationale
b. 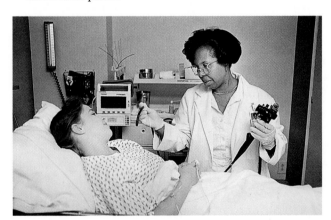 Establish IV access using large-bore cannula (see Chapter 30).	Provides access for delivery of IV fluids and/or drugs.
c. Assist client in maintaining position desired by physician: semi-Fowler's or supine (Pagana and Pagana, 1997).	Provides maximal visualization of lower airways and adequate lung expansion.
d. Instruct client not to swallow local anesthetic; provide emesis basin.	Anesthetic may be absorbed systemically and cause severe central nervous system and cardiovascular reactions.
e. Assist client through procedure by explanations.	Although premedicated and drowsy, clients need to be reminded not to change position and to cooperate.
f. Monitor electrocardiogram (ECG), pulse, and blood pressure for changes every 5 minutes during procedure.	Side effects of drugs used for IV sedation (client conscious) may include respiratory depression, decreased cardiovascular function, confusion, and diminished reflexes. Interval for assessment may be lengthened to 15 minutes if perioperative nurse determines client's condition is within normal parameters (Watson and James, 1990).
g. Assess client's respiratory status every 5 minutes during procedure: observe degree of restlessness and respiratory rate; observe capillary refill and color of nailbeds; monitor pulse oximetry (oxygen saturation).	Bronchoscope may cause feelings of suffocation; also, because airway is partially occluded, client may become hypoxic during observations. Side effects of drugs used for IV sedation (client conscious) include respiratory depression and somnolence (Watson and James, 1990).
h. Note characteristics of suctioned material.	Information used to record and report and to make further client observations.
i. Wipe client's nose to remove lubricant after bronchoscope is removed.	Promotes hygiene and comfort.
j. Assess LOC, gag reflex, pulse oximetry, respiratory rate, blood pressure, pulse, heart rate, and capillary refill after the procedure. (Use tongue depressor to touch pharynx to test for presence of gag reflex.)	Assesses for postprocedural complications.
k. Do not allow client to eat or drink until the tracheobronchial anesthesia has worn off and gag reflex returns.	Prevents aspiration of food or fluid, which could cause pneumonia.
l. Remove and discard gloves.	
8. Assist with endoscopy (see illustration).	
a. Remove client's dentures and partial bridges (if applicable).	Prevents dislodgment of dental structures during intubation phase.

Step 8

Steps	**Rationale**

b. 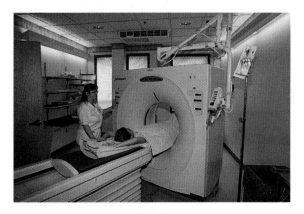 Establish IV access using large-bore cannula (see Chapter 30).

c. Assist client in maintaining left lateral position.

Unexpected change of position can cause accidental perforation of esophagus, stomach, or duodenum.

d. Assist client through procedure by anticipating needs, promoting comfort, and telling client what is happening.

Client is unable to speak after tube is passed into throat. Reassures client about procedure and how long it will last.

e. Monitor ECG, pulse, and blood pressure for changes every 5 minutes during procedure.

Side effects of drugs used for IV sedation (client conscious) may include respiratory depression, decreased cardiovascular function, confusion, and diminished reflexes. Interval for assessment may be lengthened to 15 minutes if perioperative nurse determines client's condition is within normal parameters (Watson and James, 1990).

f. Place tissue specimens in proper laboratory containers.

Ensures proper labeling and preparation of specimens for microscopic examination.

g. Suction if client begins to vomit or accumulate saliva.

Prevents aspiration of gastric contents or oral secretions.

h. Assess LOC, gag reflex, pulse oximetry, respiratory rate, blood pressure, pulse, heart rate, and capillary refill after the procedure. (Use tongue depressor to touch pharynx to test for presence of gag reflex.)

Assesses for postprocedural complications.

i. If done on an outpatient basis, provide discharge instructions.

j. Assist client to comfortable position, remove and discard gloves, and wash hands.

Promotes rest and relaxation.

9. **Assist with MRI (see illustration).**

a. If possible, show client picture of MRI machine and encourage questions.

Helps to decrease anxiety by providing information.

b. Remove all metallic objects from client, such as watch, jewelry, coins, keys, hairpins, credit cards, prosthesis, and dentures containing metal (Pagana and Pagana, 1997).

Metallic objects create artifacts on the scan, and some metal objects may be damaged by the magnetic field. Also, metallic objects may be moved by the magnetic field (see illustration).

10. Securely attach properly completed identification label and laboratory requisition to specimen(s).

Incorrect identification of specimen could result in diagnostic or therapeutic errors.

11. Send specimen immediately to laboratory.

12. See Completion Protocol (inside front cover).

• • •

NURSE ALERT

Procedure may be contraindicated if claustrophobia is severe and/or not relieved by sedation.

Clients who are medically unstable and require continuous life-support equipment (that contains metal) are not candidates for this procedure unless specially designed monitoring equipment is available.

Step 9

ALL INFORMATION IN SHADED BOXED AREA
MUST BE FILLED OUT PRIOR TO MRI

THE FOLLOWING ITEMS MAY INTERFERE WITH MAGNETIC RESONANCE IMAGING
AND SOME CAN BE POTENTIALLY HAZARDOUS. PLEASE INDICATE IF YOU HAVE
THE FOLLOWING:

Please mark on this drawing the
location of any metal inside your body.

- Cardiac Pacemaker   YES   NO
- Aneurysm Clip(s)   YES   NO
- Implanted Insulin/Drug Pump   YES   NO
- Neurostimulator (TENS Unit)   YES   NO
- Biostimulator/Bone Growth Stimulator   YES   NO
- Hearing aid/Cochlear Implant   YES   NO
- Gianturco Coil (embolus coil)   YES   NO
- Vascular Clip(s)   YES   NO
- Heart Valve Prosthesis   YES   NO
- Greenfield Vena Cava Filter   YES   NO
- Middle Ear Implant   YES   NO
- Penile Prosthesis   YES   NO
- Orbital/Eye Prosthesis   YES   NO
- Shrapnel or Bullet   YES   NO
- Wire Sutures   YES   NO
- Tattooed Eyeliner   YES   NO
- Any type of Dental Item held
  in place by a Magnet   YES   NO
- ANY OTHER IMPLANTED ITEM   YES   NO
  TYPE _____
- Diaphram/IUD   YES   NO
- Intraventricular Shunt   YES   NO
- Wire Mesh   YES   NO
- Artificial Limb or Joint   YES   NO
- Any Orthopedic Item (i.e., pins,
  rods, screws, nails, clips,
  plates, wire, etc.)   YES   NO
- Dentures   YES   NO
- Dental Braces or any other type
  of Removable Dental Item   YES   NO
- Have you ever had a surgical procedure or operation of any kind?   YES   NO
  If YES please list type of operation and the date:

_____

_____

- Are you claustrophobic   YES   NO
- Have you ever had an injury to your eye involving metal?   YES   NO
- Is there any possibility you may be pregnant?   YES   NO

I attest that the above information is correct to the best of my knowledge,
understand any risks associated with the above conditions, and consent to
undergoing this Magnetic Resonance Imaging examination.

RIGHT   LEFT

_____

(Patient's or Legal Guardian's Signature)

_____

(Witness Signature)   DATE:

Step 9b

EVALUATION

1. Ask client to state purpose and explain steps of the procedure before it is started.
2. Ask if client has questions or concerns about the procedure before it begins and later about test results. Assess nonverbal behaviors of anxiety before, during, and after procedure.
3. Ask client to demonstrate body position required for procedure. Assess client's body position throughout procedure and assist to maintain position as necessary.
4. Ask client's to describe level of comfort during and after procedure.
5. Assess client's respiratory status (rate, rhythm, and depth of respirations; symmetry of chest movement) during and after abdominal paracentesis, thoracentesis, and bronchoscopy).
6. Compare client's heart rate and blood pressure during and after procedure to preprocedure baseline. (Check hospital policy; may be as often as every 15 minutes for 2 hours.)
7. Inspect dressing over puncture site for drainage every hour after the procedure until client's condition is stable.
8. Assess client for postprocedural complications.
   a. Assess client for a decrease in blood pressure and tachycardia (could signify hemorrhage or allergic reaction to dye).
   b. Assess client for flushing, itching, and urticaria (could signify allergic reaction to dye).
   c. Assess client's respiratory status for sudden, severe shortness of breath (could signify laryngospasm and bronchospasm).
   d. Assess client for abdominal pain, fever, and bleeding (could signify perforation of abdominal structures).
   e. Assess client for low oxygen saturation, rate and/or depth of respirations, cyanosis or mottled skin, hypotension, changes in heart rate and/or rhythm (usually bradycardia), and decreased or nonpalpable peripheral pulses, reflexes, and LOC complications related to conscious sedation.
9. Ask client to describe postprocedural positioning and activity restriction for lumbar puncture, liver biopsy, and thoracentesis.

Unexpected Outcomes and Related Interventions

1. Client develops a suboccipital headache after lumbar puncture.
   a. Instruct client to lie flat in bed.
   b. Encourage fluid intake of at least 1 glass per hour if not contraindicated.
   c. Administer analgesics as prescribed.
   d. Apply ice pack to area of discomfort.
2. Client found ambulating to bathroom while on strict bed rest after liver biopsy.
   a. Instruct client to remain in bed, positioned on right side. Reinforce that this position prevents blood or bile from leaking from puncture site.
   b. Inspect dressing for blood or bile leakage.
   c. Place call light within client's reach and reinforce when to use it.
   d. Check blood pressure, pulse, and respirations.
3. Client is unable to assume correct position; moves during procedure.
   a. Reassess and instruct client on importance of maintaining position and not moving.
   b. Further assess client to determine if sedation might be necessary.
4. Client experiences tenderness and erythema at bone marrow site; decreased blood pressure and increased pulse.
   a. Continue to monitor vital signs and aspiration site.
   b. Notify physician of findings and obtain further orders.
5. Client develops shortness of breath, anxiety, and tachypnea following thoracentesis.
   a. Elevate head of bed and administer oxygen (if ordered).
   b. Monitor vital signs.
   c. Notify physician of findings and obtain further orders.
6. Client complains of lightheadedness while sitting at side of bed after abdominal paracentesis.
   a. Assist client to supine position.
   b. Check blood pressure and pulse.
   c. Inspect abdominal dressing for bleeding or peritoneal fluid.
7. One hour after gastroscopy, client attempts to drink water furnished by a family friend.
   a. Reinforce to client and friend that liquids or solid food should not be taken orally until gag reflex returns.
   b. Teach client possible complications from eating or drinking substances before gag reflex returns (aspiration pneumonia).
   c. Check gag reflex each hour.
   d. Inform client when it is appropriate to eat and drink.
8. In the recovery room after an endoscopy, client is sleepy but responds to verbal stimulation, respirations shallow at rate of 10 per minute, oxygen saturation 85%, and ECG reading normal sinus rhythm.
   a. Instruct client to take deep breaths.
   b. Administer oxygen at 2 L per nasal cannula.
   c. Elevate head of bed 30 degrees.
   d. Notify physician.

Recording and Reporting

- Record preprocedure client preparation.
- Record name of procedure, location of puncture site (if applicable), amount and color of fluid drained or specimen obtained, client's tolerance to procedure (e.g., vital signs, comfort), laboratory tests ordered, type of dressing, and drainage.
- Report to physician or charge nurse immediately:
  - Changes in vital signs or oxygen saturation status.
  - Unexpected drainage.

Sample Documentation

0930   Abdominal paracentesis completed with 1100 ml cloudy liquid aspirated. Respirations 18 with moderate depth, pulse 98, and blood pressure 138/86. Rates pain at 6 on scale of 0 to 10. 2 × 2 inch gauze dressing applied to puncture site; remains dry and intact.

0940   Demerol 50 mg given in right dorsal gluteal for abdominal pain.

1010   States pain has decreased to 2, which is tolerable. Abdominal girth measures 34 inches at umbilicus. Weight decreased to 168 pounds.

Pediatric Considerations

- Lumbar punctures are frequently done on children with cancer. The use of active coping skills, such as relaxation and imagery, have been shown to decrease children's pain perceptions during the procedure (Heiney, 1991; Broome et al., 1990).

Geriatric Considerations

- Older adults may have difficulty assuming the side-lying knee-to-chest position.
- Assess skin integrity of client after lying still on hard narrow examining table. Older adult clients are at greater risk for skin breakdown.

Home Care and Long-Term Care Considerations

- Provide written instructions to reinforce oral instructions about remaining flat and evidence of complications to report (Phipps, et al, 1995).

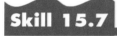

CARDIAC STUDIES (ELECTROCARDIOGRAM, EXERCISE STRESS TEST, DOBUTAMINE STRESS ECHOCARDIOGRAPHY, CARDIAC NUCLEAR SCANNING, CARDIAC CATHETERIZATION)

These procedures are performed at the client's bedside (EKG), in a specially equipped laboratory (Exercise Stress Test and Cardiac Catheterization), or in the Nuclear Medicine Radiology Department (Table 15-8). ECGs, measurement of the heart's electrical activities, are performed by either a nurse or a specially trained technician. Cardiac stress testing may be performed by a nurse or a specially trained technician (exercise stress testing), and dobutamine stress echocardiography is performed by a specially trained radiologist. Cardiac catheterization is performed by specially trained physicians, nurses, and technicians. The client tolerates all these procedures better if the he or she is well informed and aware of what will be done before the test, as well as the implications of the testing.

Exercise stress testing is a noninvasive diagnostic study that provides data regarding the client's cardiac function. During exercise stress testing, the ECG, heart rate, and blood pressure are monitored while the client engages in a form of physical activity (e.g., pedaling a stationary bike or walking on a treadmill). The goal of the test is to increase the heart rate to just below its maximal level or "target heart rate." The test is discontinued if the client reaches the "target heart rate," develops any symptoms, or has any ECG changes. The rationale for this test is based on the principle that occluded arteries will be unable to meet the heart's increased demand for blood during the test, resulting in chest pain, fatigue, dyspnea, tachycardia, and dysrhythmias (Pagana and Pagana, 1997).

Table 15-8

Cardiac Studies

Procedure	Description	Assessment Specific to Test
ECG	Graphic representation of electrical impulses generated by heart during a cardiac cycle; identifies abnormalities that interfere with electrical conduction through cardiac tissue	Assess for chest pain, dyspnea, and heart rate and rhythm. Assess blood pressure, pulse, and respirations.
Exercise stress test	A noninvasive study that provides diagnostic information about the client's cardiac function	Assess client for unstable angina, aortic valvular disease, impaired lung or motor function, serious CHF, or claudication (Pagana and Pagana, 1997). Assess blood pressure, pulse, and respirations.
Dobutamine stress echocardiography	A method to evaluate ischemic heart disease by obtaining echogardiographic images while client receives titrated doses of IV dobutamine (Thompson et al., 1996)	Assess client for aortic stenosis and unstable angina, idiopathic subaortic stenosis, ventricular tachycardia, uncontrolled atrial fibrillation, systolic blood pressure greater than 180 mm Hg, pregnancy, sensitivity to dobutamine, or recent MRI (Thompson et al., 1996). Assess blood pressure, pulse, and respirations.
Cardiac nuclear scanning	A noninvasive method of recognizing alterations of left ventricular muscle function and coronary artery blood distribution (Pagana and Pagana, 1997)	Assess if client is cooperative, pregnant, has had myocardial trauma or recent nuclear scans, or is receiving long-acting nitrates (Pagana and Pagana, 1997). Assess blood pressure, pulse, and respirations.
Cardiac catheterization	Following injection of a contrast media, studies of pressure within the heart, cardiac valvular function, and patency of coronary arteries are evaluated	Assess client for allergies to iodine contrast media, inability to lie still, uncooperativeness, pregnancy, renal disorders, and abnormal coagulation findings. Assess blood pressure, pulse, and respirations.

Dobutamine stress echocardiography is a noninvasive method that combines exercise with two-dimensional echocardiography and has been found to be a good diagnostic tool for exposing suspected coronary artery disease. Dobutamine stress echocardiography involves images before, during, and after a titrated dobutamine infusion is administered (Thompson et al., 1996).

During the cardiac nuclear scan, a radiocompound material (i.e., thallium-201) is injected intravenously while a radiation detector records and photographs images of the heart to determine left ventricular muscle functioning and coronary artery blood distribution (Pagana and Pagana, 1997).

Cardiac catheterization is a specialized form of angiography in which a catheter is passed into the heart through a peripheral vein or artery, depending on whether catheterization of the right or left side of the heart is being performed (Pagana and Pagana, 1997). Pressures within the heart, cardiac volumes, valvular function, and patency of coronary arteries are studied. A contrast medium is injected and the structures and functions of the heart assessed.

Equipment

ECG

ECG machine

Electrode paste (gel)

ECG leads or electrodes

Alcohol wipes

Razor

Stress testing

Specialized equipment in a stress testing lab

Cardiac catheterization

Special packs that contain various sizes and types of catheters for performing the procedures, as well as the necessary specialized equipment, are obtained and used in the catheterization laboratory.

Goggles

IV equipment for IV start

Diazepam, midazolam, or other sedative for IV sedation

Oxygen, resuscitative equipment, pulse oximeter, cardiac monitor for IVCS

ASSESSMENT

1. Assess client's knowledge of the procedure to determine level of health teaching required.
2. Observe verbal and nonverbal behaviors to determine client's anxiety.
3. Assess client's ability to understand and follow directions. **Rationale: Procedures require client to follow directions closely and assume proper position.**
4. Assess client's ability to assume position required for procedure and ability to remain still. **Rationale: Client must maintain position without moving, to avoid complications during needle or trochar insertion (during cardiac catheterization).**
5. Assess whether client is allergic to antiseptic, anesthetic solutions, or contrast media (cardiac catheterization). **Rationale: Common allergic reactions to anesthetic agents are central nervous system depression, respiratory difficulties, and hypotension. Allergic reactions to antiseptic solutions are usually skin irritations.**
6. Assess whether client has signed consent form (check agency policy).
7. Assess client's knowledge that no postprocedural precautions need to be taken against radioactive exposure to personnel or family. **Rationale: only trace doses of radioisotopes are used (Pagana and Pagana, 1997).**
8. Assess that client has been NPO for 6 to 8 hours before the procedure (for cardiac catheterization). Check agency guidelines for specific guidelines. **Rationale: Prevents possible aspiration because client is sedated. Excessive hydration causes dilution of the contrast medium, making structures more difficult to visualize.**
9. Assess vital signs to provide baseline data for comparison with postprocedural (cardiac catheterization, stress testing) vital signs.
10. Assess client's coagulation status (use of anticoagulants, platelet count, prothrombin time) to determine factors that can increase risk of bleeding. **Rationale: Abnormal findings may contraindicate the procedure (cardiac catheterization) at that time.**

PLANNING

Expected outcomes focus on client's knowledge of the procedure, including the need to remain still (cardiac catheterization) to prevent complications or artifacts (ECG); to participate as needed to complete the test; client's anxiety regarding procedure and results; and control of discomfort during and after the procedure.

Expected Outcomes

1. Client explains purpose and basic steps of the procedure before it is begun.
2. Client verbalizes decreased fear of procedure after the nurse reviews the procedure.
3. Client assumes the correct position and remains still throughout the procedure.
4. Client participates appropriately throughout the procedure.
5. Client has no significant changes in vital signs or peripheral pulses and no allergic response.
6. Client recovers from IVCS without respiratory complications or change in level of consciousness.
7. Client has no laboratory value changes.
8. Client is able to explain appropriate positions and activity restrictions after cardiac catheterization.
9. Client has minimal discomfort.
10. Client experiences soreness at catheter insertion site and possible backache.

DELEGATION CONSIDERATIONS

Electrocardiograms are often done by technicians specifically trained for this test. Exercise stress test and cardiac catheterization are done in a specialized setting under the direction of a cardiologist and/or radiologist usually assisted by a technician. IV conscious sedation, if used, must be administered by a RN. Monitoring routine vital signs may be delegated to AP, but assessment related to complications may not. AP must be aware of the life-threatening nature of complications.

- Stable clients may be monitored by AP including baseline and postprocedure vital signs.
- Following cardiac catheterization report any evidence of bleeding including hypotension or tachycardia, or hematoma development at the catheter insertion site.
- Following the use of dye report signs of allergic reactions including itching, hives, or respiratory distress.

IMPLEMENTATION

Steps	**Rationale**

1. See Standard Protocol (inside front cover).
2. **Perform ECG (see illustration).**
   a. Cleanse and prepare skin; wipe sites with alcohol.

   Promotes adherence of leads (electrodes) to chest or extremity.

   b. Apply electrode paste and attach leads. For 12-lead ECG:

   Position of leads promotes proper display of ECG on paper.

   (1) Chest (precordial leads)
   V_1–Fourth intercostal space (ICS) at right sternal border
   V_2–Fourth ICS at left sternal border
   V_3–Midway between V_2 and V_4
   V_4–Fifth ICS at midclavicular line
   V_5–Left anterior axillary line at level of V_4 horizontally
   V_6–Left midaxillary line at level of V_4 horizontally

   (2) Extremities: one on lower portion of each extremity
   aV_R–Right wrist
   aV_L–Left wrist
   aV_F–Left ankle

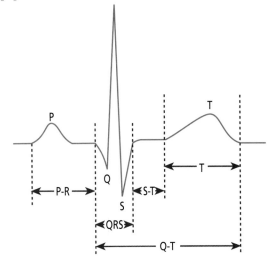

Step 2   *From Canobbio MM: Cardiovascular disorders, St Louis, 1990, Mosby.*

   c. Obtain tracing; 12-lead ECG may be obtained without removing precordial leads.

   Transfers electrocardiac conduction on ECG tracing paper for subsequent analysis by cardiologist.

   d. Disconnect leads, wipe excess electrode paste from chest, and wash hands.

   Promotes comfort and hygiene.

   e. Deliver ECG tracing to appropriate laboratory or nursing unit.

   Provides for review of ECG by cardiologist.

3. **Assist with exercise stress test.**
   a. Explain procedure to client, and obtain informed consent.
   b. Establish that client has not eaten, had fluids, or smoked for 4 hours (check agency policy for variations).
   c. Check specific orders (may vary according to agency policy) to determine if medications are to be withheld before the test.
   d. Obtain baseline vital signs.

4. **Assist with dobutamine stress test.**
   a. Obtain informed consent.
   b. Explain that the client will be receiving continuous monitoring of ECG, vital signs, pulse oximetry, and cardiac response to dobutamine (Thompson et al., 1996).
   c. Determine client's NPO status (3 to 6 hours) except for medications. Check agency policy for variations.
   d. Assist client through procedure by explanations.

COMMUNICATION TIP

Assure client that a physician usually is present during testing.

Encourage client to verbalize symptoms of chest pain, exhaustion, dyspnea, fatigue, or dizziness during the test.

COMMUNICATION TIP

Assure client that procedure is relatively complication free (Thompson et al., 1996).

Steps	Rationale

   e. Assess vital signs following procedure and compare with baseline vital signs.
   f. Prepare client for potential need for invasive cardiac testing (Thompson et al., 1996).
5. Assist with nuclear scanning.
   a. Explain procedure to client.
   b. Check agency policy to determine if short fasting period is required.
   c. Inform client that IV injection will be given in radiology department and then the scan will be performed 15 minutes to 4 hours later.
   d. Remind client to drink fluids following the test.

6. Assist with cardiac catheterization.
   a. Wash hands and apply clean gloves.
   b. For cardiac catheterization, provide IV access using large-bore cannula.
   c. Assess vital signs, obtain weight, and palpate peripheral pulses.
   d. Assist client in assuming comfortable position on x-ray table.
   e. Provide support to client throughout the procedure and as x-rays are taken, because the client may be frightened by the loud noises (Pagana and Pagana, 1997).
   f. Nurse administering IVCS monitors level of sedation and level of consciousness.
   g. Note that some clients have a tendency to cough as the catheter is placed into the pulmonary artery (Pagana and Pagana, 1997).
   h. Remove and discard gloves.
7. See Completion Protocol (inside front cover).

Aids in excretion of the radioactive substance.

> **COMMUNICATION TIP**
>
> *Tell client that the only discomfort associated with this test is the venipuncture required for injection of the radioisotope (Pagana and Pagana, 1997).*

> **COMMUNICATION TIP**
>
> *Tell client that during the injection of the dye, there may be a severe hot flash that is quite uncomfortable but lasts only a few seconds (Pagana and Pagana, 1997).*

• • •

EVALUATION
1. Ask client to describe steps of procedure.
2. Discuss anxiety and fears related to test process and results.
3. Monitor vital signs and assess peripheral pulses (compare right and left), auscultate heart and lungs if cardiac catheterizations done, and compare findings with preprocedure values.
4. Assess client for possible delayed reaction to iodine dye (if used)—dyspnea, hives, tachycardia, and rash (Pagana and Pagana, 1997); level of sedation, level of consciousness, and oxygen saturation.
5. Assess postprocedure laboratory values—CBC, prothrombin time, electrolytes, BUN, and creatinine.
6. Demonstrates correct position and activity restriction.

Unexpected Outcomes and Related Interventions
1. Client has marked changes in vital signs or peripheral pulses.
   a. Reassess to confirm findings.
   b. Follow specific postprocedural orders related to findings.
   c. Notify physician.
2. Client remains sedated with decreased respirations or blood pressure, decreased oxygen saturation, or decreased LOC.
   a. Continue monitoring as necessary.
   b. Follow specific postprocedural orders related to findings.
   c. Administer reversal agent if ordered.
   d. Notify physician.
3. Client has hematoma or hemorrhage present at catheter insertion site.

a. Apply pressure to site.
b. Follow specific postprocedural orders related to possible application of sandbag or other specific orders.
c. Notify physician.

Recording and Reporting (see Skills 15.4 and 15.6)

- Record name of procedure and laboratory where tests were sent.
- For invasive tests, record puncture site, quality of pulses, vital signs, and client's tolerance to procedure.
- Report any unexpected outcomes immediately.

Sample Documentation

1020   Returned from cardiac catheterization via stretcher. IV of 1000 ml normal saline infusing in left antecubital space at 100 ml/hr. Vital signs stable. Right groin puncture site pressure dressing remains dry and intact with sandbag in place. Right dorsalis pedis and posterior tibial pulses are 2+. Feet are warm to touch. Remains on bedrest. Voided 300 ml dark amber urine per orthopedic bedpan. Voices no complaints of pain or discomfort. Taking liquids well by mouth.

Home Care and Long-Term Care Considerations

Upon discharge, client will be instructed to contact the physician (or affiliated emergency department) if the following occurs after cardiac catheterization:

- Bleeding from the catheterization puncture site; apply gentle pressure with a clean gauze or cloth.
- Formation of a knot or lump under the skin that increases in size.
- Worsening of a bruise or its movement down the extremity rather than disappearing.
- Pain at puncture site or in the extremity used for the catheterization.
- Extremity where arterial puncture is made becomes pale and cool to touch.
- Appearance of redness, swelling, or warmth of the affected extremity.

Although bathing or showering may be allowed the day after the catheterization, the client should be cautioned to avoid slipping, because the leg (if this extremity was used) may feel stiff.

Some institutions provide written discharge instructions.

Geriatric Considerations

- Because frail older adults may be more susceptible to skin breakdown from lying in one position during this procedure, inspect bony prominences frequently.
- In the older adult, slight alterations in vital signs or behavior may be precursors to impending problems; therefore skilled observations are critical (Phipps et al., 1995).
- Older adult clients may have reduced drug clearance from decreased GFR and nephron activity or decreased hepatic function. Therefore the nurse must monitor the effects of narcotics and hypnotics that may interfere with breathing (Phipps et al., 1995).
- Offer bedpan or urinal every 2 to 3 hours in the older adult client because of age-related changes in the urinary tract.
- Be aware that NPO status in the older adult client may result in dehydration.
- Because of multiple medications the older adult client may be taking, be aware of alterations in administration schedules necessary due to NPO status for diagnostic test.

CRITICAL THINKING EXERCISES

1. Mrs. W. feared the worst when her physician recommended an MRI to test for suspected seizures. She stated, "It's not the test results I dread, it's the procedure itself. You see, I'm extremely claustrophobic." What is your response to Mrs. W?

2. The AP reports to you that Mr. X., your new admission, had a positive Hemoccult test on a stool sample. What assessments do you as the RN make on Mr. X?

3. You are to collect a clean voided specimen from your client, Mrs. W., who is an obese 76-year-old client with osteoarthritis. She is also very weak after undergoing recent chemotherapy. Describe how you would collect this specimen.

4. Mr. S. returned from the x-ray department. He had been in the process of collecting a 24-hour timed urine sample. The UAP informs you she overheard the client tell his wife that he "forgot and had to use the bathroom" while in the x-ray department. How would you respond?

REFERENCES

American Diabetes Association: 1998 Buyer's Guide to Diabetes Products, *Diabetes Forecast* 50(10): 68–71, 1997.

Beare PG, Myers JL: *Adult health nursing,* ed 3, St Louis, 1998, Mosby.

Broome ME et al: Children's medical fears, coping behaviors, and pain perceptions during a lumbar puncture, *Once Nurse Forum* 17(3):361, 1990.

Broome ME et al: The use of distraction and imagery with children during painful procedures, *Oncol Nurs Forum* 19(3):499, 1992.

Canobbio MM: *Cardiovascular disorders,* St Louis, 1990, Mosby.

Cushing M: Demystifying informed consent, *Am J Nurs* 91(11):17, 1991.

Doughty DB, Jackson DB: *Gastrointestinal disorders,* Mosby's Clinical Nursing Series, St Louis, 1993, Mosby.

Grimes D: *Infectious diseases,* Mosby's Clinical Nursing Series, St Louis, 1991, Mosby.

Heiney S: Helping children throughout painful procedures, *Am J Nurs* 91(11):20, 1991.

Occupational Safety and Health Administration: Occupational exposure to bloodborne pathogens: final rule, 29 CFR 1919: 1030, *Fed Registr* 56:64003, 1991.

Pagana KD, Pagana TJ: *Mosby's diagnostic and laboratory test reference,* St Louis, 1997, Mosby.

Phipps WJ et al, eds: Medical-surgical nursing: concepts and clinical practice, ed 5, St Louis, 1995, Mosby.

Schroeder SA et al, eds: *Current medical diagnosis and treatment,* East Norwalk, Conn, 1992, Appleton & Lange.

Society of Gastroenterology Nurses and Associates (SGNA): *Gastroenterology nursing: a core curriculum,* St Louis, 1993, Mosby.

Stanley M, Beare PG: *Gerontological nursing,* Philadelphia, 1995, FA Davis.

Thompson EJ et al: Dobutamine stress echocardiography: A new, noninvasive method for detecting ischemic heart disease, *Heart Lung* 25(2):87, 1996.

Thompson JM et al: *Mosby's clinical nursing,* ed 4, St Louis, 1997, Mosby.

Watson DS, James DS: Intravenous conscious sedation: Implications of monitoring patients receiving local anesthesia, *AORN J* 51(6):1512, 1990.

Wilkinson M: Your role in needle biopsy of the liver, *RN* 53(4):62, 1990.

Wong DL: *Whaley and Wong's nursing care of infants and children,* ed 5, St Louis, 1995, Mosby.

Wong DL: *Whaley and Wong's nursing care of infants and children,* ed 6, St Louis, 1999, Mosby.

UNIT FIVE

Administration of Medications

Chapter 16
Preparation for Medication Administration

Chapter 17
Administration of Non-Parenteral Medication

Chapter 18
Administration of Injections

CHAPTER 16

Preparation for Medication Administration

Safe and accurate administration of medications is one of the nurse's most important responsibilities. The nurse is responsible for understanding the action of the medication, dosage, desired effects, and possible adverse reactions. The nurse uses the nursing process as a framework for nursing care related to medication administration. This includes assessment and planning to identify the need for and effectiveness of medications. Nursing diagnoses help communicate concerns related to drug therapy and direct interventions for appropriate nursing care. Implementation includes administering drugs correctly, monitoring the client's response, and in many cases teaching the client how to self-administer drugs safely with an appropriate knowledge base. Evaluation involves continued monitoring of drug effectiveness. This chapter includes basic information needed when preparing to administer medications. Subsequent chapters address administration of non-parenteral medications and injections.

DRUG EFFECTS

When administering medications the nurse needs to know both the mechanism of action and the therapeutic effects of the drugs. The therapeutic effects of drugs include health maintenance, disease prevention and treatment, diagnosis, and cure. It is also important for the nurse to know possible side effects, adverse reactions, and toxic effects.

Mechanism of Action

When a drug is administered to a client, a predictable chemical reaction is expected that changes the physiological activity of the body. This most commonly occurs as the medication bonds chemically at a specific site called a *receptor site*. The reactions are possible only when the receptor site and the chemical can fit together like a key in a lock. When the chemical fits well, the chemical response is good. We call these drugs *agonists* (Skidmore-Roth, 1999). Some drugs attach at the receptor site but do not produce a new chemical reaction. These drugs are called *antagonists*. Other drugs attach and produce only a small response or prevent other reactions from occurring. These drugs are called *partial agonists* (Box 16-1).

DRUG ACTIONS

Pharmacokinetics is the study of how drugs enter the body, reach the site of action, and are metabolized and excreted from the body. *Absorption* describes how a drug enters the body and passes into body fluids and tissues and influences route of administration. *Distribution* refers to the ways drugs move to the sites of action in the body. *Metabolism* refers to the chemical reactions by which medication is broken down until it becomes chemically inactive. *Excretion* refers to the process of excretion or elimination from the body via the gastrointestinal tract, kidneys, or other body secretions (Skidmore-Roth, 1999).

A drug dose response includes onset of drug action, peak (its highest effective concentration), and duration of action (length of time the drug is present in a concentration great enough to produce a response). This information is useful in planning drug administration schedules. Most agencies have standard administration schedules (see Abbreviations and Equivalents, Appendix B) and allow for administration of the drug one half hour before or after the scheduled time without concern for altering the effectiveness of the medication. Some medications are ordered to be given as needed (prn) within certain parameters prescribed by the physician.

Box 16-1 Mechanisms of Action

Agonist: Chemical fits receptor site well; chemical response is good.
Antagonist: Drug attaches at a receptor site and then is chemically inactive; no drug response.
Partial Agonist: Drug attaches at a receptor site, and a slight chemical action is produced.

Data from Skidmore-Roth L, McKenry: *Mosby's drug guide for nurses,* ed 3, St Louis, 1999, Mosby.

Therapeutic Effects

A single medication may have many therapeutic effects. For example, aspirin creates analgesia, reduces inflammation of arthritis, reduces fever, and reduces clot formation. Other drugs have more specific therapeutic effects. For example, an antihypertensive medication has a therapeutic effect of controlling hypertension. Antibiotics are prescribed to treat a bacterial infection.

Side Effects

Predictably, a drug causes unintended secondary effects. **Side effects** may be harmless or injurious. In the example of codeine phosphate, a client may experience constipation. If the side effects are serious enough to outweigh the beneficial effects of a drug's therapeutic action, the prescriber may discontinue the drug. Clients may stop taking medications because of side effects.

Toxic Effects

After prolonged intake of high doses of medication, ingestion of drugs intended for external application, or when a drug accumulates in the blood because of impaired metabolism or excretion, a toxic effect may develop. **Toxic effects** may be lethal, depending on the drug's action. For example, morphine, a narcotic analgesic, relieves pain by depressing the central nervous system. However, toxic levels of morphine cause severe respiratory depression and death.

Idiosyncratic Reactions

Medications may cause unpredictable effects, such as an **idiosyncratic reaction** in which a client overreacts or underreacts to a drug or has a reaction different from normal. Predicting which clients will have an idiosyncratic response is impossible. For example, lorazepam, an antianxiety medication, when given to the older adult may cause agitation and delirium.

Table 16-1

Mild Allergic Reactions

Symptom	Description
Urticaria (hives)	Raised, irregularly shaped skin eruptions with varying sizes and shapes; eruptions have reddened margins and pale centers.
Eczema (rash)	Small, raised vesicles that are usually reddened; often distributed over the entire body.
Pruritus	Itching of the skin; accompanies most rashes.
Rhinitis	Inflammation of mucous membranes lining the nose, causing swelling and a clear watery discharge.
Wheezing	Constriction of smooth muscles surrounding bronchioles that decreases diameter of airways; occurs primarily on inspiration because of severely narrowed airways; development of edema in pharynx and larynx further obstructs airflow.

Allergic Reactions

Allergic reaction is another unpredictable response to a drug. Exposure to an initial dose of a medication may cause an immunological response. The drug acts as an antigen, which causes antibodies to be produced. With repeated administration the client develops an allergic response to the drug, its chemical preservatives, or a metabolite of it.

An allergic reaction may be mild or severe. Allergic symptoms vary, depending on the client and the drug. Among the different classes of drugs, antibiotics cause a high incidence of allergic reactions. Common, mild allergy symptoms are summarized in Table 16-1. Severe, or **anaphylactic,** reactions are characterized by sudden constriction of bronchiolar muscles, edema of the pharynx and larynx, and severe wheezing and shortness of breath. The client may become severely hypotensive, necessitating emergency resuscitation measures (Box 16-2, p. 406).

It is common practice for clients who are hospitalized and have a known drug allergy to have this information recorded in a clearly identifiable place so that it is easily seen by all those involved in the client's care. In many institutions this information is often recorded on the front of the client's medical record on an eye-catching sticker. Client allergies should always be recorded on the client's medication administration record. Clients cared for in other settings (e.g., home) and who have a known history of an allergy to a medication should be encouraged to

Box 16-2 Severe Allergic Reactions with Anaphylactic Shock

Constriction of bronchioles with wheezing
Edema of pharynx and larynx
Shortness of breath
Severe hypotension
In severe cases, may result in death

wear an identification bracelet or medal, which alerts all health care providers to the allergies in case the client is unconscious when receiving medical care.

Drug Tolerance and Dependence

Drug tolerance occurs when clients receive the same drug for long periods of time and require higher doses to produce the same effect. Clients who are taking various pain medications may develop tolerance over time.

Generally, clients hospitalized for acute episodes of illness do not develop tolerance. It may take a month or even longer for this phenomenon to occur (McCaffery and Ferrell, 1994). Drug tolerance is not the same as drug dependence. Two types of **drug dependence** exist: psychological (or addiction) and physical. In psychological dependence the client desires the medication for some benefit other than the intended effect. Physical dependence implies that a client will suffer some ill effect if the medication is not given. When clients receive medications for a short term (such as for postoperative pain), dependence is rare (McCaffery and Ferrell, 1994).

Drug Interactions

When one drug modifies the action of another drug, a **drug interaction** occurs. Drug interactions are common in individuals taking many medications. A drug may potentiate or diminish the action of other drugs and may alter the way in which another drug is absorbed, metabolized, or eliminated from the body.

When two drugs are given simultaneously, they can have a synergistic or additive effect. With a **synergistic reaction** the physiological action of the two drugs in combination is greater than the effect of the drugs when given separately. Alcohol is a central nervous system depressant that has a synergistic effect on antihistamines, antidepressants, and narcotic analgesics.

A drug interaction is not always undesirable. Often a physician orders combination drug therapy to create a drug interaction for therapeutic benefit. For example, a client with moderate hypertension typically receives sev-

eral drugs, such as diuretics and vasodilators, that act together to keep blood pressure at a desirable level.

Drug Dose Responses

After the nurse administers a drug, it undergoes absorption, distribution, metabolism, and excretion. These processes determine how much of the administered dose reaches the site of action. These processes are influenced by many things such as body surface area, body water content, body fat content, and protein stores.

When certain medications such as antibiotics are prescribed, the goal is to achieve a constant drug blood level within a safe therapeutic range. The client and nurse must follow regular dosage schedules and administer prescribed doses at correct intervals. Knowledge of the following time intervals of drug action also helps to anticipate a drug's effect:

1. **Onset of drug action**—Time it takes after a drug is administered for it to produce a response.
2. **Peak action**—Time it takes for a drug to reach its highest effective concentration.
3. **Duration of action**—Length of time during which the drug is present in a concentration great enough to produce a response.
4. **Plateau**—Blood serum concentration reached and maintained after repeated, fixed doses.

The therapeutic levels of certain drugs, such as antibiotics, can be monitored by laboratory testing. A blood sample is drawn to identify the peak serum level of a drug, which varies according to the specific drug involved. Blood samples for trough levels, or the lowest serum levels, are usually drawn just before the next scheduled dose of medication. Precise coordination with the laboratory is essential for obtaining meaningful information. These data allow physicians to modify drug dosages.

Routes of Administration

The route chosen for administering a drug depends on its properties and desired effect and on the client's physical and mental condition. The nurse is often the best person to judge the route most desirable for a client. Table 16-2 summarizes the routes of drug administration.

Receiving Medication Orders

A physician's order is required for all medications to be administered by the nurse (except in states where Nurse Practice Acts allow advanced practice nurses and nurse practitioners to prescribe in specific situations).

Table 16-2

Routes of Drug Administration

NON-PARENTERAL

Oral	By mouth
Sublingual	Under the tongue
Topical	On the skin (as a cream or patch), and eye/ear drops
Suppository	Into the rectum or vagina

PARENTERAL

Intramuscular	Into the muscle
Subcutaneous	Into the subcutaneous tissue
Intradermal	Into the dermis
Intravenous	Into the vein

3. The form (e.g., tabs).
4. The route (e.g., PO [by mouth]).
5. The frequency (e.g., q4h [every 4 hours]).
6. Orders for drugs to be given prn also include the reason they are to be given (e.g., for pain).
7. The signature of the prescriber.

Verbal orders and telephone orders are orders received by the nurse and written on the physician's order sheet. The name of the prescriber and the name of the nurse are included, and generally these orders are cosigned by the provider within 24 hours. In many settings there are "routine physician's orders," which are preprinted and individualized according to the client's history and circumstances. In the long-term care setting there also are "standing orders" that can be implemented when appropriate, for example, if a client needs a laxative.

A physician's order sheet (Figure 16-1) is usually a carbon form on which the physician writes the date, time, and drug order, including:

1. The name of the drug, which may be either the trade name (e.g., Percocet) or the generic name (e.g., oxycodone).
2. The dose (e.g., 5 mg).

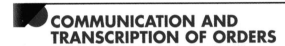

COMMUNICATION AND TRANSCRIPTION OF ORDERS

After new medication orders are written, the drugs must be obtained from the pharmacy. Usually the carbon copy of the physician's order sheet is sent to the pharmacy. The

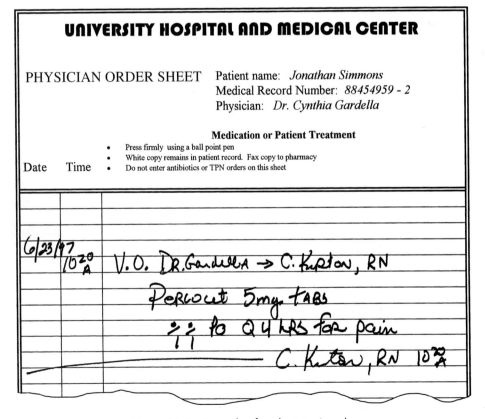

Figure 16-1 Example of a physician's order.

pharmacist is responsible for providing the correct medications and delivering them to the nursing unit.

Unit Dose System

In acute care settings each client on the nursing unit has a medication bin or drawer that contains all the medications for a 24-hour period. Many times this is in a medication cart that can be pushed from room to room to facilitate administration of medications at routine times. The cart is kept locked when not attended. In some settings the medications are kept in a locked cabinet in the client's room.

Some drugs may be distributed as floor stock. **Floor stock** are medications that are distributed to the nursing unit in bulk (either individually wrapped or in bottles). Generally, medications that are appropriate for floor stock are those that are routinely prescribed or prescribed on a prn basis. Examples of these medications are stool softeners, antacids, and antipyretics. Newer medication dispensing systems, such as computer-assisted or electronic devices, are variations of unit dose and floor stock systems. For example, the Pyxis Corporation designs the MedStation. This system can carry a variety of medications, housed in individual compartments that are accessed by the nurse after requesting the medication from a computerized screen. Medications that are frequently used, such as floor stock medications and narcotics, are often housed in the MedStation. All medications retrieved from the MedStation are recorded in the system's computer. Baxter Healthcare Corporation manufactures the Sure-Med Unit Dose Center, which provides single doses of floor stock medications.

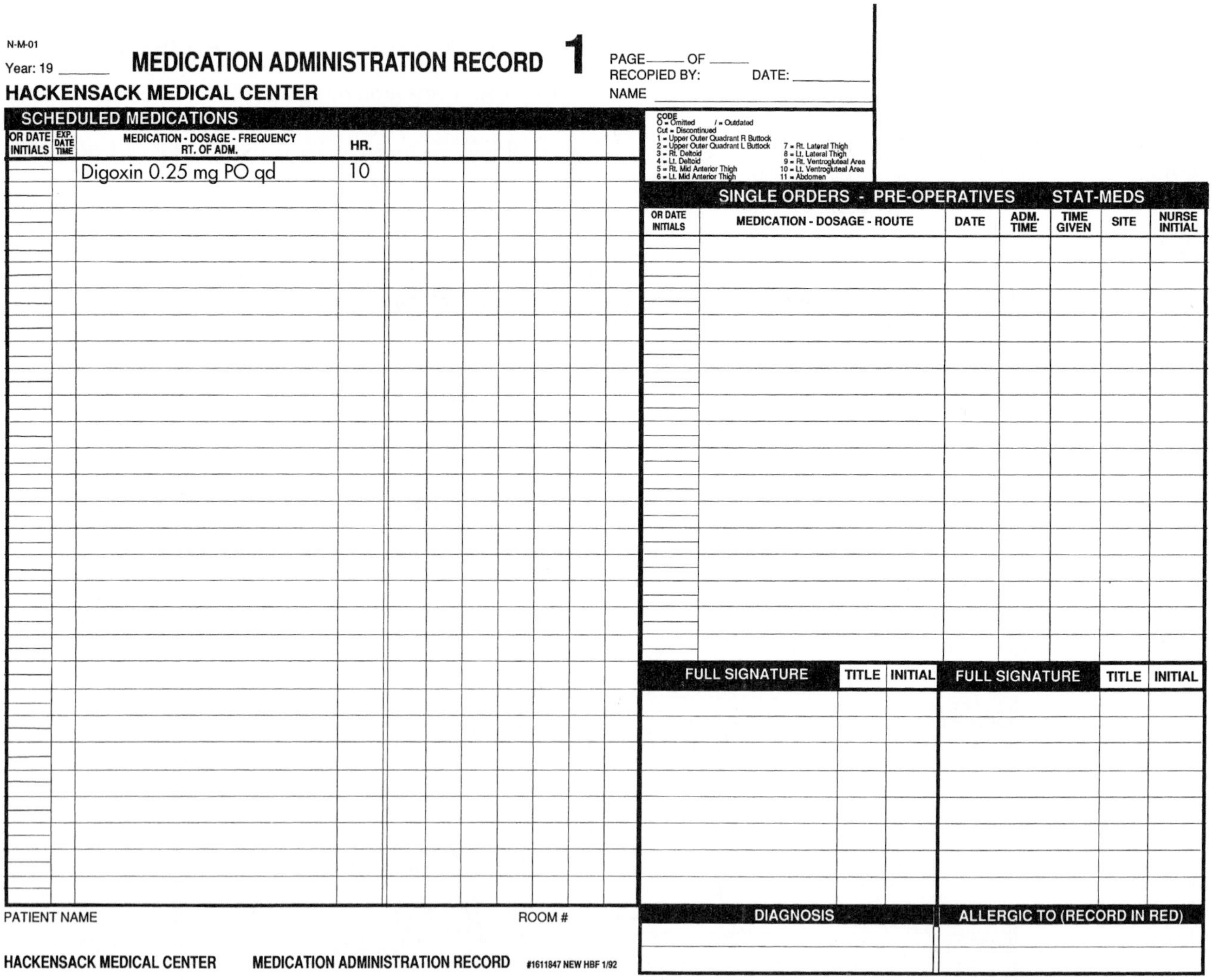
N-M-01
Year: 19 ____
MEDICATION ADMINISTRATION RECORD 1
HACKENSACK MEDICAL CENTER
PAGE ____ OF ____
RECOPIED BY: DATE: ____
NAME ____

SCHEDULED MEDICATIONS

OR DATE INITIALS	EXP. DATE TIME	MEDICATION - DOSAGE - FREQUENCY RT. OF ADM.	HR.
		Digoxin 0.25 mg PO qd	10

CODE
O = Omitted / = Outdated
Cut = Discontinued
1 = Upper Outer Quadrant R Buttock
2 = Upper Outer Quadrant L Buttock
3 = Rt. Deltoid
4 = Lt. Deltoid
5 = Rt. Mid Anterior Thigh
6 = Lt. Mid Anterior Thigh
7 = Rt. Lateral Thigh
8 = Lt. Lateral Thigh
9 = Rt. Ventrogluteal Area
10 = Lt. Ventrogluteal Area
11 = Abdomen

SINGLE ORDERS - PRE-OPERATIVES STAT-MEDS

OR DATE INITIALS	MEDICATION - DOSAGE - ROUTE	DATE	ADM. TIME	TIME GIVEN	SITE	NURSE INITIAL

FULL SIGNATURE	TITLE	INITIAL	FULL SIGNATURE	TITLE	INITIAL

PATIENT NAME ROOM #
DIAGNOSIS
ALLERGIC TO (RECORD IN RED)
HACKENSACK MEDICAL CENTER MEDICATION ADMINISTRATION RECORD #1611847 NEW HBF 1/92

Figure 16-2 Medication administration record. *Courtesy Hackensack University Medical Center, Hackensack, NJ.*

Medication Administration Record

A **medication administration record (MAR)** is a form used to verify that the right medications are being administered at the correct times (Figure 16-2). Every 24 hours an MAR is distributed for each client for that day (Figure 16-3, p. 410). The nurse is responsible for verifying that the MAR is accurate and up-to-date by comparing each medication to the original order, including drug name, dose, route of administration, and times to be given. If a medication is to be given before the computer printout is available, the nurse or a designated unit secretary writes the complete order on the MAR. The nurse who checks all transcribed orders is responsible for accuracy. If an order seems incorrect or inappropriate, the nurse needs to consult the prescriber. The nurse who gives the wrong medication or an incorrect dosage is legally responsible for the error.

The "Five Rights"

Preparing and administering medications requires accuracy and the full attention of the nurse. The *five "rights"* is a traditional checklist to promote accuracy in drug administration (Box 16-3).

Box 16-3 Five "Rights" for Administration of Medication

- Right drug
- Right dose
- Right client
- Right route
- Right time

Figure 16-2, cont'd   Medication administration record.

```
6900A-3277      THE BARNES-JEWISH HOSPITAL OF ST. LOUIS
                12:00 NN SCHEDULED MEDICATIONS DUE 6900A     03/26/00
                                              ISSUED 10:15 AM 03/26


     6901-1                                                     GIV NGIV


     HEPARIN SODIUM HEPARIN (FOR IV CATHETER IRRIGATION), (10
     UNITS/ML) 30ML VIAL, 1ML, IV PUSH, Q6H (12-6), (03/22/00
     06PM-..)                                                  --- ---


     6903-1                                                     GIV NGIV


     CEFOTAN CEFOTETAN DISODIUM INJ 1GM/10ML,   IV PIGGYBACK,
     Q12H (12-12), (03/25/00 12MN-..)                          --- ---

     HEPARIN SODIUM HEPARIN (FOR IV CATHETER IRRIGATION), (10
     UNITS/ML) 30ML VIAL, 3ML, IV PUSH, Q6H (12-6), (03/26/00
     06AM-..)                                                  --- ---


     6905-1                                                     GIV NGIV


     LACRILUBE OPHTHALMIC OINTMENT BOTH EYES(OU), Q4H (4-8-12-4-8-
     12), (03/16/00 12MN-..)                                   --- ---


     6907-1                                                     GIV NGIV


     REGLAN METOCLOPRAMIDE TAB, 10MG,, PO, Q6H (12-6), (03/26/00
     12MN-..)                                                  --- ---
```

Figure 16-3 Computer list of ordered medications. *Courtesy Barnes-Jewish Hospital, St Louis, Mo.*

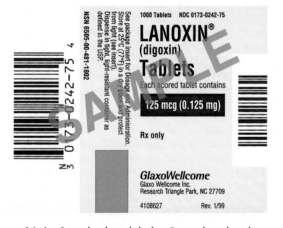

Figure 16-4 Sample drug label. *Reproduced with permission of Glaxo Welcome, Inc., Research Triangle Park, California.*

Right Drug. The nurse is responsible for verifying that the order was accurately transcribed. In many hospitals this verification is routinely done by a registered nurse (RN) on the night shift when a printed MAR is delivered to the unit for each client. It also is done by a registered nurse when new orders are handwritten on the MAR. When this is done, the MAR is initialed and signed by the RN. The nurse is also responsible for knowing the action and therapeutic effects of the drug.

The nurse compares the label of the drug with the MAR at least 3 times: (1) Before removing the drug from the storage bin; (2) before placing the drug in the medicine cup for distribution; and again (3) before giving the drug to the client. If the drug is ordered by trade name and dispensed from the pharmacy by generic name, the nurse must verify that there is no discrepancy (Figure 16-4).

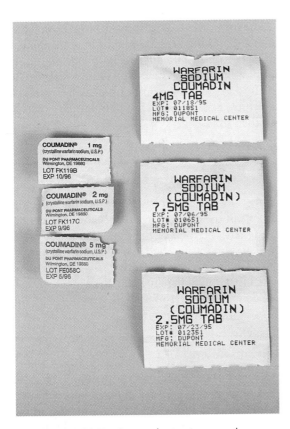

Figure 16-5   Coumadin in six strengths.

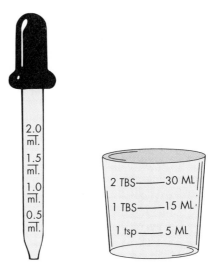

Figure 16-6   Scaled dropper for pediatric use and cup to measure oral liquids.   *From Clayton BD, Stock YN: Basic pharmacology for nurses, ed 11, St Louis, 1997, Mosby.*

If a client questions the medication, stop and recheck to be certain there is no mistake. In most cases the drug order has been changed or is manufactured by a different company than the client has been using at home. Sometimes, however, attention to a client's question is how errors are identified and prevented.

Right Dose. When a medication must be prepared from a dose other than what is ordered, the chance of errors increases. After calculating the dose, having a second nurse check the calculations is recommended, especially if it is an unusual calculation or involves a potentially toxic drug, such as coumarin (an anticoagulant preparation that can be life threatening if incorrect dose is given). Coumarin is available in a variety of strengths (Figure 16-5).

After calculating dosages, the nurse preparing the medication needs to use appropriate measuring devices. Liquid preparations may be measured using a medicine cup marked in ml (cc) or a syringe for oral use. Some pediatric medications come with a scaled dropper (Figure 16-6).

Right Client. To identify clients correctly, the nurse checks the MAR against the client's identification (ID) bracelet and asks the client to state his or her full name. In some agencies the nurse also compares the medical record number on the MAR with the ID bracelet. When student

nurses are caring for one client, this process may seem awkward; however, when a nurse is giving medications to many clients, this practice is invaluable. This is essential even after caring for the same client for several days. By forming this identification routine systematically *every single time,* it will become a good habit that can prevent serious medication errors. If the client questions the practice, the nurse should explain that this is the routine practice for making sure the client is getting the correct medication.

Right Route. The prescriber's order must designate a route of administration. If the route of administration is missing or if the specified route is not the recommended route, the nurse must consult the prescriber immediately.

When injections are administered, the nurse must use only preparations intended for parenteral use. Injection of a liquid intended for oral use can produce local complications, such as sterile abcess, or fatal systemic effects. Medication companies label parenteral medication "for injectable use only."

Right Time. Each agency has routine time schedules for medications ordered at standard intervals. For example, medications to be given tid (3 times a day) may be routinely scheduled for 0800, 1400, and 2000, or 0900, 1300, and 1900, depending on the agency policy. A drug may also be ordered q8h (every 8 hours), which is also 3 times a day; however, the medication ordered q8h needs to be given around the clock to maintain adequate therapeutic levels and would, for example, be given at 0800, 1600, and 2400. All routinely ordered medications should be given within 30 minutes before or after the scheduled time; however, nursing judgment may allow some variance, depending on the medication involved.

The medication may also be ordered for special circumstances. A preoperative medication may be ordered "Stat" (to be given immediately), "Now," which means as soon as available, usually within an hour, or "on call," which means the operating room will notify the nurse when it is the appropriate time. A drug may be ordered ac (before meals) or pc (after meals).

Some medications require the nurse's clinical judgment in determining the appropriate time. When a prn analgesic is ordered "q3–4h" the nurse needs to assess the characteristics and severity of the pain to determine whether it is given every 3 hours or less frequently. It is important to teach the client to ask for the medication when they are beginning to feel discomfort. If the client waits until the pain is severe, the medication may not be effective. A prn medication at hs (bedtime) should be given when the client is prepared for sleep.

PREPARING FOR MEDICATION ADMINISTRATION

It is legally advisable to administer only medications personally prepared. Administering a drug prepared by another nurse greatly increases the opportunity for error. The nurse who gives the wrong medication or an incorrect dose is legally responsible for the error. Physicians may order a drug using the trade name, and the pharmacist may dispense it using the generic name. Many drugs have both names on the label. The importance of checking similar names and verifying for the correct drug cannot be overemphasized.

Some medications are also available in both tablets or capsules and in liquid form. Liquid forms are appropriate when the client has difficulty swallowing or must be given medications via a nasogastric (NG) tube or gastric (G) tube (see Skill 33.2). Liquid medications include elixirs, suspensions, syrups, and tinctures. Liquids are more quickly absorbed than solids.

Interpreting Drug Labels

Drug labels include seven basic pieces of information: the trade name of the drug in large letters, the generic name in smaller letters, the form of the drug, the dosage, the expiration date, the lot number, and the name of the manufacturer. The trade name given by the manufacturer often suggests the action of the drug, and the generic name is the chemical name (Figure 16-7).

Conversions

Drugs are not always dispensed in the unit of measure in which they are ordered. Drug companies package and bottle certain standard equivalents. The nurse often must convert available units of volume and weight to desired dosages or vice versa. The nurse must know approximate equivalents in all of the measurement systems or make use of conversion tables. An example follows:

The nurse receives an order: vancomycin 1 gram IV.
The pharmacy supplies: vancomycin in 500 mg vials.
Because the drug dose on the drug label is in milligrams, conversion should be from grams to milligrams.

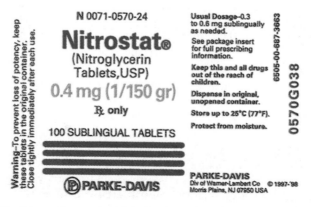

Figure 16-7   Interpreting a drug label.   *Reproduced with permission of Warner-Lambert Company.*

SYSTEMS OF DRUG MEASUREMENT

The proper administration of medication depends on the nurse's ability to compute drug dosages accurately and measure medications correctly. A careless mistake in placing a decimal point or adding a zero to a dosage can lead to a fatal error. The prescriber and client depend on the nurse to check the dosage before administering a drug. The most common system used in the measurement of medications is the metric system. The apothecary and household systems can also be used.

Metric System

As a decimal system, the metric system is the most logically organized of the measurement systems. Each basic unit of measure is organized into units of 10. Multiplying or dividing by 10 forms secondary units. In multiplication, the decimal point moves to the right; in division, the decimal moves to the left.

The basic units of measure in the metric system are the meter (length), the liter (volume), and the gram (weight). For drug calculations the nurse uses primarily volume and weight units. In the metric system small or large letters are used to designate the basic units:

> Gram = g or Gm
> Liter = 1 or L

Small letters are abbreviations for subdivisions of major units:

> Milligram = mg
> Milliliter = ml

Apothecary System

The apothecary system is one of the oldest systems of measurement. It is seldom used; however, some drug companies still include the apothecary measure in addition to the metric. The basic units of measure in the apothecary system include weight (grains) and volume (minims, drams, and ounces). The measures used in this system are approximates, and a 10% variance has become acceptable in preparation and administration of most medications. The apothecary system often uses roman numerals and fractions. The symbol "ss" is used for the fraction ½. Unlike the metric system, in the apothecary system the abbreviation or symbol for a unit of measure is written before the amount or quantity.

Household Measurements

Household measures are familiar to most people and are used when more accurate systems of measure are unnecessary. Included in household measures are drops, teaspoons, tablespoons, cups, and glasses for volume; and ounces and pounds for weight.

Prior to the actual administration of medication, the nurse may need to carry out several steps, namely, conversion of units within a system or between systems and calculation of drug dosages (Box 16-4).

NURSE ALERT

Drugs ordered in units and milliequivalents are not convertible to metric, apothecary, or household measurements

Dosage Calculations

Dosage calculations are necessary when the dose on the drug label differs from the dosage ordered. There are several methods used for calculating dosages. The most common methods are ratio-proportion or use of a formula. Dimensional analysis is becoming a popular method for dosage calculation because it involves simple multiplication and division and does not require algebra (Box 16-5, p. 414).

Box 16-4 Approximate Equivalents

> 1 gr* = 60 mg
> 1 g = 1000 mg
> 1000 mcg (μg) = 1 mg
> 1 kg = 2.2 lb
> 1 mL or ml (1 cc) = 15–16 minims*
> 5 mL = 1 tsp†
> 3 tsp = 1 tbs†
> 30 mL = 1 oz†
> 1000 mL = 1 L

*Apothecary measure.
†Household measure.

Box 16-5 Dimensional Analysis

Step 1. Identify the starting factor (amount ordered), which is the first item of the equation, and the answer label (tablets, capsules, or ml), which is the last item.

Step 2. Identify appropriate equivalents with a 1:1 ratio (e.g., 1 g = 1000 mg). Set up the equation so that labels can be canceled; for example, if mg is in the numerator, mg must be in the denominator to cancel.

Step 3. Solve the equation.
  a. Cancel labels first; the answer label should not cancel.
  b. Reduce numbers to lowest terms.
  c. Multiply/divide to solve equation.
  d. Reduce answer to lowest terms, convert to decimal, and round to a measurable quantity.

$$\text{Starting factor} \times \frac{\text{Equivalent}}{\text{Equivalent}} = \text{Answer label}$$

Example 1
When the dose ordered has the same label as the dose available:

Step 1. The starting factor is 0.5 g.
The answer label is tablets; that is, How many tablets should be given?

Step 2. Formulate the conversion equation:
The equivalent needed is 1 tablet = 0.25 g.

$$\frac{0.5 \text{ g}}{1} \times \frac{1 \text{ tab}}{0.25 \text{ g}} = 2 \text{ tabs}$$

Cancel labels (g).
NOTE: if properly written, all labels except the answer label will cancel.

Step 3. Solving the equation:
Reduce the numerical values and multiply the numerators and the denominators.

$$\frac{\overset{2}{\cancel{0.5 \text{ g}}}}{1} \times \frac{1 \text{ tab}}{\cancel{0.25 \text{ g}}} = 2 \text{ tabs}$$

Example 2
When the dose ordered has a different label than the dose available.

Dose ordered: 0.5 g
Tablets available: 250 mg per tablet

Step 1. The starting factor is 0.5 g.
The answer label is tablets: that is, How many tablets should be given?

Step 2. Formulate the conversion equation:
The equivalents needed are 1 g = 1000 mg and 1 tab = 250 mg.

$$\frac{0.5 \text{ g}}{1} \times \frac{1000 \text{ mg}}{1 \text{ g}} \times \frac{1 \text{ tab}}{250 \text{ mg}} = 2 \text{ tabs}$$

Cancel labels (g. mg).

Step 3. Solve the equation:
Reduce the values and multiply the numerators and the denominators

$$\cancel{0.5 \text{ g}} \times \frac{\overset{4}{\cancel{1000 \text{ mg}}}}{\underset{2}{\cancel{1 \text{ g}}}} \times \frac{1 \text{ tab}}{\cancel{250 \text{ mg}}} = \frac{4}{2} = 2 \text{ tabs}$$

Example 3
When the dose ordered is available in a liquid form.

Dose ordered: Keflex 250 mg PO
Available: 125 mg per 5 ml

Step 1. The starting factor is 250 mg.
The answer label is ml.

Step 2. Formulate the conversion equation:

$$\frac{250 \text{ mg}}{1} \times \frac{5 \text{ ml}}{125 \text{ mg}} = \text{ml}$$

Cancel labels (mg).

Step 3. Solve the equation:
Reduce and multiply

$$\frac{\overset{2}{\cancel{250 \text{ mg}}}}{1} \times \frac{5 \text{ ml}}{\cancel{125 \text{ mg}}} = 10 \text{ ml}$$

Example 4
When dosage is ordered based on body suface area (commonly done for pediatric dosages). The body surface area is estimated on the basis of weight, using standard charts or nomogram. The formula is a ratio of the child's body surface area compared with the body surface area of an average adult (1.7 square meters, or 1.7 m²).

$$\text{Child's dose} = \frac{\text{Surface area of child}}{1.7 \text{ m}^2} \times \text{Normal adult dose}$$

Physician orders ampicillin for a child weighing 12 kg, and the nomogram chart shows that the body surface area is 0.54 m². The normal single dose is 250 mg.

1) $\text{Child's dose} = \dfrac{0.54 \text{ m}^2}{1.7 \text{ m}^2} \times 250 \text{ mg}$

2) The m² units cancel out and can be ignored.

3) $\text{Child's dose} = \dfrac{0.54}{1.7} \times 250 \text{ mg}$

$$0.3 \times 250 \text{ mg} = 75 \text{ mg}$$

$$\text{Child's dose} = 75 \text{ mg}$$

NURSING PROCESS AND MEDICATIONS

The nurse's role extends beyond simply giving drugs to a client. The nurse is responsible for monitoring clients' responses to medications, providing education to the client and family about the medication regimen, and informing the physician when medications are effective, ineffective, or no longer necessary. The nurse uses the nursing process to integrate drug therapy into client care.

ASSESSMENT

Nursing assessment relating to drug therapy includes a history of allergies to medication. In acute care settings clients wear identification bands listing medication allergies, and allergies are conspicuously noted on the front of the chart as well as on the MAR. It is important to differentiate between allergies, such as anaphylactic shock, which can be life threatening, and drug intolerances, such as nausea and vomiting, which are uncomfortable side effects.

Nursing assessment also involves identifying drugs the client takes every day at home, including the name, purpose, dosage, route, and side effects. Often clients take many drugs and carry a list that includes this information. Clients have different levels of understanding. One client may describe a diuretic as a "water pill," whereas another describes it as a drug to minimize swelling and lower blood pressure. Still another may describe it as "the little white pill I take in the morning." By assessing the client's level of knowledge, the nurse determines the need for teaching. If a client is unable to understand or remember pertinent information, it may be necessary to involve a family member.

NURSING DIAGNOSIS

Nursing diagnoses may be identified based on therapeutic effects or side effects of specific prescribed medications or factors affecting the client's ability to self-administer drugs.

Ineffective Management of Therapeutic Regimen may be related to a knowledge deficit of the purpose of prescribed medications, the complexity of a drug schedule, or unpleasant side effects. **Health-Seeking Behaviors** is a useful nursing diagnosis when clients have a knowledge deficit and want to learn how to provide self-medication. **Noncompliance** involves a person's informed decision not to adhere to a therapeutic regime of medication administration, which may be related to economic, cultural or spiritual beliefs. Certain medications, such as chemotherapeutic agents, steroids, and anticoagulants, may contribute to **Altered Protection,** in which the client's ability to re-spond normally to infection or bleeding is decreased. **Sensory/Perceptual Alteration** may be appropriate in client's receiving eye or ear medications.

PLANNING

When a nurse assumes responsibility for administering medications, the following general goals should be met:

1. Achievement of the therapeutic effect of the prescribed medication.
2. Absence of complications related to the prescribed medication.
3. Client and/or family understanding of drug therapy.

IMPLEMENTATION

Nursing interventions focus on safe and effective drug administration. This includes careful drug preparation, accurate and timely administration, and client education.

Preadministration Activities

1. Identifying the drug action and purpose, side effects, and nursing implications for administering and monitoring. Ensure that the medication order has not expired.
2. Completing appropriate assessments, which may include and are not limited to vital signs, laboratory data, or nature and severity of symptoms. If data contraindicates medication administration, the drug should be withheld and the prescriber notified.
3. Calculate drug doses accurately and use appropriate measuring devices. Verify that the dose prescribed is appropriate for the client situation.
4. Give medications within 30 minutes before or after the scheduled time to maintain a therapeutic level. NOTE: Medications ordered STAT should be given immediately. Preoperative medications may be ordered "on call," and are given when the operating room personnel notify the nurse of the appropriate

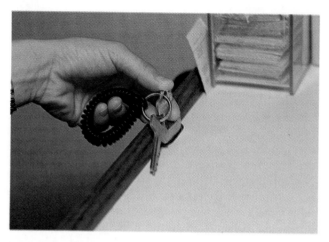

Figure 16-8 Medication carts must be kept locked when unattended.

time. Certain drugs, such as insulin, should be given at a precise interval before a meal, whereas others should be given with meals or on an empty stomach.

5. Use good handwashing technique for non-parenteral medications. Avoid touching tablets and capsules. Use sterile technique for parenteral medications.

6. Administer only those medications you personally prepare. Do not ask another person to administer drugs you prepare. Keep drugs secure (Figure 16-8).

7. When preparing medications be sure label is clear and legible and that the drug is properly mixed, has not changed in color, clarity, or consistency, and has not expired.

8. Tablets and capsules should be kept in their wrappers and opened at the client's bedside. This allows the nurse to review each drug with the client. If a client refuses medication, there is no question about which one should be withheld.

Drug Administration

1. Follow the five "rights" for medication administration (see Box 16-3 on p. 409).

2. Inform the client of each drug's name, purpose, action, and potential side effects. Evaluate the client's knowledge of the drug and provide appropriate teaching.

3. Remain with the client until the medication is taken. Provide assistance as necessary. Do not leave medication at the bedside without a prescriber's order to do so. For example, some clients may take their own vitamins or birth control pills while in the hospital.

4. Respect the client's right to refuse medication. If the medication wrapper is intact, the medication may be returned to the client's storage bin. When medication is refused, determine the reason for this, and take action accordingly. If, for example, the client has unpleasant side effects, it may be possible to

eliminate them by giving the pills with food or using a different time schedule. Refusal of medications must be documented, and the physician is notified within 24 hours.

Postadministration Activities

1. Record medications immediately according to agency policy, including drug name, dose, route, time, and signature of person administering the drug.

2. Document data pertinent to the client's response. This is particularly important when giving drugs ordered prn.

3. If a drug is refused, document that it was not given and the reason for the refusal.

EVALUATION

1. Monitor for evidence of therapeutic effects, side effects, and adverse reactions. This may involve monitoring physical response (e.g., heart rhythm, blood pressure, urine output, relief of symptoms) or laboratory results.

2. Observe injection sites for bruises, inflammation, localized pain, numbness, or bleeding.

3. Evaluate client's understanding of drug therapy and ability to self-administer medication.

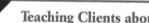

CLIENT AND FAMILY TEACHING

A properly informed client is more likely to take medications correctly. The nurse provides information about the purpose of medications, their actions, side effects, dosage schedules, and actions to take in case side or toxic effects develop. Special instructional booklets or leaflets are often available as teaching aids (Box 16-6). When teaching clients about their medications it is best to include persons identified as being significant to the client's recovery. This may include family members, partners, or home care providers.

Teaching Clients about Side Effects

All medications have side effects. The nurse teaches the client and family members about side effects associated with each medication prescribed. Because medications can have many side effects, teaching the client about all of them can overwhelm the client and impede learning; remember, client learning is a continual process. When beginning to teach a client about a new medication, evaluate each of the side effects and teach the client about the ones that are the *most likely* to occur and occur early after administration. For example, some antibiotics cause hypersensitivity reactions, hepatoxicity, nephrotoxicity, and

Box 16-6 Basic Guidelines for Drug Safety in the Home

1. Keep each drug in its original, labeled container.
2. Labels must be legible.
3. Discard any outdated medications.
4. Finish a prescribed drug unless otherwise instructed.
5. Do not save a drug for future illnesses.
6. Dispose of drugs by taking them to the pharmacy.
7. Do not place drugs in the trash or within reach of children.
8. Do not give a family member a drug prescribed for another.
9. Refrigerate medications if label indicates this is required.
10. Read labels carefully and follow all instructions.

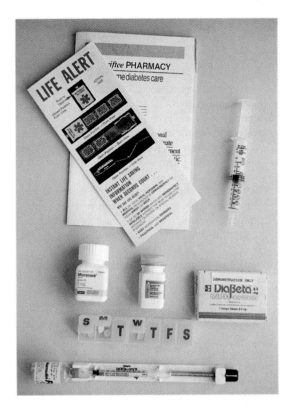

Figure 16-9 Self-help devices for managing medications at home.

platelet dysfunction. Hypersensitivity reactions are likely to occur shortly after taking a few doses of an antibiotic. The other side effects tend to occur after long-term antibiotic administration. Teach clients about side effects in terms of things that they can see, feel, touch, or hear. For example, thrombocytopenia, a reduction in the number of platelets in the blood, can be a side effect of a drug. The client cannot see, feel, touch, or hear thrombocytopenia. However, thrombocytopenia can cause bleeding. The nurse teaches the client how to *look for* evidence of bleeding. Be sure to teach the client what to do about side effects when they are discovered.

Medications and the Client's Activities of Daily Living

The nurse evaluates the client's activities of daily living and the effect they will have on the client's ability to comply with medication schedules. When medications are initiated in the acute care setting, they are often administered around the clock. In the community, it may not be reasonable to think clients can administer medications according to this schedule. In collaboration with the prescriber or the pharmacist, the nurse teaches the client and family members how to adjust medication schedules that are consistent with the client's life-style, including what to do if doses are missed.

Evaluating the effectiveness of teaching ensures that the client can administer drugs in a safe manner. One method of evaluating client understanding is to create medication cards with the name of the drug on the front of the card and all pertinent drug information on the back of the card. The nurse flashes the card in front of the client and asks the client to read the name of the medication (this also ensures that the client can read the names of the

medication). If the client correctly identifies the name of the medication, ask the client the following questions:

- Why are you taking this medication?
- How often do you take this medication?
- What side effects can occur with this medication?
- If this side effect occurs, what are you going to do about it?

It may be helpful to have actual labeled medication bottles with the drug name. Drug bottles often have fine print and may not be easily read by the client with impaired visual acuity.

Be sure to evaluate the client's sensory, motor, and cognitive functions which, when impaired, may affect the client's ability to safely self-administer medications. When impairments are assessed, family members, friends, or home health aides may be available to assist with medication administration. Many self-help devices are also available for purchase (e.g., pill boxes with times displayed, and electronic dispensers) (Figure 16-9).

SPECIAL HANDLING OF CONTROLLED II SUBSTANCES

The nurse is responsible for following legal regulations when administering controlled II substances (drugs with

Box 16-7 Storage and Accountability for Controlled Substances

- All narcotics are stored in a locked cabinet or container (Figure 16-10).
- Authorized nurses carry a set of keys or computer entry code for the narcotics cabinet.
- An inventory record is kept to record all narcotics used, including client's name, date, name of drug, and time of drug administration.
- Prior to removing any drug from the cabinet, the number actually available is compared with the number indicated on the narcotic record. If incorrect, the discrepancy must be rectified before proceeding.
- If any part of a dose of a controlled substance is discarded, a second nurse witnesses disposal of the unused portion, and the record is signed by both nurses.
- At change-of-shift one nurse going off duty counts all narcotics with a nurse coming on duty. Both nurses sign the narcotic record to indicate the count is correct. (Computerized storage has eliminated this process.)
- Discrepancies in narcotic counts are reported immediately.

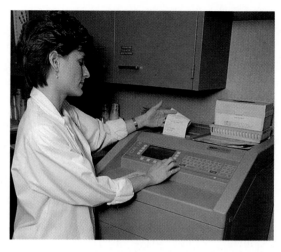

Figure 16-10   Computerized system for narcotic distribution.

potential for abuse). Violations of the Controlled Substances Act may result in fines, imprisonment, and loss of license. Health care institutions have policies for the proper storage and distribution of controlled substances, including narcotics (Box 16-7).

Medication Errors

A medication error is any event that could cause or lead to a client receiving inappropriate drug therapy or failing to receive appropriate drug therapy (Edgar, Lee, and Cousins, 1994). Medication errors can be made by anyone involved in the prescribing, transcribing, preparation, dispensing, and administration of medications. Hospital medication delivery systems are designed so that there is a system of checks that help prevent medication errors. Conscientious adherence to the five "rights" of medication administration helps prevent errors. When an error occurs, it should be acknowledged immediately and reported to the appropriate people. The nurse has an ethical and professional obligation to report the error to the physician and nurse manager. Appropriate follow-up may include administering an antidote, withholding a subsequent dose, and monitoring the effects of the drug. The client's record should include a notation including what was given, who was no-

tified, the observed effects of the drug, and follow-up measures taken.

The nurse is also responsible for completing a report describing the incident. This report provides an objective analysis of what went wrong and provides information for the risk management team to identify factors contributing to errors and ways to avoid similar errors in the future.

Special Considerations for Specific Age-Groups

Pediatric Considerations
Children vary in age, weight, and the ability to absorb, metabolize, and excrete medications. Children's dosages are lower than those of adults, and caution is needed in preparing medications. Drugs may or may not be prepared and packaged in doses appropriate for children. Preparing appropriate doses often requires calculation based on body weight. A child's parents may be helpful in determining the best way to give a child medication. Sometimes it is more effective to have the parent give the drug as the nurse stands by.

Older Adults
Individual over the age of 65 are the largest users of drugs (Ebersole and Hess, 1994). Because of physiological changes associated with the aging process, special nursing interventions are needed to promote safe and effective medication administration (Table 16-3). Be aware of the following patterns related to drug use:

1. *Polypharmacy.* The client takes many medications in an attempt to treat several disorders. This increases the risk of drug interactions with other drugs or with foods.

Table 16-3

Drug Effects in Older Adults

Drug Effect	Related Interventions
Difficulty swallowing large tablets or capsules; tissue damage related to uncoated medications such as aspirin and potassium chloride	Position client sitting upright. Give full glass of liquid (if unrestricted). Crush tablets and mix with food, or give liquid form if available.
Slowing of drug excretion; overuse and abuse of laxatives by client	Instruct client to increase fluid intake, eat high-fiber foods, and avoid daily use of laxatives.
Longer biotransformation of drugs by the liver with greater risk for drug sensitivity and toxicity	Monitor for signs of liver dysfunction (laboratory tests, jaundice, dark urine). Monitor for contra-indications in clients with known liver disease.
Risk of drug accumulation and toxicity related to altered kidney function or renal blood flow	Monitor for renal impairment (decreased urine output) and contraindications/dosage in clients with known renal disease.

2. *Self-prescribing.* Older adults often attempt to seek relief from a variety of problems with over-the-counter (OTC) preparations, folk medicines, and herbs.
3. *Misuse of drugs.* Misuse by the elderly includes overuse, underuse, erratic use, and contraindicated use.
4. *Noncompliance.* Defined as a deliberate misuse of medication. Older adults alter dose because of ineffectiveness or unpleasant side effects.

CRITICAL THINKING EXERCISES

1. A patient recovering from abdominal surgery is complaining of a pounding headache rated as 7 (scale 0 to 10). You check the MAR and find orders for Demerol 50 mg IM q3h prn for pain, last given 6 hours ago, and Tylenol with codeine 30 mg 1–2 tabs q4h prn for pain. What factors should be considered in deciding which medication to give?

2. You are preparing to give a client aspirin that is ordered 1 tab qd. When you look the drug up in the reference book, you find that aspirin can be given as an analgesic, an antipyretic, and an antiplatelet. How would you determine why this patient is getting the drug?

3. A client being admitted to the hospital states she is allergic to codeine. What information would help you differentiate between an allergic reaction and undesirable side effects not related to allergy?

REFERENCES

Clayton B, Stock Y: *Basic pharmacology for nurses,* St Louis, 1997, Mosby.

Dison N: *Simplified drugs and solutions for health care professionals,* ed 11, St Louis, 1997, Mosby.

Ebersole P, Hess P: *Toward healthy aging: human needs and nursing response,* ed 5, St Louis, 1998, Mosby.

Edgar TA, Lee DS, and Cousins DD: Experience with a national medication error reporting program, *Am J Hosp Pharm* 51:1335, 1994.

McCaffery M, Ferrell B: Understanding opiates and addiction, *Nursing 94* 24(8) 56-9, 1994.

Skidmore-Roth L: *Mosby's drug guide for nurses,* ed 2, St Louis, 1999, Mosby.

CHAPTER 17

Administration of Non-Parenteral Medication

Skill 17.1
Administering Oral Medications, 422

Skill 17.2
Applying Topical Medications, 429

Skill 17.3
Instilling Eye and Ear Medications, 433

Skill 17.4
Using Metered-Dose Inhalers, 438

Skill 17.5
Inserting Rectal and Vaginal Medications, 442

Non-parenteral medications can be given by several routes. The route chosen depends on the properties and desired effects of the medication, as well as the physical and mental condition of the client. Each route has advantages and disadvantages (Table 17-1). The nurse may encounter a variety of reasons when it becomes necessary to change one route to another. When this occurs the nurse is responsible for communicating this to the physician or pharmacist in order to meet the client's needs.

The easiest and most desirable way to administer medications is by mouth. Clients usually are able to ingest or self-administer oral drugs with a minimum of problems. Situations, however, may arise that contraindicate clients receiving medications by mouth. The primary contraindications to giving oral medications include the presence of gastrointestinal alterations, the inability of a client to swallow food or fluids, and the use of gastric suction. An important precaution to take when administering any oral preparation is to protect clients from aspiration. Aspira-

tion occurs when food, fluid, or medication intended for gastrointestinal administration inadvertently is administered into the respiratory tract. The nurse protects the client from aspiration by evaluating the client's ability to safely swallow oral medications (Box 17-1). Properly positioning the client is also essential in preventing aspiration. Unless contraindicated, the nurse positions the client in a seated position when administering oral medications. The lateral position can also be used when the client's swallow, gag, and cough are intact. A client who has difficulty swallowing should be evaluated by appropriate personnel (e.g., speech therapist) prior to receiving oral preparations.

Topical administration of medications involves applying drugs locally to skin, mucous membranes, or tissue membranes. The nurse applies medications to the skin by

---

Box 17-1 Protecting the Client from Aspiration

Evaluating the Client's Ability to Swallow
Ask the client to repeat certain sounds that require the same muscle movements as swallowing: "me-me-me" (for the lips); "la-la-la" (for the tongue); "ga-ga-ga" (for the soft palate and pharynx).

Assess the swallowing reflex by having the client slide his tongue backward along the palate.

Position your thumb and index finger on your client's larynx, ask the client to swallow. Normally the larynx elevates.

Evaluating the Client's Gag Reflex
Assess the gag reflex by stroking the posterior pharyngeal wall with a tongue blade.

Never check the gag reflex in a client who does not exhibit an intact cough or swallow reflex. To protect the airway check that the client has all three: a positive cough, gag, and swallow reflex.

Data from: Gauqitz DG: How to protect the dysphagic stroke patient, *Am J Nurs* 95:34, 1995.

Table 17-1

Non-Parenteral Routes of Administration

Route	Advantages	Disadvantages
Oral (swallowed)	Easy, comfortable, economical; may produce local or systemic effects	Some drugs are destroyed by gastric secretions. Cannot be given if client is NPO, unable to swallow, has gastric suction, or is unconscious or confused and unwilling to cooperate. May irritate lining of gastrointestinal tract, discolor teeth, or have unpleasant taste.
Skin: topical transdermal patches	Provides primarily local effect; painless; limited side effects	Extensive applications may be bulky or cause difficulty in maneuvering. May leave oily or pasty substance on skin; may soil clothing.
Mucous membranes: eyes, ears, nose; vaginal, rectal, buccal, sublingual	Prolonged systemic effects, limited side effects; local application to involved site; readily absorbed, provides rapid relief for respiratory problems	Clients with abrasions may absorb drug too rapidly, resulting in excessive systemic effects. Insertion of product may cause embarrassment. Rectal suppositories are contraindicated with rectal surgery or active rectal bleeding. More invasive, less comfortable; risk of tissue or nerve damage.
Inhalation	Provides direct effects on lung tissues and rapid relief of respiratory distress	Difficult for some clients to administer correctly.

painting, spraying, or spreading medication over an area, applying moist dressings, soaking body parts in solution, or giving medicated baths. Adhesive-backed medicated disks can also be applied to the skin to provide a continuous release of medication over several hours or days. Systemic effects from topical agents can occur if the skin is thin, if the drug concentration is high, or if contact with the skin is prolonged.

Topical administration avoids puncturing skin and lessens the risk of infection and tissue injury that may occur with injections. Gastrointestinal disturbances are encountered less frequently than with oral administration. The risk of serious side effects is generally low, but serious systemic effects can occur.

Drugs applied to membranes such as the cornea of the eye or rectal mucosa are absorbed quickly because of the membrane's vascularity. When drug concentrations are high, systemic effects can occur. For example, bradycardia may occur following atropine instillation to the eye. Mucous and other tissue membranes differ in their sensitivity to medications. The cornea of the eye, for example, is extremely sensitive to chemicals. Clients commonly experience burning sensations during administration of eye and nose drops. Medications are generally less irritating to vaginal or rectal mucosa.

Medications for topical use can be administered in the following ways:

1. Direct application of liquid—eye drops, gargling, swabbing the throat.
2. Inserting drug into body cavity—**suppository** insertion into rectum or vagina or creams and foams inserted into the vagina.
3. Instillation of fluid into body cavity (fluid is retained)—ear drops, nose drops, bladder and rectal instillation.
4. Irrigation of body cavity (fluid is not retained)—flushing eye, ear, vagina, bladder, or rectum with medicated fluid.
5. Spraying—instillation into nose or throat.
6. Inhalation of medicated aerosol spray—distributes medication throughout the **nasal** passages and tracheobronchial airway.
7. Direct application to skin or mucosa—**lotion, ointments,** creams, patches, and disk.

Skill 17.1

ADMINISTERING ORAL MEDICATIONS

The majority of medications the nurse administers are given by mouth. The nurse usually prepares the medications for the client to self-administer and prepares oral medications in an area designed for medication preparation or at the unit dose cart. Some agencies have a locked cabinet for medications in each client's room.

The ability of an oral medication to be absorbed after it is ingested depends largely on its form or preparation. Solutions and suspensions already in a liquid state (Figure 17-1) are absorbed more readily than tablets or capsules. Acidic drugs are absorbed quickly in the stomach. Some drugs are not absorbed until reaching the small intestine. Oral medications are absorbed more easily when administered between meals; when the stomach is filled with food, the contents slow the absorption process. Enteric coatings on some tablets resist dissolution in gastric juices and prevent digestion in the upper gastrointestinal (GI) tract. The coating protects the stomach lining from irritation. Enteric-coated medication should not be crushed or dissolved before administration. When effective absorption in the stomach is required for certain drugs, they should be given at least 1 hour before or 2 hours after meals or antacids.

Equipment

    Medication administration record (MAR) or computer printout

    Medication cart (Figure 17-2) or locked cabinet in client's room

    Disposable medication cups

    Glass of water, juice, or preferred liquid and drinking straw

    Device for crushing or splitting tablets (optional)

ASSESSMENT

1. Identify the drug(s) ordered: action, purpose, normal dosage and route, common side effects, time of onset and peak action, and nursing implications. **Rationale: This allows nurse to anticipate effects of drug and to observe client's response.**

2. Assess for any contraindications to oral medication, including inability to swallow, nausea/vomiting, bowel inflammation, reduced peristalsis, gastrointestinal surgery, and gastric suction.

3. Check allergies and replace any missing or faded identification bracelets. **Rationale: Identification bracelets provide positive client identification.**

4. Assess client's knowledge regarding medications to determine need for drug education and to assist in identifying client's compliance with drug therapy at home.

5. Assess client's preferences for fluids. Maintain fluid restrictions as prescribed. **Rationale: Offering fluids during drug administration is an excellent way to increase client's fluid intake. Fluids ease swallow-**

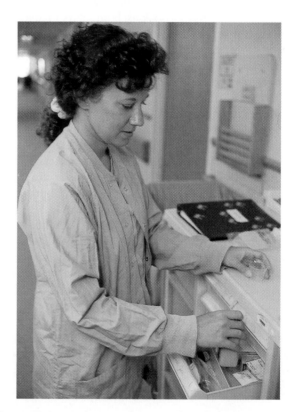

Figure 17-2 Medication drawer is kept locked when not in use.

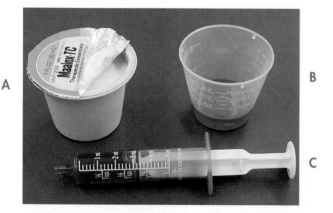

Figure 17-1 **A,** Liquid medication in single-dose package. **B,** Liquid measured in medicine cup. **C,** Oral liquid medicine in syringe.

ing and facilitate absorption from the gastrointestinal tract. However, fluid restrictions must be maintained.

PLANNING

Expected outcomes focus on safe, accurate, and effective drug therapy.

Expected Outcomes

1. Client takes medications as prescribed, with evidence of improvement in condition (e.g., relief of pain, regular heart rate, stable blood pressure).
2. Client explains purpose of medication and drug dose schedule.

DELEGATION CONSIDERATIONS

In acute care settings administration of non-parenteral medication requires professional knowledge, and delegation to assistive personnel (AP) is not appropriate. The professional nurse (RN) needs to inform unlicensed care providers about potential adverse effects of medications and to report their occurrence. In some long-term care settings AP are trained and certified to administer nonnarcotic, non-parenteral medications to stable residents; however, knowledge of desired effects and adverse reactions is very limited, therefore assessment and evaluation of medication effects remains primarily the responsibility of the professional nurse.

IMPLEMENTATION

Steps	Rationale
1. See Standard Protocol (inside front cover).	
Preparing medications	
2. Compare medication administration record with scheduled medication list. If discrepancies exist, check against original physician orders.	Physician's order is most reliable source and only legal record of drugs client is to receive. Orders should be checked at least every 24 hours and when client questions a drug order.
3. Arrange medication tray and cups in medication preparation area or move medication cart to position outside client's room.	Organization of equipment saves time and reduces error.
4. Unlock medicine drawer or cart (see illustration).	Medications are safeguarded when locked in cabinet or cart.
5. Prepare medications for one client at a time. Keep all pages of MARs or computer printouts for one client together.	Prevents preparation errors.

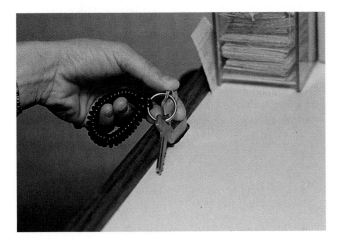

Step 4

NURSE ALERT

Review five "rights" for administering medications.

Steps	Rationale

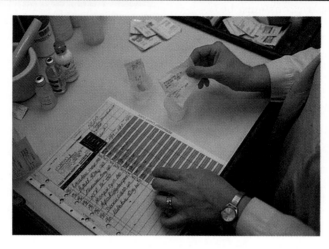

Step 6

6. Select correct drug from stock supply or unit dose drawer. Compare label of medication with MAR or computer printout (see illustration).

Reading label and comparing it against transcribed order reduces errors. **This is the first check for accuracy.**

7. Check drug dose. If label of dose differs from ordered dose, calculate correct amount to give.

Double-checking pharmacy calculations reduces risk of error. Some agencies require nurses to check calculations of certain medications with another nurse.

8. To prepare unit dose tablets or capsules, place packaged tablet or capsule directly into medicine cup without removing wrapper. Give medications only from containers with labels that are clearly marked and legible.

Wrapper identifies drug name and dosage, which can facilitate teaching.

9. To prepare tablets or capsules from a floor stock bottle, pour required number into bottle cap and transfer medication to medication cup. Do not touch medication with fingers. Extra tablets or capsules may be returned to bottle.

Floor stock bottles are often used in long-term care settings for common over-the-counter (OTC) drugs such as laxatives and nonnarcotic analgesics.

10. Check the expiration date of each drug. Return all outdated drugs to pharmacy.

Outdated drugs cannot be safely administered.

11. Place all tablets or capsules requiring preadministration assessments (e.g., pulse rate, blood pressure) in a separate cup.

Serves as a reminder to complete appropriate assessment and facilitates withholding drugs (if necessary.)

12. Medications that must be broken in order to administer half the dose can be broken using a gloved hand or cut with a cutting device. Tablets that are broken in half should be scored, as identified by a manufactured line across the center of the tablet. Unused portions of divided tablets or capsules may be discarded or returned to the original container, depending on agency policy.

Discarding prevents mislabeling by placement in the incorrect container. Returning unused portion is more cost effective.

13. When using a blister pack, "pop" medications through a foil or paper backing into a medication cup.

Many long-term care agencies use blister packs, which provide about 1 month's supply of prescription drugs for an individual client. Each "blister" usually contains a single dose. Blister packs are prepared by a pharmacist.

Steps	Rationale
14. When preparing liquids, thoroughly mix before administering. Check and discard medications that are cloudy or have changed color.	Liquid medications packaged in single-dose cups need not be poured into medicine cups.
a. Remove bottle cap from container and place cap upside down.	
b. Hold bottle with label against palm of hand while pouring.	Spilled liquid will not soil or obscure label.
c. Place medication cup at eye level on countertop or when necessary, in hand and fill to desired level (see illustration).	Ensures accurate measurement.
d. Wipe lip of bottle with paper towel.	Prevents contamination of bottle's contents and prevents bottle cap from sticking.
	Allows more accurate measurement of small amounts.
e. If giving less than 5 ml of liquids, prepare medication in a sterile syringe without a needle (see Figure 17-1, p. 422).	
15. If client has difficulty swallowing, use a mortar and pestle to grind pills or a pill-crushing device (see illustrations). Mix ground tablet in small amount of soft food (custard or applesauce.)	Ground tablet mixed with palatable soft food is usually easier to swallow.

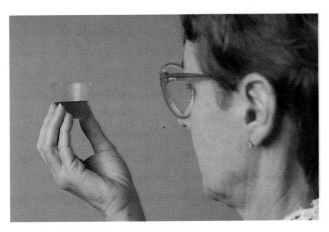

Step 14c

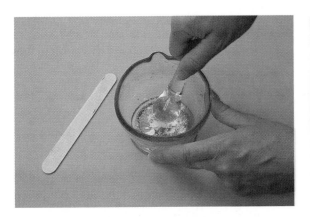
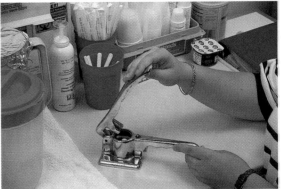

Step 15

Steps	**Rationale**
16. **Narcotic preparation.** Check narcotic record for previous drug count and compare with supply available. Narcotics may be stored in a computerized locked cart (see Chapter 16).	Controlled substance laws require careful monitoring of dispensed narcotics. In most agencies, cosignature by an RN is required when students administer narcotics.
17. Check expiration date on all medications.	Medications used past expiration date may be inactive or harmful to client.

Administering medications

18. Take medications to client within 30 minutes before or after scheduled time.	Promotes intended therapeutic effect.

19. Identify client.	
a. Compare name on MAR or computer printout with name on client's identification bracelet.	Identification bracelets are made at time of client's admission and are most reliable source of identification. **This is the second check for accuracy.**
b. Ask client to state name.	In many long-term care settings pictures are used rather than arm bands. **This is the third check for accuracy.**

20. Perform necessary preadministration assessment for specific medications (e.g., blood pressure or pulse).	Assessment data determine whether specific medications should be withheld at that time.
21. Discuss the purpose of each medication and its action with client. Allow client to ask any questions about drugs.	Client has the right to be informed, and client's understanding of purpose of each medication improves compliance with drug therapy.
22. Assist client to sitting or side-lying position.	Sitting position prevents aspiration during swallowing.

23. Administer drugs properly:	
a. Client may wish to hold solid medications in hand or cup before placing in mouth.	Client can become familiar with medications by seeing each drug.
b. If client is unable to hold medications, place medication cup to the lips and gently introduce each drug into the mouth, one at a time. Do not rush.	Administering single tablet or capsule eases swallowing and decreases risk of aspiration.

Steps	Rationale

c. Offer water or juice to help client swallow medications. Give cold carbonated water if available and not contraindicated.

Choice of fluid promotes client's comfort and can improve fluid intake. Carbonated water helps passage of tablet through esophagus.

d. For sublingual-administered drugs, have client place medication under tongue and allow it to dissolve completely. Caution client against swallowing tablet.

Drug is absorbed through blood vessels of undersurface of tongue. If swallowed, drug is destroyed by gastric juices or so rapidly detoxified by liver that therapeutic blood levels are not attained.

e. For buccal-administered drugs, have client place medication in mouth against mucous membranes of the cheek until it dissolves.

Buccal medications act locally on mucosa or systemically as they are swallowed in saliva.

NURSE ALERT

If client is to receive a combination of oral tablets, capsules, and sublingual or buccal drugs, administer tablets/capsules first and have client take sublingual and buccal medications last. Avoid administering liquids until buccal medication has dissolved.

f. Mix powdered medications with liquids at bedside and give to client to drink.

When prepared in advance, powdered drugs may thicken and even harden, making swallowing difficult.

g. Caution client against chewing or swallowing lozenges.

Drug acts through slow absorption through oral mucosa, not gastric mucosa.

h. Give effervescent powders and tablets immediately after dissolving.

Effervescence improves unpleasant taste of drug and often relieves gastrointestinal problems.

24. Stay until client has completely swallowed each medication. If concerned about ability or willingness to swallow, ask client to open mouth and inspect for presence of medication.

Nurse is responsible for ensuring that client receives ordered dosage. If left unattended, client may forget to take it, drop it, or intentionally not take dose without nurse's awareness.

25. For certain medications that should not be given on an empty stomach (e.g., aspirin), offer client nonfat snack (e.g., crackers).

Reduces gastric irritation.

26. Replenish stock such as cups and straws, return cart to medicine room, and clean work area.

Well-stocked, clean working space assists other staff in completing duties efficiently.

27. See Chapter 40 for information about discharge teaching.

28. See Completion Protocol (inside front cover).

• • •

EVALUATION

1. Return within appropriate time to determine client's response to medications, including therapeutic effects, side effects or allergy, and adverse reactions. Sublingual/buccal medications take effect in 15 minutes; most oral medications take effect in 30 to 60 minutes.

2. Ask client or family member to identify drug name and explain purpose, action, dosage schedule, and potential side effects of drug.

Unexpected Outcomes and Related Interventions

1. Client exhibits toxic effects as a result of prolonged high doses or altered excretion.
   a. Withhold further doses.
   b. Notify physician and provide supportive therapy as prescribed.

2. Tablet or capsule falls to the floor.
   a. Discard it.
   b. Repeat preparation.
   c. Replacement may need to be obtained from pharmacy with unit dose systems.

3. Client exhibits side effects common to medication.
    a. Identify comfort measures that relieve symptoms.
    b. Report severe or intolerable side effects to physician. Dosage or form of medication may be changed.
4. Client experiences allergic response that could be related to medication.
    a. Withhold further doses.
    b. Notify the physician. If symptoms are severe, drugs may be prescribed to counteract adverse effects.
5. Client is unable to explain drug information and is unable or unwilling to remember information about purpose, schedule, or adverse effects.
    a. Identify family member willing to assume responsibility.
    b. Refer to home health agency for follow-up after discharge if needed.
        Examples of learning aids: homemade calendars for each week that contain plastic bags containing medications to take at specific times, egg cartons divided into color-coded sections with medications for day, clock faces for clients who cannot read or see clearly, color coding for drug types (e.g., blue for sedative, red for pain pill).
6. Administration error is made (wrong drug, dose, client, route, or time).
    a. Acknowledge it immediately. Nurses have an ethical and professional responsibility to report the error to the client's physician.
    b. Institute measures to counteract the effects of the error if necessary.
    c. Monitor client for untoward effects according to the drug action and side effects.
    d. Complete medication error form as required by the agency. These reports can assist in preventing additional similar errors. (See Patient/Visitor Incident Report, Appendix A).

Recording and Reporting
- Record actual time each drug was administered on the MAR or computer printout. Include initials or signature (see Figure 16-3).
- If drug is withheld, record reason in nurses' notes. Circle time the drug normally would have been given on the MAR or computer printout.
- Report adverse effects/client response to nurse in charge or M.D.

Sample Documentation
0900   Apical pulse 50. Client c/o nausea. Digoxin held and Dr. Jay notified.

Pediatric Considerations

- Oral liquids available in colorful and palatable forms are preferred for administration of medications to children.
- Pediatric doses are usually calculated based on body weight. Professional nurses are responsible for verifying that the prescribed dose is safe.
- When oral medication has unpleasant taste, encourage the child to suck on ice or an ice pop before taking it to numb the tongue and minimize the taste.
- Some drugs are taken better if mixed with a small amount of syrup, jam, or sherbet. Avoid essential foods, because the child may later refuse to eat them.
- Older children may successfully take medication by holding their nose and drinking through a straw.

Geriatric Considerations

Physiological changes of aging may influence how oral medications are absorbed, distributed, and excreted. Administer with a full glass of water to minimize the following common changes:

- Loss of elasticity in oral mucosa
- Reduction in parotic gland secretion, causing dry mouth
- Delayed esophageal clearance
- Impaired swallowing
- Diminished gag reflex due to use of dentures
- Reduction in gastric acidity and stomach peristalsis
- Increased susceptibility to acidic drugs
- Reduced colon motility
- Slowed drug excretion

Skill 17.2

APPLYING TOPICAL MEDICATIONS

Topical administration of medications involves applying drugs locally to skin, mucous membranes, or tissue membranes. The client is unlikely to experience gastrointestinal (GI) disturbances, and the risk of serious side effects is generally low, although serious systemic effects can occur.

Many locally applied drugs such as lotions, patches, pastes, and ointments can create systemic and local effects if absorbed through the skin. Adhesive-backed medicated patches applied to the skin provide sustained, continuous release of medication over several hours or days. Systemic effects from topical agents can occur if the skin is thin, if drug concentration is high, or if contact with the skin is prolonged.

Skin encrustations and dead tissues harbor microorganisms and block contact of medications with the tissues to be treated. Simply applying new medications over previously applied drugs does not offer maximum therapeutic benefit. The skin should be cleansed gently and thoroughly with soap and water before applying medications.

Equipment (Figure 17-3)

Clean gloves (for intact skin) or sterile gloves (for nonintact skin)
Cotton-tipped applicators or tongue blades
Ordered agent (powder, cream, ointment, spray, patch)
Basin of warm water, washcloth, towel, nondrying soap
Sterile, dressing, tape
MAR or computer printout

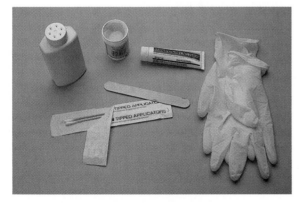

Figure 17-3 *Clockwise from right:* Clean gloves, cotton-tipped applicators or tongue blades, and topical application: powder, cream, and ointment.

ASSESSMENT

1. Review physician's order for client's name, name of drug, strength, time of administration, and site of application.
2. Review information pertinent to medication: action, purpose, side effects, and nursing implications.
3. Assess condition of client's skin. Note if client has symptoms of skin irritation, for example, pruritus or burning. Cleanse skin if necessary to visualize adequately.
4. Determine whether client has known allergy to latex or topical agent. Ask if client has had reaction to a cream or lotion applied to the skin. **Rationale: Allergic contact dermatitis is relatively common and can intensify existing dermatologic condition.**
5. Determine amount of topical agent required for application by assessing skin site, reviewing physician's order, and reading application directions carefully (a thin, even layer is usually adequate). **Rationale: An excessive amount of topical agent can cause chemical irritation of skin, negate drug's effectiveness, or cause adverse systemic effects, for example, decreased white cell counts or decreased immunity.**
6. Determine if client is physically able to apply medication by assessing grasp, hand strength, reach, and coordination. **Rationale: This is necessary if client is to self-administer drug in the home.**

PLANNING

Expected outcomes focus on safe, accurate, and effective drug therapy.

Expected Outcomes

1. Client has evidence of improvement in condition (e.g., relief of pain, inflammation, and itching).
2. Client self-administers topical medication correctly.
3. Client explains dosage schedule and possible side effects.

DELEGATION CONSIDERATIONS

Application of *some* lotions and ointments to irritated skin or for the protection of the perineum may be delegated to AP. Periodic evaluation of the affected area is the responsibility of the professional and cannot be delegated.

IMPLEMENTATION

Steps	Rationale

1. See Standard Protocol (inside front cover)
Topical creams, ointments, and oil-based lotions

NURSE ALERT

To prevent accidental exposure, the nurse must use gloves or applicators. Sterile technique is important if the client has an open wound or impaired skin integrity.

NURSE ALERT

Check client for latex sensitivity prior to glove selection.

NURSE ALERT

Review five "rights" for administering medications.

2. Expose affected area while keeping unaffected areas covered.

3. Wash affected area, removing all debris, crustations, and previous medication.

Removal of debris enhances penetration of topical drug through skin. Cleansing removes microorganisms resident in remaining debris.

4. Pat skin dry or allow area to air dry.

Excess moisture can interfere with even application of topical agent.

5. If skin is excessively dry and flaking, apply topical agent while skin is still damp.

Retains moisture within skin layers.

6. Remove gloves, and apply new clean gloves.

Sterile gloves are used when applying agents to open, noninfectious skin lesions. Disposable gloves prevent cross-contamination of infected or contagious lesions and protect nurse from drug effects.

7. In some cases, soaking may be needed using plain warm water and rinsing without soap.

Removes crusting from skin while minimizing inflammation and irritation.

8. Place approximately 1 to 2 teaspoons of medication in palm of gloved hand and soften by rubbing briskly between hands.

Softening of topical agent makes it easier to apply to skin.

9. Once medication is thin and smooth, smear it evenly over skin surface, using long, even strokes that follow direction of hair growth. Discard gloves and wash hands.

Ensures even distribution of medication. Technique prevents irritation of hair follicles.

Antianginal (nitroglycerin) ointment
10. Remove previous dosage paper.

Prevents overdose that can occur with multiple dosage papers left in place.

COMMUNICATION TIP

Tell client "Your skin will feel greasy and soothed after the topical application."

NURSE ALERT

Rotate sites to minimize skin irritation.

11. Apply desired number of inches of ointment over paper measuring guide (see illustration).
   a. Antianginal (nitroglycerin) ointments are usually ordered in inches and can be measured on small sheets of paper marked off in ½-inch markings.
   b. Unit dose packages are available. (Warning: one package equals 1 inch; smaller amount should not be measured from this package).

Application of gloves prevents absorption of antianginal ointment on the nurse's skin.

Steps	**Rationale**

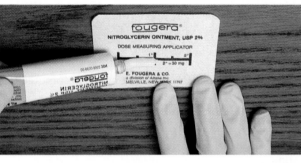

Step 11

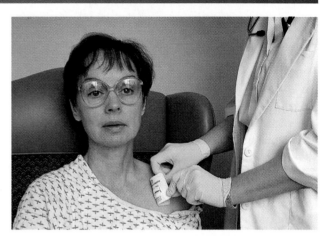

Step 13

12. Antianginal medication may be applied to the chest area, back, upper arm, or legs. Do not apply on hairy surfaces or over scar tissue. If client complains of headaches, apply ointment away from head.

13. Apply ointment to skin surface by holding edge or back of the paper wrapper and placing ointment and wrapper directly on the skin (see illustration).

Minimizes chance of ointment covering gloves and later touching nurse's hands.

14. Do not rub or massage ointment into skin. Massage increases rate of absorption.

15. Date and initial paper and note time.

Prevents missing doses.

16. Cover ointment and paper with plastic wrap and tape securely, or follow manufacturer's directions. Discard gloves and wash hands.

Prevents soiling of clothing.

Transdermal patches (e.g., analgesic, nitroglycerin, nicotine, estrogen) (Figure 17-4)

17. Choose a clean, dry area of the body that is free of hair. Do not attempt to apply the patch on skin that is oily, burned, cut, or irritated in any way.

Clients should be cautioned about using alternative forms of medications or drugs when using patches. For example, clients should not smoke while using a nicotine patch. Clients should not apply nitroglycerin ointment in addition to the patch unless specifically ordered to do so by their physician.

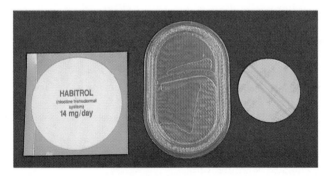

Figure 17-4 A variety of medications are available as transdermal (skin) patches.

Steps	Rationale
18. Carefully remove the patch from its protective covering. Hold the patch over lesions or by the edge without touching the adhesive edges.	Touching only the edges ensures that the patch will adhere and that the medication dosage has not been changed.
19. Immediately apply the patch, pressing firmly with the palm of one hand for 10 seconds. Make sure it sticks well, especially around the edges. Date and initial patch and note time.	Visual reminders of dose applications prevent missing doses.
20. Advise clients not to use heating pads anywhere near the site.	Heat increases circulation and the rate of absorption.
21. After appropriate time, remove the patch and fold it so the medicated side is covered and flush down the toilet. Discard gloves and wash hands.	Residual medication can be a hazard to children and pets (Willens, 1998).
22. Avoid previously used sites for at least 1 week.	Minimizes skin irritation.
Aerosol spray (e.g., local anesthetic sprays)	
23. Shake container vigorously.	Mixes contents and propellant to ensure distribution of a fine, even spray.
24. Read container's label for distance recommended to hold spray away from area, usually 15 to 30 cm (6 to 12 inches).	Proper distance ensures fine spray hits skin surface. Holding container too close results in thin, watery distribution.
25. If neck or upper chest is to be sprayed, ask client to turn face away from spray or briefly cover face with towel.	Prevents inhalation of spray.
26. Spray medication evenly over affected site (in some cases, spray is timed for period of seconds).	Entire affected area of skin should be covered with thin spray.
Suspension-based lotion	
27. Shake container vigorously.	Mixes powder throughout liquid to form well-mixed suspension.
28. Apply small amount of lotion to small gauze dressing or pad and apply to skin by stroking evenly in direction of hair growth.	Method of application leaves protective film of powder on skin after water base of suspension dries. Technique prevents irritation of hair follicles.
29. Explain to client that area will feel cool and dry.	Water evaporates to leave thin layer of powder.
Medicated powder	
30. Be sure skin surface is thoroughly dry.	Minimizes caking and crusting of powder.
31. Fully spread apart any skin folds such as between toes or under axilla.	Fully exposes skin surface for application.
32. Dust skin site lightly using dispenser so that area is covered with fine, thin layer of powder.	Thin layer of powder is more absorbent and reduces friction by increasing area of moisture evaporation.
33. Cover skin area with dressing if ordered by physician.	May help prevent agent from being rubbed off skin. Protects clothing from being stained.
34. Instruct client to dispose of applicators, patches, and similar materials into cardboard or plastic disposable containers.	Careful disposal is necessary to ensure the safety of client, others, pets, and children.
35. For all medications see Chapter 40 for information about discharge teaching.	
36. For all medications see Completion Protocol (inside front cover). Remove and dispose of gloves when appropriate.	

EVALUATION

1. Inspect condition of skin between applications to determine if skin condition improves.
2. Observe client applying lotion, ointment, or patch.
3. Ask the client or significant other to name the medication and its action, purpose, dosage, schedule, and side effects.

Unexpected Outcomes and Related Interventions

1. Skin site may appear inflamed and edematous with blistering and oozing of fluid from lesions, indicating subacute inflammation or eczema that can develop from worsening of skin lesions.
2. Client continues to complain of pruritus and tenderness.
   a. Indicates slow or impaired healing.
   b. Alternative therapies may be needed.

3. Client is unable to explain information about topical application or does not administer as prescribed.
   a. Identify possible reasons for noncompliance.
   b. Explore alternative approaches or options.

Recording and Reporting

- Describe objective data (appearance of abnormal skin, including size, shape, and characteristics of lesions).
- Include subjective data such as pain and itching.
- Report and record changes in appearance and condition of skin lesions.

Sample Documentation

0930 Skin appears dry, red, and flaky on both hands. Client complains of itching. Hydrocortisone cream 1% applied sparingly to affected areas as prescribed.

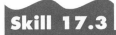

Skill 17.3

INSTILLING EYE AND EAR MEDICATIONS

EYE (OPHTHALMIC) MEDICATIONS

Eye (ophthalmic) medications commonly used by clients include both drops and ointments. Recently intraocular disks have been developed as a third type of medication delivery option. Medications delivered this way resemble a contact lens. The disk is placed into the conjunctival sac, where it remains in place for up to 1 week.

Many clients receive prescribed ophthalmic drugs after cataract extraction and for eye conditions such as glaucoma. Eye medications come in a variety of concentrations. Instilling the wrong concentration may cause local irritation to eyes, as well as systemic effects. Certain eye medications, such as mydriatics and **cycloplegics,** temporarily blur a client's vision. Use of the wrong drug concentration can prolong these undesirable effects.

Orders will indicate administration to one or both eyes, and abbreviations are often used to indicate the site. The abbreviation for right eye is OD, left eye OS, and both eyes OU.

The eye is extremely sensitive, since the cornea is richly supplied with sensitive nerve fibers that provide a protective mechanism. The conjunctival sac is much less sensitive and thus a more appropriate site for medication instillation. Care must be taken to prevent instilling medication directly onto the sensitive cornea.

Clients receiving topical eye medication should learn correct self-administration of the medication. Clients with glaucoma, for example, usually require lifelong eye drops for control of their disease. At times it may become nec-

essary for family members to learn how to administer eye drops or ointment, particularly immediately after eye surgery, when a client's vision is so impaired that it is difficult to assemble needed supplies and handle applicators correctly.

EAR MEDICATIONS (OTIC DROPS)

Internal ear structures are very sensitive to temperature extremes, and therefore solutions are administered at room temperature. When drops are instilled cold from a refrigerator, the client may experience vertigo (severe dizziness) or nausea.

Although structures of the outer ear are not sterile, it is wise to use sterile drops and solutions because the eardrum could be ruptured. Introduction of nonsterile solutions into the middle ear can cause serious infection. Forcing solution into the ear or occluding the ear canal with a medicine dropper during administration can cause pressure within the canal and injury to the eardrum.

Equipment

Medication bottle with sterile medicine dropper or ointment tube
Cotton balls or tissue
Warm water and washcloth
Disposable clean gloves
Eye patch and tape (optional)

ASSESSMENT

1. Review physician's medication order, including client's name, drug name, concentration, number of drops (if a liquid), time, and eye/ear.
2. Review information pertinent to medication, including action, purpose, side effects, and nursing implications. Tell clients receiving mydriatics that vision will be temporarily blurred. **Rationale:** *Wearing sunglasses reduces photophobia. Clients who receive cycloplegics should temporarily not drive or attempt to perform any activity that requires acute vision.*
3. Assess condition of external eye or ear structures (see Chapter 14). **Rationale: This may also be done just before drug instillation to provide a baseline to determine later if local response to medications occurs. This also indicates the need to clean the area before drug application.**
4. Determine whether client has symptoms of discomfort or hearing or visual impairment. **Rationale: Occlusion of external ear canal by swelling, drainage, or cerumen can impair hearing acuity and is painful.**
5. Determine whether client has any known allergies to medications.
6. Assess client's level of consciousness and ability to follow directions. **Rationale: If client becomes restless or combative during procedure, client may require assistance to hold still.**
7. Assess client's knowledge regarding drug therapy and desire to self-administer medication. Assess client's ability to manipulate and hold dropper. **Rationale: Client's level of understanding may indicate need for health teaching. Motivation influences teaching approach.**

PLANNING

Expected outcomes focus on relief of symptoms without unpleasant adverse reactions.

Expected Outcomes

1. Symptoms (e.g., irritation) are relieved.
2. Client denies unpleasant side effects or adverse reactions.
3. Client describes medication effects and technique of application.
4. Client correctly demonstrates self-instillation of eye drops.

DELEGATION CONSIDERATIONS

Administration of eye and ear drops requires the skills unique to a professional nurse and should not be delegated to AP.

IMPLEMENTATION

Steps	Rationale
1. See Standard Protocol (inside front cover).	
2. Compare MAR with label of eye/ear medication.	Verifies correct concentration of drug.
3. Check client's identification bracelet and ask name.	Ensures correct client receives medication.
4. Explain procedure to client. Clients experienced in self-instillation may be allowed to give drops under nurse's supervision (check agency policy).	Clients often become anxious about medication being instilled into eye because of potential discomfort.
5. For eye medications, ask client to lie supine or sit back in chair with neck slightly hyperextended.	Position provides easy access to eye/ear for medication instillation. Correct positioning minimizes drainage of eye medication into tear duct.
6. If crusts or drainage is present along eyelid margins or inner canthus, gently wash away from inner to outer canthus. If indicated, soak any crusts that are dried with a damp washcloth for several minutes.	Soaking allows easy removal of crusts. Cleansing from inner to outer canthus avoids introducing microorganisms into lacrimal ducts.

NURSE ALERT

Review five "rights" for administering medications.

NURSE ALERT

Do not hyperextend the neck of a client with a cervical neck injury.

Steps	**Rationale**

To instill eye drops

7. Hold cotton ball or clean tissue in nondominant hand on client's cheekbone just below lower eyelid.

Cotton or tissue absorbs medication that escapes eye.

8. With tissue or cotton resting below lower lid, gently press downward with thumb or forefinger against bony orbit, exposing conjunctival sac (see illustration).

Prevents pressure and trauma to eyeball and prevents fingers from touching eye.

9. Ask client to look at ceiling.

Retracts sensitive cornea up and away from conjunctival sac and reduces stimulation of blink reflex.

10. Rest dominant hand gently on client's forehead, and hold filled medication eyedropper approximately 1 to 2 cm (½ to ¾ inch) above conjunctival sac.

Helps prevent accidental contact of eyedropper with eye, reduces risk of eye injury and transfer of microorganisms to dropper (ophthalmic medications are sterile).

11. Drop prescribed number of medication drops into conjunctival sac.

Conjunctival sac normally holds 1 or 2 drops. Applying drops to sac provides even distribution of medication across eye.

12. If client blinks or closes eye or if drops land on outer lid margins, repeat procedure.

Therapeutic effect of drug is obtained only when drops enter conjunctival sac.

13. When administering drugs that cause systemic effects, apply gentle pressure to client's nasolacrimal duct with a cotton ball or tissue for 30 to 60 seconds.

Prevents overflow of medication into nasal and pharyngeal passages. Minimizes absorption into systemic circulation.

14. After instilling drops, ask client to close eye gently. Discard gloves and wash hands.

Helps to distribute medication. Squinting or squeezing of eyelids forces medication from conjunctival sac. Avoid pressure directly against client's eyeball.

Distributes medication evenly across eye and lid margin.

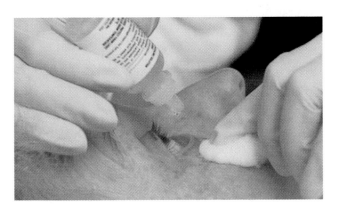

Step 8

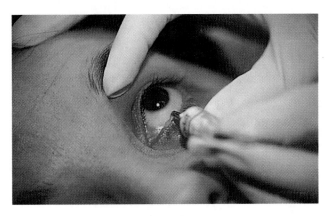

Step 16

To instill eye ointment

15. Ask client to look at ceiling.
16. Gently retract lower lid margin, using thumb or forefinger.
17. Hold ointment applicator above lid margin, and apply thin stream of ointment evenly along inside edge of lower eyelid on conjunctiva from the inner to outer canthus (see illustration).
18. Ask client to look up.
19. Apply thin stream of ointment along upper lid margin on inner conjunctiva.

Reduces blinking reflex during ointment application.
Distributes medication evenly across eye and lid margin.

Steps	Rationale
20. Have client close eye, and rub lid lightly in circular motion with cotton ball, if rubbing is not contraindicated.	Further distributes medication without traumatizing eye. Avoid pressure directly against client's eyeball.
21. If excess medication is on eyelid, gently wipe it from inner to outer canthus.	Promotes comfort and prevents trauma to eye.
22. If client has eye patch, apply clean one by placing it over affected eye so entire eye is covered. Tape securely without applying pressure to eye (see illustration).	Clean eye patch reduces chance of infection.

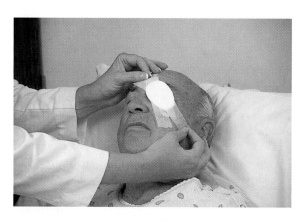

Step 22

Intraocular disk application

23. Open package containing the disk. Gently press your fingertip against the disk so that it adheres to your finger. Position the convex side of the disk on your fingertip.	Allows nurse to inspect disk for damage or deformity.
24. With your other hand, gently pull the client's lower eyelid away from his eye. Ask client to look up.	Prepares conjunctival sac for receiving medicated disk.
25. Place the disk in the conjunctival sac, so that it floats on the sclera between the iris and lower eyelid.	Ensures delivery of medication.
26. Pull the client's lower eyelid out and over the disk. Ensures accurate medication delivery.	

Removal of intraocular disk

27 . Wash hands.
28. Explain procedure to client.
29. Gently pull on the client's lower eyelid to expose the disk.
30. Using your forefinger and thumb of your opposite hand, pinch the disk and lift it out of the client's eye.

31. If excess medication is on eyelid, gently wipe it from inner to outer canthus.

32. If client had eye patch, apply clean one by placing it over affected eye so entire eye is covered. Tape securely without applying pressure to eye.

NURSE ALERT

You should not be able to see the disk at this time. Repeat Step 25 if you can see the disk.

Promotes comfort and prevents trauma to eye.

Clean eye patch reduces chance of infection.

Steps	Rationale

Ear drops
Wear gloves if drainage is present.

33. Warm ear drops to body temperature. Hold bottle in hands or place in warm water.

Ear structures are very sensitive to temperature extremes.

34. Position client on side or sitting in a chair, with affected ear facing up.

Position provides easy access to ear for instillation of medication.

35. Straighten ear canal by pulling auricle upward and outward (adult) or down and back (child) (see illustration).

Straightening of ear canal provides direct access to deeper external ear structures.

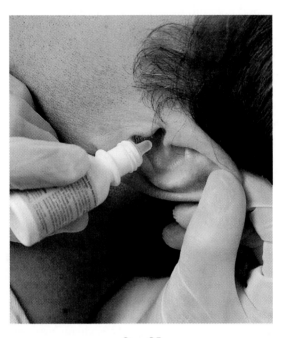

Step 35

36. If cerumen or drainage occludes outermost portion of ear canal, wipe out gently with cotton-tipped applicator, taking care not to force wax inward.

Cerumen and drainage harbor microorganisms and can block distribution of medication into canal. Occlusion blocks sound transmission.

37. Instill prescribed drops holding dropper 1 cm (½ inch) above ear canal.

38. Ask client to remain in side-lying position 2 to 3 minutes, and apply gentle massage or pressure to tragus of ear with finger.

Allows complete distribution of medication. Pressure and massage move medication inward.

39. If ordered, gently insert a portion of cotton ball into outermost part of canal.

Prevents escape of medication when client sits or stands.

40. Remove cotton after 15 minutes.

Adequate time for drug distribution and absorption.

41. Remove and discard gloves.

42. See Chapter 40 for information about discharge teaching.

43. See Completion Protocol (inside front cover).

EVALUATION

1. Observe effects of medication by assessing desired changes and noting any side effects.
2. Note client's response to instillation; ask if any discomfort was felt.
3. Ask client to discuss drug's purpose, action, side effects, and technique of administration.
4. Observe as client demonstrates self-administration of next dose.

Unexpected Outcomes and Related Interventions

1. Client complains of burning or pain after administration of eye drops.
    Use greater caution during next instillation to instill drops into conjunctival sac and not onto the cornea.
2. Client experiences local side effects, for example, headache, bloodshot eyes, and local eye irritation.
    Drug concentration and client's sensitivity both influence chances of side effects developing.
3. Client experiences systemic effects from eye drops, for example, increased heart rate and blood pressure from epinephrine or decreased heart rate and blood pressure from timolol.

Systemic absorption through tear duct can cause potentially dangerous effects. Local anesthetics and antibiotics may cause anaphylaxis.
4. Client lacks confidence or ability to instill drops without supervision.
    a. If client is unable to manipulate the dropper or is unable to see, instruct a family member in the technique.
    b. When using OTC eye drops, client should not share with family members to avoid transmission of microorganisms.

Reporting and Recording

- Include objective data related to condition of tissues involved (redness, drainage, irritation) and subjective data (discomfort, itching, altered vision or hearing).
- Include evaluation related to desired effects of medications instilled and evidence of any side effects experienced.

Sample Documentation

1300   Cyclopentolate ophthalmic 1% solution, 2 drops instilled in each eye. No side effects of tachycardia, drowsiness, or confusion apparent.

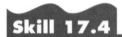

Skill 17.4

USING METERED-DOSE INHALERS

Metered-dose inhalers (MDIs) are handheld inhalers that dispense a measured dose of aerosol spray, mist, or fine powder to penetrate lung airways. The deeper passages of the respiratory tract provide a large surface area for drug absorption. The alveolar-capillary network absorbs medication rapidly.

Inhaled medications are designed to produce local effects; for example, bronchodilators open narrowed bronchioles, and mucolytic agents liquefy thick mucous secretions. However, because these medications are absorbed rapidly through the pulmonary circulation, most create systemic side effects. For example, isoproterenol (Isuprel) dilates bronchioles and can also cause cardiac dysrhythmias.

Clients who receive drugs by inhalation frequently have chronic respiratory disease, and because clients depend on medications for airway management, they need to know how to administer them safely. It is inappropriate to try to teach a client how to use an inhaler during an episode of shortness of breath, because the client's ability to learn is greatly diminished.

Drugs can be delivered by MDIs, which deliver a measured dose of drug with each push of a canister. Because use of an MDI requires coordination during the breathing cycle, clients may spray only the back of their throats and not receive a full dose. Difficulty with coordination can be resolved by the use of spacer devices or the use of a breath-activated MDI (Weilitz and VanSciver, 1996).

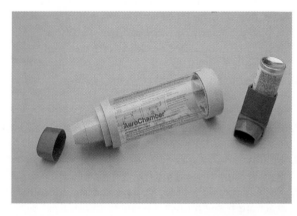

Figure 17-5   Example of a metered-dose inhaler (MDI).

Equipment (Figure 17-5)

Metered-dose inhaler with medication canister
Aerochamber spacer (optional)
Facial tissues (optional)
MAR or computer printout

ASSESSMENT

1. Assess client's ability to hold, manipulate, and depress canister and inhaler. **Rationale: Impairment of grasp or presence of tremors of hands interferes with client's ability to depress canister within inhaler.**
2. Assess client's readiness to learn: client asks questions about medication, disease, or complications; requests education in use of inhaler; is mentally alert; participates in own care.
3. Assess client's ability to learn: client should not be fatigued, in pain, or in respiratory distress; assess level of understanding of terms.
4. Assess client's knowledge and understanding of disease and purpose and action of prescribed medications.
5. Identify drug schedule and number of inhalations prescribed for each dose.

PLANNING

Expected outcomes focus on relief of symptoms and promoting knowledge for self-administration of inhalers.

Expected Outcomes

1. Client manipulates mouthpiece, canister, and inhaler correctly and cleans inhaler after use.
2. Client describes proper time during respiratory cycle to inhale spray and number of inhalations for each administration.
3. Client experiences effects of medication within 10 to 15 minutes, which validates proper administration technique.
4. Client lists side effects of medications and criteria for calling health care professional if dyspnea develops.

DELEGATION CONSIDERATIONS

Many clients self-administer metered-dose inhalers; however, because of the purpose of the prescribed medication and potential need for instructions to promote correct use of the MDI, this skill requires the unique skill of a professional nurse and should not be delegated to AP.

IMPLEMENTATION

Steps	Rationale
1. See Standard Protocol (inside front cover).	**NURSE ALERT** *Review five "rights" for administering medications.*
2. Allow client opportunity to manipulate inhaler, canister, and spacer device (aerochamber). Explain and demonstrate how canister fits into inhaler.	Familiarity with equipment enhances learning.
3. Explain what metered dose is, and warn client about overuse of inhaler, including drug side effects.	Client needs to know the dangers of excessive inhalations because of risk of serious side effects. If drug is given in recommended doses, side effects are minimal.
4. Remove mouthpiece cover from inhaler. Shake inhaler well.	Ensures that fine particles are aerosolized.
5. *Without aerochamber (spacer):* Open lips and place inhaler 1 to 2 cm (½ to 1 inch) from mouth with opening toward back of throat. Lips should not touch inhaler (see illustration, p. 440).	Avoids rapid influx of inhaled medication and subsequent airway irritation. Spacers are recommended because the device allows particles of medication to "ride" the breath into the airways rather than hit the back of the throat (Owen, 1999).
6. *With aerochamber (spacer):* Exhale fully, then grasp aerochamber mouthpiece with teeth and lips while holding inhaler with thumb at the bottom of aerochamber and fingers at the top of inhaler (see illustration, p. 440).	

Steps	Rationale

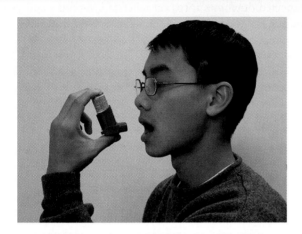

Step 5

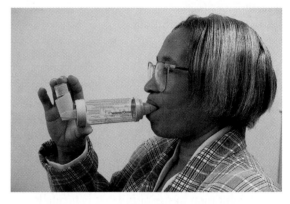

Step 6

7. Press down on inhaler to release medication while inhaling slowly and deeply through mouth.
8. Breathe in slowly for 2 to 3 seconds. Hold breath for approximately 10 seconds.

9. Exhale through pursed lips.

10. Instruct client to wait 2 to 5 minutes between puffs. More than one puff is usually prescribed.
11. If more than one type of inhaled medications are prescribed, wait 5 to 10 minutes between inhalations or as ordered by physician.
12. Instruct client to remove medication canister and clean inhaler in warm water after each use.
13. Teach client to measure the amount of medication remaining in the canister by immersing it in a large bowl or pan of water. The position the canister takes in the water determines the amount remaining (see illustration).
14. See Chapter 40 for implications for discharge teaching.
15. See Completion Protocol (inside front cover).

Medication is distributed to airways during inhalation.

As client inhales, particles of medication are delivered to airway (National Heart, Lung, and Blood Institute, 1991, 1997). Holding breath allows tiny drops of aerosol spray to reach deeper branches of airways.
Pursed-lip breathing keeps small airways open during exhalation.
First inhalation opens airways and reduces inflammation. Second or third inhalations penetrate deeper airways.
Drugs are prescribed at intervals during day to promote bronchodilation and minimize side effects.

Accumulation of spray around the mouthpiece can interfere with proper distribution during use.

COMMUNICATION TIP

Explain that there should not be a gagging sensation in the throat and that these sensations occur when inhalant is sprayed and inhaled incorrectly.

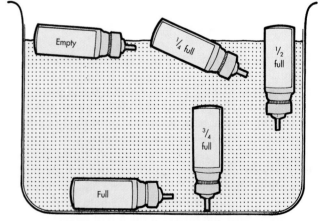

Step 13

EVALUATION

1. Have client explain and demonstrate steps in use of inhaler.
2. Ask client to explain drug schedule and dose of medication.
3. After medication instillation, assess client's respirations and auscultate lungs.
4. Ask client to list side effects and criteria for calling physician.

Unexpected Outcomes and Related Interventions

1. Client's breathing pattern is ineffective; respirations are rapid and shallow. Client's need for a bronchodilator more than every 4 hours can signal respiratory problems.
   a. Reassess type of medication or delivery method. Make sure client shakes canister before administration.
   b. Determine fullness of canister, using displacement in water.
   c. Wait adequate time between puffs to allow deeper penetration into the lungs.
   d. Observe whether the canister is releasing a spray. If not, the valve may need to be cleaned.
2. Client experiences gags or paroxysms of coughing.
   a. Client may gag or swallow medication if unable to inhale while spray is administered.
   b. Aerosolized particles irritate posterior pharynx.
3. Client is experiencing cardiac dysrhythmias. Evidence of side effects from certain medications. Signs and symptoms of overuse of xanthines and sympathomimetic drugs include tachycardia, palpitations, headache, restlessness, and insomnia.
4. Client is unable to depress medication canister because of weakened grasp or presses the canister before or after taking a breath. Both should be done simultaneously for maximum effectiveness.
   a. Client may need practice with assistance for several different steps of procedure before being able to perform each skill independently.
   b. Alternative delivery routes or methods may need to be explored.

Recording and Reporting

- Include objective data related to the desired effects of the MDI (for example, respiratory rate and pattern and breath sounds).
- Include evidence of side effects, e.g., heart rate and client's description of feelings experienced (anxiety and others).
- Include ability to demonstrate correct use of the MDI.

Sample Documentation

0900   Coughing violently and reports difficulty breathing. Wheezing noted throughout all lung fields. Resp 32/min, pulse 98. Self-administered MDI (2 puffs) correctly with no verbal coaching. Reported immediate relief from shortness of breath. Resp 24, pulse 96.

Pediatric Considerations

- Educate child and parent about the need to use inhaler during school hours. Help family find resources within the school or day care facility.

Geriatric Considerations

- Elderly client may be unable to depress medication canister because of weakened grasp.

Skill 17.5

INSERTING RECTAL AND VAGINAL MEDICATIONS

A variety of medications may be given rectally. Drugs administered rectally exert either a local effect on gastrointestinal mucosa, such as promoting defecation, or systemic effects, such as relieving nausea or providing analgesia. The rectal route is not as reliable as oral or parenteral routes in terms of drug absorption and distribution. However, the medications are relatively safe, because they rarely cause local irritation or side effects. Rectal medications are contraindicated in clients with rectal surgery or active rectal bleeding.

Female clients can often develop vaginal infections requiring topical application of antiinfective agents. Vaginal medications are available in foam, jelly, cream, or suppository form. Medicated irrigations or douches can also be given. However, their excessive use can lead to vaginal irritation.

Suppositories come individually packaged in foil wrappers and are usually stored in a refrigerator to prevent melting. *Caution:* Rectal and vaginal suppositories may be stored together in a refrigerator.

Rectal suppositories differ in shape from vaginal suppositories, being thinner and bullet shaped. The rounded end prevents anal trauma during insertion. During administration, the nurse places the suppository past the internal sphincter and against the rectal mucosa.

After a suppository is inserted into the rectum or vagina, body temperature causes the suppository to melt and be distributed. Clients may prefer self-administering suppositories and are given privacy if capable of self-administering without difficulty.

Proper placement is important to promote retention of the medication until it dissolves and is absorbed into the mucosa. Avoid placing a suppository into a mass of fecal material. If necessary, obtain a physician's order to administer a small cleansing enema to evacuate the lower bowel before the suppository is inserted.

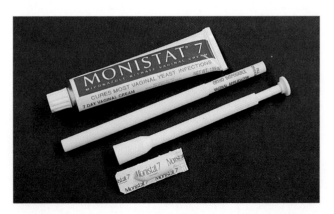

Figure 17-6 *From top:* Vaginal cream and applicator, applicator and vaginal suppository.

Equipment

Disposable clean gloves
Suppository insertion
Suppository
Lubricant (water soluble).
Vaginal creams or foam instillation (Figure 17-6)
Vaginal cream or foam in plastic tube or can
Perineal pad (optional)
MAR or computer printout

ASSESSMENT

1. Review physician's order, including client's name, drug name, form (cream or suppository), route, dosage, and time of administration.
2. Review pertinent information related to medication, including action, purpose, side effects, and nursing implications.
3. Inspect condition of external genitalia and vaginal canal or rectum (see Chapter 14). (May be done just before insertion.)
4. Ask if client is experiencing any symptoms of pruritus, burning, or discomfort.
5. Review client's knowledge of purpose of drug therapy and ability and willingness to self-administer medication.
6. Review medical record for history of rectal surgery or bleeding.

PLANNING

Expected outcomes focus on relief of symptoms without unpleasant side effects.

Expected Outcomes

1. Client reports relief of symptoms of discomfort.
2. Client has no itching or burning.
3. Client explains purpose of medication, side effects, and steps to use for proper suppository insertion.

DELEGATION CONSIDERATIONS

This skill requires assessment that uses the unique skills of a professional nurse and should not be delegated to AP. Judgment must be used regarding allowing the client to self-administer rectal or vaginal medications.

IMPLEMENTATION

Steps	Rationale

1. See Standard Protocol (inside front cover).

Rectal suppository

2. Assist client in assuming a left side-lying Sims' position with upper leg flexed upward.

Position exposes anus and helps client to relax external anal sphincter. Left side lessens the likelihood of the suppository or feces being expelled.

3. Keep client covered with only anal area exposed.

Maintains privacy and facilitates relaxation.

4. Examine condition of anus externally and palpate rectal walls as needed (see Skill 14.7).

Determines presence of active rectal bleeding. Palpation determines whether rectum is filled with feces, which may interfere with suppository placement.

5. Apply clean disposable gloves (if previous gloves were soiled and discarded).

Minimizes contact with fecal material to reduce transmission of infection.

6. Remove suppository from foil wrapper and lubricate rounded end (see illustration).

Lubrication reduces friction as suppository enters rectal canal.

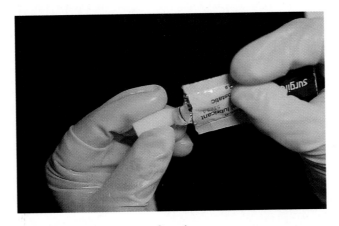

Step 6

7. Retract client's buttocks with nondominant hand. Ask client to take slow, deep breaths through mouth and to relax anal sphincter.

Forcing suppository through constricted sphincter causes discomfort.

8. With gloved index finger of dominant hand, insert suppository rounded end first gently through anus, past internal sphincter, and against rectal wall, 10 cm (4 inches) in adults.

9. Wipe client's anal area and discard gloves by turning them inside out and disposing of them in appropriate receptacle.

Inverting the gloves contains the microorganisms and prevents contamination of other articles.

10. Ask client to remain on side for 5 to 10 minutes or until urge to eliminate is strong.

Prevents expulsion of suppository. Provides sufficient time for the effects of the suppository to reach maximum effectiveness.

Steps	Rationale

11. If suppository contains laxative or fecal softener, place call light within reach so client can obtain assistance to reach bedpan or toilet.

Ability to call for assistance provides client with sense of control over elimination.

12. See Chapter 40 for implications for discharge teaching.

Vaginal suppository

13. Assist client to lie in dorsal recumbent position with abdomen and lower extremities covered.

Provides easy access to vaginal canal and allows suppository to dissolve in vagina without leaking out.

14. Be sure vaginal orifice is well illuminated.

Proper insertion requires visualization of external genitalia if not self-administered.

15. Remove suppository from foil wrapper and apply liberal amount of petroleum jelly.

Lubrication reduces friction against mucosal surfaces during insertion.

16. With nondominant gloved hand, gently retract labial folds to expose vaginal orifice.

17. Insert suppository along posterior wall of vaginal canal entire length of finger (7.5 to 10 cm, or 3 to 4 inches) (see illustration).

Proper placement of suppository ensures equal distribution of medication along walls of vaginal cavity.

18. Wipe away remaining lubricant from around orifice and labia. Remove and discard gloves.

19. Tell client there may be a small amount of discharge that is the color of medication exiting from vaginal canal. Client may wish to use disposable panty liners.

As the medication liquefies at body temperature, it is absorbed; however, small amounts may ooze from the vaginal canal.

Vaginal cream or foam

20. Fill cream or foam applicator following package directions.

Dose is instilled based on volume in applicator.

21. With nondominant gloved hand, gently retract labial folds to expose vaginal orifice.

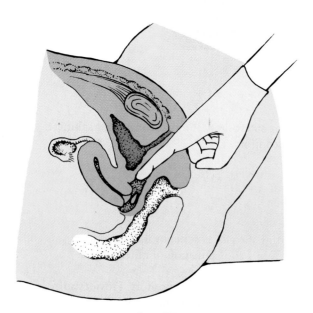

Step 17

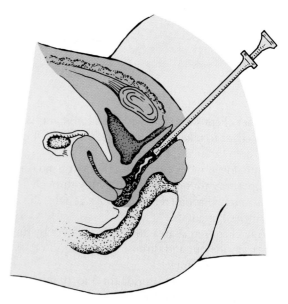

Step 22

Steps	Rationale

22. With dominant gloved hand, insert applicator approximately 5 to 7.5 cm (2 to 3 inches). Push applicator plunger to deposit medication into vagina (see illustration).

23. Withdraw applicator and place on paper towel. Wipe off residual cream from labia or vaginal orifice and remove and discard gloves.

Residual cream on applicator may contain microorganisms.

24. Instruct client who received suppository or cream to remain supine for at least 10 minutes.

Medication will be distributed and absorbed more evenly.

25. Offer disposable panty liners for use during ambulation.

Small amounts may ooze from the vaginal orifice.

Irrigation and douche

26. Place client on bedpan with absorbent pad underneath.

Allows hips to be higher than shoulders and solution will reach posterior fornix of the vagina. Bedpan will collect solution.

27. Be sure fluid is at body temperature, and run fluid through container nozzle.

Body temperature promotes the client's comfort.

28. Gently retract labial folds and direct nozzle toward the sacrum, following the floor of the vagina.

Correct angle allows nozzle access through the cervix into the uterus.

29. Raise the container approximately 30 to 50 cm (12 to 20 inches) above level of vagina. Insert the nozzle 7 to 10 cm (3 to 4 inches). Allow the solution to flow while rotating the nozzle. Administer all the irrigating solution.

Rotating the nozzle allows irrigation of all areas in the vagina.

30. Withdraw the nozzle, remove and discard gloves, and assist the client to a comfortable sitting position.

Remaining solution will drain by gravity.

31. See Completion Protocol (inside front cover).

• • •

EVALUATION

1. Ask client about relief of symptoms for which medication was prescribed.
2. Inspect condition of vagina or rectum and external genitalia between applications. Ask about the presence of itching, burning, or discomfort.
3. Ask client to discuss purpose, action, side effects, and method of administration of medication.

Unexpected Outcomes and Related Interventions

1. Thick, white, patchy, curdlike discharge clings to vaginal walls. Vaginal walls appear bright pink or inflamed, indicating yeast infection.
   a. Female clients often develop vaginal infections requiring topical application of antiinfective agents.
   b. Medications are available in foam, jelly, cream, or suppository form. Medicated irrigations or douches can also be given.
2. Client reports localized pruritus and burning, which usually indicate infection or inflammation.
   Excessive use can lead to irritation of mucous membranes.

Recording and Reporting

• Record appearance of rectum or vaginal canal and genitalia in nurses' notes and report any unusual findings.
• Record drug name, dosage, time administered, and route on MAR.
• Record and report client's response to medication.

Sample Documentation

0800 Client complains of constipation. Has not had bowel movement for 3 days. Dulcolax suppository given per rectum as ordered. Expelled large, hard, dark-brown stool.

States feeling much relieved. Encouraged to drink more fluids, to choose high-fiber foods from menu, and to ambulate as much as possible to prevent further problems. Verbalized understanding and willingness to comply.

CRITICAL THINKING EXERCISES

1. Mrs. Jones is a 76-year-old widow who has been taking eye drops 3 times a day for several months. When you observe her self-administration, you realize she often does not get the drops into the conjunctival sac. What interventions might be appropriate?

2. What are some factors that might interfere with an older client taking drugs as prescribed and keeping drugs safely stored in the home? What interventions might be helpful?

3. A client has orders for eye drops, a cough syrup, a topical cream to the perineum for itching and skin breakdown, and 4 tablets (to swallow). What is the correct sequence for administration of these medications?

REFERENCES

Gaugitz E, Werlitzm PB, DG: How to protect the dysphagic stroke patient, *Am J Nurs* 95:34, 1995.

National Heart, Lung, and Blood Institute. *Guidelines for diagnosis and management of asthma.* National Asthma Education Program, pub no 91-3042, Bethesda, Md, 1991, The Institute.

National Heart, Lung, and Blood Institute, National Education & Prevention Program. *Guidelines for the diagnosis and management of asthma.* Expert Panel Report II (NIH Pub no 97-4051), Bethesda, Md, 1997, The Institute.

Owen, CL: New directions in asthma management, *Am J Nurs* 99(3):26,1999.

Weilitz PB, VanSciver T: Obstructive pulmonary disease. In Lewis SM, Collier IC, Heitkemper MM, editors: *Medical surgical nursing: assessment and management of clinical problems,* ed 4, St Louis, 1996, Mosby.

Willens, JS: Giving fentanyl for pain outside the OR, *Am J Nurs* 98(2)24-28, 1998.

CHAPTER 18

Administration of Injections

Skill 18.1
Subcutaneous Injections (includes Insulin), 457

Skill 18.2
Intramuscular Injections, 464

Skill 18.3
Intradermal Injections, 469

Injections instill medications into body tissues for systemic absorption (Box 18-1). Injected drugs act more quickly than oral medications, and these routes may be used when clients are vomiting, cannot swallow, and/or are restricted from taking oral fluids.

Injections are invasive, and strict aseptic technique is required during preparation and administration to minimize the risk of infection. Injections involve some discomfort. Because risk of tissue or nerve damage exists, site selection is an important nursing concern. The nurse must monitor the client's response closely and be aware of potential side effects or allergic reactions.

▶ SYRINGES

Disposable syringes are packaged separately, with or without a sterile needle. The parts of a syringe are shown in Figure 18-1. Syringes come in various sizes, ranging in capacity from 0.3 to 60 ml. In selecting a syringe, it is important to choose the smallest syringe size possible to improve accuracy of medication preparation. In addition, the nurse must avoid injecting a large volume of fluid into tissues. It is unusual to use a syringe larger than 5 ml for Intramuscular injections (IM) injections. A larger volume creates discomfort. Syringes are marked in two scales along the barrel; one side is divided by minims and the other by

tenths of a milliliter (Figure 18-2, *A*). Tuberculin (TB) syringes, which are marked in hundredths, are used to measure very small dosages (Figure 18-2, *B*).

Syringes are classified as being Luer-Lok or non–Luer-Lok. Luer-Lok syringes (Figure 18-2, *A*) require special needles, which are twisted onto the tip and lock themselves in place. This prevents accidental removal of the needle. Non–Luer-Lok syringes (Figure 18-2, *B*) require needles that slip onto the tip.

Insulin syringes (Figure 18-2, *C* and *D*) hold 0.3 to 1 ml and are calibrated in units. Insulin syringes that hold 0.3 and 0.5 ml are known as low-dose syringes. These syringes are designed for more accurate dosages. Most insulin syringes are U-100s, designed for use with U-100 strength insulin. Each milliliter of solution contains 100 units of insulin. Insulin syringes are to be used only for insulin administration and are preferred over the use of TB syringes.

▶ Needles

Needles come packaged in individual sheaths to allow flexibility in choosing the right needle for a client. A needle has three parts: the *hub*, which fits onto the tip of the syringe; the *shaft*, which connects to the hub; and the *bevel*, or slanted tip (see Figure 18-1). The bevel creates a narrow slit when injected into tissue and quickly closes when the needle is removed, to prevent leakage of medication, blood, or serum. The nurse may handle the needle hub to

---

Box 18-1 Types of Injections

1. *Subcutaneous* (SQ , SC): injection into tissues just below the dermis of the skin.
2. *Intramuscular* (IM): injection into the body of a muscle.
3. *Intradermal:* injection into the dermis just under the epidermis.

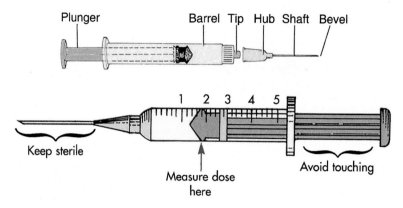

Figure 18-1   Parts of a syringe.

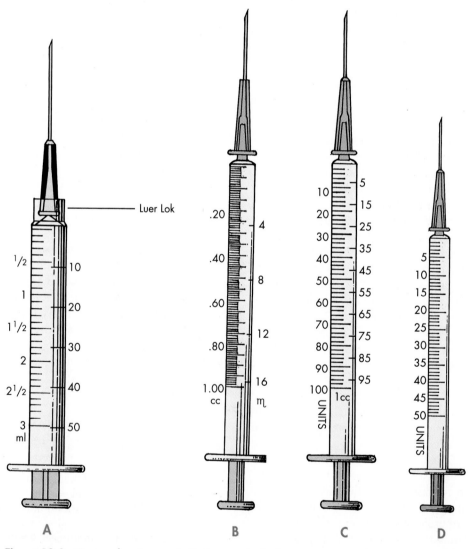

Figure 18-2   Types of syringes. **A,** Syringe with 3-ml capacity is marked in 0.1 (tenths); **B,** tuberculin syringe is marked in 0.01 (hundredths) for doses of less than 1 ml. Insulin syringes marked in units in two sizes: **C,** 100 U; or **D,** 50 U (low-dose).

ensure a tight fit on the syringe; however, the shaft and bevel must remain sterile.

Needles vary in length from $\frac{1}{4}$ to 3 inches (Figure 18-3). Often they are color-coded for ease of selection. Longer needles (1 to $1\frac{1}{2}$ inches) are used for IM injections and shorter needles ($\frac{3}{8}$ to $\frac{5}{8}$ inch) for subcutaneous (SQ) injections. The nurse chooses the needle length according to the client's size and weight and the type of tissue into which the drug is to be injected. Children and very small, thin adults generally require a shorter needle.

The smaller the needle gauge, the larger the needle diameter. The selection of a gauge depends on the viscosity of fluid to be injected. For example, a typical 22-gauge $1\frac{1}{2}$-inch needle used for IM injections is larger than a 25-gauge $\frac{5}{8}$-inch needle used for SQ injections.

Filter needles are recommended for drawing medications from vials or ampules (Beyea and Nicoll, 1995; Hahn, 1990). These needles prevent the withdrawing of glass and rubber particles. Use of a filter needle then requires the nurse to apply a new needle before the medication is given, thus preventing the tracking of medication into tissues. Needleless injection systems have specially designed vial access cannulas. The cannula allows a nurse to prepare a medication in a vial without the use of a needle.

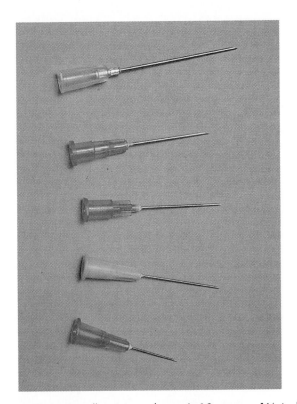

Figure 18-3   Needles *(top to bottom)*: 19 gauge, $1\frac{1}{2}$ inch-length; 20 gauge, 1 inch-length; 21 gauge, 1 inch-length; 23 gauge, 1 inch-length; and 25 gauge, $\frac{5}{8}$ inch-length.

Disposable Injection Units

Single-dose, prefilled, disposable syringes are available for some medications. The nurse must check the medication and concentration, because prefilled syringes appear very similar. With these syringes the nurse does not have to prepare medications, except perhaps to expel portions of unneeded medications or to add another drug to an existing medication. However, some clinicians transfer medication in prefilled syringes into regular syringes to verify correct doses and to avoid expelling extra medication on the needle of the prefilled syringe.

The Tubex and Carpuject injection systems include a reusable plastic mechanism that holds prefilled, disposable, sterile cartridge-needle units (Figure 18-4, p. 450). The nurse slips the cartridge into the syringe, secures it (following product directions), and checks for air bubbles in the syringe. The nurse advances the plunger to expel air and excess medication as in a regular syringe. Most cartridges have a little more medication than the label indicates; therefore, it is essential to measure the correct volume.

Needle-Stick Prevention

Increased concerns about transmission of blood-borne infections from contaminated needle sticks have resulted in special prevention techniques and equipment. Needle-stick injuries occur when nurses forget and recap needles, mishandle needles, or contact stray needles left at a client's bedside or in bed linen. Needles are packaged with plastic caps to maintain sterility before the injection. To prevent accidental needle sticks, *caps should not be replaced on the needle after the injection.* Special puncture-proof and leak-proof containers for the disposal of sharps are available on medicine carts and on the walls of client rooms throughout most health care agencies. Containers are made so that only one hand needs to be used when disposing of uncapped needles. Keeping the other hand well away from the container prevents accidental injury (Figure 18-5, p. 450). A needle should never be forced by anyone into a full needle-disposal receptacle. Used needles and syringes are never placed in any wastebasket, in the nurse's pocket, on a client's meal tray, or at the client's bedside.

Special syringes are designed with a sheath or guard that covers the needle after it is withdrawn from the skin (Figure 18-6, p. 450). The needle is immediately covered, eliminating the chance for a needle-stick injury. The sheath and syringe are disposed of together in a receptacle. The Centers for Disease Control and Prevention (CDC) and the Occupational Safety and Health Administration (OSHA) have recommended the use of safety devices to reduce the risk to health care workers of needle-stick and sharps injuries (Owens-Schwab and Fraser, 1993).

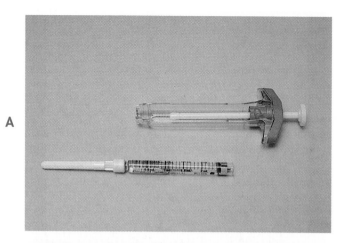

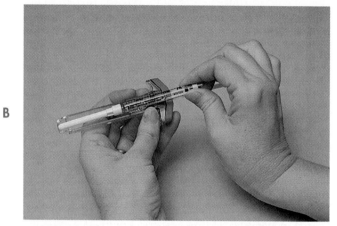

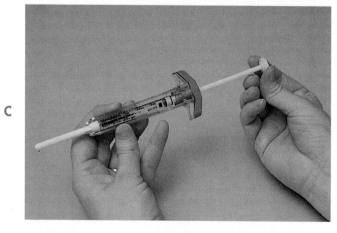

Figure 18-4 **A,** Carpuject syringe and prefilled sterile cartridge with needle. **B,** Assembling the Carpuject. **C,** Cartridge locks at needle end; plunger screws into opposite end.

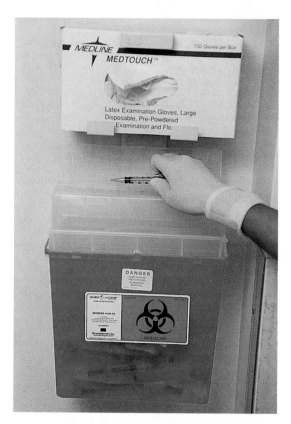

Figure 18-5 Sharps disposal using only one hand.

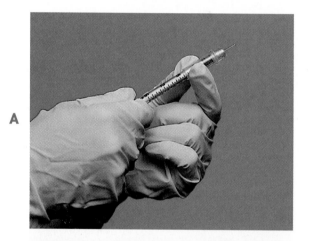

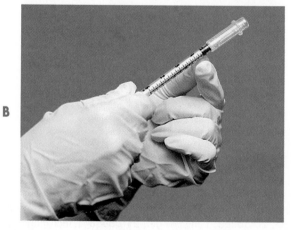

Figure 18-6 Needle with plastic guard to prevent needle sticks. **A,** Position of guard before injection. **B,** After injection the guard locks in place, covering the needle.

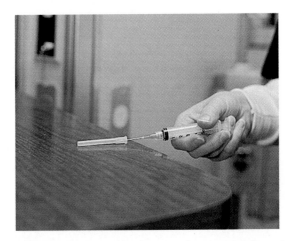

Figure 18-7 The scoop technique to prevent needle-stick injuries.

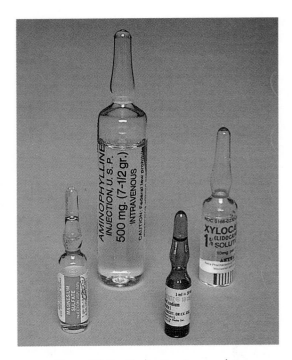

Figure 18-8 Medication in ampules.

In administering injections it may become necessary, for client safety reasons, to recap a contaminated needle. For example, the nurse may be assisting with emergency measures at the bedside and cannot reach a disposal container. If a commercially made recapping device is not available, then the nurse may use a one-handed recapping technique (Craft, 1990). The needle cap is placed on a firm surface, and using one hand only, the nurse slips the tip of the needle into the cap (Figure 18-7). The nurse then presses the syringe, needle, and cover against a flat, vertical surface (e.g., cabinet door) to get the cap firmly in place.

If a nurse is accidentally stuck with a sterile needle while preparing medication, there is no risk of infection. The contaminated needle must be replaced before proceeding with the injection. If, however, a nurse is injured with a contaminated needle, an incident report is filed, the client is asked to be tested for hepatitis and acquired immunodeficiency syndrome (AIDS), and appropriate follow-up for the nurse is required (check agency policy).

PREPARATION OF INJECTABLE MEDICATIONS

Ampules contain single doses of injectable medication in a liquid form (Figure 18-8). They are available in several sizes, from 1 ml to 10 ml or more. An ampule is made of glass with a constricted neck that must be snapped off to allow access to the medication. The fluid enters the syringe easily with aspiration because no vacuum exists within the ampule.

A vial is a single-dose or multidose container with a rubber seal at the top (Figure 18-9). A cap protects the seal until it is used and cannot be replaced. Vials may contain liquid or dry forms of medications; drugs that are unstable in solution are packaged in dry form. The vial label specifies the liquid to use to dissolve the dry drug and the

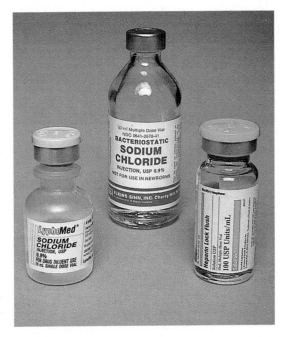

Figure 18-9 Medication in vials. Rubber top must be cleansed with alcohol when vial is reused.

amount needed to prepare a desired drug concentration. Air must be injected into the vial to permit easy withdrawal of the solution.

Tables 18-1 through 18-4 on pp. 452-456 describe the steps and rationale for drawing up medications from ampules and vials and reconstituting medication from a powder.

Table 18-1

Drawing up Medication from an Ampule

Steps	Rationale
1. Wash hands and prepare supplies.	
2. Remove fluid from neck of ampule by tapping top of ampule lightly and quickly with finger, quickly moving down in vertical direction (see illustration). Another option is to grasp the top of the ampule and shake it downward like a thermometer.	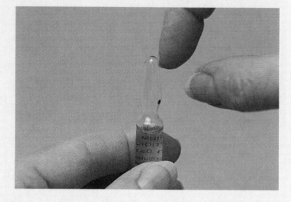
3. Place small gauze pad or alcohol swab around neck of ampule.	Protects nurse's fingers from trauma as glass tip is broken off. Avoid wrapping wet alcohol swab near neck of ampule, because alcohol may leak into ampule.
4. Break neck of ampule quickly and firmly away from hands and body (see illustration).	Prevents shattering glass toward or in nurse's fingers or face.
5. Place ampule on counter top (see illustration). Using a filter needle, draw up medication, keeping the needle tip below the surface of liquid. Tip ampule to bring fluid within reach of needle.	Filter needle prevents withdrawal of glass or rubber particulate. 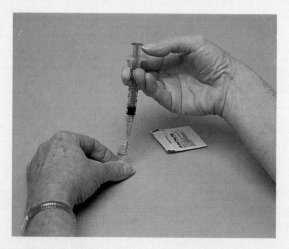
6. Aspirate medication from ampule into syringe by gently pulling back on plunger. Do not draw up the last drop in the ampule.	Leaving last drops reduces chance of withdrawing foreign particles (Beyea and Nicoll, 1995).

Table 18-1

Drawing up Medication from an Ampule—cont'd

Steps	Rationale
7. Option for holding ampule and syringe: insert filter needle into center of ampule opening and invert ampule (see illustration).	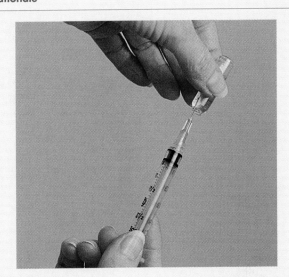
8. If air bubbles are aspirated, remove needle from ampule and hold syringe with needle pointing directly up. Tap side of syringe so that air bubbles rise toward needle (see illustration). Draw back slightly on plunger, and then push the plunger upward to eject air until 1 drop of fluid is visible on the tip of the needle.	Pulling back on plunger allows fluid within needle to enter barrel so fluid is not expelled. Air at top of barrel and within needle is then expelled.
	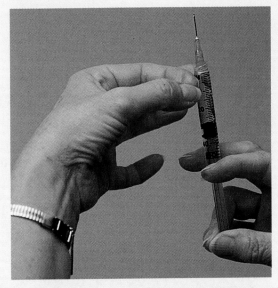
9. If syringe contains excess fluid, hold syringe vertically with needle tip up and slanted slightly toward sink or receptacle and eject excess fluid into sink. Recheck fluid level in syringe by holding it vertically to measure accurate dose.	Position of needle allows medication to be expelled without it flowing down needle shaft. If necessary, flick syringe and needle sharply to eliminate fluid from outside of needle.
10. Remove filter needle and dispose of in proper receptacle. Apply a new needle to syringe.	Prevents tracking of medication on needle through tissues, reducing pain.
11. Dispose of used supplies and take medication to client's bedside for administration.	

Table 18-2

Drawing up Medication from a Vial

Steps	Rationale
1. Wash hands and prepare supplies. Check date and time of any opened vials.	Drugs cannot be used after expiration dates (check agency policy).
2. Remove cap covering top of unused vial to expose sterile rubber seal, keeping seal sterile. If using a multidose vial that has been used before, firmly wipe off surface of rubber seal with alcohol swab using friction.	Vial comes packaged with cap to maintain sterility of rubber seal. Cap cannot be replaced after removal. Alcohol removes surface contaminants.
3. Pick up syringe, remove needle, and apply a filler needle. Pull back on plunger to draw amount of air into syringe equivalent to volume of medication to be aspirated from vial.	Prevents buildup of negative pressure in vial when aspirating medication.
4. Insert tip of needle through center of rubber seal (see illustration).	Center of seal is thinner and easier to penetrate.
5. Inject air into vial, holding on to plunger.	Plunger may be forced backward by air pressure within vial.
6. Invert vial while keeping firm hold on syringe and plunger (see illustration).	Allows fluid to settle in lower half of container.
7. Keep tip of needle below fluid level.	Prevents aspiration of air.
8. Allow air pressure to fill syringe gradually with medication, or pull back slightly on plunger.	Positive pressure within vial forces fluid into syringe.
9. Tap side of syringe barrel carefully to dislodge any air bubbles, and eject any air remaining at top of syringe into vial.	Accumulation of air displaces medication and may cause dosage errors. Draw up the exact volume of medication.
10. When correct volume is obtained, remove needle from vial by pulling on barrel of syringe.	Pulling plunger rather than barrel causes separation from barrel and loss of medication.
11. Remove and discard filler needle in appropriate receptacle. Apply new needle to syringe.	
12. Label multidose vial with date, time, and initials.	Check agency policy for expiration regulations.

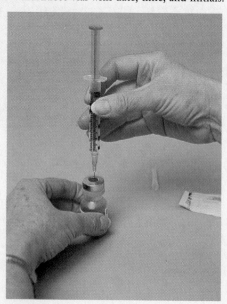

Step 4

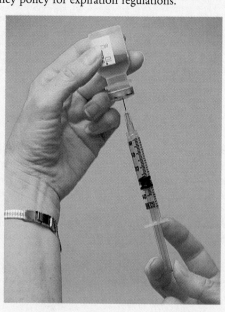

Step 6

Table 18-3

Reconstituting Medications from a Powder

Steps	Rationale
1. Remove metal cap covering vial containing powdered medication and vial containing diluent.	Cap prevents contamination of rubber seal.
2. Draw up diluent into syringe as before (see Table 18-2, Steps 3 to 10).	Label may specify use of sterile water, normal saline, or special diluent provided with the medication.
3. Insert tip of syringe needle through center of rubber seal of vial of powdered medication. Inject diluent into vial. Remove needle.	Diluent begins to dissolve and reconstitute medication.
4. Mix medication by gently rolling vial between hands until completely dissolved.	Dry, powdered drugs usually dissolve easily. Shaking vigorously tends to produce bubbles.
5. Once diluent has been added, concentration of medication (mg/ml) determines dose to be given (see illustration).	
	Step 5 *From Brown M, Mulholland JL: Drug calculations: process and problems for clinical practice, St Louis, 1996, Mosby.*
6. Change needle on syringe before administering medication.	Multiple insertions of needle through rubber seal dulls needle.

Mixing Medications in One Syringe

To avoid giving two injections at one time, some medications can be mixed in the same syringe. It is essential that any medications mixed be compatible. Compatibility charts are available in most pharmacology books or the central pharmacy. When mixing medications, observe for changes in the appearance of the solution, which suggests incompatibility. When using multidose vials, it is essential to avoid injecting the vial's contents into medication from another vial or ampule. When mixing medications from a vial and ampule, always prepare the vial first. Then withdraw medication from the ampule.

To mix medications when one of the two is in a prefilled cartridge, draw back on the plunger of the syringe. Remove the needle from the syringe. Fill the syringe with the correct volume of medication from the prefilled cartridge by inserting the cartridge needle into the syringe tip.

NURSING DIAGNOSES

Nursing diagnoses may be identified based on therapeutic effects or side effects of specific prescribed medications and effect of injection into tissues. **Risk for impaired skin integrity** related to heparin injections refers to the bruising that can develop with injections. **Pain** is a diagnosis that may be appropriate when clients have received multiple injections. **Anxiety** is a common diagnosis for clients who are uncomfortable with having injections. **Knowledge deficit** regarding self-administration of medications is appropriate for clients newly prescribed or in need for review of injection techniques.

Table 18-4

Mixing Medications from Vials

Steps	Rationale
1. Cleanse tops of both vials with alcohol wipe.	
2. Take syringe and aspirate volume of air equivalent to first medication's dosage (vial A).	Air introduced into vial prevents a vacuum when medication is withdrawn.
3. Inject air into vial A, making sure needle does not touch solution. Withdraw needle (see illustration).	Prevents cross-contamination.

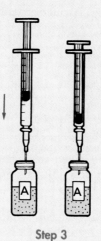

Step 3

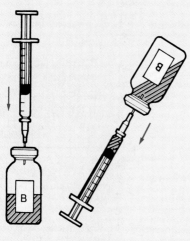

Step 4

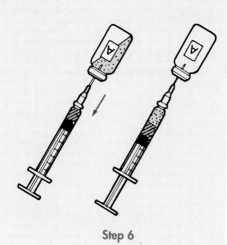

Step 6

4. Repeat with vial B. Without removing needle from vial B, fill syringe with proper volume of medication from vial (see illustration).

5. Calculate total volume of medication by adding volume of both prescribed medications.

6. Insert needle of syringe into vial A, being careful not to push plunger and expel medication into vial. Invert vial and carefully withdraw the exact amount of medication required into syringe (see illustration).

  Exact measurement is essential because medications are now mixed and cannot be readjusted without discarding entire amount and starting again.

7. Needleless syringe units that utilize vial access cannulas do not permit mixing of medications. The plastic cannula cannot be removed once the rubber stopper is punctured. Prepare both doses separately and then mix by adding each to a new sterile syringe.

Skill 18.1

SUBCUTANEOUS INJECTIONS (INCLUDES INSULIN)

A subcutaneous (SQ) injection involves depositing medication into the loose connective tissue underlying the dermis (Figure 18-10). Subcutaneous tissue is not as richly supplied with blood vessels as muscle; thus drugs are absorbed more slowly than those given IM. Drugs commonly given SQ include insulin, heparin, and allergy medications. This skill focuses on insulin and heparin administration.

The rate of absorption is affected by anything affecting blood flow to tissues, such as physical exercise or the local application of hot or cold compresses. Conditions such as circulatory shock or occlusive vascular disease impair client's blood flow and may prevent or delay absorption (Newton, Newton, and Fudin, 1992).

Only small doses of medications (0.3 to 1 ml) should be given SQ. The subcutaneous tissue is sensitive to irritating solutions and large volumes of medications. Medications collecting within the tissues can cause sterile abscesses, which appear as hardened, painful lumps.

The best sites for SQ injections include vascular areas around the outer aspect of the upper arms, the abdomen from below the costal margins to the iliac crests, and the anterior aspect of the thighs (Figure 18-11). These areas are easily accessible, especially for clients who must self-administer medications. Fahs and Kinney (1991) demonstrated that there was no statistically significant difference in level of heparinization among these three sites. Similarly, there was not significant differences among bruise occurrence for the three injection sites. When using the abdominal site it is important to administer the injection within a 2-inch diameter of the umbilicus because of the vascularity of this area. Other sites include the scapular areas of the upper back and the upper ventral or dorsal gluteal areas.

Injection sites should be free of infection, skin lesions, scars, bony prominences, and large underlying muscles or nerves. Rotation of insulin injections from major site to major site, once a common practice, is no longer necessary when clients use human insulin. Human insulins are now almost exclusively prescribed for clients. Clients can choose one region (e.g., the abdomen) and must be sure to systematically rotate sites within that region, thus maintaining consistency in absorption from day to day (American Diabetes Association, 1997). Rotation prevents the formation of lipohypertrophy or lipoatrophy in the skin.

Body weight influences the depth of the SQ layer and is the criterion for selecting needle length and angle of insertion. Generally, a 25-gauge $\frac{5}{8}$-inch needle with a medium bevel inserted at a 90-degree angle (see Figure 18-10) deposits medication into the SQ tissue of a normal size client. If a client is obese, the nurse pinches the tissue and uses a needle long enough to insert through the fatty tissue at the base of the skinfold. The preferred needle length is one half the width of the skinfold. A $\frac{7}{8}$-inch needle is the longest needle for SQ use. Insulin is injected into the abdomen usually at a 90-degree angle. To ensure medication reaches SQ tissue, follow this rule: If 2 inches of tissue can be grasped, insert the needle at a 90-degree an-

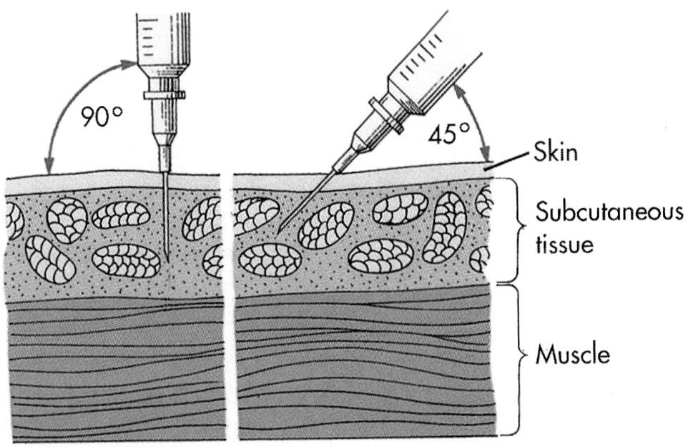

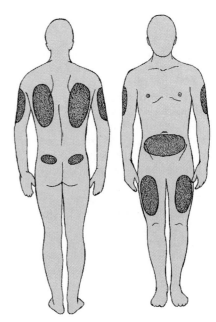

Figure 18-11 Sites recommended for subcutaneous injections.

Figure 18-10 Subcutaneous injection. Angle and needle length depend on the thickness of skinfold.

Table 18-5

Characteristics of Insulin Preparations after Subcutaneous Administration

Insulins*	Onset (Hours)	Peak Effect (Hours)	Duration of Action (Hours)
RAPID ACTING			
Insulin injection (regular insulin)†	$\frac{1}{2}$–1	2–4	5–7
Prompt insulin zinc suspension (Semilente)	1–3	2–8	12–16
INTERMEDIATE ACTING			
Insulin zinc suspension (Lente insulin)	1–3	8–12	18–28
Isophane insulin suspension (NPH insulin)	3–4	6–12	18–28
Isophane insulin suspension (70%) plus insulin injection (30%) (Mixtard, Novolin 70/30)	1/2	4–8	24
LONG ACTING			
Extended insulin zinc suspension (Ultralente)	4–6	18–24	36
Protamine zinc insulin suspension (PZI)	4–6	14–24	36

From McKenry LM, Salerno E: *Pharmacology in nursing,* St Louis, 1995, Mosby.
*All above insulins, with the exception of Mixtard and Novolin combinations, are available in 100-unit strengths. Beef, pork, beef-pork, and human insulins are available in rapid-acting insulins and the three insulins listed under intermediate acting.
†This is the only insulin for IV use. Intravenously, the onset of action is within $\frac{1}{6}$ to $\frac{1}{2}$ hour, peak effect within $\frac{1}{4}$ to $\frac{1}{2}$ hour, and duration of action within $\frac{1}{2}$ to 1 hour.

Box 18-2 General Guidelines for Insulin Administration

- Vials of insulin not in use should be refrigerated. Insulin may be kept at room temperature for 30 days from the date opened. Always time and date a vial when it is first opened.
- Inspect a vial of insulin before each use for changes (e.g., clumping, frosting, precipitation, change in clarity or color) that may signify a loss in potency.
- Be certain the correct form of insulin is prepared. Do not interchange insulin species or types without the approval of the prescriber.
- Rapid-acting insulin should be injected within 15 minutes before a meal. The most commonly recommended interval between injection of short-acting insulin and a meal is 30 minutes.
- If client is NPO for diagnostic tests, insulin may be withheld depending on the time of the test and the client's blood sugar. Check with prescriber about insulin administration before surgery or diagnostic tests.
- Before administering insulin, review available laboratory data (e.g., serum glucose, blood glucose monitoring–normal range is 80 to 120 for nonpregnant adults). Abnormal results may indicate need for dosage adjustment.

- When a dose of insulin is being adjusted, watch for signs of hypoglycemia or hyperglycemia and encourage the client to report symptoms (e.g., weakness, shakiness, sweating, headache, visual disturbances).
- All individuals requiring insulin should carry at least 15 g carbohydrate to be eaten or taken in liquid form in the event of a hypoglycemic reaction (e.g., 4 oz juice, 8 oz milk).
- Administer mixed insulin (e.g., regular and NPH) within 5 minutes of preparation. Regular insulin binds with NPH, which reduces the action of the regular insulin.
- When mixing insulin, be sure to inject sufficient air into both vials before drawing up the dose. When mixing rapid- or short-acting insulin with intermediate- or long-acting insulin, the clear rapid or short-acting insulin should be drawn into the syringe first (see Table 18-4).

Source: Modified from American Diabetes Association: Position statement: Insulin administration, *Diabet Care* 20(suppl 1):S46–S49, 1997.

gle; if 1 inch of tissue can be grasped, insert the needle at a 45-degree angle.

Aspiration of medication following insertion of a needle into SQ tissues is not recommended for SQ insulin or heparin administration (American Diabetes Association, 1997; Fahs and Kinney, 1991; Winslow and Jacobson, 1997). The literature suggests that there is no evidence that SQ injections, when given correctly, enter blood vessels. Instead, the amount of adipose tissue rather than the presence of major blood vessels at the site is the key to SQ injection errors (Thow & Home, 1992).

SPECIAL CONSIDERATIONS FOR ADMINISTRATION OF INSULIN

Insulin is the hormone used to treat diabetes mellitus. Clients with diabetes often receive a combination of different types of insulin to control their blood sugar levels. Regular, short-acting, unmodified insulin comes in a clear solution. The other intermediate-acting insulins (e.g., Lente, NPH) are cloudy solutions because of the addition of a protein, which slows absorption. Table 18-5 compares effects of various insulin preparations. General guidelines related to insulin administration are listed in Box 18-2.

SPECIAL CONSIDERATIONS FOR ADMINISTRATION OF HEPARIN

Heparin therapy is used to provide therapeutic anticoagulation to reduce the risk of thrombus formation in immobilized clients, clients with cardiovascular disease, and clients with cancer. It is administered subcutaneously or intravenously. Heparin suppresses clot formation and is therefore a major risk for bleeding. Nurses should be alert for signs of bleeding (e.g., bleeding gums, hematemesis, hematuria, melena) in clients receiving long-term anticoagulation therapy. A blood test measuring activated partial thromboplastin time (APTT) may be used in monitoring the desired therapeutic range for heparinization.

Equipment

Insulin administration
    Syringe (0.3 to 1 ml)
    Needle (27 to 25 gauge, $3/8$ to $5/8$ inch)
Heparin administration
    Tuberculin or 1- to 3-ml syringe
    Needles (25 to 26 gauge, $1/2$ to $5/8$ inch)
Small gauze pad
Alcohol swab
Medication ampule or vial
Disposable gloves
Medication administration record (MAR) or computer printout

ASSESSMENT

1. Review physician's medication order for client's name, drug name, dose, and time and route of administration.
2. Gather information pertinent to drug(s) ordered: action, purpose, appropriate route, time of onset and peak action, normal dosage, common side effects, and nursing implications.
3. Check expiration date of medication.
4. Assess for factors that may contraindicate SQ injections, such as circulatory shock or reduced local tissue perfusion.
5. Assess indications for SQ injections: unconscious or confused client; client who is unable to swallow or has GI disturbances; presence of gastric suction.
6. Assess client's medical history, history of allergies, and medication history.
7. Assess adequacy of adipose tissue; note presence of hardening or reduction in amount of tissue. **Rationale: Physiological changes of aging or repeated injections may create changes in SQ tissue.**
8. Assess client's knowledge regarding medication to be received. **Rationale: Information may pose implications for client education.**
9. Observe client's verbal and nonverbal response toward injection. **Rationale: Injections can be painful, causing anxiety, which may increase pain.**
10. Ask if client prefers to administer own injection if accustomed to doing so. If learning to do own injections, reinforce learning process.
11. Assess for preexisting conditions that may contraindicate the use of SQ heparin, including threatened abortion, cerebral or aortic aneurysm, cerebrovascular hemorrhage, severe hypertension, blood dyscrasias, and recent ophthalmic surgery or neurosurgery (McKenry and Salerno, 1995).
12. For heparin administration, assess for conditions in which increased risk of hemorrhage is present: recent childbirth, severe diabetes, severe renal disease, liver disease, severe trauma, vasculitis, and active ulcers or lesions of the gastrointestinal (GI), gastrourinary (GU) or respiratory tract (McKenry and Salerno, 1995).
13. Review client's current medication regimen for possible drug interactions with heparin: aspirin, NSAIDs, cephalasporins, antithyroid agents, probenecid, and thrombolytics (McKenry and Salerno, 1995). **Rationale: Drugs can interfere with normal clotting mechanisms, prolonging or enhancing heparin's anticoagulant effect.**

PLANNING

Expected outcomes focus on safe, effective administration of injections with minimal anxiety and discomfort.

Expected Outcomes

1. Client demonstrates improved clinical condition after medication administration.
2. Client experiences mild burning at injection site.
3. No allergies or undesired effects of medication occur.
4. Client's tissues remain soft and supple at injection site.
5. Client explains purpose, dosage, and effects of medication.

For insulin

6. Client maintains serum glucose levels between 80 and 120 mg/dl or an individualized targeted range.
7. Client describes symptoms of hypoglycemia to report to physician.

For heparin

8. Client describes symptoms of bleeding to report to physician.
9. Client shows no evidence of abnormal bleeding.
10. Client maintains laboratory values within therapeutic range.

DELEGATION CONSIDERATIONS

The skill of administering SQ injections requires problem solving and knowledge application unique to a professional nurse. Delegation is inappropriate. Be sure assistive personnel (AP) know to report unexpected changes in client's condition to an RN as soon as possible.

IMPLEMENTATION

Steps	Rationale
1. See Standard Protocol (inside front cover).	**NURSE ALERT** *Review five "rights" for administration of medications.*
2. Before drawing up insulin, gently roll vial in palm of hands. Do not shake. For other medications, mixing is unnecessary.	Resuspends insulin. Exception: do not mix rapid- or short-acting insulin (ADA, 1997).
3. Prepare medication in syringe.	
4. Select appropriate injection site. Inspect skin's surface over sites for bruises, inflammation, or edema. Palpate site for masses, edema, or tenderness.	
5. Rotate injection within one area. Refer to nurses' notes for previous site location.	Rotating within one area is recommended rather than rotating to a different area with each injection. This may decrease variability in absorption from day to day (ADA, 1997).
6. Be sure needle size is correct by grasping skinfold at site with thumb and forefinger. Measure skinfold from top to bottom, and be sure needle is approximately one-half this length.	Ensures that needle will be injected into SQ tissue.
7. Assist client to comfortable position and ask client to relax arm, leg, or abdomen depending on site chosen for injection.	Relaxation of area minimizes discomfort during injection. Promoting client's comfort through positioning and distraction helps reduce anxiety.
8. Talk with client about subject of interest. Keep syringe out of line of vision.	Minimizes anxiety.
9. Relocate site using anatomical landmarks (see Figure 18-11).	Correct site avoids injury to underlying nerves, bone, or blood vessels.

Steps	**Rationale**
10. Cleanse site with an antiseptic swab. Apply swab at center of site and rotate outward in circular direction for about 5 cm (2 inches) (see illustration).	Mechanical action removes microorganisms.
11. Hold swab or square of gauze between fingers of nondominant hand or place near site.	
12. Remove needle cap or sheath from needle by pulling it straight off.	
13. Hold syringe between thumb and forefinger of dominant hand as if grasping dart (see illustration), or hold syringe across tops of fingertips.	Quick, smooth injection requires proper manipulation of syringe parts.

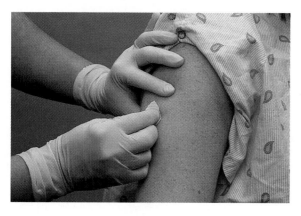

Step 10

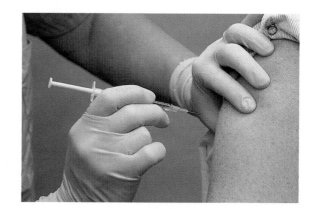

Step 13

14. *Average-size client*	
a. Gently grasp a roll of tissue.	Ensures medication enters SQ tissue.
b. Inject needle quickly and firmly at 90-degree angle.	
15. *Thin client*	
a. Gently grasp a roll of tissue.	
b. Inject needle quickly and firmly at 45-degree angle.	Angle ensures that medication reaches SQ tissue rather than muscle.
16. *Obese client*	
a. Grasp tissue at site and inject needle *below* tissue fold.	Obese clients have fatty layer of tissue above SQ layer. Pinching elevates SQ tissue.
b. Angle of insertion may be between 45 and 90 degrees to ensure medication reaches SQ tissues.	
(1) If 5 cm (2 inches) of tissue can be grasped, needle is inserted at 90-degree angle.	
(2) If 2.5 cm (1 inch) of tissue can be graped, needle is inserted at 45-degree angle.	
17. After needle enters site, grasp lower end of syringe barrel with nondominant hand. Move dominant hand to end of plunger. Avoid moving syringe.	Movement of syringe may displace needle and cause discomfort.

Steps	Rationale

NURSE ALERT

Do not aspirate medication.

18. With dominant hand, inject medication slowly but smoothly.
19. Withdraw needle quickly while placing antiseptic swab or sterile gauze gently above or over site.

20. Apply gentle pressure to site.

Slow injection reduces pain and trauma.

Supporting tissues around injection site minimizes discomfort during needle withdrawal. Dry gauze may lessen discomfort associated with alcohol on nonintact skin.

Aids absorption.

NURSE ALERT

When giving heparin, hold site 1 to 2 minutes and do not massage so as to minimize bruising.

21. Discard uncapped needle or needle enclosed in safety shield in appropriately labeled receptacle. Discard gloves and wash hands.
22. See Completion Protocol (inside front cover).

Prevents injury to client and health care personnel. CDC (1988) warns that capping needles increases risk of needle-stick injury.

COMMUNICATION TIP

Use this time with client to ask if client has questions regarding medication and its effects. Explain what to expect from a medication. If caring for client who has self-administered insulin, give immediate feedback regarding how well the injection was performed.

• • •

EVALUATION

1. Observe client's response to medication 30 minutes after injection to determine effectiveness of drug.
2. Identify any indications of side effects or adverse reactions.
3. Inspect and palpate injection site for lumps, tenderness, or swelling.
4. Have client describe purpose, dosage, intended effects, and side effects of medication.

For insulin
5. Monitor blood glucose readings before meals, at bedtime or as ordered, and when possibility of hypoglycemia is evident.
6. Ask client to list the signs and symptoms of hypoglycemia.

For heparin
7. Have client describe symptoms of bleeding to report.

8. Routinely monitor character of drainage in drainage tubes and on surgical or topical dressings.
9. Monitor related laboratory values and report levels above or below therapeutic range.

Recording and Reporting
- See medication administration record (MAR) and Diabetic Management Record, Appendix A.
- If client has unexpected outcome, describe symptoms and actions taken in nurses' notes.

Unexpected Outcomes and Related Interventions
1. Client complains of localized pain or continued burning at injection site.
   a. Indicates potential injury to nerve or tissues.
   b. Provide warm or cool compresses for comfort.
2. Client displays signs of urticaria, eczema, pruritus, wheezing, and dyspnea.
   a. Indicates possible allergy.
   b. Report to physician for treatment of symptoms and change in medication orders.
3. Client develops bleeding internally or externally.
   a. Withhold the heparin dose and notify physician immediately.
   b. Be prepared to administer protamine sulfate for treatment of spontaneous bleeding.

Sample Documentation
0900   Bruise (4 cm in diameter) noted on RLQ of abdomen, deep purple, soft and nontender. Urine and stool clear; negative for occult blood.

Home Care and Long Term Care Considerations

- Clients should always have available a spare bottle of each type of insulin used. A slight loss in potency may occur after the bottle has been in use for more than 30 days (ADA, 1997).
- Home care agencies can usually provide puncture-proof containers for needle and syringe disposal. Local trash-disposal authorities should be consulted to determine appropriate disposition of containers.
- It is safe and practical for clients to reuse syringes in the home. The syringe should be discarded when the needle becomes dull, has been bent, or has contacted any surface other than the client's skin (ADA, 1997).
- Clients with inadequate personal hygiene, an acute concurrent illness, open wounds on the hands, or decreased resistance to infection should not reuse a syringe (ADA, 1997).
- Family members, friends, and co-workers should be instructed in use of glucagon for situations when the individual cannot take carbohydrate orally for hypoglycemia.
- Instruct clients receiving heparin to read labels of over-the-counter (OTC) medications that may contain ibuprofen, aspirin, and other salicylates.
- Clients on daily insulin or heparin doses at home should wear a Medic Alert bracelet.
- Fall prevention can be important for clients receiving heparin therapy.

Geriatric Considerations

- Visual and dexterity impairment may make it difficult for an older adult to prepare and administer an injection. This can be aggravated during times of illness. A friend or family member should be taught how to administer injections.
- Jet injectors are available for insulin administration. These devices may improve accuracy of insulin administration in clients with visual impairment or dexterity problems. However, the cost of the injectors is high and they may cause trauma to the skin if used incorrectly. Several penlike devices and insulin-containing cartridges are available that deliver insulin through a needle (ADA, 1997).
- Clients over the age of 60, especially women, are more susceptible to the hemorrhagic effects of heparin (McKenry and Salerno, 1995).

Skill 18.2

INTRAMUSCULAR INJECTIONS

An injection given by the IM route deposits medication into deep muscle tissue. The vascularity of muscle results in rapid drug absorption. An aqueous solution is absorbed in 10 to 30 minutes, as opposed to at least 30 minutes when given subcutaneously (McConnell, 1982). A larger volume of drug (up to 4 ml) can be injected into the well-developed muscles of adults because fluid spreads rapidly through the muscle's elastic fibers (Beyea and Nicoll, 1995; Farley et al, 1986). A volume of 1 to 2 ml is generally recommended for individuals with less well-developed muscles (Beyea and Nicoll, 1995). Older infants and children under the age of 2 receiving IM injection should receive no more than 1 ml of medication (Wong, 1995).

The IM site is preferred for irritating drugs or more rapid or strong effects. IM injections require a longer and larger-gauge needle to penetrate deep muscle tissue. Generally, for the average adult, a 21- to 23-gauge, 1½-inch needle inserted at a 90-degree angle will pass through SQ tissue and enter deep muscle (Beyea and Nicoll, 1995). Older adults, cachetic clients, and children require smaller needles. The size of the syringe is determined by the volume of medication and should correspond as closely as possible to the amount to be administered. Volumes of less than 0.5 ml should be given with a low-dose syringe to ensure dosage accuracy (Zenk, 1982, 1993).

The Z-track technique is recommended for IM injections (Keen, 1982, 1986). The Z-track technique, pulling the skin either downward or laterally before injection, reduces leakage of medication into SQ tissue and minimizes pain.

A topic debated in many nursing texts is the use of an air bubble in a syringe. Beyea and Nicoll (1995) note that use of an air bubble is outdated, unnecessary, and potentially dangerous to a client. Modern syringes are calibrated to deliver an accurate dose of medication without an air bubble. Use of an air bubble has been reported to affect dosage of medication by a factor of 5% to 100% (Chaplin, Shull, and Welk, 1985; Zenk, 1982). However, Quartermaine and Taylor (1995) reported on a study comparing air bubble and Z-track technique for skin seepage of medication. Their research showed that the air-bubble method controlled seepage better than the Z-track method. A subjective measure was used to estimate medication seepage. This text does not describe the air-bubble technique.

INTRAMUSCULAR (IM) SITE SELECTION

When selecting an IM site, the nurse considers the following: Is the area free of infection or necrosis? Are there local areas of bruising or abrasions? What is the location of underlying bones, nerves, and major blood vessels? What volume of medication is to be given? Each site has certain advantages and disadvantages (Box 18-3).

Location of an appropriate site for IM injection involves the ability to palpate anatomical landmarks accurately and knowledge of the location of underlying nerves and major blood vessels. Presence of excessive fatty tissue may make location of bony structures difficult; with experience, however, accurate site location is achieved. Correct techniques for locating standard IM sites for injection are described in Table 18-6.

Equipment

Syringe (1 to 5 ml)
Needle (1 to 1½ inch, 21 to 23 gauge)
Medication ampule or vial
Alcohol swab
Dry sterile gauze
Disposable gloves
MAR or computer printout

Box 18-3 Advantages and Disadvantages of Intramuscular Injection Sites

- *Ventrogluteal*—Muscle is situated deep and away from major nerves and blood vessels. Provides most consistent layer of adipose tissue. Preferred injection site for adults and anyone over 7 months old (Beyea and Nicoll, 1995).
- *Vastus Lateralis*—Muscle is thick and well developed. Recommended site for adults and infants under 7 months of age. Has small nerve endings resulting in discomfort after injection.
- *Deltoid*—Easily accessible muscle. Used only for small medication volumes (0.5 to 1.0 ml) or when other sites are inaccessible because of dressings or casts. Muscle is not well developed in many adults. Hepatitis-B vaccine should be given only in the deltoid (Beyea and Nicoll, 1995).
- *Dorsogluteal*—A traditional site for IM injections. No longer recommended because of the risk of causing injury to sciatic nerve and the fact that the layer of subcutaneous fat overlying the muscle is inconsistent and frequently results in medication not being deposited in the muscle (Beyea and Nicoll, 1995).

Table 18-6

Locating Sites for Intramuscular Injections

Site/Steps	Figure

VENTROGLUTEAL SITE

1. Position client on either side, with knee bent and upper leg slightly ahead of the bottom leg. Client may also remain supine or may be lying on abdomen. Instruct client to relax muscles to be injected.

2. Palpate the greater trochanter at the head of the femur and the anterior superior iliac spine. To locate the proper site, use the left hand when the client lies on the left side and the right hand when the client lies on the right side (see illustration).

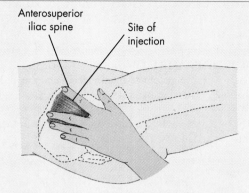

Step 2

3. Place the palm of the hand over the greater trochanter and index finger on the anterior superior iliac spine. Point the thumb toward the client's groin and fingers toward the client's head (see illustration).

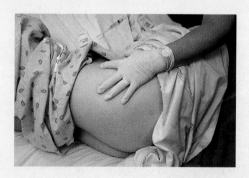

Step 3

4. Spread the middle finger back along the iliac crest toward the buttock as far as possible.

5. The injection site is the center of the triangle formed by your index and middle fingers.

6. Change hands as needed to spread skin taut to give injection. Use dominant hand to give injection (see illustration).

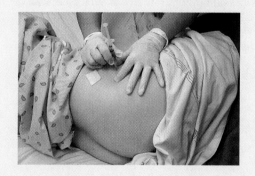

Step 6

VASTUS LATERALIS SITE

1. Client may be lying supine or sitting with site well exposed. If supine, have client flex knee on side where medication will be given.

2. Place one hand above the knee and one hand below the greater trochanter of the femur (see illustration).

3. Locate the midline of the anterior thigh and the midline of

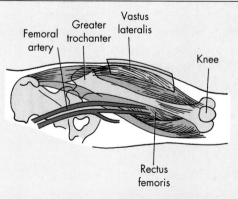

Step 2

Continued

Table 18-6

Locating Sites for Intramuscular Injections—cont'd

Site/Steps	Figure

VASTUS LATERALIS SITE—cont'd

3. Locate the midline of the anterior thigh and the midline of the thigh's lateral (outer) side.

4. The injection site is located within a rectangle formed by these boundaries (see illustration).

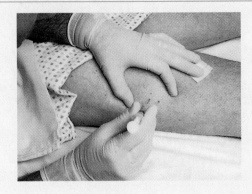

Step 4

DELTOID SITE

1. Client may be sitting or lying down, exposing the upper arm and shoulder. A tight-fitting sleeve should be removed rather than rolled up.

2. Ask client to relax the arm at the side with the elbow flexed.

3. Palpate the lower edge of the acromion process, which forms the base of a triangle (see illustration).

4. Place four fingers across the deltoid muscle, with the top finger along the acromion process.

5. The injection site is in the center of the triangle, three finger-widths or 2.5 to 5 cm (1 to 2 inches) below the acromion process (see illustration).

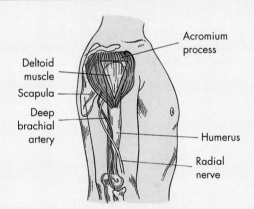

Step 3

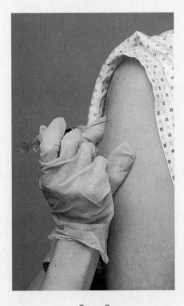

Step 5

ASSESSMENT

1. Review physician's medication order for client's name, drug name, dose, time, and route of administration.
2. Gather information pertinent to drug(s) ordered: action, purpose, appropriate route, time of onset and peak action, normal dose, common side effects, and nursing implications.
3. Check expiration date of medication.
4. Consider factors that may contraindicate IM injection (e.g., muscle atrophy, reduced blood flow, circulatory shock).
5. Assess client's medical history, history of allergies, and medication history.
6. Assess client's knowledge regarding medication and dosage schedule.
7. Observe client's verbal and nonverbal responses toward receiving injection.

PLANNING

Expected outcomes focus on safe, effective administration of injection with minimal anxiety and discomfort.

Expected Outcomes

1. Client demonstrates effects of medication within 30 to 60 minutes.
2. Client has no evidence of adverse effects from medication or injection.

DELEGATION CONSIDERATIONS

The skill of administering IM injections requires problem solving and knowledge application unique to a professional nurse. Delegation is inappropriate. Inform AP of possible side effects to report immediately to the RN.

IMPLEMENTATION

Steps	Rationale

1. See Standard Protocol (inside front cover).

NURSE ALERT

Review the five "rights" for administration of medications.

Steps	Rationale
2. Check expiration date of medication, and prepare medication in syringe.	
3. Change needle on syringe.	Prevents tracking of irritating substances as needle passes into muscle.
4. Explain procedure, location of injection site, and how positioning lessens discomfort. Proceed in calm manner.	Allows client to anticipate injection so as to lessen anxiety.
5. Choose appropriate IM injection site (ventrogluteal preferred) by assessing size and integrity of muscle. Palpate for areas of tenderness or hardness. Note presence of bruising or area of infection.	Muscle is soft when relaxed and firm when tense; absence of tenderness or bruising indicates healthy tissue.
6. Assist client to comfortable position, depending on site (see Table 18-6).	Minimizes discomfort of injection.
7. ✋ Relocate site using anatomical landmarks.	Injection into correct anatomical site prevents injury to nerves, bones, and blood vessels.
8. Carefully remove cap or sheath from needle.	
9. With nondominant hand, pull the skin 2.5 to 3.5 cm (1 to 1½ inches) laterally down so as to administer the injection in a Z-track manner. Hold the skin taut.	Z-track technique reduces discomfort and incidence of lesions.
10. Cleanse site with an antiseptic swab beginning at the center of the site and moving outward in a circular direction for about 5 cm (2 inches). Allow alcohol to dry.	Cleansing reduces surface pathogens, reducing risk of infecting deep tissues.

Steps	Rationale

11. Hold swab or gauze square between fingers of nondominant hand or place near site.

Swab remains accessible when needle is withdrawn.

12. Hold syringe between thumb and forefinger of dominant hand as if holding a dart, with palm down at 90-degree angle to client's skin.

Needle must be injected at 90-degree angle to enter muscle.

13. Insert needle with a steady pressure (see illustration). Hold syringe and aspirate with one hand for at least 5 to 10 seconds. If no blood appears in syringe, inject medication slowly at a rate of 1 ml every 10 seconds. If blood appears, remove needle and dispose of medication and syringe. Repeat preparation procedure.

Aspirating for 5 to 10 seconds is adequate to ensure needle is not in a small blood vessel. A slow, steady injection rate promotes comfort and minimizes tissue damage (Beyea and Nicoll, 1995).

14. Wait 10 seconds after injecting the medication before withdrawing the needle.

Allows medication to deposit into muscle and to begin to diffuse (Keen, 1990).

15. Smoothly and steadily withdraw the needle and release the skin (see illustration). Apply gentle pressure at site with dry sponge or swab.

Minimizes tissue injury. Leaves a zig-zag path that seals the needle track where tissue planes slide across each other. Massaging site can cause tissue irritation (Beyea and Nicoll, 1995).

16. Place small adhesive bandage over puncture site if bleeding is noted.

17. Discard uncapped needle and attached syringe into appropriate receptacle. Discard gloves and wash hands.

Prevents injury to clients and health care personnel.

18. See Completion Protocol (inside front cover).

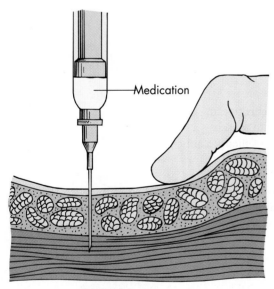

During Injection

Step 13

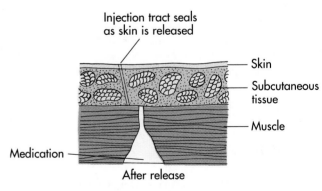

After release

Step 15

EVALUATION

1. Observe for effects of prescribed IM medication within 30 to 60 minutes.
2. Assess the injection site 2 to 4 hours after injection for redness, swelling, pain, or other effects.

Unexpected Outcomes and Related Interventions

1. Client develops signs and symptoms of allergy or side effects.
   a. Notify physician for treatment of symptoms and to change medication.
   b. Be sure client wears allergy bracelet indicating medications and substances to which client is allergic.
2. Client insists on selecting site using incorrect criteria.
   a. Clients requiring regular injections (e.g., vitamin B$_{12}$) should learn how to rotate and select sites.
   b. Instruct client and primary caregiver on how to observe injection sites for complications.

Recording and Reporting

* See MAR, Appendix A. Include description of site used.

Geriatric Considerations

* Older adults are prone to muscle atrophy, requiring careful assessment and selection of injection sites.

Home Care and Long Term Care Considerations

* Clients requiring regular injections (e.g., vitamin B$_{12}$) should learn importance of rotating sites. Injections may be given by family members, client, or home health nurse. Instruction will be necessary on proper injection preparation and administration, as well as disposal of syringes and needles.

Skill 18.3

INTRADERMAL INJECTIONS

Intradermal injections are used for administering small amounts of local anesthetic and skin testing, such as in tuberculosis (TB) screening and allergy tests. This skill focuses on skin testing and TB screening. Because these medications are potent, they are injected in small amounts into the dermis, where blood supply is reduced and drug absorption occurs slowly. A client may have an anaphylactic reaction if the medication enters the circulation too rapidly. For clients with a history of numerous allergies, the physician may perform skin testing.

Skin testing requires clear identification of injection sites for changes in color and tissue integrity. Intradermal sites should be lightly pigmented, free of lesions, and relatively hairless. The inner forearm and upper back are ideal locations.

A TB or 1-ml syringe with a short ($\frac{1}{4}$- to $\frac{1}{2}$-inch), fine-gauge (26 or 27) needle is used for skin testing. Very small amounts of medication (0.01 to 0.1 ml) are injected intradermally. If a bleb does not appear or if the site bleeds after needle withdrawal, the medication may enter SQ tissues. In this case, skin test results will not be valid.

Equipment

1-ml TB syringe with 26- or 27-gauge ($\frac{1}{4}$- to $\frac{1}{2}$-inch) needle
Alcohol swabs
Dry sterile gauze
Vial or ampule of skin test solution
Disposable gloves
MAR or computer printout

ASSESSMENT

1. Review physician's medication order for client's name, drug name, dose, time, and route of administration.
2. Know information regarding drug action, purpose, normal route, dosage, and expected reaction when testing skin with specific allergen or medication.
3. Assess client's history of allergies, substance to which client is allergic, and normal allergic reaction.
4. Determine if client has had previous reaction to skin testing. **Rationale: Can prevent a major allergic response.**

5. Check date of expiration for medication vial or ampule.
6. Assess client's knowledge of purpose and reactions of skin testing.

PLANNING

Expected outcomes focus on safe administration and the identification of allergies or exposure to tuberculosis.

Expected Outcomes

1. Client remains free from systemic allergic reaction.
2. Client describes purpose and expected skin reactions.
3. Client observes for skin reaction and notifies health care provider as instructed including:
   a. Erythema
   b. Induration

IMPLEMENTATION

Steps	Rationale

1. See Standard Protocol (inside front cover).

NURSE ALERT

Review the five "rights" for administration of medications.

2. Check expiration date of test solution and prepare in syringe.
3. Select appropriate injection site:
   a. *TB testing:* three to four fingerwidths below antecubital space and handwidth above wrist.
   b. *Skin testing:* inner forearm and upper back.

Injection sites should be free of abnormalities that may interfere with drug absorption. An intradermal site should be clear so results of skin test can be seen and read correctly.

NURSE ALERT

Avoid bruises, areas of inflammation, edema, lesions, or discolorations of forearm.

4. Assist client to comfortable position with elbow and forearm extended and supported on flat surface.

Stabilizes injection site for easiest accessibility.

5. Cleanse site with an antiseptic swab, beginning at center of the site and rotating outward in a circular direction for about 5 cm (2 inches). Allow to dry.

Mechanical action of swab removes secretions containing microorganisms. Drying prevents antiseptic from affecting test results.

6. Hold swab or square of sterile gauze between fingers of nondominant hand.

Swab or gauze remains readily accessible when needle is withdrawn.

7. Remove needle cap or sheath from needle by pulling it straight off.

Preventing needle from touching sides of cap prevents contamination.

8. Hold syringe between thumb and forefinger of dominant hand with bevel of needle pointing up.

Bevel up facilitates correct needle placement.

9. With nondominant hand, stretch skin over site with forefinger or thumb.

Needle pierces tight skin more easily.

Steps	**Rationale**

10. With needle almost against client's skin, insert it carefully at a 5- to 15-degree angle until resistance is felt, and advance needle through epidermis to approximately 3 mm (⅛ inch) below skin surface. Needle tip can be seen through skin (see illustration).

11. Inject medication slowly. It is not necessary to aspirate, because dermis is relatively avascular. Normally, resistance is felt. If not, needle is too deep; remove and begin again.

Slow injection minimizes discomfort at site. Dermal layer is tight and does not expand easily when solution is injected.

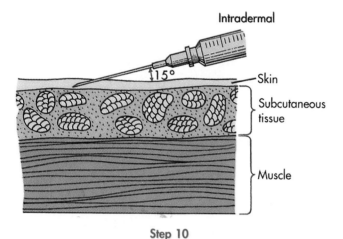

Step 10

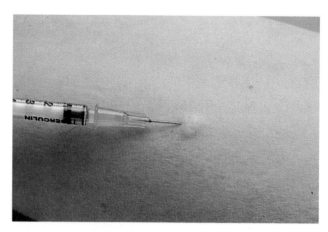

Step 12

12. While injecting medication, a light-colored bleb resembling a mosquito bite approximately 6 mm (¼ inch) in diameter forms at site and gradually disappears (see illustration). Minimal bruising may be present.

Medication is in dermis and is eventually absorbed. Bruising is a result of minor bleeding from capillaries.

COMMUNICATION TIP

During this time, explain to client what the skin will look like: Normally the skin will remain clear or you might notice a needle mark. If the test is positive, you will notice redness and a lump at the site.

13. Withdraw needle while applying alcohol swab or gauze gently over site.

14. Do not massage site.

Support of tissue around injection site minimizes discomfort during needle withdrawal.

Massage may disperse medication into underlying tissue layers and alter test results.

15. Discard uncapped needle and syringe in appropriately labeled receptacle. Discard gloves and wash hands.

Prevents injury to client and health care personnel.

16. Use skin pencil and draw circle around perimeter of injection site. Tell client not to wash off markings around injection site.

Identifies site for testing to be read in 48 to 72 hours

17. After skin testing have the client wait for 30 minutes.

Allows for observation of development of any allergic reaction.

18. When clients are tested in a clinic or other outpatient setting, have them call in results to physician.

19. See Completion Protocol (inside front cover).

EVALUATION

1. Observe for any allergic reactions.
2. Ask client to describe implications of skin testing and signs of expected skin reaction/hypersensitivity.
3. There is a prescribed wait of 20 minutes to several days (depending on the antigen) before the local reaction should be evaluated for positive test (McKenry and Salerno, 1995).
    a. Inspect site for erythema:

(Trace)	Faint discoloration
+ (1 plus)	Pink
++ (2 plus)	Red
+++ (3 plus)	Purplish red
++++ (4 plus)	Vesiculation or necrosis

    b. Inspect site for induration (area of hardness):

(Trace)	Barely palpable
+ (1 plus)	Palpable, but not visible
++ (2 plus)	Easily palpable and visible; indurated area buckles when squeezed gently
+++ (3 plus)	Easily palpable and visible; does not buckle when squeezed gently
++++ (4 plus)	Vesiculation or necrosis

Unexpected Outcomes and Related Interventions

1. Occasionally a highly positive reaction will result in vesiculation and necrosis of overlying skin (McKenry and Salerno, 1995).
    a. Physician may order corticosteroids.
2. Systemic allergic reaction of urticaria, sneezing, or dyspnea may develop. More likely occurring if hyposensitization therapy to allergens has begun.
    a. Have epinephrine available if necessary.
3. Positive TB reaction is indicated by induration 9 mm or more of injection site. Five to 9 mm is a questionable result. Test is read at 48 to 72 hours.
    a. Positive TB test indicates exposure, not active disease. Further testing for diagnosis is required.
    b. A person who has contact with an individual with tuberculosis and whose initial TB reaction (induration) is more than 5 mm should have a chest x-ray film and be considered for preventive therapy (American Thoracic Society, 1992).
    c. Contacts who initially have negative skin test results should receive a repeat skin test 10 to 12 weeks after the initial test (American Thoracic Society, 1992).

Recording and Reporting

- Record amount, type of medication, site of injection, and date and time on medication record.
- In progress notes, describe appearance of injection site; note size, color, skin texture, and appearance of lesions.

Sample Documentation

1000   PPD injection site in left lower forearm read at 72 hours; test site is clear, without redness or induration.

Geriatric Considerations

- TB skin testing in older adults is an unreliable indicator of tuberculosis. Older adults often display a false-negative skin test as a result of reduced immune system activity (Lueckenotte, 1996).
- If skin testing is used, it is recommended that the standard 5-TU Mantoux technique test be given and then repeated for a booster effect (Morris, 1990).

CRITICAL THINKING EXERCISES

1. Mrs. Thomas has been admitted after an automobile accident. She is 45 years old, 5 feet 6 inches tall, and weighs 140 pounds. She is in a traction apparatus to immobilize her right leg. She cannot turn to her side and must remain supine. What is the best site to use in administering an IM injection to Mrs. Thomas?

2. You see a colleague demonstrating insulin injection to a client. The nurse administers the medication in the client's outer arm. If you were instructing the client, what might you do differently?

3. Mr. Schwartz is a 68-year-old client with arthritis. He has been recently admitted to the hospital for a deep vein thrombosis. Mr. Schwartz will be discharged home tomorrow on regular doses of heparin for 1 week. He takes NSAIDs for his arthritis and daily vitamin supplements. What client education and consultation are necessary for Mr. Schwartz?

REFERENCES

American Diabetes Association: Position statement: Insulin administration, *Diabet Care* 20(suppl 1):S46–S49, 1997.

American Thoracic Society: Control of tuberculosis in the United States, *Am Rev Respir Dis* 146(16):1623, 1992.

Beyea SC, Nicoll LH: Administration of medications via the intramuscular route: An integrative review of the literature and research-based protocol for the procedure, *Appl Nurs Res* 8(1):23–33, 1995.

Centers for Disease Control and Prevention: Update: universal precautions for prevention of transmission of HIV, hepatitis-B virus, and other bloodborne pathogens in health care settings, *MMWR* 37:377, 1988.

Chaplin G, Shull H, Welk PC: How safe is the air-bubble technique for IM injections? *Nurs 85* 6:7, 1985.

Craft K: Do you really know how to handle sharps? *RN 53* (8):33, 1990.

Fahs PS, Kinney MR: The abdomen, thigh, and arm as sites for subcutaneous sodium heparin injections, *Nurs Res* 40:204–207, 1991.

Farley F et al: Will that IM needle reach the muscle? *Am J Nurs* 86(12):1327–1328, 1986.

Gray D: *Calculate with confidence*, St Louis, 1994, Mosby.

Hahn K: Brush up on your injection technique, *Nurs 90* 20(9):54–58, 1990.

Keen MF: Comparison of two intramuscular injection techniques on the incidence and severity of discomfort and lesions at the injection site, *Dissertation Abstracts International* (University Microfilms No 8120152), 42(4):1394B, 1982.

Keen MF: Comparison of intramuscular injection techniques to reduce site discomfort and lesions, *Nurs Res* 35:207–210, 1986.

Keen MF: Get on the right track with Z-track injections, *Nurs 90* 20(8):59, 1990.

Lueckenotte A: *Gerontologic nursing*, St Louis, Mosby, 1996.

McConnell EA: The subtle art of really good injections, *RN* 45:24, 1982.

McKenry LM, Salerno E: *Pharmacology in nursing*, ed 19, St Louis, 1995, Mosby.

Morris JF: Pulmonary diseases. In Casssel CK et al: *Geriatric medicine*, ed 2, New York, 1990, Springer.

Newton M, Newton D, Fudin J: Reviewing the "big three" injection routes, *Nurs 92* 22(2):34–42, 1992.

Owens-Schwab E, Fraser VJ: Needles and needle protection devices: a second look at efficacy and selection, *Infect Control Hosp Epidemiol* 14(11):657, 1993.

Quartermaine S, Taylor R: A comparative study of depot injection techniques, *Nurs Times* 91(30):36–39, 1995.

Thow JC, Coulthard A, Home PD: Insulin injection site tissue depths and localization of a simulated insulin bolus using a novel air contrast ultrasonographic technique in insulin treated diabetic subjects, *Diabet Med* 9(10):915–920, 1992, Dec.

Winslow EH, Jacobson AF: Research for practice, *Am J Nurs* 97(5):71–72, 1997.

Wong DL: *Whaley and Wong's nursing care of infants and children*, ed 5, St Louis, 1995, Mosby.

Zenk KE: Improving the accuracy of mini-volume injections, *Infusion* 6(1):7–12, 1982.

Zenk KE: Beware of overdose, *Nurs 93* 23(3):28–29, 1993.

UNIT 6

Perioperative Nursing Care

Chapter 19
Preparing the Client for Surgery

Chapter 20
Intraoperative Techniques

Chapter 21
Caring for the Postoperative Client

Chapter 22
Pain Management

Chapter 23
Therapeutic Use of Heat and Cold

CHAPTER 19

Preparing the Client for Surgery

Skill 19.1
Preoperative Assessment, 476

Skill 19.2
Preoperative Teaching, 480

Skill 19.3
Physical Preparation, 485

with surgery. Many clients return home the same day, and the family members may be unsure about their role in the client's recovery. Before the client undergoes surgery, and again before discharge, the nurse teaches the client and family what to expect and what they can do to assist in the recovery process.

Physically preparing the client to undergo surgery and anesthesia involves important skills for the nurse. Regardless of the surgery, safety measures, such as verifying the procedure and consent, are critical. Other steps, such as urinary catheterization or special laboratory tests, are completed only for specific surgical procedures. Physical preparation focused on minimizing the risks involved with surgery and anesthesia places the client in the best condition possible.

Surgery is a stressful experience for the client, both psychologically and physiologically. The client has little control over the situation or the outcome. This results in feelings of anxiety, fear, and powerlessness. As with trauma, the surgery itself is a physiological stressor affecting the major body systems. Preoperative care can reduce this stress and place the client in the best condition possible to undergo the surgery. The nurse thoroughly assesses the client's condition, teaches the client and family what to expect, and physically prepares the client for surgery.

For any surgical procedure, it is important for the nurse to complete a thorough preoperative assessment. For clients who are already hospitalized, this may occur the day before surgery. In an outpatient setting, the preoperative assessment may begin several days before surgery and be completed the morning of surgery. Regardless of the setting, the preoperative assessment forms the basis for a plan of care for the client during and after surgery.

Often the client is unsure what to expect and has concerns about the amount of pain or disfigurement involved

NURSING DIAGNOSES

Nursing diagnoses associated with the surgical experience include **Risk for Infection** related to the surgical wound, urinary catheter, and invasive lines and **Risk for Injury** related to inadequate identification and communication of risks. The risk for injury is also related to surgical positioning and electrical equipment used in the operating room. The risk of hypoxemia is related to hypoventilation from anesthesia, surgical positions, and incisions. Psychological states such as **Knowledge Deficit** and **Anxiety** often result when a client is unsure what to expect before, during, and after the surgery. The inability to control the situation often results in **Powerlessness,** and the inability to accept the situation may result in **Ineffective Coping.** During and after surgery using general anesthesia, the client's cough and gag reflexes are suppressed. This results in a risk for **Ineffective Airway Clearance** related to the presence of secretions.

Skill 19.1

PREOPERATIVE ASSESSMENT

To identify risks and plan for the client's care during and after surgery and anesthesia, the nurse performs a thorough preoperative assessment of the client's physiological and psychological condition. To provide efficient services, the assessment is frequently begun before the day of surgery and completed 1 to 2 hours before the scheduled time of surgery. This provides time for the nurse to follow up on any unexpected outcomes. Before beginning this assessment, the nurse establishes a trusting relationship with the client. It is not unusual for the client to remember and report facts to the nurse at this time that were not told to the physician earlier. To encourage open communication, the nurse provides privacy and a location free of interruption.

Equipment

- Stethoscope
- Blood pressure cuff
- Pulse oximeter
- Thermometer
- Watch or clock
- Scale
- Preoperative assessment form (Figure 19-1)

PLANNING

Expected outcomes of the preoperative assessment focus on obtaining accurate information and identifying risk factors related to the intended surgery.

Expected Outcomes

1. Client provides the information required to establish a plan of care.
2. Client assists the nurse in completing the assessment.

DELEGATION CONSIDERATIONS

The skills of assessment that are part of preparing the client for surgery require problem solving and knowledge application unique to a professional nurse. For these skills delegation is inappropriate. Assistive personnel (AP) may obtain vital signs and weight and height measurements. Instruct personnel on proper steps and precautions for delegated procedures.

IMPLEMENTATION

Steps	Rationale
1. See Standard Protocol (inside front cover).	
2. Determine if the client has any communication impairment (e.g., blindness, hearing loss), ability to understand English, and if the client is mentally competent.	
3. Assess the client's understanding of the intended surgery and anesthesia.	
4. Obtain a nursing history:	
a. Condition leading to surgery	
b. The need for isolation precautions (e.g., for infectious disease or compromised immunity).	
c. Chronic illnesses	Some chronic conditions increase the risk of complications from surgery and anesthesia (e.g., hypertension-bleeding and stroke; asthma-impaired ventilation; hiatal hernia–aspiration).
d. Last menstrual period (for female clients in childbearing years)	Anesthetic agents and other medications could injure the fetus.
e. Previous hospitalizations	

A-1c4 NURSE'S DETAILED PERIOPERATIVE NOTE

DATE *12 – 1 – XX*

HOSP. # *23-6694-93*

NAME *John Doe*

BIRTH DATE

ADDRESS

SS#

IF NOT IMPRINTED, PLEASE PRINT DATE, HOSP. #, NAME AND LOCATION

1. Place initials in the space preceding the appropriate response (YES/NO, MET/NOT MET, NOT APPLICABLE)
2. Explain any "NO" or "NOT MET" in the space provided adjacent to the item or in the comment section provided, except for * items.
3. Record additional information in the comment section.
4. Record initials immediately following narrative entry.

PERIOPERATIVE TRANSPORT BY:	*MM*	METHOD: *W/C*	PREOPERATIVE UNIT/AREA:
TIME RECEIVED IN PRESURGICAL CARE UNIT:	*0830*	TIME RECEIVED IN OR:	*0915*

PATIENT ASSESSMENT/PREPARATION	YES	NO	COMMENT
PATIENT IDENTIFIED	X X		ID Band Location Ⓡ *WRIST*
BLOOD BAND PRESENT*	X X		#/Location Ⓡ *WRIST, ABC 000*
ALLERGIES* (If yes, please list)	X X		*PCN, SULFA*
LATEX PRECAUTIONS INDICATED*		X X	
CONSENT	X X		*In chart*
NPO	X		*since 0030*
HEALTH CHANGED SINCE LAST APPT		X	If Yes, Specify: Physician Notified:
INFECTIONS, PROBLEMS WITH HEART OR LUNGS		X	If Yes, Specify: Physician Notified:
TAKING ANY NEW MEDICATIONS		X	If Yes, Specify: Physician Notified:
PREOPERATIVE ORDERS COMPLETED	X		
SKIN ASSESSMENT COMPLETED	X		*intact*
VITALS OBTAINED DAY OF SURGERY	X		
HISTORY AND PHYSICAL PRESENT	X		
LAB VALUES REVIEWED	X		*WNL*
LEVEL OF CONSCIOUSNESS—Answers questions/responds appropriately for age	X X		*ORIENTED X 3*
IMPLANTS/PROSTHESIS* (If yes, please list)		X X	

Nursing Comments: *IV infusing LFA*

NURSING DIAGNOSIS	NURSING ORDERS/INTERVENTIONS	EXPECTED PATIENT OUTCOMES
ANXIETY—Potential for, Related to Surgical Intervention and Outcomes	1. Psychologic & physiologic comfort measures are provided. ⊾ Yes ___ No	The patient reports and/or demonstrates a reduction in anxiety. ⊾ MET ___ NOT MET
KNOWLEDGE DEFICIT—Potential for, Related to Surgical Intervention	1. The patient's understanding is assessed and questions/concerns are addressed by the appropriate individuals. ⊾ Yes ___No *Reviewed operative exercises*	The patient's (guardian's) description of surgery corresponds with the Operative Consent (G-2d). ⊾ MET ___ NOT MET
INJURY—Potential for, Related to Tubes, Catheters, Lines ___ Not Applicable	1. Integrity of tubes, catheters, and lines is maintained. ⊾ Yes ___ No Catheters/Tubes/Drains/Lines: *IV in* Ⓛ *forearm*	The patient's risk for injury related to care and management of tubes, catheters, and lines is minimized. ⊾ MET ___ NOT MET

Initials	Standards Implemented By:	Initials	Standards Implemented By:
MM	*Marilyn Moss, RN*		

88976/10-98/MH05659

THE UNIVERSITY OF IOWA HOSPITALS AND CLINICS

A -1c4

B CLIN. NOTES

C LABORATORY

D X-RAY EXAM

E CONSULTATION

F SPEC. EXAM

G THERAPY

H PATHOLOGY

I DIAGNOSIS

Figure 19-1 Preoperative assessment form. *Courtesy University of Iowa Hospitals and Clinics.*

Steps	Rationale
f. Medication history, including prescription and over-the-counter (OTC), and date/time of last doses	Client may not report OTC medications unless specifically asked. The client may be instructed to take any routine blood pressure, cardiac, or seizure medications.
g. Previous experience with surgery and anesthesia	
h. Family history of complications from surgery or anesthesia	A family history of reactions to anesthetic agents may indicate a familial condition, malignant hyperthermia, which is life threatening.
i. Allergies to medications or food, including specific questions about natural rubber latex	Reactions to latex can be life threatening, and prevention in sensitized clients requires specific precautions. Many clients do not understand that rubber and latex are the same. Using both words will help obtain accurate information (Steelman, 1997).
j. Physical impairment	
k. Prostheses and implants (e.g., dentures, hearing aid, pacemaker, internal defibrillator, hip prosthesis)	These devices could become damaged or malfunction from electrical equipment used during surgery. This information should be communicated to the operating room nurse.
l. Smoking, alcohol, and drug use	
m. Occupation	

COMMUNICATION TIP

- *Speaking in a clear, slow voice helps reduce the client's anxiety.*
- *When asking the client about allergies, ask a specific question about reactions or problems the client might have had to natural rubber latex. Most clients do not know that rubber is latex. Using both words with the examples of balloons and gloves has been found to obtain otherwise missed information.*

- *Allow the client to wear eyeglasses, dentures, or hearing aid as long as possible before surgery. These aids facilitate client cooperation by ensuring that the client has clear vision and maximal auditory perception throughout the preoperative phase.*

5. Assess client's weight (see Skill 8.3), height, and vital signs (see Skill 13.1).	Height and weight are used to calculate drug dosages.
6. Assess client's respiratory status, including character and rate of respirations, oxygen saturation, ability to breathe lying flat, and chest x-ray report.	
7. Evaluate client's circulatory status, including apical pulse, electrocardiogram (ECG) report, and peripheral pulses (see Skills 13.3 and 14.6).	
8. Determine client's neurological status, including level of consciousness (LOC) (see Skill 13.9)	
9. Evaluate client's musculoskeletal system, including range of motion (ROM) of joints (see Skill 13.10).	If the ROM is limited, extra care will be needed to prevent injury related to positioning in surgery.
10. Examine client's skin; identify any breaks in skin integrity and determine level of hydration (see Skill 24.1)	If skin is thin, broken, or bruised, extra padding will be needed in surgery.
11. Evaluate client's emotional status, including level of anxiety, coping ability, and family support.	

Steps	**Rationale**
12. Review the results of laboratory tests, including complete blood count (CBC), electrolytes, urinalysis, and other diagnostic tests.	Laboratory work provides an assessment of major body systems.
13. Ask if client has an advanced directive (see Chapter 38).	Advanced directives protect client's rights by communicating client's desires.
14. Identify the time of client's last intake of food or drink.	With client under general anesthesia, the esophageal sphincter relaxes and the stomach contents can be aspirated.
15. See Completion Protocol (inside front cover).	

• • •

EVALUATION

1. Determine if client has provided the information requested.
2. Evaluate client's ability to cooperate (e.g., eye contact, answers appropriately).

Unexpected Outcomes and Related Interventions

1. The client does not understand English.
   Obtain an interpreter.
2. The client is not mentally competent.
   Determine who is legally authorized to consent for surgery (see agency policy).
3. Client does not understand what surgery will be performed.
   Notify the surgeon.
4. The client reports a hiatal hernia.
   Notify the anesthesiologist.
5. The client may be pregnant.
   Notify surgeon and anesthesiologist.
6. The client has been taking anticoagulants.
   Notify the surgeon.
7. The client reports excessive vomiting after a previous surgery.
   Notify the anesthesiologist.
8. The client reports a family history of serious complications associated with previous surgery or anesthesia.
   Notify the anesthesiologist.
9. Client reports having a cold or upper respiratory infection.
   Notify surgeon and anesthesiologist/nurse anesthetist.
10. Client reports an allergy to latex.
    a. Remove all supplies containing latex from client's room.
    b. Post a latex precautions sign on the door or stretcher.
    c. Notify surgeon, anesthesiologist/nurse anesthetist, and operating room nurse (Steelman, 1997).

11. Client reports recent chest pain.
    Notify anesthesiologist/nurse anesthetist.
12. Appropriate laboratory tests were not ordered or completed.
    Notify surgeon and anesthesiologist/nurse anesthetist, and make arrangements for tests to be completed.
13. Chest x-ray report, ECG, or laboratory tests show abnormal findings.
    Notify anesthesiologist/nurse anesthetist.
14. Client has a blister, abrasion, or boil near the incision site.
    Notify surgeon.

Recording and Reporting

- Document findings on the Preoperative portion of the nurses' detailed preoperative notes (see Figure 19-1) or other designated agency form.
- Report abnormal laboratory values or other concerns to the surgeon or anesthesiologist.

Geriatric Considerations

- The older adult client may have some limitation in range of joint motion. If this limitation is significant, notify the operating room nurse so that surgical position can be modified.

Skill 19.2

PREOPERATIVE TEACHING

Preoperative client teaching involves assisting a client to understand and mentally prepare for the surgical experience (Iowa Intervention Project, 1996). Clients and their families are often very anxious about impending surgery. This anxiety increases heart rate and blood pressure after surgery, which can contribute to bleeding and complications. Postoperatively, high anxiety can lead to negative psychological and physiological outcomes. Preoperative information about expected perioperative sensations has been shown to decrease the distress associated with surgery. By teaching the client preoperatively, the nurse can make a significant contribution to the success of surgery and to the client's postoperative recovery (Butcher, 1997).

Equipment

Stretcher or bed
Pillow
Incentive spirometer
Preoperative education flow sheet (Figure 19-2)

ASSESSMENT

1. Ask about client's previous experiences with surgery and anesthesia. **Rationale: This provides information that the nurse may use to individualize teaching and address specific concerns of the client.**
2. Determine client and family's understanding of surgery. **Rationale: This information determines if correction of misunderstanding is necessary.**
3. Identify the client's cognitive level, language, and culture. **Rationale: These factors may alter the client's ability to understand the meaning of surgery.**
4. Assess client's anxiety related to surgery. **Rationale: This information directs the nurse to provide additional emotional support and indicates the client's readiness to learn.**

PLANNING

Based on the preoperative assessment, the nurse plans preoperative teaching. Every attempt should be made to ensure privacy for the client. The best learning method for the client should be selected. In many settings, a videotape and written materials are available to assist the nurse. Whenever possible, the family should be present. Later, they serve as coaches and assist the client in performing exercises. Expected outcomes of preoperative teaching focus on reducing the anxiety level of the client and family and demonstrations of their understanding of key information and specific skills necessary to prevent complications.

Expected Outcomes

1. Expected outcomes focus on demonstrating an understanding of skills taught. Client demonstrates eye contact and asks and answers questions appropriately.
2. Client correctly performs breathing exercises and leg exercises.
3. Family identifies the location of the waiting room.
4. Family verbalizes the ability to care for client at home.
5. Family provides emotional support for client preoperatively.
6. Client and family demonstrate appropriate coping skills.

DELEGATION CONSIDERATIONS

The skills of preoperative teaching require problem solving and knowledge application unique to a professional nurse. AP can reinforce and assist clients in performing postoperative exercises.

- Review with AP any precautions unique for a particular client.
- Be sure staff know when to inform the nurse if the client is unable to perform the exercises correctly.

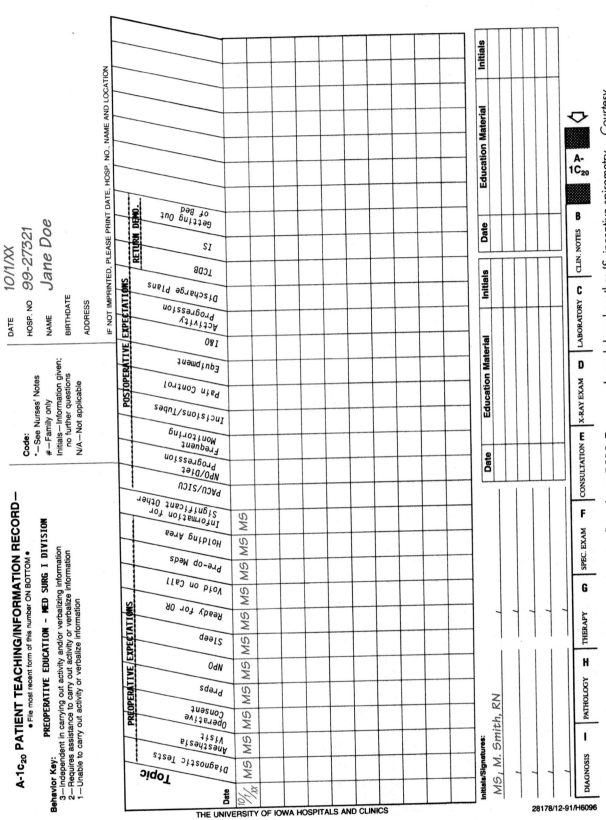

Figure 19-2 Preoperative education flow sheet. *TCDB,* Turn, cough, and deep breathe; *IS,* incentive spirometry. *Courtesy University of Iowa Hospitals and Clinics.*

IMPLEMENTATION

Steps	Rationale

1. See Standard Protocol (inside front cover).
2. Inform client and family of date, time, location of surgery, and where to wait.

    Accurate information helps reduce the stress associated with surgery.

3. Inform client and family about the anticipated length of time of surgery.
4. Answer questions client and family ask.
5. Describe perioperative routines (e.g., intravenous [IV] therapy, urinary catheterization, enema, hair removal, laboratory tests, transport to operating room).
6. Describe preoperative medications.
7. Review which routine medications are to be discontinued before surgery.

    Some medications are discontinued before surgery. For example, anticoagulants may increase bleeding and are usually discontinued several days before surgery. Insulin dosages are usually adjusted because of the reduced intake of food preoperatively.

8. Describe perioperative sensations (e.g., blood pressure cuff tightening, ECG leads, cool room, beep of monitor).

    Describing what sensations client will experience has been shown to reduce distress associated with the experience.

9. Describe pain-control methods. Many clients have a patient-controlled analgesia (PCA) pump (see Chapter 22).

    Clients are fearful of postoperative pain. Explaining pain-management techniques will reduce this fear.

10. Describe what client will experience postoperatively (e.g., frequent vital signs, turning, catheters, drains, tubes).
11. Instruct client in splinting. Hold pillow to abdomen for support while sitting up or coughing (see illustration).
12. **Instruct client on turning and sitting up.**
    a. Flex knees.
    b. Splint incision with left arm and pillow (see illustration).
    c. Push on the mattress with right arm and swing feet over the edge of the bed.

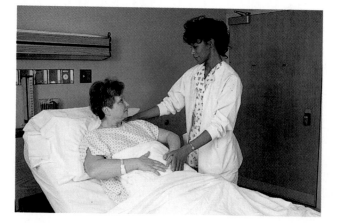

Step 11

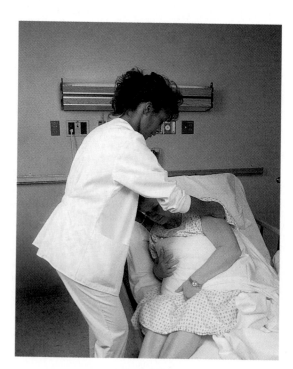

Step 12b

Steps

Rationale

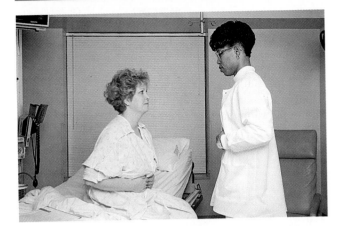

Step 13

13. **Instruct client in deep breathing and coughing (see illustration).**

Client may be unable or reluctant to deep breathe because of weakness or pain, resulting in secretions remaining in the base of the lungs. This collection of secretions increases the risk of pulmonary complications such as pneumonia.

   a. Assist client to sitting position.
   b. Instruct client to place palms of hands over the lower border of the rib cage with third fingers touching.
   c. Have client take slow, deep breaths and feel fingers separate.
   d. Have client hold the breath for 3 seconds and exhale through the mouth slowly, as if blowing out a candle.
   e. Instruct client to cough forcefully.
   f. Have the client practice several times.
   g. Instruct client to perform turn, cough, and deep breathing every 2 hours.

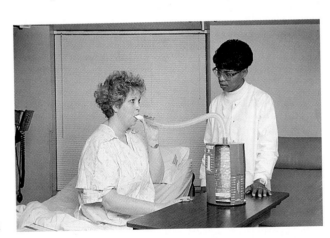

Step 14

14. **Instruct client in use of an incentive spirometer (see illustration).**
   a. Position in a setting or reclining position.
   b. Instruct client to exhale completely, then place mouthpiece so that lips completely cover it and inhale slowly, maintaining constant flow through unit.

Encourages deep breathing and loosens secretions in lung bases.

Promotes complete inflation of lungs and minimizes atelectasis.

Steps	Rationale

c. After maximum inspiration, client should hold breath for 2 to 3 seconds, then exhale slowly.

d. Instruct client to breathe normally for a short period, then repeat process.

Prevents hyperventilation and fatigue.

15. Instruct client on three leg exercises.

Leg exercises encourage circulation in the lower extremities and reduce the risk of circulatory complications such as an embolism.

a. Rotate each ankle in a complete circle.

b. Instruct client to draw imaginary circles with the big toe 5 times.

c. Alternate dorsiflexion and plantar flexion while instructing client to feel calf muscles tighten and relax. Repeat 5 times (see illustration).

d. Instruct client to alternate flexing and extending knees one leg at a time. Repeat 5 times (see illustration).

e. Instruct client to alternate straight leg raises. Repeat 5 times.

f. Instruct client to perform these three leg exercises every 2 hours while awake.

16. Verify that client's expectations of surgery are realistic. Correct expectations as needed.

17. Reinforce therapeutic coping strategies. If ineffective, encourage alternatives.

18. See Completion Protocol (inside front cover).

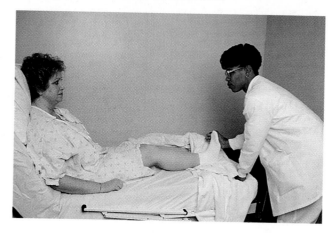

Step 15c

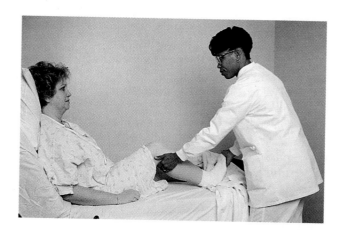

Step 15d

• • •

EVALUATION

1. Ask client to repeat key information.

2. Ask client to demonstrate splinting, deep breathing, and leg exercises.

3. Ask family to identify location of the waiting room.

4. Ask family if they are able to care for client at home after discharge.

5. Observe the level of emotional support family provides client.

6. Observe client and family coping strategies.

Unexpected Outcomes and Related Interventions

1. Client identifies an incorrect date, time, or location of surgery.

   Provide the correct information verbally and in writing for client and family.

2. Client questions the importance of not drinking the morning of surgery.

   Explain that under anesthesia, the fluid can come up from the stomach and go into the lung.

3. Client is withdrawn.
   a. Explain that it is normal to feel anxious about surgery.
   b. Ask how client feels about the surgery.
4. Client incorrectly performs breathing exercises.
   a. Explain the correct breathing technique.
   b. Explain the importance of postoperative breathing.
   c. Instruct client to repeat the demonstration.
5. Family verbalizes anxiety about care for client at home.
   a. Explain that these feelings are normal.
   b. Provide written instructions.
   c. Provide a telephone number for contact if there are further questions.
6. Family indicates that they are unable to care for client at home.
   Contact physician and discuss the alternative of a home health care referral.

Recording and Reporting

Record preoperative teaching on the preoperative education flow sheet (see Figure 19-2) or designated agency form.

Geriatric Considerations

Aging causes changes in the central nervous system, inhibiting short-term memory and making learning more difficult (Smith, Gurkowski, and Bracken, 1995). The elderly client may retain verbal information better than nonverbal information. The room should be well lighted and free of distractions. Presenting one idea at a time and reinforcing information verbally will aid in learning (Daley, 1996).

Skill 19.3

PHYSICAL PREPARATION

Physical preparation of the client for surgery involves providing care immediately before surgery, verification of required procedures and tests, and documentation in the client's record (Iowa Intervention Project, 1996). This preparation minimizes the risks of infection and injury related to surgery and anesthesia (Jepsen and Bruttomesso, 1993). Specific steps are taken to prepare every client. These steps depend on the type of surgery being performed and the risks involved. For example, antiembolism stockings and/or sequential compression stockings may be used for adult clients undergoing surgery that will last several hours and require a long period of immobilization afterward (Dalen and Hersh, 1995). The bowel may need to be prepped with an enema or by drinking a purgative (this may be done at home by clients admitted the morning of surgery) even for abdominal surgery on or near the intestine. Hair near the incision site may need to be removed. It is important to check the physician's orders to determine what steps are needed for the surgical client. Regardless of the type of surgery, the goal of physical preparation is to place the client in the best condition possible to minimize the risks of the surgery that is planned.

Equipment

Hospital gown
IV solution, tubing, catheter, tourniquet, alcohol swab, and IV tape
Antiembolism stockings (when ordered)
Sequential compression device (when ordered)
Clippers, gloves, disposable towel
Preoperative checklist (Figure 19-3, p. 486).

ASSESSMENT

The preoperative assessment forms the basis for physical preparation of the client for surgery (see Skill 19.1).

PLANNING

Expected outcomes focus on the physical preparation of the client for surgery.

Expected Outcomes

1. Client cooperates during preparatory measures (e.g., starting an IV, laboratory tests).
2. Client undergoes measures to reduce the risk of infection (e.g., preoperative antibiotic, skin preparation).

A-1c PREOPERATIVE CHECKLIST

● File with other A-1c's of same date ●

1. Place initials in appropriate box: YES, NO. Each item must have an entry.
2. Explain any "No." This can be done in the space after the item or in the "Comments" section. Use back of form, if needed.
3. To give more information on any item, use the space after the item. If more space needed, use the "Comments" section on back of form.

DATE **8/1/XX**

HOSP. # **99-23764-1**

NAME **James Lee**

BIRTH DATE

ADDRESS

SS #

IF NOT IMPRINTED, PLEASE PRINT DATE, HOSP. #, NAME AND LOCATION

YES	NO	NA		
X/ML			**Special Information/Transport Needs** (e.g., blind, O_2, monitoring) *Mr. Lee is very hard of hearing*	A-1c
ML			Preoperative orders written.	
ML			Consent complete and in medical record.	
	ML		**Specify Allergies:** *NKA*	B
	ML		Allergies (or NKA) labeled on cover of medical record.	
	ML		Latex precautions indicated.	
	ML		Isolation label on cover of medical record. **Specify Type:**	
	ML		Has health changed since last appt? **If Yes, Specify:**	
	ML		Infections, problems with heart or lungs? **If Yes, Specify:**	
	ML		Taking any new medications? **If Yes, Specify:**	C
ML			Teaching completed and documented.	
ML			Chest X-ray completed ___*7/30/XX*___ Ordered labs completed ___*7/30/XX*___ EKG completed ___*7/30/XX*___	
ML			Forms completed and filed in medical record.	
ML			Anesthesia preop evaluation in medical record.	
ML			NPO since: *0015*	D
ML			Vitals (Obtain Day of Surgery) T_*98⁶*_ P_*100*_ R_*24*_ BP_*110*_/_*70*_	
ML			Jewelry absent. Specify item(s) removed and disposition of jewelry/valuables. *valuables are at home*	
		ML	Prostheses removed: hearing aid, eye glasses, contact lenses (circle).	
		ML	Other: Disposition:	
ML			Identification band on patient and legible. **Specify location:** *(R) wrist*	E
ML			Type and cross screen (circle) done. Date drawn: *7/30/XX*	
ML			Blood band on patient and legible. **Specify location:** *(R) wrist*	
ML			Anti-embolism stockings with patient.	
		ML	Sequential compression device sleeve on per orders.	
ML			Preps/tests completed as ordered. **Specify:** *Routine LAB, EKG results in medical record*	
ML			Voided/catheterized (circle). Time: *0730*	F
ML			Level of consciousness—Answers questions/responds appropriately for age	
ML			Medication(s) given.	
		ML	Medication(s) sent with patient. **Specify:**	
		ML	Article(s) sent with patient. **Specify:**	
ML			Addressograph plate with medical record. All volumes with patient.	

COMMENTS: | | | | | G

(Right margin tabs from top to bottom: A-1c | B CLIN. NOTES | C LABORATORY | D X-RAY EXAM | E CONSULTATION | F SPEC. EXAM | G THERAPY | H PATHOLOGY | I DIAGNOSIS)

Initials	Signature and Title of Individuals Filing Out Form	Initials	Signature and Title of Individuals Filing Out Form
ML	*Margaret Lenz*		

88574/10-98/MH07528

THE UNIVERSITY OF IOWA HOSPITALS AND CLINICS

Figure 19-3 Preoperative checklist. *Courtesy University of Iowa Hospitals and Clinics.*

DELEGATION CONSIDERATIONS

Preparing the client for surgery requires problem solving and knowledge application unique to a professional nurse. For this skill delegation is inappropriate. Assistive personnel may administer an enema or a douche, obtain vital signs, apply antiembolic stockings, and assist client in removing clothing, jewelry, and prostheses.

- Instruct AP on proper steps amd precautions when preparing a client for surgery.
- Instruct AP on proper observations and precautions if the client has an intravenous catheter in place.

IMPLEMENTATION

Steps	Rationale

1. See Standard Protocol (inside front cover).
2. Assist client to put on hospital gown and remove personal items.
3. Instruct client to remove makeup, nail polish, hairpins, and jewelry.

During and after surgery, the skin is assessed to determine tissue perfusion. (In some settings, clients are allowed to have a ring taped and to remove polish from only one nail.)

4. Ensure that money and valuables have been locked up or given to a family member.
5. Verify that client's identification and blood band are correct and legible.

In outpatient settings, these bands are applied at this time.

6. Ensure that client has had nothing to eat or drink during the past 8 hours.

Under general anesthesia, the sphincters in the stomach relax, and contents can reflux into the esophagus and into the trachea. (Some settings now use a shorter time frame.)

7. Verify that client has taken medications as instructed.
8. Verify that a bowel preparation (e.g., purgative, enema) has been completed if ordered.

For clients admitted the morning of surgery, this may have been performed at home.

9. Ensure that a medical history and physical examination results are in client's record.
10. Verify that surgical consent is complete (see illustration, p. 488).

Ensuring that the client has consented to the intended procedure is essential. In most settings, the surgeon obtains the consent and the nurse verifies that it is complete and consistent with the client's understanding (refer to agency policy).

11. Ensure that necessary laboratory work, ECG, and chest x-ray studies have been completed.
12. Check that type and crossmatch has been completed if ordered by the physician and that blood transfusions are available as needed.
13. Ask if client has an advanced directive. If so, place it in client's record.
14. Assess and record client's heart rate, blood pressure, respiratory rate, oxygen saturation, and temperature.
15. Administer purgatives or enemas if ordered (see Skill 34).

Enemas are used when surgery is near the lower intestine.

G-2d₂ CONSENT FOR OPERATION OR PROCEDURE

(See reverse for Monitored Telephone Call)

• File most recent sheet ON BOTTOM •

DATE

HOSP. NO.

NAME

BIRTHDATE

ADDRESS

IF NOT IMPRINTED, PLEASE PRINT DATE, HOSP. NO., NAME AND LOCATION

1. I hereby authorize Doctors _____ , and such other associates
(Attending and Resident Physician[s]/Dentist[s])
as may be selected by the attending doctor to perform upon _____
(Myself or Name of Patient)
the following operation/procedure: _____
(Technical name, followed by description in lay language)

_____

_____

_____

_____

_____

2. In the event developments indicate that further operations/procedures may be necessary, I authorize the physicians to use their own judgment and do whatever they deem advisable during the operation/procedure for the patient's best interests, except the following: _____

_____
(List any exclusions. If none, write "none.")

3. I consent to the administration of such anesthetics as may be considered necessary or advisable by the anesthetist, with the exception of: _____

_____
(List any exclusions. If none, write "none.")

4. The nature of my condition, the nature and purpose of the operation/procedure, possible alternative methods of treatment, the risks involved, and the possible consequences and complications have been explained to me by Doctor _____ . My questions concerning the operation/procedure and its possible outcome have been answered to my satisfaction.

5. I am aware that the practice of dentistry, medicine, and surgery is not an exact science and acknowledge that no guarantees have been made to me by anyone concerning the results of the operation/procedure.

6. Any tissues surgically removed may be disposed by the Hospital in accordance with accustomed practice,

including use in research studies, except as follows: _____

_____
(If none, write "none.")

Signature: _____
(Patient or person authorized to consent for patient)

I declare that I have personally explained to _____ the nature of the patient's
(Patient or Representative)
condition, the procedures to be undertaken, the risks involved, and the alternatives, as set forth in 1 and 4 above,

on_____at_____a.m. _____
      (Date)   (Time)   p.m.   (Signature of Physician/Dentist)

—Continued On Reverse—

29365/7-84/H1575   **THE UNIVERSITY OF IOWA HOSPITALS AND CLINICS**

Step 10   *Courtesy University of Iowa Hospitals and Clinics.*

Steps	Rationale

16. Instruct client to void.
17. Start an IV line; refer to unit standards or physician's orders (see Skill 30.1).
18. Administer preoperative medications as ordered.
19. **Apply antiembolism stockings.**

    Antiembolism stockings promote circulation during periods of immobilization, reducing the risk of an embolism.

   a. Measure client while standing, from gluteal fold to the floor, circumference of largest part of the calf (refer to agency policy).
   b. With the client lying down, invert the stocking and slip it over the foot (see illustrations).
   c. Ease the stocking snugly over the leg (see illustration).

20. **Apply sequential compression stockings if ordered.**
   a. Measure around the largest part of the thigh.

    Sequential compression stockings promote circulation by sequentially compressing the legs from the ankle upward.

   b. Wrap stockings around the leg, starting at the ankle, with the opening over the patella (see illustration, p. 490).
   c. Attach the stockings to the insufflator, and verify that the intermittent pressure is between 35 and 45 mm Hg.

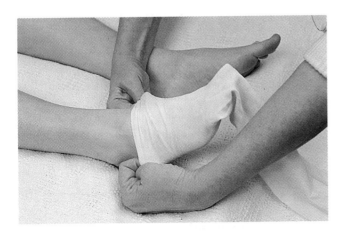

Step 19b

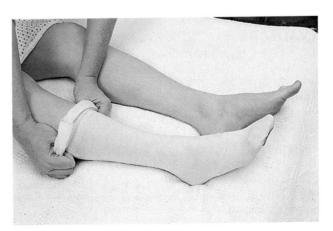

Step 19c

| **Steps** | **Rationale** |

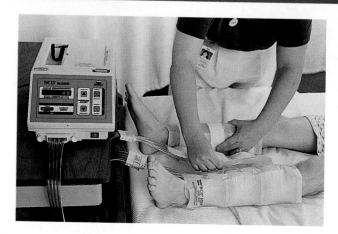

Step 20b

21. Clip hair at incision site.
   a. Inspect the general condition of the skin.
   b. Explain the purpose of hair removal to client.
   c. Apply towels along edges of area.
   d. Clip hair with an electric clipper.
   e. Remove hair with disposable towels.

If abrasions or signs of skin infection are present, the risk of surgical wound infection increases. If hair removal is necessary, clipping the morning of surgery has been associated with the lowest infection rates. Shaving increases the risk of infection (Jepsen and Bruttomesso, 1993). Clients may be instructed to shower with an antimicrobial soap the evening before surgery.

22. Insert a urinary catheter if ordered. See Skill 35.1.
23. Remove contact lenses, eyeglasses, hairpieces, and dentures.

In some settings, dentures are left in place.

24. Place a cap on client's head.

The cap contains the hair and minimizes operating room contamination during surgery. Plastic or reflective caps reduce heat loss during surgery.

25. Assist client onto stretcher for transport to operating room.
26. See Completion Protocol (inside front cover).

Some abulatory surgery clients walk to operating room.

• • •

EVALUATION
1. Observe client's level of cooperation during preparation.
2. Ask client to assist with measures to reduce the risk of infection (preoperative antibiotics, skin preparation).

Unexpected Outcomes and Related Interventions
1. Client reports having eaten breakfast or drinking fluids.
   Notify surgeon and anesthesiologist/nurse anesthetist.
2. Client refuses to go to surgery until contacting a family member.
   a. Notify surgeon.
   b. Assist client to contact family member.
3. Consent is incomplete or incorrect.
   Notify surgeon and anesthesiologist/nurse anesthetist.
4. Client did not follow instructions regarding medications.
   Notify surgeon.
5. Client has a reaction to a preoperative medication.
   a. Discontinue the medication.
   b. Treat the reaction as per policy in the setting.
   c. Notify surgeon.
6. Client is scheduled to be discharged postoperatively and does not have an accompanying adult.

a. Notify surgeon and anesthesiologist/nurse anesthetist.
b. Assist client in contacting someone to provide care at home.

Recording and Reporting

Preoperative physical preparation is frequently documented in a form called a *preoperative checklist* (see Figure 19-3, p. 486).

Geriatric Considerations

Older adult clients may have limited ROM. When preparing the client, the nurse is careful not to force any joint beyond what is comfortable for the client.

CRITICAL THINKING EXERCISES

1. Evaluate each of the following situations. For each, decide if further action is required on the part of the nurse. If so, what action should be taken?
   a. While you are reviewing Mrs. Bates' chart preoperatively, you notice that her last chest x-ray was 6 months ago, even though one was ordered 4 days ago.
   b. While reviewing the operative consent form, you notice that it says "surgery will be on the left knee." Mr. Jones tells you it will be on the right knee.
   c. When asked about the last time she had anything to eat or drink the morning of surgery with general anesthesia. Ms. Baker says she had "just a cup of coffee this morning at 5:00."
   d. While reviewing the laboratory results preoperatively, you notice that Mr. Davis' white blood cell count is higher than normal.
   e. When asked preoperatively, if he has any prostheses or implants, Mr. Perez reports that he has an internal defibrillator.

2. Maria is scheduled for abdominal surgery in the morning. After you apply the sequential compression stockings, she states that she does not have varicose veins and doesn't understand why this is necessary,
   a. How should you respond to Maria's comment?
   b. Maria appears anxious and asks if you think she is going to have problems after surgery. How would you respond to Maria's question?

3. The morning of surgery, Mrs. Martinez accompanies 5-year-old José. When asked if she has any questions, she reports that José was exposed to chicken pox at school and had a slight fever and runny nasal discharge 2 days

REFERENCES

Butcher L: Teaching: Preoperative. In Bulechek GM, McCloskey JC, eds: *Nursing interventions: Effective nursing treatments,* ed 3, St Louis, 1997, Mosby.

Butts JD, Wolford ET: Timing of preoperative antibiotic administration, *AORN J* 65(10):109–115, 1997.

Dalen JE, Hersh J: Prevention of venous thromboembolism, *Chest* 108(suppl):312S–334S, 1995.

Daley K: Learning theory. In *Core curriculum for geriatric nurses,* Baltimore, Md, 1996, Mosby.

Iowa Intervention Project: *Nursing interventions classification,* ed 2, St Louis, 1996, Mosby.

Jepsen OB, Bruttomesso KA: The effectiveness of preoperative skin preparations: An integrated review of the literature, *AORN J* 58(3):477, 1993.

Smith RB, Gurkowski MA, Bracken C: *Anesthesia and pain control in the geriatric patient,* New York, 1995, McGraw-Hill.

Steelman V: Latex allergy precautions: A research based protocol. In Bulechek GM, McCloskey JC, eds: *Nursing interventions: Effective nursing treatments,* ed 3, St Louis, 1997, Mosby.

CHAPTER 20

Intraoperative Techniques

Skill 20.1
Surgical Hand Scrub,   493

Skill 20.2
Sterile Gowning and Closed Gloving,   497

The intraoperative phase starts when the client enters the operating room suite and ends with admission to the postanesthesia care unit or recovery area. During this intraoperative phase, the perioperative nurse applies the nursing process to coordinate each client's care, keeping in mind safety, comfort, and support.

Members of the surgical team include the surgeon and assistant(s), certified registered nurse anesthetist (CRNA) and/or physician anesthesiologist, circulating nurse, and scrub nurse or surgical technologist. A few examples of more specialized team members include a cardiopulmonary perfusionist, blood (cell) saver technologist, or orthopedic technician.

The perioperative nurse assumes one of two roles in the operating room. The *circulating nurse* is always a registered nurse (RN) and is considered to be the charge nurse in the room (AORN, 1998c). The circulator assists the scrubbed personnel by linking the team to the unsterile environment and assumes responsibility and accountability for the delivery of safe, quality client care (Box 20-1).

The *scrub nurse,* who may be an RN, licensed practical nurse (LPN), or surgical technologist, passes instruments and supplies to the surgeons and assistants and maintains the sterile field (Box 20-2). Both the circulating and the scrub nurses monitor for and enforce strict adherence to the principles of aseptic technique (see Chapter 4), ensuring optimum client protection against contamination of microorganisms during the surgical procedure.

It is essential that perioperative nurses fully understand and follow the principles of aseptic technique and are willing to develop a sterile conscience. A sterile conscience requires knowledge of the principles of aseptic

technique; self-discipline; good communication skills to identify, address, and correct any breaks in sterile technique; and the maturity to overcome personal preferences (Perry and Potter, 1998).

Box 20-1 Role of the Circulating Nurse

- Organizes and prepares operating room before start of case; checks to see equipment works properly.
- Gathers supplies for case and opens sterile supplies for scrub nurse.
- Counts sponges, sharps, and instruments with scrub nurse before incision is made.
- Sends for client at appropriate time.
- Conducts preoperative client assessment, including:
  Explains role and identifies client.
  Reviews medical record and verifies procedure and consents.
  Confirms client's allergies, NPO status, laboratory values, electrocardiogram (ECG), and x-ray studies.
- Safely transfers client to operating table, and positions client according to surgeon's preference and procedure type.
- Applies conductive pad to client if electrocautery used; may prepare client's skin; may apply ECG electrodes for local case.
- Explains briefly to the client what the circulating nurse and scrub nurse are doing.
- Assists surgical team by tying gowns and arranging tables.
- Assists anesthesiologist during induction and extubation.
- Continuously monitors procedure for any breaks in aseptic technique or to anticipate needs of the team; opens additional sterile supplies for scrub nurse.
- Handles surgical specimens per institutional policy.
- Documents on perioperative nurses' notes.
- Performs sponge, sharp, and instrument counts with scrub nurse before the case, at beginning of wound closure, and at the end.

Box 20-2 Role of the Scrub Nurse

- Assists circulating nurse in preparing operating room.
- Performs surgical hand scrub and wears sterile gown and gloves.
- Sets up sterile field with procedure-appropriate supplies and instruments, verifying all are in working order.
- Performs sponge, sharp, and instrument counts with circulating nurse before incision.
- Gowns and gloves surgeons and assistants as they enter the operating room.
- Assists surgeons with sterile draping of client.
- Keeps sterile field orderly and monitors progress of procedure and any breaks in aseptic technique.
- Passes instruments and supplies to surgeons and assistants.
- Handles surgical specimens per institutional policy.
- Constantly monitors location of all sponges and sharps in the field and performs closing sponge, sharp, and instrument counts with circulating nurse.

If any question exists about sterility, the item must be considered to be unsterile. A sterile gown that touches the floor while being put on is discarded and exchanged for a new one; the surgeon who touches an unsterile area with a gloved hand changes the affected glove; the scrub nurse who accidentally touches the faucet with one hand while rinsing rescrubs. These are all examples of following one's sterile conscience and being committed to safe, quality client care.

Although not directly related to aseptic technique, most clients who undergo surgery are unfamiliar with the operating room environment and what to expect. The perioperative nurse must assess and document the client's emotional status and understanding of the surgical procedure to be performed.

NURSING DIAGNOSES

Risk for Infection is the most appropriate nursing diagnosis for clients undergoing invasive procedures. When the surgical procedure involves an incision or entrance into a sterile body cavity, such as the bowel or bladder, prevention of infection is a major nursing responsibility. Even when aseptic technique is followed, some clients will have a greater-than-average risk for infection (see Chapters 21 and 24).

Skill 20.1

SURGICAL HAND SCRUB

The surgical hand scrub is an essential skill to achieving surgical asepsis. Although the skin cannot be sterilized, the number of microorganisms can be greatly reduced by chemical, physical, and mechanical means. The surgical hand scrub removes debris and transient microorganisms from the nails, hands, and forearms; reduces the resident microbial count to a minimum; and inhibits rapid/rebound growth of microorganisms (AORN, 1998b). Antimicrobials such as Betadine, Hibiclens, and Septisol improve removal of bacteria from hands and arms (Perry and Potter, 1998).

Surgical attire (scrubs) should be worn in the operating room to reduce the chance for contamination from personnel to clients, and vice versa. Fingernails should be short, clean, and free of polish and/or artificial nails, which can harbor bacteria and fungi (AORN, 1998b). All rings, watches, and bracelets are removed before the surgical scrub.

The AORN recommends a 5- to 10-minute hand scrub with an approved antimicrobial agent for all surgical procedures. The institution should standardize the surgical hand scrub procedure for all staff using either the anatomical timed scrub or the counted stroke method (AORN, 1998b) (see agency policy). Some procedures require a vigorous hand wash but not necessarily a surgical scrub. Some examples of clean procedures are laryngoscopy, esophagoscopy, and proctoscopy.

Equipment

Deep sink with foot or knee controls for dispensing water and soap
Antimicrobial agent (approved by facility)
Surgical scrub brush with plastic nail file
Paper mask and cap or hood
Sterile towel
Proper scrub attire
Protective eyewear

ASSESSMENT

1. Determine type and length of time for hand wash or scrub (check agency policy).
2. Remove bracelets, rings, and watches.
3. Inspect fingernails, which must be short, clean, and healthy. Artificial nails should be removed. Nail polish should be removed if chipped or worn longer than 4 days. **Rationale: Long nails and chipped or old polish increases number of bacteria residing on nails. Long fingernails can puncture gloves, causing contamination. Artificial nails are known to harbor gram-negative microorganisms and fungus.**
4. Inspect skin and cuticles of hands and arms for abrasions, cuts, or open lesions.

PLANNING

Expected outcomes should focus on prevention of infection resulting from breaks in aseptic technique.

Expected Outcome
Client does not develop signs of surgical wound infection.

DELEGATION CONSIDERATIONS

The role of the scrub nurse can be delegated to a surgical technologist or LPN. Assistive personnel (AP) can assist the RN in the circulating role by opening sterile supplies, setting up sterile fields, and running errands under the direction of the RN.

IMPLEMENTATION

Steps	Rationale

1. Put on surgical shoe covers, cap or hood, face mask, and protective eyewear.
2. Turn water on using foot or knee control and adjust to comfortable temperature.
3. Rinse hands and arms, keeping arms flexed with hands pointed upward, allowing the water to flow off at the elbows.

    Water runs from fingertips to elbows by gravity, thus keeping the hands the cleanest part of the upper extremity.

4. Clean under nails of both hands with file under running water, then discard file (see illustration).

    Removes dirt and organic materials that harbor a large number of microorganisms.

5. Wet brush and apply antimicrobial agent. Scrub the nails of one hand with 15 strokes (see illustration). Scrub the palm, each side of thumb and fingers, and the posterior side of the hand with 10 strokes each (see illustration). The arm is mentally divided into thirds, and each third is scrubbed 10 times (Perry and Potter, 1998). Some agencies may scrub by time rather than 10 strokes.
6. Discard brush; flex arms and rinse from fingertips to elbows in one continuous motion, allowing water to run off at elbow (see illustration).
7. Turn off water with foot or knee control and back into room with hands elevated in front and away from body.

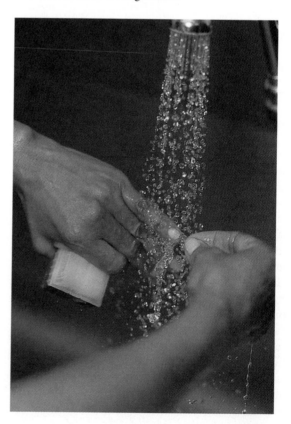

Step 4

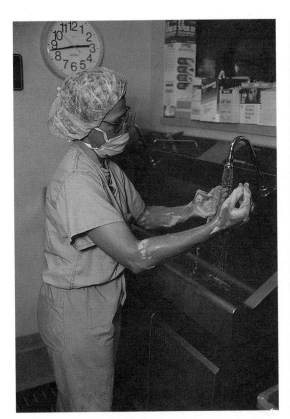

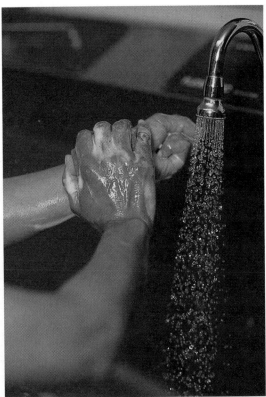

Step 5

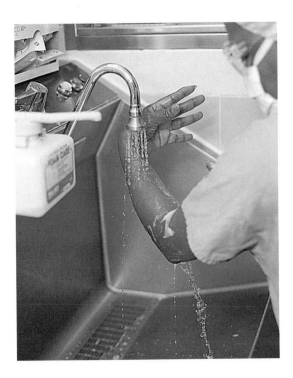

Step 6

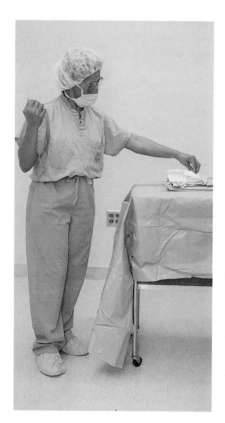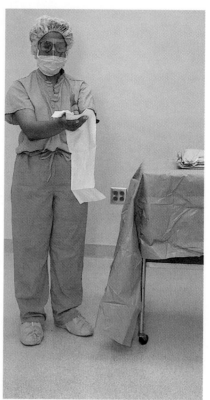

Step 8

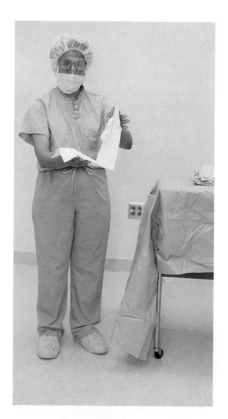

Step 9

Steps	Rationale
8. Go to sterile setup and grasp sterile towel, taking care not to drip water on the sterile field (see illustration). Bending slightly at the waist, use a sterile towel to dry one hand thoroughly, moving from fingers to elbow in a rotating motion (see illustration).	Dry from cleanest (hands) to least clean (elbows).
9. Use the opposite end of the towel to dry the other hand (see illustration).	Avoids transfer of microorganisms from elbow to opposite hand.
10. Drop towel into linen hamper or into circulating nurse's hands.	

• • •

EVALUATION

Monitor postoperative client for signs of surgical wound infection, including redness, tenderness, and purulent drainage.

Unexpected Outcome and Related Interventions

Client develops postoperative surgical wound infection. Interventions should be individualized to client situation (e.g., wound care, antibiotic therapy).

Skill 20.2

STERILE GOWNING AND CLOSED GLOVING

Immediately following a surgical scrub, a sterile gown should be applied, followed by application of sterile gloves. All members of the surgical team that will work around the sterile field must prepare in this manner before entering the sterile field. Once applied, the surgical gown is considered sterile in front from chest to waist or table level. The sleeves are considered sterile from 5 cm (2 inches) above the elbow to fingertips. The back of the gown is no longer considered sterile.

Surgical gowns should cover all garments worn underneath. All sterile gowns and drapes made of materials that are free of tears, punctures, strain, and abrasion provide an effective barrier against microorganisms passing between unsterile and sterile areas (AORN, 1998a).

Nursing personnel should use the closed-glove method when initially entering the sterile field. If a glove becomes contaminated during the surgery, the circulating nurse, wearing protective unsterile gloves, grasps the outside of the glove and pulls off the glove inside out, leaving the stockinette cuff in place. Another sterile team member can assist in regloving, or the open-glove method can be used. If both the scrub nurse's gloves become contaminated, it is recommended to regown and reglove using the closed-glove method.

Equipment

Package of proper-size sterile gloves
Sterile pack containing sterile gown

Clean, flat, dry surface (table or Mayo stand) on which to open gown and gloves
Surgical cap, mask, eyewear, and footwear
Protective eyewear

ASSESSMENT

1. Select proper size and type of sterile gloves. Proper fit ensures care of handling supplies.
2. Select proper size and type of sterile surgical gown.

PLANNING

Expected outcome focuses on prevention of infection resulting from breaks in aseptic technique.

Expected Outcome

Client does not develop signs of surgical wound infection.

DELEGATION CONSIDERATIONS

The skills of sterile gowning and gloving can be delegated to surgical technicians who have received the proper training.

IMPLEMENTATION

Steps	Rationale
1. Perform surgical hand scrub (see Skill 20.1). Nurse will have protective garments applied.	
2. Have circulating nurse open sterile gown and glove package on a clean, dry, flat surface (see illustrations).	
3. Enter operating suite after surgical scrub (see Skill 20.1), keeping elbows bent and hands above waist. Pick up gown (folded inside out) from sterile package, grasping the inside surface of gown at the collar.	Prevents hands from touching contaminated object.
4. Lift folded gown directly upward and away from the table.	
5. Locate neckband; with both hands, grasp the inside front of gown just below neckline.	Clean hands may touch inside of gown without contaminating outer surface.
6. Allow gown to open, keeping at arm's length away from body with the inside of gown toward body (see illustration on p. 500). Do not touch outside of gown or allow it to touch the floor.	Outside of gown remains sterile.
7. Slip both arms into armholes simultaneously (do not allow hands to move through cuff opening), keeping hands at shoulder level.	
8. Have circulating nurse pull on gown by reaching inside arm seams. Gown is pulled on, leaving sleeves covering hands.	
9. Have circulating nurse tie gown at neck and waist (see illustration on p. 500). If wraparound gown, sterile flap is not touched until sterile gloves have been applied.	

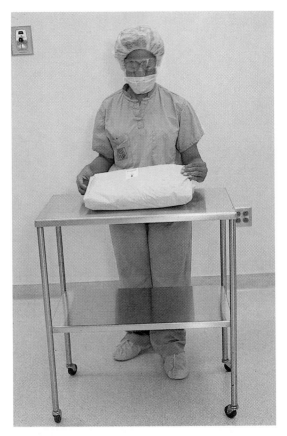

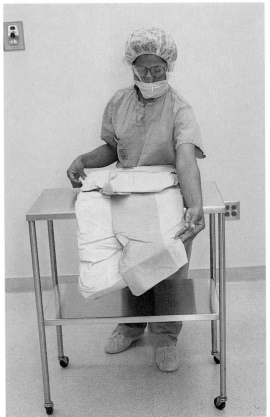

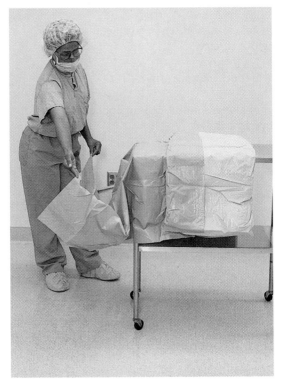

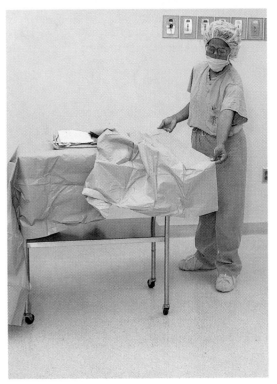

Step 2

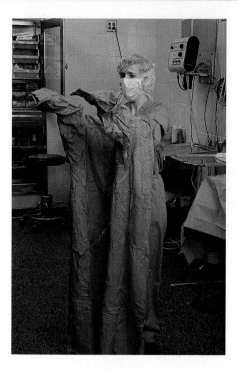

Step 6

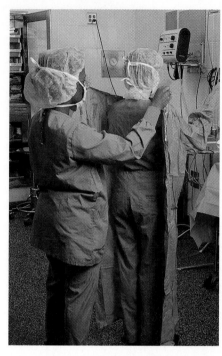

Step 9

10. Apply gloves using the closed-glove method.
    a. With hands covered by gown cuffs and sleeves, open inner sterile glove package (see illustration on p. 501).

    b. Grasp folded cuff of glove for dominant hand with the nondominant hand.

    c. Extend dominant forearm forward with palm up, and place palm of glove against palm of dominant hand. Gloved fingers point toward elbow.

    d. Grasp cuff edges with thumb and forefingers of dominant hand. Grasp back of glove cuff with nondominant hand, and turn cuff over dominant hand (see illustration on p. 501). Extend fingers into glove and pull glove over cuff.

    e. Glove nondominant hand in same manner with gloved, dominant hand (see illustrations on p. 501). Keep hand inside sleeve. Be sure fingers are fully extended into both gloves.

Hands remain clean, and sterile gown cuff will touch sterile glove surface.

Sterile gown touches sterile glove.

Open end of glove is positioned for application over cuff-covered hand.

Steps	Rationale

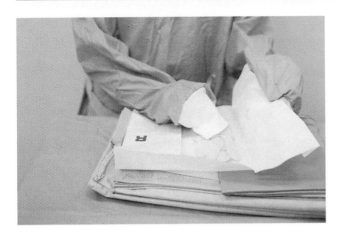

Step 10a

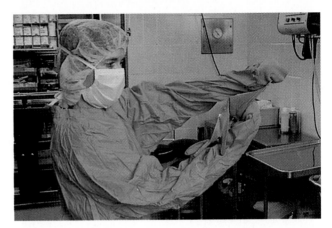

Step 10d

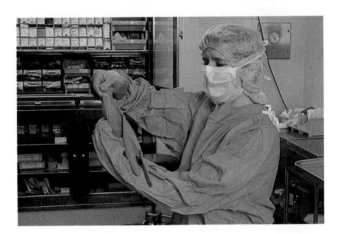

Step 10e

11. For wraparound gown:
  a. Grasp sterile waist tie with gloved hands and untie.
  b. Pass tie to another sterile team member, who stands still, or wrap tie in sterile towel and pass to circulating nurse. Keep gown tie in left hand.
  c. Allowing margin of safety, turn to the left one-half turn, covering back with extended gown flap. Retrieve tie only from team member, and secure both ties in place.
  NOTE: On disposable sterile gowns, there is often a tab attached to the tie that can be passed to a nonsterile team member for turning, and then is pulled off and discarded (see illustration on p. 502).
12. Stand in a position to maintain sterility.

Front of gown is sterile.

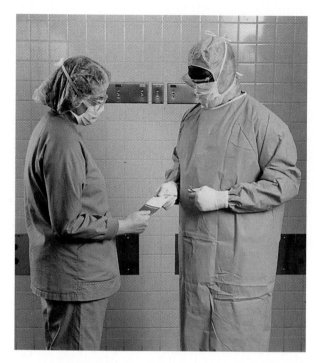

Step 11c

• • •

EVALUATION

Monitor postoperative client for signs of surgical wound infection; inspect wound and palpate for tenderness.

Unexpected Outcome and Related Interventions

Client develops postoperative surgical wound infection. Interventions should be individualized to client situation (e.g., wound care, antibiotic therapy).

Sample Documentation

Documentation is entered on an OR record, including details about intraoperative events including times client entered and left the OR; sponge, needle, and instrument counts; sutures and dressings used; members of OR team, etc.

CRITICAL THINKING EXERCISES

1. You are the circulating nurse in a radical prostatectomy. Josie is the scrub technician assigned to this case. She has scrubbed on these cases before, but has worked primarily for the past few years in the cystoscopy suites. While scrubbing for the case, you notice she does not pay attention to what she is doing and has missed scrubbing several areas on her hands and forearms, and has even bumped her hand against the back of the sink. What would you do?

2. Jack is assigned to be the scrub nurse for a total knee replacement. Because this is his first week out of orientation, he is eager to keep up with this fast-paced surgical team. As Jack prepares to scrub, he realizes he forgot to open his sterile surgical gown and gloves. The circulating nurse and anesthesiologist have gone to get the client. Jack hurries to open his gown and gloves, accidentally dropping the outer package of the gloves onto the sterile gown. This was the last sterile gown pack in the room. The client is being transported to the operating room suite, and no one saw Jack contaminate the gown. Jack looks at the clock, discards the contaminated gown and gloves, and runs to the supply room to obtain a new, sterile gown pack.
   a. What do Jack's actions demonstrate?
   b. What principle of aseptic technique has Jack violated?
   c. How could this situation have been handled differently?

REFERENCES

Association of Operating Room Nurses: Recommended practices for protective barrier materials for surgical gowns and drapes. In *AORN standards and recommended practices for perioperative nursing,* Denver, 1998a, AORN.

Association of Operating Room Nurses: Recommended practices for surgical hand scrubs. In *AORN standards and recommended practices for perioperative nursing,* Denver, 1998b, AORN.

Association of Operating Room Nurses: Statement on mandate for the registered nurse as circulator in the operating room. In *AORN standards and recommended practices for perioperative nursing,* Denver, 1998c, AORN.

Perry A, Potter P: *Clinical nursing skills and techniques,* ed 4, St Louis, 1998, Mosby.

CHAPTER 21

Caring for the Postoperative Client

Skill 21.1
Providing Immediate Postoperative Care in Postanesthesia Care Unit, 506

Skill 21.2
Providing Comfort Measures During Phase II (Convalescent Phase), 512

Skill 21.3
Providing Surgical Wound Care, 516

Skill 21.4
Monitoring and Measuring Drainage Devices, 520

Skill 21.5
Removing Staples and Sutures (including applying SteriStrips), 524

The care of postoperative clients may be divided into two phases: the immediate postanesthesia recovery and the convalescent phase. Phase I extends from the time the client leaves the operating room (OR) to the time of transfer from the postanesthesia care unit (PACU) to the nursing division. This phase requires 2 or more hours. Phase II, the convalescent phase, involves several days or weeks for the initial healing process. The client with a chronic medical condition, such as chronic respiratory disease or diabetes, may require even longer.

Cost-containment measures and reimbursement policies have dramatically changed routines for surgical procedures. Many surgical procedures that once required an overnight hospital admission are not reimbursed by insurance for inpatient services. Newer equipment, such as laser and laparoscopy, are less invasive and also decrease the need for inpatient admission. Many clients are admitted the morning of surgery rather than receiving inpatient preparation for surgery. The current trend involves more ambulatory outpatient surgery and shorter hospitalizations to achieve cost containment. In addition, clients often recover better at home.

PACUs, in many respects, are critical care units that require professional nurses with specific education and experience to recognize and help manage anesthesia-related and surgery-related complications (ASPAN, 1995).

The client is accompanied to the PACU by a member of the anesthesia care team, who provides a verbal report, including postoperative status (e.g., vital signs, oxygen saturation, allergies); length of anesthesia and technique (general, regional, or local); anesthesia, muscle relaxant, narcotic, and reversal agents used; current vital signs; intravenous (IV) fluids or blood products used in surgery; presence of drains; estimated blood loss and replacement; and complications that occurred during surgery (ASPAN, 1995).

Preoperative orders typically are canceled by surgery, in which case postoperative orders may include a statement to "Continue all preoperative orders." Postoperative orders usually specify frequency of vital signs and special assessments, types of IV fluids and infusion rate, postoperative medications, fluids or foods allowed by mouth, level of activity or type of positioning, intake and output, laboratory tests or x-ray studies to be done, and special interventions such as dressing changes, an immobilizing device, or an incentive spirometer.

The immediate postoperative recovery phase requires frequent assessments for potentially life-threatening complications resulting from anesthesia or surgery. It is important to emphasize the ABCs: *A* is for airway, *B* is for breathing, and *C* is for circulation (Table 21-1). Postopera-

tive clients have a tendency to be hypoxic, oxygen saturation levels are routinely monitored, and supplemental oxygen is given.

Size, location, and depth of a wound influence type and amount of drainage. It is important to know what type of drainage is expected (Table 21-2). Nurses can estimate drainage by counting the number of saturated gauze sponges. Hemorrhage is loss of large amounts of blood either externally or internally in a short time and will result in shock if uncontrolled. Arterial bleeding is bright red and gushes forth in waves related to heart rhythm; or if a vessel is very deep, flow will be steady. Venous bleeding is

Table 21-1

Complications of Anesthesia

Condition	Interventions
AIRWAY	
Mechanical obstruction: decreased level of consciousness and muscle relaxants resulting in flaccid muscles and tongue blocking airway	Hyperextend neck; pull mandible forward; use nasal or oral airway; encourage deep breathing.
Retained thick secretions: irritation from anesthesia; anticholinergic medications: history of smoking	Suction; encourage coughing.
Laryngospasm: stridor from excessive secretions or airway irritation	Provide positive-pressure ventilation with oxygen, small dose of muscle relaxant, and intubation.
Laryngeal edema: allergic reaction, irritation from endotracheal tube, fluid overload	Administer oxygen, antihistamines, steroids, sedatives, and intubation.
Bronchospasm: preexisting asthma, anesthetic irritation (expiratory wheeze)	Administer bronchodilators as ordered.
Aspiration: vomiting from hypotension, accumulated gastric secretions and delayed gastric emptying, pain, fear, position changes	Position on side; suction airway; administer antiemetic as ordered.
BREATHING: HYPOVENTILATION/HYPOXEMIA	
Central nervous system depression: anesthesia, analgesics, muscle relaxants (respiratory rate shallow)	Encourage to cough and deep breathe; use mechanical ventilator; administer narcotic antagonist, muscle relaxant reversal agent; reposition; give analgesic; loosen cast or dressings; provide nasogastric intubation.
Mechanical restriction: obesity, tight cast or dressings, abdominal distention, pain	
CIRCULATION	
Hypovolemia: blood loss, dehydration	Elevate legs; give oxygen, IV fluids, or blood replacement; administer vasopressors; monitor I&O, stimulation, hemoglobin and hematocrit.
Hypotension: Anesthesia/drug effects, spinal anesthesia may cause vasodilation; narcotics	
Cardiac failure: preexisting cardiac disease; circulatory overload; excessive/too-rapid fluid replacement	Provide digitalization, diuretics; monitor electrocardiogram (ECG).
Cardiac arrhythmias: hypoxemia; myocardial infarct; hypokalemia, hypothermia; imbalance of potassium, calcium, magnesium	Provide IV fluid replacement; monitor ECG, urine output; identify and treat cause.
Hypertension: pain, distended bladder, preexisting hypertension, vasopressor drugs	Compare to preoperative baseline; identify and determine cause.
Compartment syndrome: pressure from edema causing enough compression to obstruct arterial and venous circulation resulting in ischemia, permanent numbness, loss of function; forearm and lower leg most common sites	Elevate extremity no more than 5 inches above the heart, apply ice, remove or loosen bandage or cast to relieve compression; if left untreated, amputation may be required.

Table 21-2

Expected Drainage from Tubes and Catheters

Substance	Daily Amount	Color	Odor	Consistency
INDWELLING CATHETER				
Urine	500–700 ml, 1–2 days postoperatively; 1500–2500 ml thereafter	Clear, yellow	Ammonia	Watery
NASOGASTRIC OR GASTROSTOMY TUBE				
Gastric contents	Up to 1500 ml/day	Pale, yellow-green Bloody following gastrointestinal (GI) surgery	Sour	Watery
HEMOVAC				
Wound drainage	Varies with procedure	Varies with procedure Usually serosanguineous	Same as wound dressing	Variable
T TUBE				
Bile	500 ml	Bright yellow to dark green	Acid	Thick

Modified from Lewis SM, Collier IC: *Medical-surgical nursing: assessment and management of clinical problems,* ed 4, St Louis, 1996, Mosby.

dark red and flows smoothly. Capillary bleeding is oozing of dark red blood; self-sealing controls this bleeding. Some bloody drainage is expected through chest tubes. Bloody drainage exceeding 100 to 200 ml/hr must be reported.

Some surgical wounds have gauze dressings or are covered with a clear, transparent dressing. Some are left open to air (OTA). Physician's orders will specify type and frequency of dressing changes. If excessive drainage is noted, the physician must be notified.

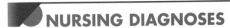 **NURSING DIAGNOSES**

High-risk nursing diagnoses are appropriate relating to the prevention of complications of surgery and anesthesia. Some incisional pain is expected and can increase the risk for postoperative complications. Risk for **Ineffective Airway Clearance** related to incisional pain and increased secretions secondary to general anesthesia and history of smoking could be appropriate. This directs interventions of pain control and removal of secretions from the airway. Risk for or actual **Ineffective Breathing Pattern** related to sedation secondary to general anesthesia could be appropriate for clients who need stimulation to promote respiratory effort and tend to hypoventilate. **Risk for Aspiration** related to depressed cough/gag reflex secondary to anesthesia focuses interventions on prevention of airway

obstruction. **Impaired Physical Mobility** related to incisional pain is useful when the focus of increasing mobility is facilitated by adequate pain control. Risk for **Decreased Cardiac Output** may be used to identify the risk for hemorrhage caused by slipping of suture, inadequate clotting, or excessive blood or fluid loss for any reason. **Fluid Volume Deficit** is also related to excessive loss of fluid and blood from wound drainage or from inadequate fluid replacement. Risk for **Altered Tissue Perfusion** related to venous stasis or vessel trauma may be indicated after surgery of the legs, abdomen, pelvis, and major blood vessels. This is also appropriate when blood coagulation studies indicate increased coagulation and when clients are immobilized, have chronic hypoxia, or use oral contraceptives containing estrogen.

Risk for Infection related to surgical incision (specify location) is appropriate when the client has lowered resistance to infection for any reason including conditions such as obesity, advanced age, impaired circulation, diabetes, immunosuppression, radiation, smoking, poor cellular nutrition, very deep wounds, or wounds healing by secondary intention result in increased risk of infection. **Risk for Altered Health Maintenance** related to inadequate knowledge of postoperative self-care may be appropriate for clients who have not had surgery previously or who require an extended convalescence because of the nature of the surgery. Teaching needs should be considered for all postoperative clients.

Skill 21.1

PROVIDING IMMEDIATE POSTOPERATIVE CARE IN POSTANESTHESIA CARE UNIT

The first phase of postoperative care takes place during the immediate recovery period, which extends from the time the client leaves the OR to the time the client has stabilized in the recovery room (RR) or PACU and has been transferred to the nursing division.

The first 1 to 2 hours are the most critical for assessing aftereffects of anesthesia, including airway clearance, cardiovascular complications, temperature control, and neurological function. The client's condition can change rapidly, and assessments must be timely, knowledgeable, and accurate. Quick judgment regarding the most appropriate interventions is essential. The client is usually considered ready for discharge to the general unit when specific standardized criteria are met. REACT is one of several scoring systems for assessment. It uses parameters of *r*espiration, *e*nergy, *a*lertness, *c*irculation, and *t*emperature (Table 21-3). A score of 10 indicates a fully recovered client.

Recovery from ambulatory surgery requires the same assessments; however, the depth of general anesthesia may be less because the surgery is less involved and of shorter duration. Some clients have only IV sedation, for which less monitoring is usually required. As soon as the client is stable and alert, instructions for home care are given to the client and caregiver. Demonstrations and written instructions are provided. Encourage the client not to drive and to postpone making important decisions for 24 hours. Adequate support for home care must be established.

Equipment

Stethoscope, sphygmomanometer, pulse oximeter, cardiac monitor, thermometer
Oxygen equipment such as mask, oxygen regulator and tubing, and positive-pressure delivery system
Suction equipment
Dressing supplies
Warmed blanket or active rewarming device
Emergency equipment
Emergency medications

ASSESSMENT

1. Review client's pre-existing conditions during operative procedure, including baseline and intraoperative vital signs, oxygen saturation, blood volume or fluid loss, fluid replacement, type of anesthesia, type of airway and size, and extent of surgical wound, including presence of surgical drains. **Rationale: This**

Table 21-3

Postanesthesia Recovery Scoring System (REACT)

Category	Criterion	Score*
Respiration	Requires ventilator	0
	Artificial airway; spontaneous respirations	1
	Spontaneous respirations; rate <10 without support	2
Energy	Does not move legs, even with stimulation	0
	Moves legs, cannot keep head up	1
	Moves legs, can keep head up	2
Alertness	Awakens when vigorously stimulated	0
	Awakens when gently stimulated	1
	Usually awake, dozes occasionally	2
Circulation	Systolic blood pressure (BP) <80, pulse weak	0
	Systolic BP between 80 and preoperative level, pulse strong	1
	Systolic BP at or above preoperative resting level, pulse strong	2
Axillary temperature	<35° C (95° F)	0
	35° C (95° F) to 35.5° C (95° F to 96° F)	1
	>35.5° C (96° F)	2

*Scoring: fully recovered, 10; some residual effects of anesthesia, 9; continuous close monitoring required, 8 or less.

determines client's general status and allows nurse to anticipate need for special equipment, nursing care, and activities in PACU.

2. On client's arrival in PACU, obtain report from circulating nurse and anesthesiologist or nurse anesthetist that provides review of client's physiological status and baseline data to determine any change in condition.

3. Consider the effects of the client's type of surgery and anesthesia and restrictions to movement. **Rationale: This information influences type of assessments nurse initiates, type of complications to observe for, and specific nursing interventions.**

PLANNING

Expected outcomes focus on early detection of complications from surgery or anesthesia and adequate pain control by the time of transfer (usually 1 to 2 hours).

Expected Outcomes

1. Client's airway remains clear, and respirations are deep, regular, and within normal limits by the time of transfer.

2. Client's blood pressure, pulse, and temperature remain within previous baseline or normal expected range by the time of transfer.

3. Dressings are clean, dry, and intact by discharge from recovery.

4. Intake and output are within expected parameters by discharge from recovery.

5. Client reports relief of discomfort after analgesia or other pain relief measures by the time of transfer from the immediate recovery area (usually 1 to 2 hours).

6. Client's postoperative assessments are within expected normal postoperative parameters.

DELEGATION CONSIDERATIONS

The skill of initiating and managing postoperative care of the client requires problem solving and knowledge application unique to a professional nurse. Assistive personnel (AP) may obtain vital signs, apply nasal cannula or oxygen mask, and provide comfort and hygiene measures.

IMPLEMENTATION

Steps	Rationale
1. See Standard Protocol (inside front cover).	
2. As client enters RR or PACU on stretcher, immediately attach oxygen tubing to regulator and check IV flow rates. Connect any drainage tubes to intermittent suction.	Inhaled oxygen promotes tissue oxygenation during recovery from anesthesia. IV fluids maintain circulatory volume and provide route for emergency drugs. Drainage tubes must remain patent to prevent pressure within wound cavity.
3. Compare vital signs with client's preoperative baseline. Continue assessing vital signs at least every 5 to 15 minutes until stable.	Vital signs can reveal respiratory depression, cardiac irregularity, hypotension, or hypothermia.
4. ⬛ Maintain airway after general anesthesia.	
a. If client is supine, elevate head of bed slightly, support neck extension, and turn head to side unless contraindicated. Initially, client may need to be reminded to breathe (see illustration, p. 508).	Opens airway while client has decreased level of consciousness (LOC).
b. Suction artificial airway and oral cavity if secretions accumulate (see Chapter 31). Assist client to spit out oral airway (see illustration, p. 508) as gag reflex returns.	Indicates client can clear airway independently.
5. Call client by name in normal tone of voice. If there is no response, attempt to arouse client by touching or gently moving a body part. Explain that surgery is over and you are in the RR.	Determines client's LOC and ability to follow commands. Assists client to be oriented to place.
6. Encourage client to cough and deep breathe every 15 minutes (see Chapter 19).	Promotes lung expansion, elimination of inhalation anesthetic, and expectoration of mucous secretions. A mucous plug will result in collapsed alveoli and atelectasis (see illustration in step 4b).

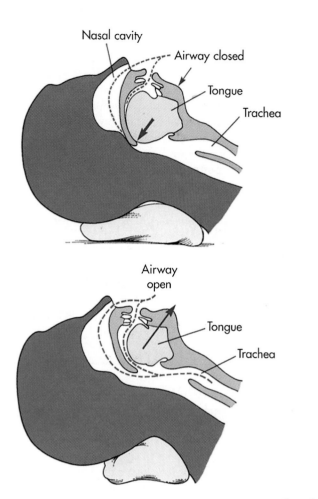

Nasal cavity

Airway closed

Tongue

Trachea

Airway open

Tongue

Trachea

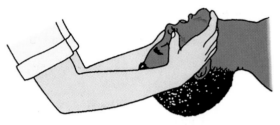

Step 4a

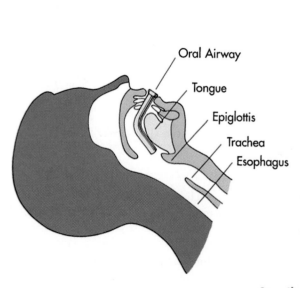

Oral Airway

Tongue

Epiglottis

Trachea

Esophagus

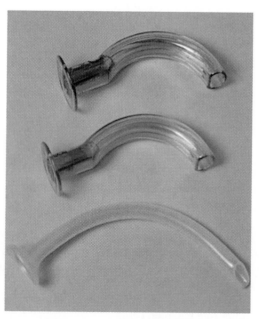

Step 4b

Steps	Rationale
7. Inspect color of nailbeds and skin. Palpate for skin temperature.	Indicators of peripheral tissue perfusion.
8. Assess closely for potential cardiovascular complications of anesthesia (see Table 21-1).	
9. Provide care after spinal anesthesia.	
a. Monitor for hypotension, bradycardia, and nausea and vomiting.	Blockade of sympathetic nervous system may result in vasodilation of major vessels and systemic hypotension.
b. Maintain adequate IV infusion.	Maintains blood pressure by increasing fluid volume and fills temporarily expended vascular space.
c. Keep client flat and maintain position.	Minimizes risk of post–spinal anesthesia headache from leakage of spinal fluid at injection site, with increased pressures induced by elevation of upper body. (Incidence of headache is less with use of smaller-gauge spinal needles [Lewis and Collier, 1996].)
d. Clients are observed in PACU until movement has been regained in extremities. Inform client that loss of extremity sensation and movement is temporary and usually requires several hours to be restored to normal.	Clients often fear permanent loss of function.
e. Assess respiratory status, level of sensation, and mobility in lower extremities. Following IV sedation, drowsiness will be apparent.	Spinal block should be set within 20 minutes of onset. However, if level of anesthesia moves above sixth thoracic vertebra (T6), respiratory distress may require mechanical ventilation (see illustration).

COMMUNICATION TIP

- *If client had general anesthesia: as client arouses, introduce yourself and orient client to surroundings.*
- *If client has spinal anesthesia: remind client that loss of extremity movements is normal for several hours.*

NURSE ALERT

In an emergency situation, document interventions and evaluation as reported to physician, including maintenance of airway and bleeding control, distal pulses, vital signs, IV line, LOC, oxygenation or hypoxia, and anxiety level.

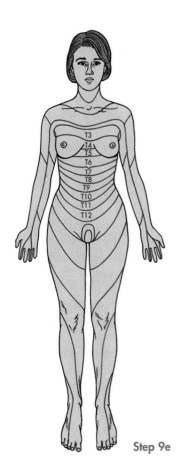

Step 9e

Steps	Rationale

10. Monitor drainage.

   a. Observe dressing and drains for any evidence of bright red blood. Also, look underneath client for any pooling of bloody drainage.

Hemorrhage from a surgical wound is most likely within first few hours, indicating inadequate hemostasis during surgery. As a dressing becomes saturated, blood may ooze down client's side and collect under client.

   b. Inform physician of unexpected bloody drainage, and reinforce dressing as indicated. Monitor for decreased blood pressure and increased pulse.

Dressing maintains hemostasis and absorbs drainage. First dressing changes usually occur 24 hours postoperatively and are done by the surgeon unless otherwise ordered.

   c. Inspect condition and contents of any drainage tubes and collecting devices. Note character and volume of drainage (see Chapter 24).

Determines drainage tube patency and extent of wound drainage.

   d. Observe amount, color, and appearance of urine from indwelling Foley catheter (if present).

Urine output of less than 30 ml/hr may indicate decreased renal perfusion or altered renal function (see Table 21-2).

   e. If nasogastric (NG) tube is present, assess drainage. If not draining, check placement and irrigate if necessary with normal saline (see Chapter 32).

Maintains patency of tube to ensure gastric decompression. Expected drainage may be dark or pale, yellow, green, and 100 to 200 ml/hr. Bloody drainage may be expected after some surgeries.

   f. Monitor IV fluid rates. Observe IV site for signs of infiltration (see Chapter 30).

Provides adequate hydration and circulatory function.

11. Promote comfort.

   a. Provide mouth care by placing moistened washcloth to lips, swabbing oral mucosa with dampened swab, or apply petrolatum to lips.

Mouth may be dry from nothing-by-mouth (NPO) status and preoperative anticholinergics such as atropine.

   b. Provide a warm blanket or active rewarming therapy to promote warmth and minimize shivering.

General anesthesia impairs thermoregulation, the OR environment is cold, and exposure of the body cavity may result in internal heat loss. Shivering can increase oxygen consumption and predispose client to arrhythmias and hypertension (Einhorn and Chant, 1994).

12. Assess pain as client awakens, including quality, severity, and location. Do not assume postoperative pain is incisional pain.

Pain may not be directly related to the surgical procedure, for example, chest pain (myocardial infarction/pulmonary emboli) or muscle pain (trauma from positioning). Referred pain (in shoulder) often occurs after a laparoscopy.

13. Provide pain medication as ordered and when vital signs have stabilized.

Clients in pain often have increased blood pressure and occasionally decreased blood pressure. Pain medication can influence anesthesia effects.

14. Explain client's condition to client, and inform of plans for transfer to nursing division or discharge home.

15. When client's condition is stabilized, contact anesthesiologist to approve transfer to clinical unit or release to home (see Table 21-3).

A physician is responsible for authorizing transfer or discharge.

16. Before discharge to home from the ambulatory surgery unit (ASU), provide verbal and written instructions.

Clients and home care providers must be aware of potential complications and follow-up care.

   a. Signs and symptoms of possible complications.

   b. Do not drive for 24 hours.

   c. Avoid important legal decisions for 24 hours.

   d. Care for surgical site.

   e. Restrict activities.

   f. Control pain.

   g. Plan for follow-up visit.

   h. Clarify reasons to call physician and number to call.

17. See Completion Protocol (inside front cover).

EVALUATION

1. Observe respirations: rate, depth and rhythm. Auscultate breath sounds.
2. Compare all blood pressure, pulse, and temperature readings with client's baseline and expected normal values.
3. Inspect dressings for drainage.
4. Measure intake and output. Urine output is at least 30 to 50 ml/hr.
5. Ask client to rate pain on scale of 0 to 10, and determine location and characteristics.
6. Conduct physical assessments according to client's unique type of surgery, for example:
   a. Craniotomy–neurological assessment
   b. Neck surgery–airway status
   c. Vascular surgery–circulation and bleeding
   d. Orthopedic surgery–immobility or positioning

Unexpected Outcomes and Related Interventions

These include alterations from effects of anesthesia or surgical complications.

1. Client exhibits respiratory depression (pulse oximetry less than 92, respiratory rate less than 10 and/or shallow).
   a. Administer oxygen at 6 to 10 L/min by mask.
   b. Encourage deep breathing every 5 to 15 minutes.
   c. Position to promote chest expansion (on side or semi-Fowler's).
   d. Administer prescribed medications (epinephrine, muscle relaxant, or narcotic reversal agent).
2. Client exhibits respiratory obstruction (abnormal lung sounds, snoring, stridor or crowing sounds, wheezing).
   a. Reposition to open airway.
   b. Administer oxygen at 6 to 10 L/min by mask.
   c. Encourage to cough and deep breathe.
   d. Suction if needed.
   e. Notify anesthesiologist if unresponsive to interventions; may need to be reintubated if severe.
3. Client exhibits signs of hypovolemia related to internal or incisional hemorrhage.
   a. Client's legs should be elevated enough to maintain a downward slope toward the trunk of the body. The head should not be lowered past flat position, which would increase respiratory effort and potentially decrease cerebral perfusion.
   b. Administer oxygen at 6 to 10 L/min by mask.

   c. Increase rate of IV fluid or administer blood products.
   d. Monitor blood pressure and pulse every 5 to 15 minutes.
   e. Apply pressure dressings as follows.
      (1) *Abdominal dressing.* Cover bleeding area with several thicknesses of gauze compresses, and place tape 7 to 10 cm (3 to 4 inches) beyond width of dressing with firm even pressure on both sides close to bleeding source. Maintain pressure as entire dressing is taped to maximize pressure at the source of bleeding.
      (2) *Dressing on extremity.* Apply rolled gauze, pressing gauze compress over bleeding site. Tape must *not* be continued around entire extremity. Assess frequently to ensure blood flow to distal tissues, and identify compartment syndrome resulting from edema that creates sufficient pressure to cause ischemia (see Unexpected Outcome 4).
      (3) *Dressing in neck region.* Assess every 5 to 15 minutes for evidence of airway obstruction.
   f. Client should remain NPO, because it may be necessary to return to surgery for control of bleeding.
   g. Report to physician present status of client's bleeding control, time bleeding was discovered, estimated blood loss, nursing interventions (including effectiveness of applied pressure bandage), apical and distal pulses, blood pressure, level of consciousness (LOC), and signs of restlessness.
4. Client complains of severe incisional pain.
   a. The earliest symptom of compartment syndrome is pain unrelieved by analgesics. Other symptoms include numbness, tingling, pallor, coolness, and absent peripheral pulses. The physician should be notified, the extremity elevated to improve venous return, and ice applied to minimize edema (Lewis and Collier, 1996).
   b. Nurse should administer analgesics before the pain is severe. It is not necessary to wait for client to request pain medication.
   c. Pain can sometimes lower blood pressure; thus analgesia may restore vital signs to normal. Monitor vital signs carefully.
   d. For clients with patient-controlled analgesia (PCA), be sure client is using device correctly.
5. Client has hypothermia (temperature less than 34.5° C [94° F]) resulting from effects of anesthesia or loss of body heat from surgical exposure. Shiver-

ing can increase oxygen consumption and predispose client to arrhythmias and hypertension.

    a. Use warm blankets or active rewarming device.

    b. Monitor temperature every 30 to 60 minutes.

Recording and Reporting

- Document in progress notes the client's arrival time at PACU; describe vital signs, including LOC; assessment findings, including the dressings, tubes, and drainage; and all nursing measures initiated.
- Record vital signs and intake and output on appropriate flow sheets.
- Report any abnormal assessment findings and signs of complications to physician.

Sample Documentation

1000   Client received from OR via stretcher. Alert and oriented × 3. BP 110/60, temp 97° F, pulse 98, respirations 22, pulse ox. 96%. Oxygen administered at 3 L/nasal cannula. Abdominal dressing saturated with bright red blood and pad under client saturated, 12 × 20 cm area. Dressing reinforced with pressure dressing. IV infusing with lactated Ringer's at 150 ml/hr. Dr. J notified. Client is NPO. Warm blanket applied.

Geriatric Considerations

- The ability of the elderly to tolerate surgery depends on the extent of physiological changes that have occurred with aging, the presence of any chronic diseases, and the duration of the surgical procedure.
- When communicating with the elderly, be aware of any auditory, visual, or cognitive impairment that may be present.

Home Care and Long Term Care Considerations

- Teach primary caregiver about any postoperative exercises, home modifications, or activity limitations.
- If client is discharged with dressing changes, bedroom or bathroom is usually ideal for procedure. Have primary caregiver perform return demonstration of dressing change.

Skill 21.2

PROVIDING COMFORT MEASURES DURING PHASE II (CONVALESCENT PHASE)

Phase II of postoperative recovery is the convalescent period. This period extends from the time the client is discharged from the RR or PACU to the time the client is discharged from the hospital. Clients who have outpatient surgery undergo convalescence at home. Nursing care must be individualized depending on the type of surgery, preexisting medical conditions, the risk or development of complications, and the rate of recovery. Teaching promotes the client's independence, educates the client about any limitations, and provides resources needed for the client to achieve an optimal state of wellness.

Equipment

    Postoperative bed (recliner in ASU)
    Stethoscope, sphygmomanometer, thermometer
    IV fluid poles
    Emesis basin
    Washcloth and towel
    Waterproof pads
    Equipment for oral hygiene
    Pillows

    Facial tissue
    Oxygen equipment
    Suction equipment (to suction airway)
    Dressing supplies
    Intermittent suction (to connect to NG or wound drainage tubes)
    Orthopedic appliances (if needed)

ASSESSMENT

1. Obtain phone report from nurse in PACU. **Rationale: A preliminary report allows nurse to prepare hospital room with necessary supplies and equipment for client's special needs.**
2. On arrival, assist with transfer and complete initial assessment. Review chart to identify type of surgery, preoperative medical risks, and baseline vital signs. **Rationale: Data provide baseline to detect any change in client's condition.**
3. Review surgeon's postoperative orders.

PLANNING

Expected outcomes focus on prevention of complications, maintenance of pain control adequate for recovery activities, and teaching to promote optimal wellness.

Expected Outcomes

1. Client's breath sounds remain clear.
2. Client's vital signs remain within normal limits compared with preoperative baseline.
3. Client describes pain as less than 3 (scale 1 to 10) while engaged in moderate activity by discharge.
4. Fluid balance is evident by intake and output records.
5. Normal bowel sounds present after bowel surgery or general anesthesia within 48 to 72 hours postoperatively.
6. Incisional wound edges are well approximated; no drainage is noted.
7. Client (or caregiver) describes plans for coping with stress of surgery (altered function or body image).
8. Client (or caregiver) describes evidence of complications that should be reported to physician by discharge.
9. Client (or caregiver) describes or demonstrates incision care and activity restriction and plans follow-up visit.

DELEGATION CONSIDERATIONS

The skill of initiating and managing postoperative care of the client requires problem solving and knowledge application unique to a professional nurse. AP may obtain vital signs, apply nasal cannula or oxygen mask, and provide comfort and hygiene measures.

IMPLEMENTATION

Steps	Rationale
1. See Standard Protocol (inside front cover).	
Initial postoperative care	
2. Prepare bed in high position (level with the stretcher), with sheet folded to side with room for a stretcher to be easily placed beside bed (see illustration) (see Chapter 6).	Arrangement of equipment ensures smooth transfer process.
3. Assist transport staff to move client from stretcher to bed (see Chapter 6).	
4. Attach any existing oxygen tubing, position IV fluids, check IV flow rate, and check drainage tubes (Foley catheter or wound drainage).	
5. Maintain airway. If client remains sleepy or lethargic, keep head extended and support in side-lying position (see Skill 21.1).	Minimizes chances of aspiration and obstruction of airway with tongue.

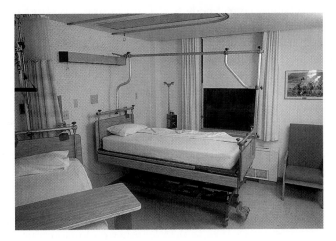

Step 2

Steps	Rationale

6. Take vital signs and compare findings with vital signs in recovery area as well as client's baseline values. Continue monitoring as ordered.

During transfer, client's status may change. Movement of client and pain level can influence stability of vital signs.

7. Encourage coughing and deep breathing (see Chapter 19).

Anesthesia, medications, and intubation irritate airways, resulting in secretions and atelectasis (see illustration).

8. If NG tube is present, check placement (see Chapter 32) and connect to proper drainage device. Connect all drainage tubes to appropriate suction device as indicated, and secure to prevent tension.

Transfer and movement may dislodge tube, which would interfere with drainage.

9. Assess client's surgical dressing for appearance and presence and character of drainage. Unless contraindicated by physician, outline drainage along the edges with a pen and reassess in 1 hour for increase. If no dressing present, inspect condition of wound (see Chapter 24).

Hemorrhage is most likely to occur on the day of surgery. Dressing should be clean, dry, and intact.

10. Assess client for bladder distention. If Foley catheter is present, check placement and be sure it is draining freely and properly secured. Client may have continuous bladder irrigations or suprapubic catheter for urinary drainage (see Chapter 35).

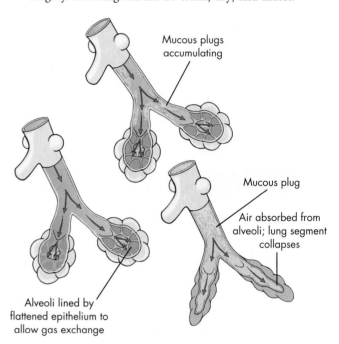

Step 7   Atelectasis can result from accumulating mucus. *From Lewis, et al: Medical-sugical nursing: assessment and management of clinical problems, ed 3, St Louis, 1996, Mosby.*

11. Measure all sources of fluid intake and output (including estimated blood loss during surgery). Remove and discard gloves and wash hands.

Altered fluid and electrolyte balance is a potential complication of major surgery (see Chapter 37).

12. Describe the purpose of equipment and frequent observations to client and significant others.

Unfamiliar sights (equipment, client's appearance) can be anxiety provoking.

13. Position client for comfort, maintaining correct body alignment. Avoid tension on surgical wound site.

Reduces stress on suture line. Helps client relax and promotes comfort.

14. Place call light within reach and raise side rail. Instruct client to call for assistance to get out of bed.

Promotes client's safety as effects of anesthesia continue to diminish.

15. Assess the need for pain medication based on client's level of discomfort and last time analgesic was given. PCA may be used for pain control (see Chapter 10).

Client should be medicated freely every 3 to 4 hours during the first 24 to 48 hours. Adequate pain control is needed to permit client to participate with breathing exercises, coughing, and ambulation.

Continued postoperative care

16. Assess vital signs at least every 4 hours or as ordered.

Temperature above 38° C (100.4° F) in the first 48 hours may indicate atelectasis, the normal inflammatory response, or dehydration. Elevation above 37.7° C on the third day or after may indicate wound infection, pneumonia, or phlebitis (Lewis and Collier, 1996). Altered blood pressure and/or pulse may indicate cardiovascular complications (see Table 21-1).

Steps	Rationale
17. Provide oral care at least every 2 hours as needed. If permitted, offer ice chips.	Medication given preoperatively, such as atropine (anticholinergic), makes mouth dry. Oral care and ice chips promote comfort.
18. Encourage to turn, cough, and deep breathe at least every 2 hours.	Benefits clients with history of smoking or pneumonia along with chronic obstructive pulmonary disease (COPD), or confined to bed rest.
19. Encourage use of incentive spirometer as ordered (see Chapter 19).	
20. If no urinary drainage system is present, explain that voiding within 8 hours postoperatively is expected. Male clients may void successfully if allowed to stand.	After spinal or epidural anesthesia, risk for urinary retention is increased. Many clients are unable to feel the urge to void. If client is unable to void and bladder is distended, catheterization may be required.
21. Promote ambulation and activity as ordered. Assess vital signs before and after activity to assess tolerance. Clients often are encouraged to be up in a chair the evening of surgery or the following morning and progress to walking in room or hallway.	Ambulation is the most significant nursing intervention to prevent postoperative complications. Mobility promotes circulation, lung expansion, and peristalsis. Sudden position changes can cause postural hypotension.
22. Progress from clear liquids to regular diet progressively as tolerated if nausea and vomiting do not occur.	Nausea and vomiting are associated with anesthesia and surgery. IV fluids are usually discontinued when oral intake is tolerated. Some clients must be NPO for several days until bowel sounds are heard.
23. If possible, include client and family in decision making and answer questions as they arise.	Promotes client's sense of control and independence and improves self-esteem.
24. Provide opportunity for clients who must adjust to a change in body appearance or function to verbalize feelings.	Radical surgery (mastectomy, colostomy), amputation, or inoperable cancer may result in anxiety and depression. The grief response to loss of a body organ (e.g., the uterus) is common and should be expected.
25. Discuss plans for discharge with client and caregivers, including wound care, medications, activity restrictions, and complications that warrant notifying the physician. Clarify follow-up appointments and encourage quick access to emergency telephone numbers.	
26. See Completion Protocol (inside front cover).	

• • •

EVALUATION
1. Auscultate breath sounds.
2. Obtain vital signs.
3. Ask client to describe pain (scale 1 to 10) after moderate activity.
4. Evaluate intake and output records.
5. Auscultate bowel sounds.
6. Inspect incision (wound edges well approximated, no drainage is noted).
7. Ask client to describe ability to cope with stress of surgery (altered function or body image).
8. Ask client (or caregiver) to indicate complications that should be reported to the physician by discharge.
9. Have client (or caregiver) describe incision care, activity restrictions, and plans for follow-up visit.

Unexpected Outcomes and Related Interventions
1. Vital signs are above or below client's baseline or expected range. This could be related to anesthesia efforts, pain, hypovolemic shock, airway obstruction, fluid and electrolyte imbalance, or hypothermia.
   a. Identify contributing factors.
   b. Notify the physician.
2. Bowel sounds are absent or decreased. Client experiences nausea and vomiting. Client is unable to pass flatus, and abdomen is hard and distended. Paralytic ileus is a common complication after bowel surgery. Intestinal motility may return slowly.
   a. Report to physician.
   b. Placement of an NG tube may be required (see Chapter 31).

Recording and Reporting

- Document client's arrival at nursing unit; describe vital signs, assessment findings, and all nursing measures initiated in progress note. Document every 4 h or more frequently as client condition warrants.
- Record vital signs and intake and output (I&O) on appropriate flow sheet.
- Report any abnormal assessment findings and signs of complications to physician.

Sample Documentation

Third postoperative day after abdominal surgery:

1800   Client vomited 300 ml dark green mucus × 2 since 1600. Abdomen firm and distended. No bowel sounds heard. Not passing flatus. Rates pain at 7 (scale 1 to 10). Morphine Sulfate 10 mg given IM. Instructed not to eat or drink anything.

1910   Vomited 200 ml dark green material and c/o being "very nauseated." Abdominal pain now rated at 6 (scale 1 to 10). Dr. K notified. NG tube inserted and connected to low intermittent suction as ordered with return of 400 ml dark green material within 15 minutes. Phenergan 5 mg given IM for nausea.

1950   Resting comfortably. Denies nausea. Pain now rated at 4 (scale 0 to 10). NG draining large amount of dark green drainage.

Geriatric Considerations

- For Geriatric Considerations, see Skill 21.1.

Home Care and Long Term Care Considerations

- Teach client and primary caregiver about any postoperative exercises, home modifications, activity limitations, medications, and nutritional needs.
- If client is discharged with dressing changes, bedroom or bathroom is usually ideal for procedure. Have client and primary care giver perform return demonstration of dressing change.

Skill 21.3

PROVIDING SURGICAL WOUND CARE

Proper wound care is necessary to promote healing after a surgical incision. Risk of local or systemic infection, impaired circulation, and breakdown of tissue is directly influenced by the ability of the dermal layer to heal. Factors that influence wound healing include age, nutrition, circulation, chronic illness, and drug therapy (Box 21-1).

The stages of healing and interventions related to dressings are described in Chapter 24. Types of healing include healing by primary intention and healing by secondary intention. Healing by *primary intention* is expected when the edges of a clean surgical incision remain close together, tissue loss is minimal or absent, and the client has less risk for developing an infection. The skin cells quickly regenerate, capillary walls stretch across under the suture line to form a smooth surface as they join, and inflammation is absent or minimized. A healing ridge can be palpated beneath the incision, extending about 1 cm on each side between day 5 and day 9 after surgery. If no ridge is apparent, the risk of dehiscence (separation) is increased by the eighth postoperative day (Bryant, 1992).

Healing by *secondary intention* often accompanies traumatic open wounds with tissue loss, jagged edges, and granulation tissue gradually filling in the area of the scar. This process is typical of severe laceration or massive surgical intervention with skin loss. The risk of infection is directly related to the length of time it takes for the body surface to be covered with an intact skin covering.

When drainage is expected within the wound, a Penrose drain (Figure 21-1) may be used to help prevent complications. This type of drain is a soft tube that may be "advanced" or pulled out in stages as the wound heals from the inside out. A safety pin is inserted through this drain, not the skin, to prevent the tubing from moving into the wound. Nursing interventions protect skin surfaces in direct contact with the drainage, especially if it is irritating to the skin. Other types of drains are described in Skill 21.4.

Meticulous handwashing and infection control procedures relating to wound care limit the risk of nosocomial infection. Antiseptic swabs are used to clean, beginning at the cleanest area to avoid transmitting microorganisms from one area to another. The presence of wound exudate is an expected stage of epithelial cell growth. After the third postoperative day, increasing inflammation and a

Box 21-1 Factors that Influence Healing of an Incision

1. With increasing age, blood vessels become less elastic, collagen tissue is less pliable, and scar tissue is tighter.
2. Inadequate nutrition, including proteins, carbohydrates, lipids, vitamins, and minerals, delays tissue repair and increases risk for infection. Nutrition requirements can double in presence of infection.
3. Obese client has greater risk for wound infection and dehiscence or evisceration. Fatty tissue has less vascularization, which decreases transport of nutrients and cellular elements required for healing.
4. Tissue repair is negatively influenced by a hematocrit value below 33% and a hemoglobin value below 10 g/dl. Oxygen delivery is decreased with both. Oxygen release to tissues is reduced in smokers.
5. Diabetes alters tissue perfusion and interferes with release of oxygen to tissues. Uncontrolled hypoglycemia interferes with phagocytosis of the leukocytes.
6. Radiation therapy results in vascular scarring and fibrosis within 4 to 6 weeks and influences tissue healing. Chemotherapy depresses bone marrow function and resistance to infection.
7. Long-term steroid therapy may reduce inflammatory response and interfere with wound healing.

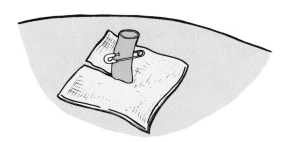

Figure 21-1 Penrose drain with drain dressing. *From Lewis SM, Collier IC:* Medical-surgical nursing: assessment and management of clinical problems, *ed 4, St Louis, 1996, Mosby.*

temperature above 37.7° C (100.4° F) with or without apparent drainage indicate possible wound infection. Wound infection, particularly from aerobic organisms, is often accompanied by a fever that spikes in the afternoon or evening and returns to near-normal levels in the morning.

Intermittent high fever accompanied by shaking chills and diaphoresis suggests septicemia, a systemic infection with microorganisms in the bloodstream. The source of microorganisms may be the wound site, a urinary infection, phlebitis, or peritonitis (Table 21-4). Wound culture reveals the type of organisms causing infection. Sensitivity reports indicate which antibiotics will be effective for the specific microorganism present.

Table 21-4

Some Common Pathogenic Organisms that Cause Wound Infections

Microorganism	Possible Sources/Comments
GRAM POSITIVE	
Staphylococcus aureus	Skin infections, pneumonia, urinary tract infections. Methicillin-resistant *S. aureus* (MRSA) is a common nosocomial infection resistant to many antibiotics and very difficult to treat.
Streptococcus faecalis	Genitourinary infection, common infection in surgical wounds.

Modified from Lewis SM, Collier IC: *Medical-surgical nursing: assessment and management of critical problems,* St Louis, 1996, Mosby.

Equipment

Clean gloves
Sterile gloves
Waterproof underpad, if needed
Dressing supplies (unless incision is OTA)
Disposable waterproof bag
Gown, if risk of spray
Goggles, if risk of spray

ASSESSMENT

1. Identify the wound's location, its size (measure depth, length, width), type of incision, presence of drains, and type of dressing. **Rationale: Assists nurse to plan for proper types and amount of supplies needed.**
2. Review documentation related to healing of the incision, including approximation of wound edges and drainage from wound (amount, color), to provide basis for comparison. **Rationale: Amount decreases as healing takes place; serous drainage is clear; presence of small amounts is normal; bright red drainage indicates fresh bleeding; purulent drainage is thick and yellow, pale green, or white.**
3. Review culture reports to identify presence of pathogenic organisms (Table 20-4).
4. Assess client's comfort level and identify symptoms of anxiety. Administer prescribed analgesic 30 to 45 minutes before changing dressing if appropriate. **Rationale: Discomfort may be related directly to wound or indirectly to muscle tension and immobility. Anxiety may result from outcome of surgery, awaiting pathology reports, anticipation of pain, or other factors.**
5. Identify client's history of allergies. **Rationale: Known allergies suggest application of a sample of prescribed antiseptic as skin test and avoidance of certain types of tape.**

PLANNING

Expected outcomes focus on prevention and early detection of infection.

Expected Outcomes

1. Client's incision shows wound edges well approximated.
2. Client's incision shows absence of drainage or drainage begins to diminish in amount.
3. Wound drain, if present, is patent and intact. Skin around drain is free of irritation.
4. Client verbalizes pain at less than 4 (scale 0 to 10).

IMPLEMENTATION

Steps	Rationale
1. See Standard Protocol (inside front cover).	
2. Form cuff on waterproof bag and place it near bed.	
3. Remove dressing, pull tape toward suture line.	Prevents tension on suture line.
4. Inspect dressing for drainage. A small amount of serous drainage is normal. Discard soiled dressings and gloves directly into appropriate receptacle.	
5. Inspect incision for inflammation and healing and describe appearance to client. Client may want to see incision. Provide a mirror if desired. Remove and discard gloves and wash hands.	Inflammation is evidenced by pink area and slight swelling, which confirms increased circulation to enhance healing. Incision edges should be well approximated and may be stapled or closed with visible or subcutaneous sutures.
6. Open sterile supplies for dressing and antiseptic swabs using aseptic technique. Position for easy access without reaching over the sterile field.	

COMMUNICATION TIP

1. Explain expected wound appearance and review how to provide wound care (if appropriate).

2. Instruct client and primary caregiver about signs of improper wound healing, wound infection, and what should be reported.

Steps	Rationale
7. Put on sterile gloves.	
8. Cleanse the suture line from top to bottom. Discard the antiseptic swab (see illustration).	Avoids introducing microorganisms from surrounding skin into the incision.
9. Then cleanse the skin along each side of the incision using a single, sterile antiseptic swab for each stroke.	
10. To cleanse a drain site, use a circular stroke starting with the area immediately next to the drain and moving out from the drain (see illustration).	
11. Apply dry, sterile dressing and secure with tape with ends folded under 0.5 cm (¼ inch). Remove and discard gloves and wash hands.	Facilitates removal of tape with minimal trauma to skin.
12. See Completion Protocol (inside front cover).	

| Steps | Rationale |

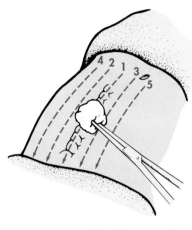

Step 8

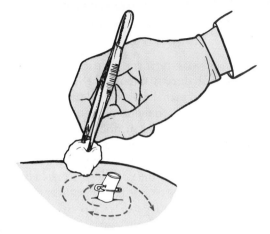

Step 10

EVALUATION

1. Inspect incision with each dressing change.
2. Note amount, color, and consistency of drainage.
3. If drain is present, inspect skin integrity. Drainage may be irritating to skin.
4. Ask client to describe pain (scale of 0 to 10) and indicate quality, location, and factors that intensify or relieve it.

Unexpected Outcomes and Related Interventions

1. Client develops increased tenderness and pain at wound site
   a. Monitor for temperature above 37.7° C (100° F) and increased white blood cell count.
   b. Observe for purulent drainage; a culture and sensitivity test can identify infectious microorganisms and appropriate antibiotic therapy (see Chapter 15).

Recording and Reporting

- Report and record in the progress notes:
  a. Appearance of wound and drainage
  b. Change in wound characteristics or wound drainage
  c. Type of dressing applied
- Record subjective data related to level of discomfort.

Sample Documentation

0930   Abdominal dressing changed. Two 4 X 4's saturated with serosanguineous drainage at site of Penrose drain. Sutures intact, wound edges well approximated. Three 4 X 4's and ABD applied and secured with nylon tape. Client describes pain as 3 (scale 0 to 10) and denies need for analgesic. Resting comfortably on right side.

Geriatric Considerations

- Prevent injury to older skin by avoiding skin tears from tape removal or products that can cause skin injury. Older skin is more easily damaged.
- Compensate for any auditory, visual, or cognitive impairment the client has when performing a dressing change.

Home Care and Long Term Care Considerations

- If client is discharged with dressing changes, bedroom or bathroom is usually ideal for procedure. Have primary caregiver perform return demonstration of dressing change.
- Assess client's home environment to determine adequacy of facilities for performing wound care; check especially for adequate lighting, running water, and storage of supplies.

Skill 21.4

MONITORING AND MEASURING DRAINAGE DEVICES

When drainage may interfere with healing, the surgeon will insert a drain directly through the suture line into the wound or through a small stab wound near the suture line into the wound. Two common types of drainage devices are portable, self-contained suction units that connect to drainage tubes within the wound and provide constant low-pressure suction to remove and collect drainage without wall suction. When the container is one-half to two-thirds full, it should be emptied and reset to apply suction. A Jackson-Pratt drain (Figure 21-2) is used when small amounts (100 to 200 ml) of drainage are anticipated. A Hemovac drainage system can be used for larger amounts (up to 500 ml) of drainage.

Equipment

Measuring container (size varies)
Alcohol sponge
Gauze sponges
Sterile specimen container, if needed
Sterile dressings, if drain needed
Gloves

ASSESSMENT

1. Identify placement of closed wound drain or type of drainage system when client returns from surgery. System may include one straight tube or a Y-tube arrangement with two tube insertion sites and one drainage container. **Rationale: Drainage tubing may be placed within wound or through small surgical incision near major wound. Awareness of drain placement is needed to plan skin care and identify quantity of sterile dressing and supplies required.**

2. Inspect for tube patency by observing drainage movement through tubing in direction of the reservoir, and look for intact connection sites. **Rationale: Properly functioning system maintains suction until reservoir is filled; drainage is no longer being produced or accumulated. Tension on drainage tubing increases injury to skin and underlying muscle.**

PLANNING

Expected outcomes focus on promoting wound healing and comfort by maintaining adequate suction and preventing infection.

Expected Outcomes

1. Quantity and appearance of wound drainage remain within expected guidelines based on type of surgery.
2. Client's drainage device is properly located and intact.
3. Client denies discomfort from presence of drainage device.

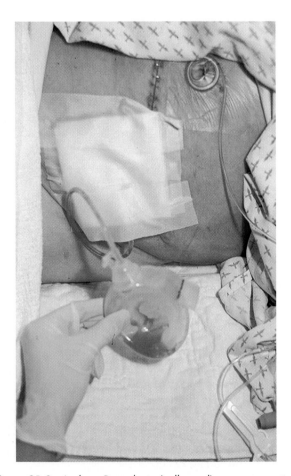

Figure 21-2 Jackson-Pratt drain (collapsed) to create suction.

DELEGATION CONSIDERATIONS

Assessment of wound drainage and maintenance of drains and the drainage system requires problem solving and knowledge application unique to a professional nurse. However, delegation to AP may be appropriate for emptying a closed drainage container, measuring the amount of drainage, and reporting the amount on the client's intake and output (I&O) record.

IMPLEMENTATION

Steps	Rationale

1. See Standard Protocol (inside front cover).

2. **Empty Hemovac, VacuDrain, or Constavac.**
   a. Open plug on port for emptying drainage reservoir, and slowly squeeze two flat surfaces together, tilting container in that direction.
   b. Drain contents into sterile measuring container (see illustration).
   c. Place container on a flat surface and press downward until bottom and top are in contact (see illustration).
   d. Hold surfaces together with one hand, cleanse opening with alcohol swab and plug with other hand, and immediately replace plug. Remove and discard gloves and wash hands.
   e. Check for patency of drainage tubing and absence of tension on tubing.

3. **Empty Hemovac with wall suction.**
   a. Turn suction **off**.
   b. Disconnect suction tubing from Hemovac port.

Vacuum is broken and reservoir pulls air in until chamber is fully expanded.

Prevents splashing of contaminated drainage.

Cleansing of plug reduces transmission of microorganisms. Compression of surface of Hemovac creates vacuum.

Facilitates wound drainage and prevents pressure and trauma to tissues.

COMMUNICATION TIP

- *Instruct client on anticipated postoperative drainage, expected progress of wound healing, drainage volume, and estimated date of drainage removal.*
- *Remind client to keep drain lower than the wound level when ambulating, sitting, or laying down.*

Step 2b

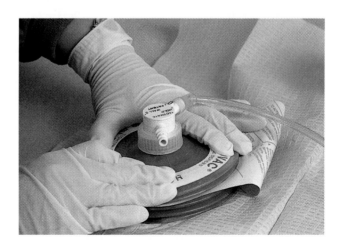

Step 2c

Steps	**Rationale**

c. Empty Hemovac as described in Step 2.

d. Reconnect tubing with connection to open port of Hemovac. Tape securely, if needed.

e. Set suction level as prescribed or on **low** if physician does not specify suction level. Remove and discard and wash hands.

4.   **Empty Jackson-Pratt drain.**

a. Open port on the end of bulb-shaped reservoir (see illustration).

b. Hold bulb over drainage container to empty drainage (see illustration). Compress bulb to reestablish vacuum (see Figure 21-2, p. 520).

c. Cleanse ends of emptying port with alcohol sponge. Replace cap immediately.

d. Note characteristics of drainage; measure volume and discard by flushing down the commode.

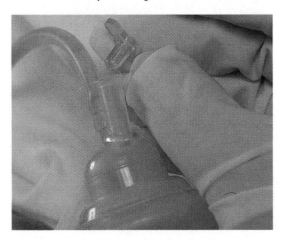

Step 4a

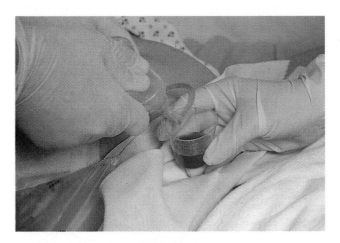

Step 4b

e. Proceed with inspection of skin and dressing change using drain sponges. Place the bulk of the dressings below the drain, depending on client's usual position. Remove and discard gloves and wash hands.

f. Instruct client about anticipated postoperative drainage, expected progress of wound healing and drainage volume, and estimated date of removal of drain as volume diminishes.

g. Instruct client to keep drain lower than waist level when ambulating, sitting, and lying down.

h. Instruct client not to pull or tug on tubing; secure drain below incision to dressing with tape and safety pin.

5.   **Remove drains (Penrose, Jackson-Pratt, Hemovac).**

a. Remove dressings, discard in receptacle, and clean the area around the drain (see Skill 21.4).

b. If removing a Jackson-Pratt or Hemovac drain, release the suction on the drainage device by opening the drainage port.

Drainage may be irritating to skin and may cause skin breakdown. Application of protective barrier may be indicated.

Unexplained bloody drainage is worrisome to any client. Knowing what to expect reduces anxiety.

Facilitates drainage.

NURSE ALERT

Be sure there is slack in the tubing from the reservoir to the wound so that it allows for client movement and does not pull on the insertion site.

Continued suction increases the tension required for drain removal and the risk of tissue damage and bleeding.

Steps	Rationale
c. Inform client that there will be a pulling sensation as the drain is removed.	Gains cooperation and alleviates anxiety.
d. Place a disposable drape adjacent to the area to receive the drain after removal.	Allows immediate enclosure of drain and prevents spread of microorganisms.
e. Clip and remove the suture if present (see Skill 21.5). Remove clean gloves and put on sterile gloves.	
f. Grasp the drain with sterile forceps or sterile gloved fingers and gently remove the drain. Inform client that momentary increased tension is felt just before completion of the removal.	Jackson-Pratt drains have a wide flat area (see illustration) that must be pulled through the stab wound with more force.
g. Immediately cover the stab wound with a 4 × 4 dressing.	Some drainage may continue for a few hours.
h. Instruct client to notify you if dressing becomes saturated with drainage. Remove and discard gloves and wash hands.	Dressing may need to be changed.
6. See Completion Protocol (inside front cover).	

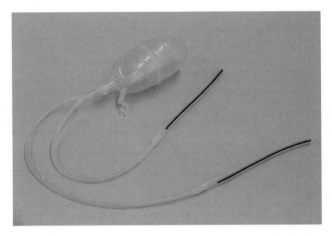

Step 5f

• • •

EVALUATION

1. Routinely empty container every 8 hours and sooner if half to two-thirds full. Compare amount and characteristics of drainage with what is expected to determine patency of tubing and functioning of drainage evacuator.
2. Inspect wound for drainage around the tubing, which may indicate obstruction of drainage system.
3. Ask client to describe level of comfort in relation to drainage tubing.

Unexpected Outcomes and Related Interventions
1. Drainage is not accumulating in drainage system.
   a. Position tubing to enhance gravity flow and eliminate kinks or pressure on tubing.
   b. Gently "milk" tubing to release any clots that may have blocked tubing.

2. Drainage containers expand rapidly:
   a. Check all connections for leakage.
   b. Tape or otherwise eliminate leaks in system.
3. Excessive amount of bright bloody drainage accumulates over a short time (e.g., 4 hours). Drainage that is bright red in large amounts may indicate hemorrhage.
   a. Report excessive bright red drainage to the surgeon.
   b. Keep client NPO, because it may be necessary to return to surgery for suturing of a bleeding vessel.
4. Wound infection develops as evidenced by unexpected purulence or foul odor.
   a. Collect diagnostic specimen for culture and sensitivity.

b. Assess for additional indications of infection, including fever, elevated white blood cell count, redness, swelling, and increasing pain.

c. Report findings to physician.

5. Pain can result from manipulation of drainage device or accumulation of drainage within the wound. After a time, infection accompanied by inflammation and edema may increase pain.

a. Secure tubing to minimize irritation from moving or pulling at the insertion site.

b. Report unrelieved increasing pain to the physician.

Recording and Reporting

Emptying drain and dressing change:

- Record results of emptying wound drainage system and dressing change on progress notes and I&O record. Note characteristics of insertion site and drainage; measure volume and discard.
- Record subjective data related to discomfort.
- Report presence of functioning drainage system and emptying frequency at end-of-shift report to nurse.

Drain removal:

- Record number and type of drain(s) removed from client on progress notes. Note characteristics of the insertion site and drainage. Note the type of dressing applied to the insertion site.
- Record subjective data related to discomfort.

Sample Documentation

Emptying drain and dressing change:

1300   Dark red drainage (700 ml) emptied from Hemovac and dressing changed around insertion site. Site is pink. Quarter-size spot of serosanguineous drainage noted. Drain is securely sutured with one stitch. 4 × 4 drain dressings applied over drain site. Client reports no discomfort with dressing change.

Drain removal:

1020   Hemovac drain and 1 suture removed as ordered. Site pink (1 cm around perimeter), covered with 4 × 4. Client reports no discomfort. No drainage apparent on dressing.

Geriatric Considerations

- Be aware that clients with large amounts of drainage will need additional fluid intake to prevent dehydration.
- Measures may need to be taken to prevent a confused client from pulling out the drain.

Home Care and Long Term Care Considerations

- Instruct primary caregiver and client on how to change dressings located around old drain site or stab wound. Have primary caregiver perform return demonstration of dressing change.
- Assess client's home environment to determine adequacy of facilities for performing wound care; check especially for adequate lighting, running water, and storage of supplies. Dispose of dressings in a plastic bag before disposing in appropriate waste container.
- Instruct caregiver to wear clean gloves and wash hands after procedure.

Skill 21.5

REMOVING STAPLES AND SUTURES (INCLUDING APPLYING STERISTRIPS)

Sutures are threads used for closure of a surgical wound both within tissue layers in deep wounds and for the skin layer. The client's history of wound healing, site of wound, tissues involved, and the purpose of the sutures determine the closure material selected. Deep sutures may be a material that is absorbed or an inert wire that remains indefinitely. Sutures are available in silk, steel, cotton, linen, wire, nylon, and Dacron. Skin sutures that are removed may be interrupted or continuous. *Interrupted* sutures are separate stitches, each with its own knot (Figure 21-3, *A*). A *continuous* suture is one long "thread" that spirals along the entire suture line at evenly spaced intervals. The surface appearance is very similar to a line of interrupted sutures, except that each section crossing the incision line does not have a knot (Figure 21-3, *B*). Another type of continuous stitch is *blanket* continuous suture. This

A   B   C   D

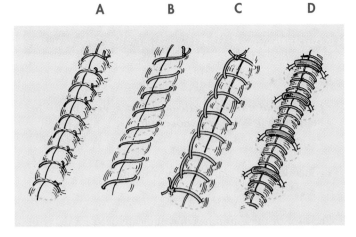

Figure 21-3

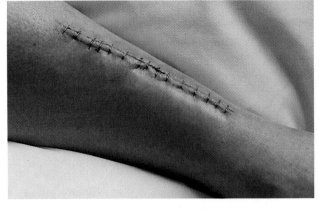

Figure 21-4

spirals along the incision with each turn pulled over to one side. The suture is looped around the thread of the previous stitch before making the next turn in spiral (Figure 21-3, *C*).

When appearance and minimal scarring are important, very fine Dacron or subcutaneous sutures beneath the skin are used. An obese client with abdominal surgery may have retention (wire) sutures covered with rubber tubing to provide greater strength (Figure 21-3, *D*). Wire sutures are usually removed by the physician.

Staples are made of stainless steel wire, are quick to use, and provide ample strength. They are popular for skin closure of abdominal incisions and orthopedic surgery when appearance of the incision is not critical (Figure 21-4). The time of removal is based on the stage of incisional healing and extent of surgery. Sutures and staples are generally removed within 7 to 10 days after surgery if healing is adequate. Retention sutures are left in place longer (14 days or more). Leaving sutures in too long makes removal more difficult and increases the risk of infection. The physician determines the time for removal of sutures or staples.

Routinely, every other suture or staple is removed first, with the rest removed if the incision remains securely closed. If any sign of suture line separation is evident during the removal process, the remaining sutures are left in place and a description is documented and reported to the physician. In some cases, these sutures are left to be removed several days to a week later.

Equipment

Disposable waterproof bag
Sterile suture removal set (forceps and scissors) or sterile staple remover
Sterile applicators or antiseptic swabs
SteriStrips (optional)
Clean gloves
Sterile gloves (optional)

ASSESSMENT

1. Review physician's orders for specific directions related to suture or staple removal, including which sutures are to be removed. **Rationale: Indicates specifically which sutures are to be removed (e.g., every other suture).**
2. Check for allergies to antiseptic solutions or tape.
3. Consider conditions that may interfere with healing, including advanced age, cardiovascular disease, diabetes, immunosuppression, radiation, obesity, smoking, poor cellular nutrition, very deep wounds, and infection.
4. Inspect skin integrity of suture line for uniform closure of wound edges, normal color, and absence of drainage and inflammation. **Rationale: Adequate healing needs to take place before removal of sutures or staples.**

PLANNING

Expected outcomes focus on maintaining skin integrity, preventing infection, and promoting comfort.

Expected Outcomes

1. Client's incision is intact with edges well approximated after suture/staple removal.
2. Client describes pain as less than 2 (scale 0 to 10) during suture removal.
3. Client demonstrates ability to perform self-care related to promoting wound healing by discharge.

DELEGATION CONSIDERATIONS

The skill of suture removal requires problem solving and knowledge unique to a professional nurse. For this skill, delegation is inappropriate.

IMPLEMENTATION

Steps	Rationale

1. See Standard Protocol (inside front cover).
2. Prepare sterile field with suture or staple removal instruments, sterile antiseptic swabs, and SteriStrips.

3. 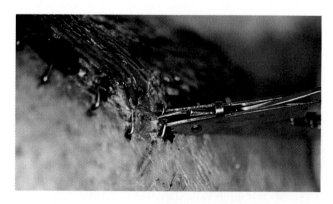 Remove dressing and discard in proper receptacle. Remove gloves and dispose in same receptacle.

   Reduces transmission of microorganisms.

4. Inspect wound for approximation of wound edges and absence of drainage and inflammation (redness, warmth, swelling).

   Presence of these findings may indicate need for delay of suture/staple removal.

5. Apply sterile gloves if required by policy.

   Use of sterile instruments can provide adequate protection from infection when incision is healing well. If drainage is anticipated, such as with drain removal, sterile gloves are advisable.

6. Cleanse sutures or staples and healed incision with antiseptic swabs.

   Removes surface bacteria from incision and sutures or staples. Softens dry crusting and facilitates gentle removal.

7. **Remove staples.**
   a. Place lower tips of staple remover under first staple (see illustration).
   b. Squeeze handles together all the way (without lifting).

      Releases the ends of staple from the skin with minimal suture line pressure and pain.

   c. When both ends of staple are visible, gently lift it away from skin surface. If necessary, alter the angle and remove one end at a time (see illustration).
   d. Release handles of staple remover over container.

      Allows staple to drop into refuse container.

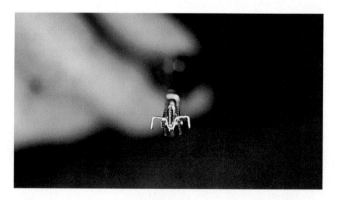

Step 7a

Step 7c

Steps	Rationale

e. Repeat steps for every other staple.

f. Assess for healing ridge and secure approximation of incision edges before remaining staples are removed.

Minimizes risk of separation of wound edges.

If edges separate, staple removal should be discontinued.

8. Remove interrupted sutures.

a. Hold scissors in dominant hand and forceps (clamp) in nondominant hand. Note position of indented tip of scissors.

b. Grasp knot of suture with forceps and gently pull while slipping tip of scissors under suture near skin (see illustrations).

c. Snip suture as close to skin as possible and pull the suture through from the other side.

d. Gently remove suture and place it on sterile gauze.

Portion of the suture on the skin's surface harbors microorganisms and debris, which could lead to infection if pulled through the underlying tissue.

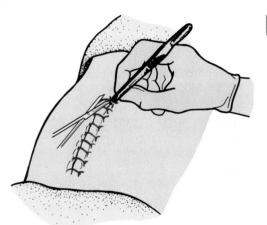

NURSE ALERT

Placement of scissors and forceps is very important. Avoid pinching the skin around the wound when lifting up the suture. Also, avoid cutting the skin around the wound by accident when snipping the suture.

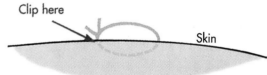

Step 8b

COMMUNICATION TIP

- *Teach client how to apply own dressing and inspect suture line for continued healing.*
- *Instruct client on resumption of shower activities, prevention of abdominal strain during defecation, and ambulation.*
- *Instruct client on adequate nutrition for wound healing.*

NURSE ALERT

Never snip suture on opposite side; there will be no way to remove half of a suture situated below surface.

e. Repeat steps until every other suture has been removed.

f. Assess for healing ridge and secure approximation of incision edges before remaining sutures are removed.

If edges separate, suture removal should be discontinued.

9. Remove continuous sutures (see Figure 21-3, *B*, p. 525).

a. Snip suture close to skin surface at end distal to knot.

b. Snip second "suture" on same side.

Avoids tension to suture line.

Steps	Rationale

c. Grasp knot and gently pull with continuous smooth action, removing suture from beneath the skin. Place suture on gauze.

d. Grasp and lift next suture, and snip with tip of scissors close to skin.

e. Grasp suture and gently remove loop of suture.

f. Repeat these steps until the end knot is reached. Cut the last one and remove it by grasping and pulling the knot.

10. **Remove blanket continuous suture (see Figure 21-3, C, p. 525).**

a. Cut the suture opposite the looped blanket edge.

b. Remove each "suture" by grasping at the looped end.

11. **Apply SteriStrips.**

a. Gently cleanse suture line with antiseptic swab.

b. Using a strong light, carefully inspect incision to be sure all sutures are removed.

c. Apply tincture of benzoin to the skin on each side of the suture line over an area 4 to 5 cm (1½ to 2 inches) wide, and allow to dry a few minutes until tacky.

Makes SteriStrips adhere more securely.

d. Cut SteriStrips to allow strips to extend 4 to 5 cm (1½ to 2 inches) on each side of the incision (see illustration).

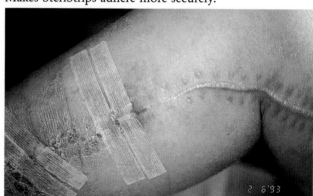

Step 11d

e. Remove backing and apply across incision.

f. Apply light dressing if drainage is apparent or if clothing may rub and irritate the suture line, or the incision may be left OTA.

g. Inform client to take showers rather than soak in bathtub according to physician's preference.

SteriStrips are not removed and are allowed to fall off gradually.

12. Review local and systemic indications of infection. Instruct client to notify physician if these occur after discharge.

13. Inform client to minimize abdominal strain during defecation and show how to support the incision with pillow or bath blanket.

Minimizes tension on sutures and discomfort.

14. Encourage good nutrition (protein, vitamins).

Enhances healing process.

15. Encourage ambulation.

Promotes circulation and healing.

16. Follow physician's instructions for limiting activity.

Heavy lifting, driving, and stair climbing may need to be avoided for a time.

17. Provide written instructions, as well as verbal instructions, allowing opportunity to answer questions as they arise.

18. See Completion Protocol (inside front cover).

EVALUATION
1. Inspect incision for approximation of wound edges.
2. Ask client to rate pain using a scale of 0 to 10.
3. Ask client to explain self-care guidelines before discharge.

Unexpected Outcomes and Related Interventions
Predisposition to delayed wound healing includes diabetes, immunosuppression, radiation, wound stress, inadequate cellular nutrition and tissue oxygenation, obesity, smoking, depth of wound, and length of surgical procedure.

1. Client exhibits wound dehiscence (separation of wound or incision edges).
   a. Client reports feeling something "gave way."
   b. Increased serosanguineous drainage is noted.
2. Evisceration is seen, involving protrusion of visceral organs through wound opening. This is a serious emergency because blood supply to tissues may be compromised when organs protrude.
   a. Organs must be kept moist by applying sterile towels that have been saturated in warm sterile saline solution.
   b. Notify surgeon so that surgical intervention can be arranged.

Recording and Reporting
- Record number of sutures or staples removed on the client's progress note. Indicate that the entire suture was removed, if appropriate.
- Record time, level of healing of wound, and client's response to suture removal.
- Notify physician immediately of any of the following findings: suture line separation, dehiscence, evisceration, bleeding, or purulent drainage.

Sample Documentation
1030   Wound edges well approximated. Healing ridge palpated. All sutures removed from abdominal incision, and SteriStrips applied and left OTA. No redness, swelling, or drainage. Client instructed to shower, avoid tension on incision, and avoid heavy lifting.

Home Care and Long Term Care Considerations

- Instruct primary caregiver and client on how to maintain clean technique when changing dressings.
- Wear clean gloves and wash hands after procedure.

CRITICAL THINKING EXERCISES

1. Mr. Palmer is a 68-year-old retired banker who has just undergone a partial gastrectomy.
   a. On the nursing unit, the nurse is aware that it has been 8 hours since surgery and Mr. Palmer has not voided. What action should the nurse take?
   b. Later in the evening the nurse notices that the abdominal dressing is saturated with bright red blood. What action should the nurse take?

2. Mrs. Smith is a 64-year-old at 5 days after abdominal hysterectomy. She has abdominal interrupted sutures that are ordered to be removed.
   a. What nursing assessments should be made before removing the sutures?
   b. How should the nurse proceed during the suture removal?

3. Mr. Sellers is admitted to the Ambulatory Surgery Unit (ASU) after a right shoulder arthroplasty. His respirations are labored, and he has secretions accumulating around his oral airway and in his pharynx.
   a. What action should the nurse do first? Why?
   b. Mr. Sellers is now awake, alert, and oriented. Before discharge to home from the ASU, what instructions should the nurse provide?

Geriatric Considerations

- Older adults may need reassurance about the suture removal procedure. Assess mental status for comprehension of the procedure.
- Older skin may be at higher risk for dehiscence after sutures are removed.

REFERENCES
American Society of Post Anesthesia Nurses: *Standards of post anesthesia nursing practice*, Richmond, Va. 1995, ASPAN.

Bryant RA, ed: *Acute and chronic wounds*, St Louis, 1992, Mosby.

Einhorn GW, Chant P: Practical points: postanesthesia care unit dilemmas: prompt assessment and treatment, *J Post Anesth Nurs* 9(1):28, 1994.

Lewis SM, Collier IC: *Medical-surgical nursing: assessment and management of clinical problems*, ed 3, St Louis, 1996, Mosby.

CHAPTER 22

Pain Management

Skill 22.1
Nonpharmacological Pain Management, 533

Skill 22.2
Pharmacological Pain Management, 537

Skill 22.3
Patient-Controlled Analgesia (PCA), 539

Skill 22.4
Epidural Analgesia, 544

Pain can be described as an unpleasant sensory, perceptual, and emotional experience resulting from tissue damage. It may be caused by disease, trauma, surgery, or certain therapeutic procedures (Lewis, Collier, and Heitkemper, 1996). Pain response is varied and is influenced by the individual's psychosocial, economic, and cultural experiences (Allcock, 1996).

Pain is classified as acute, chronic nonmalignant, or malignant. These classifications are differentiated according to onset, duration, and cause. *Acute pain* usually has a sudden onset associated with occurrence of an injury or disease and continues until healing occurs. It may progress to a chronic state if it does not respond to treatment (Lewis et al, 1996). *Chronic nonmalignant pain* is a continuous or regularly recurring pain that lasts a prolonged period. It is associated with prolonged healing of an acute injury or disease. Clients may become anxious, frustrated, and depressed in response to chronic nonmalignant pain (Lewis

et al, 1996). *Malignant pain* is a response to a malignant process such as arthritis or cancer. This pain manifests itself as recurrent episodes of acute pain, chronic pain that continues, or a combination of both. Clients with malignant pain state it interferes with all aspects of their lives (Lewis et al, 1996).

Managing a client's discomfort can be a challenging and rewarding experience when the nurse is skilled and knowledgeable about a variety of management options. Because freedom from pain is not always a realistic option, the goal of pain management may need to be pain control rather than pain relief. In 1992 the Agency for Health Care Policy and Research (AHCPR) issued a guideline for effective pain management for clients with acute pain after surgery, medical procedures, or trauma (AHCPR, 1992). This guideline is designed to help care givers, clients, and their families understand the assessment and treatment of acute pain in both adults and children and has four major goals:

1. Reduction of incidence and severity of client's postoperative or posttraumatic pain
2. Education of clients about the need to communicate unrelieved pain so that they can receive prompt evaluation and effective treatment
3. Enhancement of client comfort and satisfaction
4. Decrease in postoperative complications to achieve shorter stays after surgical procedures

The flow chart (Figure 22-1) offers a guide for decision making about acute pain management. It must be emphasized that pain is a unique experience for each client, and multiple strategies may be needed for successful management. No single therapy can provide relief for all clients all the time. The AHCPR guidelines advocate a range and combination of approaches to pain management, including nonpharmacological (Table 22-1) and pharmacological interventions (Table 22-1, p. 532).

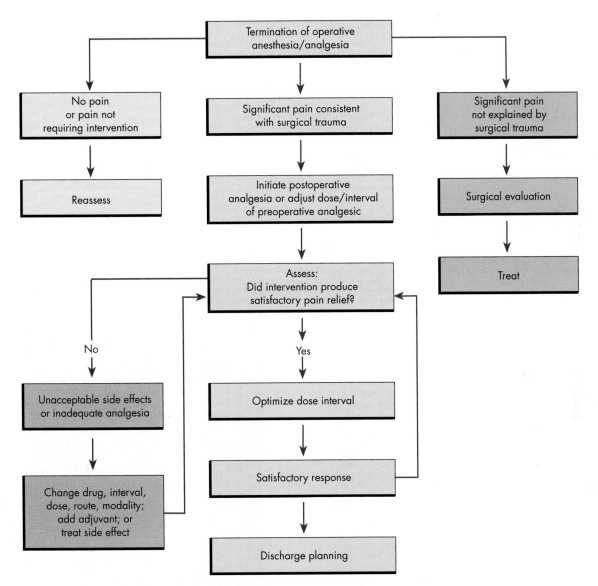

Figure 22-1   Pain treatment flow chart: postoperative phase.   *From Acute pain management guideline panel. Acute pain management: operative or medical procedures and trauma, Clinical practice guideline, AHCPR Pub No 92-0032, Rockville, Md, AHCPR, Public Health Service, USDHHS, Feb. 1992.*

Table 22-1

Nonpharmacological Interventions for Pain

Interventions	Comments
Progressive muscle relaxation	Reduces mild to moderate pain. Use as an adjunct to analgesics for clients interested in relaxation. Requires 3 to 5 minutes of staff time for instruction.
Music	Simple relaxation. Best taught preoperatively. Both client preferred and "easy listening" music effective for mild to moderate pain.
Biofeedback	Effective in reducing mild to moderate pain and operative site muscle tension. Requires skilled personnel and special equipment.
Imagery	Effective for reduction of mild to moderate pain. Requires skilled personnel.
Education	Effective for reduction of all types of pain. Should include sensory and procedural information and instruction aimed at reducing activity-related pain. Requires 5 to 15 minutes of staff time.
Massage	Effective for reduction of mild to moderate discomfort. May be firm, gentle, or light stroking of the body part involved or the opposite extremity. Requires 3 to 10 minutes of staff time.
Cold or heat applications	Selection of heat vs. cold varies with the situation. Moist heat relieves stiffness of arthritis and relaxes muscles. Cold applications reduce acute pain associated with inflammation from arthritis or from acute injury.
Transcutaneous electrical nerve stimulation (TENS)	Effective in reducing mild to moderate pain by stimulating the skin with mild electrical current. Electrodes are placed over or near the site of pain. Requires special equipment (Figure 22-2).

NURSING DIAGNOSES

Impaired Physical Mobility related to pain applies to clients who have limited independent physical movement resulting from painful conditions. **Fatigue** related to pain applies to clients who experience a decreased capacity for physical and mental work. **Risk for Disuse Syndrome** is a state in which a client is at risk for deterioration of body systems resulting from inactivity associated with severe pain. Other nursing diagnoses may include **Anxiety, Ineffective (Individual) Coping,** or **Powerlessness** when pain compromises a client's emotional resources. **Pain** and **Chronic Pain** are nursing diagnoses in which the focus of care is on pain control rather than on the client's response to pain.

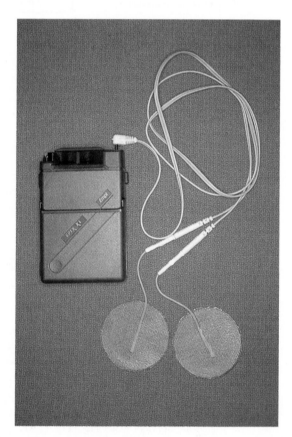

Figure 22-2   Transcutaneous electrical nerve stimulation (TENS) unit.

Table 22-2

Pharmacological Interventions

Pharmacological Agents	Route	Comments
Nonsteroidal antiinflammatory drugs (NSAIDs)	Oral	Effective for mild to moderate pain. Begin preoperatively. May mask fever.
	Parenteral	Effective for moderate to severe pain.
Narcotics	Oral	As effective as parenteral in appropriate doses. Route of choice as soon as oral medication is tolerated.
	Transdermal patch	Noninvasive and relatively stable plasma drug level.
	Intramuscular	Has been the standard parenteral route, but injections are painful and absorption unreliable. Avoid this route when possible.
	Intravenous	Parenteral route of choice after major surgery. Suitable for titrated bolus or continuous administration, including PCA.
	PCA	Intravenous or subcutaneous routes recommended. Good steady level of analgesia. Requires special infusion pumps and staff education.
	Epidural	When suitable, provides good analgesia. Risk of respiratory depression. Requires careful monitoring.

Modified from Pharmacologic interventions. In Acute Pain Management Guideline Panel: *Acute pain management in infants, children and adolescents: operative or medical procedures and trauma,* Clinical practice guideline, AHCPR Pub No 92-0032, Rockville, Md, 1992, Public Health Service, US Department of Health and Human Services, AHCPR.

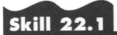

Skill 22.1

NONPHARMACOLOGICAL PAIN MANAGEMENT

Controlling pain and promoting comfort are two of the most important aspects of nursing practice. All clients experience some form of physical or emotional discomfort or pain, and attention to providing comfort must be considered in every client interaction. When possible, the nurse should design interventions to achieve satisfactory pain relief using nonpharmacological pain relief measures.

ASSESSMENT

1. Identify factors that cause discomfort/pain. Alterations in comfort may be acute (postoperative, associated with labor of childbirth, traumatic wounds, burns) or chronic (associated with cancer, migraine headaches, low back pain).
2. Assess factors that influence tolerance of discomfort/pain. **Rationale: Fatigue, loneliness, anxiety, and fear are examples of influences that significantly reduce client's ability to cope with pain.**
3. Assess client's perception of the discomfort/pain.
   a. *Onset:* sudden or gradual.

   b. *Precipitating factors:* position, movement, inability to move, edema, constricting dressings, tubes or drains, invasive procedures, or distended bladder.
   c. *Quality:* sharp, dull, burning, nagging, stabbing, aching, throbbing, or crushing.
   d. *Region:* localized, radiating, or generalized. Have client point to area of body affected.
   e. *Severity:* have client rate on a scale as established by agency policy. See Figure 22-3. For children ages 3 years and older, use Wong-Baker Faces Scale to assess severity of pain (Figure 22-3, p. 534).
   f. *Duration:* constant or intermittent.
      Rationale: Assessment is more accurate if clients describe the sensation with their own words.
4. Assess physiological and psychological responses to acute or chronic pain (Table 22-3, p. 534). **Rationale: Signs of sympathetic nervous system stimulation (fight or flight) are often, but not always, present. Persons with chronic pain are less likely to show overt physical responses because of physiological adaptation, and psychological distress is often evident.**

Numerical										
0	1	2	3	4	5	6	7	8	9	10
No pain										Severe pain

Descriptive				
No pain	Mild pain	Moderate pain	Severe pain	Unbearable pain

Visual analog	
No pain	Unbearable pain

Client designates a point on the scale corresponding to his perception of the pain's severity at the time of assessment.

Figure 22-3   Sample pain scales.   *From Potter PA, Perry AG: Basic Nursing, ed 4, 1999, Mosby, Inc.*

Table 22-3

Physiological and Psychological Responses to Acute and Chronic Pain

Mild to Moderate Acute Pain	Severe Acute Pain	Chronic Pain
Tachycardia	Decreased heart rate	Fatigue
Tachypnea		Insomnia
Increased blood pressure	Rapid, irregular respirations	Anorexia
Diaphoresis	Decreased blood pressure	Weight loss
Increased serum glucose levels		Impaired mobility
Dilated pupils	Weakness	Depression
Pallor	Nausea/vomiting	Anger
Increased muscle tension	Muscle tension	Hopelessness
Decreased gastrointestinal (GI) motility	Pallor	Despair
	Exhaustion	Fear
	Dilated pupils	Anxiety
	Stoicism	Isolation
Anxiety	Powerlessness	

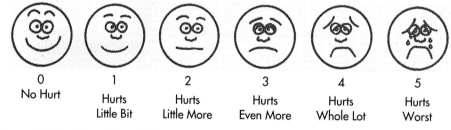

0	1	2	3	4	5
No Hurt	Hurts Little Bit	Hurts Little More	Hurts Even More	Hurts Whole Lot	Hurts Worst

Figure 22-4   Wong-Baker FACES Pain Rating Scale.   *From Wong D: Whaley & Wong's Nursing care of infants and children, ed 6, St Louis, 1999, Mosby.*

Table 22-4

Behavioral Indicators of Pain

Motor	Affective
Facial expression	Moaning
Posture	Crying
Gait	Withdrawal
Decreased activity level	Irritability
Guarding	Restlessness
Muscle tension	

Modified from Lewis SM, Collier IC, Heitkemper MM: Medical-surgical nursing: assessment and management of clinical problems, ed 4, St Louis, 1996, Mosby.

5. Assess behavioral responses to pain (Table 22-4). **Rationale: Nonverbal behavior may be useful in describing pain experienced by clients.**

6. Assess environment for factors such as noise or bright lights that may aggravate the client's perception or tolerance of pain. **Rationale: Environmental factors that may intensify discomfort.**

7. Assess affected body part by inspection, palpation, auscultation, or percussion as indicated. **Rationale: Further assessment may suggest the nature of the pain and appropriate interventions.**

8. Determine what relieves the discomfort or what the client believes will help. Consider client's experience with over-the-counter drugs that have helped to reduce pain in the past. Consider physician's orders regarding activity, oral intake, and prescribed medication.

PLANNING

Expected outcomes focus on adequate pain management rather than elimination of pain.

Expected Outcomes

1. Client rates pain less than assessed value on a scale 0 to 10.
2. Client identifies factors that increase pain.
3. Client asks for assistance in repositioning when needed.
4. Client ambulates three times a day with pain level rated as less than 4 (scale 0 to 10) by second postoperative day.

DELEGATION CONSIDERATIONS

The nurse, in collaboration with the client, is responsible for the assessment, planning, initial implementation, and evaluation of needed comfort measures. The following information is necessary when delegating skills to assistive personnel (AP) or family members:

- Assess and report to RN changes in client's condition.
- Identify and eliminate environmental conditions that might enhance pain.
- Provide maximum rest periods.
- Instruct AP on any turning or positioning limitations for client.

IMPLEMENTATION

Steps	Rationale
1. See Standard Protocol (inside front cover).	
2. Remove or reduce painful stimuli.	
a. Reposition using pillows as needed for support and to prevent pressure areas.	Repositioning reduces stimulation of pain and pressure receptors.
b. Reapply dressings if wet or constricting (see Skill 24.3).	Clean, dry dressings minimize irritation to surrounding tissues and improve circulation.
c. Reapply or adjust equipment as needed: blood pressure (BP) cuff, intravenous (IV) armboard, Ace bandages, tubes, drains, or identification bands.	
3. Reduce or eliminate factors that increase the pain experience.	Fear or anxiety may cause muscle tension and vasoconstriction, which intensify the pain experience.
a. Relate acceptance and acknowledge the reality of the pain experience.	
b. Explain the cause of pain (if known), providing accurate information.	

COMMUNICATION TIP

- *This is a good time to use open-ended statements, such as, "Tell me what your discomfort feels like," or "What makes your pain feel better (or worse)?"*
- *If the client is unable to describe the quality of the pain, suggest examples, such as sharp, dull, burning, nagging, stabbing, aching, throbbing, or crushing.*

Steps	Rationale

4. Assist client to splint painful area using firm pressure over a bath blanket or pillow during coughing, deep breathing, and turning (see Skill 19.2).

Splinting reduces pain by minimizing muscle movement.

5. Massage painful area gently or firmly.

6. Encourage relaxation using imagery, progressive relaxation, or deep rhythmical breathing (see Chapter 10).

Cutaneous stimulation alters conscious awareness of pain.

NURSE ALERT

Do not massage in the presence of abnormal reactive hyperemia. Massage may cause tissue damage (see Chapter 24).

7. Direct client's attention to something else that increases pain tolerance. Possible distractions include:
   a. Singing or music
   b. Praying
   c. Describing pictures
   d. Discussing pleasant memories
8. If worn, remove and dispose of gloves.
9. See Completion Protocol (inside front cover).

The reticular activating system (RAS) in the brain, which is essential for concentration, inhibits painful stimuli if a person receives sufficient or excessive sensory input. With meaningful sensory input a person can ignore the pain. Pleasurable stimuli also increase endorphins, which relieve pain.

EVALUATION

1. Ask client to rate pain using a scale of 0 to 10. Assess location and characteristics of pain.
2. Ask client what intensifies or alleviates pain.
3. Observe client's position, mobility, relaxation, and ability to rest and sleep.
4. Ask client to rate pain using a scale of 0 to 10 before and after ambulation.

Unexpected Outcome and Related Interventions

1. Client continues to display nonverbal behaviors reflecting pain.
2. Discomfort that is unrelieved or is worse may indicate need for additional diagnostic, medical, or surgical intervention.

Recording and Reporting

• Report change in quality or increased intensity of pain, presence of bright red blood saturating dressing, constriction of casted extremity, or change in vital signs to nurse in charge or to physician.

• Record findings of ongoing assessment, interventions completed (including notification of physician, if done), and client's response to interventions.

Sample Documentation

0700   Client continues to rate pain in left foot at 6 (scale 0 to 10). Repositioned with foot elevated and gentle massage of ankle and knee for 5 minutes. Body more relaxed, and client stated pain decreased to 3 (scale 0 to 10). Refused pain medication at this time.

Geriatric Considerations

• Pain may be difficult to assess in older adults. Cognitive impairment or dementia may affect their ability to report pain using a numeric pain intensity scale.

• Pain is not a normal part of the aging process. Such a belief can lead to underreporting of pain by these clients.

• Pain assessment in older adults should include an evaluation of the effect of pain on the client's quality of life (Lueckenotte, 1996).

• Many older clients tend to have multiple sources of pain.

• Visual, hearing, cognitive, and motor impairments may make it difficult for older adults to be able to effectively use procedures such as distraction, relaxation, or guided imagery (Acute Pain Management Guideline Panel, 1992).

Home Care and Long Term Care Considerations

• A supportive bed and quiet environment will enhance sleep and promote the control of pain.

Skill 22.2

PHARMACOLOGICAL PAIN MANAGEMENT

Analgesics are the most common method of pain relief. There are, however, misconceptions about the dangers and effects of analgesics. Until recently concerns about addiction and misinformation about client behaviors in relation to pain have resulted in inadequate management of pain.

Nonnarcotic analgesics and nonsteroidal antiinflammatory drugs (NSAIDs) provide relief for mild to moderate pain, such as that associated with arthritis, minor surgery and dental procedures, and low back problems. These act primarily on peripheral receptors to diminish transmission of pain stimuli. Most inhibit the synthesis of prostaglandins at the site of injury. See Table 22-5 for commonly used nonnarcotic analgesics and NSAIDs.

Narcotic analgesics are used for severe pain, such as malignant pain, and are given orally or by injection acting on higher centers of the brain and modifying perception of and reaction to pain. Opiates may cause respiratory depression and result in side effects such as nausea, vomiting, constipation, and drowsiness. See Table 22-6 for commonly used narcotic analgesics.

Sedatives, antianxiety agents, and muscle relaxants are adjuncts often prescribed to minimize responses to pain and other signs and symptoms associated with pain, such as depression and nausea. These drugs can cause drowsiness and impaired coordination, judgment, and mental alertness.

Table 22-5

Commonly Used Nonnarcotic Analgesics and NSAIDs

Acetaminophen (Anacin-3,* Panadol,* Tempra,* Tylenol*)
Aspirin (acetylsalicylic acid) (ASA,* Aspergum,* Bayer Aspirin,* Ecotrin,* Empirin*)
Ibuprofen (Advil,* Children's Advil, Excedrin-IB,* Midol-200,* Motrin, Motrin IB,* Nuprin*)
Indomethacin (Indocin, Indocin SR)
Ketorolac tromethamine (Toradol)
Naproxen (Naprosyn)
Naproxen sodium (Aleve,* Anaprox)
Piroxicam (Feldene)
Sulindac (Clinoril)

*The trade named drugs that are immediately followed by an asterisk may be purchased without a prescription.

Table 22-6

Commonly Used Narcotic Analgesics

Codeine sulfate
Fentanyl citrate (Sublimaze)
Fentanyl transdermal system (Duragesic)
Hydromorphone hydrochloride (Dilaudid)
Meperidine hydrochloride (Demerol)
Morphine sulfate (Duramorph, MS Contin, Roxanol)
Oxycodone hydrochloride (Roxicodone, also found in Percocet, Percodan, Tylox)
Propoxyphene hydrochloride (Darvon)
Proposyphene napsylate (Darvon-N)

Equipment
Prescribed medication
Necessary administration device (see Chapter 18)
Narcotic control sheet (for controlled substances only)

ASSESSMENT
1. Perform complete assessment as for Skill 22.1.
2. Determine time of administration of previously administered medications, including dose, length of time, and degree of relief experienced.
3. Determine if client has allergies to medications.
4. Determine analgesics prescribed, route, and frequency. Nonnarcotics can be alternated with narcotics. Injectable medications act within 1 hour; oral medications may require up to 2 hours to take effect. **Rationale: Allows for planning pain relief measures with client activities.**

PLANNING
Expected outcomes focus on reduction of pain and return to optimal functioning with minimal side effects.

Expected Outcomes
1. Client rates pain less than 4 (scale 0 to 10).
2. Client identifies factors that increase pain.
3. Client asks for assistance in repositioning when needed.
4. Client ambulates 3 times a day with pain level rated as less than assessed value (scale 0 to 10).

DELEGATION CONSIDERATIONS

The skill of administration of nonnarcotic and narcotic analgesics usually requires problem solving and knowledge application unique to a professional nurse. For this skill, delegation is inappropriate. However, AP should know the signs of unrelieved pain and notify the nurse when they occur.

IMPLEMENTATION

Steps	Rationale

1. See Standard Protocol (inside front cover).

NURSE ALERT

Review five "rights" for administration of medications.

2. Administer analgesics (see Chapters 16, 17, and 18).
   a. As soon as pain occurs
   b. Before pain increases in severity
   c. Before pain-producing procedures or activities
   d. As routinely scheduled

   Nonnarcotic analgesics may be administered with narcotic analgesics to increase efficacy of the narcotic agent.

   Routinely administering analgesics often prevents pain from reoccurring.

3. Include nonpharmacological pain control measures in addition to analgesics (see Skill 22.1).

   Increases effectiveness of pain control.

4. Identify expected time for peak effects and usual duration of action of analgesics.

   Effects vary depending on the type of medication used.

5. Coordinate nursing care measures to maximize effectiveness (i.e., encourage to turn, cough, and deep breathe while medication effects are best).
6. Remove and dispose of gloves.
7. See Completion Protocol (inside front cover).

• • •

EVALUATION

1. Ask client to rate pain using a scale of 0 to 10. Assess location and characteristics of pain.
2. Ask client what intensifies or alleviates pain.
3. Observe client's position, mobility, relaxation, and ability to rest and sleep.
4. Ask client to rate pain using a scale of 0 to 10 before and after ambulation.

Unexpected Outcome and Related Interventions
See Skill 22.1.

Recording and Reporting
• Record in nurses' notes client's pain rating, procedure and technique, preparation given to client, client's response to procedure or technique, and further comfort needs related to event. Incorporate pain-relief technique in nursing care plan.

• Record alterations in client's condition (e.g., changes in blood pressure, pulse, respiration, condition of client's skin, complaints of dizziness).
• Report client's response to procedure or technique to charge nurse and to staff at change of shift.
• Report any unusual responses to techniques (e.g., uncontrolled or aggravated pain) to nurse in charge or physician.

Sample Documentation

0800 Client complains of severe aching pain in lower back, 9 on scale of 0 to 10. Unable to obtain relief in any position, lying, sitting or standing. Morphine 10 mg given IM. Positioned on side with legs supported and back in alignment.

0845 Is relaxed now and drowsy. Pain now described as 6 (scale 0 to 10). Encouraged to rest.

◆
Geriatric Considerations

- Pain may be difficult to assess in older adults. Cognitive impairment or dementia may affect their ability to report pain severity on a visual analog scale or numerical scale. Behavioral observations (e.g., agitation, restlessness, groaning) for pain may be confused with signs of dementia (Acute Pain Management Guideline Panel, 1992).
- If older adults have liver or kidney impairment, they may experience an increased effect from some analgesic agents because of the increased time it takes for these agents to be cleared from the body. Dosage and frequency of analgesic administration should be titrated to the client's response to the specific analgesic agent (McHenry & Salerno, 1995; Luekenotte, 1996).

◆
***Home Care and
Long Term Care Considerations***

- Family members may need to collaborate planning time to reduce noise and other stimuli in the home to promote client's relaxation.
- Family members may need to be taught how to administer analgesic agents to clients living at home.

Skill 22.3

PATIENT-CONTROLLED ANALGESIA (PCA)

Patient-controlled analgesia (PCA) is based on the theory that clients are the best judges of their pain; it allows them to take active roles in controlling that pain (Pasero, 1996). PCA allows clients to self-administer small, frequent prescribed doses of IV narcotics such as morphine as they feel the need.

The equipment used includes a portable infusion pump with a timing device that can be set to limit the amount and frequency of medication. Most are battery operated, have locking doors to prevent tampering and overdosing, and have digital readouts that describe functions and store information about the amount of medication actually used.

PCA enables a client to self-administer prescribed doses of analgesic intermittently on demand or through the continuous infusion feature. Both features may be used simultaneously to control severe pain. Clients must be able to understand the use of the PCA equipment and be physically able to locate and press the button to deliver the dose. Instructions are best given when the client is not experiencing intense pain or sedated from anesthesia. If surgery is the reason for PCA analgesia, teaching should be done preoperatively. The client should be aware that the analgesia may not eliminate all discomfort but will allow reasonable comfort to allow rest and movement with minimal pain.

Not all clients are suitable candidates for PCA. Older adults and debilitated and cognitively impaired clients should be carefully assessed before initiating therapy. In addition, PCA is not appropriate for clients with a history of narcotic addiction or abuse, neurological disease, hypovolemia, or impaired renal or pulmonary function (Lazzara, 1993). Several models of PCA devices are available; therefore the nurse must read the manufacturer's guide to obtain specific guidelines.

Equipment

PCA system and tubing (Figure 22-5, p. 540)
Prescribed medication in a 30-ml vial (e.g., morphine, 1 mg/ml) (Preparations vary with pump design.)
Tape

ASSESSMENT

1. Check physician's orders for prescribed medication, dosage, and lockout settings. Verify that client is not allergic to prescribed medication.
2. Verify patency of the IV site and compatibility with the solution currently infusing. **Rationale: Other medication and blood transfusions are not compatible. If necessary, start another IV infusion.**
3. Determine client's physical ability to manipulate PCA device and cognitive ability to understand directions.
4. Assess client's severity of pain (scale 0 to 10).

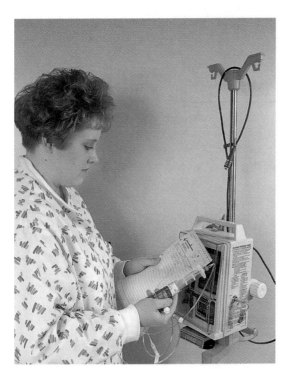

Figure 22-5 PCA system and tubing.

PLANNING

Planning focuses on proper use of PCA device and adequate pain control without oversedation.

Expected Outcomes

1. Client demonstrates how to operate PCA device correctly.
2. Client rates pain less than assessed value (scale 0 to 10).
3. Client remains cooperative and responsive to verbal instructions.
4. Client maintains respirations of greater than 12/min.

DELEGATION CONSIDERATIONS

The skill of PCA administration requires problem solving and knowledge application unique to a professional nurse. For this skill, delegation is inappropriate. However, AP should know the signs of unrelieved pain and notify the nurse when they occur. AP should also notify the nurse if the client is confused about operating the PCA pump, if the PCA syringe is almost empty, or if it is suspected that the PCA pump is not working properly. AP should *never* administer a PCA dose for the client.

IMPLEMENTATION

Steps	Rationale
1. See Standard Protocol (inside front cover).	
2. Teach the client before the therapy is initiated, including:	Ensures client understands how to manipulate device and implications of therapy.
a. The advantages of self-initiated control of medication delivery.	
b. How to initiate a dose of medication using the control button.	
c. That the lockout feature prevents risk of overdose.	
d. Possible side effects, based on the medication prescribed.	
e. To notify the nurse if relief is not being obtained, severity or location of pain changes, alarms sound, or questions arise.	
3. Prime the unit.	
a. Remove protective caps from prefilled vial and connect to plunger (see illustration). Eject air from the vial.	
b. Attach PCA tubing to the vial (see illustration).	
c. Flush the tubing as far as the Y branch and clamp the tubing.	

COMMUNICATION TIP

- *"You may feel a sting when I inject the medication."*
- *"I will assist you in coughing and deep breathing exercises after your pain medication has decreased your pain."*
- *"If you use your pillow to splint your abdominal incision when coughing and deep breathing, it will help to decrease the pain in addition to the pain injection I gave you."*

Steps	**Rationale**

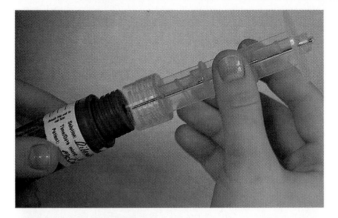

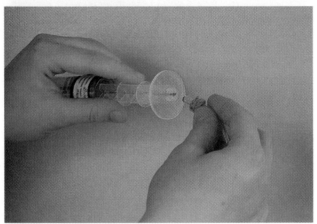

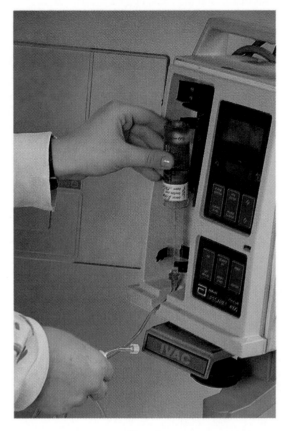

Step 3a & b

Step 4

4. Insert the vial into the drive mechanism of the pump (see illustration).
   a. Insert key and open door.
   b. Pinch the spring-loaded lever, and clamp vial securely in place until it clicks. Close door.
5. Transport equipment to client's room and plug into electrical outlet.
6. Verify client identity by checking identification band and asking client to state name.

7. ⬛ Attach assembly to client's IV tubing.
   a. Clamp off maintenance fluids and disconnect from connecting tubing, being sure to maintain sterility.
   b. Remove protective cap from Y site on PCA tubing and attach maintenance fluids.
   c. Prime tubing.
   d. Insert PCA tubing directly into hub of intracath or connecting tubing.
   e. Open slide clamps on both PCA tubing and tubing for IV maintenance fluids.
   f. Secure with tape.
   g. Remove gloves and wash hands.
   h. Place control device within easy reach of client.

Battery backup is intended for transport only.

Following the five "rights" is essential for client safety.

Steps	Rationale

8. Reinforce previous teaching of proper use of PCA pump. Assist client to self-administer initial dose by pressing button (see illustration).

VOLUME DELIVERED will display as each dose is delivered. LOCKOUT INTERVAL will display until allotted time has passed. Repeating instructions reinforces learning.

9. Encourage client to self-administer medication without delay whenever discomfort is felt.
10. Instruct family to support and assist client, but not to administer medication independently while client is sleeping.

Effectiveness and appropriate dosage are able to be determined only with participation of client. Oversedation can occur.

11. To discontinue PCA:
    a. Clamp off maintenance fluids.
    b. Disconnect maintenance fluid tubing from Y site on PCA tubing, being sure to maintain sterility.
    c. Disconnect PCA tubing from hub of intracath or connection tubing.
    d. Attach maintenance fluid tubing to hub on intracath or connection tubing.
    e. Unclamp maintenance fluid tubing.
12. If worn, remove and dispose of gloves.
13. See Completion Protocol (inside front cover).

COMMUNICATION TIP

- *"Press the PCA button to deliver a small dose of pain medication into your IV. Because you are administering your pain medication, you will not need to wait for a nurse to draw up and administer a pain shot; therefore your pain will be decreased sooner. There is a lockout time between doses to prevent an overdose."*
- *"Giving yourself a dose of pain medication before you walk or cough and deep breathe will make these activities less painful for you."*
- *"If you believe your PCA pump is not relieving your pain as you think it should, contact your nurse."*

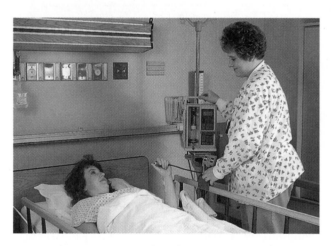

Step 8

NURSE ALERT

If pump is discontinued before syringe is completely empty, waste must be witnessed by another RN, with a notation on the PCA medication record regarding date, time, amount wasted, and reason. Federal regulations specify guidelines for recording use and waste of controlled substances in the Controlled Substances Act.

• • •

EVALUATION
1. Observe client manipulate control button.
2. Ask client to describe pain control level using a scale of 0 to 10. Compare to the number representing this individual client's satisfactory comfort level.
3. Observe client's ability to cooperate and respond to verbal instructions.
4. Evaluate client's respiratory rate regularly.

Unexpected Outcomes and Related Interventions
1. Client does not achieve adequate comfort level.
   a. Physician may need to adjust the dosage parameters. (Blood levels of analgesics need to remain stable to be effective. A continuous rate of administration may need to be added to provide coverage during hours of sleep. The PCA dose may need to be increased. See manufacturer's in-

MEMORIAL MEDICAL CENTER
Springfield, Illinois
PATIENT CONTROLLED ANALGESIA (PCA)
FLOW SHEET

Drug Used: ☒ Morphine   ☐ Morphine   ☐ Other_____
            1mg/ml-30ml   5mg/ml-30ml   ___mg/ml-30ml

Instructions: - Record one syringe only per flow sheet. Syringes must be changed q 48-72 h, tubing q 72 h.
                 - Chart all appropriate information q 4 h.

Date	10 – 15 – XX	10/15	10/15	10/15														
Time		1300	1700	2100														
Mode: P=PCA C=Continuous P+C=PCA+Cont.		PCA + C	PCA + C	PCA + C														
PCA Dose (mg)		2 mg	2 mg	2 mg														
Lockout Interval (min)		15	15	15														
Continuous Dose (mg/hr)		0.5	0.5	0.5														
4 hr. Limit		8 mg	8 mg	8 mg														
Loading Dose (mg)		3mg																
TOTAL DELIVERED		3mg	3mg	3mg														
Tubing Change																		
Sedation Level		2	3	2														
Analgesic Level		3	2	2														
RN Initial		RM	RM	RM														
RN Signature		R. Martinez, RN																

Sedation Level
1=wide awake   4=mostly sleeping
2=drowsy   5=awaken only when aroused
3=dozing intermittently

Analgesic Level
1=asleep   4=pain
2=comfortable   5=bad pain
3=mild discomfort 6=very bad pain

		Record of waste & Spoilage		
Date	Quantity	Describe in Detail	Signature #1	Signature #2

16756
Order #7408

Return carbon copy to pharmacy

Figure 22-6 Patient Controlled Analgesia (PCA) Flow Sheet. *Courtesy Memorial Medical Center, Springfield, Ill.*

structions to change PCA dose or start continuous administration.)

b. Use other pain-relieving interventions (e.g., positioning, relaxation, distraction).

2. The venipuncture site shows evidence of infiltration or inflammation.

a. Restart a new IV site.

3. Client is too sedated and unable to participate in recovery activities (turning, coughing, deep breathing, ambulation). Adverse reactions to medication occur, including hypotension, dizziness, nausea, vomiting, constipation, or shallow respirations at a rate less than 12 per minute.

a. Determine how frequently the pump has been used and total dose administered.

b. Dosage parameters may need to be adjusted by the physician. (The physician may decrease the PCA dose, decrease the continuous rate, and/or increase the lockout interval. See manufacturer's instructions for changing these parameters.)

4. Client is unable to manipulate device to maintain pain control.

a. Reposition the PCA button.

b. Use an alternative form of analgesia.

Recording and Reporting

Record drug, concentration, dose, time started, and lockout time. Many institutions have a separate flow sheet for PCA documentation (Figure 22-6). Dose calculation includes adding PCA dose, continuous dose, and loading dose. The following example is documented on a PCA flow sheet; see Figure 22-6. A PCA pump is initiated at 1300 with the following parameters: loading dose 3 mg, PCA dose 2 mg, continuous dose 0.5 mg, lockout interval 15 minutes, and 4-hour limit 15 mg. At 1300, the total amount of drug administered was 3 mg (the amount of the loading dose administered). At 1700, the total amount of drug administered was 6 mg (2 mg from continuous dose of 0.5 mg/hr and 4 mg from PCA doses administered by the client).

Sample Documentation

1700   Client reports abdominal pain at level of 4. Sleeping at intervals. IV infusing in left forearm without signs of infiltration. Morphine 6 mg infused in last 4 hours.

Geriatric Considerations

- Older adults are more likely to be undermedicated than are middle-age adults because of ungrounded fears of respiratory depression. Older clients may not need to be medicated as frequently because of likelihood of delayed excretion of narcotic; however, their dose should still be large enough to achieve pain relief (McCaffery and Ferrell, 1992).

Skill 22.4

EPIDURAL ANALGESIA

The administration of narcotics into the epidural space has become an increasingly popular technique for managing acute postoperative pain. Epidural narcotic infusions may also be used to control chronic pain, especially for clients with cancer. An epidural narcotic infusion reduces the total amount of narcotic required to control pain while producing fewer side effects.

The epidural space is located between the vertebral column and the dura mater, the outermost protective layer of the spinal cord. When a narcotic is injected into the epidural space, it diffuses slowly into the cerebrospinal fluid (CSF) of the subarachnoid space, where it binds to opiate receptors located on the dorsal horn of the spinal cord. The binding of the narcotic on the dorsal horn results in a block of pain impulse transmission to the cerebral cortex.

The anesthesiologist or nurse anesthetist places a catheter into the epidural space, usually in the lower lumbar region, to administer analgesics. Usually, opiates such as morphine sulfate or fentanyl citrate (Sublimaze) are used. When the epidural catheter is intended for short-term use, it does not need to be sutured in place and exits from the insertion site on the back (Figure 22-7). A catheter used for long-term use, however, is tunneled under the subcutaneous tissue and exits on the side of the body or the abdomen (Figure 22-8). Tunneling reduces the risk of infection and dislodging of the catheter. In both cases the catheter is secured with a sterile occlusive dressing (Figure 22-9).

Although the use of epidural narcotics for control of pain has many advantages for the client, it also requires astute nursing observation and care. The epidural catheter poses a threat to client safety because of its anatomical lo-

cation, its potential for migration through the dura, and its proximity to spinal nerves and vessels. In many hospitals, anesthesiologists and nurse anesthetists are the only health care professionals who may initiate an epidural narcotic infusion or administer a bolus. Some hospitals have nurses who have successfully completed a certification program that enables them to initiate the epidural narcotic infusion or administer a bolus once the catheter has been placed (review agency policy).

Equipment

Gloves
Bolus medication:
    10- to 12-ml syringe
    Filter needle
    20-gauge, 1-inch needle
    Povidone-iodine swabs
    Prediluted preservative-free narcotic as prescribed by physician
    Label (for injection port)
Continuous infusion:
    Prediluted preservative-free narcotic as prescribed by physician and prepared for use in IV infusion pump (usually prepared by pharmacy)
    Infusion pump
    Infusion pump–compatible IV tubing *without* Y ports
    Tape
    Label (for tubing)

ASSESSMENT

1. Assess client's comfort level (see Skill 22.1). Certain conditions make epidural analgesia the method of

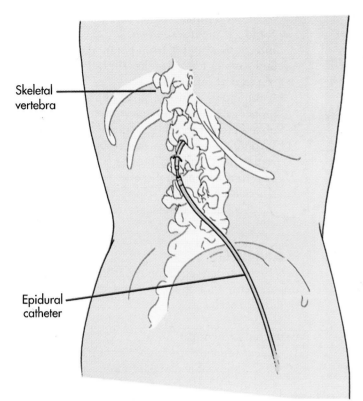
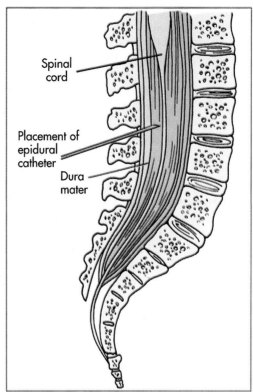

Skeletal
vertebra

Epidural
catheter

Spinal
cord

Placement of
epidural
catheter

Dura
mater

Figure 22-7 Epidural catheter.

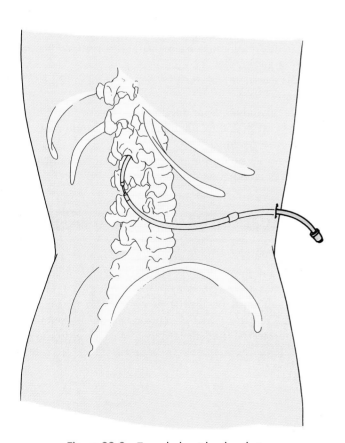

Figure 22-8 Tunneled epidural catheter.

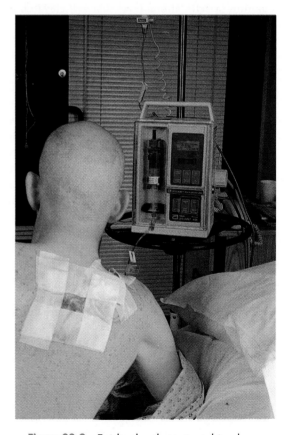

Figure 22-9 Epidural catheter taped in place.

choice for clients experiencing pain: postoperative states, trauma, and advanced cancer.

2. Assess client's nonverbal response. **Rationale: Signs of sympathetic nervous stimulation are often, but not universally, seen in clients experiencing acute pain of mild to moderate intensity or superficial pain (McCaffery and Ferrell, 1992). Clients with chronic pain often do not show overt signs and symptoms of acute pain.**

3. Assess characteristics and client's perceived intensity of pain (see Skill 22-1, Assessment) **Rationale: Objective indicators are not as reliable as client's expression of pain (McCaffery, 1992; Allcock, 1996).**

4. Assess sedation level of client, including level of consciousness (LOC), to establish a baseline before first dose. **Rationale: The first sign of altered respiratory function from opioid use is most often a change in LOC (Wild and Coyne, 1992).**

5. Check rate, depth, and pattern of respirations to establish a baseline. **Rationale: Slow, shallow, and irregular respirations are signs of respiratory depression, which may occur as late as 24 hours after epidural injection (Wild and Coyne, 1992; Naber et al, 1994).**

6. Check blood pressure to establish a baseline. Small drop in blood pressure may be seen in the first hour after epidural injection. **Rationale: Hypotension after opioid use usually results from a decreased circulating catecholamine level that was elevated in response to pain (Wild and Coyne, 1992).**

7. Assess mobility and motor/sensory function (see Chapter 14) before assisting client into or out of bed. Check for motor weakness and numbness and tingling of lower extremities (paresthesias). **Rationale: Prevents injury from falling that may occur from weakness, sedation, or postural hypotension. In addition, rapid onset of motor weakness is an indication that the epidural catheter may have migrated from the dura into the subarachnoid space (Wild and Coyne, 1992; Youngstrom et al, 1996); if the catheter puts pressure on spinal nerves, paresthesias can result (Jurf and Nirschl, 1993; Youngstrom et al, 1996).**

8. Check to see if epidural catheter is secured to client's skin. **Rationale: Prevents dislodging or migration of catheter.**

9. Assess epidural catheter insertion site for redness, warmth, tenderness, swelling, and drainage. **Rationale: Local inflammation and a superficial skin infection at the insertion site are the most common infections resulting from epidural catheters (Wild and Coyne, 1992; Brooks, 1997). Purulent drainage is a sign of infection.**

10. If continuous infusion, check infusion pump for proper calibration and operation to ensure client will obtain prescribed analgesic dose.

11. If continuous infusion, check patency of IV tubing. **Rationale: IV tubing must be patent for medication to reach epidural space.**

12. Check client's history of drug allergies to avoid placing client at risk for allergic reaction.

PLANNING

Expected outcomes focus on the achievement of pain control or relief and the prevention of complications of epidural analgesia.

Expected Outcomes

1. Client verbalizes pain relief within 30 to 60 minutes of initiation of epidural infusion.

2. Client's epidural dressing remains dry and intact.

3. Client does not have headache while epidural catheter is in place or up to 72 hours after removal.

4. Client experiences no redness, warmth, exudate, tenderness, or swelling at catheter insertion site during time epidural catheter is in place. The client is afebrile.

5. Client's respirations are regular, unlabored, and equal to or greater than 12/min.

6. Client is alert and oriented to person, place, and time.

7. Client voids without difficulty and in adequate amounts of 250 to 500 ml after administration of epidural narcotic.

8. Client has no or minimal pruritus after administration of epidural narcotic.

DELEGATION CONSIDERATIONS

Administration of epidural analgesia requires problem solving and knowledge application unique to a professional nurse. Delegation to AP is inappropriate. However, staff must be instructed on how to reposition clients so as to prevent disruption of the catheter and to report to RN immediately any drainage on dressing.

IMPLEMENTATION

Steps	Rationale

1. See Standard Protocol (inside front cover).

2. **Administer bolus injection.**

   a. Attach "epidural line" label close to injection cap on epidural catheter.

   b. Using a large syringe, draw up prediluted preservative-free narcotic solution through a filter needle.

   c. Change from filter needle to regular 20-gauge needle.

   d. Clean injection cap with povidone-iodine. (Do *not* use alcohol.)

   e. Dry the injection cap with sterile 2 × 2 gauze.

   f. Insert needle into injection cap. Aspirate.

Labeling helps to ensure narcotic analgesic is administered into correct line and into epidural space.

A large volume of fluid permits narcotic to contact the optimal number of receptors (Wild and Coyne, 1992). Preservative may be toxic to neural tissue and could result in nerve damage (Naber, Jones, and Halm, 1994). Filter needle removes any microscopic glass particles.

Changing to regular needle is necessary to allow medication to be injected.

Cleaning agent prevents introduction of microorganisms during needle insertion. Alcohol causes pain and is toxic to neural tissue.

Aspiration of clear fluid of less than 1 ml is indicative of epidural catheter placement.

   g. If less than 1 ml clear fluid returns, inject drug slowly (see Chapter 30). (Administer a bolus of a narcotic via a pump at a rate of 1 ml/30 sec.)

   h. Remove needle from injection cap.

   i. Dispose of uncapped needle and syringe in "sharps" container. Remove and discard gloves and wash hands.

Slow injection helps prevent client discomfort by lowering the pressure exerted by fluid as it exits the catheter (Wild and Coyne, 1992).

3. **Administer continuous infusion.**

   a. Attach "epidural line" label to IV tubing connected to epidural catheter. Use tubing without Y ports.

   b. Attach container of diluted preservative-free narcotic to infusion pump tubing and prime.

   c. Attach proximal end of tubing to pump and distal end to epidural catheter. Tape all connections. Start infusion. (See Chapter 30 for use of infusion pump.)

   d. Check infusion pump for proper calibration and operation.

Tubing should be filled with solution and free of air bubbles to avoid air embolus.

Infusion pump propels fluid through tubing. Taping maintains a secure, closed system to help prevent infection.

Maintains patency and ensures client is receiving proper dose and pain relief.

Steps	Rationale

4. Remove and dispose of gloves.
5. See Completion Protocol (inside front cover).

COMMUNICATION TIP

- *"Some potential side effects of epidural analgesia include respiratory depression, urine retention, and itching. We will be monitoring your respiratory and urinary status routinely. Please contact a nurse if you experience any itching."*
- *"If your pain level increases, contact your nurse."*
- *"If your epidural catheter dressing feels wet or it starts to peel off, contact your nurse."*

• • •

EVALUATION

1. Ask client if pain is relieved.
2. Inspect epidural dressing for dryness and intactness.
3. Ask client if headache is present. Note nonverbal expression.
4. Assess catheter insertion site for redness, warmth, exudate, tenderness, or swelling.
5. Assess rate, depth, and pattern of respirations. (When infusion started or if a bolus is given, check respiratory rate, depth, and pattern every 15 minutes for 2 hours, then every 30 minutes for 2 hours, then every 1 hour for 1 hour, then every 2 hours.)
6. Assess LOC and orientation.
7. Assess client's voiding pattern and amount. If voiding in amounts less than 150 ml and is experiencing frequency, palpate for bladder distention.
8. Ask client if pruritus is present.

Unexpected Outcomes and Related Interventions

1. Client's respirations decrease to 6/min and are shallow. Client is not easily aroused with verbal stimulation.
   a. Follow institution's policy, which may include:
      (1) Stop epidural infusion.
      (2) Administer naloxone (Narcan), 0.4 mg IV.
      (3) Notify anesthesiologist/nurse anesthetist.
      (4) Assess respiratory rate, rhythm, and depth every 15 minutes for 2 hours, every 30 minutes for 2 hours, every hour for 1 hour, then every 2 hours.
   b. Do not give other narcotics or central nervous system depressants except as prescribed by the anesthesiologist/nurse anesthetist responsible for epidural analgesia.
2. Client states pain is not controlled.
   a. Check infusion pump for malfunction if receiving a continuous infusion.
   b. Check tubing for kinks.
   c. Teach client other pain management strategies that may supplement or enhance pharmacological intervention (e.g., imagery, distraction, relaxation).

d. Explain that pain relief begins within 30 to 60 minutes after epidural injection and may last between 6 and 24 hours.

3. Client experiences redness, warmth, tenderness, swelling, or exudate at catheter insertion site. Client is febrile.
   Notify anesthesiologist/nurse anesthetist.
4. Client complains of headache. Clear drainage is present on epidural dressing or more than 1 ml can be aspirated from catheter.
   a. Stop infusion or bolus injection.
   b. Notify anesthesiologist/nurse anesthetist.

Reporting and Recording

- Record drug, dose, and time given (if injection) or time begun and ended (if infusion) on appropriate medication record. Specify concentration and diluent.
- Record any supplemental analgesic requirements.
- Record medication on narcotic record.
- With continuous infusion, obtain and record pump "readout" hourly for first 24 hours after infusion is begun and then every 4 hours.
- Record regular periodic assessments of client's status in nurses' notes or on appropriate flow sheets (Figure 22-10). Indicate:
   a. Vital signs
   b. Intake and output
   c. Sedation level
   d. Pain status
   e. Neurological status
   f. Status of epidural site
   g. Presence or absence of adverse reactions to medication
   h. Presence or absence of complications resulting from placement and maintenance of epidural catheter
- Report any adverse reactions or complications to physician.

MEMORIAL MEDICAL CENTER
Springfield, Illinois

EPIDURAL ANALGESIA FLOW SHEET

Analgesic Drug Used:

____ Duramorph (_____ mcg/ml)
✓ Fentanyl (10 mcg/ml)
____ Hydromorphone (_____ mcg/ml)
____ Sufentanil (_____ mcg/ml)

Device In Use:

_____ Abbott PCA (mcg units)
_____ Bard PCA (ml units)

Date	5/3	5/3														
Time	09	13														
Mode: B = Bolus / P = PCA / C = Continuous / P+C = PCA + Continuous	P+C	P+C														
Manual Bolus by MD (Drug/Dose)	3mcg	—														
Volume in Bag	100	60														
Volume Infused	—	40														
Concentration	0.0	0.0	0.0	0.0	0.0	0.0	0.0	0.0	0.0	0.0	0.0	0.0	0.0	0.0	0.0	
PCA Dose (ml)	1.0	1.0														
Delay (min)	20	20														
Basal Rate	10	10														
One Hour Limit	13	13														
Sedation Level	2	3														
Analgesic Level	7	3														
Complications	—	—														
Initials	JD	JD														
RN Signature	J Davenport, RN															

Sedation Level		Analgesic Level	Complications	
1=wide awake	4=mostly sleeping	1 2 3 4 5 6 7 8 9 10	1=nausea	5=headache
2=drowsy	5=awakens only when aroused	no worst	2=vomiting	6=respiratory depression
3=dozing intermittently		pain pain imaginable	3=pruritis 4=unable to void	7=ileus

Record of Waste & Spoilage				
Date	Quantity	Describe in Detail	Signature #1	Signature #2

White copy to chart   Yellow copy to Pharmacy   Pink copy to Anesthesia Pain Service   Page 1 of 1

Figure 22-10 Epidural Analgesia Flow Sheet. *Courtesy Memorial Medical Center, Springfield, Ill.*

Sample Documentation

0800 2000 µg fentanyl in 500 ml 0.9 normal saline infusing at 15 ml/hr into epidural catheter via infusion pump. Respiratory rate 10 with moderate depth and regular pattern. States abdominal surgical pain relieved.

1000 Respiratory rate 6 with shallow depth and periods of apnea. Arouses with verbal stimulation. Epidural infusion stopped. Narcan 0.2 mg IV push given. Anesthesiologist notified.

1005 Respiratory rate 8, shallow depth, and regular pattern. Alert.

1020 Respiratory rate 12, moderate depth, regular pattern. Rates abdominal surgical pain a 4 on a 0 to 10 scale.

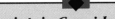

Geriatric Considerations

- If supplemental IV or IM dosages of narcotics need to be used for breakthrough pain or inadequate analgesia, they must be administered and titrated carefully because of possible additive or synergistic interactions, especially in older adults who are sensitive to narcotics. The anesthesiologist/nurse anesthetist responsible for the epidural analgesia should also write the orders for the supplemental dosages of narcotics.

◆◆

Home Care and Long Term Care Considerations

- Clients needing long-term therapy are discharged with a tunneled catheter (see Figure 22-8, p. 545). Before consideration of catheter placement in preparation for discharge and care in the home, several variables must be assessed, including fine motor skills, cognitive ability, stage of disease and prognosis, and degree of involvement of family or significant others.
- Teach client and caregiver proper dosage and administration of medication. Evaluating client's technique for catheter care and administering medication, as well as reinforcing instructions, are priorities.
- Teach client and caregiver aseptic technique for narcotic administration and for all catheter care procedures, including dressing changes. Teach signs and symptoms of infection and to report these signs and symptoms to the nurse or physician immediately.
- Teach client and caregiver about signs and symptoms of adverse reactions to narcotic being used (respiratory depression, urinary retention, and pruritus) and actions to be taken.
- Inform client and caregiver how to contact clinician for increase in narcotic dosage if highest level prescribed is ineffective, if signs and symptoms of infection develop, or if signs and symptoms of adverse reactions to the narcotic being used occur.

CRITICAL THINKING EXERCISES

1. A 56-year-old man had abdominal surgery 2 days ago. He complains of pain rated 4 on a scale of 0 to 10. How would you determine if pharmacological pain management is appropriate for this client?

2. A 63-year-old woman underwent a colon resection and has just returned from the postanesthesia care unit (PACU) at 1300. Assessment reveals pain rated a 3 (on a scale of 0 to 10), which the client states is adequate for her at this time. Morphine sulfate is being administered via PCA, which was initiated by the PACU nursing staff.
   a. When is the best time to teach this client how to use PCA?
   b. The client uses the PCA appropriately for pain control and maintains a pain level of 4 or less until 2330 when she awakens and complains of severe pain rated an 8. What interventions should the nurse implement to assist this client in gaining control over her pain?

3. A 72-year-old man has a continuous epidural analgesia infusion for pain management following a radical prostatectomy.
   a. What nursing interventions are associated with the use of an epidural analgesia in the care of this client?
   b. If this client's respiratory rate decreases to 6/min and he arouses easily with verbal stimulation, what should the nurse's response be?

REFERENCES

Agency for Health Care Policy and Research: Acute Pain Management Guideline Panel: *Acute pain management in infants, children and adolescents: operative or medical procedures and trauma,* Clinical practice guideline, AHCPR Pub No 92-0032, Rockville, Md, 1992, Public Health Service, US Department of Health and Human Services, AHCPR.

Allcock N: Factors affecting the assessment of postoperative pain: A literature review, *J Adv Nurs* 24:1144, 1996.

Brooks K: Reducing epidural catheter infections: proven techniques to keep your patient safe, *Nursing 97* 27(5):15, 1997.

Jurf J, Nirschl A: Acute postoperative pain management: a comprehensive review and update, *Crit Care Nurse Q* 16(1):8, 1993.

Lazzara D: Patient-controlled analgesia in the intensive care unit, *Crit Care Nurs Q* 16(1):26, 1993.

Lewis SM, Collier IC, Heitkemper MM: *Medical-surgical nursing: assessment and management of clinical problems,* ed 4, St Louis, 1996, Mosby.

Lueckenotte A: *Gerontologic nursing,* St Louis, 1996, Mosby.

McCaffery M: RN's assessment is critical in pain control, *Am Nurs* 42(2):4, 12, 1992.

McCaffery M, Ferrell BR: How vital are vital signs, *Nurs '92* 22(1):42, 1992.

McHenry LM, Salerno E: *Mosby's pharmacology in nursing,* ed 19, St Louis, 1995, Mosby.

Naber L, Jones G, Halm M: Epidural analgesia for effective pain control, *Crit Care Nurs* 14(5):69, 1994.

Pasero CL: Pain control, *AJN* 96(9):22, 1996.

Wild L, Coyne C: The basics and beyond: epidural analgesia, *Am J Nurs* 92(4):26, 1992.

Wong D: *Whaley and Wong's essentials of pediatric nursing,* eds, St Louis, 1995, Mosby.

Youngstrom P, Baker SW, Miller JL: Epidurals redefined in analgesia and anesthesia: a distinction with a difference, *JOGNN* 25(4):3350, 1996.

CHAPTER 23

Therapeutic Use of Heat and Cold

Skill 23.1
Moist Heat,   553

Skill 23.2
Dry Heat,   556

Skill 23.3
Cold Compresses and Ice Bags,   559

There are benefits and risks to the therapeutic use of heat and cold. Local heat produces vasodilation, which decreases tissue congestion by improving blood flow. Improved circulation leads to healing, exudate consolidation, and analgesia (Perry and Potter, 1998). Also, heat reduces tissue viscosity, which increases blood flow. Thus there is decreased stiffness and greater mobility and healing (Lindsey, 1990). Risks after heat treatments are burns, bleeding, chilling, dehydration, and maceration.

Local cold application results in vasoconstriction, thus reducing soft tissue bleeding and edema. Also, cooling slows nerve conduction, relieving pain (Kaul et al, 1994) (Table 23-1, p. 552). Improperly applied cold treatments can result in ischemia and even frostbite.

Clients at greatest risk for adverse reactions to local heat and cold therapies are those with circulation and sensation problems (Lindsey, 1990). This would include clients with peripheral vascular disease, diabetes, and Raynaud's phenomenon. Also at risk are clients with any known sensitivity to heat or cold (McDowell et al, 1994). Others at risk are very young or elderly clients and those who are confused or debilitated because of the reduced perception of temperature extremes (Perry and Potter, 1998).

Sensory receptors adapt to temperature changes, preventing awareness of those changes before damage occurs. Therefore it is imperative to verify safe temperatures of hot and cold treatments to prevent tissue burns and ischemia (Table 23-2, p. 552).

NURSING DIAGNOSES

Reasons for implementing hot and cold therapies may include **Pain, Impaired Tissue Integrity, Impaired Skin Integrity,** and **Impaired Physical Immobility** related to an inflammatory process or injury. When using these therapies, there is a **Risk for Injury, Impaired Skin Integrity,** or **Hypothermia.** Each of these risks is greatest for clients with **Altered Peripheral Tissue Perfusion, Tactile Sensory/Perceptual Alterations,** or **Acute** or **Chronic Confusion.** The nurse should teach about heat and cold treatments if the client has a **Knowledge Deficit** about these treatments, especially if they are to be used at home.

Table 23-1

Therapeutic Effects of Heat and Cold Applications

Therapy	Physiological response	Therapeutic benefit	Examples of conditions treated
Heat	Vasodilation	Improves blood flow to injured body part, promotes delivery of nutrients and removal of wastes, lessens venous congestion in injured tissues.	Inflamed or edematous body part; new surgical wound; infected wound; arthritis, degenerative joint disease; localized joint pain, muscle strains; low back pain, menstrual cramping; hemorrhoidal, perianal, and vaginal inflammation; local abscesses
	Reduced blood viscosity	Improves delivery of leukocytes and antibiotics to wound site.	
	Reduced muscle tension	Promotes muscle relaxation and reduces pain from spasm or stiffness.	
	Increased tissue metabolism	Increases blood flow; provides local warmth.	
	Increased capillary permeability	Promotes movement of waste products and nutrients.	
Cold	Vasoconstriction	Reduces blood flow to injured body part, prevents edema formation, reduces inflammation.	Immediately after direct trauma such as musculoskeletal sprains, or strains, fractures, muscle spasms; after superficial laceration or puncture wound; after minor burn; when malignancy is suspected in area of injury or pain; after injections; for arthritis, joint trauma
	Local anesthesia	Reduces localized pain.	
	Reduced cell metabolism	Reduces oxygen needs of tissues.	
	Increased blood viscosity	Promotes blood coagulation at injury site.	
	Decreased muscle tension	Relieves pain.	

Table 23-2

Temperature Ranges for Hot and Cold Applications

Temperature	Centigrade range	Fahrenheit range
Very hot	41° to 46° C	105° to 115° F
Hot	37° to 41° C	98° to 105° F
Warm	34° to 37° C	93° to 98° F
Tepid	26° to 34° C	80° to 93° F
Cool	18° to 26° C	65° to 80° F
Cold	10° to 18° C	50° to 65° F

Skill 23.1

MOIST HEAT

Moist heat therapy is most easily implemented by applying a compress to the skin or wound (Lindsey, 1990). The compress can be a clean or sterile gauze or small towel moistened with a heated solution. Commercially packaged sterile premoistened compresses can be heated in a compress heater or with an infrared lamp. A body part can be immersed in a warm solution. This can be done with basin soaks, sitz baths, and whirlpool treatments (Figure 23-1).

Moist heat penetrates quickly and deeply. To protect the client from burns and maceration, the duration and temperature of a treatment are critical; microwave ovens must never be used to heat compresses. This is because the temperatures achieved are unreliable. Burns can result easily.

Covering the client will prevent chilling. Clothing or blankets can be used.

Equipment

All moist heat:
Bath blanket
Warmed prescribed solution
Dry bath towel
Bath thermometer for clean treatments
Compresses:
Waterproof pad
Ties or cloth tape
Compress heater or infrared lamp
Aquathermia
Clean compress
Clean basin
Clean gauze or towel
Sterile compress

Sterile basin
Sterile gauze or towel
Clean gloves
Sterile gloves
Hazardous waste bag
Soak or sitz bath
Clean or sterile basin or sitz bath
Hazardous waste bag

ASSESSMENT

1. Inspect wound dimensions and character, presence of pain and drainage amount, color consistency, and odor. **Rationale: This provides baseline to determine changes in wound following heat application.**
2. Assess skin around wound and in area for integrity, color, temperature, edema, pain, and sensitivity to touch. **Rationale: This provides baseline to determine changes in skin during heat application.**
3. Measure joint range of motion. **Rationale: This provides baseline to determine changes in joint mobility.**

PLANNING

Expected outcomes focus on increasing mobility and decreasing pain and other signs of inflammation while at the same time preventing burns.

Expected Outcomes

1. Client's wound size and character are improved after multiple treatments.
2. Client's skin remains intact, and skin color, temperature, edema, pain, and sensitivity to touch improve after multiple treatments. Client's skin might be slightly red and warm immediately after treatment.
3. Client's joint mobility improves.

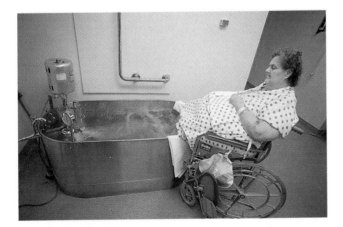

Figure 23-1 Whirlpool moist heat therapy.

DELEGATION CONSIDERATIONS

This skill can be delegated to assistive personnel (AP).

- Be sure personnel can perform skill competently.
- Caution personnel to maintain proper temperature of the application.

IMPLEMENTATION

Steps	Rationale

1. See Standard Protocol (inside front cover).
2. Provide warmth for client.
      Prevents chilling by preventing heat loss.
3. Place waterproof pad under area (except for sitz bath).
4. Apply moist compress.
   a. Clean moist compress to intact skin.
      (1) Pour solution into clean basin.
      (2) Test solution temperature using bath thermometer.
         Prevents burns by ensuring proper temperature.
      (3) Place gauze or towel into solution.
      (4) Remove gauze or towel from basin.

   b. Sterile moist compress to open skin.
      (1) Pour solution into sterile basin.
      (2) Test solution temperature by pouring small amount over inside of forearm. Solution should feel warm but not uncomfortably so.
      (3) Place sterile gauze into solution. Open package and pour into solution.
      (4) Remove dressing and dispose of it and gloves.
      (5) Put on sterile gloves.
      (6) Remove gauze from basin.

   c. Sterile moist compress to open area using premoistened sterile compresses.
      (1) Place up to 10 packages of premoistened sterile gauze into compress heater or under special infrared lamp.
      (2) Cover heater, turn on, and wait until red light is on. Compresses are left under infrared lamp up to time they are used (follow manufacturer's directions).
      (3) Remove dressing and dispose of it and gloves.
      (4) Put on sterile gloves.
      (5) Remove bottom compress from heater or top compress from under infrared lamp.
5. Wring excess moisture out of compress and place lightly on area.
6. Cover with clean or sterile dry dressing and then a dry bath towel.
7. Secure with tape or ties.
8. Repeat steps 1 to 7 every 5 minutes or as ordered.
9. Provide warm soak to intact or open skin.
   a. Cleanse intact skin or skin around open area with clean cloth and soap and water or sterile gauze and sterile water.
   b. Pour heated solution into clean or sterile basin.
   c. Remove dressing and dispose of it and gloves.
   d. Immerse area into solution.
   e. Every 10 minutes empty solution and replace with new.

NURSE ALERT

If there is bleeding, redness, underlying inflammation, or elevated body temperature, do not apply heat because it may exacerbate the problem (Perry and Potter, 1998). If there is an open wound, use sterile supplies to prevent infection.

COMMUNICATION TIP

Tell the client that the treatment should feel warm, but that the nurse should be notified if it feels uncomfortably so and then stop the treatment.

Signifies compress is at proper temperature.

Steps 7 and 9 maintain constant temperature of treatment (McConnell, 1991).

Steps	Rationale

10. Provide sitz bath to intact or open skin.

Sitz bath may be disposable type or special device with circulating water and temperature controls (see illustration).

a. Set sitz bath under toilet seat, hang bag above the level of the toilet seat, and connect tubing into sitz bath.

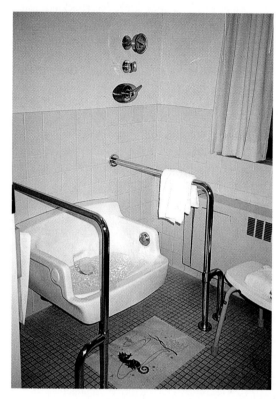

Step 10

NURSE ALERT

Test temperature of solution by pouring small amount over forearm.

b. Pour solution into bag.
c. Fill sitz bath one-third full of solution from the bag by opening the clamp on tubing.
d. If there is a dressing, remove it and dispose of it and gloves.
e. Assist client to sit in solution.

11. Every 5 to 10 minutes, assess client for tolerance of treatment.

12. Remove treatment after a total of 20 minutes. For positive therapeutic effects, the sitz bath may be repeated after the client has been out of the bath for 15 minutes (Perry and Potter, 1998).

13. See Completion Protocol (inside front cover).

NURSE ALERT

Clients with a history of cardiac difficulty may develop hypotension. Be alert for dizziness and light-headedness. Monitor blood pressure.

• • •

EVALUATION

1. Assess wound size and character, pain and drainage amount, color, consistency, and odor.
2. Assess skin area for integrity, color, temperature, sensitivity to touch, and blisters.
3. Measure range of motion of joint.

Unexpected Outcomes and Related Interventions

1. Client's wound remains the same size or is larger, has the same or increased amount of drainage of a different color, consistency, and amount.
   a. Report to physician.
   b. In collaboration with other health care team members, evaluate effectiveness of concurrent therapies and plan alternative treatments.

2. Client's skin area is broken, erythematous and warm, hypersensitive to touch, and blistered either during treatment or up to 30 minutes after treatment.
   a. Stop treatment.
   b. Report to physician.
   c. Ensure proper temperatures or check equipment for proper functioning.
   d. Collaborate with physician to treat complications.
   e. Investigate performance of the procedure, report appropriately, and follow through with disciplinary action.
3. Client's range of motion remains the same or is decreased.
   a. Report to physician.
   b. In collaboration with other health care team members, evaluate concurrent therapy effectiveness and plan other treatments.

Recording and Reporting
- Wound dimensions and character, pain and drainage amount, color, consistency, and odor.
- Skin integrity, color, temperature, and sensitivity to touch during treatment and up to 30 minutes afterward.
- Range of motion of joint.
- Temperature and duration of treatment.
- Client's subjective report of tolerance of treatment.

Sample Documentation
0930   Sterile water sitz bath for complaint of perirectal pain 8 on scale of 0 to 10 secondary to third-degree enterocele erosion. Red area 2.5 cm long, 5 cm wide, slightly raised, no drainage. Perirectal skin red extending about 10 cm around anus. States pain worse since having liquid stool this morning. Remaining skin intact, pink, warm, no blisters. States feels touch of hand.

1000   Discontinued sitz bath. Enterocele erosion and perirectal redness unchanged from 0930 entry. Remaining skin pink to red, warm. States feels touch of hand, skin feels "warm, not hot," and pain 2 on scale of 0 to 10.
1030   Skin of buttocks pink, warm.

◆

Geriatric Considerations

- Older clients have thinner, more fragile skin, especially those undergoing long-term steroid therapy.
- Check skin after 2 minutes and every 5 minutes thereafter.
- Ask for client's subjective pain assessment whenever assessing skin.

◆◆

Home Care and Long-Term Care Considerations

- Any clean basin or cloth can be used for clean moist compresses or soaks.
- The bathtub can be used for sitz baths, provided the client is safe and the tub is cleaned with antiseptic before and after each treatment.
- A towel immersed in warmed water is a good clean warm compress.
- A warm gentle shower substitutes for a warm soak or soak (Lindsey, 1990).
- Careful teaching is needed about temperature control, assessment of the skin, and length of treatment.
- Remind clients to never use a microwave oven to heat compresses. Burns can easily result.

Skill 23.2

DRY HEAT

Dry heat can be applied directly to the skin with an Aquathermia pad (Figure 23-2), an electric heating pad, or a commercial heat pack.

Dry heat treatments penetrate superficially but maintain temperature changes longer than moist heat treatments. Therefore temperature and duration of these treatments must be controlled carefully. It is important to protect the client from burns, skin dryness, and loss of body fluids through diaphoresis.

Equipment
Aquathermia pad, electric heating pad, or commercial chemical heat pack
Bath towel
Ties or tape

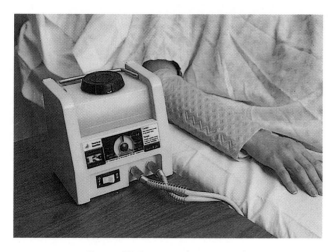

Figure 23-2 Aquathermia pad.

ASSESSMENT

1. Ask client to report pain level on scale of 0 to 10. **Rationale: This provides baseline to determine if pain relief is achieved.**
2. Assess range of motion of body part. **Rationale: This provides baseline to determine changes in joint mobility.**
3. Assess client's skin for integrity, color, temperature, sensitivity to touch, blistering, and excessive dryness. **Rationale: Establishes baseline for condition of skin.**
4. Check temperature level of external heating device, to make sure it functions properly.

PLANNING

Expected outcomes focus on decreasing pain and improving mobility while preventing burns and dehydration.

Expected Outcomes

1. Client reports decreased level of pain.
2. Client's range of motion increases.
3. Client's skin remains intact, pink, warm, and sensitive to touch, with no excessive dryness and no blisters. Immediately after treatment, skin may be pink to red and warm.

DELEGATION CONSIDERATIONS

The skill of dry heat application requires the RN to assess and evaluate the condition of the client's skin. Application of heat can be delegated to AP.

- Be sure AP can perform skill competently.
- Caution AP to maintain proper temperature of the application.
- Caution AP to maintain application for only the length of time ordered by the physician.
- Caution AP to check client's skin for excessive redness and pain during application and to report any such adverse reactions to the nurse.
- Ask AP to report to the nurse when the treatment is completed so that the evaluation of the client's response can be made.

IMPLEMENTATION

Steps	Rationale
1. See Standard Protocol (inside front cover).	
2. Prepare heat application.	
a. Aquathermia pad	**COMMUNICATION TIP**
(1) Turn Aquathermia unit on. Most units used in acute care settings have the temperature preset at 105° F, or 40.5° to 43° C. (Perry and Potter, 1998).	*Tell client that it is normal for treatment to feel warm, but that if it feels uncomfortably so, the nurse should be notified so the treatment can be stopped.*
(2) If uncovered, wrap with towel.	Prevents heated surface from touching client's skin.
b. Electric heating pad	
(1) Turn pad on. Set temperature to low or medium.	**NURSE ALERT**
(2) If uncovered, wrap pad with towel.	*A higher setting, over 105° F, should never be used (Perry and Potter, 1998). Avoid placing heat source under body part. Never position client directly on pad.*
c. Commercial heat pack	
(1) Break pouch inside larger pack.	
(2) Knead to mix chemicals.	
(3) Wrap pack in washcloth or soft cloth.	

Steps	Rationale

3. Place heat application on intact skin.
4. Secure with cloth tape or ties.
5. Monitor condition of site every 5 minutes, assessing client's tolerance of treatment.
6. Remove treatment after 20 to 30 minutes (or time ordered by physician).
7. See Completion Protocol (inside front cover).

Applications deliver warm heat to injured tissues.

Determines if heat exposure is resulting in burn.

• • •

EVALUATION
1. Ask client to rate pain level on scale of 0 to 10.
2. Measure client's range of motion.
3. Assess client's skin for integrity, color, temperature, dryness, and blistering. Evaluate again after 30 minutes.
4. Assess client's skin turgor to determine hydration status.

Unexpected Outcomes and Related Interventions
1. Client reports increased pain.
    a. Stop treatment.
    b. Assess skin for signs of burns.
    c. Report to physician.
    d. Reduce temperatures for susceptible client.
    e. Check for proper function of equipment.
2. Client's range of motion is decreased.
    a. Report to physician.
    b. In collaboration with other health care team members, evaluate effectiveness of concurrent therapies and plan new treatments.
3. Client's skin is broken, red, excessively warm, dry, and blistered.
    a. Stop treatment.
    b. Report to physician.
    c. In collaboration with physician, begin treatment of complications.
4. Client's skin turgor is inelastic.
    a. Assess client's vital signs and fluid I & O.

    b. Begin measuring fluid intake and output if not ordered.
    c. Report vital signs, I & O, and skin turgor to physician.
    d. Prepare to encourage fluids or administer intravenous fluids as ordered by physician.

Reporting and Recording
• Pain level.
• Range of motion of body part.
• Skin integrity, color, temperature, sensitivity to touch, dryness, and blistering.
• Skin turgor.
• Temperature and duration of treatment.
• Client tolerance of treatment.

Sample Documentation
1630   Heating pad set on low, applied to right shoulder for complaint of pain severity at level 6 on scale of 0 to 10 when moving it. Flexion and abduction 135°, external rotation 45°, hyperextension 30°. Skin intact, pink, warm, turgor elastic.

1650   Heating pad removed. Right shoulder area pink to red warm, no blistering, turgor elastic. States feels touch of hand. States pain 1 on scale of 0 to 10. Flexion and abduction 145°, external rotation 70°, hyperextension 30°.

1700   Right shoulder area pink, warm.

Geriatric Considerations

- Older clients have thinner, more fragile skin that burns more easily.
- Older clients are less sensitive to pain.
- Check skin 2 minutes after beginning heat application and every 5 minutes thereafter.
- Ask for client's subjective pain assessment whenever assessing the skin.
- Use extreme caution with electric heat pads in older clients.
- The safest dry heat treatment for older clients is one with good temperature control, such as an Aquathermia with the temperature set lower at 100°.

Home Care and Long-Term Care Considerations

- Client teaching is very important to prevent burns. Teaching should emphasize the purpose of the treatment, the temperature and duration of treatment, demonstration of treatment, and the importance of frequent skin assessments.
- Assess client's use of alternative treatments at home. These might be rice socks or herb packs. Educate clients in proper use of such treatments.
- Remind clients that the microwave oven must never be used to heat compresses. Burns can result easily.

Skill 23.3

COLD COMPRESSES AND ICE BAGS

Cold treatments have been used for a long time for acute athletic injuries. Halvorsen (1990) recommends that ice be applied during the first 48 to 72 hours after such an injury to prevent bruising, edema, and pain.

Rest, compression bandages such as snug elastic wraps, and elevation of the injured area are all helpful adjunct therapies to the vasoconstriction provided by ice. All contribute to the decreased blood flow, which prevents bruising, edema, and pain. The acronym RICE helps in remembering these elements of care (McDowell et al, 1994) (Box 23-1).

Another suggested acronym, RECIPE, adds the element of proper exercise to the treatment of acute athletic injury (Box 23-2). The exercise should be directed by physical therapists to speed healing (Lindsey, 1980).

To deliver cold treatments, simple ice bags or compresses work well. Commercial reusable gel packs and instant disposable chemical ice packs are available, as are electrically controlled cooling devices.

Box 23-1 RICE Acronym
R est
I ce
C ompression
E levation

Box 23-2 RECIPE Acronym
R est
E levation
C ompression
I ce
P roper
E xercise

Equipment

All compresses, bags, and packs
Soft cloth covering, towel, or pillowcase
Cloth tapes or ties
Bath towel
Bath blanket for warmth
Cold compress
Toweling or gauze
Prescribed solution, ice
Basin
Bath thermometer for clean compress
Ice bag
Ice bag
Ice chips and water
Reusable commercial gel pack
Disposable commercial chemical cold pack
Electrically controlled cooling device
Gauze roll or elastic wrap

ASSESSMENT

1. Assess client's pain on scale of 0 to 10. **Rationale: Provides baseline to determine pain relief.**
2. Assess area of injury for edema and bleeding.
3. Assess surrounding skin for integrity, color, temperature, and sensitivity to touch. **Rationale: This provides baseline for determining change in condition of injured tissues.**

PLANNING

Expected outcomes focus on decreasing pain, edema, bleeding, and bruising while preventing ischemia.

Expected Outcomes

1. Client will report decreased pain.
2. Client's skin or area of injury will have less edema and bleeding.
3. Client's surrounding skin will remain intact, be pink and warm, and remain sensitive to touch. Immediately after treatment the client's skin may be pale, cool, and less sensitive to touch.

IMPLEMENTATION

Steps	Rationale
1. See Standard Protocol (inside front cover).	
2. Provide warm covering for client.	
3. Position client carefully, keeping affected body part in proper alignment and exposing only the area to be treated.	Prevents further injury to area. Avoids unnecessary exposure of body parts, maintaining client's warmth, comfort, and privacy.
4. Prepare cold application.	
a. Cold compress	
(1) Place ice and water into basin.	
(2) Test temperature of solution.	
(a) Clean compress: use bath thermometer.	
(b) Sterile compress: pour a small amount over back of hand. It should feel cold, but not uncomfortably so.	
(3) Place gauze or towel into solution.	
(4) Wring excess solution from compress.	
b. Ice pack	
(1) Fill bag with water, then empty.	
(2) Fill bag two-thirds full with ice and water.	
(3) Express air from bag.	Prevents maceration by testing for leaks.
(4) Secure closure.	
(5) Wipe bag dry.	
(6) Wrap with towel or pillowcase.	
c. Commercial gel pack	
(1) Remove pack from freezer.	
(2) Wrap pack in towel or pillowcase (optional if client's skin is covered).	
(3) Cover client's skin with towel (see illustration).	

DELEGATION CONSIDERATIONS

The skill of cold compress application requires the RN to assess and evaluate the condition of the client's injury. Applying cold can be delegated to AP.

- Be sure AP can perform skill competently.
- Caution AP to maintain proper temperature of the application.
- Caution AP to maintain application for only the length of time as ordered by the physician.
- Caution AP to check client's skin for excessive redness or pain, and report any such adverse reactions to the nurse.
- Ask AP to report to the nurse when the treatment is complete so that the evaluation of the client can be made.

COMMUNICATION TIP

Tell client that there is a normal progression of sensation change during cold therapy: cold, then pain relief followed by burning skin pain, and finally numbness. To avoid frostnip, the treatment should be removed when the area feels numb (Stamford, 1996).

NURSE ALERT

Sterile supplies must be used with open skin wounds.

Steps	Rationale

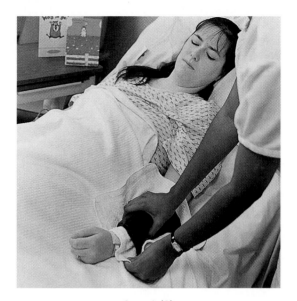

Step 4c(3)

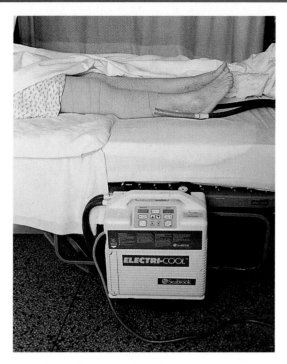

Step 4d

   d. Electrically controlled cooling device (see illustration).
     (1) Make sure all connections are intact and temperature is set. (See agency policy, physician's order, and manufacturer's directions.)
     (2) Wrap cool water flow pad around body part.
     (3) Wrap pad with gauze or elastic bandage.

5. If skin is uncovered, or if application has not been covered, apply towel, or sterile towel, over injured area, then apply cold application to skin (see illustration).
6. Secure with cloth tape or ties.
7. Remove treatment when the area feels numb to the client (Stamford, 1996). The actual duration of treatment may vary. Lindsay (1990) recommends removing treatment after as few as 10 minutes. McDowell et al (1994) state that leaving a cold treatment on longer than 30 minutes can lead to frostnip or cold nerve palsy.
8. See Completion Protocol (inside front cover).

Direct cold applications should never be placed directly on the skin because damage can occur to underlying tissues from direct exposure to cold. Applications deliver cold to injured tissues.

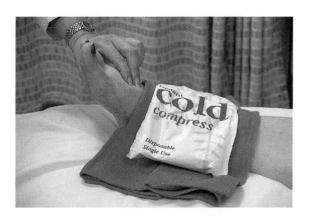

Step 5

EVALUATION

1. Ask client to report pain level on scale of 0 to 10.
2. Inspect tissue or wound for edema, bruising, and bleeding.
3. Assess surrounding tissues for integrity, color, temperature, and sensitivity to touch. Reevaluate after 30 minutes.

Unexpected Outcomes and Related Interventions

1. Client expresses increased pain in tissues.
   a. Remove treatment.
   b. Maintain immobility and good alignment.
   c. Report to physician.
   d. Collaborate with other health care team members to determine effectiveness of concurrent therapies and diagnostic tests. Together plan revised diagnostics and care.
2. Client has increased bleeding, bruising, and edema.
   a. Remove treatment.
   b. Apply compression for bleeding or bruising.
   c. Elevate edematous area if not contraindicated.
   d. Report to physician if symptoms excessive or if they persist for more than 30 minutes.
3. Client's skin is mottled, reddened, or bluish-purple, and cold with breaks.
   a. Remove treatment.
   b. Position tissues in dependent position if not contraindicated.
   c. Apply warm blanket (McDowell et al, 1994).
   d. Report to physician if symptoms are excessive or if they persist for more than 30 minutes.

Recording and Reporting

- Pain level.
- Bleeding, bruising, and edema.
- Skin: integrity, color, temperature, and sensitivity to touch.
- Temperature and duration of treatment.

Sample Documentation

0930 Left upper arm edematous, measuring 33 cm around, 7 cm proximal to elbow. Ecchymosis approximately 8 cm diameter at medial upper arm approximately 7 cm proximal to antecubital space. States pain to touch is at level 8 on scale of 0 to 10. Skin around ecchymosis pink, warm, intact; states feels touch of hand. Cold compress applied, temperature 60° F.

1000 Cold compress removed. Left upper arm measures 33 cm around, states pain level 1 on scale of 0 to 10. Ecchymosis approximately 8 cm in diameter. Skin pale pink, cool; states barely feels touch of hand.

1030 Left upper arm measures 32 cm around. Skin pink, warm; states feels touch of hand. States pain level 2 on scale of 0 to 10. Tylenol #3 given.

Geriatric Considerations

- Older clients are more sensitive to cold.
- Stay with client for first 5 minutes of treatment to assess subjective response.
- Anticipate shortening duration of treatment.
- Assess skin every 2 to 3 minutes after the first 10 minutes of treatment.
- Older clients may require more covering for warmth.

Home Care and Long-Term Care Considerations

- Gel packs kept in the freezer at home make easy cold treatments.
- Teach clients that cold blocks used in freezer chests for food/beverages should never be used on skin (Lindsey, 1990).
- A bucket filled with ice and water can be used to immerse a foot, hand, or elbow. A bath thermometer should be used to test temperature (Lindsey, 1990).
- A styrofoam cup of water frozen in it can be used to treat a sprain or strain. Peel the rim off the cup and apply ice in a circular motion (Lindsey, 1990).
- A bag of frozen vegetables conforms readily to a body part needing cold therapy for a brief time (Stamford, 1990).
- Putting ice and water in a zipper locked bag can make a quick ice bag for home use (Perry and Potter, 1998).

CRITICAL THINKING EXERCISES

1. As the nurse caring for the following clients, how would you respond?

   a. John is using an electric heating pad at home for his lower back pain. He says it doesn't feel warm to him after about 10 minutes, so he turns the pad to high heat. He tells you he fell asleep with the pad on last night and that he feels this was really an efficient way to treat his back, especially because his back feels so much better today.

   b. Portia injured her ankle about 30 minutes ago during a high school field hockey practice. She is crying as two of her classmates assist her into the emergency room. You are the registered nurse. You assist Portia to lie on a treatment cart, splint her ankle, and elevate it on a pillow, extending the edges of the pillow a couple of inches proximal to the knee for good alignment. An x-ray confirms that her ankle is sprained, not fractured. The doctor orders ice bags, elevation, elastic wrap compression, and Tylenol #3, 2 tablets every 3 to 4 hours as needed for pain.

2. The nurse should exercise caution when using heat and cold treatments for clients with certain medical problems. What are the types of primary problems? Discuss precautions the nurse should take and why.

3. The registered nurse is assigning a warm water sitz bath treatment to a licensed practical nurse. The client is a 39-year-old female who just had a hemorrhoidectomy. She complains that it hurts when she sits down. She did have a myocardial infarction 2 years ago and tires easily. What points of care should the nurse review with the practical nurse?

REFERENCES

Halvorsen GA: Therapeutic heat and cold for athletic injuries, *The Physician and Sports Medicine* 18(5):87–94, 1990.

Kaul MP et al: Superficial heat and cold. How to maximize the benefits, *The Physician and Sports Medicine* 22(12):69–72, 74, 1994.

Lindsey B: Patient care guidelines. Cold and heat application in musculoskeletal injury, *Journal of Emergency Nursing* 16(1):54–57, 1990.

McDowell JH et al: Use of cryotherapy for orthopaedic patients, *Orthopaedic Nursing* 13(5):21–30, 1994.

McConnel EA: Using an aquathermia pad safely, *Nursing '91* 21(12):72, 1991.

Perry A, Potter P: *Clinical nursing skills and techniques,* ed 4, St Louis, 1998, Mosby.

Stamford B: Giving injuries the cold treatment, *The Physician and Sports Medicine* 24(3):99–103, 1996.

UNIT SEVEN

Managing Immobilized Clients

Chapter 24
Pressure Ulcers and Wound Care Management

Chapter 25
Special Mattresses and Beds

Chapter 26
Promoting Range of Motion

Chapter 27
Traction

Chapter 28
Cast Care

Chapter 29
Assistive Devices for Ambulation

CHAPTER 24

Pressure Ulcers and Wound Care Management

Skill 24.1
Pressure Ulcer Risk Assessment and Prevention Strategies, 568

Skill 24.2
Treatment of Pressure Ulcers and Wound Management, 577

Skill 24.3
Applying Dressings, 585

Skill 24.4
Changing Transparent Dressings, 592

Skill 24.5
Applying Binders and Bandages, 594

PRESSURE ULCERS

Pressure ulcers are defined as "localized areas of tissue necrosis that develop when soft tissue is compressed between a bony prominence and an external surface for a prolonged period of time" (National Pressure Ulcer Advisory Panel [NPUAP], 1989). Formerly called *decubitus ulcers,* it is now known that these ulcers develop when clients are in positions other than bed rest. Pressure ulcers can occur when clients are in the sitting position. Pressure points over bony prominences where pressure ulcers develop in sitting and lying positions are shown in Figures 6-1, *A* and *B*. Some of the most common sites are the sacrum, heels, elbow, lateral malleoli, greater trochanters, and ischial tuberosities (Meehan, 1994). Three elements are the cornerstone of pressure ulcer development: (1) intensity of pressure, (2) duration of pressure, and (3) tissue tolerance. Many risk factors such as friction, shear, poor nutrition, altered sensory perception, incontinence, and moisture have been proposed (Bergstrom, Demuth, and Braden, 1987). Fat and muscle tissue do not tolerate decreased blood flow and are therefore less resistant to pressure than skin. Maklebust and Sieggreen (1996) describe the two models of **pressure ulcer** formation that have been proposed. The traditional model is that the tissue destruction first occurs in the epidermis of the skin and then later in the deeper layers of tissue. The other model suggests that the tissue nearest to the bone or muscle is injured first, before signs of tissue damage can be seen on the skin surface. Ischemia may be evident by skin discoloration such as a red spot in clients with light skin. If pressure is unrelieved or repeated, tissues will continue to break down relative to the client's general health and tolerance for pressure. This pressure, if not relieved, can cause irreversible tissue damage in as little as 90 minutes.

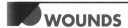

WOUNDS

Unbroken skin is a protective barrier against disease-causing organisms and a sensory organ for pain, temperature, and touch. Injury to the skin poses risks for infection and triggers a complex healing response. Knowing the normal healing pattern helps the nurse recognize alterations that require intervention. The nurse's main responsibilities are to prevent infection and to support the body's defenses for healing. When choosing dressings, the nurse considers the type of wound, the pain associated with it, conditions that affect healing, and the client's psychological responses.

Physiologically, wound healing occurs in the same way for all clients, with skin cells and some tissues (including the vascular tissues) regenerating quickly and others regenerating slowly or not at all. The latter group includes cells of the liver, renal tubules, and central nervous system neurons.

Wound healing involves a series of physiological processes (Box 24-1). These processes can be affected by the location, severity, and extent of the injury. The ability of cells and tissues to regenerate, return to normal structure, or resume normal functioning also affects healing.

Most surgical incisions and some traumatic injuries heal by *primary intention*, because tissue is cleanly cut and the edges are well approximated. New capillary circulation bridges the wound in 3 to 4 days, and once normal tissue oxygenation is achieved, the wound is considered to be healed. Susceptibility to infection is greatest during the first 4 days.

Burns, infected wounds, and deep pressure ulcers heal by *secondary intention*. The wound is left open (not sutured). Granulation tissue and epithelialization close the defect. This healing occurs much more slowly.

Wound infection is the second most common nosocomial infection. The chances of wound infection are greater when the wound contains dead or necrotic tissue, when there are foreign bodies in or near the wound, and when blood supply and local tissue defenses are reduced. Many factors may delay healing and increase risk of infection (Table 24-1). According to the Centers for Disease Control and Prevention (CDC), a wound is infected if purulent material drains from it (Table 24-2), even if a culture has negative results or is not taken. A sample of drainage from an infected wound may not reveal bacteria in a culture because of inadequate technique or previous treatment with antibiotics. Positive cultures may contain colonies of noninfective resident bacteria.

Box 24-1 Stages of Wound Healing

Defensive or Inflammatory Stage

Starts when skin integrity is impaired and continues for 4 to 6 days.

- Hemostasis—Blood vessels constrict, gathering of platelets stops bleeding. Clots form a fibrin matrix. Scab forms, preventing entry of infectious organisms.
- Inflammatory response—Increases blood flow to wound and vascular permeability to plasma, resulting in localized redness and edema.
- White blood cells arrive at wound.
  Neutrophils ingest bacteria and small debris, then die in a few days and leave enzyme exudate, which either attacks bacteria *or* interferes with tissue repair.
  Monocytes become macrophages.
  Macrophages clean cell of debris by phagocytosis; aid in wound repair by recycling normal amino acids and sugars.
- Epithelial cells move from wound margins to base of clot or scab (for period of approximately 48 hours).

Reconstruction or Proliferative Stage

Closure begins on day 3 or 4 of defensive stage and continues for 2 to 3 weeks.

- Fibroblasts—Function with help of vitamins B and C; oxygen and amino acids synthesize collagen.
- Collagen—Provides strength and structural integrity to the wound.
- Epithelial cells—Differentiate to duplicate damaged cells (e.g., intestinal mucosal cells acquire their columnar appearance).

Maturation Stage

This final healing stage may continue for 1 year or more as collagen scar strengthens.

A contaminated or traumatic wound may show signs of infection within 2 to 3 days. A surgical wound infection usually develops on the fourth or fifth day. The client will have fever, tenderness, and increasing pain at the wound site and an elevated white blood cell (WBC) count. The edges of the wound appear inflamed (red and swollen). Drainage, if visible, is purulent, is odorous, and has a yellow, green, or brown color, depending on the causative organism (Table 24-2).

Table 24-1

Factors that Delay Wound Healing and Increase Risk for Infection

Factor	Reason for Increased Risk
Older adult	Physiological changes of aging alter the immune system, resulting in decreased resistance to pathogens, and loss of subcutaneous tissue as well.
Obesity	Fatty subcutaneous tissue has diminished vascularity. Fatty tissue makes approximation of wound edges difficult and creates tension on the wound.
Diabetes	Associated vascular changes reduce blood flow to peripheral tissues; leukocyte malfunction results from hyperglycemia.
Compromised circulation	Results in inadequate supply of nutrients, blood cells, and oxygen to wound.
Malnutrition	Chronic illness or alcoholism often results in malnutrition, which impairs the normal inflammatory process and formation of new tissue.
Immunosuppressive therapy	Decreases inflammatory response and collagen synthesis.
Chemotherapy	Interferes with leukocyte production and immune response.
Steroids	Slows rate of tissue growth and development of new capillaries.
Radiation	Radiation in area of wound decreases blood supply to tissues.
High levels of stress	Increased cortisol levels reduce number of lymphocytes and decrease inflammatory response.

Table 24-2

Types of Wound Drainage

Type	Appearance
A. Serous	Clear, watery plasma
B. Purulent	Thick, yellow, green, tan, or brown
C. Serosanguineous	Pale, red, watery: mixture of serous and sanguineous
D. Sanguineous	Bright red: indicates active bleeding

NURSING DIAGNOSES

Nursing diagnoses that are associated with prevention of pressure ulcers include **Impaired Skin Integrity** related to physical immobilization and/or altered circulation. Related nursing diagnoses using the web of causation model (Figure 24-1, p. 568) might include **Risk for Impaired Skin Integrity** related to restricted movement; decreased strength and endurance; prolonged bed rest, or external devices such as casts, splints, braces, or tubing; **Incontinence; Altered Nutrition: Less than Body Requirements; Altered Peripheral Tissue Perfusion; Altered Body Temperature; and Hyperthermia.**

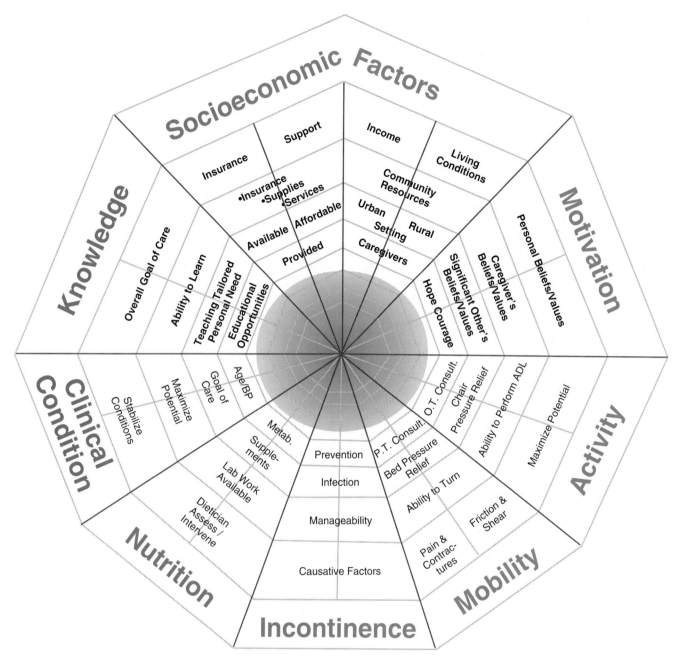

Figure 24-1 Web of causation for pressure ulcers. ©1992 Barbara Oot-Giromini. Reprinted with permission.

Skill 24.1

PRESSURE ULCER RISK ASSESSMENT AND PREVENTION STRATEGIES

Pressure ulcer risk assessment should be done systematically (Agency for Health Care Policy and Research [AHCPR], 1984; NPUAP, 1989). An assessment tool that is validated for a specific type of client population is recommended. There are several published pressure ulcer risk assessment tools, including the Braden scale.

The Braden scale (Table 24-3) has the following six parameters: sensory perception (recognition of pressure), friction and shear, ability to change and control body position, skin moisture, nutritional intake, and physical activity (Bergstrom et al, 1987). It is important to understand how to interpret the meaning of the client's total score.

Table 24-3

Braden Scale for Predicting Pressure Sore Risk

Patient's Name _____ Evaluator's Name _____ Date of Assessment

SENSORY PERCEPTION Ability to respond meaningfully to pressure-related discomfort	1. Completely Limited Unresponsive (does not moan, flinch, or grasp) to painful stimuli because of diminished level of consciousness or sedation. OR Limited ability to feel pain over most of body surface.	2. Very Limited Responds only to painful stimuli. Cannot communicate discomfort except by moaning or restlessness. OR Has a sensory impairment that limits the ability to feel pain or discomfort over $\frac{1}{2}$ of body.	3. Slightly Limited Responds to verbal commands, but cannot always communicate discomfort or need to be turned. OR Has some sensory impairment that limits ability to feel pain or discomfort in one or two extremities.	4. No Impairment Responds to verbal commands. Has no sensory deficit that would limit ability to feel or voice pain or discomfort.
MOISTURE Degree to which skin is exposed to moisture	1. Constantly Moist Skin is kept moist almost constantly by perspiration, urine, etc. Dampness is detected every time patient is moved or turned.	2. Very Moist Skin is often, but not always, moist. Linen must be changed at least once a shift.	3. Occasionally Moist Skin is occasionally moist, requiring an extra linen change approximately once a day.	4. Rarely Moist Skin is usually dry. Linen only requires changing at routine intervals.
ACTIVITY Degree of physical activity	1. Bedfast Confined to bed.	2. Chairfast Ability to walk severely limited or nonexistent. Cannot bear own weight and/or must be assisted into chair or wheelchair.	3. Walks Occasionally Walks occasionally during day, but for very short distances, with or without assistance. Spends majority of each shift in bed or chair.	4. Walks Frequently Walks outside the room at least twice a day and inside room at least once every 2 hours during waking hours.
MOBILITY Ability to change and control body position	1. Completely Immobile Does not make even slight changes in body or extremity position without assistance.	2. Very Limited Makes occasional slight changes in body or extremity position but unable to make frequent or significant changes independently.	3. Slightly Limited Makes frequent though slight changes in body or extremity position independently.	4. No Limitations Makes major and frequent changes in position without assistance.

Continued

Table 24-3

Braden Scale for Predicting Pressure Sore Risk—cont'd

Patient's Name _____ Evaluator's Name _____ Date of Assessment

NUTRITION *Usual* food intake pattern	1. Very Poor Never eats a complete meal. Rarely eats more than $\frac{1}{3}$ of any food offered. Eats 2 servings or less of protein (meat or dairy products) per day. Takes fluids poorly. Does not take a liquid dietary supplement. OR Is NPO and/or maintained on clear liquids or IV for more than 5 days.	2. Probably Inadequate Rarely eats a complete meal and generally eats only about $\frac{1}{2}$ of any food offered. Protein intake includes only 3 servings of meat or dairy products per day. Occasionally will take a dietary supplement. OR Receives less than optimum amount of liquid diet or tube feeding.	3. Adequate Eats over half of most meals. Eats a total of 4 servings of protein (meat, dairy products) each day. Occasionally will refuse a meal, but will usually take a supplement if offered. OR Is on a tube feeding or TPN regimen that probably meets most of nutritional needs.	4. Excellent Eats most of every meal. Never refuses a meal. Usually eats a total of 4 or more servings of meat and dairy products. Occasionally eats between meals. Does not require supplementation.
FRICTION AND SHEAR	1. Problem Requires moderate to maximum assistance in moving. Complete lifting without sliding against sheets is impossible. Frequently slides down in bed or chair, requiring frequent repositioning with maximum assistance. Spasticity, contractures, or agitation leads to almost constant friction.	2. Potential Problem Moves feebly or requires minimum assistance. During a move skin probably slides to some extent against sheets, chair, restraints, or other devices. Maintains relatively good position in chair or bed most of the time but occasionally slides down.	3. No Apparent Problem Moves in bed and in chair independently and has sufficient muscle strength to lift up completely during move. Maintains good position in bed or chair at all times.	

Total Score

© 1988 Barbara Braden and Nancy Bergstrom. Used with permission.

INSTRUCTIONS: Score client in each of the six subscales. Maximum score is 23, indicating little or no risk. A score of ≤16 indicates "at risk"; ≤9 indicates high risk.

Equipment

Risk assessment tool
Client's documentation record
AHCPR booklet: *Preventing Pressure Ulcers: A Patient's Guide*

ASSESSMENT

1. Select which pressure ulcer risk assessment tool will be used in your client setting. **Rationale: A validated risk assessment tool is recommended by AHCPR and NPUAP.**

Box 24-2 Cultural Considerations for Skin Assessment for Pressure Ulcers: The Client with Intact Darkly Pigmented Skin

Assess Localized Skin Color Changes
Any of the following may appear:

- Skin color changes
- Color darker than surrounding skin, purplish, bluish, eggplant
- Taut
- Shiny
- Induration

Assess for Edema (Nonpitting Swelling)

Importance of Lighting for Skin Assessment

- Use natural or halogen light
- Avoid fluorescent lamps, which can give the skin a bluish tone

Assess Skin Temperature

- Initially may feel warmer than surrounding skin
- Subsequently may feel cooler than surrounding skin
- Use the back of your hand and fingers and, if client condition permits, no gloves when doing this assessment

Based on Bennett MA: Report of the Task Force on the Implications for Darkly Pigmented Intact Skin in the Prediction and Prevention of Pressure Ulcers, *Adv Wound Care* 8(6):34, 1995.

2. Identify client's risk for pressure ulcer formation by assessing the factors for each client according to the selected tool. This information will yield a risk assessment score. Compare the obtained score for client with the established scores that indicate high risk for skin breakdown with the selected risk assessment tool. **Rationale: To prevent pressure ulcers, individuals at risk must be identified so that risk factors can be reduced through intervention (AHCPR, 1992b, 1994).**

3. Assess condition of client's skin, especially over areas at high risk for breakdown, such as bony prominences. Indicators other than color, such as temperature, "orange peel" pore appearance, firmness or tightness, and hardness, may be helpful in early assessment of clients with dark skin (Graves, 1990; Maklebust and Sieggreen, 1991). Skin discoloration may vary (Box 24-2). Redness is present in light-tone skin; however, purple or bluish discoloration is present in darkly pigmented skin (Bennett, 1995). **Rationale: "Skin inspection is fundamental to any plan for preventing pressure ulcers" (AHCPR, 1992b).**

4. Assess client for additional areas of potential pressure: nares (nasogastric [NG] tubes, oxygen cannula); tongue and lips (oral airway, endotracheal tube); skin next to drainage tubes or beneath orthopedic devices (braces, casts). **Rationale: Clients at high risk have multiple sites for pressure necrosis in addition to bony prominences.**

5. Observe client for preferred positions when in bed or chair. **Rationale: Weight of body will be placed on certain bony prominence. Presence of contractures may result in pressure in unexpected places.**

6. Observe ability of client to initiate and assist with position changes. **Rationale: Potential for friction and shear increases when client is completely dependent on others for position changes.**

7. Assess client's and support person's understanding of risks for pressure ulcers and knowledge of skin care. **Rationale: "Patient and family are integral to prevention and management of pressure ulcers" (AHCPR, 1992b).**

PLANNING

Expected outcomes focus on identifying clients at risk for skin breakdown and prevention of skin breakdown.

Expected Outcomes
1. Client's skin remains intact and without discoloration.
2. Peripheral circulation is maintained.
3. Client's risk assessment score on Braden scale is 16-23.

DELEGATION CONSIDERATIONS

This skill requires problem solving and knowledge application unique to a professional nurse. For this skill, delegation is inappropriate.

IMPLEMENTATION

Steps	Rationale
1. See Standard Protocol (inside front cover).	
2. Inspect skin at least once a day.	"Skin inspection provides the information essential for designing interventions to reduce risk and for evaluating the outcomes of those interventions" (AHCPR, 1992).

COMMUNICATION TIP

Assessment for pressure ulcer risk is a good time to discuss skin care with client and family.

- *Inform client and family about risks for pressure ulcer development and alert family to manifestations of impaired skin integrity.*

- *Explain the 30-degree lateral position so that the client will understand its value in maintaining skin integrity.*
- *Discuss the impact of prolonged exposure to moisture and secretion on the client's skin.*

3. Cleanse skin with warm water and a mild cleansing agent.	Hot water and soap can dry and irritate the skin.
4. Apply moisturizers after bathing and do not massage reddened bony prominences (AHCPR, 1992; Olson, 1989).	Prevents drying of skin. Massage may lead to tissue trauma.
5. Maintain adequate humidity in environment.	Low humidity (less than 40%), can dry the skin.
6. Manage incontinence.	Skin exposed to moisture from incontinence is more susceptible to injury (Table 24-4 lists interventions designed to reduce the risk of pressure ulcer development resulting from tube-feeding–related diarrhea).

Table 24-4

Measures to Reduce Risk of Pressure Ulcers: Practical Management of Loose Bowel Movements Related to Tube Feeding*

Possible Cause(s)	Treatment
Antibiotic use	Lactobacilli per feeding tube (2 packets tid × 3 doses)
Lactose intolerance	Use lactose-free liquid diet
Choleretic diarrhea	Questran, 1 g q6–8h and/or Titralac tabs, 2 q6–8h
Mild enterotoxigenic pathogens	Pepto-Bismol, 30 ml q6–8h
Severe enterotoxigenic pathogens with WBCs in stool– on Gram stain	Selected antibiotic per stool culture and sensitivity testing
Insufficient fiber	Fiber supplement, 3 g q6–8h
Idiopathic	Lomotil, Imodium, paregoric (Warning: This may cause reactive constipation.)

From Bergstrom N et al: *Treatment of pressure ulcers*, AHCPR Pub No 95-0652, Rockville, Md, 1994, DHHS, PHS, AHCPR.
*Any or all treatments may be indicated. *tid*, Three times daily; *q*, every; *h*, hours; *WBCs*, white blood cells.

Steps	Rationale

7. Turn and reposition: (AHCPR, 1992a).
  a. Perform full position changes every 2 hours.

Prolonged, unrelieved pressure on an area can lead to skin breakdown (Knox, Anderson, and Anderson, 1994).

  b. Use 30-degree lateral position rather than side-lying position directly on the trochanter (see Skill 6.1, Step 5j).

Higher pressures when positioned directly on the trochanters can lead to their breakdown.

  c. Perform small shift of body weight changes every 15 minutes.

Relief of pressure is needed at shorter intervals to prevent tissue breakdown, especially for clients in the sitting position.

  d. When needed, use pillow bridging (see illustration).

Use of pillows will prevent direct contact between bony prominences.

8. Palpate any area of discoloration or mottling. Skin temperature changes may be an important early indicator of stage I (Table 24-5, p. 575) pressure ulcer in clients with darkly pigmented skin.

Early detection of pressure indicates need for more frequent position changes.

9. Monitor length of time any area of discoloration persists.
  a. Determine appropriate turning interval.

Redness usually persists for 50% of the time hypoxia occurred (see Step 9a).

If turning interval is 2 hours and redness lasts 15 minutes, then hypoxia was approximately 30 minutes. Recommended turning interval should be the turning interval minus hypoxia time: 2 hours − 30 minutes = 1½ hours.

  b. A turning interval of less than 1½ to 2 hours may not be realistic. Therefore use of a pressure relief device would be recommended (see Chapter 25).

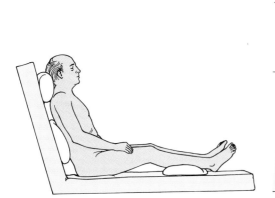

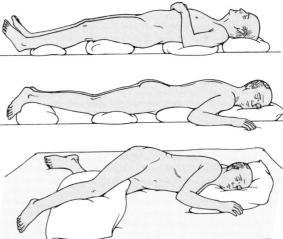

Step 7d

Steps	Rationale
10. Keep head of bed at less than 30 degrees, except as required for care (e.g., feeding).	Limiting the amount of time that the head of the bed is elevated will reduce tissue injury from shearing forces.
11. Use protective devices and support surfaces (see Chapter 25).	Pressure-reducing devices can decrease the incidence and severity of pressure ulcers (Flemister, 1991; Johnson et al., 1991; Lazzara and Buschmann, 1991).
12. Encourage range of motion and ambulation (see Chapters 26 and 29).	Improving mobility and activity levels can reduce risk of pressure ulcers.
13. Evaluate client's nutritional status (see Chapter 8). Nutritional assessment of clients with a pressure ulcer includes review of weight pattern and serum albumin and total lymphocyte laboratory values. Clinically significant malnutrition is present if serum albumin is less than 3.5 mg/dl, total lymphocyte count less than 1800 mm^3, or weight loss greater than 15%. This should be done at least every 3 months. Also observe the mouth and skin for signs of vitamin or mineral deficiencies.	Assessment of nutritional intake and nutritional support is suggested to maintain skin integrity and prevent pressure ulcers (AHCPR, 1992b, p. 21). Malnutrition is a risk factor for formation of pressure ulcers. Stage of pressure ulcer correlates with serum albumin levels (Bergstrom et al., 1994).
14. Provide client and support person education about pressure ulcer risk and prevention (Maklebust and Magnan, 1992). Use of the AHCPR booklet *Preventing Pressure Ulcers: A Patient's Guide* (AHCPR, 1992b) can be a helpful teaching tool (Ayello, 1993) (Table 24-6, p. 576).	Effective pressure ulcer prevention depends on the coordinated efforts of health care professionals in health care facilities and continued implementation of preventive interventions by family and the patient in the home (AHCPR, 1992a).
15. See Completion Protocol (inside front cover).	

• • •

EVALUATION

1. Observe client's skin for areas at risk for change in color or texture.
2. Observe tolerance of client for position change.
3. Compare subsequent risk assessment scores.

Unexpected Outcomes and Related Interventions

1. Skin becomes mottled reddened, purplish, or bluish.
   a. These are early signs of pressure.
   b. Increase frequency of turning schedule.
   c. Obtain physician's order for a pressure relief device.
2. Areas under pressure develop persistent discoloration, induration, or temperature changes.
   a. These signs indicate damage to the skin and underlying tissue resulting from pressure.
   b. Institute interventions listed in Step 1.
   c. Provide wound care according to pressure ulcer stage (see Skill 24.2).

Recording and Reporting

• Record client's risk score.
• Record appearance of skin under pressure.
• Describe position, turning intervals, pressure-relieving support devices, and other prevention measures.
• Report any need for additional consultations for the high-risk client.

Sample Documentation

1500   Braden scale assessment completed on admission. Client score = 12; therefore client is at high risk for skin breakdown. Inspection of client's skin reveals intact skin, pressure ulcer prevention protocol implemented.

Table 24-5

Staging of Pressure Ulcers

Definition

Stage I
Nonblanchable erythema of intact skin; the heralding lesion of skin ulceration. In individuals with darker skin, discoloration of the skin, warmth, edema, induration, or hardness may also be indicators (Bergstrom et al., 1994).

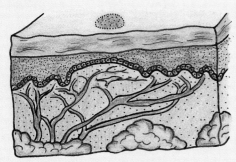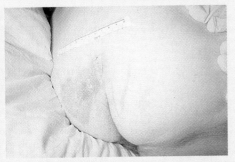

Stage II
Partial-thickness skin loss involving epidermis and/or dermis. The ulcer is superficial and presents clinically as an abrasion, blister, or shallow crater.

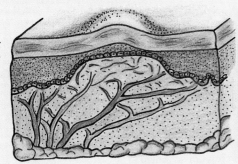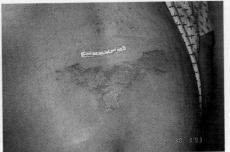

Stage III
Full-thickness skin loss involving damage or necrosis of subcutaneous tissue that may extend down to, but not through, underlying fascia. The ulcer presents clinically as a deep crater with or without undermining of adjacent tissue.

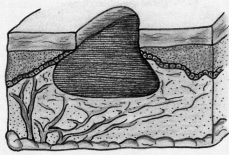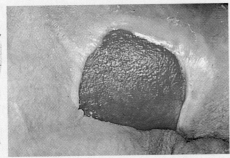

Stage IV
Full-thickness skin loss with extensive destruction, tissue necrosis, or damage to muscle, bone, or supporting structures, for example, tendon or joint capsule. (NOTE: Undermining and sinus tracts may also be associated with stage IV pressure ulcers.)

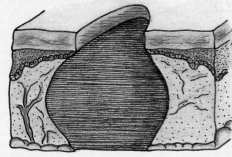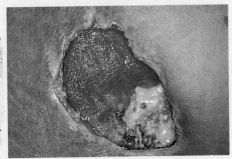

Staging definitions recognize these assessment limitations:
1. Identification of stage I pressure ulcers may be difficult in patients with darkly pigmented skin.
2. When eschar is present, accurate staging of the pressure ulcer is not possible until the eschar has sloughed or the wound has been debrided.

Table 24-6

Care of Pressure Ulcers by Risk Factors

Risk Factor	Preventive Actions

Bed or chair confinement	Inspect skin at least once a day.
	Bathe when needed for comfort or cleanliness.
	Prevent dry skin.
	For client in bed:
	    Change position at least every 2 hours.
	    Use a special mattress that contains foam, air, gel, or water.
	    Raise the head of bed as little and for as short a time as possible.
	For client in a chair:
	    Change position every hour.
	    Use foam, gel, or air cushion to relieve pressure.
	Reduce friction by:
	    Lifting rather than dragging when repositioning.
	    Using cornstarch on skin.
	Avoid use of donut-shaped cushions.
	Participate in a rehabilitation program.

Inability to move	Clients confined to chairs should be repositioned every hour if unable to do so themselves. For client in a chair who is able to shift his or her own weight, change position at least every 15 minutes. Use pillows or wedges to keep knees or ankles from touching each other. When in bed, place pillow under legs from midcalf to ankle to keep heels off the bed.

Loss of bowel or bladder control	Clean skin as soon as soiled.
	Assess and treat urine leaks.
	If moisture cannot be controlled:
	    Use absorbent pads and/or briefs with a quick-drying surface.
	    Protect skin with a cream or ointment.

Poor nutrition	Eat a balanced diet. If a normal diet is not possible, talk to health care provider about nutritional supplements.
Lowered mental awareness	Choose preventive actions that apply to client with lowered mental awareness. For example, if the client is confined to chair, refer to the specific preventive actions outlined in first risk factor.

Data from Agency for Health Care Policy and Research (AHCPR): *Preventing pressure ulcers: a patient's guide,* Pub No 92-0048, Rockville, Md, 1992, US Department of Health and Human Services, Public Health Service.

Geriatric Considerations

- A score of 17 or 18 (rather than the usual 16) on the Braden scale may be a more efficient predictor of pressure ulcer risk in older adults (Bergstrom et al, 1998).
- In the older adult, the epidermal-dermal junction becomes flatter, putting the client at increased risk for epidermal peel as a result of shearing (Loescher, 1995).

Home Care and Long-Term Care Considerations

- The 30-degree lateral and prone positions may be useful at night to prolong the time between position changes, resulting in less sleep disruption for the client and caregiver.

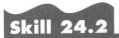

TREATMENT OF PRESSURE ULCERS AND WOUND MANAGEMENT

Treatment of clients with pressure ulcers and wounds requires a holistic approach that uses the expertise of several multidisciplinary health care professionals. Besides the nurse, this can include the physician, physical therapist, occupational therapist, nutritionist, and pharmacist (Rodeheaver et al., 1994). Aspects of pressure ulcer treatment include the local care of the wound, which is described in this skill, and supportive measures such as adequate nutrients and relief of pressure (see Skill 24-1).

A thorough description of the pressure ulcer (see Table 24-5) provides the basis for the decision-making tree for the treatment plan (Maklebust and Sieggreen, 1991). Principles of local wound care include debridement, cleansing, and dressing application. Removal of necrotic tissue is necessary to rid the ulcer of a source of infection, enable visualization of the wound bed to stage the ulcer accurately, and to provide a clean base necessary for healing (Rodeheaver et al., 1994). Methods of debridement include mechanical, autolytic, chemical/enzymatic, and surgical. Pressure ulcers should be cleansed with solutions such as normal saline or commercial wound cleansers that will not damage fibroblasts and healing tissue. To avoid tissue trauma, care must be taken not to use pressure forces above 15 pounds per square inch (psi) in cleaning or irrigating the pressure ulcer. The choice of dressing depends on the characteristics of the ulcer identified during the pressure ulcer assessment and the goal of the treatment plan. It will change as the ulcer heals. For example, for a necrotic wound, a membrane dressing may be used initially to debride the wound by autolysis. Afterward, pressure ulcers staged III or IV that had large amounts of exudate would require a dressing with absorptive ability. *Clean* dressings, rather than sterile dressings, can be used to treat pressure ulcers (Bergstrom et al., 1994).

All pressure ulcers are colonized; therefore swab cultures should not be used to diagnose wound infection. Quantitative bacterial cultures of the wound fluid or of the soft tissue is recommended by AHCPR (1994) (Bergstrom et al., 1994).

The new AHCPR pressure ulcer treatment guidelines (1994) recommend that *clean* gloves be used when doing pressure ulcer care. One set of gloves can be used on the same client with multiple pressure ulcers. When treating multiple ulcers on the same client attend to the most contaminated ulcer last (e.g., in the perianal region). Remove gloves and wash hands between clients (Bergstrom et al., 1994).

Besides local wound treatment, other methods such as electromagnetic energy have been used to foster ulcer healing (Itoh et al., 1991). Education (Maklebust and Magnan, 1992) and understanding of the client and experience of the support person are helpful (Baharestani, 1994). The AHCPR treatment guidelines released in December 1994 are an additional resource for clinicians to use for client care management (Bergstrom et al., 1994).

Equipment

Disposable gloves (clean)
Plastic bag for dressing disposal
Tracing film, wound measuring device, cotton-tipped applicators
Topical agent as ordered
Normal saline or cleansing agent
Wash basin, warm water, soap, washcloths, towels
Dressings as ordered
Skin protectant
Tape, if needed
35 ml syringe
19-gauge needle or angiocath

ASSESSMENT

1. Assess client's level of comfort and need for pain management. **Rationale: Dressing change procedure is better tolerated if pain is controlled.**

2. Assess condition of client's skin, especially over areas at high risk for breakdown, such as bony prominences. **Rationale: Bony prominences are the most common sites for pressure ulcer development.**

3. Determine if client has allergies to topical agents. **Rationale: Topical agents contain elements that may cause localized skin reactions.**

4. Review physician's order for topical agent or dressing. **Rationale: Ensures that proper medication and treatment are administered.**

5. Assess each of the client's wounds and pressure ulcer(s) and surrounding skin to determine ulcer characteristics, including stage (see Tables 24-5 and 24-7, pp. 575 and 578-579). **Rationale: Staging is a way of classifying a pressure ulcer based on the depth of destruction of the tissue.**

6. Minimum characteristics to include in assessing the wound are as follows: location, stage, size, sinus tracts, exudate, necrotic tissue (black, hard tissue is called *eschar*), granulation tissue, and epithelization. All pressure ulcers should be reassessed at least weekly (AHCPR, 1994).

   a. Note color, temperature, edema, moisture, and appearance of skin around the ulcer and of the ulcer itself. Remember to modify the assessment technique based on the client's individual skin color (see Box 24-2, p. 571). **Rationale: Skin condition may indicate progressive tissue damage. Retained moisture causes maceration.**

b. Measure two maximum perpendicular diameters. It is important to have the client in the same position each time pressure ulcer measurements are taken. Obtain the wound's length first and then its width (Surface area = Length × Width). Use either a tape or circular pressure ulcer measuring device (Figure 24-2, p. 580). **Rationale: Provides an objective measure of wound size. May influence size and type of dressing selected. Provides consistency so that subsequent measurements can be compared for changes in size.**

c. Measure depth of pressure ulcer using sterile cotton-tipped applicator or other device that will allow measurement of wound depth. **Rationale: Depth measure is important for determining wound volume. While surface area adequately represents tissue loss in stage I and II ulcers, volume more adequately represents tissue loss in deeper stage III and IV wounds.**

Volume = $2(L × D) + 2(W × D) + (L + D)$

d. Measure depth (d) of undermining skin by lateral tissue necrosis. Use a cotton-tipped applicator to gently probe under skin edges. **Rationale: Undermining represents the loss of the underlying tissues (subcutaneous and muscle) to a greater extent than the skin. Undermining may indicate progressive tissue necrosis.**

7. Assessment of the entire client is necessary in developing a pressure ulcer treatment plan. According to the AHCPR (1994), this assessment should include (a) a complete history and physical examination, (b) the identification of complications and comorbid conditions, (c) a nutritional assessment, (d) an assessment of pain, (e) a psychosocial assessment, and (f) an evaluation of the individual's risks for additional pressure ulcers.

8. The client's nutritional status should be assessed at least every 3 months. Clinically significant malnutrition is present if (a) serum albumin is less than 3.5 g/dl, (b) lymphocyte count is less than 1800/mm^3, or (c) body weight decreases more than 15% (AHCPR, 1994). Observe the client's mouth and skin for signs of vitamin and mineral deficiencies.

9. Assess client's and support persons' understanding of pressure ulcer characteristics and purpose of treatment (AHCPR, 1994). **Rationale: Explanations relieve anxiety and promote cooperation during procedure.**

Table 24-7

Wound Classifications

Type and Description	Causes	Implications for Healing
STATUS OF SKIN INTEGRITY		
Open wound involving break in skin or mucous membranes	Trauma by sharp object (e.g., surgical incision, venipuncture, gunshot wound)	Exposes body to invasion by microorganisms
		Loss of blood and body fluids through wound
		Reduces function of body part
Closed wound involving no break in skin integrity	Part of body being struck by blunt object	May predispose person to internal hemorrhage
	Twisting, straining, or deceleration force against body (e.g., bone fracture or tear of visceral organ)	Reduces function of affected body part
CAUSE		
Intentional wound resulting from therapy	Surgical incision Introduction of needle into body part	Usually performed under aseptic technique, which minimizes chances of infection
		Wound edges usually smooth and clean
Unintentional wound occurring unexpectedly	Traumatic injury (e.g., knife wound, burn, pressure ulcer)	Occurs under unsterile conditions Wound edges often jagged

Table 24-7

Wound Classifications—cont'd

SEVERITY OF INJURY

Superficial wound involving only epidermal layer of skin	Result of friction applied to skin surface (e.g., abrasion, first-degree burn)	Creates risk of infection Does not involve underlying injury to tissues or organs Blood supply to area intact
Penetrating wound involving break in epidermal skin layer and dermis and deeper tissues or organs	Foreign object or instrument entering deep into body tissues, usually unintentional (e.g., gunshot wound, stab wound)	High risk of infection because foreign object is contaminated May cause internal and external hemorrhage Damage to organs causes temporary or permanent loss of function
Perforating penetrating wound in which foreign object enters and exits internal organ	Same as penetrating wound	High risk of infection Nature of injury depends on organ perforated: 　Lung—compromised oxygenation 　Major vessel—serious hemorrhage 　Intestine—contamination of abdominal cavity by feces

CLEANLINESS

Clean wound containing no pathogenic organisms	Surgical wound that does not enter the gastrointestinal tract, respiratory tract, or oropharyngeal cavity	Low risk of infection
Clean-contaminated wound made under aseptic conditions but involving entrance into body cavity that normally harbors microorganisms	Surgical wound entering gastrointestinal or respiratory tract or oropharyngeal cavity	Greater risk of infection than with clean wound
Contaminated wound existing under conditions in which presence of microorganisms is likely	Open, traumatic wounds Surgical wound in which break in asepsis occurred	Tissues often not healthy and show inflammation High risk of infection
Infected wound involving bacterial organisms in wound site	Any wound that does not properly heal and grows organisms Old traumatic wound Surgical incision into area infected (e.g., ruptured bowel)	Wound presents signs of infection (e.g., inflammation, purulent drainage, skin separation)
Colonized wound containing microorganisms (usually multiple)	Chronic wound (e.g., vascular wound or stasis or pressure ulcer)	Wound healing slow High risk of infection

DESCRIPTIVE QUALITIES

Laceration: tearing of tissues with irregular wound edges	Severe traumatic injury (e.g., knife wound, industrial accident involving machinery, tissues cut by broken glass)	Wound usually created by contaminated object Depth determines other complications Painful from exposure of superficial nerves
Abrasion: superficial wound involving scraping or rubbing of skin's surface by friction	Fall (e.g., skinned knee or elbow) Dermatological procedure for removing scar tissue	Deeper tissues uninvolved Risk of infection from exposure to contaminated surface
Contusion: closed wound caused by blow by blunt object; contusion by bruise characterized by swelling, discoloration, and pain	Bleeding in underlying tissues caused by blunt force against body part	More severe if internal organ contused May cause temporary loss of function of body part Localized bleeding into tissues may form hematoma, or collection of blood

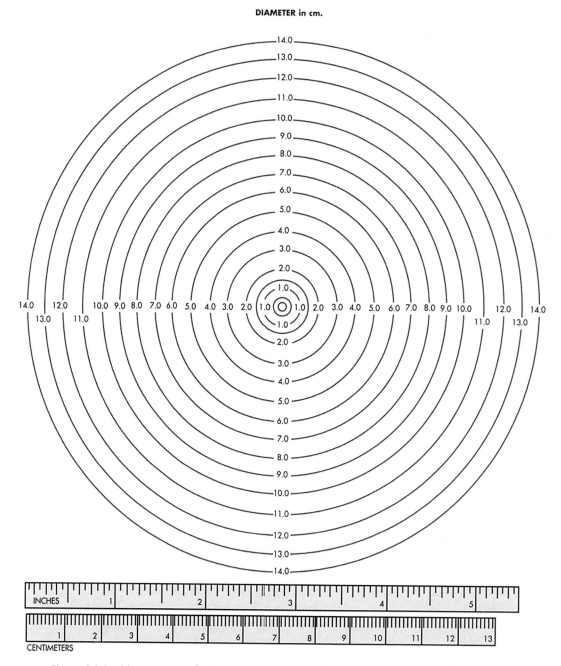

DIAMETER in cm.

Figure 24-2 Measuring guide. Center over wound to be measured. *Adapted from Maklebust J, Sieggreen M: Pressure ulcers: guidelines for prevention and nursing management, ed 2, Springhouse, Pa, 1996, Springhouse Corp.*

PLANNING

Expected outcomes focus on healing of the ulcer and prevention of further skin breakdown.

Expected Outcomes

1. Client's ulcer drainage decreases.
2. Measurements and tracings of client's ulcer are progressively smaller.
3. Skin surrounding ulcer remains healthy and intact.
4. Client remains afebrile.

IMPLEMENTATION

Steps	Rationale
1. See Standard Protocol (inside front cover).	
2. Consider selecting pressure ulcer management based on identified stage and other factors. Principles of local wound care:	The use of a decision tree may be useful in determining pressure ulcer care.
a. Debride wound.	
b. Clean wound.	
c. Dress wound.	
d. Relieve pressure.	

DELEGATION CONSIDERATIONS

This skill requires problem solving and knowledge application unique to a professional nurse. For this skill, delegation is inappropriate.

NURSE ALERT

To correctly stage a pressure ulcer, the nurse must be able to see its base. Therefore, pressure ulcers that are covered with necrotic tissue cannot be staged until the eschar is debrided (AHCPR, 1994).

Steps	Rationale
3. Remove any necrotic tissue in the pressure ulcer (see physician's orders). Discard gloves and wash hands.	Necrotic tissue provides a source for infection; a clean wound base free of devitalized tissue is necessary for healing.
4. Select an appropriate dressing (Table 24-8, p. 583) based on the pressure ulcer characteristics, purpose for which the dressing is intended, and client care setting.	The dressing should maintain a moist environment for the wound while keeping the surrounding skin dry (AHCPR, 1994).
a. Gauze type: 4 × 4 pads, fluffs	Applied over ulcers treated with enzymes, mechanical debridement with a wet to dry normal saline dressing, or dextranomer beads.
b. Transparent membrane dressings	Applied over superficial ulcers and skin subjected to shear.

NURSE ALERT

Transparent membrane dressings can also be used for autolytic debridement of noninfected pressure ulcers.

Steps	Rationale
c. Hydrocolloid	Maintains moist environment to facilitate wound healing.

NURSE ALERT

Hydrocolloid dressings also protect skin from friction and shear. Custom shapes are available for specific anatomical parts of the body. Make sure dressing near anus remains intact (AHCPR, 1994).

Steps	Rationale
d. Hydrogel	Maintains moist environment to facilitate wound healing. Very soothing to clients with painful wounds.

Steps	**Rationale**
e. Calcium alginate	Highly absorbent of wound **exudate** in heavily draining wounds.
f. Exudate absorbers	Highly absorbent of wound exudate.
g. Foam	Protective and will prevent wound dehydration; also absorbs small to moderate amounts of drainage.
h. Hypoallergenic tape or adhesive dressing sheet (Hypofix)	Used to secure nonadherent dressing. Prevents skin irritation and tearing.
5. Open sterile packages and topical solution containers. (Goggles and moisture-proof cover gown should be worn if potential for contamination from spray exists when cleansing the wound.)	Supplies should be ready for easy application so that nurse can use supplies without contaminating them; reduces transmission of microorganisms.
6. Remove bed linen and client's gown to expose ulcer and surrounding skin. Keep remaining body parts draped.	Prevents unnecessary exposure of body parts.
7. Thoroughly clean with warm water and mild soap, rinse, and dry skin surrounding ulcer. Discard gloves and wash hands.	Cleansing skin surface reduces bacteria. Retained moisture causes maceration of skin layers, leading to further skin breakdown
8. Apply sterile gloves (check agency policy). Cleanse ulcer thoroughly with normal saline or prescribed wound cleansing agent. Use an adequate amount of pressure (measured in psi) to effectively clean the wound, but do not use so much pressure that you injure the wound tissue.	In a nonnecrotic wound, a psi between 4 and 15 is considered safe and effective for cleaning a pressure ulcer (AHCPR, 1994).
a. Use a 19-gauge needle (or angiocath) with a 35-ml syringe to clean most pressure ulcers, especially deep ulcers (see illustration).	The psi of this type of wound cleaning system is 8, which will not harm the fragile healing tissue in the pressure ulcer (AHCPR, 1994).
b. Cleansing in the shower may be done with a handheld shower head.	

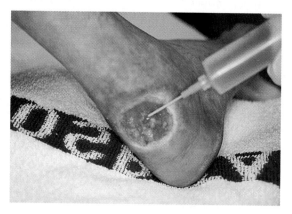

Step 8a

COMMUNICATION TIP

When caring for a wound or applying dressings use the time to communicate to client:

- *Sensations client may perceive during dressing change*
- *Progress of wound healing*
- *Changes in treatment regimen*
- *Role of nutrition in promoting wound healing*
- *How the client may independently manage the wound*

---

9. Whirlpool treatments may be used to assist with wound debridement. Keep the wound away from the direct pressure of the water jets.	Removes wound debris. Previously applied enzymes may require soaking for removal.
10. Apply topical agents, as prescribed:	Topical agents should be changed as wound heals or worsens.
a. Enzymes:	Thick layer of ointment is not necessary. Thin layer absorbs and acts more effectively. Excess medication can irritate surrounding skin. Apply only to necrotic areas.

Table 24-8

Treatment Options by Ulcer Stage

Ulcer Stage	Ulcer Status	Dressing	Comments*	Expected Change	Adjuvants
I	Intact	None	Allows visual assessment.	Resolves slowly without epidermal loss over 7 to 14 days.	Turning schedule. Support hydration. Nutritional support. Silicone-based lotion to decrease shear. Pressure relief mattress or chair cushion.
		Film, adherent	Protects from shear.		
		Hydrocolloid	May not allow visual assessment.		
II	Clean	Composite film	Viasorb, film plus telfa, Exudry. Limits shear.	Heals through reepithelialization and epithelial budding.	See previous stage. Manage incontinence.
		Hydrocolloid	Change every 7 days if occlusive seal.		
		Hydrogel sheet	Absorbent, requires secondary dressing of gauze or adherent film.		
III	Clean	Hydrocolloid	See stage II.	Heals through granulation and reepithelialization. (Note: does not become a stage II ulcer as it heals.)	See previous stages. Electrical stimulation. Evaluate pressure relief needs.
		Hydrogel foam	Apply ¼-inch thick, cover with gauze or hydrocolloid.		
		Exudate absorbers calcium alginate wound pastes	Change when strike through is noted on secondary dressing. Cover with gauze or hydrocolloid.		
		Gauze, fluffy	Use with normal saline.		
		Growth factors	Use with gauze.		
IV	Clean	Hydrogel	See stage III Clean.	Heals through granulation and reepithelialization. Because of contraction, surface may close more rapidly than base, leaving wound cavity.	Surgical consult for closure. See stages I, II, and III Clean.
		Hydrocolloid plus hydrocolloid paste/beads	See stage III Clean; critical to treat areas of undermining.		
		Calcium alginate	See stage III Clean.		
		Gauze	Pack deeply undermined ulcers.		
		Growth factors	Use with gauze.		
	Eschar	Adherent film	Will facilitate softening of eschar.	Eschar will lift at the edges as healing progresses. Cross-hatching central area of eschar with a small blade will facilitate release from center.	See previous stages. Surgical consult for debridement. Enzymes covered with gauze dressing may be used to debride ulcer.
		Hydrocolloid	Will facilitate softening of eschar.		
		Gauze plus ordered solution	Absorb drainage and control odor if Dakin's is used.		
		None	Rarely, if eschar is dry and intact, no dressing is used, allowing eschar to act as physiological cover.		

*As with *all* occlusive dressings, wounds should *not* be clinically infected.

Steps	Rationale
(1) Apply thin, even layer of ointment over necrotic areas of ulcer. Do not apply enzyme to surrounding skin.	Proper distribution of ointment ensures effective action. Enzyme can cause burning, paresthesia, and dermatitis to surrounding skin.
(2) Apply gauze dressing directly over ulcer.	Protects wound.
(3) Tape securely in place.	Prevents bacteria from entering moist dressing.
b. Hydrocolloid beads or paste:	
(1) Fill ulcer defect to approximately half of the total depth with hydrocolloid beads or paste.	Hydrocolloid beads or paste assist in absorbing wound drainage. Highly draining wounds are best treated with hydrocolloid beads or granules.
(2) Cover with hydrocolloid dressing; extend dressing 1 to 1½ inches beyond edges of wound.	Maintains wound humidity. May be left in place 7 days. Not effective on dry eschar (Bryant, 1992).
c. Hydrogel agents:	
(1) Cover surface of ulcer with hydrogel using applicator or gloved hand.	Provides maintenance of wound humidity while absorbing excess drainage. May be used as carrier for topical agents.
(2) Apply dry fluffy gauze or hydrocolloid or transparent dressing over gel to completely cover ulcer.	Holds hydrogel against wound surface; is absorbent.
d. Calcium alginates:	
(1) Pack wound with alginate using applicator or gloved hand.	Provides maintenance of wound humidity while absorbing excess drainage.
(2) Apply dry gauze, foam, or hydrocolloid over alginate.	Holds alginate against wound surface.
11. Reposition client comfortably off wound.	Avoids pressure on an area of impaired skin integrity and accidental removal of dressing.
12. See Completion Protocol (inside front cover).	

NURSE ALERT

A clean wound should show evidence of some healing within 2 to 3 days. A clean pressure ulcer should show some evidence of healing within 2 to 4 weeks. Do not use the pressure ulcer staging system to measure pressure ulcer healing.

• • •

EVALUATION

1. Observe skin surrounding wound or ulcer for inflammation, edema, and tenderness.
2. Inspect dressings and exposed wounds, observing for drainage, foul odor, and tissue necrosis. Monitor client for signs and symptoms of infection, including fever and elevated white blood cell count.
3. Compare subsequent wound or ulcer measurements (Figure 24-3).

Unexpected Outcomes and Related Nursing Interventions

1. Skin surrounding ulcer becomes macerated.
   a. Reduce exposure of surrounding skin to topical agents and moisture.

2. Ulcer becomes deeper with increased drainage and/or development of necrotic tissue.
   a. Notify physician for possible change in pressure ulcer management.
   b. Additional consults, for example a wound care nurse specialist, may be needed.
   c. Obtain necessary wound cultures.
3. Pressure extends beyond original margins.
   a. Increase types of pressure reduction interventions.
   b. Alter turning schedule to decrease duration of time in one position.

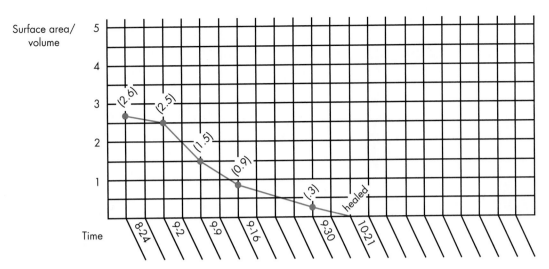

Figure 24-3   Graph of wound surface area or volume measurements over time.

Recording and Reporting
- Record appearance of ulcer and character of drainage in client's record.
- Describe type of topical agent used, dressing applied, and client's response.
- Report any deterioration in ulcer appearance.

Sample Documentation
2300   Sacral stage III pressure ulcer is 2 by 3 cm irregular shape. Pale pink subcutaneous tissue visible, no drainage present. Wound edges are rolled, surrounding skin is intact. Wound cleansed with normal saline and hydrocolloid dressing applied. Client and family have read AHCPR booklets *Preventing Pressure Ulcers: A Patient's Guide* and *Pressure Sore Treatment* and are practicing positioning techniques.

Geriatric Considerations
- Wound healing may be slower in the older adult.
- Because the skin in older adults has a slower and less intense inflammatory reaction, older clients must be monitored more closely for altered responses to skin irritants.

Home Care and Long-Term Care Considerations
- Medicare regulations limit reimbursement of some types of pressure relief equipment for stage III and IV pressure ulcers.
- Disposal of contaminated dressings in the home should be done in a manner consistent with local regulations (AHCPR, 1994).

Skill 24.3

APPLYING DRESSINGS

Dry dressings protect the wound from injury, prevent introduction and spread of bacteria, reduce discomfort, and speed healing. Drainage from surgical or traumatic wounds may be serous, sanguineous, or serosanguineous (Table 24-2, p. 567). Dressings promote hemostasis by direct pressure and absorption of drainage. Dressings also may support or immobilize a body part. The ideal dressing is easy to apply, conforms to body contours, is durable but flexible, is able to absorb or contain exudate, is easily removed without damage to the healing surface, and is acceptable in appearance (Boston, Rijswijk and Braden, 1999).

Dry dressings are most often used for abrasions and

A

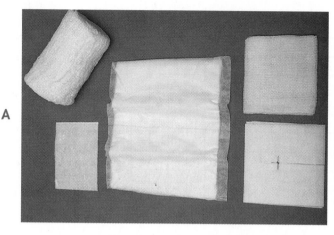

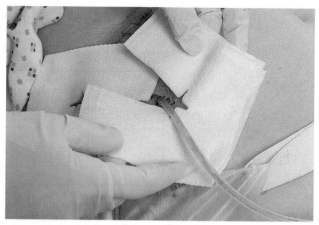

B

Figure 24-4   **A,** Types of dressings. *Left to right:* Rolled gauze, telfa, ABD, 4 × 4, and drain dressing. **B,** Applying a drain dressing.

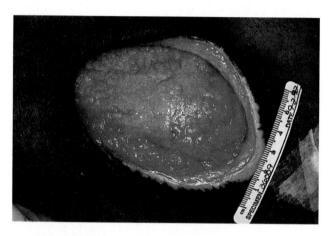

Figure 24-5   Granulation tissue in an open wound.

postoperative incisions when minimal drainage is anticipated. Gauze dressings come in a variety of sizes, such as 4 × 4 (16 inches square), 4 × 8 (rectangle), precut drain sponge, and rolls. Telfa gauze dressings contain a shiny, nonadherent surface on one side that does not stick to the wound. Drainage passes through the nonadherent surface to the outer gauze dressing (Figure 24-4). If a dry dressing adheres to a wound, the nurse should moisten the dressing with sterile normal saline or sterile water before removing the gauze to minimize trauma to the wound as it is removed.

Moist dressings are often used for helping to heal full-thickness wounds that look like craters. Granulation tissue and new capillary networks must form to fill in the defect (Figure 24-5).

Wet-to-dry dressings are used for wounds requiring debridement. The nurse moistens the contact dressing layer that touches the wound surface. The moistened gauze increases the absorptive ability of the dressing to collect exudate and wound debris. This layer dries and adheres to dead cells and debrides the wound when the dressing is removed.

An outer absorbent layer is a dry dressing to protect the wound from invasive microorganisms (Johnson, 1992).

Wet-to-damp dressings are appropriate for wounds that are healing with granulation tissue without significant amounts of ischemic or necrotic tissue or large amounts of drainage. Because granulation tissue is fragile and bleeds easily, damp dressings are less likely to result in tissue damage as old dressings are removed. The outermost layer is dry for this type of dressing as well (Krasner, 1991).

The most frequently used solution is normal saline, which is an isotonic solution. Some other solutions may be ordered. Lactated Ringer's solution contains electrolytes that create an environment conducive to tissue growth (Doughty, 1992). Solutions are available in 250- to 1000-cc (ml) containers. At the time the container is opened, the label should be clearly marked with the date and time, and unused portions should be discarded 24 hours after opening. Extended use can harbor growth of microorganisms.

Most dressings are secured with tape, which may be paper, plastic, woven, or elastic material with adhesive. Some clients are allergic to the adhesive. Frequent removal of tape for dressing changes is irritating to the skin. These dressings should be secured with Montgomery straps, which use ties that allow changing the dressing without changing the tape each time. Dressings on an extremity may be secured with rolls of gauze (Table 24-9). The dressing is secured by several turns around the extremity (Figure 24-6, *A*), continuing with a figure-eight method of application (Figure 24-6, *B*).

Equipment
    Unsterile and sterile gloves
    Sterile dressing set (scissors and forceps)
    Sterile drape (optional)
    Thin, fine-mesh gauze, dressings, and pads
    Sterile normal saline (or prescribed solution)

Table 24-9

Principles for Wrapping an Extremity

Action	Rationale
Position body part in comfortable position of normal alignment.	Reduces risk of deformity or injury.
Prevent friction between and against skin surfaces by placing gauze or cotton padding (e.g., between toes).	Skin surfaces that touch may cause friction or skin breakdown.
Apply securely to prevent slipping, beginning at distal end and moving toward trunk.	Promotes venous return and minimizes edema or circulatory impairment.
Observe areas distal to bandage for signs of circulatory impairment (cool, pale, swollen, numbness, tingling, slow capillary refill).	Prompt attention to circulatory impairment prevents serious complications.
Avoid complete wrap at distal parts of extremities.	Provides exposure for assessment of peripheral circulation of extremity.

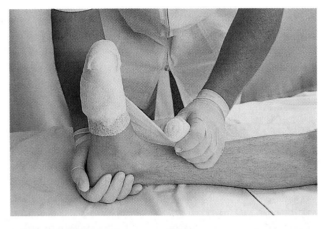

A

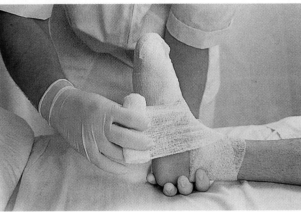

B

Figure 24-6 Applying circular dressings to an extremity.

Protective underpad
Waterproof bag
Moisture-proof gown, goggles, and mask (optional)
Cleansing agents as ordered
Measuring guide (optional)

ASSESSMENT

1. Assess size and location of wound to be dressed. **Rationale: This assists nurse in planning for proper type and amount of supplies needed (see Skill 24.2, Assessment, Steps 1–9).**
2. Ask client to rate pain using a scale of 0 to 10. **Rationale: Client may require pain medication before dressing change to allow drug's peak effect during procedure.**
3. Assess client's knowledge of purpose of dressing change. **Rationale: Determines level of support and explanation required.**
4. Determine the need for client or family member to participate in dressing wound. **Rationale: Prepares client or family member if dressing will be changed at home.**

PLANNING

Expected outcomes focus on preventing infection, promoting healing, pain control, and client and family education.

Expected Outcomes

1. Client's wound shows evidence of healing by smaller size and less drainage, redness, or swelling.
2. Client reports pain less than client's assessed level (scale of 0 to 10) during and after dressing changes.
3. Client or family demonstrates correct method of dressing changes.

DELEGATION CONSIDERATIONS

Controversy about delegating wound care to other personnel exists. Nurses should check their specific state practice act as to what interventions are considered within the scope of nursing practice and which can be delegated to others, including assistive personnel (AP). In some states, aspects of wound care such as dressing change can be delegated. This may include the changing of dressings using *clean* technique for chronic wounds. The care of acute new wounds and those that require sterile technique for dressing change generally remain within the domain of professional nursing practice. The *assessment* of the wound remains within the scope of the professional nurse even if the dressing change is delegated to others.

IMPLEMENTATION

Steps	Rationale
1. See Standard Protocol (inside front cover).	
2. Expose wound site, preventing unnecessary client exposure. Instruct client not to touch wound or sterile supplies.	Provides access to the wound but minimizes unnecessary exposure.

NURSE ALERT

If evidence of highly contagious infection is suspected, it may be necessary to place client in a private room (Chapter 3). First postoperative dressings are often changed by the physician. If excessive drainage is *noted, the dressing is reinforced (added to) without removing existing dressings (check agency policy). Subsequent changes are done by staff as ordered.*

3. Place disposable waterproof bag within reach of work area with top folded to make a cuff (see illustration).	Facilitates safe disposal of soiled dressings.
4. Remove tape: pull parallel to skin, toward dressing. If over hairy areas, remove in the direction of hair growth. Secure client permission to shave area (check agency policy).	Reduces stress on suture line or wound edges and reduces irritation and discomfort.

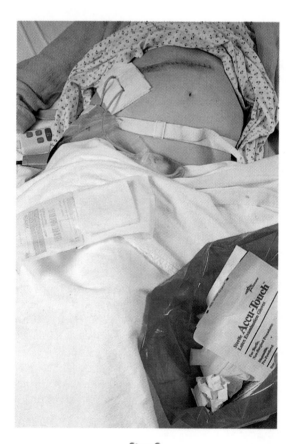

Step 3

Steps	Rationale

5. With clean gloves, remove dressings one layer at a time, observing appearance and drainage on dressing. Use caution to avoid tension on any drains that are present.

Determine dressings needed for replacement. More or less may be appropriate depending on the degree of saturation. Drains may or may not be sutured in place.

6. Consider client's needs with regard to looking at the wound or drainage.

Clients may or may not want to see wound or drainage.

7. Inspect wound for appearance, size, depth, drainage, integrity (wound edges are together), or granulation tissue.

Indicates status of healing.

8. Fold dressings with drainage contained inside and remove gloves inside out. With small dressings, remove gloves inside out over dressing (see illustration). Dispose of gloves and soiled dressings in waterproof bag. Wash hands.

Provides containment of soiled dressings and prevents contact of nurse's hands with drainage.

9. Create a sterile field with a sterile dressing tray or individually wrapped sterile supplies on overbed table. Pour necessary prescribed solution into sterile basin.

Sterile dressings remain sterile while on or within sterile area.

10. Use sterile gloves or no-touch technique with sterile forceps, which maintain sterility of all items in direct contact with the wound (Krasner and Kennedy, 1994).

Sterile gloves may be used for more complex situations with extensive drainage.

11. Cleanse wound using a separate swab for each cleansing stroke and cleaning from least contaminated area to most contaminated (see illustrations).

Prevents transfer of organisms from one area to another.

12. Cleanse around drain (if present), using a circular stroke starting near the drain and moving outward.

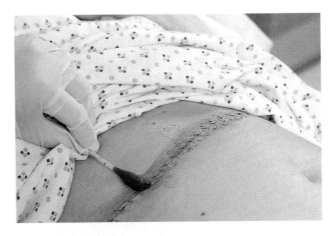

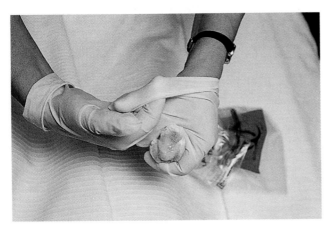

Step 8

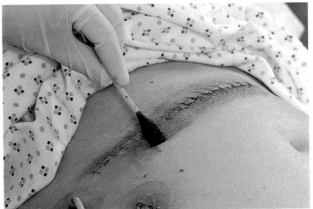

Step 11

IMPLEMENTATION

Steps	Rationale

13. Apply dressing.

   a. Dry dressing:

     (1) Apply loose, woven gauze as contact layer. Promotes proper absorption of drainage.

     (2) Cut 4 × 4 gauze flat to fit around drain, if present. Precut gauze is also available.

     (3) Apply second layer of gauze.

     (4) Apply thicker woven pad.

   b. Wet-to-dry dressing:

     (1) Place fine-mesh gauze in container of sterile solution. Squeeze out excess solution.

     (2) Apply moist fine-mesh gauze as a single layer directly onto wound surface. If wound is deep, gently pack gauze into wound with forceps until all wound surfaces are in contact with moist gauze (see illustration).

     (3) Apply dry, sterile 4 × 4 gauze over moist gauze.

     (4) Cover with ABD pad, Surgipad, or gauze.

14. Secure dressing.

   a. Montgomery ties

     (1) A protective skin barrier is recommended.

     (2) Place adhesive so that edges are 5 to 8 cm (2 to 3 inches) apart at the center (see illustration).

     (3) Secure dressing by lacing ties across dressing snugly enough to hold dressings secure but without pressure on the skin (see illustration).

   b. Circumferential dressing on an extremity, dressing is secured with roller gauze (see Figure 24-6) or Surgiflex elastic net (see illustration).

15. Remove gloves inside out and dispose of them in a waterproof container. Wash hands.

16. See Completion Protocol (inside front cover).

Rationale (right column)

Secures drain and promotes drainage absorption at site.
Ensures proper coverage and optimal absorption.
Protects wound from external environment.
Protects wound from microorganisms.

Contact layer must be totally moistened to increase dressing's absorptive abilities.
Absorbs drainage and adheres to debris. Wound should be loosely packed to facilitate wicking of drainage into absorbent outer layer of dressing.

Pulls moisture from wound.
Protects wound from the entrance of microorganisms.

Skin barrier (Stomahesive) protects intact skin from stretch and tension of adhesive tape.

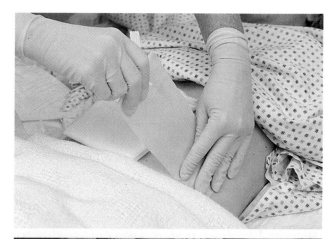

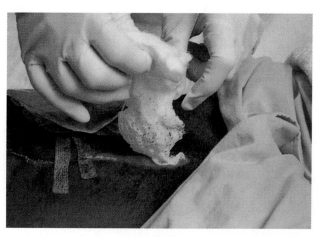

Step 13b(2)

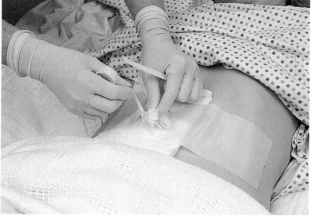

Step 14a(2,3)

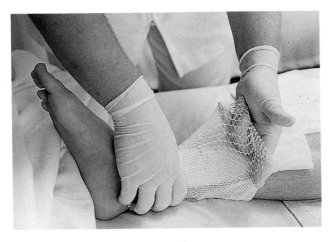

Step 14b

• • •

EVALUATION

1. Compare appearance of wound with previous assessment.
2. Ask client to rate pain using a scale of 0 to 10.
3. Observe client or caregiver's ability to perform dressing change.

Unexpected Outcomes and Related Nursing Interventions

1. Wound appears inflamed and tender, drainage is present, and an odor is present.
   a. Monitor client for signs of infection, for example, fever, increased WBC count.
   b. Notify physician.
   c. Obtain wound cultures as ordered.
2. Wound bleeds during dressing change.
   a. Observe color and amount of drainage. If excessive, may need to apply direct pressure.
   b. Inspect area along dressing and directly underneath client to determine the amount of bleeding.
   c. Obtain vital signs as needed.
   d. Notify physician of findings.
3. Client reports a sensation that "something has given way under the dressing."
   a. Observe wound for dehiscence (partial or total separation of wound layers) or evisceration (total separation of wound layers and protrusion of viscera through the wound opening).
   b. Protect wound. Cover wound with sterile moist dressing.
   c. Instruct client to lie still.
   d. Notify physician.
4. Client or caregiver is unable to perform dressing change.
   a. Provide additional teaching and support.
   b. Obtain services of home care agency as needed.

Recording and Reporting

- Record appearance of wound, color, characteristics of drainage, response to dressing change in nurse's notes.
- Write date and time dressing applied in ink (not marker) on outer tape.
- Report brisk, bright bleeding or evidence of wound dehiscence or evisceration to physician immediately.

Sample Documentation

1000 Wet-to-dry dressing on right ankle changed using normal saline and sterile technique. First layer of gauze had pea-sized spot of light-yellow drainage. Ulceration is 4 cm in diameter, 0.5 cm deep, with pinpoint spots of yellow drainage along the border; erythema noted on surrounding area. Used one moist and one dry 4 × 4 gauze and wrapped with Kling gauze. Client denied pain during procedure.

Geriatric Considerations

- Adhesive tape may be too irritating to older adults' skin and cause skin tears. Use paper tape and adhesive remover as needed.

Home Care and Long-Term Care Considerations

- Some wounds may be cleansed in the shower. Have client verify this practice with physician prior to discharge.
- Clean dressings may be used in the home environment.
- Disposal of contaminated dressings should be done in a manner consistent with local regulations (AHCPR, 1994).

Skill 24.4

CHANGING TRANSPARENT DRESSINGS

Transparent dressings are thin, self-adhesive elastic films (e.g., Op-site or Tegaderm). This synthetic permeable membrane acts as a temporary second skin, adheres to undamaged skin to contain exudate and minimize wound contamination, and allows the wound surface to "breathe." The nurse is able to assess the wound without removing the film. This dressing conforms well to body contours with less restriction of movement. It promotes a moist environment, which speeds epithelial cell growth, and can be removed without damaging underlying tissues (Krasner, 1992). The film is ideal for small, superficial wounds and as a dressing over an intravenous (IV) catheter site. Transparent dressings may be with or without adhesives and may stay in place up to 7 days, if complete occlusion is maintained.

For best results, these dressings are used on clean, debrided wounds that are not actively bleeding. The film is applied wrinkle free but not stretched over the skin and may be used over another smaller dressing (e.g., Telfa) cut to fit area of wound. Topical medications may be applied over nonadhesive transparent dressings without disturbing the dressing. Nonadhesive transparent dressings will fall off as wound heals. If removal is needed, moisten with normal saline. If approved by physician, the client may shower or bathe with dressing in place.

Equipment
    Clean disposable gloves
    Sterile gloves (optional)
    Sterile scissors and forceps (optional)
    Sterile saline, or other wound cleanser (as ordered)

Transparent dressing (size as needed) and sterile gauze pads (2 × 2)
Waterproof bag for disposal
Moisture-proof gown, goggles, and mask (if risk of splashing is present)

ASSESSMENT
1. Assess location, appearance, and size of wound (see Skill 24.2) to be dressed to allow nurse to determine supplies and assistance needed.
2. Assess client's comfort level using a scale of 0 to 10.

PLANNING
Expected outcomes focus on promoting wound healing.

Expected Outcomes
1. Client's wound shows reduction or absence of drainage.
2. Skin surrounding the wound remains clean and intact.
3. Client reports less pain during and after dressing change.

DELEGATION CONSIDERATIONS

This skill requires problem solving and knowledge unique to a professional nurse. Delegation is inappropriate.

IMPLEMENTATION

Steps	Rationale
1. See Standard Protocol (inside front cover).	
2. Cuff top of disposable waterproof bag to prevent contamination of outer bag. Place within easy reach of work area.	
3. Remove old dressing by pulling back slowly across dressing in direction of hair growth and toward the center.	Reduces excoriation, pain, and irritation of skin after dressing removal.
4. Remove disposable gloves by pulling them inside out over soiled dressings and dispose of them in waterproof bag.	
5. Inspect wound for color, odor, and drainage; measure if indicated.	Appearance indicates state of wound healing.

Steps	Rationale

6. Cleanse area gently, swabbing toward area of most exudate, or spray with cleanser (check agency policy and physician preference).

> Reduces transmission of organisms from contaminated area to cleaner site.

7. Reapply sterile (or clean) gloves (check agency policy.

> Prevents risk of exposure to body secretions if present.

8. Dry skin around wound thoroughly with sterile gauze. Make sure skin surface is dry.

> Transparent dressing with adhesive backing will not adhere to damp surface. Nonadhesive transparent dressing will cling to moist wound surface.

9. Apply transparent dressing according to manufacturer's directions.

    a. Remove paper backing, taking care not to allow adhesive areas to touch each other (see illustration).

> Results in wrinkles and may be impossible to use.

    b. Place film smoothly over wound without stretching (see illustration).

> Wrinkles can provide tunnel for drainage.

    c. Label with date, initials, and time if required by agency policy (see illustration).

10. Remove gloves, discard in waterproof bag, and wash hands.

11. See Completion Protocol (inside front cover).

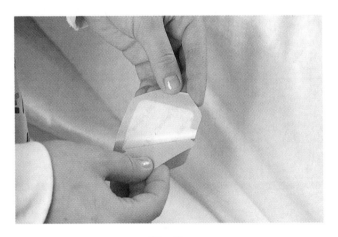

Step 9a

NURSE ALERT

Dressing should be clean and dry, and incision/wound should be protected by dressing.

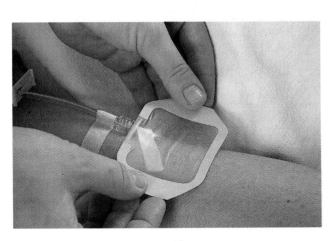

Step 9b

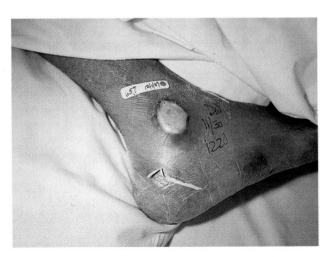

Step 9c

EVALUATION

1. Inspect appearance of wound and amount of drainage and compare with previous assessment.
2. Inspect condition of skin around the wound.
3. Ask client to rate pain using a scale of 0 to 10.

Unexpected Outcomes and Related Nursing Interventions

1. Wound appears inflamed and tender, drainage is present, and an odor is present.
   a. Remove dressing and obtain wound culture according to agency policy.
   b. A different type of dressing and more frequent dressing changes may be ordered.
2. Dressing does not stay in place.
   a. Evaluate size of dressing used for adequate (1 to 1½ inches) margin.
   b. Dry client's skin thoroughly before reapplication.
3. Outer layer of skin tears on removal of dressing.
   a. Adhesive backing may be too strong for fragile skin.
   b. Use non–adhesive backed transparent dressing.

Recording and Reporting

- Record appearance of wound, color, characteristics of drainage, response to dressing change.
- Write date and time dressing applied in ink (not marker) on outer label.

Sample Documentation

1000   Transparent dressing changed. Wound on left thigh is 6 × 10 cm, with oozing serosanguineous drainage. Area very tender to touch. Client describes pain as 2 (on a scale of 0 to 10). Refusing medication at this time.

Geriatric Considerations

- Adhesive tape may be too irritating to older adults' skin and cause skin tears. Use paper tape and adhesive remover as needed.

Home Care and Long-Term Care Considerations

Disposal of contaminated dressings should be done in a manner consistent with local regulations (AHCPR, 1994).

Skill 24.5

APPLYING BINDERS AND BANDAGES

Binder and bandages applied over or around dressings can provide extra protection and therapeutic benefits by:

1. Creating pressure over a body part (e.g., an elastic pressure bandage applied over an arterial puncture site).
2. Immobilizing a body part (e.g., an elastic bandage applied around a sprained ankle).
3. Supporting a wound (e.g., an abdominal binder applied over a large abdominal incision and dressing).
4. Reducing or preventing edema (e.g., a breast binder used to minimize swelling between skin and tissue layers after a mastectomy).
5. Securing a splint (e.g., a bandage applied around hand splints for correction of deformities).
6. Securing dressings (e.g., elastic webbing applied around leg dressings after a vein stripping).
7. Maintaining the position of special equipment for applying traction (e.g., Buck's extension).
8. Enabling the client to participate in effective respiratory functions of deep breathing, coughing, and clearing of airway secretions; for example, a breast or abdominal binder supports local incisions, reducing the pain from respiratory maneuvers.

Bandages are available in rolls of various widths and materials, including gauze, elasticized knit, elastic webbing, flannel, and muslin. Gauze bandages are lightweight and inexpensive, mold easily around contours of the body, and permit air circulation to prevent skin maceration. **Elastic bandages** conform well to body parts but can also be used to exert pressure over a body part. Elastic bandages are used to secure dressings on extremities, stumps, and the hand (Table 24-10). Flannel and muslin bandages are thicker than gauze and thus stronger for supporting or applying pressure. A flannel bandage also insulates to provide warmth.

Table 24-10

Types of Bandage Turns

Type	Description	Purpose or Use
Circular	Bandage turn overlapping previous turn completely	Anchors bandage at the first and final turn; covers small part (finger, toe)
Spiral	Bandage ascending body part, with each turn overlapping previous one by one-half or two-thirds width of bandage	Covers cylindrical body parts such as wrist or upper arm
Spiral–reverse	Turn requiring twist (reversal) of bandage halfway through each turn	Covers cone-shaped body parts such as the forearm, thigh, or calf; useful with nonstretching bandages such as gauze or flannel
Figure eight	Oblique overlapping turns alternately ascending and descending over bandaged part, each turn crossing previous one to form figure eight	Covers joints; snug fit provides excellent immobilization
Recurrent	Bandage first secured with two circular turns around proximal end of body part; half turn made perpendicular up from bandage edge; body of bandage brought over distal end of body part to be covered with each turn folded back over on itself	Covers uneven body parts such as head or stump

Binders are bandages made of large pieces of material specially designed to fit a specific body part. Most binders are made of elastic, cotton, muslin, or flannel. The most common types of binders are the breast binder, abdominal binder, and T-binder.

A breast binder looks like a tight-fitting sleeveless vest. It conforms to the shape of the chest wall and is available in different sizes. Breast binders can provide support after breast surgery.

An abdominal binder supports large abdominal incisions that are vulnerable to tension or stress as the client moves or coughs (Figure 24-7). The nurse secures a binder with Velcro strips, metal fasteners, or safety pins.

As the name implies, the **T-binder** looks like the letter T (Figure 24-8) and is used to secure rectal or perineal dressings. The single-T-binder fits female clients, and the double-T-binder fits male clients.

The belt of the T-binder fits securely around the client's waist, with the tail passing between the client's legs from back to front and attaching to the belt's front. The nurse should be sure the tail fits smoothly and against the dressing. T-binders become soiled easily and require frequent changing. Irritation to the urethra or scrotum must be avoided.

Correctly applied bandages and binders do not cause injury to underlying and nearby body parts or create discomfort for the client. For example, an abdominal binder must be applied correctly to allow for normal chest expansion.

Equipment
Clean gloves, if wound drainage is present
Correct type and size of binder
Safety pins (unless Velcro closure is available)

ASSESSMENT
1. Observe client with need for support of thorax or abdomen. Observe ability to breathe deeply and cough effectively. **Rationale: Baseline assessment determines client's ability to breathe and cough. Impaired ventilation of lungs can lead to alveolar collapse (atelectasis) and inadequate arterial oxygenation.**
2. Review medical record for order of binder type. **Rationale: Application of supportive binders may be used based on a nursing judgment. In some situations a physician's order may be required (check agency policy).**
3. Inspect skin for actual or potential alterations in integrity. Observe for irritation, abrasion, skin surfaces that rub together, or allergic response to adhesive tape. **Rationale: Actual impairments in skin integrity can be worsened with the application of a binder. Binders can cause pressure and excoriation.**
4. Inspect surgical dressing. **Rationale: Dressing replacement or reinforcement precedes application of any binder.**

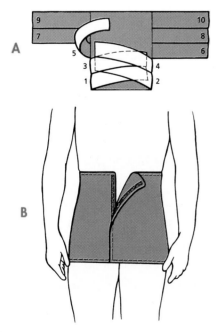

Figure 24-7 Abdominal binders. **A,** Scultetus. **B,** Straight.

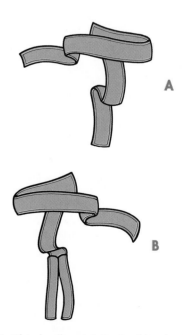

Figure 24-8 **A,** T-binder (female). **B,** Double T-binder (male).

5. Assess client's comfort level, using a scale of 0 to 10 and noting any objective signs and symptoms. **Rationale: Data will determine effectiveness of binder placement to support underlying tissues.**

PLANNING

Expected outcomes focus on improving client's comfort level, maintaining baseline respiratory functioning, securing underlying dressing, and maintaining underlying skin integrity.

Expected Outcomes

1. Client reports pain less than 3 on a scale of 0 to 10.
2. Client's respiratory rate remains within 3 breaths of baselines.
3. Underlying surgical dressing remain intact.
4. Client does not have any impairment in skin integrity on tissue underneath and surrounding binder.

IMPLEMENTATION

Steps	Rationale

1. See Standard Protocol (inside front cover).

NURSE ALERT

Cover any exposed areas of incision or wound with sterile dressing.

2. Apply binder:
   a. Abdominal binder:

Steps	Rationale
(1) Position client in supine position with head slightly elevated and knees slightly flexed.	Minimizes muscular tension on abdominal organs.
(2) Fanfold far side of binder toward midline of binder.	Reduces time client remains in uncomfortable position.
(3) Instruct and assist client to roll away from nurse toward raised side rail while firmly supporting abdominal incision and dressing with hands.	Reduces pain and discomfort.
(4) Place fanfolded ends of binder under client.	Permits placement and centering of binder with minimal discomfort.
(5) Instruct or assist client to roll over folded ends.	
(6) Unfold and stretch ends out smoothly on far side of bed.	Maintains skin integrity and comfort.
(7) Instruct client to roll back into supine position.	Facilitates chest expansion and adequate wound support when the binder is closed.
(8) Adjust binder so that supine client is centered over binder using symphysis pubis and costal margins as lower and upper landmarks.	Centers support from binder over abdominal structures, which reduces incidence of decreased lung expansion.
(9) Close binder. Pull one end of binder over center of client's abdomen. While maintaining tension on that end of binder, pull opposite end of binder over center and secure with Velcro closure tabs, metal fasteners, or horizontally placed safety pins.	Provides continuous wound support and comfort.

DELEGATION CONSIDERATIONS

The skills of applying a binder (abdominal, T, or breast) can be delegated to AP.

- The nurse completes an assessment of the client's ability to breathe deeply, cough effectively, and move independently; of skin for irritation/abrasion; of incision/wound and dressing; and of comfort level before a binder or sling is applied for the first time. (See assessment criteria under individual skill.)
- The nurse evaluates the client's response to binder application.

Steps	**Rationale**
(10) Assess client's comfort level.	Helps determine effectiveness of binder placement.
(11) Adjust binder as necessary.	Promotes comfort and chest expansion.
b. Single-T and double-T binders (see Figure 24-10):	
(1) Assist client to dorsal recumbent position, with lower extremities slightly flexed and hips rotated slightly outward.	Minimizes muscular tension on perineal organs.
(2) Have client raise hips and place horizontal band around client's waist (or above iliac crests) with vertical tails extending past buttocks. Overlap waistband in front and secure with safety pins.	Facilitates placement of binder. Secures binder around client.
(3) Complete binder application:	
(a) T-binder: Bring remaining vertical strip over perineal dressing and continue up and under center front of horizontal band. Bring ends over waistband and secure all thicknesses with safety pin.	Single-T and double-T binders provide support to perineal muscles and organs and help maintain placement of perineal or suprapubic dressing.
(b) Double-T binder: Bring remaining vertical strips over perineal or suprapubic dressing, with each tail supporting one side of scrotum and proceeding upward on either side of penis. Continue drawing ends behind and then downward in front of horizontal band. Secure all thicknesses with one horizontally placed safety pin.	

NURSE ALERT

Binder should hold perineal or suprapubic dressing in place as the client ambulates, without applying pressure to urethra or scrotum.

(4) Assess client's comfort level with client in lying, sitting, and standing positions. Readjust front pins and tails as necessary, ensuring that tails are not too tight. Increase padding if any area rubs against surrounding tissues.	Determines efficacy of binder to maintain dressings and support perineal structures.
(5) Instruct client regarding removal of binder before defecating or urinating and need to replace binder after performing these bodily functions.	Cleanliness of binder reduces infection risk.
c. Breast binder:	
(1) Assist client in placing arms through binder's armholes.	Eases binder placement process.
(2) Assist client to supine position in bed.	Supine positioning facilitates normal anatomical position of breasts; facilitates healing and comfort.
(3) Pad area under breasts if necessary.	Prevents skin contact with undersurface.
(4) Using Velcro closure tabs or horizontally placed safety pins, secure binder at nipple level first. Continue closure process above and then below nipple line until entire binder is closed.	Horizontal placement of pins may reduce risk of uneven pressure or localized irritation.
(5) Make appropriate adjustments, including individualizing fit of shoulder straps and pinning waistline darts to reduce binder size.	Maintains support to client's breasts.
(6) Instruct and observe skill development in self-care related to reapplying breast binder.	Self-care is integral aspect of discharge planning. Skin integrity and comfort level goals are ensured.

Steps	Rationale

3. Remove binder at scheduled intervals to assess underlying skin integrity (check agency policy).

Promotes timely identification of impaired skin integrity.

4. See Completion Protocol (inside front cover).

EVALUATION

1. Ask client to rate pain on a scale of 0 to 10.
2. Observe client's respiratory status when using an abdominal binder.
3. Observe site to be sure underlying dressings are intact.
4. Remove binder and observe underlying and surrounding skin.

Unexpected Outcomes and Related Nursing Interventions

1. Client's pain increases.
   a. Remove binder and assess wound site.
   b. Reapply binder using less pressure.
2. Client's respiratory rate decreases.
   a. Remove binder.
   b. Encourage client to cough and deep breathe.
3. Dressing becomes dislodged.
   a. Remove binder.
   b. Reinforce underlying dressings.
4. Client develops a break in the skin because of binder application.
   a. Remove binder.
   b. Initiate measures to heal affected area.

Recording and Reporting

- Record baseline data about client's respiratory status, level of comfort, status of dressings, and skin integrity.
- Following use of binder, record information pertaining to client's level of comfort, respiratory status, tolerance to binder, and status of underlying wound and skin.
- Report client's tolerance to binder application and the prescribed duration of the application.

Sample Documentation

1000   Client complains of "pulling" sensation around abdominal incision line. Pulling sensation increases with ambulation. Vital signs stable. Dressings to abdominal wound dry and intact. Underlying skin intact. Abdominal binder applied. Client rates pain as 1 on scale, able to ambulate with ease.

Geriatric Considerations

- The increased fragility of the skin of an older adult may contraindicate the use of a binder. Assess skin thoroughly prior to any binder application. May want to observe underlying skin more frequently for this population.

Home Care and Long-Term Care Considerations

Client should be instructed to have two binders. Because binders are washable and need to be "line dried," the client has one to wear and one that is in the process of being washed or dried.

CRITICAL THINKING EXERCISES

1. A client with a left trochanter wound was just admitted to a chronic wound service. The wound is 2×3 cm, edges are red, drainage is yellow.
   a. What other assessments must you make about this wound?
   b. What are the immediate 10-day goals for this client?

2. Compare and contrast techniques for securing dressings for the following clients:
   a. Client with an open wound on the anterior aspect of leg
   b. Client with an abdominal wound
   c. Client with a scalp wound

3. You are delivering home care and client instruction to a client family unit. The client has a stage II clean sacral pressure ulcer. How will you instruct family members to care for this wound? What instruction will you provide regarding progression of wound?

REFERENCES

Agency for Health Care Policy and Research (AHCPR): *Pressure ulcers in adults: a patient's guide,* Pub No 92-0048, Rockville, Md, 1992a, US Department of Health and Human Services, Public Health Service.

Agency for Health Care Policy and Research (AHCPR): *Pressure ulcers in adults: prediction and prevention,* Pub Nos 92-0047 and 92-0050, Rockville, Md, 1992b, US Department of Health and Human Services, Public Health Service.

Agency for Health Care Policy and Research (AHCPR) Panel for the Prediction and Prevention of Pressure Ulcers in Adults: *Pressure ulcers in adults: prediction and prevention,* Clinical practice guideline no 15, Pub No 95-0653, Rockville, Md, 1994, US Department of Health and Human Services, Public Health Service.

Ayello EA: A critique of the AHCPR's "Preventing pressure ulcers: a patient's guide" as a written instructional tool, *Decubitus* 6(3):44, 1993.

Baharestani MM: The lived experience of wives caring for their frail, home bound, elderly husbands with pressure ulcers, *Adv Wound Care* 7(3):40, 1994.

Bennett MA: Report of the Task Force on the Implications for Darkly Pigmented Intact Skin in the Prediction and Prevention of Pressure Ulcers, *Adv Wound Care* 8(6):34, 1995.

Bergstrom N, Demuth PJ, Braden B: A clinical trial of the Braden scale for predicting pressure sore risk, *Nurs Clin North Am* 22(2):417, 1987.

Bergstrom N et al: *Treatment of pressure ulcers,* AHCPR Pub No 95-0652, Rockville, Md, 1994, US Department of Health and Human Services, Public Health Service, Agency for Health Care Policy and Research.

Bergstrom N et al: Predicting pressure ulcer risk: a multisite study of the predictive validity of the Braden Scale, *Nurs Res* 1998 Sept-Oct 47(5).

Bryant RA: *Acute and chronic wounds,* St Louis, 1992, Mosby.

Doughty DB: Principles of wound healing and wound management. In Bryant R, editor: *Acute and chronic wounds,* St Louis, 1992, Mosby.

Flemister BG: A pilot study of interface pressure with heel protectors used for pressure reduction, *J ET Nurs* 18:158, 1991.

Graves DJ: Stage I in ebony complexion, *Decubitus* 3(4):4, 1990 (letter).

Itoh M et al.: Accelerated wound healing of pressure ulcers by pulsed high peak power electromagnetic energy (Diapulse), *Decubitus* 4(1):24, 1993.

Johnson A: A short history of wound dressings, *Ostomy/Wound Manage* 38(2):36, 1992.

Johnson G, Daily C, Franciscus V: A clinical study of hospital replacement mattresses, *J ET Nurs* 18:153, 1991.

Kaminski MV, Pinchocofsky-Devin G, Williams SD: Nutritional management of decubitus ulcers in the elderly, *Decubitus* 2(4):20, 1989.

Knox MD, Anderson TM, Anderson PS: Effects of different turn intervals on skin of healthy older adults, *Adv Wound Care* 7(1):48, 1994.

Krasner D: Wound care update 91: new packing trends, *Nursing '91* 21(4):50, 1991.

Krasner D: Resolving the dressing dilemma: selecting wound dressings by category, *Plast Surg Nurs* 12(1):22, 1992.

Krasner D, Kennedy KL: Using the no touch technique to change a dressing, *Nursing* 24(9):50, 1994.

Lazzara DJ, Buschmann MT: Prevention of pressure ulcers in elderly nursing home residents: are special support surfaces the answer? *Decubitus* 4(4):42, 1991.

Maklebust J, Magnan MA: Approaches to patient and family education for pressure ulcer management, *Decubitus* 5(4):18, 1992.

Maklebust J, Sieggreen M: *Pressure ulcers: guidelines for prevention and nursing management,* West Dundee, Ill, 1991, S-N Publications.

Maklebust J, Sieggreen M: *Pressure ulcers: guidelines for prevention and nursing management,* ed 2, Springhouse, Pa, 1996, Springhouse.

McKnight's Survey: Data watch: pressure sores, *McKnight's Long Term Care News* 26, 1992.

Meehan M: National Pressure Ulcer Prevalence Survey, *Adv Wound Care* 7(3):27, 1994.

National Pressure Ulcer Advisory Panel: Pressure ulcer prevalence, cost and risk assessment: consensus development conference statement, *Decubitus* 2(2):24, 1989.

National Pressure Ulcer Advisory Panel: Position on reverse staging of pressure ulcers, *Adv Wound Care* 8(6):32, 1995.

Olson B: Effects of massage for prevention of pressure ulcers, *Decubitus* 2(4):32, 1989.

Panel for Urinary Incontinence Guideline: *Urinary incontinence in adults,* AHCPR Pub No 920038, Rockville, Md, 1992, Public Health Service, US Department of Health and Human Services, Agency for Health Care Policy and Research.

Rodeheaver G et al: Wound healing and wound management: focus on debridement, *Adv Wound Care* 7(1):22, 1994.

U.S. Dept of Health and Human Services, Centers for Disease Control and Prevention, National Center for Health Statistics. *Vital and Health Statistics, Detailed Diagnosis and Procedures,* National Hospital Discharge Survey, 1994, Series 13, Hyattsville, Md, DHHS Pub No 127, 1997.

van Rijswijk L, Braden BJ: Pressure ulcer patient and wound assessment: an AHCPR clinical practice guideline update, *Ostomy Wound Manage,* 1999, Jan 45.

CHAPTER 25

Special Mattresses and Beds

Skill 25.1
Using a Support Surface Mattress, 602

Skill 25.2
Using an Air-Suspension Bed, 605

Skill 25.3
Using an Air-Fluidized Bed, 608

Skill 25.4
Using a Rotokinetic Bed, 611

Skill 25.5
Using a Bariatric Bed, 614

Nurses have a variety of special mattresses and beds to use as adjuncts to their care. These support surfaces have differing purposes, including pressure reduction, pressure relief, repositioning, and support of the morbidly obese client. These support surfaces are used in acute, rehabilitative, long-term, and home care settings.

Pressure reduction or relief is a common nursing concern in the client with reduced mobility. A person can be bedridden, but not immobile. It is decreased mobility which increases client risk of pressure. Tissue damage occurs when the pressure exerted on the capillaries is high enough to close the capillaries. According to Bryant (1992), 12 to 32 mm Hg is considered the normal pressure exerted on the capillaries. When the capillary closing pressure (the pressure needed to close capillaries) is exceeded, the capillaries begin to collapse and thrombose. In a normal healthy adult, high capillary pressures stimulate a shifting of body weight to relieve pressure on the affected tissue. Repositioning distributes pressure among tissues, avoiding tissue compression and subsequent ischemia. When immobility prevents these natural shifts in weight,

the client's tissue becomes compressed between his or her skeletal structure and the bed. This compression decreases circulating blood supply, leading to tissue anoxia and damage.

For clients with restricted mobility, those with chronic diseases, and elderly clients, pressure management is a significant nursing concern because these clients lack the ability to reposition themselves. Special support mattresses and beds are frequently used to reduce or relieve pressure on tissues.

Support surfaces designed for pressure management may also incorporate rotational therapy to aid in pulmonary management, pulsation to improve cutaneous circulation, and pressure management. Support surfaces designed for use other than pressure management include the Rotokinetic bed and the bariatric bed. The Rotokinetic bed (see Skill 25.4) provides skeletal alignment with constant side-to-side rotation up to 90 degrees. The bariatric bed, also called an *obesity bed*, is wider and sturdier than standard hospital beds. It is useful in the care of the morbidly obese client because it accommodates weights up to 850 pounds and improves access to the client in a manner safe for the client and caregiver.

▶ NURSING DIAGNOSES

Multiple conditions (e.g., cerebrovascular accident [CVA], head injury, multiple sclerosis, chronic illness) may limit mobility and necessitate the use of specialty beds. When a client has **Impaired Physical Mobility,** pressure reduction/relief or rotational beds may lessen the effects of immobility. Clients with actual or high risk for **Impaired Skin Integrity** may benefit from the use of pressure reduction/relief surfaces to counteract the combined effects of immobility and pressure.

Anxiety and **Fear** may surface, especially with the use of kinetic beds. The constant turning and rigid structure of the Rotokinetic bed may contribute to sympathetic stimulation, restlessness, increased tension, and apprehension.

Skill 25.1

USING A SUPPORT SURFACE MATTRESS

Support surfaces are widely used to reduce pressure on tissue underlying bony prominences. These surfaces may be used to actually replace the standard hospital mattress or as an overlay that rests on top of the hospital mattress. It is important to understand the difference between a pressure reduction mattress, a pressure relieving support system, and a surface used for comfort.

Although special beds and mattresses have been designed to reduce the hazards of immobility to the skin and musculoskeletal system, no bed or mattress totally eliminates the need for meticulous nursing care. It is estimated that pressure on the skin is multiplied three times at the bone–soft tissue interface! The 3 purposes of support surfaces are comfort, postural control, and pressure management (Krouskop and van Rijswijk, 1995).

Foam and air are the two prevalent types of support surfaces. A foam mattress overlay (Figure 25-1), commonly called an *egg crate* because of its appearance, is designed with foam peaks. The egg crate is used for client comfort because it has minimal pressure reduction capabilities.

Foam replacement mattresses are denser, thicker, and more resilient to weight and actually decrease pressure to a much greater degree than the foam overlay.

These replacement mattresses have built-in foam, gel, or fluid sections that can be customized to a specific client's need.

The air mattress overlay rests over the mattress. It may be inflated once by the use of a blower, or it may use a pressure cycling device to inflate and deflate intermittently the air pressure among various segments of the mattress. Another available option is an air mattress that replaces the conventional mattress. These mattresses may also be fully integrated into the bed (Figure 25-2).

Use of support surfaces simply aids in pressure reduction. Clients still must be repositioned regularly to avoid complications of immobility such as pulmonary congestion and contractures.

Equipment

Risk assessment tool (see Chapter 24)
Mattress support surface of choice: bed with integrated surface, replacement mattress, or overlay
Sheet(s)
Disposable gloves (if soiled linen is being handled)
Standard bed frame (with mattress if overlay is to be used)

ASSESSMENT

1. Determine client's risk for pressure ulcer formation using a validated assessment tool. **Rationale: Use of a validated instrument is suggested by the AHCPR guidelines. Using an assessment tool provides an objective measure of risk consistent between evaluators.**

2. Perform skin assessment, especially over dependent sites and bony prominences. Look for changes in color (erythema or pallor), texture (edema or induration), temperature (warmth or coolness), blistering, or ulceration. **Rationale: Provides a baseline to determine change in skin integrity or change in existing pressure ulcer.**

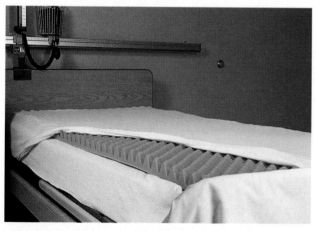

Figure 25-1 "Egg-crate" foam overlay is primarily for comfort.

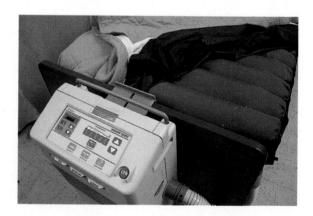

Figure 25-2 Integrated air mattress.

3. Assess client's level of comfort and presence of pain. **Rationale: Client may require pain medication to tolerate movement to another bed/mattress surface. Inadequate pain control may limit client's tolerance of position changes.**
4. Assess client's understanding of purposes of support surfaces. **Rationale: Misconceptions can affect client's cooperation in use of mattress.**
5. Verify physician's order for surface. **Rationale: A physician's order is required to ensure third-party payment of the support surface. NOTE: A physician's order is not required in Canada.**

PLANNING

Expected outcomes focus on maintenance of skin integrity and client comfort.

Expected Outcomes

1. Client's skin remains intact without evidence of abnormal reactive hyperemia or mottling.
2. Existing pressure ulcers show evidence of healing by formation of granulation tissue.
3. Client rates comfort as a 4 (on a scale of 0 to 10).

DELEGATION CONSIDERATIONS

The skills of applying support surface mattresses or preparation of an alternative bed can be delegated to assistive personnel (AP).

- Inform and assist care provider in proper method of applying support surface to bed.
- Encourage care provider to obtain assistance when positioning client to reduce risk of friction and shear and to prevent self-injury.
- Explain to care provider the rationale for client to be routinely repositioned even though on support surfaces.
- Caution care provider to routinely inspect bony prominences and heels for signs of pressure and to notify RN to conduct assessment when abnormalities are noted.
- Caution care provider to wear gloves when inspecting mattress surfaces for wetness.
- Educate care provider on importance of maintaining adequate nutritional and fluid status in the client.
- Inform care providers to replace soiled bed linens or straighten wrinkled sheets.
- Explain to care provider how to clean and monitor special mattresses and beds.
- Explain to care provider how to determine if air mattress needs to be reinflated.

IMPLEMENTATION

Steps	Rationale
1. See Standard Protocol (inside front cover).	
2. Close room door or bedside curtain.	Provides client privacy during application of mattress to bed or transfer to alternate bed.
3. Apply support surface to bed or prepare alternate bed (bed may be occupied or unoccupied).	
a. Mattress replacement:	
(1) Apply mattress to bed frame after removing standard hospital mattress.	Hospital mattress needs to be stored. In some instances, mattress replacements may be standard procedure.
(2) Apply sheet over mattress.	Sheet reduces soiling.
b. Air mattress/overlay:	
(1) Apply deflated mattress flat over surface of bed mattress. (There may be directions on pad indicating which side to place up.)	Provides smooth, even surface.

NURSE ALERT

Avoid use of sharp objects near mattress.

COMMUNICATION TIP

Tell client that the mattress may inflate and deflate periodically, may feel cool, and may require a period of adjustment.

Steps	Rationale
(2) Bring any plastic strips or flaps around corners of bed mattress.	Secures air mattress in place.
(3) Attach connector on air mattress to inflation device. Inflate mattress to proper air pressure determined by air pump or blower.	Mattresses vary as to requiring one-time or continuous inflation cycle. Manufacturer's directions indicate desired air pressure designed to distribute client's body weight evenly. Directions are included with each mattress.
(4) Place sheet over air mattress, being sure to eliminate all wrinkles.	Prevents soiling of mattress and reduces direct contact of skin against plastic surface.
(5) Check air pumps to be sure pressure cycle alternates.	Alternating air-flow mattress produces intermittent cycling, inflating only parts of mattress at any one time. Intermittent cycle continually alternates pressure against skin and soft tissue.
c. Integrated air-surface bed: (1) Obtain and make bed.	In some instances bed may be available in all client rooms; if not, an ordering system exists to obtain one as needed (see agency policy).
(2) Place switch in the "Prevention" mode.	In the "Prevention" mode, surface pressures change automatically with client position to equalize pressure and eliminate points of pressure.
d. Water mattress (supplemental and self-contained): (1) Apply unfilled supplemental mattress flat over the surface of standard bed mattress. (Self-contained water mattress would replace bed mattress.)	Provides a smooth, even surface.
(2) Bring any plastic strips or flaps around corners of bed mattress.	Secures water mattress in place.
(3) Attach connector on water mattress to water source and fill mattress to level recommended by manufacturer. Follow manufacturer's directions regarding temperature of water. Mattress should be filled in close proximity to water source.	Manufacturer's directions (enclosed with mattress) indicate desired water level designed to distribute client's body weight evenly (usually determined by client weight or height and weight).
(4) Place sheet over water mattress, being sure to eliminate all wrinkles.	Reduces soiling of mattress and prevents direct contact of skin against plastic surface.
4. Position client comfortably as desired over support surface. Reposition routinely.	Location of existing pressure sore might influence type of positioning.
5. Reposition regularly for comfort.	
6. Reassess the client's level of risk for skin breakdown, and periodically verify the bed or mattress is still appropriate and necessary.	

NURSE ALERT

Support surfaces do not alter the need for regular turning.

Steps	Rationale
7. Instruct the client to call for assistance to get into and out of the bed.	The height of the bed is different, and the mattress overlay may make getting into and out of bed difficult.
8. See Completion Protocol (inside front cover).	

• • • •

EVALUATION

1. Inspect condition of skin every 8 hours to determine changes in skin and effectiveness of support mattress.
2. Inspect client's pressure ulcers for evidence of healing.
3. Ask client to rate comfort on a 0 to 10 scale.

Unexpected Outcomes and Related Interventions

1. Client develops localized areas of abnormal reactive hyperemia for longer that 30 minutes, mottling, swelling, and tenderness with evidence of breakdown. Existing pressure ulcers fail to heal or increase in size.
   a. Revise turning schedule for more frequent position changes.
   b. Avoid prolonged exposure on any one side.
   c. Keep skin clean and dry. Keep linens free of wrinkles.
   d. Notify physician. Advancement of existing pressure ulcers may be related to infection, nutritional deficiencies, or an exacerbation of other systemic factors.
   e. Evaluate need for alternative surface.
2. Client expresses or demonstrates discomfort.
   a. Evaluate air level of surface.
   b. Evaluate need for alternative surface.
   c. Reposition client more frequently.
   d. Unless contraindicated, provide back massage. Do not massage reddened areas, because this contributes to skin breakdown.
3. Support surface develops a leak.
   a. Take corrective action in accordance with institutional policies.

Recording and Reporting

- Record type of support surface applied, extent to which client tolerated procedure, and condition of client's skin in nurse's notes or skin assessment flow sheet.

- Report evidence of pressure ulcer formation to nurse in charge or to physician.

Sample Documentation

1000   Air mattress overlay applied to bed. Client's skin dry and intact without erythema.

Geriatric Considerations

- Implement preventive measures for older adults, because the aging process causes their skin to become drier, thinner, and less pressure sensitive, increasing the risk of skin breakdown.
- Adding a mattress overlay changes bed height. Care should be taken when transferring client in and out of bed.

Home Care and Long-Term Care Considerations

- Most of the devices covered in this section may be adapted for home use on a standard twin bed or hospital bed.
- Selection should be based on client needs and environmental audit. For example:
  - The client on total bed rest who smokes would not be an ideal candidate for a foam mattress because of the potential for fire.
  - The client with pets that sleep in the bed may not be suited for a water- or air-filled mattress because of the risk of puncture.
- Reimbursement varies by surface type and payer source.

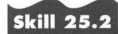

USING AN AIR-SUSPENSION BED

Air-suspension beds are useful in promoting skin integrity in the immobile or bedridden client. These beds reduce the effects of shear, friction, maceration, and pressure. Air-filled cushions support and redistribute weight (Figure 25-3, p. 606). A controlled amount of air is continually lost through the surface of the bed cushions. This air loss has a drying effect on the skin, which decreases the effects of maceration without dehydrating the client. Special high-air-loss cushions may also be used to draw moisture from a certain area.

It is also possible to adapt the air-suspension beds to individual client needs with specialty cushions for positioning, foot support, and lateral arm supports. Another adaptation of the air-suspension bed is the kinetic low-air-loss bed. This bed is marketed widely to intensive care areas and has the ability to provide a pressure-relief surface

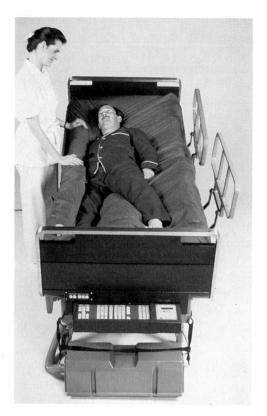

Figure 25-3 Air-suspension bed. *Courtesy Kinetic Concepts, Inc [KCI], San Antonio, Tex.*

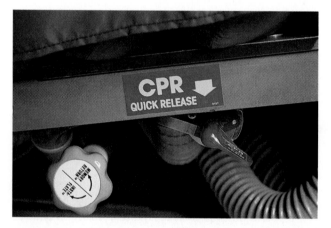

Figure 25-4 Cardiopulmonary resuscitation switch deflates air-suspension bed to provide hard surface.

while rotating approximately 30 to 35 degrees. This surface should not be used with a client who has an unstable spinal cord or who is in traction. A pediatric version also exists.

These beds have cardiopulmonary resuscitation (CPR) switches (Figure 25-4), which permit immediate deflation to provide a hard surface for chest compressions. Scales may be built into the bed for ease in weighing. A battery system is necessary to maintain inflation during interruptions of power or during transport.

Equipment
Air-suspension bed (see Figure 25-3)
Gortex sheet (supplied by distributor)
Disposable bed pads, if indicated
Disposable gloves (optional)

ASSESSMENT
1. Use a validated instrument to determine client's risk for pressure ulcer formation.
2. Carefully inspect the skin for erythema, especially over bony prominences. **Rationale: These data provide a baseline for monitoring changes in client's skin.**
3. Assess client's level of comfort and presence of pain.
4. Assess client's understanding of the air-suspension bed.

PLANNING
Expected outcomes focus on the maintenance of skin integrity and comfort for the patient.

Expected Outcomes
1. Client's skin remains intact without evidence of abnormal reactive hyperemia or mottling.
2. Existing pressure ulcers show evidence of healing.
3. Client rates comfort as a 4 (on a scale of 0 to 10).
4. Client remains alert and oriented.

DELEGATION CONSIDERATIONS

The skill of applying a support surface mattress or preparation of an alternative bed can be delegated to AP; however, assessment of the need for a special support surface, choice of the type to use, and evaluation of its effectiveness is not. When delegating the care of a client on a special surface mattress/bed, emphasize the importance of regular turning and routine inspection of the skin for changes. The AP needs to notify the professional nurse of changes in skin condition.

IMPLEMENTATION

Steps	Rationale
1. See Standard Protocol (inside front cover).	
2. Close client's room door or bedside curtain.	Maintains client's privacy during transfer.
3. Explain steps of transfer.	Reduces anxiety and helps client be a part of decision making during maneuvering.
4. Transfer client to bed using appropriate transfer techniques.	Appropriate transfer techniques maintain alignment and reduce risk of injury during procedure. Company representative will adjust bed to client's height and weight.
5. Turn bed on by depressing switch; regulate temperature.	Suspension minimizes pressure against skin's surface and reduces friction and shear force when client moves (Seila and Stahelin, 1992).
6. Position client and perform range-of-motion (ROM) exercises as appropriate.	Promotes comfort and reduces contracture formation. The bed reduces pressure on skin, but clients must still be turned and exercised to avoid joint deformity or contractures.
7. To turn clients, position bedpans, or perform other therapies, set instaflate. Once procedure is completed, release instaflate.	Instaflate firms the bed surface to facilitate turning and handling client.

8. There are a number of special features available for air-suspension beds. When requesting a bed of this type, you will need to specify what special features may be required. Special features include:
   a. Scales for patient weight.
   b. Portable transport units to maintain inflation when primary power source is interrupted.
   c. Specialty cushions to allow patient to lie in the prone position.
   d. Kinetic (turning) features that allow approximately 30 degrees of turning while maintaining a pressure-relief surface.
9. Provide adequate fluid intake because the bed surface may be drying and contributes to dehydration.
10. See Completion Protocol (inside front cover).

NURSE ALERT

Client will not receive pressure relief when bed is firm for procedures. Activate CPR switch to quickly deflate the bed in an emergency (see Figure 25-4).

• • •

EVALUATION

1. Inspect condition of skin periodically to determine changes in skin and effectiveness of air-suspension mattress.
2. Inspect client's pressure ulcers for evidence of healing.
3. Ask client to rate comfort on a 0 to 10 scale.
4. Observe client's level of consciousness and orientation.

Unexpected Outcomes and Related Interventions

1. Client develops areas of breakdown, or existing areas of breakdown worsen.
   a. Evaluate and revise turning schedule as needed.
   b. Avoid prolonged exposure on any one side.
   c. Keep skin clean and dry and linens wrinkle free.
   d. Notify physician. Advancement of existing pressure ulcer may be related to tissue necrosis, infection, nutritional deficiencies, or exacerbation of other systemic factors. Surgical debridement may be required.
   e. Evaluate need for alternative therapy.
2. Client experiences restlessness or nausea or becomes disoriented because of constant flotation.
   a. Reposition patient for comfort.
   b. Notify physician. Symptomatic treatment may be required while adjusting to the bed.
   c. If unable to adjust to flotation, evaluate the need for alternative support mattress.

3. Bed malfunctions.
   a. Follow institutional policies to obtain replacement. Client may need to be transferred to hospital bed in the interim.

Recording and Reporting

- Record transfer of client to bed, tolerance of procedure, and condition of skin in nurse's notes or skin assessment flow sheet.
- Report changes in condition of skin and electrolyte levels to physician.
- Report restlessness or change in orientation.

Sample Documentation

1000   Client transferred onto air-suspension bed without injury. Skin warm, dry, and intact without erythema or breakdown. Denies dizziness. Rates comfort as an 8 on a scale of 0 to 10.

Geriatric Considerations

- When hospitalized, older adult clients may experience significant misperceptions of their environment. This type of sensory perceptual change may be intensified by the constant flotation of the air-suspension bed.

Home Care and Long-Term Care Considerations

- A version of the bed is available for home use for rent or purchase.
- Instruct family on importance of maintaining client hydration.
- Instruct family regarding the need to provide client's skin care.

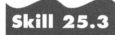

Skill 25.3

USING AN AIR-FLUIDIZED BED

An **air-fluidized bed** (Fig. 25-5) is designed to distribute a client's weight evenly over its support surface. The bed minimizes pressure and reduces shear force and friction through the principle of fluidization. Fluidization is created by forcing a gentle flow of temperature-controlled air upward through a mass of fine ceramic microspheres. The microspheres fluidize and take on the appearance of boiling milk and all the properties of a fluid. The client lies directly on a polyester filter sheet that allows air to pass through but does not allow the microspheres to escape. Clients feel as though they are floating on a surface like a warm waterbed. The contact pressure of the client's body against the filter sheet stays at 11 to 16 mm Hg.

Air-fluidized beds are useful in the care of clients who require minimal movement to prevent skin damage by shearing force and for clients who experience significant pain when being turned or positioned. Clients who can benefit from the bed include burn clients, those who have undergone extensive skin grafts or who have existing pressure ulcers, and victims of multiple trauma. Clients tend to perspire and lose body fluids while on the bed (Bryant 1992; Fowler, 1987). The surface of the filter sheet warms; as clients perspire, moisture is quickly absorbed into the circulating microspheres. Diaphoresis can go undetected, and thus insensible fluid loss may not be noticed until a client develops fluid and electrolyte imbalances.

Conventional fluidized beds do not allow for head-of-bed position changes. Foam wedges are used to elevate the head. There are also combination fluidized–air-suspension beds that allow head-of-bed elevation. These beds use air to lift the upper body, while the lower body stays in a fluidized bed surface. The weight of the bed structure makes transport extremely difficult. A pediatric version of the bed is available.

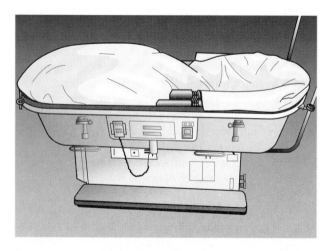

Figure 25-5 Clinitron bed.

Equipment

Air-fluidized bed

Foam positioning wedges, if indicated

Filter sheet (supplied by the distributor)

ASSESSMENT

1. Use a validated risk assessment tool to determine client's risk for pressure ulcer formation. **Rationale: Immobilized clients are particularly vulnerable.**

2. Carefully inspect the skin for evidence of pressure and impending breakdown. **Rationale: These data provide a baseline to determine changes in client's skin.**

3. Review client's temperature and serum electrolytes. **Rationale: Body fluids may be lost through diaphoresis.**

4. Assess client's emotional response and level of orientation. **Rationale: Flotation effect may cause altered sensory perceptions.**

5. Identify clients at risk for complications of air-fluidized therapy:

   a. Older adult clients may become dehydrated from the airflow, which may increase insensible fluid losses.

   b. Clients receiving enteric tube feedings are at risk for aspiration because of the inability to elevate head of bed, which is limited to placing foam wedges under client's head and shoulders.

   c. Clients who have limited ability to change positions and who are susceptible to dehydration may have tenacious pulmonary secretions that are difficult to remove.

PLANNING

Expected outcomes focus on maintenance of skin integrity and adequate electrolyte balance and the client's comfort.

Expected Outcomes

1. Skin remains warm, clean, and intact, or there is evidence of healing of pressure ulcers.

2. Client rates comfort level as acceptable.

3. Skin remains well hydrated, with good turgor; mucous membranes are moist; and electrolytes are in normal range.

4. Client remains alert and oriented or shows no change in level of consciousness.

IMPLEMENTATION

Steps	Rationale
NURSE ALERT *Review manufacturer's instructions. (Company representative may be in attendance.)* *Premedicate client 30 minutes before transfer if needed. Obtain additional personnel as needed.*	Ensures proper and safe use of bed. Promotes comfort during transfer for those clients in moderate to severe pain. Aids in ensuring client's safety. Company representatives ensure proper functioning of bed.
1. See Standard Protocol (inside front cover). 2. Transfer client onto air-fluidized bed using appropriate transfer techniques (see Chapter 6). A slide or lift may be used.	A slide or lift is needed to maneuver client over the rigid sides of the bed.
COMMUNICATION TIP *Tell client that there may be a sensation of floating or nausea when first placed on the bed. Encourage client to move and use upper extremities and participate in ROM exercise because fluidization accelerates muscle weakness.*	
3. Depress *on* switch to begin fluidization; regulate temperature.	Fluidization relieves pressure on the skin.
4. Position client and perform ROM exercises routinely. Foam wedges may be needed to place client in a Fowler's position.	Positioning and ROM exercises are necessary to prevent pulmonary complications and contractures.

Steps	**Rationale**
5. Use fluidization switch to harden bed for turning, positioning bedpans, and other procedures. Remember to reactivate fluidization after procedure.	When fluidization is stopped, the bed becomes firm, allowing for ease in positioning. Reactivation of fluidization is necessary to minimize pressure.

NURSE ALERT

Activate CPR switch when resuscitation is necessary.

NURSE ALERT

Allows for hard surface to perform manual chest compressions.

6. Obtain assistance when positioning client.	Reduces risk of friction and shear forces, as well as preventing self-injury.
7. Use of a wedge facilitates elevating the head of the client for position changes. Areas supported by the foam wedge are not getting any benefit of the special bed.	Air-fluidized bed does not have capacity to raise head of bed.
8. Inspect bony prominences and heels for signs of pressure every 8 to 12 hours. Avoid use of underpads.	Underpads interfere with the therapeutic effects of the bed.
9. Replace soiled sheets as needed; soiled sheets are sent to the rental company for cleaning.	
10. Maintain adequate nutritional and fluid intake.	Promotes tissue healing and helps prevent skin breakdown (see Chapter 24).
11. See Completion Protocol (inside front cover).	

• • • •

EVALUATION

1. Inspect condition of skin periodically to determine changes in skin and effectiveness of air-fluidized therapy.
2. Ask client to rate level of comfort on a scale of 0 to 10.
3. Observe moisture of client's skin and mucous membranes and skin turgor. Monitor client's temperature and laboratory serum electrolytes
4. Evaluate client's emotional response and orientation to flotation. Assess client's level of orientation.

Unexpected Outcomes and Related Interventions

1. Client develops areas of breakdown, or existing areas of breakdown worsen.
   a. Evaluate and revise turning schedule as needed.
   b. Keep skin clean and dry.
   c. Reevaluate the client's risk factors affecting wound healing.
   d. Notify physician. Advancement of existing pressure ulcer may be related to tissue necrosis, infection, nutritional deficiencies, or other systemic factors.

2. Client experiences agitation, restlessness, or disorientation related to flotation.
   a. Reposition for comfort.
   b. Provide reassurance and emotional support. Encourage client to verbalize concerns.
   c. Notify physician. Symptomatic treatment may be necessary while adjusting to constant flotation.
   d. If unable to adjust to flotation, evaluate the need for alternative measures.
3. Client's skin and mucous membranes are dehydrated and serum electrolytes are abnormal related to the temperature and evaporative effects of the bed.
   a. Evaluate nutritional and fluid status, including intake and output.
   b. Increase fluid intake unless contraindicated.
   c. Collaborate with physician for other treatment modalities.
4. The filter sheet tears, expelling small sandlike particles in the air.
   a. Cover the puncture site to prevent particles from getting on client and wounds.
   b. Promptly follow the institution's policy to obtain a replacement. Client may need to be transferred to another bed while corrective measures are taking place.

Recording and Reporting

1. Record transfer of client to bed, tolerance to procedure, and condition of skin in nurse's notes or skin assessment flow sheet.
2. Report changes in condition of skin and electrolyte levels to nurse in charge or to physician.
3. Report change in orientation.

Sample Documentation

1600   Client transferred onto air-fluidized bed without incident. Skin warm, dry, and intact. Mucous membranes moist. A 3-cm reddened area noted to sacrum with brisk capillary refill. Client oriented to person, place, and time. Rates comfort as 6 on a scale of 0 to 10.

Geriatric Considerations

- Older adult clients are at increased risk for dehydration.
- When hospitalized, older adult clients may experience intensified flotation of the air-fluidized bed or air-suspension bed.

Home Care and Long-Term Care Considerations

- Beds weigh between 1700 and 2100 pounds; therefore the rental company leasing the bed needs to inspect the home for accessibility and structural support.
- Rental company is responsible for cleaning the tank of microspheres at regular intervals, usually every 1 to 4 weeks, depending on need as body fluids drain into bed.

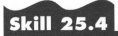

USING A ROTOKINETIC BED

The Rotokinetic bed is used to maintain skeletal alignment while providing constant rotation. It is used in the care of spinal cord–injured and multitrauma clients. The support structure of the bed outlines the body parts and maintains proper alignment when secured properly. The bed rotates from side to side at a 60- to 90-degree angle every 7 minutes. Turning angles may be adjusted to meet the client's needs. Constant rotation reduces pressure ulcer development and stimulates body systems. It is recommended that the bed stay in the rotation mode for at least 20 hours a day. There is an emergency gatch that can quickly interrupt rotation when needed.

The constant motion may lead to sensory distress for the client, especially older adults. This may be associated with the constant kinetic stimulation, the limited visual field, and inner ear disequilibrium. The nurse must be mindful of these complications and provide necessary emotional support.

A physician's order is required for third-party payment.

Equipment

Rotokinetic bed with support packs, bolsters, and safety straps (Figure 25-6, p. 612)
Top sheet
Pillowcases for bolsters

ASSESSMENT

1. Identify clients who require complete immobilization and continuous skeletal alignment.
2. Carefully inspect the skin for evidence of pressure. **Rationale: Proper position is critical to hold position and prevent pressure and shear.**
3. Assess the client's level of consciousness, orientation, and anxiety.
4. Assess client's breath sounds, blood pressure, height, and weight.
5. Assess the client's and family members' understanding of and response to the Rotokinetic bed.

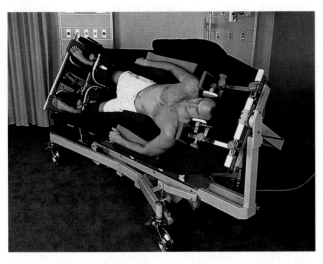

Figure 25-6 Rotokinetic bed. *Courtesy Kinetic Concepts, Inc [KCI], San Antonio, Tex.*

PLANNING

Expected outcomes are concerned with maintaining skin integrity and proper body alignment, promoting client comfort, decreasing client's anxiety, preventing pulmonary congestion, and maintaining skin integrity.

Expected Outcomes

1. Client's skin remains intact without evidence of abnormal reactive hyperemia or mottling.
2. Existing pressure ulcers show evidence of healing.
3. Client's musculoskeletal system is properly aligned and free of contractures.
4. Client's breath sounds improve from baseline assessment or remain clear to auscultation.
5. Client remains alert, oriented, and cooperative.
6. Client denies nausea or dizziness.
7. Client's blood pressure remains consistent with baseline vital signs.

DELEGATION CONSIDERATIONS

The skill of preparation of a Rotokinetic bed can be delegated to AP; however, assessment, teaching, and evaluation are not. When delegating the care of a client on a Rotokinetic bed, stress the importance of maintaining bed rotation and routine inspection of the skin for tissue trauma. The AP needs to notify the professional nurse of changes in skin condition and concerns expressed by the client.

IMPLEMENTATION

Steps	Rationale

NURSE ALERT

Review manufacturer's instructions. (Company representatives may be in attendance.)

Steps	Rationale
1. See Standard Protocol (inside front cover).	
2. Premedicate client 30 minutes before transfer if needed.	Promotes comfort during transfer.
3. Place Rotokinetic bed in horizontal position and remove all bolsters, straps, and supports. Close posterior hatches.	
4. Unplug electrical cord. Lock gatch.	Prevents accidental rotation during transfer.
5. Maintaining proper alignment, transfer client to Rotokinetic bed.	Reduces risk of further tissue injury during transfer. May need physician available to assist in transfer.
6. Secure thoracic panels, bolsters, head and knee packs, and safety straps.	Maintains proper alignment and prevents sliding during rotation.
7. Cover client with top sheet.	
8. Plug bed in.	
9. Have company representative set rotational angle as ordered by the physician. May gradually increase rotation.	Rotational angle is determined by the physician based on the client's overall condition and tolerance to constant motion. Gradually increasing rotation may prevent nausea and dizziness.

Steps	Rationale

10. Increase degree of rotation gradually according to client's ability to tolerate it.
11. It is difficult to maintain eye contact when talking with clients during rotation. Provide adequate space for caregivers and family to move around the bed to facilitate communication.
12. The bed may be stopped for assessment and procedures. To stop the bed, permit bed to rotate to the desired position, turn the motor off, and push knob into a lock position. If necessary the bed can be manually repositioned.
13. See Completion Protocol (inside front cover).

COMMUNICATION TIP

Tell the client that there may be a sensation of light headedness or falling. However the client will not fall because the pads are positioned to prevent this and are checked by two people to ensure proper placement.

NURSE ALERT

Manual rotation may cause nausea or dizziness if done too rapidly. Keep bed stopped for no longer than 30 minutes at a time.

• • •

EVALUATION

1. Inspect condition of skin (occiput, ears, axillae, elbows, sacrum, groin, and heels) and musculoskeletal alignment every 2 hours to determine changes in skin and effectiveness of Rotokinetic therapy.
2. Inspect client's pressure ulcers for evidence of healing.
3. Observe alignment and range of motion of all joints.
4. Auscultate lung sounds every shift and compare with baseline.
5. Determine client's level of orientation once per shift while on the bed.
6. Ask whether client is experiencing nausea or dizziness.
7. Monitor blood pressure for orthostatic hypotension.

Unexpected Outcomes and Related Interventions

1. Client develops areas of breakdown, or existing areas of breakdown worsen.
   a. Evaluate rotation schedule, because bed should stay in rotation for 20 hours a day to prevent breakdown.
   b. Keep skin clean and dry. Change linen on bolsters as needed.
2. Client experiences orthostatic hypotension.
   a. If severe drop in blood pressure, stop rotation. Notify physician. Monitor vital signs every 5 minutes.
   b. For less severe blood pressure changes, decrease the rotational angle. Gradually increase the rotational angle as client adjusts to rotation.
3. Client becomes disoriented, confused, or uncooperative related to sensory/perceptual distortion.
   a. Reorient client to person, place, and time.
   b. Provide audio simulation via radio or tape recorder.
   c. Provide TV secured to bed frame (available from manufacturer).

   d. Hang mirror on ceiling so that client may view surroundings.
   e. Notify physician. Symptomatic treatment for motion sickness may be helpful.
4. Client develops crackles in lung fields.
   a. Have client cough and deep breathe every 2 hours.
   b. Notify physician. Incentive spirometry or other treatment measures may be warranted.
5. Bed malfunctions or fails to rotate.
   a. Ensure safety of client.
   b. Follow institutional policies to correct situation. Client may need to be transferred to conventional hospital bed in the interim.

Recording and Reporting

• Describe the condition of skin prior to placement on the Rotokinetic bed. A photograph may be taken to document skin condition and provide a baseline for later assessments for progress in healing.
• Time of transfer to Rotokinetic bed and the degree of rotation.
• Subjective data indicating response to the constant rotation and presence/absence of dizziness, nausea, or blood pressure changes.
• A flow sheet may be used to document routine assessment and care, including the length of time the bed rotation is stopped. The bed needs to be rotating at least 20 hours out of every 24 hours and stopped for no more than 30 minutes at a time.

Sample Documentation

0930 Client transferred to a Rotokinetic bed to prevent skin breakdown. Skin intact. An area of redness noted on sacrum 4 inches in diameter, and both heels are reddened. Initial rotation begun at 30 degrees without c/o nausea or dizziness. BP stable at 130/74.

Skill 25.5

USING A BARIATRIC BED

A **morbidly obese** client (a person who weighs more than 100 pounds above ideal weight) may benefit from a bariatric bed. The **bariatric bed** is capable of allowing upright or sitting positioning, client transport, and in-bed scales (Figure 25-7). The bed is equipped with hand controls that allow self-positioning and facilitate independence for the obese client. Because the bariatric bed is capable of supporting weights up to 850 pounds, it provides a stable, balanced surface.

The full-function hand controls allow the nurse caring for the obese client to change the bed position and thus facilitate care while reducing risk of staff injury in moving the client. The in-bed scale provides the nurse with a means of obtaining accurate weights, which is frequently a problem with the obese client, and thus improves health care and client dignity. The bed is slightly wider than a standard hospital bed, yet it is within the guidelines for standard door width and allows movement into and out of a room without difficulty.

The at-risk obese client should have some type of pressure-relief mattress placed on the bariatric bed. Choices for pressure relief may include static air or gel-type mattresses. Several manufacturers have low-air-loss mattress overlays and low-air-loss mattress replacement systems for the bariatric bed.

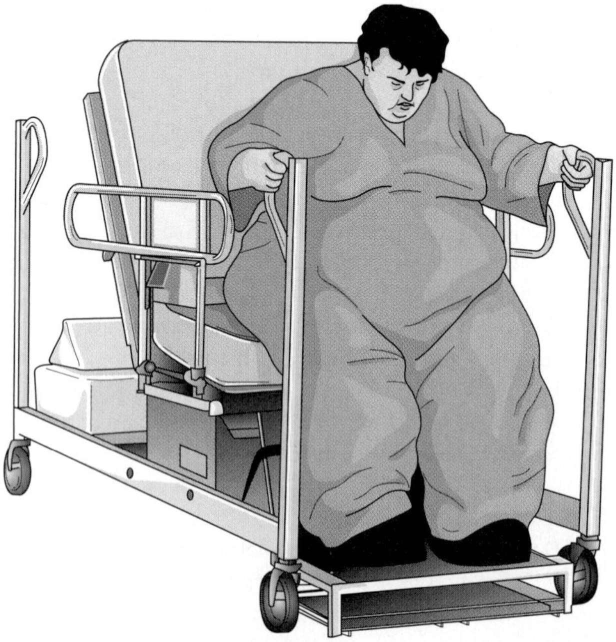

Another type of bed for the bariatric client is a full or double-wide bed. These beds are available for rent or purchase and are equipped to accommodate a patient weighing up to 1000 pounds. The extrawide bed is usually constructed from two or three pieces in a client's room. Because this bed will not move through a doorway, another means of moving the client from the room in case of emergency must be available. Available for rent with the oversized bed are extrawide heavy-duty wheelchairs, commodes, lift equipment, scales, and walkers. This "room of furniture" generally requires a private room for the client and is made to maximize the client's independence with staff and client safety in mind.

Equipment

Bariatric bed
Pressure relief overlay
Sheets
Overhead frame (optional)
Heavy-duty lift (optional)

ASSESSMENT

1. Determine client's need for bed based on height and weight. **Rationale: Morbidly obese clients who have the potential for independent positioning with assistance of a stable surface will benefit from the use of a bariatric bed.**
2. Assess condition of skin. Note condition of skin between skinfolds. Note potential pressure sites. **Rationale: Determine need for client to have a low-air-loss or other pressure-relieving surface on the bed.**
3. Assess client's and family members' understanding of purpose of bed.
4. Review client's medical orders. **Rationale: A physician's order is required to obtain reimbursement in the United States.**

PLANNING

Expected outcomes are concerned with safety, maximum independence, and maintaining skin integrity.

Expected Outcomes

1. Client is able to reposition independently for comfort.
2. Client remains free of injury.
3. Client's skin remains intact without abnormal reactive hyperemia.

Figure 25-7 The bariatric bed eliminates unnecessary patient transfers. *Courtesy Burke, Inc, Mission, Kan.*

DELEGATION CONSIDERATIONS

The skill of preparation for a bariatric bed may be delegated to AP. Be sure adequate assistance is available to reduce risk of friction and shearing forces and to prevent injury to client and care givers.

IMPLEMENTATION

Steps	Rationale
1. See Standard Protocol (Inside front cover).	
2. Position four to six persons around the stretcher or bed to allow a distribution of the client's weight during the lift.	
3. Place a pull sheet under the client and transfer safely.	Minimizes trauma to client's skin from shearing forces as client is moved.
4. Position the client for comfort with hand controls and trapeze bar within reach.	Encourages maximum independence and mobility.
5. Encourage client to initiate frequent position changes and to move about in the bed as much as possible. It may be helpful to suggest linking movement to some external cue (such as commercials on TV).	
6. See Completion Protocol (inside front cover).	

NURSE ALERT

Consider the use of a heavy-duty lift. For clients over 850 pounds cargo netting may be used (available from the local fire department).

• • •

EVALUATION
1. Observe client's ability to manipulate the bed and change positions independently for comfort.
2. Assess client's risk for injury.
3. Inspect client's skin every 8 hours for evidence of breakdown.

Unexpected Outcomes and Related Interventions
1. Client is unable to operate bed independently.
   a. Assist client as needed.
   b. Consult physician regarding physical therapy or occupational therapy evaluation to increase mobility or to provide facilitative devices.
2. Client develops areas of skin breakdown, or existing areas worsen.
   a. Reevaluate need for support surface in use.
   b. Evaluate turning schedule. May need to change or shift position more frequently than every 2 hours.

Recording and Reporting
• Record transfer of client to bed, subjective response, and condition of skin in nurse's notes or skin assessment flow sheet.
• Report changes in condition of skin.

Sample Documentation
1000   Transferred to bariatric bed. Client demonstrated use of hand controls and trapeze bar. Skin without erythema or evidence of breakdown.

Home Care and Long-Term Care Considerations

• Full-size bariatric (Size-Wise, Equitron, etc.) bed and room of equipment is well suited for the long-term care and rehabilitation setting and is available for purchase for use in the home.
• Persons of extreme obesity who are immobile should alert their local emergency service personnel. This will ensure that in case of an emergency they will have adequate equipment and personnel available to meet the client's needs.

CRITICAL THINKING EXERCISES

1. Mrs. C. is a thin 69-year-old bedridden client admitted today from home. You perform a risk assessment for skin breakdown and find her risk for breakdown is high. Mrs. C. and her husband prefer a "firm" mattress.
   a. What category of mattress/bed should you consider for a patient at high risk for breakdown?
   b. You know that pressure relief mattresses and beds are not typically "firm." How and what will you present to Mr. and Mrs. C.?

2. Mr. M. has been on an air-fluidized bed for management of a large sacral pressure ulcer. The wound has improved, and Mr. M. is ready to begin rehabilitation to optimize his independence. Today his risk assessment for skin breakdown has improved to "at risk."
   a. What features of the air-fluidized bed will provide a challenge to beginning rehabilitation and attaining independence?
   b. What bed/mattress might you recommend to the physician for Mr. M.?

3. In addition to skin assessment, what information should you gather when caring for a client placed on an air-fluidized bed?

4. You are caring for a 17-year-old client who sustained a cervical spine injury after diving into a shallow stream. He is on a Rotokinetic bed. What can you do to facilitate his adjustment to the bed and provide some distraction?

5. You are caring for a toddler with a 60% body burn. The burn is largely over the toddler's back and buttocks, making positioning difficult. What special bed/mattress might be considered for this toddler during grafting and healing?

REFERENCES

Bryant, RA: *Acute and chronic wounds: nursing management,* St Louis, 1992, Mosby.

Fowler EM: Equipment and products used in management and treatment of pressure ulcers, *Nurs Clin North Am* 22(7):449, 1987.

Krouskop T, van Rijswijk L: Standardizing performance-based criteria for support surfaces, *Ostomy/Wound Manage* 41(1):34, 1995.

Panel for the Prediction and Prevention of Pressure Ulcers in Adults: *Pressure ulcers in adults: prediction and prevention,* Clinical practice guideline AHCPR Pub No 92-0047, Rockville, Md, 1992, US Department of Health and Human Services, Agency for Health Care Policy and Research.

Seila WO, Stahelin HB: Efficient pressure ulcer prevention using a new automatic pressure relieving mattress system, *Wounds* 4(3):108, 1992.

CHAPTER 26

Promoting Range of Motion

Skill 26.1
Range-of-Motion Exercises,   618

Skill 26.2
**Continuous Passive Motion (CPM) Machine
(for Client with Total Knee Replacement),   632**

The range of motion of a joint is the maximum movement that is possible for that joint. Each person's range is determined by genetic inheritance, developmental patterns, the presence or absence of disease, and the person's normal amount of physical activity.

Range-of-motion (ROM) exercises have a number of purposes: (1) to restore or maintain strength of the muscles; (2) to maintain or increase the flexibility of the joints; (3) to maintain or promote the growth of bones through application of physical stressors; (4) to improve the functioning of other body systems, such as the cardiovascular and gastrointestinal systems, and (5) to prevent contractures.

Altered health status increases a client's risk for impaired mobility. Each system may then be at risk for impairment. Examples of conditions that can alter mobility are musculoskeletal conditions such as fractured extremities or muscle sprains, neurological conditions such as spinal cord trauma, degenerative neurological conditions such as myasthenia gravis, and head injuries. Some clients may not actually be immobilized by an injury or musculoskeletal problem but are prescribed bed rest or restricted ambulation for therapeutic conditions or medical problems (Perry and Potter, 1998).

Regardless of whether the causes of immobility are permanent or temporary, the immobilized client must receive some type of exercise to prevent excessive muscle atrophy and joint contracture.

Nurses need to assess clients for individual mobility levels. If the client is mobile and can move about freely, the client can independently perform activities of daily living (ADLs) and ROM exercises. If the client is partially immobile or unable to move about freely (paraplegic, quadriplegic), the nurse or a mechanical device is needed to assist the client with ROM exercises.

Nurses are responsible for assessing the need for and implementing interventions to prevent pulmonary and circulatory complications associated with immobility. Nursing measures attempt to maintain and/or restore optimal mobility and to decrease the hazards associated with immobility (Hamilton and Lyon, 1995). Frequent interventions used to prevent complications include coughing and deep-breathing exercises, frequent repositioning and turning to prevent problems with skin integrity, upper and lower extremity exercises to prevent contracture of the joint and shortening of the muscle, adequate hydration, and well-balanced meals to maintain muscle strength and endurance. It is important to initiate ROM exercises early. The client will profit by actively participating in the level of care, which decreases length of stay and the risk for further impairment in body functions (Beare and Myers, 1998).

NURSING DIAGNOSES

Risk for Impaired Physical Mobility is appropriate when the inability to move independently could result in the development of contractures or decreased strength and endurance. **Altered Health Maintenance** may be related to lack of knowledge or difficulty following through with prescribed ROM exercises.

Skill 26.1

RANGE-OF-MOTION EXERCISES

Range-of-motion exercises may be active, passive, or active assisted or resisted. They are *active* if the client is able to perform the exercise independently and *passive* if the exercises are performed for the client by someone else.

Active assisted ROM exercises are performed by a client with some assistance (Dawe and Curran-Smith, 1994). A client who is weak or partially paralyzed may be able to move a limb partially through its ROM. In this case the nurse can help the client perform active-assisted ROM exercises by helping the client finish the full ROM. Another form of active-assisted ROM exercise is when a client uses the strong arm to exercise the weaker or paralyzed arm.

The nurse should always encourage the client to be as independent as possible. Active ROM exercises should be encouraged and supervised every day by the nurse. Active ROM exercises can be incorporated into the client's ADLs (Table 26-1).

Equipment

No mechanical or physical equipment is needed.

ASSESSMENT

1. Review client's chart for nurse's physical assessment, physician orders, medical diagnosis, medical history, and progress. **Rationale: Any joint or cardiac conditions aggravated by energy expenditure or joint movement indicate need for nursing judgment whether to consult the physician before beginning exercises.**

2. Assess client's or caregiver's readiness to learn. Explain all rationales for the ROM exercises and describe exercises to be performed. **Rationale: Allows client time to express questions and concerns before the implementation begins.**

3. Assess client's level of comfort (on a scale of 0 to 10) before exercises. **Rationale: Determines if client will need an analgesic before exercising.**

4. Assess client's ROM for joints to be exercised. **Rationale: Provides baseline to determine changes in ROM.**

Table 26-1

Incorporating Active ROM Exercises into Activities of Daily Living

Joint Exercised	Activity of Daily Living	Movement
Neck	Nodding head yes	Flexion
	Shaking head no	Rotation
	Moving right ear to right shoulder	Lateral flexion
	Moving left ear to left shoulder	Lateral flexion
Shoulder	Reaching to turn on overhead light	Flexion
	Reaching to bedside stand for book	Extension
	Applying deodorant	Abduction
	Combing hair	Flexion
Elbow	Eating, bathing, shaving, grooming	Flexion, extension
Wrist	Eating, bathing, shaving, grooming	Flexion, extension, abduction, adduction
Fingers and thumb	All activities requiring fine motor coordination (e.g., writing, eating, hobbies)	Flexion, extension, abduction, adduction, opposition
Hip	Walking	Flexion, extension
	Moving to side-lying position	Flexion, extension, abduction
	Moving from side-lying position	Extension, adduction
	Rolling feet inward	Internal rotation
	Rolling feet outward	External rotation
Knee	Walking	Flexion, extension
	Moving to and from side-lying position	Flexion, extension
Ankle	Walking	Dorsiflexion, plantar flexion
	Moving toe toward head of bed	Dorsiflexion
	Moving toe toward foot of bed	Plantar flexion
Toes	Walking	Extension, flexion
	Wiggling toes	Abduction, adduction

PLANNING

Expected outcomes focus on maintaining joint ROM and client's physical and emotional ability to perform exercises.

Expected Outcomes

1. Client's range of joint motion remains within normal or maintains baseline range.
2. Client denies discomfort during exercises.
3. Client demonstrates ROM during activities of daily living.
4. Significant other correctly performs passive ROM on client by discharge.

DELEGATION CONSIDERATIONS

The skill of performing range of motion exercises can be delegated to assistive personnel (AP). Clients with spinal cord or orthopedic trauma usually require exercise by professional nurses or physical therapists. The following information is needed when delegating this skill to nursing staff or family members:

- Perform exercises slowly.
- Provide adequate support to joint being exercised.
- Do not exercise joints beyond the point of resistance or to the point of fatigue or pain.

IMPLEMENTATION

Steps	Rationale

1. See Standard Protocol (inside front cover).
2. Wear gloves (only if there is wound drainage or skin lesions).
3. Assist the client to a comfortable position, preferably sitting or lying down.
4. When performing active-assisted or passive ROM exercises, support joint by holding distal and proximal areas adjacent to joint (see illustrations), by cradling distal portion of extremity, or by using cupped hand to support joint.

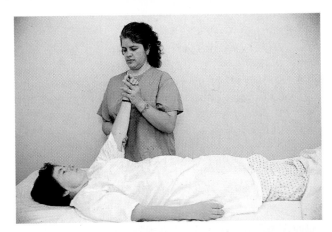

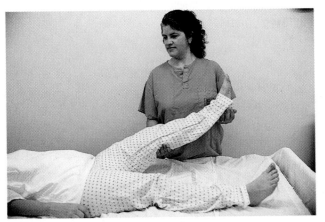

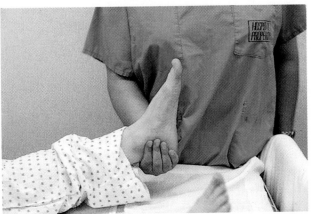

Step 4

Steps	Rationale

COMMUNICATION TIPS

- *Inform client how to incorporate ROM exercises into activities of daily living, such as grooming, bathing, etc. (see Table 26-1 on p. 618).*
- *When chronic mobility problems exist, discuss with client which exercises need to be performed, and the limitation of joint mobility for the affected area.*

- *If client has had recent orthopedic injury or surgery, reinforce how the ROM should feel and how the ROM for the affected joint(s) should progress.*

5. Begin following exercises in sequence outlined. Each movement should be repeated 5 times during exercise period.
    a. **Neck**
        (1) *Flexion:* Bring chin to rest on chest (ROM: 45°) (see illustration).

It is easiest to perform exercises in head-to-toe format.

Adequate ROM in all directions permits satisfactory visual fields and increased level of independence. If flexion contracture of neck occurs, client's neck is permanently flexed with chin toward or actually touching chest. Ultimately, client's total body alignment is altered, visual field is changed, and overall level of independent functioning is decreased.

NURSE ALERT

Discontinue exercise if client complains of discomfort or if there is resistance or muscle spasm. Ranges are measured in degrees (e.g., ROM: 45°).

(2) *Extension:* Return head to erect position (ROM: 45°).
(3) *Hyperextension:* Gently bend head back (ROM: 10°) (see illustration).
(4) *Lateral flexion:* Tilt head toward each shoulder (ROM: 40° to 45°) (see illustration).

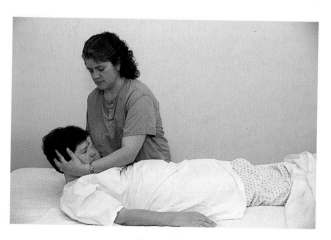

Step 5a(1)

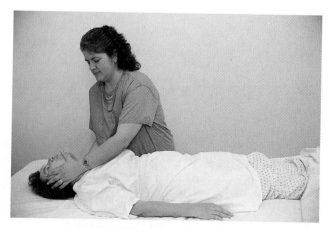

Step 5a(3)

Steps	Rationale

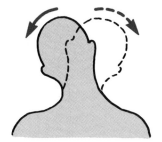

Step 5a(4)

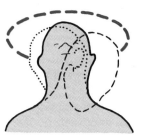

Step 5a(5)

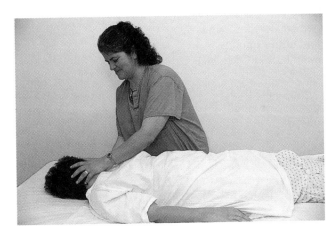

Step 5a(6)

(5) *Rotation:* Rotate head in circular motion (ROM: 360°) (best done in sitting position) (see illustration).

(6) Turn head side to side (see illustration).

b. **Shoulder**

(1) *Flexion:* Raise arm from side position forward to above head (ROM: 180°) (see illustration).

(2) *Extension:* Return arm to position at side of body (ROM: 180°).

Exercising shoulder actively increases power of deltoid muscle and facilitates use of crutches or a walker.

A frozen shoulder makes it impossible to reach overhead and makes dressing difficult.

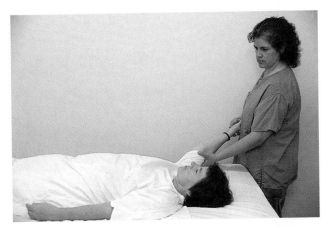

Step 5b(1)

Steps   **Rationale**

(3) *Hyperextension:* Move arm behind body, keeping elbow straight (ROM: 45° to 60°) (see illustration).

(4) *Abduction:* Raise arm to side to position above head with palm away from head (ROM: 180°) (see illustration).

(5) *Adduction:* Lower arm sideways and across body as far as possible (ROM: 320°) (see illustration).

(6) *External rotation:* With elbow flexed, move arm until thumb is upward and lateral to head (ROM: 90°) (see illustration).

(7) *Internal rotation:* With elbow flexed, rotate shoulder by moving arm until thumb is turned inward and toward back (ROM: 90°) (see illustration).

(8) *Circumduction:* Move arm in full circle. Circumduction is a combination of all movements of ball-and-socket joint (ROM: 360°) (see illustration).

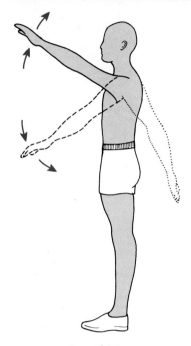

Step 5b(3)

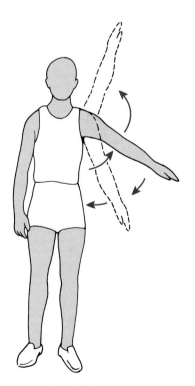

Step 5b(4)

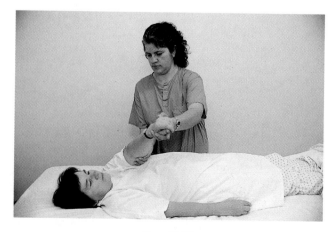

Step 5b(5)

Steps	Rationale

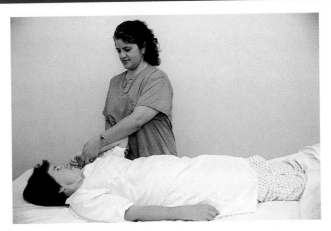

Step 5b(6)

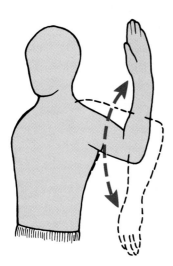

Step 5b(7)

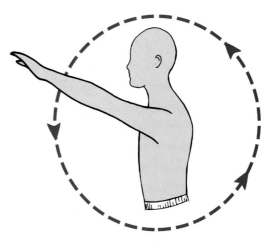

Step 5b(8)

c. **Elbow**
  (1) *Flexion:* Bend elbow so that lower arm moves toward its shoulder joint and hand is level with shoulder (ROM: 150°) (see illustration).
  (2) *Extension:* Straighten elbow by lowering hand (ROM: 150°) (see illustration).
  (3) *Hyperextension:* With arm extended bend lower arm back (ROM: 10° to 20°).

Elbow fixed in full extension or full flexion is very disabling and limits client's independence.

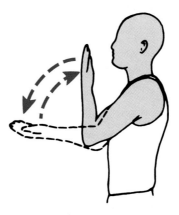

Step 5c(1,2)

Steps	Rationale

d. **Forearm**

(1) *Supination:* Turn lower arm and hand so that palm is up (ROM: 70° to 90°) (see illustration).

(2) *Pronation:* Turn lower arm so that palm is down (ROM: 70° to 90°) (see illustration).

Forearm rotates from supination to pronation.

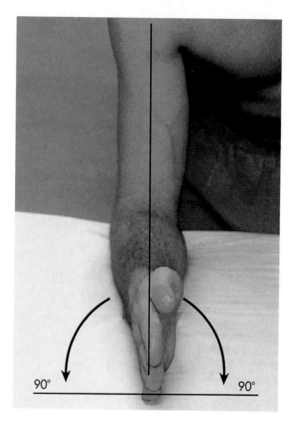

Step 5d(1,2) *From Mourad LA: Orthopedic disorders, Mosby's clinical nursing series, St Louis, 1991, Mosby.*

Steps	**Rationale**

e. **Wrist**

(1) *Flexion:* Move palm toward inner aspect of forearm (ROM: 80° to 90°) (see illustration).

(2) *Extension:* Move palm so fingers, hands, and forearm are in the same plane (ROM: 80° to 90°).

(3) *Hyperextension:* Gently bring dorsal surface of hand back (ROM: 80° to 90°) (see illustration).

(4) *Abduction (radial flexion):* Bend wrist medially toward thumb (ROM: up to 30°) (see illustration).

(5) *Adduction (ulnar flexion):* Bend wrist laterally toward fifth finger (ROM: 30° to 50°) (see illustration).

If wrist becomes fixed in even slightly flexed position, client's grasp is weakened. Wrist strength is necessary to be able to use crutches.

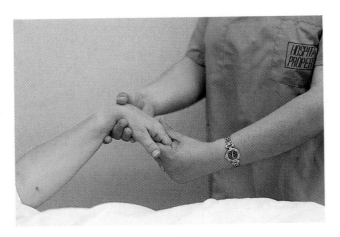

Step 5e(1)

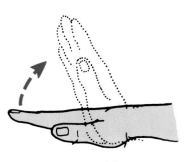

Step 5e(3)

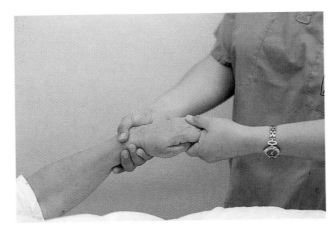

Step 5e(4)

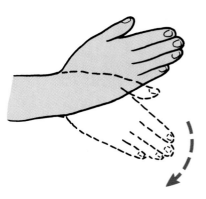

Step 5e(5)

Steps	Rationale

f. **Fingers**

(1) *Flexion:* Make fist (ROM: 90°) (see illustration).

(2) *Extension:* Straighten fingers (ROM: 90°).

(3) *Hyperextension:* Gently bend fingers back (ROM: 30° to 60°) (see illustration).

(4) *Abduction:* Spread fingers apart (ROM: 30°) (see illustration).

(5) *Adduction:* Bring fingers together (ROM: 30°) (see illustration).

Flexibility of fingers and thumb is necessary to grasp items (e.g., holding onto a crutch or using feeding utensils).

If not stretched into extension, natural tendency is for flexion. (In between ROM sessions, client with cerebrovascular accident [CVA] may need a firm device placed in hand to prevent full flexion.)

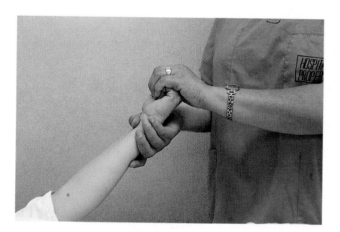

Step 5f(1)

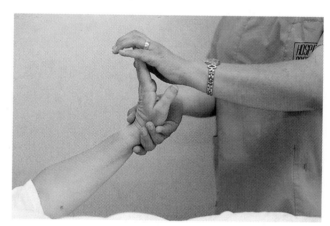

Step 5f(3)

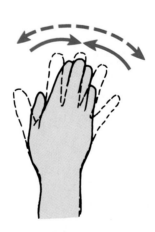

Step 5f(4,5)

Steps	Rationale

g. **Thumb**

(1) *Flexion:* Move thumb across palmar surface of hand (ROM: 90°) (see illustration).

(2) *Extension:* Move thumb straight away from hand (ROM: 90°).

(3) *Abduction:* Extend thumb laterally (usually done when placing fingers in abduction and adduction) (ROM: 30°).

(4) *Adduction:* Move thumb back toward hand (ROM: 30°).

(5) *Opposition:* Touch thumb to each finger of same hand (see illustration).

Flexibility of thumb maintains coordination for fine motor activities.

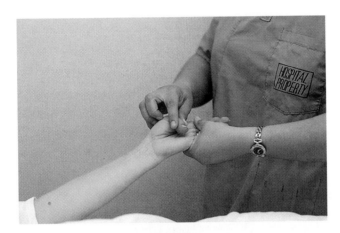

Step 5g(1)

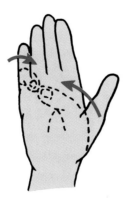

Step 5g(5)

Steps	Rationale

h. **Hip**

   (1) *Flexion:* Move leg forward and up (ROM: 90° to 120°) (see illustration).

   (2) *Extension:* Move leg back beside other leg (ROM: 90° to 120°).

   (3) *Hyperextension:* Move leg behind body (best done standing or lying on abdomen) (ROM: 30° to 50°) (see illustration).

   (4) *Abduction:* Move leg laterally away from body (ROM: 30° to 50°) (see illustration).

   (5) *Adduction:* Move leg back toward medial position and beyond if possible (ROM: 30° to 50°) (see illustration).

   (6) *Internal rotation:* Turn foot and leg toward other leg (ROM: 90°) (see illustration).

   (7) *External rotation:* Turn foot and leg away from other leg (ROM: 90°).

   (8) *Circumduction:* Move leg in circle (ROM: 360°) (see illustration).

Adequate ROM in lower extremities (i.e., hip, knee, ankle, foot) allows client to walk with stable gait. Contracture of hip can cause unsteady gait or difficulty ambulating.

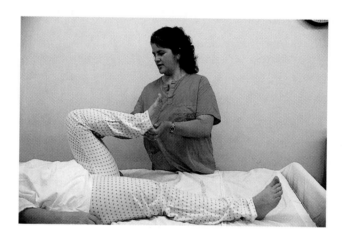

Step 5h(1)

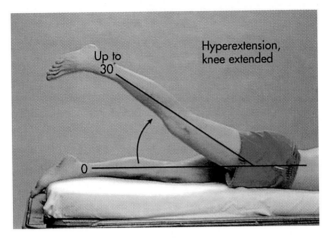

Step 5h(3) *From Mourad LA: Orthopedic disorders, Mosby's clinical nursing series, St Louis, 1991, Mosby.*

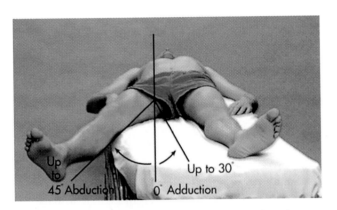

Step 5h(4,5) *From Mourad LA: Orthopedic disorders, Mosby's clinical nursing series, St Louis, 1991, Mosby.*

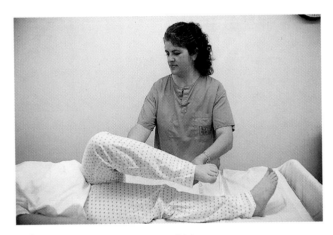

Step 5h(6)

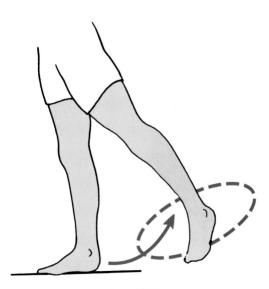

Step 5h(8)

Steps	Rationale

i. **Knee**
  (1) *Flexion:* Bring heel toward back of thigh (done with hip flexion) (ROM: 120° to 130°) (see illustration).
  (2) *Extension:* Return leg to straight position on bed (ROM: 120° to 130°) (see illustration).

Stiff knee can result in severe disability, degree of which depends on position in which knee is stiffened. If knee is fixed in full extension, client must sit with leg thrust straight out in front. If knee is fixed in any flexed position, client limps when walking or may be unable to "touch down" with foot.

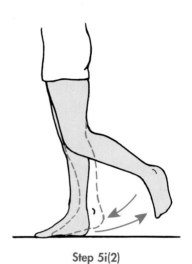

Step 5i(2)

j. **Ankle**
  (1) *Plantar flexion:* Move foot so toes are pointed downward (ROM: 45° to 50°) (see illustration).
  (2) *Dorsal flexion:* Move foot so toes are pointed upward (ROM: 20° to 30°) (see illustration).

Deformity of ankle can impair client's ability to walk.

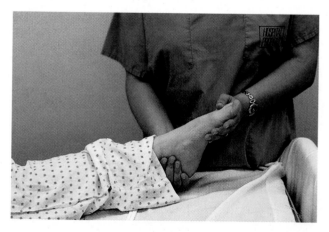

Step 5j(1)

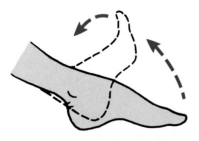

Step 5j(2)

Steps | Rationale

k. **Foot**
   (1) *Inversion:* Turn sole of foot medially (ROM: 10° or less) (see illustration).
   (2) *Eversion:* Turn sole of foot laterally (ROM: 10° or less) (see illustration).
   (3) *Flexion:* Curl toes downward (ROM: 30° to 60°).
   (4) *Extension:* Straighten toes (ROM: 30° to 60°).
   (5) *Abduction:* Spread toes apart (ROM: 15° or less).
   (6) *Adduction:* Bring toes together (ROM: 15° or less).
6. See Completion Protocol (inside front cover).

Adequate ROM of foot permits steady gait and stable base of support.
Adequate ROM in lower extremities allows client to walk.

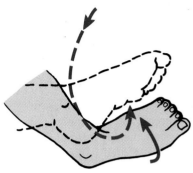

Step 5k(1,2)

• • •

EVALUATION
1. Observe client performing ROM activities; measure ROM as needed.
2. Ask client to rate any discomfort on a scale from 0 to 10.
3. Ask client to demonstrate active ROM exercises during selected ADLs.
4. Observe caregiver performing passive ROM exercises on client.

Unexpected Outcomes and Related Interventions
1. Client experiences discomfort with ROM exercises.
   a. Reposition client to a comfortable position.
   b. Premedicate client 30 minutes before ROM exercises begin, if necessary.
   c. Determine cause of discomfort.
2. Client cannot perform ROM exercises correctly.
   a. Assess joint ROM and note any limitations.
   b. Demonstrate specific exercises to client caregiver thoroughly.

Recording and Reporting
• Record joints exercised, type of exercise, degree of joint motion, any joint abnormalities, and client's activity tolerance.
• Report immediately any resistance to range of joint motion; pain on ROM; swelling, heat or redness in joint.

Sample Documentation
090   Client able to correctly perform hip flexion > 90 degrees 5 times without sign of fatigue.

1300   Client incorrectly performed hip flexion exercises. Client reinstructed on correct technique; was able to correctly perform hip flexion exercises > 90 degrees 5 times without signs of fatigue. Client verbalized understanding of the correct and incorrect way to perform the specific ROM exercises.

Geriatric Considerations
• Older adults who have chronic illnesses may need ROM exercises in two or more sessions to control fatigue.

Home Care and Long-Term Care Considerations
• Assess family member or primary caregiver's ability, availability, and motivation to assist client with exercises client is unable to perform independently.
• Assist family or primary caregiver to arrange home environment to promote exercise program (e.g., space allocation, lighting, temperature, safety precautions).
• Consult physical therapist for additional assistance or exercises and client's response to exercise program.

Skill 26.2

CONTINUOUS PASSIVE MOTION (CPM) MACHINE (FOR CLIENT WITH TOTAL KNEE REPLACEMENT)

The continuous passive motion (CPM) machines are designed to exercise many different joints, including the hip, ankle, shoulder, wrist, and fingers. Orthopedic surgeons routinely order a knee CPM machine postoperatively for a total knee arthroplasty (replacement). Continuous passive motion may be initiated on the day of surgery or on the first postoperative day, according to individual surgeon's preference. CPM machines are also used often in outpatient physical therapy or home health settings. The most common CPM used is the knee CPM (Lawrence, 1996).

The purpose of the CPM machine is to mobilize the knee joint to prevent contracture, muscle atrophy, venous stasis, and thromboembolism. Passive movement of the joint can replace more strenuous exercises during the first few postoperative days. Properly used, the CPM can decrease complications and shorten a client's hospital stay. If initiated on the day of surgery, heavier wound drainage should be expected (Johnson, 1993; Montgomery and Eliasson, 1996).

The electronically controlled CPM machine flexes and extends the knee to a desired degree and at a set speed as ordered by the physician. There are many different brands and models. They differ slightly, but each includes a full-length leg cradle hinged at the knee and ankle, a foot support, a motor controller, an electric plug, and an on/off switch. The foot support and the cradle frame adjust to fit the length of the client's thigh and calf. The frame is metal or plastic. Sheepskin or liners are available from most manufacturers. Velcro straps attached to the liner loosely strap the leg to the cradle. When the device is turned on, the frame slides slowly back and forth, gently moving the joint through preset ROM (Birdsall, 1986).

Before the CPM can be adjusted, it is applied to the client's affected lower extremity. This process will take two hospital personnel because the CPM is heavy and weighs approximately 20 to 25 pounds. Using two hospital personnel will (1) prevent damage to the client's knee and (2) prevent unnecessary strain on the staff's backs.

Equipment
CPM machine and sheepskin that is applied to the CPM (Figure 26-1).

ASSESSMENT
1. Check the machine for electrical safety.
2. Assess the setup of the machine before placing on bed: check the stability of the frame, the flexion/extension controls, speed controls, and the on/off switch. **Rationale: This ensures that all pieces of the equipment are operational and will prevent damage to the client's knee.**
3. Assess the client for comfort before and during use. **Rationale: This determines if the client will be able to tolerate the CPM at the ordered flexion and extension.**
4. Assess the client's ability and willingness to learn about the CPM machine.
5. Assess client's ROM before therapy begins.

PLANNING
Expected outcomes focus on improving joint ROM, maintaining physical mobility, and skin integrity.

Expected Outcomes
1. Client increases length of time in CPM machine by 2 hours every day with no evidence of increased heart rate or increased blood pressure.
2. Client increases flexion 6 to 7 degrees daily (Chiarello, Gunderson, and O'Halloran, 1997).
3. Client maintains intact skin throughout use of CPM.

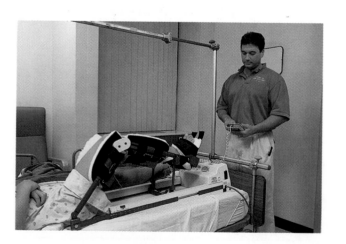

Figure 26-1

DELEGATION CONSIDERATIONS

The skill of using the CPM machine requires problem solving and knowledge unique to a professional nurse and should not be delegated. The RN should inform AP about potential side effects of the CPM, for example, increased pain, skin breakdown, joint inflammation, and to report their occurrence.

IMPLEMENTATION

Steps	Rationale
1. See Standard Protocol (inside front cover).	
2. 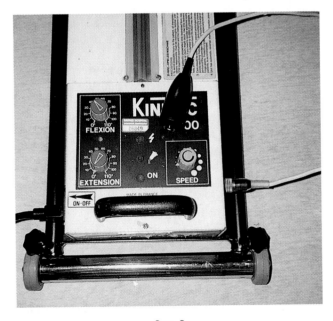 Wear gloves (if wound drainage is present).	
3. Test all CPM controls to make sure they are functional (see illustration).	Testing equipment first saves time for nurse and client. A malfunctioning machine can cause damage to client's knee and may increase client's pain.
4. Stop the machine in full extension.	This position allows correct fit of client's leg.
5. Place client's leg in the machine, being sure to support above, below, and at knee.	Two nurses perform this step to prevent damage or injury to client or nurse.
6. Fit CPM machine to client by lengthening and shortening appropriate section of the CPM frame.	Ensures a proper fit.
7. Align client's knee joint (bend of the knee) with the machine knee hinge, then position the client's knee 2 cm below knee joint line of the CPM.	This is extremely important because if the client's new knee is not properly aligned, the knee may be damaged.
8. Center client's leg in the machine to avoid pressure on the lateral and medial aspects of the knee joint. Adjust the foot support to approximately 20 degrees of dorsiflexion to prevent footdrop.	Footdrop is an abnormal condition caused by damage of the peroneal nerve and can cause abnormal gait.

COMMUNICATION TIP

- *Before initiating CPM it may be helpful to demonstrate the actual functioning of the machine.*
- *Before initiating CPM discuss diversional activities with client that he might do during CPM, for example, read, watch TV, hobbies, etc. Ensure that materials for these activities are in easy reach of the client.*

Step 3

Steps	Rationale
9. When client's leg is in correct position, secure the Velcro straps across lower extremity (thigh) and top of foot (see illustration).	Correct placement of the thigh and foot straps prevents friction and skin breakdown.
10. Start CPM machine. Watch at least two full cycles of prescribed flexion and extension. Remove and discard gloves, if worn, and wash hands.	Ensures that CPM machine is fully operational at the preset flexion and extension modes (Sheppard, Westlake, and McQuarrie, 1995).
11. Make sure client is comfortable. Provide client with the on/off switch. Instruct to use only if CPM seems to be malfunctioning.	Allows client to stop the machine if the degree of flexion/extension or speed changes, creating intolerable discomfort.
12. See Completion Protocol (inside front cover).	

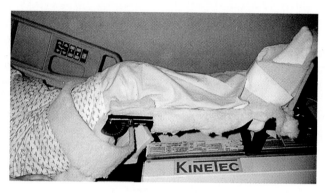

Step 9

• • • •

EVALUATION

1. Ask client to keep a log of when the CPM machine is in use, with times and dates.
2. Observe client at the initial onset of an increase in the flexion of the machine.
3. Measure joint ROM achieved with CPM machine.
4. Observe skin every 2 hours for signs of breakdown.

Unexpected Outcomes and Related Interventions

NOTE: Because of new insurance guidelines regarding length of stay in the hospital, most clients are discharged after a relatively short period. If the client needs additional physical therapy to maintain function of the new knee replacement and to increase flexion, client may be placed in a temporary rehabilitation facility or be sent home with a CPM machine.

1. Client cannot increase flexion.
   a. Increase activities throughout the day to improve muscle strength (e.g., ambulation, physical therapy exercises).
   b. Give "time out" periods throughout the day to rest the leg.
   c. Sit client in chair and have gravity assist with increasing knee flexion.

2. Client experiences increased pain when in CPM machine.
   a. Provide analgesic as prescribed.
   b. Release leg out of CPM until pain subsides.
   c. Determine cause of increased pain.
3. Client develops reddened areas on heel from foot support.
   a. Readjust foot in CPM machine at least every 2 hours.
   b. Pad the foot support more.

Recording and Reporting

• Record joint exercised, degree of joint motion, time of CPM use, pain and need for analgesia, any joint abnormalities, and client's activity tolerance.
• Report immediately any resistance to range of joint motion; increased pain with CPM; swelling, heat, or redness in joint.

Sample Documentation

1000   Functional CPM applied to client's left leg. Client able to tolerate 0 degrees extension and 40 degrees flexion at slow speed. Prescribed analgesic offered to client and given 2 Tylenol with codeine #3 tabs. Skin dry and intact, without evidence of breakdown.

1200 Client tolerating CPM well at 0–40 degrees. Stated the Tylenol with codeine tablets took care of his pain in the left knee. Skin assessed for breakdown, top of left foot slightly red under CPM foot strap. Foot repositioned in CPM and strap readjusted to a secure but loose position. Reassessment will be done in 1 hour.

Geriatric Considerations

- Older adults who have chronic illnesses may need rehabilitation care to continue CPM because they are not able to manage the equipment in their home.
- Older adults have increased risk of skin breakdown because of decreased elasticity and increased fragility of the skin. Pressure from the CPM increases the risk of pressure ulcer development on the older adult's heel.

Home Care and Long-Term Care Considerations

- Home care physical therapist may assist client/family in continuing CPM in the home.
- Be sure client/family have specific instructions regarding use of the CPM device, length of time for each session, expected outcomes, and what to do if the client experiences increased pain, the client is unable to tolerate the CPM sessions, or the equipment malfunctions.

CRITICAL THINKING EXERCISES

1. Mr. Kline is a 58-year-old who has left hemiplegia following a stroke. He has a prescription for ROM to the affected side, and he also receives physical therapy in the home. The home care nurse has taught Mrs. Kline to do the exercises and has encouraged Mrs. Kline to let her husband do his own exercises. She is reluctant to do so and is unwilling to have him continue with physical therapy in a free-standing physical therapy agency. She feels that she can adequately care for her husband. How would you intervene?

2. Ms. Isaac is a 50-year-old independent single woman who is having decreased range of motion in her hands and fingers as a result of arthritis. When you see her in a clinic setting, Ms. Isaac feels that the doctor's prescription for pain is sufficient, but she wants to increase her ROM in her hands so that she can quilt and sew. How would you assess her ROM in relation to these activities?

3. You are caring for Jim Butler, a 23-year-old athlete who has had a knee replacement procedure. He receives CPM to increase mobility of the joint. As an RN you are responsible for the CPM activities, but caregiver is responsible for Mr. Butler's hygiene and skin care. What information is needed by the caregiver about the CPM?

REFERENCES

Beare P, Myers J: *Principles and practices of adult nursing*, ed 3, St Louis, 1998, Mosby.

Birdsall C: How do you use the continuous passive motion device? *Am J Nurs* 86(6):657, 1986.

Chiarello CM, Gunderson L, O'Halloran T: The effect of continuous passive motion duration and increment on range of motion in total knee arthroplasty patients. *J Orthop Sports Phys Ther* 25(2):119, 1997.

Dawe D, Curran-Smith J: Going through the motions, *Can Nurs* 90(1):31, 1994

Hamilton L, Lyon P: A nursing driven program to preserve and restore functional ability in hospitalized elderly patients. *J Orthop Nurs Assoc* 25(4):30, 1995.

Johnson RL: Total shoulder arthroplasty *Orthop Nurs* 12(1):14, 1993.

Lawrence BR: The dose effect of continuous passive motion in postoperative rehabilitation of the first metatarsophalangeal joint. *J Foot Ankle Surg* 35(2):155, 1996.

Montgomery F, Eliasson M: Continuous passive motion compared to active physical therapy after knee arthroplasty: similar hospitalization times in a randomized study of 68 patients, *Acta Orthop Scand* 67(1):7, 1996.

Mourad L: *Orthopedic disorders*, St Louis, 1991, Mosby.

Perry A, Potter P: *Clinical nursing skills and techniques*, ed. 4, St Louis, 1998, Mosby.

Rada S: Nursing assessment: musculoskeletal system. In Lewis S, Collier I, Heitkemper M, editors: *Medical-Surgical nursing: assessment and management of clinical problems*, ed. 4., St Louis, 1996, Mosby.

Sheppard MS, Westlake SM, McQuarrie A: Continuous passive motion—where are we now? *Physiotherapy Canada* 47(1):36, 1995.

CHAPTER 27

Traction

Skill 27.1
Maintaining Skin Traction,   639

Skill 27.2
Skeletal Traction Assessment and Pin Site Care,   642

Traction, as with a cast, is a means by which a part of the body is immobilized. Unlike a cast, however, traction involves a pulling force through weights that is applied to a part of the body while a second force, called *countertraction,* pulls in the opposite direction. Too much force can cause damage to nerves and tissues and prevent callus formation; too little force can produce painful muscle spasms, impair healing, and result in malunion and nonunion (Folcik, Carini-Garcia, and Birmingham, 1994).

The pulling force of traction is provided through a system of pulleys, ropes, and weights attached to the client; the countertraction is often achieved by elevating the foot or head of the bed and therefore is supplied by the client's body. In *balanced* traction, the amount of force in the traction is equal to the amount of force in the countertraction. A *suspension* is a mechanism that suspends a body part by using traction equipment, but it does not involve a pulling force. However, traction may be added to a suspension. In *straight* or *running* traction, the traction force pulls against the long axis of the body, and the countertraction is supplied by the client's body. In a *suspension* or *balanced* traction, the affected part is supported by a sling, hammock, or the body and partly by a system of weights attached to an overhead frame with pulleys and ropes (Perry and Potter, 1998).

Traction is prescribed for one or more of the following general uses: (1) correction of deformities, (2) gradual correction or improvement of a joint contracture, (3) treat-ment of a joint dislocation, (4) reduction, immobilization, and alignment of a fracture, (5) prevention and management of muscle spasms, (6) prevention of further soft tissue damage, (7) preoperative and postoperative positioning and alignment, and (8) rest of a diseased joint (Folcik, Carini-Garcia, and Birmingham, 1994).

SKIN TRACTION

Skin traction applies pull to an affected body structure by straps attached to the skin around the structure. To be effective, there must be a pull in the opposite direction, which is referred to as *countertraction.* Countertraction is achieved by using the weight of the client's body or by elevating part of the bed toward the traction.

One form of skin traction, Buck's extension, is used to reduce muscle spasms, contractures, and dislocations and occasionally for lumbosacral muscle spasms causing low back pain (Figure 27-1). It may be applied to one or both legs using straps or a commercially prepared foam boot with Velcro straps. Dunlop's traction is another form of Buck's extension applied to the forearm to treat fractures of the humerus (Figure 27-2).

Cervical traction using a head halter involves a halter with a cutout for the ears and face (Figure 27-3). The halter cups the chin and has straps leading to a bar attached to ropes, pulleys, and weights. This is used for arthritic conditions of the cervical vertebrae, not fractures. It can be removed occasionally.

Pelvic belt traction consists of a girdlelike belt that fits around the lumbosacral and abdominal areas with straps attached to a board connected to ropes, pulleys, and weights (Figure 27-4). This is used for clients with low back pain, muscle spasms, and ruptured or herniated disk. This traction helps relieve inflammation and irritation of injured nerves and muscles.

Bryant's traction is skin traction used to immobilize fractures of the femur for children weighing less than 40 pounds (Figure 27-5, p. 638). Traction to both legs is maintained with the legs in a vertical position for 7 to 10 days, and then a spica cast is used to continue recovery.

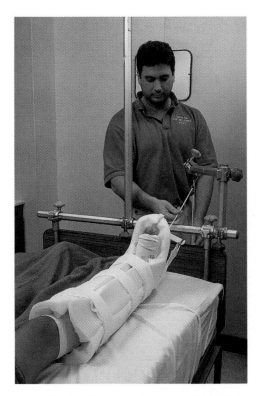

Figure 27-1   Buck's extension.

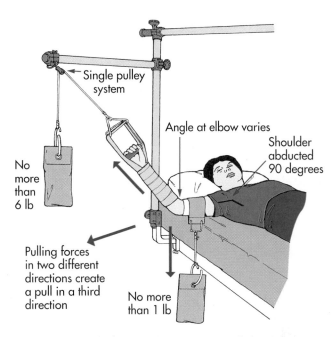

Figure 27-2   Dunlop's traction. *From Folcik MA, Carini-Garcia G, Birmingham JJ: Traction: assessment and management, St Louis, 1994, Mosby.*

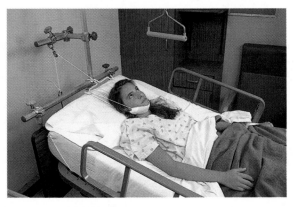

Figure 27-3   Cervical traction.

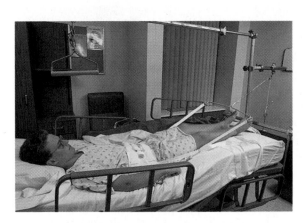

Figure 27-4   Pelvic belt traction.

SKELETAL TRACTION

Skeletal traction is a type of traction applied by a physician under sterile conditions and used for treatment of fractures. It involves placement of a pin, wire, or nail through the bone. Weights are then attached to the device using ropes and pulleys. The amount of the weights is determined by the age and condition of the client and the purpose of the traction. Skeletal traction is used to immobilize fractures of the femur below the trochanter, fractures of the cervical spine, and some fractures of the bones of the arm or ankle and is used for longer periods (6 to 8 weeks) to allow for healing. When skeletal traction is used,

the skin is punctured at the site where the pin enters and exits and in the case of external fixation or halo traction, where the device attaches to the bone. This provides a site for microorganisms to enter the soft tissues and bone. Meticulous care needs to be taken to prevent the development of infection at these sites.

Clients in skeletal traction often are immobilized for weeks or sometimes months until healing occurs. Nursing care involves supporting activities of daily living (ADLs), maintenance of the traction, and prevention of complications of immobility, such as skin breakdown and pulmonary or fat emboli. Although there are many types of traction for different parts of the body, five general princi-

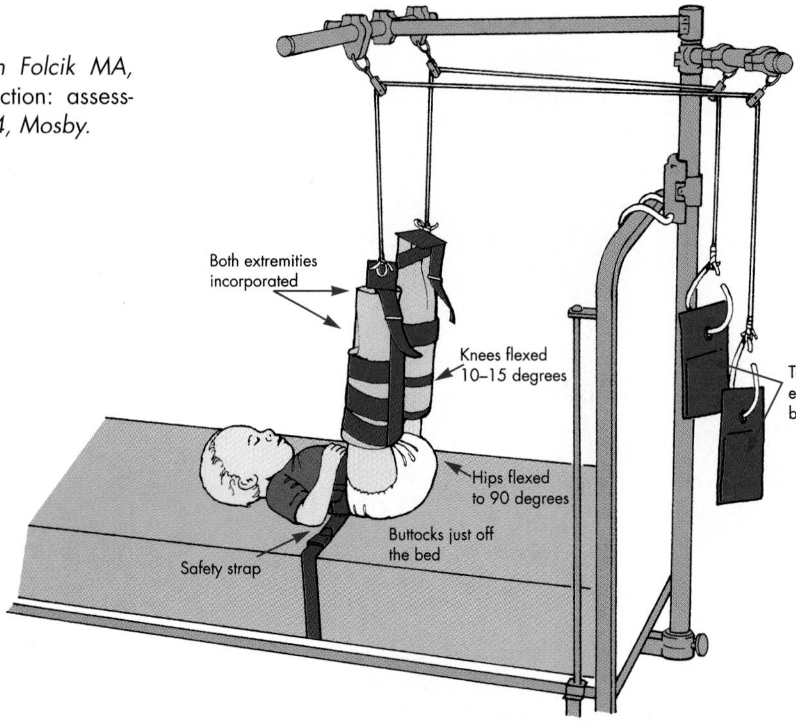

Figure 27-5 Bryant's traction. *From Folcik MA, Carini-Garcia G, Birmingham JJ:* Traction: assessment and management, *St Louis, 1994, Mosby.*

Box 27-1 Assessment of Neurovascular Function (The Five P's)

Pain
Pallor
Pulselessness
Paresthesia
Paralysis

Box 27-2 The Four P's of Traction Maintenance

Pounds–Is the correct weight in place?
Pull–Is the direction of pull aligned with the long axis of the bone?
Pulleys–Is the rope riding over the pulley and gliding smoothly?
Pressure–Is each clamp and connection tight?

ples apply: (1) maintain the established line of pull, (2) prevent friction on the skin, (3) maintain countertraction, (4) maintain continuous traction unless ordered otherwise, and (5) maintain correct body alignment (Beare and Myers, 1998).

Circulation and neurological function may be affected by swelling from soft tissue trauma in the presence of a fracture. In addition, pressure exerted from skin traction wraps may result in neurovascular deficits. Sensory complaints such as pain, numbness, and tingling and motor changes such as weakness or inability to move the extremity distal to the traction may indicate a developing neurovascular problem (Box 27-1).

When caring for a client in traction it is essential that the traction device is checked initially and regularly for correct maintenance. Hospital policy may specify a frequency of checks, which needs to be at least every 4 to 8 hours. Traction maintenance involves checking the weights, the direction of pull, the ropes and pulleys, and all connections. An acronym to remember is the four P's (Box 27-2).

NURSING DIAGNOSES

Nursing diagnoses for clients in traction focus on comfort and prevention of complications. **Anxiety** related to pain and/or immobility is appropriate when the traction results in muscle spasms or if immobilization creates feelings of isolation, apprehension, and helplessness. **Risk for Impaired Skin Integrity; Bathing, Hygiene, Dressing and Grooming Self-Care Deficit; Impaired Physical Mobility; and Pain** are appropriate if traction is maintained continuously for days to weeks. **Risk for Peripheral Neurovascular Dysfunction** is appropriate when there is soft tissue swelling and/or skin wraps, as in skin traction. **Risk for infection** is related to pin sites for the client having skeletal traction, external fixation, or halo traction. All nursing diagnoses related to immobility should also be considered.

Skill 27.1

MAINTAINING SKIN TRACTION

Skin traction is the application of a pulling force directly to the skin and soft tissue that indirectly pulls on the skeletal system. The purposes of skin traction include relief of muscle spasms, restriction of movement, promoting alignment in cervical disk disease, hip and pelvic fractures, and spinal deformities (Folik, Carini-Garcia, and Birmingham, 1994). Skin traction may be used intermittently to relieve low back pain associated with sciatica or continuously to treat a fracture and relieve muscle spasms. Skin traction usually provides temporary immobilization until open reduction and internal fixation (ORIF) or skeletal traction can be implemented.

There are several types of skin traction. The most common type of adult skin traction is Buck's traction, which is applied to the lower leg to immobilize a fractured femur or hip (see Figure 27-1, p. 637). The more weight applied to the traction, the greater the chance of skin breakdown; therefore, no more than 7 pounds is used for Buck's traction. Cervical traction may use 7 to 10 pounds, and 15 to 30 pounds is used for pelvic traction.

Skin traction may be contraindicated for clients with skin problems such as ulcers, dermatitis, burns, or abrasions. Elderly clients and clients with diabetes are also at increased risk of skin breakdown.

Equipment for Buck's Traction

Overhead frame
Traction bar
Cross clamp and pulley
Rope
Buck's traction boot or moleskin and elastic bandages
1- to 5-pound weights
Spreader bar

ASSESSMENT

1. Assess client's knowledge of the reason for traction. **Rationale: Determines concerns, fears, and need for further teaching.**
2. Assess integrity and condition of skin to be placed in traction. **Rationale: Determines ability of local tissues to tolerate traction's pulling forces.**
3. Assess client's overall health condition, including degree of mobility, ability to perform ADLs, and current medical conditions. **Rationale: Determines client's health state and ability to tolerate traction.**
4. Assess client's position in bed: supine, perpendicular to the ends of the bed, with the affected limb in proper body alignment.
5. Assess client's level of pain and need for analgesics before procedure begins. **Rationale: Analgesics decrease client's discomfort while applying skin traction, and assessment also serves as the baseline for later comparison.**
6. Following application, assess traction setup: weights hanging freely, ordered amount of weight applied, ropes moving freely through pulleys, all knots tight in ropes and away from pulleys. **Rationale: This ensure accurate function of traction.**
7. Assess neurovascular status of extremity distal to the traction, including skin color, temperature, capillary refill, presence of distal pulses, sensation, and client's ability to move digits every 30 minutes times 2, then every 4 hours. **Rationale: This provides necessary baseline information and detects neurovascular complications.**

PLANNING

Expected outcomes focus on client's mental status, skin integrity, ADLs, comfort level, neurovascular status, and mobility.

Expected Outcomes

1. Client will experience reduced anxiety levels as evidenced by a decrease in symptoms of apprehension, irritability, and/or helplessness.
2. Skin under traction boot or elastic wrap remains intact, without redness or breakdown.
3. Client will participate in ADLs as much as possible within limitations.
4. Client will verbalize a sense of comfort on a 0 to 10 scale after repositioning and administration of analgesics.
5. Client will demonstrate no neurovascular deficit following application of circumferential dressing or boot.
6. Client will move all extremities independently by date of discharge.

DELEGATION CONSIDERATIONS

The skill of assisting with application of skin traction may be delegated to assistive personnel (AP) who have had specific training and supervised practice.

- Inform and assist care provider in proper method of aiding in application of skin traction.
- Instruct AP to inform the nurse of clinical manifestations of neurovascular deficit.

IMPLEMENTATION

Steps	Rationale

1. See Standard Protocol (inside front cover).
2. Position client supine and nearly flat with no more than 30 degrees elevation, with the affected leg halfway between the edge of the bed and middle of the bed.
3. Wash affected leg (or legs) gently and pat dry.

COMMUNICATION TIP

Tell the client you will hold the extremity using slight tension to minimize discomfort as traction is applied.

NURSE ALERT

Skin traction is not placed over irritated, damaged, or broken skin.

NURSE ALERT

Clients should have written orders for specific traction weights, bed position, and turning regimen.

4. Apply cross clamp and pulley to overhead frame (see illustration).
5. Apply foam boot, moleskin, or elastic bandages to affected leg, proceeding from distal to the proximal, making sure it is neither too loose and slips or too tight and constricts circulation.

NURSE ALERT

Skin traction that is too tight puts pressure on nerves and vascular structures that could result in an irreversible neurovascular deficit.

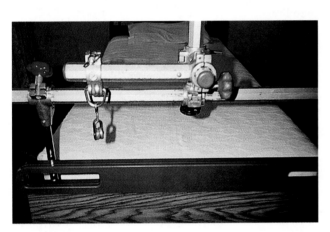

Step 4

NURSE ALERT

When applying Buck's traction, avoid pressure to the peroneal nerve at the neck of the fibula. Decreased sensation in the web space between the great toe and second toe, as well as inability to dorsiflex the foot and extend the toes, may indicate pressure to the nerve. Be alert to pressure over bony prominences about the ankle or the back of the heel.

6. Apply rope to boot and through pulley. Ropes are tied securely in knots, passed through grooves of pulleys to weights, and are not frayed.
7. Tie rope to weight and hang weight gradually and gently at end of the bed.
8. Assess neurovascular status of extremity distal to the traction, including skin color and temperature, capillary refill, presence of distal pulses, sensation, and client's ability to move digits every 30 minutes times 2, and every 4 hours while traction is in place.
9. Lower bed only to point that ensures that weights hang freely.
10. Release traction boot every 4 to 8 hours and provide skin care according to physician's orders.
11. See Completion Protocol (inside front cover).

NURSE ALERT

If tissues distal to skin traction are cold or cool, or if capillary refill is greater than 3 seconds, then compare with unaffected extremity to determine if deficit is related to traction wrap.

EVALUATION

1. Evaluate traction setup: knots tied, not frayed, ropes in pulleys, weights hanging freely.
2. Inspect skin tissues for signs of pressure, color changes, edema, or tenderness.
3. Determine client's participation in ADLs.
4. Ask client to rate discomfort on a scale of 0 to 10 and to report muscle spasms.
5. Evaluate neurovascular status and report deficits.
6. Observe client's use of trapeze and overhead frame with unaffected limbs to reposition self correctly.

Unexpected Outcomes and Related Interventions

1. Client complains of increased pain after Buck's traction is applied.
   a. Take the traction off (if allowed by physician), reposition client, and then reapply the traction.
   b. Administer analgesics as prescribed.
   c. Realign body and/or limb.
   d. If increased pain continues or pain occurs upon passive motion, then notify physician of possible neurovascular deficit.
2. Client has reddened areas on leg or heel under Buck's traction boot.
   a. Take foam boot off for 1 hour to relieve pressure if ordered by physician.
   b. Foam boot should always be applied securely (nurse should be able to insert one finger between client's skin and Buck's traction boot). Recheck correct tightness frequently.
   c. Increase skin checks to every hour.
   d. Apply protective barrier agent (e.g., Aloe Vista or Sween cream) to affected limb for protection against breakdown.
   e. Ensure heels do not rest on bed or pillow.

Recording and Reporting

- Record assessment of skin integrity beneath traction and nursing interventions implemented to maintain skin integrity.
- Record neurovascular assessment every 2 hours for the first 24 hours and, if no deficit, then every 4 hours thereafter.
- Report any neurovascular deficits to physician immediately.
- Record length of time client is in or out of specific traction.

Sample Documentation

0900 Buck's traction applied to client's left leg using a 5-lb weight. No c/o pain, tingling, or numbness. Capillary refill <3 seconds in nailbeds of toes bilaterally, able to wiggle toes, skin warm and pink to lower left leg. Side rails up, bed down, 5-lb weights hanging freely. Knots tied, rope in pulley. Client in supine position with left leg in proper alignment.

1100 Client assessed for comfort. States he is "hurting a lot"—an 8 on a 0–10 scale. Medicated with 5 mg morphine sulfate IM. Buck's boot taken off. Skin assessed and no breakdown evident. Buck's reapplied. Client repositioned. No skin breakdown noted to heels, coccyx, or back.

1200 Client reassessed for comfort. Verbalized that pain medication helped and that pain is almost gone. Client resting comfortably at present.

Gerontologic Considerations

- Older adults may have keratoses, rashes, or other lesions that could become irritated in skin traction.
- Older adults may have long-standing conditions of musculoskeletal tissues such as arthritis or gout that could lead to inflamed tissues and skin breakdown.
- Older and chronically ill clients may have increased need for position changes resulting from limitations from osteoporosis, osteomalacia, weakened muscles, or increased risk of skin breakdown.

Home Care and Long-Term Care Considerations

- If client is to be discharged to home, relatives or caregivers should be instructed on care needs (including home traction) and mode of ambulation.
- Integrity of traction should be inspected daily—weights hang freely, traction ropes rest in groove of pulley, and client's body is not allowed to interfere with countertraction. In many cases the client's body is the countertraction.

Skill 27.2

SKELETAL TRACTION ASSESSMENT AND PIN SITE CARE

A common form of skeletal traction is balanced-suspension skeletal traction (BSST), usually used for a fractured femur (Figure 27-6). Balanced suspension brings relief of muscle spasms, realignment of the fracture fragments, and callus formation, that is, development of new supportive bone around the injured site. This is now primarily used temporarily while stabilizing client condition for surgical insertion of an internal fixation device such as a plate or nail. Balanced suspension involves splints under the leg and a Steinmann pin or Kirschner wire supplying the traction (Figure 27-7). Sufficient weight to overcome the quadriceps and hamstring muscle spasms may be 30 to 40 pounds.

Other common forms of skeletal traction are side-arm traction (with a pin drilled through the lower humerus [Figure 27-8]), external fixation (used for comminuted fractures with soft tissue injury, skull and facial fractures, and pelvic bones [Figure 27-9]). For cervical spine fractures, Crutchfield or Gardner-Wells tongs are inserted into the skull. Halo traction is frequently used for neurologically intact clients, preventing further injury to the spinal cord (Figure 27-10).

External fixation is a form of skeletal traction that consists of a frame or apparatus to hold pins placed into or through bones above and below a fracture site. External fixation devices promote early ambulation and use of other joints while maintaining immobilization of affected bones. A variety of external fixation frames are used for skull and facial fractures, ribs, bones of the extremities, and pelvic bones (Perry and Potter, 1998).

All skeletal traction involves placement of a device through the skin, called a *pin site*. Procedures for pin site care must be kept current with infection control guidelines established by the Centers for Disease Control and Prevention (CDC). Some institutions have policies outlining pin site care, and others require specific physician's orders to specify frequency of pin site care and cleansing agent to use. Clients discharged with an external fixation device need to be given specific guidelines for continued care of the pin sites and assessment for potential problems.

Equipment
Balanced suspension skeletal traction (BSST) (see Figure 27-6)
  Ropes, pulleys, weights
  Thomas splint
  Pearson attachment with sheepskin padding
  Footplate
  Trapeze
Halo traction (see Figure 27-10)
  Halo ring with four pins
  Molded vest jacket
  Vertical metal bars connecting ring to jacket
  Tracheostomy tray (for emergency resuscitation)
  Allen wrench (allows removal of screws for resuscitation)

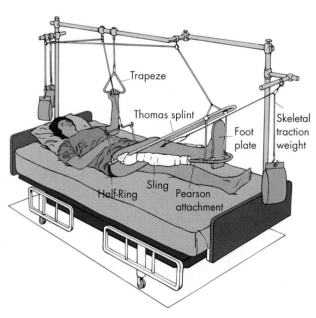

Figure 27-6 Balanced-suspension skeletal traction. Traction in long axis of right thigh is applied by means of Kirschner wire through proximal portion of tibia. Limb is supported by Thomas splint beneath thigh and Pearson attachment beneath leg. Footplate attachment prevents footdrop. Weights apply countertraction to upper end of Thomas splint and suspend its lower end. By using the left arm and leg as shown, client can shift position of the hips without change in amount of traction.

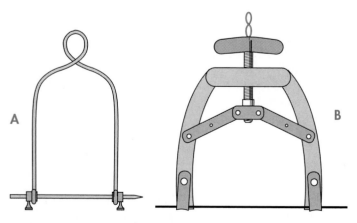

Figure 27-7 **A,** Kirschner wire and tractor. **B,** Steinmann pin and holder.

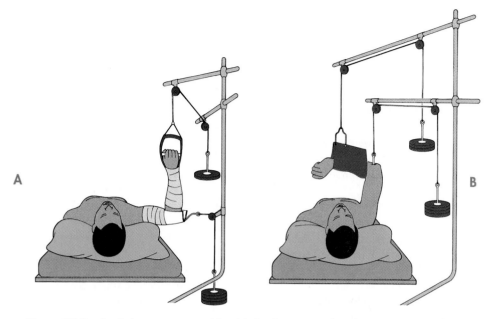

Figure 27-8 A, Side-arm traction (skin/skeletal). **B,** Overhead 90-90 traction (skeletal). *From Beare PG, Myers JL: Principles and practice of adult health nursing, ed 2, St Louis, 1994, Mosby.*

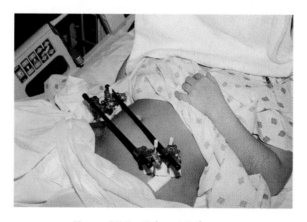

Figure 27-9   Pelvic AO fixator.

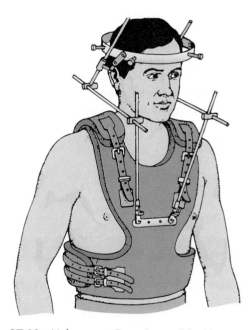

Figure 27-10   Halo vest.   *From Beare PG, Myers JL: Adult health nursing, ed 3, St Louis, 1998, Mosby.*

Pin site care supplies
  Sterile cotton-tipped applicators
  Sterile normal saline
  Sterile hydrogen peroxide
  Antiseptic ointment
  Split 2 × 2 dressings
  Disposable gloves

ASSESSMENT

1. Assess client's knowledge of the reason for traction, including nonverbal behavior and responses. **Rationale: Determines concerns, anxiety, and need for further teaching.**

2. Assess integrity and condition of skin over bony prominences and under devices in use. **Rationale: Determines baseline status of local tissues at risk for pressure ischemia.**

3. Assess client's overall health condition, including degree of mobility, ability to perform ADLs, and cur-

rent medical conditions. **Rationale: Determines client's health state and serves as baseline for further reference.**

4. Assess client's level of pain and need for analgesics before procedure begins. **Rationale: This decreases client's discomfort while applying traction and also serves as baseline for later comparison.**

5. Following application, assess traction setup: weights hanging freely, ordered amount of weight applied, ropes moving freely through pulleys, all knots tight in ropes and away from pulleys. **Rationale: This ensure accurate function of traction.**

6. Assess neurovascular status of extremity distal to the traction, including skin color, temperature, capillary refill, presence of distal pulses, sensation, and client's ability to move digits. **Rationale: This provides necessary baseline information and detects neurovascular complications.**

7. Assess client's mobility. **Rationale: This determines client's ability to participate in repositioning and ADLs.**

8. Assess pin sites for redness, edema, discharge, or odor. **Rationale: This determines presence of infection.**

9. Assess for respiratory dysfunction. **Rationale: Pulmonary embolus can occur with the client who has associated spinal cord injury or who is on prolonged bed rest. Halo vests are not recommended for clients with respiratory insufficiency because of the restricted chest expansion.**

10. Client demonstrates no evidence of complications of immobility or infection.

PLANNING

Expected outcomes focus on client's anxiety level, skin integrity, self-care abilities, comfort and mobility level, neurovascular status, infection risks, and pulmonary status.

Expected Outcomes

1. Client will experience reduced anxiety levels as evidenced by a decrease in symptoms of apprehension, irritability, and or helplessness.

2. Skin over bony prominences or under halo vest remains intact, without redness or breakdown.

3. Client performs ADLs independently to all unaffected areas.

4. Client verbalizes a sense of comfort on a 0 to 10 scale after repositioning and administration of analgesics.

5. Client demonstrates no neurovascular deficit following application of traction.

6. Skin around pin sites shows no evidence of redness, swelling, or drainage.

DELEGATION CONSIDERATIONS

Skeletal traction is applied by the physician. The skill of assisting with insertion of skeletal pins and pin site care may be delegated to AP who are adequately trained in principles of surgical asepsis.

- Instruct personnel in signs and symptoms associated with infection or inflammation at pin insertion site.

IMPLEMENTATION

Steps	Rationale

1. See Standard Protocol (inside front cover).
2. Inspect traction setup: knots secure; ropes in pulleys; weights hanging freely, not caught on bed or resting on floor, and bedclothes not interfering with traction apparatus. Check the four P's of traction (Box 27-2) maintenance:
3. Monitor neurovascular status of distal aspects of involved extremities in comparison with corresponding body part every 2 hours for the first 24 hours and every 4 to 12 hours thereafter (according to agency policy).
   a. Inspect color and temperature. Pink, warm tissues are adequately oxygenated. Whitish tissue indicates decreased arterial supply, and bluish color signifies venous stasis.

NURSE ALERT

Irreversible tissue death occurs within 4 to 12 hours.

Steps	Rationale

b. Monitor for edema resulting from tissue trauma or venous stasis.

c. Assess capillary refill by pressing on toe or fingernail, releasing, and noting "pinking" on nail within 3 seconds.

4. Provide pin site care according to hospital policy or physician's orders.

   a. Remove gauze dressings from around pins and discard in receptacle.

   b. Inspect sites for drainage or inflammation.

   c. Prepare supplies and apply new gloves.

   d. Clean each pin site with prescribed solution by placing sterile applicator close to the pin and cleaning away from the insertion site. Dispose of applicator.

   e. Continue process for each pin site.

   f. Using a sterile applicator, apply a small amount of topical antibiotic ointment (check for physician's orders or hospital policy).

   g. Cover with a sterile 2 × 2 split gauze dressing or leave site open to air (OTA) as prescribed or according to hospital policy. Remove and discard gloves and wash hands.

NURSE ALERT

Never touch one pin site with material used on another.

5. Inspect skin (bony prominences, heels, elbows, sacrum, and under appliances) for signs of pressure, and lightly massage pressure areas every 2 hours unless evidence of beginning skin breakdown is evident (tenderness, reactive hyperemia).

Light massage increases circulation to area. Massage to compromised tissues increases tissue breakdown.

6. Monitor respiratory status every shift (see Chapter 14). Assess for possible fat embolism syndrome, including hypoxia, restlessness, mental changes, tachycardia, tachypnea, dyspnea, low blood pressure, and petechial rash over upper chest and neck.

Clients with fractures of long bones are at especially high risk for fat embolism. All immobilized clients are at high risk for atelectasis and pulmonary emboli.

7. Assess level of discomfort and provide nonpharmacological and pharmacological relief as indicated (Chapter 22).

Pain may result from the traumatic injury and muscle spasms

NURSE ALERT

Clients at risk for pressure ulcers may benefit from special bed or mattress. If appropriate obtain order for pressure relief bed (see Chapter 25).

NURSE ALERT

Never ignore a client's complaint. Follow through and check it out.

8. Encourage active and passive exercises (Chapter 6) and use of unaffected extremities for ADLs. Encourage use of trapeze bar for repositioning in bed.

Prevents muscle atrophy and maintains muscle tone for later ambulation.

9. For elimination provide a fracture pan.

Smaller bedpan is more comfortable for the client and easier to place under client.

10. See Completion Protocol (inside front cover).

• • • •

EVALUATION

1. Determine client's anxiety level in response to traction and immobilization.
2. Inspect skin for evidence of breakdown.
3. Observe participation in ADLs and use of unaffected extremities.
4. Evaluate level of pain and discomfort from muscle spasms.
5. Evaluate neurovascular status and peripheral tissue perfusion.
6. Evaluate for local and systemic indications of infection, including drainage and inflammation at pin sites, fever, elevated white blood cell count, continuous dull aching pain, redness, or warmth in extremity (possible osteomyelitis, i.e., bone infection).

Unexpected Outcomes and Related Interventions

1. Client has severe edema, marked increase in pain, inability to actively move joint or increased pain on passive movement, indicating compartment syndrome, which leads to decreased venous perfusion and increased venous stasis; tissue anoxia may be developing with the potential for loss of function.
   a. Prompt management is critical. Notify physician.
   b. Apply ice and elevate if possible.
   c. Reduce or eliminate compression caused by therapeutic devices.
2. Redness, increased swelling, and drainage develop at pin site(s) or fracture site (osteomyelitis).
   a. Cultures may be indicated to identify infecting organism. (Physician's order is not usually required, see agency policy.)
   b. Notify physician for antibiotic orders.
3. Signs of osteomyelitis or systemic infection develop, including fever, elevated white blood cell count, general malaise. This is especially a concern with open fractures and extensive soft tissue injury.
   a. Notify physician. Orders may include irrigation of the site with antibiotic solution and/or intravenous (IV) antibiotics.
   b. Encourage fluid intake and provide comfort measures for fever.
4. Evidence of nerve damage develops from pressure or trauma to nerves, depending upon type of traction in place. For example peroneal nerve; footdrop may develop with inability to evert and dorsiflex foot; radial or median nerve at wrist: inability to approximate thumb and fingers (radial) and numbness and tingling of thumb, index, middle fingers (medial) with wrist drop.
   a. Eliminate pressure if possible according to type of traction in place.
   b. Notify physician.
5. Client experiences fat embolism (more common in fractures of long bones) with symptoms of anoxia, restlessness, mental changes, tachycardia, tachypnea, dyspnea, low blood pressure, and petechial rash over upper chest and neck.
   a. This is a life-threatening emergency—50% of persons with fat emboli die.
   b. Notify physician and initiate major resuscitation efforts.

Recording and Reporting

- Record in nurse's notes type of traction, site to which traction is applied, amount of weights, and client's response.
- Often a flow sheet is used that specifies specific routine assessments and frequency of assessment.

Geriatric Considerations

- Older adults are particularly prone to the development of altered skin integrity when they are bedridden and not repositioned frequently. This tendency results from a decreased amount of subcutaneous fat and skin that is less elastic, thinner, drier, and more fragile than that of a younger adult.
- Older adults may have long-standing conditions of musculoskeletal tissues such as arthritis or gout that could lead to inflamed tissues and skin breakdown.
- Older and chronically ill clients may have increased need for position changes resulting from limitations from osteoporosis, osteomalacia, or weakened muscles.
- Severe varicose veins will prevent the use of skin traction in the elderly because of the risk of skin breakdown.

Home Care and Long-Term Care Considerations

- Client is taught to ambulate slowly within medical guidelines, gradually increasing length of time out of bed and distance walked.
- Client is taught to notify physician of undesirable signs, such as marked increase in pain, muscle spasms, and increased numbness. Symptoms may signify reinjury or insufficient healing.
- Family members are taught to apply skin traction correctly if it is prescribed for home use.
- Client and family members are taught the use of muscle relaxants and analgesics if prescribed for home use.

CRITICAL THINKING EXERCISES

1. Jewell Cleveland, age 76, fell at home and broke her left hip. She has been admitted to the nursing unit to await hip pinning and is in Buck's skin traction. The nurse performs a baseline assessment and finds cold left toes, capillary refill of 5 seconds, and weak dorsalis pedis pulse.
   a. What should the nurse do?
   b. Following ORIF, Mrs. Cleveland is experiencing muscle spasms. Dr. Morrison orders a muscle relaxant and reapplication of the Buck's traction. Mrs. Cleveland tells you she doesn't understand why.
   c. In assessing her skin, the nurse notices a small reddened area on her left heel. What does the nurse do?

2. Fred Russell was admitted to the orthopedic unit following a motor vehicle accident. He is placed in balanced skeletal traction. The nursing technician asks the nurse how to "change the bed with all those ropes and weights."
   a. What should the nurse do?
   b. Mr. Russell needs to defecate. How does the nurse assist the client?
   c. Dr. Morrison orders pin care to the Steinmann pin. The nurse notices a small amount of clear drainage at the medial pin. What does the nurse do?

3. Lorraine Michelle is admitted to the emergency department with a dislocation of the C6 vertebra. The nurse assists Dr. Morrison in applying halo traction.
   a. What equipment does the nurse gather?
   b. Lorraine is neurologically intact but is very scared. What should the nurse say?
   c. Lorraine is being discharged after several days on the nursing unit. What instructions does the nurse give her?

REFERENCES

Beare PG, Myers JL: *Principles and practice of adult health nursing,* ed. 3, St Louis, 1998, Mosby

Folcik MA, Carini-Garcia G, Birmingham JJ: *Traction: assessment and management,* St Louis, 1994, Mosby.

Jones-Walton P: Clinical standards in skeletal traction pin site care, *Orthop Nurs* 10(2):12, 1991.

Perry A, Potter P: *Clinical nursing skills and techniques,* ed 4, St Louis, 1998, Mosby.

CHAPTER 28

Cast Care

Skill 28.1
Cast Application, Assessment, and Care, 650

Skill 28.2
Cast Removal, 655

sists of removing the cast and padding, followed by skin care to the affected area. The cast is removed by use of a cast saw. The saw is noisy, but the procedure is painless because the saw will not cut the skin. It is necessary, however, to prepare the client adequately for cast removal. A small child or confused adult may require gentle restraint during removal to avoid any injury. Careful removal of a synthetic cast (with gore lining) is important to prevent burns.

A cast is an immobilization device applied externally to hold injured or deformed musculoskeletal tissues in proper position to promote healing. A cast prevents movement of injured tissues. Therefore correct application of the cast, with tissue structures in optimal position for healing, is imperative. Casts are used in many different ways (Figure 28-1). The use and application materials required depends on the anatomical area of injury.

One of two types of cast materials, plaster of Paris or synthetic, may be used. The type of cast material selected depends on physician preference, number of cast changes anticipated, and type of musculoskeletal injury. Plaster of Paris is composed of open-weave cotton covered with calcium sulfate crystals. This material molds easily during application, but requires 48 hours to dry before weight bearing or external pressure can be applied. During the period of drying, the cast must be well supported on firm surfaces to avoid indentations such as fingerprints. Lifting the cast by supporting the joints above and below the casted area, prevents injury to underlying soft tissues. This type of cast is heavier compared with the synthetic cast.

Synthetic casting materials are composed of polyester and cotton covered with a polyurethane resin that is activated by water. This cast sets very quickly, in approximately 15 minutes, and can withstand pressure or weight bearing in 30 minutes (Table 28-1, p. 650). Different colors of this casting material are also available, ranging from fluorescent pink to navy blue. Colors are often more appealing to children and aid in maintaining the appearance of the cast (Figure 28-2).

When caring for clients with casts, it is also important to understand the techniques for cast removal, which con-

NURSING DIAGNOSES

Nursing diagnoses associated with cast application include **Bathing/Hygiene Self-Care Deficit, Dressing/Grooming Self-Care Deficit,** and **Toileting Self-Care Deficit,** in which clients with a cast applied to an extremity or body portion (body spica cast) experience difficulty in performing activities of daily living (ADLs). These clients are also at a high risk for **Impaired Skin Integrity** relating to the skin condition before, during, and after cast application. Because of the rigidity of the cast and the swelling of inflammation that accompanies injury, **Risk for Peripheral Neurovascular Dysfunction** should be considered.

When a client is at home with a cast, **Impaired Home Maintenance Management** is a possibility, depending on the client's degree of independence, self-care, and assistance required. **Knowledge Deficit** regarding cast care is important in these clients, especially regarding contact with water, restrictions in activity, and positioning. **Pain** may be a significant concern in fractures and musculoskeletal injuries. Finally, if the cast is on a lower extremity or torso, **Risk for Injury** or **Impaired Physical Immobility** may be appropriate as a result of gait disturbances or the client's need for ambulatory assistive devices.

Nursing diagnoses associated with cast removal include **Anxiety,** in which clients are concerned about how the procedure is performed, and **Impaired Skin Integrity** resulting from pressure points within the cast, previous skin conditions before the casting, or presence of surgical incisions under the cast. **Knowledge Deficit** regarding cast removal should also be considered.

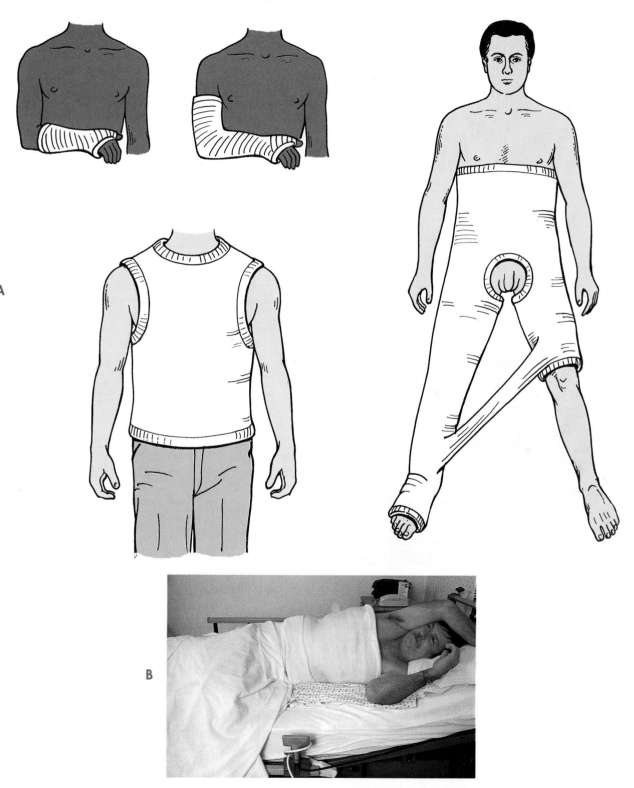

Figure 28-1 **A,** Types of casts. *Top left,* short arm cast; *top center,* long arm cast; *bottom left,* plaster body jacket cast; *far right,* one and one-half hip spica cast. **B,** Client in body cast.

Table 28-1

Comparison of Casting Materials

	Plaster of Paris	Synthetic
Indications	Unstable fractures, edema, frequent cast changes	Stable fractures, long-term cast
Drying time	At least 24 hours	7–15 minutes; can be weight bearing in 30 minutes
Drying method	Air dry	Air dry
Radiolucent	Minimal	Yes
Weight of cast	Heavy	Lightweight
Durability	Can crumble and flake	Very durable
Bathing/immersibility	Must be kept from moisture	Can be immersed, as in swimming and bathing; *must be thoroughly dried after exposure to water*
Choice of colors	No	Yes
Surface area	Smooth	Rough
Allergic reactions	Possible	Possible
Molding	Greater moldability	Limited moldability
Special equipment	None	May need special cast saw for cast removal
Padding	Natural fiber padding and stockinette	Synthetic nonabsorbent lining
Cost	Inexpensive (usually requires more rolls)	Expensive
Strength	Strong	Stronger than plaster of Paris

Data from Slye D, Theis I: *An introduction to orthopaedic nursing: an orientation module,* Pitman, NJ, 1991, Anthony J Jannetti.

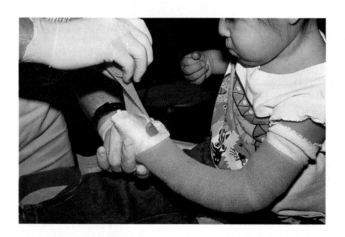

Figure 28-2 Synthetic casting materials are available in different colors that are appealing to children.

Skill 28.1

CAST APPLICATION, ASSESSMENT, AND CARE

This skill includes assessment parameters before, during, and after cast application, including peripheral neurovascular status. Assisting with the application of the cast is also discussed. It is important to follow guidelines for care after application with respect to pressure against cast and weight bearing.

Equipment (may be on cast cart) (Figure 28-3)
Plaster cast
Plaster rolls: sizes 2, 3, 4, or 6 inch
Padding material (felt, sheet wadding, Webril, stockinette, or gore lining)
Gloves, apron, or protective cover
Plastic-lined bucket or basin
Water warmed at time of application
Cart, chair, or fracture table scissors
Paper or plastic sheets

Synthetic cast
Synthetic rolls: 2, 3, or 4 inch
Pail with water to dampen rolls
Padding materials (sheet wadding, stockinette, Webril)
Gloves, apron, or protective cover
Elastic bandages or cast cutter (to trim or core edges of cast, if needed)

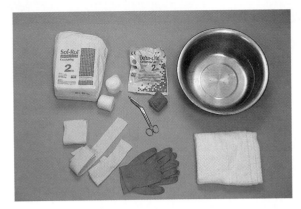

Figure 28-3

ASSESSMENT

1. Assess client's health status, focusing on factors that may affect wound healing, such as diabetes, poor nutritional status, or steroid medication use. **Rationale: Healing of the injured tissues may be slower in these clients, or additional nutritional supplements may be required.**
2. Assess client's ability to cooperate and level of understanding concerning the casting procedure. **Rationale: Sudden movement during procedure could cause injury.**
3. Assess condition of the skin that will be under the cast. Specifically, note any areas of skin breakdown, rashes present, or incisional wound.
4. Assess neurovascular status of the area to be casted. Specifically, note presence or absence of motor and sensory function, skin color, temperature, and capillary refill. Compare with opposite extremity or surrounding tissues. **Rationale: Changes in neurovascular status may occur after casting, possibly further compromising already injured tissues. It is important to note the baseline neurovascular status so that these changes, if they occur, can be readily assessed.**
5. Assess client's pain status using a scale of 0 to 10.
6. Consult with physician to determine the extent to which client will be able to use the casted body part. **Rationale: Determines extent to which self-care will be impaired.**

PLANNING

Expected outcomes focus on skin integrity, comfort, self-care, mobility, prevention of neurovascular complications, and maintenance of cast integrity.

Expected Outcomes

1. Client's exposed skin distal to cast is warm and pink, with capillary refill less than 3 seconds.
2. Pulses distal to the cast are palpable, strong, and regular.
3. Cast remains clean, without indentions or fraying, until removal.
4. Client has edema of 1 plus or less and demonstrates less than 25% decrease in active range of motion (ROM) of affected extremity after cast application.
5. Client verbalizes satisfactory pain control after analgesic administration 20 to 30 minutes before the procedure.
6. Client requires minimal assistance with ADLs after an extremity is casted.
7. Client verbalizes correct activities related to cast care.
8. Client demonstrates proper cast care.

DELEGATION CONSIDERATIONS

The registered nurse should complete a thorough assessment of the client. The skill of assisting with cast application may be delegated to assistive personnel (AP).

- Inform care provider in method to assist in positioning specific client.

IMPLEMENTATION

Steps	Rationale
1. Administer analgesic before cast application: orally (PO) 30 to 40 minutes before; intramuscularly (IM) 20 to 30 minutes before; intravenously (IV) 2 to 5 minutes before.	Reduces pain during cast application. Provides optimal analgesic effect.
2. See Standard Protocol (inside front cover).	
3. Assist physician or certified technician in positioning client and injured extremity as desired, depending on type of cast to be used and area to be casted.	The parts to be casted must be supported and in optimal alignment.

Steps	Rationale

4. Prepare skin that will be enclosed in the cast. Change any dressing (if present), and cleanse the skin with mild soap and water.

Assists in maintaining skin integrity.

COMMUNICATION TIP

Explain that client may experience warmth during the cast application process.

5. Assist with application of padding material around body part to be casted (see illustration). Avoid wrinkles or uneven thicknesses.
6. Hold body part or parts to be casted *or* assist with preparation of casting materials.
   a. Plaster cast: Mark the end of the roll by folding one corner of the material under itself. Hold plaster roll under water in a plastic-lined bucket or basin until bubbles stop, then squeeze slightly and hand roll to person applying the cast.
   b. Synthetic cast: Submerge cast roll in lukewarm water for 10 to 15 seconds. Squeeze to remove excess water.

Decreases complications to the skin and prevents pressure points under the cast. Plaster gives off heat from a chemical reaction when drying.

Support of body part may require application of slight manual traction.

Once dampened, the end of the casting tape may be difficult to find. Dampened plaster rolls are unrolled and molded to fit the extremity or body part to be casted.

Submersion in water initiates the chemical reaction, which will eventually result in hardening of the cast.

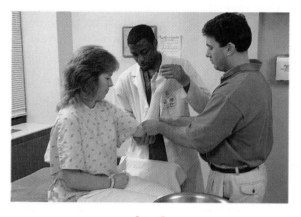

Step 5

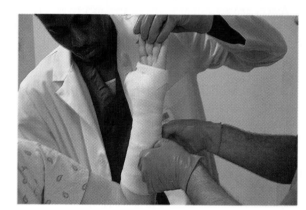

Step 7

7. Continue to hold the body parts as necessary as the cast is applied (see illustration) or supply additional rolls of casting tape as needed.
8. Provide walking heel, brace, bar, or other material to stabilize the cast as requested by the physician.

Thickness of the plaster determines strength of the cast.

After cast has dried, ambulation may be permitted with partial weight bearing on the affected extremity. This is facilitated by the use of a walking heel or sole. Bars or wooden posts may be used to stabilize a spica cast. Braces are often incorporated into a cast to assist in joint motion and mobility.

9. Assist with "finishing" the cast by folding the edge of the stockinette down over the cast to provide a smooth edge. A dampened plaster roll is unrolled over the stockinette to hold it in place.
10. Using scissors, trim the cast around fingers, toes, or the thumb as necessary. Remove and discard gloves and wash hands.
11. Elevate the casted tissues on cloth-covered pillows or in a sling. Avoid complete encasing of the cast.

Smooth edges decrease the chance for skin irritation or tissue injury.

The cast should not restrict joint movement or constrict circulation.

Pillows or other soft areas prevent indentation or other undesirable hardening of the cast. Covering of the cast delays drying.

Steps	Rationale

12. Assist client with transfer to stretcher or wheelchair for return to unit, or prepare for discharge.

Additional personnel may be required to transfer client safely, especially with client in a spica or other large body cast. Pillows, restraints, and side rails may also be needed to maintain principles of safe transport.

NURSE ALERT

Client with wet large-limb or wet spica cast requires three people to assist in turning and transfer. Proper assistance prevents undue pressure on cast and prevents client injury.

13. Review all home care instructions (Box 28-1) with client and significant other.

Box 28-1 Cast Care Instructions

The First 24 Hours

Follow the doctor's instructions. Your cast needs at least 24 hours to dry if it is plaster. Avoid handling it as much as possible. When you do have to move the cast, such as when you change your body position, use only the palms of your hands and support the cast under your joints. You want to avoid putting indentations in the cast that will put pressure on the skin inside. You may use a fan placed 18 to 24 inches from the cast to aid its drying in the first 24 hours. You should be sure to expose the whole cast for drying, and do not cover it with linen for the first 24 hours.

If you have a fiberglass cast you may be able to continue a more normal life-style, for example, bathing or swimming, if your doctor approves. A fiberglass cast can become wet.

Keep the cast and extremity above the level of the heart for at least 48 hours by propping your cast up on firm pillows. Put ice directly over the fractured area for 24 hours, but be sure to enclose the ice in a plastic bag to keep the cast dry. Move the parts of your body above and below the cast regularly to aid circulation and relieve stiffness. Massaging the joints and extremities around the cast will also improve circulation.

How to Care for Your Cast
Plaster

If you have a plaster cast, do not get the cast wet because it will lose its strength. If cast does become wet, dry immediately. Use a towel to blot moisture off the cast, then dry it with a hair dryer set on low. When your cast does not feel cold and damp, it is dry. To keep the cast clean and dry, you should cover it with plastic when bathing, using the toilet (if it is a spica cast), or going out in rain or snow. You may use a damp cloth and scouring powder to clean soiled spots on the cast. Be sure to brush away plaster crumbs or other objects from the edges of the cast, but do not remove or rearrange any padding. Do not break off or trim cast edges.

Synthetic

If you have a synthetic or fiberglass cast and you do not have any wounds under the cast, your doctor may allow you to bathe and swim with it. You should use only a small amount of mild soap around your cast and should rinse under your cast thoroughly. If you swim in a pool or a lake, be sure to rinse both the inside and outside of the cast to flush out any dirt and chemicals.

Washing or rinsing inside your fiberglass cast may reduce odor and irritation and improve the overall skin condition of the cast area. You may use a spray nozzle at a sink or a flexible shower head to rinse inside your cast with warm water. *Never insert any object into your cast for any purpose.* No special drying procedures are necessary after wetting, but you may want to lightly towel off excess water. Do not cover the cast while it is drying.

Skin Care

Skin care is very important during the time a cast is worn. Routinely inspect the skin condition around the cast. Do not insert objects under the cast, because you could scrape the skin or add pressure and cause an infection or sore under the cast. You should use powders and lotions only outside the cast so that the skin stays clean and soft. Powder inside a cast can cake and cause sore areas.

Activity

Do not walk on a leg cast for the first 48 hours. If you are allowed to walk on it, be sure to walk on the walking heel. If your arm is in a cast, be sure to use your sling for support and comfort.

Contact Your Doctor if

- You have pain, burning, or swelling
- You feel a blister or sore developing inside the cast
- You notice an unusual odor coming from the cast
- You experience numbness or persistent tingling
- Your cast becomes badly soiled
- Your cast breaks, cracks, or develops soft spots
- Your cast becomes too loose
- You develop skin problems at the cast edges
- You develop a fever
- You have any questions regarding your treatment

Steps	Rationale
14. Clean used equipment and return to usual storage area.	Expedites use of equipment for the next client and maintains principles of infection control.
15. Explain to client the need to keep cast exposed until drying is complete and the use of elevation or ice.	Casts must dry from the inside out for thorough drying. Elevation and application of ice assist in decreasing edema formation.
16. Have client turn every 2 to 3 hours when a body jacket or a hip spica cast is applied.	Avoids indentation and prevents continuous pressure to one area.
17. See Completion Protocol (inside front cover).	

• • •

EVALUATION

1. Inspect exposed skin and assess capillary refill by pressing on toe or finger if the cast is on an extremity (Figure 28-4).
2. Inspect condition of the cast.
3. Palpate the temperature of tissues around the casted area for warmth.
4. Palpate any accessible pulses distal to the cast.
5. Observe for edema of tissues distal to the cast for signs of vascular compromise (whitish or bluish coloration).
6. Observe client for signs of pain or anxiety (hyperventilation, tachycardia, blood pressure increases).
7. Observe client performing ADLs and ROM.
8. Ask client to describe cast care.
9. Observe client perform cast care.

Unexpected Outcomes and Related Interventions

1. Client experiences impaired physical mobility related to the cast.
   a. Assist client with ROM exercises every 3 to 4 hours.
   b. Teach isometric exercises.

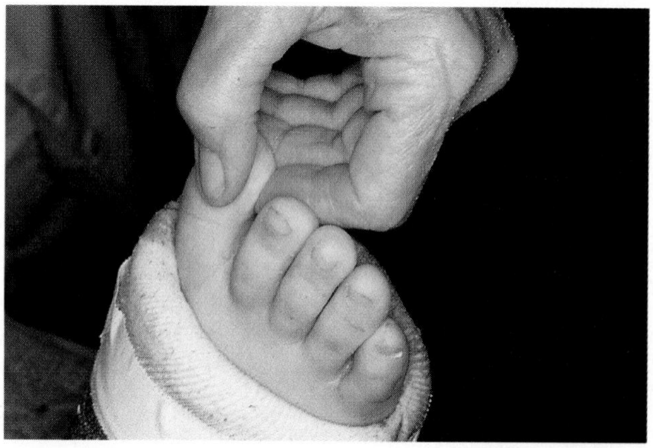

Figure 28-4 Inspecting toe to assess capillary refill.

2. Client complains of pain after application of the cast.
   a. Assess description, amount, type, and severity.
   b. Reposition casted extremity or client. Adjust elevation of pillows as necessary.
   c. Apply ice bags as needed.
   d. Administer analgesics as ordered to maintain client's comfort level.
   e. Perform neurovascular checks.
   f. Assess tightness of the cast by checking with fingers around the edges and checking with client.
   g. If pain continues, notify MD.
3. Client develops compartmental syndrome, a condition in which increased pressure within a limited space compromises the circulation and function of tissues within that space.
   a. Assess for severe pain (usually more severe than explained by injury).
   b. Assess change in neurovascular status, such as numbness, tingling, or decreased movement in distal skin and tissues.
   c. Assess for pulse in area distal to casted extremity (pulselessness develops late in the syndrome).
4. Client is unable to describe cast care.
   a. Reinforce the rationale for correct skin care measures with the cast.
   b. Reinstruct client concerning cast care.

Recording and Reporting

- Record application of cast and condition of skin and circulation. Report abnormal or untoward findings from neurovascular checks; report the following *immediately:* bluish color to distal parts, marked increase in edema or pain, delayed capillary refill (longer than 3 seconds), inability to palpate distal peripheral pulses if originally palpable, increased numbness or tingling, cold tissues, and inability to move tissues actively.

Sample Documentation

0900   Left long arm synthetic cast applied and left arm placed in shoulder sling by Dr. Miller. Capillary refill of left index finger is 2 seconds. Client able to move all fingers of left hand, fingers warm to touch, nailbeds pink, no swelling noted. No complaints of pain or discomfort at this time.

0930   Left long arm cast intact and sling readjusted. Capillary refill of left index finger unchanged. Client moves all fingers of left hand, fingers warm to touch, denies any numbness or tingling present. No edema noted. Denies any pain or discomfort.

Geriatric Considerations

- Lightweight, synthetic casts are better for older adult clients. Cast is less restrictive, and light weight helps clients maintain better balance.
- Plaster of Paris casts on older adults may have less plaster, to aid in moving or lifting.
- Older adult clients may have reduced sensation and be less able to detect compression (Lewis and Knortz, 1993).
- Older adult clients may take longer for bone healing than younger clients.

Home Care and Long-Term Care Considerations

- Reinforce cast care instruction (see Box 28-1).
- Client must inspect cast daily for foul odor, which indicates skin excoriation or infection under cast.
- Client must inspect skin daily for pressure or friction areas.
- Client must inspect cast daily for cracks or changes in alignment.

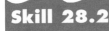

Skill 28.2

CAST REMOVAL

This skill includes gathering the equipment necessary for cast removal, adequate client preparation, and providing skin care to the casted area after cast removal. After cast removal, the client may experience tenderness, soreness, or muscle weakness.

Equipment

Cast saw (Figure 28-5)
Plastic sheets or paper
Cold water enzyme wash
Skin lotion
Basin, water, washcloth, towels
Scissors

ASSESSMENT

1. Assess client's understanding and ability to cooperate with cast removal. **Rationale: Cast removal may require a cast saw. Client needs to understand that the saw is noisy but does not cut skin.**
2. Assess client's readiness for cast removal (physician's orders, x-ray results, physical findings).
3. Ask if client feels itching or burning under the cast. **Rationale: Skin dryness or irritation may be present.**

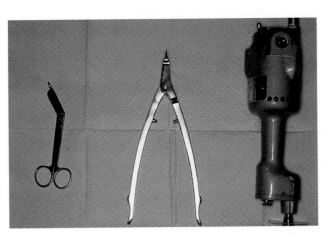

Figure 28-5

PLANNING

Expected outcomes focus on skin integrity of the underlying skin and client understanding of the cast removal procedure.

Expected Outcomes

1. Client is able to describe and demonstrate levels of activity and weight-bearing limitations.
2. There is no underlying tissue damage after cast removal.
3. Client can describe skin care measures and perform ADLs as appropriate.

DELEGATION CONSIDERATIONS

The skill of assisting with cast removal may be delegated to AP.

- Review with care provider proper method of cast removal.

IMPLEMENTATION

Steps	Rationale

1. See Standard Protocol (inside cover).
2. Assist with positioning of client.

Prevents injury.

NURSE ALERT

Proper positioning techniques prevent accidental injury to the skin during cast removal.

3. Describe the physical sensations to expect during cast removal (vibration of cast saw and generation of heat) (see illustration).

Knowledge of the procedure decreases level of anxiety.

4. Describe the expected appearance of the extremity.

Skin under cast becomes scaly, and dead cells that normally slough off accumulate.

5. Explain the loud noise of the cast saw.
6. Stay with client, and explain progress of procedure as cast is removed (see illustration).
7. Inspect tissues underlying the cast after removal.

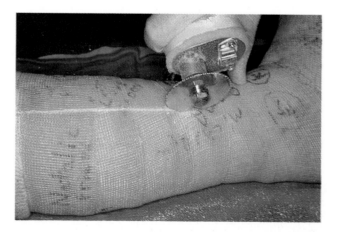

Step 3

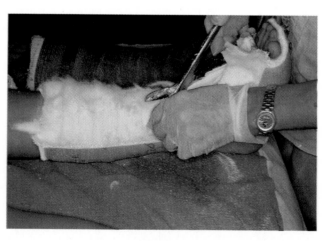

Step 6

Steps	Rationale

8. If skin is intact, apply cold water enzyme wash (if available) to skin and leave on for 15 to 20 minutes. Mild soap and water may also be used. Do not scrub the skin.

Enzyme washes assist in dissolving dead cells and fatty deposits.

9. Gently wash off enzyme wash. Immerse tissues in basin or tub, if possible, to assist in dead cell removal.

10. *Pat* extremity dry, remove and discard gloves, wash hands, and apply thin coat of skin lotion.

Rubbing may further traumatize the tissues.

11. After cast removal explain and write out skin care procedures for client (Box 28-2).

Provides ongoing home care instruction for client and family.

12. Obtain physician's order to perform active and passive ROM, and clarify level of activity allowed.

After immobilization, the involved joints and muscles will be weak and ROM may be limited. Activity must be resumed slowly.

13. Assist in transfer of client for return to unit or discharge.

14. Clean all equipment. Dispose of cast and materials according to standard precautions.

Prevents spread of infection.

15. See Completion Protocol (inside cover).

• • •

Box 28-2 Skin Care after Cast Removal

Instructions on skin care and strategies to relieve the pain, edema, and muscle weakness should be given in writing before discharge.

Instructions Related to Skin Care
- Wash the areas with full-strength cold water wash solution with enzymes such as Woolite or Delicare. Apply the solution liberally and leave in place for at least 20 minutes. The enzymes in the solution loosen dead cells and help emulsify fatty or crusty lesions but cause no skin irritation.
- After 20 minutes, immerse the area in warm water and gently wash away all the debris. Caution client not to rub or scrub the skin areas but to gently rinse off the areas with a soft cloth.
- Rinse with clear warm water and **pat** dry.
- Apply a moisturizing skin lotion, gently massaging it in to help maintain the integrity of the cells.
- Instruct client to repeat the above steps in 24 hours, after which the area should need no special care.

Instructions for Relieving Edema
- Apply ice bags if the edema is marked.
- Wrap (or have the edematous tissues wrapped) from distal to proximal areas with elastic bandages.
- Elevate the affected tissues for the next 24 hours.

Instructions for Tenderness, Soreness, or Pain
- Take prescribed nonnarcotic analgesic every 3 to 4 hours to build a therapeutic blood level, and continue the medication for 24 to 48 hours.
- Immerse the part or entire body in warm water and gently exercise muscles under water.
- Begin to reuse affected tissues and muscles slowly to avoid frank pain. Explain that usually it takes twice as long to regain full function because the part was in the cast. Thus it would take 8 weeks to regain full function of a part that was in a cast for 4 weeks.
- Perform prescribed muscle exercises with 5 to 10 repetitions every 4 hours to aid in regaining muscle strength. If muscle soreness persists, continue intake of prescribed nonnarcotic analgesic and preexercise soaking in warm water. Soreness should lessen as the muscle regains strength.

Instructions for Exercise
Consult with therapist to prescribe scheduled exercises to increase mobility and strength.

From Mourad L: Orthopedic disorders, Mosby's clinical nursing series, St. Louis, 1991, Mosby.

EVALUATION

1. Ask client to explain and demonstrate activity level and ROM exercises prescribed.
2. Inspect underlying skin for pressure areas, erythema (redness), or other signs of irritation or trauma.
3. Observe client perform skin care.

Unexpected Outcomes and Related Interventions

1. Client becomes very tense and is unable to cooperate during the cast removal.
   a. Offer reassurance and support.
   b. Reexplain the cast removal procedure and expected sensations during removal.
2. Client experiences edema, pain, and difficulty moving affected tissues after removal of cast.
   a. Assess neurovascular status of involved tissues.
   b. Assess the type, length, site, amount, and severity of the pain, including onset.
   c. Assess ability to perform active and passive ROM.
   d. Contact physician with findings.
3. Client has scratch on underlying skin.
   a. Inspect skin edges and severity of scratch.
   b. Cleanse area and apply water-soluble lotion or ointment as ordered.
4. Client is unable to explain self-care measures or skin care.
   a. Reassure client as necessary.
   b. Reinstruct client in self-care after cast removal.
   c. Instruct client in skin care measures, including gentle cleansing of the casted area (avoid scrubbing) and patting the area dry (avoid rubbing). Apply a water-soluble lotion or ointment to any scratches as ordered.

Recording and Reporting

- Record cast removal, condition of tissues formerly in cast, and person removing cast in nurse's notes.

Sample Documentation

1000   Left long arm cast removed without difficulty. Skin dry, intact. Left arm soaking in basin of enzyme wash, rinsed.
1030   Skin on left arm remains dry, lotion applied.

Geriatric Considerations

- Older adult clients may experience marked stiffness or weakened muscles, depending on length of time in cast.
- Older adult client's skin is drier, thinner, and more fragile than that of a baby, child, or younger adult.

Home Care and Long-Term Care Considerations

- Client should have chair or bed with pillows to elevate extremity for intermittent edema.
- Suggest regular use of moisturizers for dry, scaly skin of casted extremity.
- Assess client's environment for potential safety risks.

CRITICAL THINKING EXERCISES

1. Two weeks after Mrs. Wilson had a cast applied to her lower right arm, she comes to the clinic for a checkup. Her cast, made of plaster, is badly frayed at the top edge. While moving your hand along the length of the cast, you notice a soft spot, up toward the upper arm. With these findings, what would you assess further with Mrs. Wilson? What instructions might be necessary?

2. Mr. Limon had a long leg cast applied 2 hours ago. During your rounds on the orthopedic unit, you assess Mr. Limon's skin condition and neurovascular status. The skin of the feet is warm and pink, with capillary refill of less than 3 seconds. You can palpate a strong dorsalis pedis pulse. Mr. Limon complains of some swelling in the foot, but denies burning or discomfort. When you check the sensation of both lower extremities, Mr. Limon is able to distinguish a pin prick. What do your findings indicate?

3. Mr. Wang's cast of the lower leg has been on for approximately 2 weeks. During your assessment, you notice a foul odor coming from the cast. What might this indicate?

REFERENCES

Adkins LM: Cast changes: synthetic vs plaster, *Pediatr Nurs* 23(4), 1997.

Haze AJ: Fiberglass and its potential health risks related to casting, National Association of Orthopedic Technologists. *Journal* (Winter 1995–1996): 4–5.

Johnson & Johnson Orthopedics: *Delta cast elite and Flashcast elite,* Raynham, Mass, 1994.

Lewis CB, Knortz KA: *Orthopedic assessment and treatment of the geriatric patient,* St Louis, 1993, Mosby.

Lewis SM, Heitkemper MM, Dirksen SR: *Medical-Surgical nursing,* ed 5, St Louis, 1999, Mosby.

Perry A, Potter P: *Clinical Nursing Skills and Techniques,* ed 4, St Louis, 1998, Mosby.

Richard, RE: Fracture immobilization polymers. In JC Salamone, editor: *The polymeric materials encyclopedia,* pp 1–13, Raynham, Mass, CRC Press.

Thompson JM et al.: *Mosby's clinical nursing,* ed 4, St Louis, 1998, Mosby.

Wolff CR, James P: The prevention of skin excoriation under children's hip spica casts using cortex pantaloon, *J Pediatr Orthop* 15:386, 1995.

CHAPTER 29

Assistive Devices for Ambulation

Skill 29.1
Preventing Falls, 662

Skill 29.2
Teaching Use of Cane, Crutches, and Walker, 665

Skill 29.3
Caring for the Client with an Orthotic Device (Brace/Splint), 677

Several ambulation aids are available to assist the client with mobility and to maintain stability, either with or without weight bearing on an injured lower extremity. Assistive devices also help the client assume a more active role in health care practices. However, the use of an ambulation aid may place a client at greater risk for injury from falls. The client's physical status, mental status, medications, and devices used to ambulate are assessed to determine the degree of risk (see Chapter 5).

An assistive device may be ordered to increase stability, to support a weak extremity, or to reduce the load on weight-bearing structures such as hips, knees, or ankles. These devices range from standard canes, which provide minimal support, to crutches and walkers, which can be used by clients who are unable to bear complete weight on their lower extremities. If a client is unable to bear weight on both lower extremities, a wheelchair is often used for mobility. Selection of the appropriate device depends on the client's age, diagnosis, muscular coordination, ease of maneuverability, weight-bearing status, and functional status before the injury. Use of assistive devices may be temporary, such as during recuperation from a fractured extremity or orthopedic surgery, or permanent, such as for a client with paralysis or permanent weakness of the lower extremities.

Canes are lightweight, easily movable devices that reach about waist high and are made of wood or metal.

Canes help maintain balance by widening the base of support. They are indicated to assist clients with a slightly unsteady gait, hemiparesis, or minor knee or hip injuries or to ease strain on weight-bearing joints. Canes are not recommended for clients with bilateral leg weakness; crutches or walkers are more appropriate. Three types of canes are typically used. The *standard* cane (Figure 29-1, *A*, p. 660) provides the least support and is used by clients requiring only slight assistance to walk. It has a half-circle handle, which allows it to be hooked over chairs. The *T handle* cane (Figure 29-1, *B*) has a bent shaft and a straight-shaped handle with grips, which makes it easier to hold. It provides greater stability than the standard cane and is especially useful for clients with hand weakness. The *quad* cane (four legs) (Figure 29-2, p. 660) or tripod (pyramid cane) provide a wide base of support. This type of cane is useful for clients with unilateral or partial paralysis who need a little extra support. It also has the advantage in that it stands alone, freeing the arms to help the client rise from a chair (Borgman-Gainer, 1996). Metallic canes are usually heavier than their wooden counterparts and are frequently adjustable, which is not possible with wooden canes.

Crutches are used to support weight from one or both legs. They are used by clients who must transfer more weight to their arms than is possible with canes. There are three types of crutches: the axillary, the Lofstrand or Canadian, and the platform crutch. The *axillary* crutch is frequently used by clients of all ages on a short-term basis (Figure 29-3, p. 660). The *Lofstrand* crutch has a handgrip and a metal band that fits around the client's forearm. Both the metal band and the handgrip are adjusted to fit the client's height (Figure 29-4, p. 661). This type of crutch is useful for clients with a permanent disability, such as paraplegic or cerebral palsy clients. The metal arm band stabilizes and assists in guiding the crutch and allows clients to use their hands for other activities, such as opening doors, without dropping the crutches. The anterior opening of the band allows clients to free themselves of the crutches if a fall occurs. The *Canadian* crutch is similar to the Lofstrand, but it has an additional cuff for the upper arm to give added support. The *platform* crutch is used by clients who are unable to bear weight on their wrists. It has a horizontal trough on which the clients can rest their

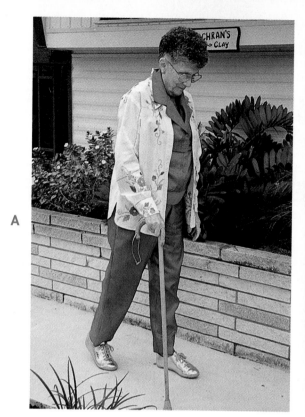
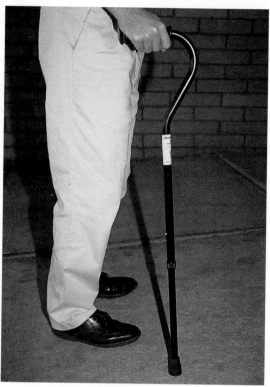

Figure 29-1 **A,** Standard cane. **B,** T-handle cane.

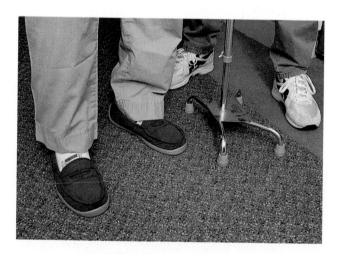

Figure 29-2 Quad cane (four legs).

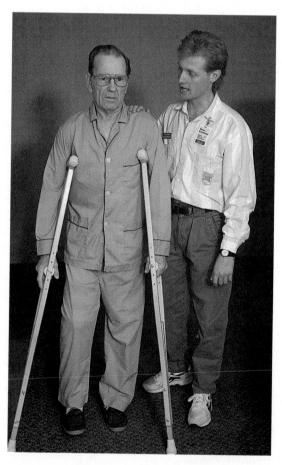

Figure 29-3 Axillary crutches.

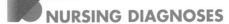

forearms and wrists and a vertical handle for the clients to grip (Borgman-Gainer, 1996). A platform can also be attached to a standard walker if the client requires more stability than that provided by platform crutches.

A walker is an extremely light, movable device, about waist high, consisting of a metal frame with handgrips, four widely placed sturdy legs, and one open side. Because it has a wide base of support, the walker provides the greatest stability and security. A walker can be used by a client who is weak or who has balance problems (Figure 29-5). Variations include a foldable version that is easier to transport and store, one with a fold-down seat, and one with wheels on the front legs. Walkers with wheels are useful for clients who have difficulty lifting the walker as they walk because of limited balance or endurance. The disadvantage, however, is that the walker can roll forward when weight is applied (Borgman-Gainer, 1996).

NURSING DIAGNOSES

Nursing diagnoses associated with teaching the use of assistive devices include **Health-Seeking Behaviors** or **Knowledge Deficit** related to a client's unfamiliarity with use of the assistive device and related safety precautions. **Risk for injury** is appropriate when the focus involves prevention of falls related to unsteady gait while using an assistive device. **Impaired Physical Mobility** related to limited range of motion (ROM) or decreased muscle strength, control, or coordination may be appropriate after traumatic injury or surgery (see Chapter 14). **Activity Intolerance** related to weakness and fatigue from prolonged bed rest is appropriate when activity alters vital signs (e.g., pulse, respirations, blood pressure). Psychological factors such as **Fear** related to a history of falling also result in a client's refusal to ambulate.

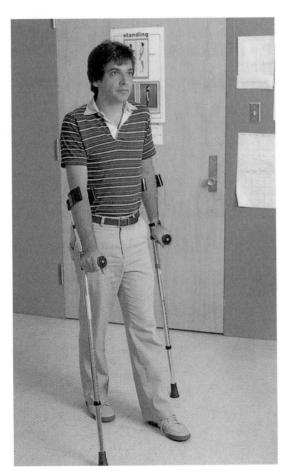

Figure 29-4   Lofstrand crutches.

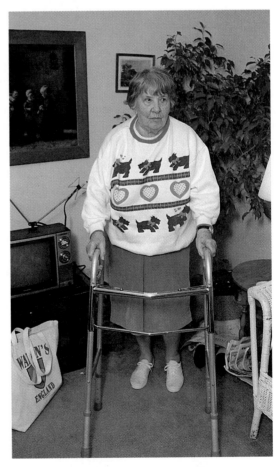

Figure 29-5   Standard walker.

Skill 29.1

PREVENTING FALLS

It is estimated that about 30% of adults age 65 years and older fall at least once each year (Clinical News, 1995). Falls account for up to 90% of all reported hospital incidents, with the risk for the older adults significantly greater (Brady et al., 1993). It is therefore essential for nurses to accurately assess clients for risk factors in the home, health care facility, and community environment. In this way, measures may be instituted to reduce or eliminate hazards before client injury occurs.

In the home, older adult clients are more likely to fall in the bedroom, bathroom, and kitchen. These falls most often occur while transferring from beds, chairs, and toilets; getting into or out of bathtubs; tripping over carpet edges or doorway thresholds; slipping on wet surfaces; and descending stairs. A home hazard assessment (see Chapter 40) can be used to assess the client's environment for potential hazards. In the hospital setting, the Risk for Falls Assessment Tool may be used to identify a client at risk for falling (see Chapter 5). Clients with a history of falls who also have an altered mental status, weakness, dizziness, or unsteady gait are at greater risk for falls. The use of an ambulation assistive device, particularly when used incorrectly, can further increase clients' risk for falls or injury. Based on an individual client's condition and environment, nursing measures are instituted to ensure safety.

At home or in the health care setting, it is important that clients have adequate footwear when ambulating. Clients should have well-fitting sturdy shoes or slippers with nonskid rubber soles. A walking shoe or sneaker is recommended. In addition, clients should wear cotton socks, which absorb moisture and prevent friction. Many physical hazards can be minimized by adequate lighting, removal of clutter and throw rugs, and installation of safety features, such as grip bars and nonslip floor surfaces. In addition, safety in the hospital or long-term care setting is enhanced by the presence of call bells or other signaling devices and side rails.

Equipment

Home safety checklist (see Chapter 40)
Risk for Falls Assessment Tool (see Chapter 5)
Hospital bed with side rails
Call bell

ASSESSMENT

1. Assess client's motor, sensory, and cognitive status, including medical history and medications. **Rationale: This reveals client's physical risk factors for falls.**
2. Assess environment for potential threats to client's safety (e.g., cluttered pathways, wet floors, poor lighting). **Rationale: This reveals client's environmental risk factors for falls.**
3. Assess the degree of assistance client needs by observing client ambulate. Look for signs of grabbing for support, swaying, stumbling, hesitancy, and dizziness while pivoting. **Rationale: This promotes client independence and determines whether client needs assistance to ambulate.**

PLANNING

Expected Outcomes focus on preventing client injury and improving client's knowledge of safety risks.

Expected Outcomes

1. Client's environment is free of hazards.
2. Client is able to identify at least three safety risks.
3. Client does not suffer a fall or injury.

DELEGATION CONSIDERATIONS

Fall prevention is the responsibility of all caregivers, including assistive personnel (AP).

- Be sure to inform care provider of client's mobility limitations.
- Review environmental safety precautions (e.g., bed locked and in low position, call bell and personal items within reach, nonskid footwear).
- Review what to do when a client starts to fall while being assisted with ambulation (i.e., ease client into a sitting position in a chair or on the floor, and alert the nurse).

IMPLEMENTATION

Steps	Rationale

1. See Standard Protocol (inside front cover).
2. Provide adequate, nonglare lighting throughout care area.

   Reduces likelihood of falling over objects or bumping into them. Glare is a major problem for older adults. Eliminates potential hazards.

3. Remove unnecessary objects from rooms, hallways, and stairs. Pay particular attention to items outside client's field of vision.
4. Arrange necessary care items in a logical way, placing them in easy-to-reach locations.

   Allows client to carry out self-care activities safely.

5. Place bed in low position with wheels locked.
6. Explain and demonstrate how to turn call bell on and off at bedside and in bathroom.

   Knowledge of location and use of call bell are essential to client safety.

7. Explain to client reasons for using side rails: preventing falls and as an aid to turn self in bed.
   a. Check agency policies regarding side rail use.
   b. Leave one side rail up, leave the side rail down on the side where the oriented and ambulatory client gets out of bed.

   Client can use the side rail to raise to a sitting position in bed.

8. Explain to client specific safety measures to prevent falls (e.g., dangle feet for a few minutes before standing, walk slowly, call for help if dizzy or weak).
9. While standing next to the client's weak side, have the client take a few steps with the assistive device being used. If no assistive device is being used, stand next to the client's stronger side.
10. Support client by placing arm closest to client on safety belt or around client's waist and other arm around inferior aspect of client's upper arm.

    Providing constant contact by nurse reduces the risk of falls or injury.

11. Take a few steps forward with client, assessing client's strength and balance.

    Ensures client has satisfactory strength and balance to continue.
    Prevents fall to floor.

12. If client becomes weak or dizzy, return the client to bed or chair, whichever is closer.
13. See Completion Protocol (inside front cover).

COMMUNICATION TIP

- *At this time, talk to the client about risks for falls: "You should know that some medications, tests, or procedures and long periods of immobility may make you feel dizzy or weak. Always ask for assistance before trying to walk under these conditions." "Falls can be prevented if safety measures are instituted."*
- *Also let the client who has a fear of falling know that confidence can be regained with continued practice.*

• • • •

EVALUATION

1. Observe client's environment for physical hazards.
2. Ask the client to identify at least three safety risks.
3. Observe client ambulate within living or care area to determine need for further instructions or assistance.

Unexpected Outcomes and Related Interventions

1. Client starts to fall while ambulating with a caregiver.
   a. Put both arms around client's waist or grasp gait belt.
   b. Stand with feet apart to provide broad base of support (Figure 29-6, *A*).
   c. Extend one leg and let client slide against it to the floor (Figure 29-6, *B*).
   d. Bend knees to lower body as client slides to floor (Figure 29-6, *C*).
2. Client suffers a fall while ambulating.
   a. Call for assistance.
   b. Assess client for injury.
   c. Stay with the client until assistance arrives to help lift client to bed or to a wheelchair.
   d. Notify physician.
   e. Note pertinent events related to fall and resultant treatment in medical record.
   f. Follow institution's incident reporting policy.
   g. Reassess client and environment to determine if fall could have been prevented.

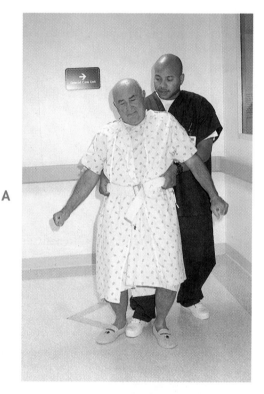
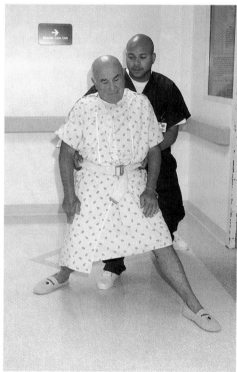
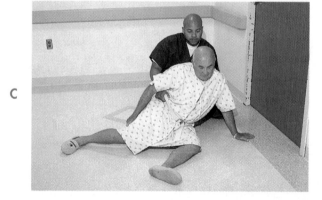

Figure 29-6 **A,** Stand with feet apart to provide broad base of support. **B,** Extend one leg and let client slide against it to the floor. **C,** Bend knees to lower body as client slides to floor.

Recording and Reporting

- Record specific interventions to prevent falls and promote safety in progress notes.
- Report to all health care personnel specific risks to client's safety and measures taken to reduce risks.
- Report immediately if client sustains a fall or an injury.
- Document instructions given to client and any information related to the use of side rails or call bell.

Sample Documentation

1615   *Client assessed for fall risk using the Risk for Falls Assessment Tool. Placed on fall precautions because of history of falls and weakness: call bell within reach, side rails up × 4 at night, hourly room checks, night-light on at all times, bedside commode in place. Instructed on safety measures and instructed to call for help when ambulating. Client voiced understanding.*

0900   *Found client on floor in bathroom after responding to emergency call light. Client stated "I slipped on the wet floor." Alert and oriented × 3. Assisted back to bed with assistance of two personnel. Assessed for injury. No apparent injury noted from fall. BP 110/74, P 82 and regular, R 20. Instructed not to get out of bed without assistance of hospital personnel. Call bell placed within client's reach. Side rails up × 4. Physician notified of client's fall.*

Geriatric Considerations

- Older clients, especially those with a history of falls and/or sensory perception and mobility problems, are prone to falls (Lueckenotte, 1996).
- Older adults, especially postmenopausal women, are at risk for fractured hips. Fractures can cause independent clients to become more dependent or immobilized (Lueckenotte, 1996).

Home Care and Long-Term Care Considerations

- The home care and long-term care environment should be assessed carefully (see Chapter 40).
- Night-lights, grip bars, hand rails, and raised toilet seats should be used.
- Items should be kept in their familiar positions.
- Carpeting, mats, and tile should be secured and nonskid backing placed under area rugs.
- Client should have well-fitting, flat footwear with nonskid soles.

Skill 29.2

TEACHING USE OF CANE, CRUTCHES, AND WALKER

Assistive devices (i.e., canes, crutches, walkers) are usually recommended for clients who cannot bear full weight on one or more joints of the lower extremities. Other indications for their use are instability, poor balance, or pain in weight bearing. Nurses are expected to supervise clients to use their assistive devices correctly (Phipps et al., 1995). It is important for the nurse to know the client's weight-bearing status and any specific movement precautions ordered by the physician. The wrong weight-bearing status or improper movement can cause further damage to the injured extremity.

Non–weight-bearing status requires the client to support weight on the assistive device and the unaffected limb. The affected leg is kept off the floor at all times. Partial or touch-down weight bearing is similar to that for non–weight bearing, but either limb can be advanced initially. Partial weight bearing more closely approximates normal walking except that less weight is placed on the affected limb. Total weight bearing allows the client to distribute equal weight between each limb with minimal weight on the assistive device. Muscle-strengthening exercises such as knee-and-foot extension (kicking leg straight out while sitting in a chair) or hip flexion (marching while sitting in a chair) and walking in parallel bars help the client increase strength and confidence before using an assistive device.

Rubber tips on the ends of assistive devices prevent slipping when using any of the aids. Teaching to lift rather than slide the device lessens the possibility of catching the tips, which could cause the user to lose balance, trip, or fall. Personnel should attend to clients when using an assistive device until they are assured that the client's understanding and strength are sufficient for safe solo ambulation. Observing unaccompanied clients on their walks may reveal a need for attendance and/or additional or continued reminding about the amount of weight permitted or the distance covered. One of the pleasures of being a member of the health profession is assisting clients in regaining mobility with an assistive device after trauma to a foot, leg, knee, or hip, then "graduating" to unassisted walking and moving when possible (Mourad and Droste, 1993).

Canes

Canes primarily increase the person's security and balance by increasing the base of support. Canes also absorb or take the body weight when necessary for mobility during partial weight-bearing periods. Instruction for use of cane-assisted ambulation is required to assess the client's balance, strength, and confidence (Mourad and Droste, 1993). When canes are unilaterally used, they are most often used opposite the weak or injured side and are advanced forward with the injured or affected limb.

Crutches

Persons using one or two crutches as aids for ambulation are frequently seen. The user's proficiency varies with age, condition, degree or extent of injury, musculoskeletal functions, and so on. Use of crutches may be a temporary aid for persons with sprains, in a cast, or following surgical treatments; or crutches may be routinely and continuously used for those with congenital or acquired musculoskeletal anomalies, neuromuscular weakness, or paralysis; or they may be used after amputations.

Placing the crutches in an easily accessible and safe location is the first requirement when crutches are used to rise to a standing position. Accessible sites are on the back or side of the chair or upright against a near cabinet or wall. The handrests of the crutches may be used for bracing while rising if the chair is solid and heavy enough to preclude tipping, and if only one arm is to be used with the crutches for bracing while rising. If the chair is lightweight, both armrests should be used for even bracing while rising, and then the crutches placed for ambulating. When sitting down or rising, the client should be instructed to use either both armrests, or one armrest and both crutches together, to maintain balance. Balance can be lost or chairs can be tipped from uneven or one-sided pressure.

Walkers

Constructed of aluminum or metallic alloys, walkers are lightweight aids strong enough to withstand prolonged use. Heights are adjustable for individual needs. The use of a walker facilitates partial, full, or non–weight bearing. Before using a walker, the client should understand the specific amount of weight bearing permitted or non–weight bearing to be maintained and how to use and care for the walker. Demonstrating the technique to be used for a particular client is beneficial, because techniques vary for non–weight bearing on one extremity vs. partial weight bearing. For both walking activities, the assistant supports the client to prevent loss of balance, tipping, or uneven balance on the walker. The affected limbs should be re-

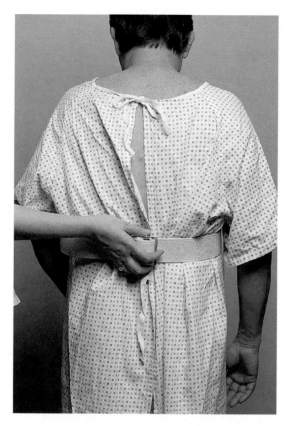

Figure 29-7   Safety belt (gait belt).

ferred to as "left or right" or "strong or weak," not as "good or bad," because those words are physiologically distressing to many persons (Mourad and Droste, 1993).

Equipment

Ambulation device (cane, crutches, walker)
Well-fitting, flat shoes or slippers with non-skid soles
Robe; well-fitting pants or dress
Safety belt (gait belt) (Figure 29-7)

ASSESSMENT

1. Review client's chart, including medical history, previous activity level, and current activity order. **Rationale: Reveals client's current and previous health status.**
2. Assess client's physical readiness: vital signs and orientation to time, place, and person. **Rationale: Baseline vital signs offer a means of comparison after exercise. Level of orientation may reveal risk for fall.**
3. Assess ROM and muscle strength or the presence of foot deformities. **Rationale: Determines if assistance is needed for client to ambulate safely.**

4. Assess client for any visual, perceptual, or sensory deficits. **Rationale: Determines if client can use assistive device safely.**

5. Assess environment for potential threats to client safety (e.g., bed brake, bed position, objects in pathway). Make sure floor is dry and area is well lighted.

6. Assess client for discomfort. **Rationale: Determines if client needs prescribed analgesic before exercise.**

7. Assess client's understanding of technique of ambulation to be used. **Rationale: Allows client to verbalize concerns.**

8. Determine optimal time for ambulation.

PLANNING

Expected outcomes focus on improving mobility, minimizing activity intolerance, preventing risk for injury, minimizing fatigue, and improving client's knowledge.

Expected Outcomes

1. Client demonstrates correct use of assistive device.
2. Client demonstrates correct gait pattern and weight-bearing status.
3. Client rates pain/discomfort as 4 or less on a scale of 0 to 10 during ambulation.
4. Client performs activities with return of vital signs to baseline 3 to 5 minutes after rest.
5. Client independently performs all activities of daily living (ADLs) using assistive device safely.

DELEGATION CONSIDERATIONS

The skill of assisting the client with ambulation may be delegated to AP. The following information is needed when delegating this skill to nursing staff or family members:

- Have client wear shoes with a nonskid surface during ambulation.
- Be sure the area is free of clutter, wet areas, and rugs that may slide or buckle.
- Make sure client uses the correct gait and weight bearing during ambulation.
- Ease client to a sitting position in a chair or on the floor if he or she becomes dizzy or faint.
- Alert the nurse if client becomes dizzy or lightheaded or suffers a fall.

IMPLEMENTATION

Steps	Rationale
1. See Standard Protocol (inside front cover).	**NURSE ALERT** *Make sure that surface client will walk on is clean, dry, and well lighted. Remove objects that might obstruct the pathway.*
2. Prepare client for procedure.	
a. Explain reasons for exercise and demonstrate specific gait technique to client or caregiver.	Teaching and demonstration enhance learning, reduce anxiety, and encourage cooperation.
b. Decide with client how far to ambulate.	Determines mutual goal.
c. Schedule ambulation around client's other activities.	Avoids client fatigue.
d. Place bed in low position.	Reduces risk of injury.

Steps	Rationale

    e. Help client put on well-fitting, flat shoes or slippers.

    f. Slowly assist client from a lying to a sitting or standing position. Assist client to stand stationary until balance is maintained. Check blood pressure as appropriate.

Prevents orthostatic hypotension.

3. Make sure that the assistive device is the appropriate height.

Wrong height causes client to expend more energy, experience greater discomfort, and feel unable to achieve adequate weight transmission through the arms (Hale, Clark, and Harrison, 1990).

4. Make sure assistive device has rubber tips.

Rubber tips increase surface tension and reduce the risk of the assistive device slipping.

5. Apply safety belt if unsure of client's stability. Safety belt encircles client's waist and has space for nurse to hold while client walks. Assist client to standing position and observe balance. If client appears weak or unsteady, return client to bed. Grasp safety belt in middle of client's back, or place hands at client's waist if safety belt is not available.

Providing constant contact by nurse reduces risk of fall or injury.

COMMUNICATION TIP

- *Let the client know that use of the ambulation device may seem awkward at first. Independence will be gained after practice.*
- *Instruct the client to use good posture and always look ahead while using the ambulation device.*

6. **Cane**

    a. Client should hold cane on uninvolved side 4 to 6 inches (10 to 15 cm) to side of foot. Cane should extend from greater trochanter to floor. Allow approximately 15 to 30 degrees elbow flexion.

Offers most support when on stronger side of body. Cane and weaker leg work together with each step. If cane is too short, client will have difficulty supporting weight and be bent over and uncomfortable. As weight is taken on by hands and affected leg is lifted off floor, complete extension of elbow is necessary.

    b. Assist client in ambulating with cane. (Same steps are taught whether standard or quad canes are used.)

    c. Begin by placing cane on the side opposite the involved leg.

Provides added support for the weak or impaired side.

Steps	Rationale

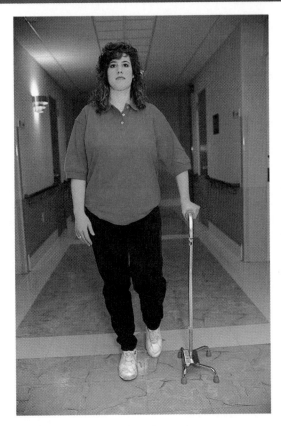

Step 6e

d. Place cane forward 6 to 10 inches (15 to 25 cm), keeping body weight on both legs.

Distributes body weight equally.

e. Move involved leg forward, even with the cane (see illustration).

Body weight is supported by cane and uninvolved leg.

f. Advance uninvolved leg past cane.

g. Move involved leg forward, even with uninvolved leg.

Aligns client's center of gravity. Returns client body weight to equal distribution.

h. Repeat these steps.

7. **Crutches**

a. Crutch measurement includes three areas: client's height, distance between crutch pad and axilla, and angle of elbow flexion. Measurements may be taken with client standing or lying down. Make sure shoes are on before performing measurements.

Measurement promotes optimal support and stability. Radial nerves that pass under axilla are superficial. If crutch is too long, it can cause pressure on axilla. Injury to nerve causes paralysis of elbow and wrist extensors, commonly called *crutch palsy*. If crutch is too long, shoulders are forced upward and client cannot push body off the ground. If ambulation device is too short, client will be bent over and uncomfortable.

Steps	Rationale

(1) *Standing.* Position crutches with crutch tips at point 4 to 6 inches (10 to 15 cm) to side and 4 to 6 inches in front of client's feet. Position crutch pads 1½ to 2 inches (4 to 5 cm) below axilla. Two or three fingers should fit between top of crutch and axilla (see illustration).

(2) *Supine.* Crutch pad should be 3 to 4 finger widths under axilla, with crutch tips positioned 6 inches (15 cm) lateral to client's heel (see illustration).

(3) Elbow flexion is verified with goniometer (see illustration). Handgrip should be adjusted so that client's elbow is flexed 15 to 20 degrees.

b. To use crutches, client supports self with hands and arms. Therefore strength in arm and shoulder muscles, ability to balance body in upright position, and stamina are necessary. Type of gait client uses in crutch walking depends on amount of weight client is able to support with one or both legs.

NURSE ALERT

Instruct client to report any tingling or numbness in upper torso. This may mean crutches are being used incorrectly or that they are wrong size.

Low handgrips cause radial nerve damage. High handgrips cause client's elbow to be sharply flexed, and strength and stability of arms are decreased.

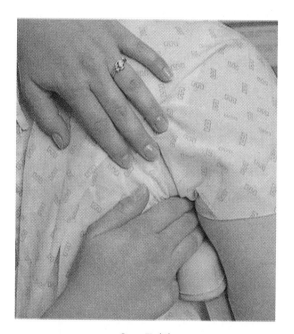

Step 7a(1)

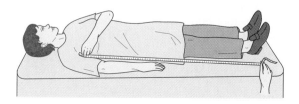

Step 7a(2)

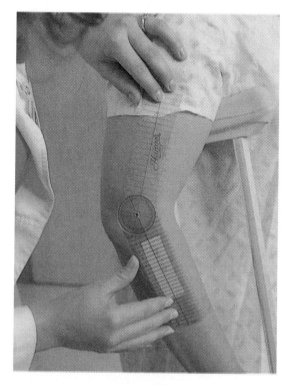

Step 7a(3)

Steps	**Rationale**

c. Have client stand up from a sitting position.
  (1) Move to the edge of the chair, with the strong leg slightly under chair seat.
  (2) Place both of the crutches in the hand on the affected side. If chair has armrests and is heavy and solid enough to avoid tipping, one armrest and both crutches may be used for bracing while rising. If the chair is lightweight, both armrests should be used for even bracing (see illustration).

Balance can be lost or chairs tipped with uneven or one-sided pressure.

  (3) Push down on the crutch handrests while raising the body to a standing position.

d. Choose appropriate crutch gait (darkened areas indicate movement).
  (1) *Four-point gait*
    (a) Begin in tripod position (see illustration). Crutches are placed 6 inches (15 cm) in front and 6 inches to side of each foot. Posture should be erect head and neck, straight vertebrae, and extended hips and knees.

Most stable of crutch gaits because it provides at least three points of support at all times. Requires weight bearing on both legs. Often used when client has paralysis, as in spastic children with cerebral palsy (Whaley and Wong, 1995). May also be used for arthritic clients. Improves client's balance by providing wider base of support.

    (b) Move right crutch forward 4 to 6 inches (10 to 15 cm) (see illustration, *a*).
    (c) Move left foot forward to level of left crutch (see illustration, *b*).
    (d) Move left crutch forward 4 to 6 inches (see illustration, *c*).
    (e) Move right foot forward to level of right crutch (see illustration, *d*).
    (f) Repeat sequence.

Crutch and foot position are similar to arm and foot position during normal walking.

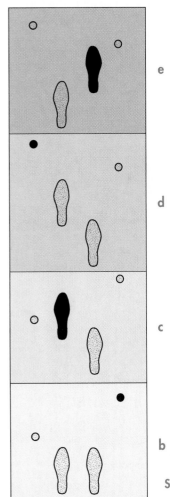

Step 7d(b-e) Four-point gait.

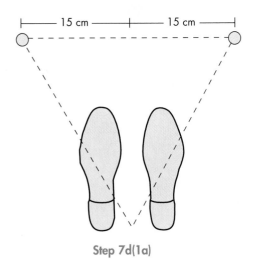

Step 7d(1a)

Steps	Rationale

(2) *Three-point gait*
   Requires client to bear all weight on one foot. Weight is borne on uninvolved leg, then on both crutches. Affected leg does not touch ground during early phase of three-point gait. May be useful for client with broken leg or sprained ankle.
   (a) Begin in tripod position.

   (b) Advance both crutches and affected leg (see illustration).
   (c) Move stronger leg forward.
   (d) Repeat sequence.

(3) *Two-point gait*
   Requires at least partial weight bearing on each foot. Is faster than the four-point gait. Requires more balance because only two points support body at one time.
   (a) Begin in tripod position.

   (b) Move left crutch and right foot forward (see illustration).
   (c) Move right crutch and left foot forward.
   (d) Repeat sequence.

Improves client's balance by providing wide base of support.

Improves client's balance by providing wider base of support.
Crutch movements are similar to arm movement during normal walking.

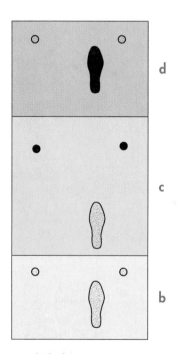

Step 7d(2b-d) Three-point gait.

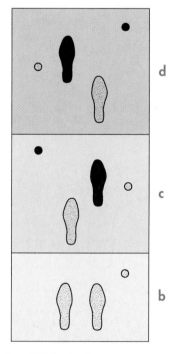

Step 7d(3b-d) Two-point gait.

Steps	**Rationale**
(4) *Swing-to gait*	Frequently used by clients whose lower extremities are paralyzed or who wear weight-supporting braces on their legs.
	This is the easier of the two swinging gaits. It requires the ability to bear body weight partially on both legs.
(a) Move both crutches forward.	
(b) Lift and swing legs to crutches, letting crutches support body weight.	
(c) Repeat two previous steps.	
(5) *Swing-through gait*	
Requires that client have the ability to sustain partial weight bearing on both feet.	
(a) Move both crutches forward.	Increases client's base of support so that when the body swings forward, client is moving the center of gravity toward the additional support provided by crutches.
(b) Lift and swing legs through and beyond crutches.	
(6) *Climbing stairs with crutches*	
(a) Begin in tripod position.	Improves client's balance by providing wider base of support.
(b) Client transfers body weight to crutches (see illustration).	Prepares client to transfer weight to unaffected leg when ascending first stair.
(c) Advance unaffected leg onto the step (see illustration).	Crutch adds support to affected leg. Client then shifts weight from crutches to unaffected leg.

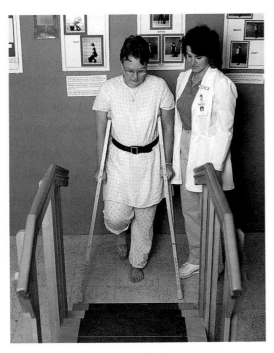

Step 7d(6b)

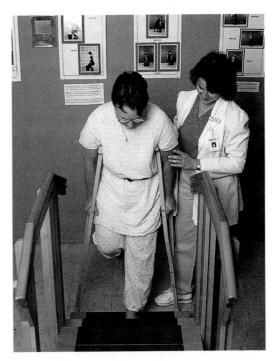

Step 7d(6c)

Steps	**Rationale**

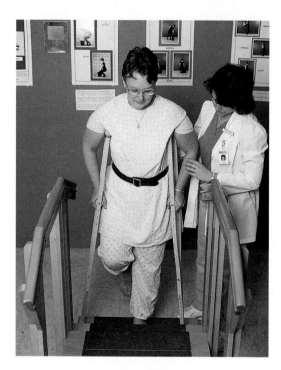

Step 7d(6d)

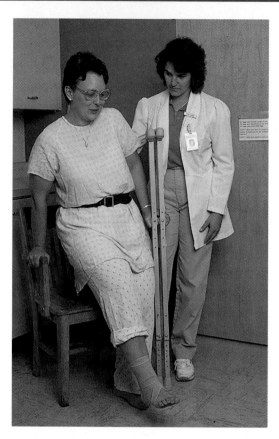

Step 7e(2)

(d) Align both crutches with the unaffected leg on the step (see illustration).

(e) Repeat sequence until client reaches top of stairs.

(7) *Descending stairs with crutches*

  (a) Begin in tripod position.

  (b) Transfer body weight to unaffected leg.

  (c) Move crutches to stair below, and instruct client to transfer body weight to crutches and move affected leg forward.

  (d) Move unaffected leg to stair below and align with crutches.

  (e) Repeat sequence until client reaches bottom step.

e. Teach client to sit in a chair.

  (1) Transfer both crutches to the same hand and transfer weight to crutches and unaffected leg.

  (2) Grasp arm of chair with free hand and extend the affected leg out while lowering into chair (see illustration).

Maintains balance and provides wide base of support.

Improves client's balance by providing wider base of support.

Prepares client to release support of body weight maintained by crutches.

Maintains client's balance and base of support.

Maintains balance and provides base of support.

The non–weight-bearing client should be able to balance on one leg before transferring both crutches to the same hand.

Steps	Rationale

8. Walker

  a. Upper bar of walker should be slightly below client's waist. Elbows should be flexed at approximately 15 to 30 degrees when standing with walker, with hands on handgrips.

  b. Assist client in ambulating.

Walkers without wheels must be picked up and moved forward. Client must have sufficient strength to be able to move walker. A four-wheeled walker, which does not have to be picked up, is not as stable and may cause injury.

Client balances self before attempting to walk.

   (1) Have client stand in center of walker and grasp handgrips on upper bars.

   (2) Lift walker, moving it 6 to 8 inches (15 to 20 cm) forward, making sure all four feet of walker stay on the floor. Take a step forward with either foot. Then follow through with the other foot (see illustrations). If there is unilateral weakness after walker is advanced, instruct client to step forward with the weaker leg, support self with the arms, and follow through with the uninvolved leg. If client is unable to bear full weight on the weaker leg after advancing walker, have client swing the stronger leg through while supporting weight on hands. Instruct the client not to advance the lower extremity past the front bar of the walker.

Provides broad base of support between walker and client. Client then moves center of gravity toward the walker. Keeping all four feet of the walker on the floor is necessary to prevent tipping of the walker.

Providing constant contact by nurse reduces the risk of fall or injury.

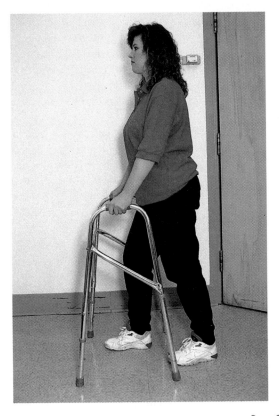 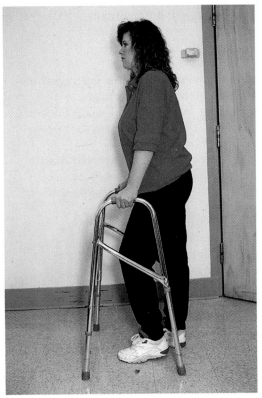

Step 8b(2)

Steps	Rationale
9. Have client take a few steps with the assistive device being used. If client is hemiplegic (one-sided paralysis) or has hemiparesis (one-sided weakness), stand next to client's unaffected side. Then support client by placing arm closest to client on safety belt or around client's waist and other arm around inferior aspect of client's upper arm.	
10. Take a few steps forward with client. Then assess for strength and balance.	Ensures client has satisfactory strength and balance to continue.
11. If client becomes weak or dizzy, return to bed or chair, whichever is closer.	Allows client to rest.
12. See Completion Protocol (inside front cover).	

• • •

EVALUATION
1. Observe client using assistive device.
2. Inspect hands and axillae for redness, swelling, or skin irritation caused by using assistive device.
3. Ask client to rate level of discomfort after ambulating.
4. Monitor client for postural hypotension; increased heart rate, blood pressure, respirations or shortness of breath during and after ambulation.
5. Ask client/family about the ease with which ADLs are performed using assistive device.

Unexpected Outcomes and Related Interventions
1. Client is unable to ambulate correctly.
   a. Reassess client for correct fit of assistive device.
   b. Have added assistance nearby to ensure safety.
   c. Reassess comfort level.
   d. Reassess muscle strength in uninvolved extremities. Alternative device may be needed.
   e. Obtain referral for physical therapy to assist with gait training.
2. Client becomes dizzy and lightheaded.
   a. Call for assistance.
   b. Have client sit or lie down on nearest chair or bed.
   c. Assess client's vital signs.
   d. Allow client to rest thoroughly before resuming activity.
   e. Ask if client is ready to continue.

Recording and Reporting
• Record type of gait the client used, weight-bearing status, amount of assistance required, tolerance of activity, and distance walked in progress notes.

• Document instructions given to client and family.
• Immediately report any injury sustained during attempts to ambulate, alteration in vital signs, or inability to ambulate.

Sample Documentation
Cane
0900 Client able to ambulate 20 feet correctly using quad cane, standby assist of one, and partial weight bearing on right lower extremity. Requested pain pills. Rates pain in right knee at 6 (scale 0 to 10). Returned to bed. Side rails up × 4.
0910 Prescribed analgesic given.
0930 Resting quietly in bed. Denies discomfort.
Crutches
0900 Client able to ambulate 40 feet using axillary crutches and standby assist of one. Gait slow and steady, maintaining non–weight-bearing status on right leg. Able to ambulate up and down stairs correctly using axillary crutches; standby assistance of two needed to steady gait. Voiced no complaints of pain. Returned to bed. Side rails up × 4. Client instructed not to get out of bed without assistance of hospital personnel. Voiced understanding.
Walker
0900 Client able to ambulate 20 feet correctly using walker, with full weight-bearing status. Became dizzy and lightheaded. Assisted to chair with assistance of two personnel. Vital signs: BP 126/70, P 78, R 18. Client rested 5 minutes and then continued ambulating back to bed. Side rails up × 4. Vital signs: BP 124/80, P 72, R 16. Denies dizziness or discomfort.

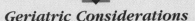

Skill 29.3

CARING FOR THE CLIENT WITH AN ORTHOTIC DEVICE (BRACE/SPLINT)

An orthotic device is applied externally to the body to support, stabilize, or immobilize a body part. Orthotic devices are also used to prevent deformity, protect against injury, relieve pain and muscle spasm, maintain position until healing is complete, or assist with function. Orthotic devices are available in many variations, ranging from arm slings to back braces and finger splints. They may be made from a variety of materials, including rubber, leather, metal, fabric, canvas, and plastic. They are usually designed by an orthotist, physical therapist, or occupational therapist. Orthotic wearers include clients in all age groups, although they are more prevalent in the pediatric and gerontological populations (Shurr and Cook, 1990). Nursing care of the client wearing an orthotic device focuses on maintenance of skin integrity, prevention of neurovascular compromise to the affected area, and education of the client and caregiver regarding application, removal, schedule of wear, activity limitations, and care of the brace/splint. The ability to move freely affects a client's physiological and psychological well-being.

Splints are generally used to immobilize and protect an injured part of the body. Temporary splints prevent further motion and tissue destruction immediately after an injury such as a fracture or sprain. Cloth and foam splints, called *immobilizers*, provide long-term immobilization for such injuries as sprains and dislocations that do not require complete, continuous immobilization in a cast or traction. Velcro or buckle closures permit splints to be adjusted to fit a body part of almost any shape and size. These splints are often used after surgery. Immobilizers are available for almost any body part, including the jaw, shoulder, knee, wrist, clavicle, and cervical vertebrae. The abductor splint, commonly used after hip surgery, maintains the client's legs in an abducted position, allowing the client to be turned without changing the healing limb's position. The device is easily removed for skin care, dressing changes, neurovascular checks, and physical therapy. Other common types of immobilizers include cervical collars (soft or hard), belt-type shoulder immobilizers, and vinyl wrist forearm splints. Molded splints are made of plastic and are used by clients with chronic injuries or diseases such as arthritis. They maintain the body part in a functional position to prevent contractures and muscle atrophy during the period of disuse.

Braces are designed to support weakened structures during weight bearing. For this reason, they are made of sturdy materials such as leather, metal, and molded plastic. Chest and abdominal braces, such as the Milwaukee brace, hold the thoracic and lumbar vertebral column to correct scoliosis (curvature of the spine). They are made of a strong, lightweight material and extend from a chin cup to the pelvis. Lumbar braces hold lumbar and sacral tissues after spinal surgery or fusion. Leg braces hold the thigh, leg, and foot in functional positions for weight bearing and ambulation (Figure 29-8, p. 678). Some of the more common types of braces for the lower extremities include short leg and long leg. These devices are used to support weak leg muscles, to aid in control of involuntary muscle movement, or to maintain surgical correction during the postoperative healing process. They are commonly used for clients with cerebral palsy, muscular dystrophy, multiple sclerosis, and fractures (Shurr and Cook, 1990).

Equipment

Brace/splint
Cotton shirt or gown

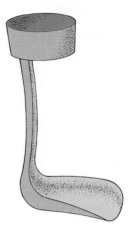

Figure 29-8 Ankle-foot orthosis (AFO). *Modified from Sorrentino SA: Assisting with patient care, St Louis, 1999, Mosby.*

ASSESSMENT

1. Review client's chart, including medical history, previous and current activity level, and description of the condition requiring bracing or splinting. **Rationale: Reveals client's current and previous health status and purpose for the brace/splint.**
2. Assess client's previous experience with braces or splints. **Rationale: Reveals client's baseline knowledge.**
3. Assess client's understanding of reason for brace/splint, care of, application of, and schedule of wear.
4. Assess client's risk for skin breakdown because of bracing/splinting or immobilization. Look at area of skin to be in contact with support device. **Rationale: Immobile and older adult clients are particularly vulnerable.**
5. Refer to occupational or physical therapy consult to determine type of brace to be used, desired position, and amount of activity and movement permitted.

6. Assess client's additional need for an assistive device such as a cane, walker, or crutches. **Rationale: An assistive device may be needed to provide support and promote balance during ambulation.**

PLANNING

Expected outcomes focus on maintaining skin integrity, improving client's knowledge, and preventing risk for injury.

Expected Outcomes

1. Client's skin remains in good condition without circulatory impairment.
2. Client/significant other understands purpose, correct application, and care of the device.
3. Client rates comfort of >8 (scale 0-10).
4. Circulation and sensation distal to brace/splint is maintained.
5. Client uses the device correctly, including schedule of wear, activity limitations, and positioning.

DELEGATION CONSIDERATIONS

The skill of caring for the client wearing a brace or splint may be delegated to AP. The following information is needed when delegating this skill to nursing staff or family members:

- Review the purpose of the brace/splint.
- Review correct application of the brace/splint and positioning of any ties or straps.
- Review prescribed schedule of wear and activities permitted while in the brace.
- Have staff alert the nurse if client complains of pain, rubbing, or pressure from the brace or splint or if a change occurs in client's skin condition.

IMPLEMENTATION

Steps	Rationale
1. See Standard Protocol (inside front cover).	
2. Explain reasons for the brace or splint, and demonstrate how the device works.	Teaching and demonstration enhance learning, reduce anxiety, and encourage cooperation.
3. Assist the client to a comfortable position, preferably sitting or lying down.	Client's position will depend on the type of brace/splint being used. Upper-extremity braces/splints might be applied best with the client sitting upright. Lower-extremity braces may be applied best with the client lying down.

Steps	Rationale

4. Prepare the skin that will be enclosed in the brace/splint by cleaning the skin with soap and water; rinse, pat dry, and change any dressings (if present). If applying a back brace, put a thin cotton shirt or gown on the client.

This protects the skin, absorbs moisture, and keeps the brace clean.

COMMUNICATION TIP

Tell the client, "Be sure to let us know if you feel pressure, pain, numbness, rubbing, or if the skin becomes reddened."

5. Inspect the device for wear, damage, or rough edges.

Potential for skin breakdown is decreased and correct alignment is maintained.

6. Apply the brace/splint as directed by physician, orthotist, physical therapist, or occupational therapist.

Proper application of the brace/splint is important to avoid skin breakdown, pressure ulcers, neurovascular compromise, calluses, or worsening of the deformity.

7. Teach the client the prescribed schedule of wear and allowed activities while in the brace/splint as directed by physician, physical therapist, or occupational therapist.

Proper use of the brace/splint will facilitate healing and mobility and reduce pain and stress.

8. Reinforce the signs of skin breakdown, pressure, or rubbing to report.

Brace/splint may need to be adjusted. Changes may also be required because of growth or atrophy, when muscles regain or lose strength, or after reconstructive surgery. Particular attention should be given to insensitive areas of the body.

9. Teach the client how to care for the brace/splint.
   a. When not in use, store brace/splint in a safe but easily accessible location.

Metal braces should be stored upright. Splints of molded materials should be stored away from heat. Leather materials should be treated with a leather preservative to prevent drying or cracking.

   b. Keep the brace clean, dry, and in good working order.

Plastic parts are cleaned with a damp cloth and thoroughly dried. Metal joints can be cleaned with a pipe cleaner and should be oiled weekly. Remove rust with steel wool, and clean metal parts with a solvent.

10. Assist client to ambulate with brace/splint in place. This will determine if client is able to ambulate safely.

11. Have the client apply and remove the brace/splint. Promotes client independence; demonstration confirms level of learning skill.

12. See Completion Protocol (inside front cover).

COMMUNICATION TIP

Let the client know that the brace/splint may seem awkward at first. Tell the client, "After you have had practice in using it you will feel more comfortable and better able to move about." Also let the client know that assistance may be needed to apply and remove the brace/splint.

• • • •

EVALUATION

1. Inspect areas of the skin underneath the brace/splint for signs of pressure, including redness or breakdown.
2. Observe the client using the brace/splint.
3. Ask the client to rate level of comfort while the brace/splint is in place.
4. Palpate pulse and test sensation of extremity distal to position of brace/splint.
5. Ask the client/family the ease with which ADLs are performed with the brace/splint on.

Unexpected Outcomes and Related Interventions

1. Client is unable to use the brace/splint correctly.
   a. Reassess client for correct fit.
   b. Reassess level of comfort.
   c. Reassess muscle strength in uninvolved extremities.
   d. Obtain referral for physical or occupational therapy.
2. Client develops areas of pressure, redness, or skin breakdown.
   a. Assess device for proper fit and positioning.
   b. Inspect brace/splint for damage, wear, or rough edges.
   c. Inform the physician.
   d. Inform the orthotist, physical therapist, or occupational therapist so that adjustments to brace/splint can be made.
   e. Do not allow the client to use the brace/splint until adjustments are made.
   f. If necessary, temporarily pad the area of incorrect fit rather than the reddened or irritated area.
3. Circulation to the affected extremity is altered because of improper fit.
   a. Remove the device immediately.
   b. Notify physician.

Recording and Reporting

- Document type of brace/splint applied, schedule of wear, activity level and movement permitted, and client's tolerance of procedure in progress notes.
- Record specific assessments related to skin integrity and neurovascular status.
- Document instructions given to client and family.
- Record observations regarding client's ability to apply, ambulate with and remove the brace/splint.
- Immediately report any injury sustained while using the brace/splint.

Sample Documentation

0900 Knee immobilizer placed on client's right lower extremity. Client instructed on proper application and positioning of the device. Instructed to keep immobilizer on at all times when ambulating with crutches and to maintain partial weight-bearing status on the right leg. Areas of skin assessed for signs of redness or breakdown. Skin dry and intact. Dorsalis pedis pulse present. Brisk capillary refill in all toes. Positive sensation and movement of right foot. No complaints of pain or discomfort at this time.

1100 Velcro straps readjusted to a secure but loose position after client complained of slight pressure on the knee. Skin assessed for redness and breakdown. Toes warm to touch; client denies any numbness, tingling, or pain.

Geriatric Considerations

- Integrity of the older adult's skin should be monitored closely.
- Older adults may experience stiffness or weakened muscles, depending on length of time in the orthotic device.
- Older adults with limited mobility may need assistance with application of the brace/splint.

Home Care and Long-Term Care Considerations

- Prolonged immobility in a brace/splint may cause decreased ROM or contractures.
- Assess the ability and willingness of the client and primary caregiver regarding care required for the brace/splint.
- Braces/splints should be inspected and cleaned weekly.
- Remove the brace/splint when bathing or showering.
- Assist clients with adapting clothing so that an acceptable appearance can be maintained.
- Assess for environmental factors in the home that may interfere with safe ambulation.
- It is important that the client and caregiver are aware of signs and symptoms of impaired skin integrity.

CRITICAL THINKING EXERCISES

1. Anna is a 72-year-old female who is being discharged tomorrow, assisted by her husband. She had surgery to repair her fractured right hip, which she suffered after falling down the steps in her two-story home. Anna has since been using a walker to ambulate. For the past 2 days she has needed the assistance of only one person to stand. Anna has a history of hypertension, which is treated with an antihypertensive.
   a. What factors place this client at risk for falls in the home?
   b. What instructions would be given to the client and her husband to reduce her risk for injury?

2. You are making your nightly rounds and suddenly hear Mr. James, who was admitted earlier today, calling out for help from his room. As you enter his dark room you find him on the floor in the hall between the bathroom and bed. He states, "I couldn't reach my cane so I tried to make it to the bathroom without it." He is also complaining of right arm pain.
   a. How should you proceed?
   b. What actions could have prevented this fall from occurring?

3. Jason is a 19-year-old construction worker who broke his right leg after falling from a roof. He underwent surgery to repair the fracture and has a full cast on his right leg. Physician orders for today are to begin axillary crutch ambulation with non–weight-bearing status on the right leg. On your morning rounds, Jason shows you a pair of wooden, axillary crutches his family brought in last evening, which he used 2 years ago when he sprained his ankle. He asks you if it is okay to use them. How would you respond?

4. What aspects of client care remain the same regardless of the type of orthotic device applied?

REFERENCES

Borgman-Gainer M: Independent function: movement and mobility. In Hoeman S, editor: *Rehabilitation nursing: process and application*, ed 2, St Louis, 1996, Mosby.

Brady R et al: Geriatric falls: prevention strategies for the staff, *J Gerontol Nurs* 19(9):26, 1993.

Clinical News: Falls in the home: the price of prevention, *Am J Nurs* 95(2):10, 1995.

Hale J, Clark A, Harrison R: Guidelines for prescription walking frames, *Physiotherapy* 76(2):118, 1990.

Lueckenotte A: *Gerontologic nursing*, St Louis, 1996, Mosby.

Mourad L, Droste M: *The nursing process in care of adults with orthopedic conditions*, ed 3, Albany, NY, 1993, Delmar.

Phipps W et al: *Medical-surgical nursing: concepts and clinical practice*, ed 5, St Louis, 1995, Mosby.

Shurr D, Cook T: *Prosthetics and orthotics*, Norwalk, CT, 1990, Appleton and Lange.

Sorrentino SA: *Assisting with patient care*, St Louis, 1998, Mosby.

Whaley L, Wong D: *Nursing care of infants and children*, ed 4, St Louis, 1995, Mosby.

UNIT 8

Managing Complex Nursing Interventions

Chapter 30
Intravenous Therapy

Chapter 31
Promoting Oxygenation

Chapter 32
Gastrointestinal Intubation for Suction

Chapter 33
Enteral Tube Feedings

Chapter 34
Altered Bowel Elimination

Chapter 35
Altered Urinary Elimination

Chapter 36
Altered Sensory Perception

Chapter 37
Fluid, Electrolyte, and Acid-Base Balance

Chapter 38
Emergency Measures for Life Support in the Hospital Setting

Chapter 39
Care of the Clients with Special Needs

Chapter 40
Discharge Teaching and Home Health Management

CHAPTER 30

Intravenous Therapy

Skill 30.1
Basic IV Insertion Techniques (Intermittent and Continuous Infusion), 684

Skill 30.2
Regulating Flow Rates, 696

Skill 30.3
Maintenance of IV Site, 703

Skill 30.4
Administering IV Medications, 711

Skill 30.5
Transfusions with Blood Products, 720

Delivery of infusion therapy is an essential element in the treatment of clients and requires a nurse's professional accountability and skill. The nurse applies the nursing process when assessing and choosing the most appropriate vascular access site and device, preparing the client, using proper insertion technique, and closely monitoring the infusion until the completion of therapy. Because of the extensive use of intravenous (IV) therapy, the professional nurse plays a primary role in safely and efficiently delivering IV medications and fluids, as well as protecting the client from the potential complications associated with IV therapy.

Nurses should follow institutional policy and procedure when managing IV therapy. Individual practitioners should know the various Nurse Practice Act regulations in their state regarding care and insertion of IV devices for short-duration and long-duration therapy. These may vary from state to state.

National standards guide nursing practice in safeguarding the client, the nurse, and the institution. The *In-travenous Nursing Standards of Practice,* published by the Intravenous Nurses Society (INS), establishes the scope of practice, competencies, and educational requirements for the administration of infusion therapy (INS, 1998). Additional guidelines supporting quality client care in this high-technology arena are published by the Oncology Nursing Society and the Centers for Disease Control and Prevention (CDC) (Camp-Sorrell, 1996; Pearson, 1996).

A nurse must be highly skilled with IV therapy. An IV device is invasive, increasing the risk of infection. Pain is associated with any IV insertion. A client's previous experience with IV therapy also affects how the nurse approaches care. The nurse's skill and expertise directly influence the client's response to the initiation of therapy.

Assessment of a client who requires IV therapy should be comprehensive. The nurse considers anatomy and physiology, fluid and electrolyte balance, chemistry, pathophysiology, and the client's response to illness. Assessment also extends to the observation of the client's venous anatomy of the upper extremities, assessment of mobility or immobility, and previous attempts or experiences of IV therapy. The goal of all IV therapy is to restore, prevent, or correct fluid and electrolyte imbalance without complications associated with the delivery of IV medications or fluids.

NURSING DIAGNOSES

Nursing diagnoses for clients receiving IV therapy may include **Risk for Infection** related to an invasive procedure. The client with an IV line is also at risk for **Impaired Skin Integrity.** For the client receiving IV therapy for correction of fluid and electrolyte imbalance or with potential or existing alterations in regulatory mechanisms of hydration, actual or potential **Fluid Volume Excess** or actual or potential **Fluid Volume Deficit** may be appropriate. **Risk for Injury** is created by the presence of an IV catheter acting as a foreign body and adverse events related to IV medications. **Knowledge Deficits** are seen in most clients receiving IV therapy because of a lack of experience with this type of therapy. In addition, home care clients may misinterpret or have a lack of interest in information pertaining to care of IV devices. **Noncompliance,** especially in home care, is seen with failure to comply with medication administration, flushing, or tubing change procedures.

Psychological factors such as **Fear** related to the client's previous experience with IV therapy or perceived **Pain** associated with the actual procedure may result in apprehension. Tension and **Anxiety** may cause sympathetic stimulation, resulting in venous constriction, making venipuncture more difficult and painful.

For clients receiving care in the home, nursing diagnoses may include **Impaired Home Maintenance Management.** The client's home could be insufficiently cleaned, lack adequate lighting or proper medication and supply storage, or fail to have a telephone for emergency situations. **Ineffective Management of the Therapeutic Regimen** could result from the complexity of the IV therapy or excessive demands made on the individual or family.

Skill 30.1

BASIC IV INSERTION TECHNIQUES (INTERMITTENT AND CONTINUOUS INFUSION)

To maintain fluid and electrolyte balance, isotonic, hypotonic, or hypertonic fluids are delivered through a variety of IV methods using continuous intermittent infusion and direct injection. IV therapy also provides access to the venous system to deliver various medications in emergent and nonemergent situations and to infuse blood or blood products. Reliable access for IV administration is one of the most essential features of current medical care.

Successful delivery of peripheral IV therapy depends on client preparation, vein selection, selection of an appropriate catheter, and skilled catheter insertion. Several vascular access devices are available for use in peripheral veins (Table 30-1). Because potential for exposure to blood-borne pathogens is high during insertion and care of IV devices, adherence to asepsis and standard precautions is required (see Chapters 3 and 4).

Concern for the personal safety of nurses during the delivery of IV therapy has gained importance in recent years because of the possibility of transmission of organisms such as hepatitis B virus (HBV) and human immunodeficiency virus (HIV). The most common cause of exposure of nurses to blood during IV therapy is by needle stick, with the highest risk occurring from stylets used to puncture the vein wall (Ippolito, 1997). To decrease this risk, safety products are available on over-the-needle catheters (ONCs) and winged butterfly needles and catheters.

Equipment

Tourniquets (single client use or disinfected after each use) or blood pressure cuff
Disposable gloves
Prepping agent(s) (70% alcohol, povidone-iodine, tincture of iodine)
IV fluids with time tape attached (if applicable)
Tubing (if applicable)

PRN adapter (intermittent infusion injection cap)
3-ml syringe
Sterile tape, 1/2-inch wide
Flush solution (e.g., sterile normal saline [NS] or heparin)
Transparent membrane dressing or sterile 2 × 2 and tape
IV pole
Appropriate IV catheter (gauge appropriate to type of solution infused) (see Table 30-1)

ASSESSMENT

1. Assess client's previous or perceived experience with IV therapy and arm placement preference. **Rationale: Determines level of emotional support and instruction necessary.**
2. Determine if client is to undergo any planned surgeries. **Rationale: Allows nurse to place an adequate-size catheter (i.e., 18 or 16 gauge for surgery) and avoids placement in an area that will interfere with medical procedures.**
3. Assess client's activities of daily living (ADLs). **Rationale: Ensures placement will not impair therapy or interfere with mobility and improves client's comfort and tolerance of IV therapy.**
4. Assess the type and duration of IV therapy as ordered by the physician. **Rationale: Assists in selection of an appropriate access device and early placement of longer-term infusion devices and minimizes multiple venipunctures.**
5. Assess laboratory data and client's history of allergies. **Rationale: May reveal information that affects insertion of devices, such as fluid volume deficit or allergy to iodine, adhesive, or latex.**

Table 30-1

IV Access Device Options

Type	Use
Winged infusion butterfly needle	One-time infusion, IV push administration

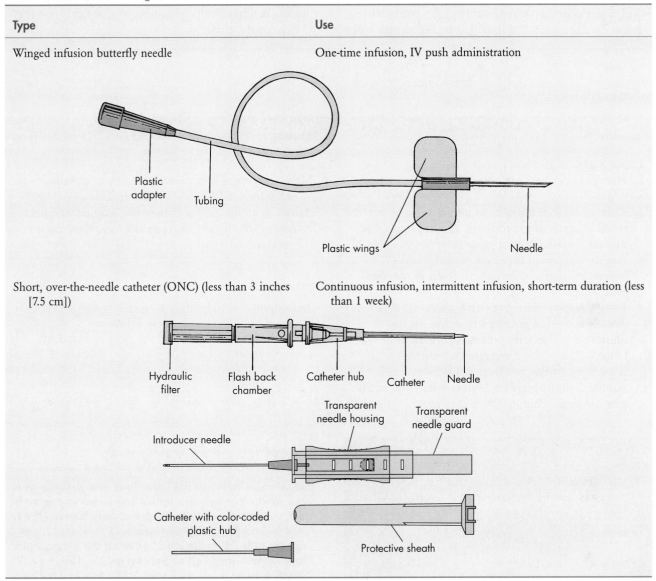

Short, over-the-needle catheter (ONC) (less than 3 inches [7.5 cm])

Continuous infusion, intermittent infusion, short-term duration (less than 1 week)

6. Assess client's medical history for chronic illnesses and all medications. **Rationale: Chronic cardiac or renal diseases and subsequent medications (e.g., diuretics) indicate the need for electronic control of the infusion (see Skill 30.2).**

PLANNING

Expected outcomes focus on minimal complications from IV therapy, minimal discomfort to the client, restoration of normal fluid and electrolyte balance, and client's ability to verbalize complications that require immediate nursing intervention.

Expected Outcomes

1. Client remains free of vasovagal reaction during the procedure.
2. Client remains free of complications associated with the presence of the catheter, including absence of pain, swelling, or redness.
3. Client verbalizes comfort and minimal restrictions to activities of daily living (ADLs) immediately after catheter insertion.
4. Client identifies one symptom of infiltration (e.g., swelling), phlebitis (e.g., redness), and occlusion (e.g., stoppage of flow).
5. Client notifies the health care provider when symptoms are found.

DELEGATION CONSIDERATIONS

The skill of basic IV insertion requires problem solving and knowledge application unique to a professional nurse. In many states, this skill is included within the scope of practice for licensed practical (vocational) nurses. For this skill, delegation to assistive personnel (AP) is inappropriate.

IMPLEMENTATION

Steps	Rationale
1. See Standard Protocol (inside front cover).	
2. Place client in a supine position.	Minimizes the risk of vasovagal reactions during venipuncture (Pavlin et al., 1993; Rapp et al., 1993).
3. Assist client in techniques to minimize anxiety: visual imagery, deep breathing, and not looking at the site. Explain steps of procedure.	Assists in minimizing apprehension, sympathetic nervous system stimulation, and possible vasovagal reaction to venipuncture.
4. Prepare equipment for insertion and prime IV tubing, maintaining sterility of closed system (see Skill 30.2).	
5. Apply tourniquet 4 to 6 inches (10 to 15 cm) above the proposed insertion site (see illustration). Check for presence of radial pulse. OPTION: Apply blood pressure cuff instead of tourniquet. Inflate to a level just below client's normal diastolic pressure. Maintain inflation at that pressure until venipuncture is completed.	Tourniquet should be tight enough to impede venous return but *not* occlude arterial flow.

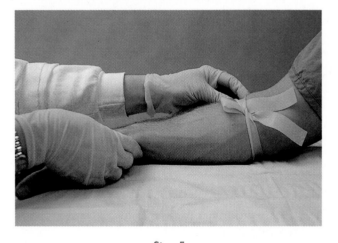

Step 5

COMMUNICATION TIP

Encourage client to ask questions and provide honest, forthright answers with a calm, reassuring manner. Tell the client, "The stick will hurt a little bit but will be less painful if you can hold very still. It's OK to move the opposite arm." After all the preparation and immediately before puncturing the skin, say, "It is going to be a big stick now," then proceed immediately to insert the catheter. Keep reminding the client to take slow deep breaths, especially if you have difficulty entering the vein. Distract the client by talking about other subjects.

6. Select the vein.	
a. Use the most distal site in the nondominant arm, if possible (see illustrations).	Venipuncture should be performed distal to proximal, which increases the availability of other sites for future IV therapy.
b. Avoid areas that are painful to palpation.	
c. Select a vein large enough for catheter placement.	Prevents interruption of venous flow while allowing adequate blood flow around the catheter.
d. Choose a site that will not interfere with client's ADLs or planned procedures.	

Steps	Rationale

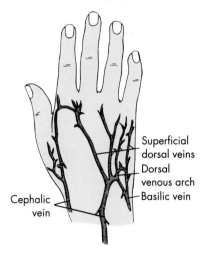

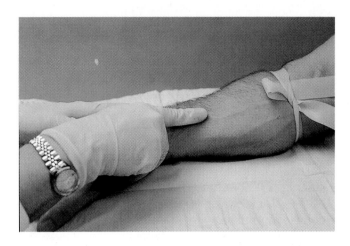

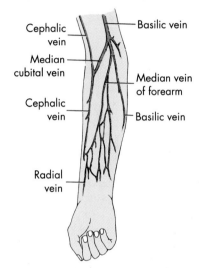

Step 6a

e. Palpate the vein by pressing downward and noting the resilient, soft, bouncy feeling as the pressure is released. Always use the same finger to palpate.

Use of the same finger causes a development of sensitivity to better assess the vein condition (Perucca, 1995).

f. Promote venous distention by instructing the client to open and close the fist several times, lowering the client's arm in a dependent position, and rubbing or stroking the client's arm.

g. Avoid sites distal to previous venipuncture site, sclerosed or hardened cordlike veins, infiltrated site or phlebotic vessels, bruised areas, and areas of venous valves or bifurcation.

Such sites cause infiltration of newly placed IV line and excessive vessel damage.

h. Avoid fragile dorsal veins in older adult clients and vessels in an extremity with compromised circulation (e.g., in cases of mastectomy, dialysis graft, or paralysis).

Venous alterations can increase risk of complications (e.g., infiltration and decreased catheter dwell time).

NURSE ALERT

In clients with fragile veins or engorged veins (e.g., client with congestive heart failure [CHF]) or those receiving anticoagulants, tourniquets should be avoided. Light pressure can be applied by the hand of another nurse and released as soon as the catheter has punctured the vein wall. This decreases the chance of excessive vein wall tearing and hematoma formation (Fabian, 1995).

Steps	Rationale
7. Options for venous distention in clients with limited peripheral venous sites or sclerosed veins:	
a. Apply warm packs to arm for 10 to 20 minutes.	Heat causes vasodilation.
b. Apply one tourniquet on mid–upper arm and stroke downward toward hand. After 1 to 2 minutes, apply a second tourniquet slightly below the antecubital fossa and stroke downward.	Gradually forces blood to distend smaller veins (Fabian, 1995).
8. Release tourniquet temporarily and carefully. Clip arm hair with scissors. Avoid shaving the area.	Hair impedes venipuncture or adherence of the dressing. Shaving can cause microabrasions and predispose client to infection.
9. Cleanse the insertion site using a circular motion moving from the insertion site outward in concentric circles. Use 70% alcohol, povidone-iodine, or tincture of iodine and allow to dry (see illustration). Reprep the skin if touched after preparation.	Drying prevents chemical reactions between agents and allows time for maximum microbicidal activity of agents.
10. Reapply tourniquet.	
11. Stabilize the vein by pulling the skin taut opposite the direction of the venipuncture (see illustration) Instruct client to relax hand.	
12. Warn client of a sharp, quick stick. Puncture the skin and vein, holding the catheter at a 10- to 30-degree angle (see illustration).	Superficial veins require a smaller angle. Deeper veins require a greater angle.

NURSE ALERT

Use a direct approach for large, easily seen veins: catheter punctures skin and vein wall simultaneously.

Use an indirect approach for small, fragile, or deeper veins: catheter punctures skin, vein is relocated, then catheter punctures vein wall.

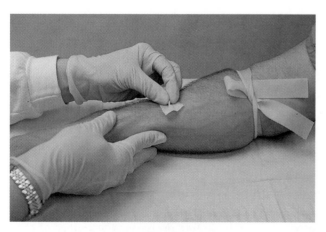

Step 9

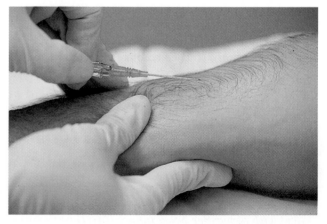

Step 11

Steps	Rationale

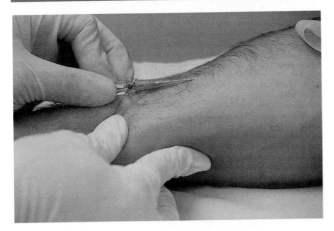

Step 12

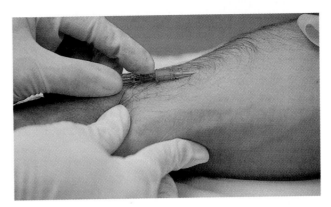

Step 14

13. Observe for a "flashback" of blood in the catheter's stylet, lower the catheter until almost flush with the skin, and slowly advance another ⅛ to ¼ inch.

14. Advance the catheter off the stylet while continuing to hold skin taut (see illustration).

15. Release tourniquet or blood pressure cuff.

16. After catheter is fully advanced, apply pressure with index finger of nondominant hand 1¼ inches (3 cm) above the insertion site. Remove the stylet.

17. **Intermittent Infusion**
    Hold the cannula firmly with nondominant hand and attach sterile injection cap; clean with alcohol. Insert prefilled syringe containing flush solution into injection cap. Flush injection cap slowly with flush solution. Withdraw the syringe, while still flushing.

18. **Continuous infusion**
    Connect IV tubing (see illustration) primed with fluid, maintaining sterile technique.
    Begin the infusion by slowly opening the slide clamp or adjusting the roller clamp of the IV tubing.

Allows for full penetration of the vein wall, placement of the catheter in the vein's inner lumen, and easy advancement of the catheter off the stylet.

Restores blood flow to arm.
Obstructs venous flow, minimizing blood loss.

"Positive pressure flushing" allows fluid to displace the removed needle, creates positive pressure in the catheter, and prevents reflux of blood during flushing. Stabilizing the cannula prevents accident withdrawal or dislodgement.

Initiates flow of fluid through IV catheter, preventing clotting.

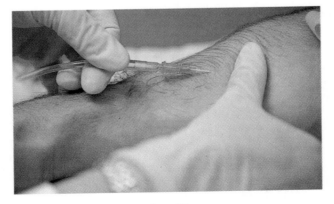

Step 18

Steps	**Rationale**

19. Tape or secure catheter.

    a. If applying a gauze dressing, tape the IV catheter. Place narrow piece (½ inch) of tape under hub of catheter with adhesive side up and cross tape over hub (see illustration).

    Place tape only on the catheter, *never* over the insertion site. Secure the site to allow easy visual inspection and early recognition of infiltration and phlebitis. Avoid applying tape around the extremity.

    b. If applying transparent dressing, secure catheter with nondominant hand while preparing to apply dressing.

Securing the catheter and tubing prevents movement and tension on the device, reducing mechanical irritation and possible phlebitis or infection.

Taping around extremity could result in a "tourniquet effect" and impede venous return.

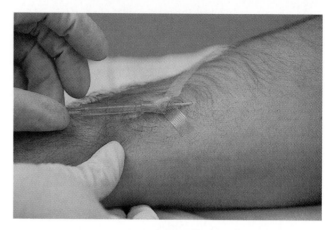

Step 19a

20. Apply sterile dressing over site.

    a. Transparent dressing

      (1) Carefully remove adherent backing. Apply one edge of dressing and then gently smooth remaining dressing over IV site, leaving end of catheter hub uncovered (see illustrations).

      (2) Fold a 2 × 2 gauze in half and cover with a 1-inch-wide tape extending about an inch from each side. Place under the tubing/catheter hub junction. Curl a loop of tubing alongside the arm and place a second piece of tape directly over the padded 2 × 2, securing tubing in two places.

Tape on top of tape makes it easier to access hub/tubing junction. Securing loop of tubing reduces risk of dislodging catheter from accidental pull.

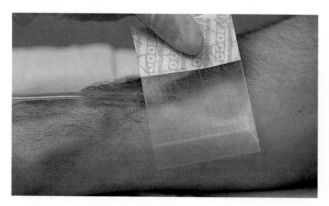 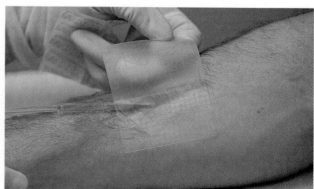

Step 20a

Steps	Rationale

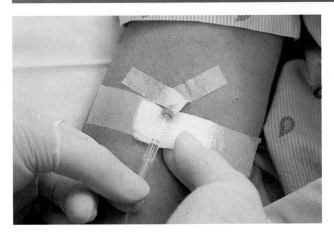 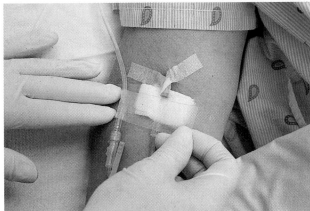

Step 20b(1)

b. Sterile gauze dressing
   (1) Follow Step 20a(2) (see illustrations).
   (2) Place 2 × 2 gauze pad over venipuncture site and catheter hub. Secure all edges with tape. Do not cover connection between IV tubing and catheter hub.
21. Remove and dispose of gloves.
22. Label the dressing, including the date, time, catheter gauge size and length, and nurse's initials.

Allows for easy recognition of type of device and time interval for site rotation. INS standard for site rotation of IV access devices every 48 hours (INS, 1998). Check agency policy.

23. Instruct client on how to move about in and out of bed without dislodging IV line.
24. Dispose of uncapped needle(s) and stylet in appropriate "sharps" container as soon as device is secured.
25. See Completion Protocol (inside front cover).

NURSE ALERT

If venipuncture is unsuccessful, always obtain a new catheter before a second attempt. Never reinsert the stylet into the catheter, because this may cause injury to the catheter and potential catheter embolism.

• • •

EVALUATION
1. Monitor client's intake and output (I & O), daily weights as indicated, skin turgor, mucous membranes, and vital signs for evidence of normal fluid volume.
2. Inspect client's IV site and extremity every 2 to 4 hours for the absence of pain, swelling, heat, or redness during the infusion. Aspirate for blood return if necessary.
3. On completion of IV insertion and during IV infusion, ask if client is comfortable. Observe client during activity for restrictions to mobility.
4. Ask client to describe one symptom of infiltration, phlebitis, and occluded infusion device complications (e.g., swelling, pain, tenderness, reduced flow).
5. Ask client to explain what steps to take if symptoms are noticed.

Table 30-2

Phlebitis Scale

Score	Clinical Signs
0	No clinical symptoms
1+	Erythema with or without pain
	Edema may or may not be present
	No streak formation
	No palpable cord
2+	Erythema with or without pain
	Edema may or may not be present
	Streak formation
	No palpable cord
3+	Erythema with or without pain
	Edema may or may not be present
	Streak formation
	Palpable cord

From Intravenous Nurses Society: Intravenous nursing standards of practice, *J Intraven Nurs* 21(15):535, 1998.

Unexpected Outcomes and Related Interventions

1. *Phlebitis.* Client complains of pain and tenderness at IV site with erythema at site or along path of vein. Insertion site is warm to touch, and rate of infusion may stop.
   a. Discontinue existing IV and restart in another site, preferably in opposite extremity, with new IV tubing and fluids.
   b. Document degree of phlebitis and nursing interventions per agency policy and procedure (Table 30-2).
2. *Infiltration.* Client's rate of infusion slows; site of insertion becomes swollen, cool to touch, pale, and painful.
   a. Discontinue existing IV line and restart in another site, preferably in opposite extremity.
   b. Monitor previous insertion site every 4 hours until resolution of swelling.
   c. Document degree of infiltration and nursing intervention (Table 30-3).
3. Client experiences burning, irritation, redness, or pain during infusion without phlebitis or infiltration.
   a. Slow the infusion to deliver in maximum time for best therapeutic response.
   b. Assess client's tolerance to prescribed therapy. Discuss with client and physician insertion of midline or peripherally inserted central catheter as an option if duration of therapy and venous access permit.
4. Infusion is completed before or after appropriate time frame.
   a. Evaluate access device for position and patency, and restart as necessary.

Table 30-3

Infiltration Scale

Score	Clinical Signs
0	No symptoms
1	Skin blanched
	Edema less than 1 inch
	Cool to touch
	With or without pain
2	Skin blanched
	Edema 1 to 6 inches on skin surface
	Cool to touch
	With or without pain
3	Skin blanched, translucent
	Gross edema greater than 6 inches on skin surface
	Cool to touch
	Mild to moderate pain
	Possible numbness
4	Skin blanched, translucent
	Skin tight, leaking
	Skin discolored, bruised, swollen
	Gross edema greater than 6 inches on skin surface
	Deep pitting tissue edema (+3, +4)
	Circulatory impairment
	Moderate to severe pain
	Infiltration of any amount of blood product, irritant, or vesicant

   b. Monitor client for too-rapid infusion or fluid overload. Check vital signs, respiratory status, and I&O.
   c. Monitor client for signs and symptoms of drug toxicity.
   d. Notify physician.
   e. Reregulate remainder of infusion to infuse over prescribed time. Assess need for electronic flow-control device.
5. *Positional IV infusion:* Client's flow rate is altered and changes with position of extremity.
   a. Apply arm board (Figure 30-1).
   b. Remove dressing, apply additional prepping agents, and resecure devices.
   c. If catheter device has been withdrawn from vessel, do not reinsert exposed portion of catheter.
   d. Continue hourly monitoring for proper rate of infusion.
6. *Infection:* Client complains of chills, fever, and malaise; IV site may show purulent drainage.
   a. Discontinue IV by prepping site first with alcohol (removes resident bacteria). Allow to dry. Then place dry sterile gauze over insertion site and remove catheter.

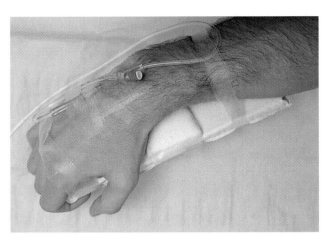

Figure 30-1   IV arm board.

b. Retain previous IV catheter for possible culture (follow agency policy) and notify physician.

c. Document nursing intervention as delineated in agency policy and procedure.

Recording and Reporting

*   Record in nurses' notes number of attempts for insertion, type of fluid, insertion site by vessel, flow rate, size and type catheter or needle, and when infusion was begun. A special parenteral therapy flow sheet may be used (Figure 30-2, p. 694).
*   Record client's response to IV fluid, amount infused, and integrity and patency of system every 4 hours or according to agency policy.
*   Report to oncoming nursing staff: type of fluid, flow rate, status of venipuncture site, amount of fluid remaining in present solution, expected time to hang next IV bag or bottle, and any side effects.
*   Report to physician immediately any adverse reactions such as pulmonary congestion, shock, or thrombophlebitis.

Sample Documentation

Documentation may be recorded on an IV Maintenance Record (see pp. 694 to 695).

1500   After procedure explained and site prepped with alcohol and Betadine, left cephalic vein accessed with 20-gauge 1¼-inch insyte catheter. Positive blood return after full advancement. Catheter flushed with 1 ml NS, and saline lock attached for IV antibiotics. Client stated insertion was nonpainful and "felt fine" after insertion.

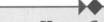

Home Care and
Long-Term Care Considerations

*   Ensure that the client/caregiver is able and willing to administer IV therapy.
*   Determine the client's ability to obtain help; for example, availability of caregiver, and presence of and ability to use telephone.
*   Ensure that all needles and equipment contaminated by blood are disposed of in puncture-resistant containers with lids; for example, plastic milk cartons or coffee cans. Some suppliers will provide sharps containers for needle disposal (see Chapter 41).
*   Instruct client and primary caregiver about procedures of IV therapy, including handwashing and sterile technique while manipulating syringes and other supplies.
*   Teach client and primary caregiver to recognize potential problems at insertion site and appropriate reaction to problems.

*   Teach primary caregiver to apply pressure with sterile gauze if catheter falls out, and, if client is on anticoagulant therapy, to tape several pieces of sterile gauze in place for at least 20 minutes or until bleeding stops.
*   Teach client and primary caregiver to take tub bath but not to let IV dressing touch water and to unplug pump first if one is used. If showering is mandatory, the client must insert hand and forearm into a plastic bag. Tape bag in place to ensure that IV site is completely covered.
*   Instruct client to wear clothes with wide sleeves.
*   Teach client about activity restrictions; for example, avoiding strenuous exercise of the arm with the IV.
*   In addition, for home care clients, teach client and family to monitor I&O using household measuring devices.

ST. JOHN'S HOSPITAL
Springfield, Illinois
I.V. MAINTENANCE RECORD

I.V. FLUID & I.V. MEDICATION

Site Code
R.J. or L.J. – Right or Left Jugular
R.S.V. or L.S.V. – Right or Left Subclavian Vein
R.L.L. or L.L.L. – Right or Left Lower Leg
R.H. or L.H. – Right or Left Hand
R.F.A. or L.F.A. – Right or Left Forearm
R.U.A. or L.U.A. – Right or Left Upperarm
R.F. or L.F. – Right or Left Foot
R.S., L.S. or M.S.– Right, Left or Mid Scalp
R.F.V. or L.F.V. – Right or Left Femoral Vein
R.A.C. or L.A.C. – Right or Left Antecubital
R.W. or L.W. – Right or Left Wrist

K.V.O. – Keep Vein Open
H.L. – Heparin Lock
P.B. – Piggyback
P. – Push

Triple Lumen Catheter

Proximal - 18 gauge (White)	Middle - 18 gauge (Blue)	Distal - 16 gauge (Brown)
Draw blood, Blood Adm. Medications	TPN Medications	Blood Adm. Colloids Viscous Fluids CVP Monitoring Medications

Signature:

Allergy:

No. of last I.V. _____ Letter of last expander _____
No. of last Blood/Component _____

DATE			
Night Nurse			
Day Nurse			
Evening Nurse			

Order Date		Amount, Solution, Infusing Time or Rate, Medication, Dose, Time	Site(s)			Pump	Time	Time
		One Time I.V. Meds.						
	No.	I.V. Fluids						
		I.V. TUBING CHANGE. (Indicate I.V. No. & Time)						
	Stop Date	Intermittent & PRN I.V. Meds.						
		I.V.P.B. TUBING CHANGE (Indicate Drug & Time)						

#1005
(1 of 2)

I.V. MAINTENANCE RECORD

Figure 30-2   IV Maintenance Record.   *Courtesy St John's Hospital, Springfield, Ill.*

I.V. SITE ASSESSMENT		
SITE CODE		**TYPE CODE**

SITE CODE		TYPE CODE	
R.J. or L.J. – Right or Left Jugular		M.C. – Medicut	H.C. – Hickman Catheter
R.S.V. or L.S.V. – Right or Left Subclavian Vein K.V.O. – Keep Vein Open		A.C. – Angiocath	B.C. – Broviac Catheter
R.L.L. or L.L.L. – Right or Left Lower Leg H.L. – Heparin Lock		S.V. – Scalpvein	M.L.C. – Multi-lumen Catheter
R.H. or L.H. – Right or Left Hand P.B. – Piggyback		A.S. – Angio-set	M.L.P. – Multi-lumen Proximal
R.F.A. or L.F.A. – Right or Left Forearm P. – Push			
R.U.A. or L.U.A. – Right or Left Upperarm Cath – Catheter		C.D. – Cutdown	M.L.M. – Multi-lumen Middle
R.F. or L.F. – Right or Left Foot		I.C. – Intracath	M.L.D. – Multi-lumen Distal
R.S., L.S. or M.S. – Right, Left or Mid Scalp			
R.F.V. or L.F.V. – Right or Left Femoral Vein		I.P.. – Infuse A Port	I. – Introducer
R.A.C. or L.A.C. – Right or Left Antecubital			
R.W. or L.W. – Right or Left Wrist NA – Not Applicable			

Document on each site once each shift & P.R.N.   No space is to be left blank.   Place "NA" in spaces which do not apply.

Date	Time	I.V. Site Start	d/c	Site Code	Cath Size	Type Code	Site Day	Cap Change	Dressing Change	I.V. Site: s̄ tenderness redness, edema, drainage	Signature

Figure 30-2, cont'd   IV Maintenance Record.

Geriatric Considerations

- Older adults veins are very fragile. Avoid sites that are easily moved or bumped. (Use commercial protective device to protect site.)
- In older clients, use the smallest gauge possible, for example, 22, 24, or 26 gauge. This is less traumatizing to the vein and allows better blood flow to provide increased hemodilution of the IV fluids or medications (Fabian, 1995).
- If possible, avoid the back of the older adult's hand or the dominant arm for venipuncture because these sites greatly interfere with the older adult's independence.

- If the older adult has fragile skin and veins, use minimal tourniquet pressure or no tourniquet at all.
- When the older adult has lost subcutaneous tissue, the veins lose stability and roll away from the needle. To stabilize the vein, apply traction to the skin below the projected insertion point (Fabian, 1995).
- Using an angle of 5 to 15 degrees on insertion is helpful because the older adult's veins are more superficial (Fabian, 1995).

Skill 30.2

REGULATING FLOW RATES

The ability to establish accurate infusion rates in IV therapy is essential to deliver prescribed infusion volumes and medications. Complications associated with IV therapy (e.g., infiltration, phlebitis, clotting of device, circulatory overload) can be reduced or eliminated with a properly regulated IV infusion. Various factors can interfere with infusion rates (Table 30-4). Observation of the flow rate and IV system should occur hourly to achieve the desired therapeutic response.

Numerous methods are used to ensure an accurate hourly infusion rate for IV therapy. Fluids that run by gravity are adjusted through use of a flow control/regulator clamp. Fluids infused by an electronic infusion device or rate controller are regulated by a mechanical pump set at the prescribed rate. Physicians usually order the volume of fluid a client is to receive within a specific time frame. For example, "Administer 1 liter of D_5NS over 8 hours." The nurse must be able to calculate hourly flow rates to ensure the prescribed amount of fluid infuses over 8 hours. Regardless of gravity infusion or infusion via an electronic device, the nurse must assess infusion rates hourly.

Infusion pumps are necessary when administering low, hourly volumes, (e.g. 5 ml/hr or less, 20 ml/hr, etc.) to neonatal or pediatric clients or clients who are at risk for volume overload. In addition, when infusing high volumes of IV fluids (more than 150 ml/hr) to clients with impaired renal clearance, older adults, or pediatric clients, or when infusing drugs or IV fluids that require specific hourly volumes, electronic infusion pumps permit accurate, on-time infusion. Electronic infusion devices deliver the infusion via positive pressure. A rate controller used on gravity infusions regulates the infusion but, unlike the electronic pump, can be affected by many mechanical and client factors. Recent advances in infusion technology have resulted in a variety of devices available for use to ensure accurate delivery.

Many devices have operating and programming capabilities that allow for single- and multiple-solution infusions at different rates (Figure 30-3, *A*). A variety of detectors and alarms respond to air in IV lines, completion of infusion, high and low pressure, low battery power, occlusion, and the inability to deliver at a preset rate. An anti–free flow safeguard (preventing bolus infusion in the event of machine malfunction) is an important element of an electronic infusion pump. Most pumps may be used for IV infusions. Manufacturer's recommendations for specific device features should always be checked.

Clients in alternative care settings achieve infusion accuracy with ambulatory infusion pumps. Most pumps weigh less than 6 pounds and range from palm size to backpack size. They function on battery power, allowing the client freedom to return to normal life. Programming capabilities include automatic rate adjustments, remote site adjustments via a telephone modem, and therapy-specific settings such as patient-controlled analgesia (PCA) (Figure 30-3, *B*). Follow the manufacturer's recommendations for specific device features.

Equipment

Watch with a second hand
Paper and pencil (or calculator)
IV tubing, macro drip or micro drip, depending on rate ordered by physician and manufacturer specifications (some machines only use micro drip)
Electronic infusion control device (optional)
Volume control device (optional)
Tape
Label

ASSESSMENT

1. Review client's medical record for physician's order, stating type, amount, and rate or duration of IV fluid order or IV medications.
2. Assess client's understanding of purpose of therapy and knowledge of how positioning affects flow rate.

Table 30-4

Alterations in Flow Rates

Client Factors	Mechanical Factors
Change in client position	Height of parenteral
Flexion of involved extremity	container (should be
Partial or complete occlusion	higher than 36 inches
of IV device	[90 cm] above heart)
Venous spasm	Positional access device
Vein trauma (phlebitis)	Viscosity or temperature of
Manipulated by client or	IV solution
visitor	Occluded air vent
	Occluded in-line filter
	Improperly placed restraints
	Crimped administration set
	tubing
	Tubing dangling below bed
	Low battery of an electronic
	device

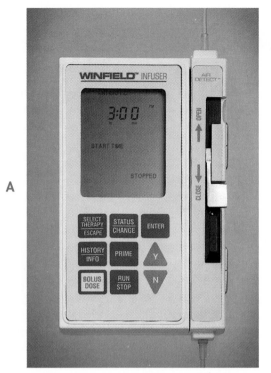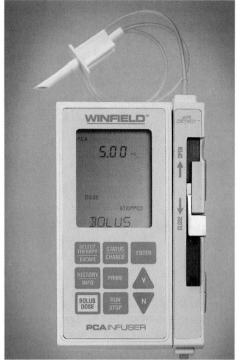

Figure 30-3   A, Electronic infusion device. **B,** Ambulatory infusion pump with patient-controlled analgesia (PCA).

3. Identify client's risk for fluid imbalance (e.g., pediatric, older adult, history of heart failure or renal failure). **Rationale: Strict control of infusion volumes may be required.**
4. Determine the presence of any client or mechanical factor that may alter ordered fluid rates (client confusion, ability of client to cooperate, diuretic therapy, electrolyte imbalance, etc.). **Rationale: Decreases the risk of IV infusion complications.**
5. Obtain information from pharmacology references about specific infusion requirements of IV medication, admixture, or device. **Rationale: Reinforces "5 rights" of medication administration, determines length of infusion time.**
6. Assess patency of IV device.

PLANNING

Expected outcomes focus on normal fluid and electrolyte balance and administration of IV fluids at the prescribed rate and correct dosage.

Expected Outcomes

1. Client receives prescribed volume of fluid within appropriate time frame, as evidenced by moist mucous membranes, adequate skin turgor, and balanced I&O.
2. Client's medications are administered over appropriate time frame with achievement of therapeutic response.

DELEGATION CONSIDERATIONS

The skill of regulating IV flow rates requires problem solving and knowledge application unique to a professional nurse. In many states, this skill is included within the scope of practice for licensed practical (vocational) nurses. Calculating and adjusting flow rates on gravity or electronic controlling devices is inappropriate for AP to perform. However, AP can be delegated to inform the nurse when a fluid container is almost empty, when the client complains of any discomfort, and when an electronic controlling device sounds an alarm.

IMPLEMENTATION

Steps	Rationale

1. See Standard Protocol (inside front cover).
2. Obtain IV fluid and appropriate tubing.
   a. *Macro drip:* Delivers rates *greater than* 100 ml/hr. (Drip factor is 10 to 15 gtt/ml depending on equipment used. Drop factor is printed on box.)
      Travenol Laboratories: 10 gtt/ml
      Abbott Laboratories: 15 gtt/ml
      McGraw Laboratories: 15 gtt/ml
   b. *Micro drip:* Delivers rates *less than* 100 ml/hr.
      Micro drip: 60 gtt/ml

Use of correct tubing ensures more accurate infusion delivery. Macro drip tubing allows for higher infusion volumes. Micro drip tubing is used for slow delivery and lower volumes.

3. Calculate desired flow rate (hourly volume) of prescribed infusion:

Flow rate (ml/hr) =

$$\frac{\text{Total infusion (volume in ml)}}{\text{Hours of infusion (time to be infused)}}$$

Example: $\dfrac{1000 \text{ ml}}{8 \text{ hr}} = \dfrac{125 \text{ ml}}{1 \text{ hr}}$

4. Calculate the drop rate based on drops per minute.

$$\frac{\text{gtt factor}}{60} \times \frac{\text{Flow rate}}{1} = \text{Drop rate}$$

Examples: Infuse 120 ml/hr via 10 gtt/ml drop factor:

$$\frac{10}{60} \times \frac{120}{1} = 20 \text{ gtt/min}$$

Via 15 gtt/ml:

$$\frac{15}{60} \times \frac{120}{1} = 30 \text{ gtt/min}$$

Via 20 gtt/ml:

$$\frac{20}{60} \times \frac{120}{1} = 40 \text{ gtt/min}$$

Via 60 gtt/ml (microgtt):

$$\frac{60}{60} \times \frac{120}{1} = 120 \text{ gtt/ml}$$

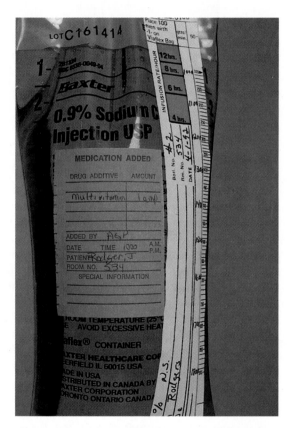

Step 6

5. Optional method for calculation:
   If drop factor is 10 gtt/ml, take ordered rate per hour and divide by 6.
   If drop factor is 15 gtt/ml, take ordered rate per hour and divide by 4.
   If drop factor is 20 gtt/ml, take ordered rate per hour and divide by 3.
   If drop factor is 60 gtt/ml, take ordered rate per hour and divide by 1.

Steps	Rationale

6. Time-tape the IV bottle or bag by securing adhesive tape or fluid indicator tape along side of fluid container (see illustration). Document each IV fluid bag sequentially, and note type of fluid, client's name, infusion span, and beginning and expected end of infusion.

Gives a visual scale to assess progress of infusion hourly. Avoid use of felt-tip pens or permanent markers on plastic bag; these can contaminate IV solutions (INS, 1998). In some agencies all fluids, including those on pumps, should be labeled and time-taped (see agency policy).

7. Close rate-controlling clamp on IV tubing.

8. Insert infusion set into fluid bag. Remove protective cover from IV bag without touching opening. Remove cap from spike and insert spike into opening of IV bag (see illustrations). Hang bag from IV pole.

Maintains sterility of solution.

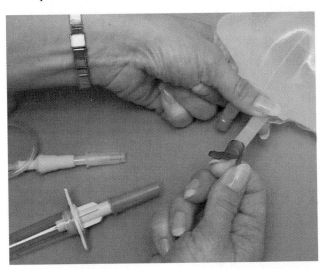 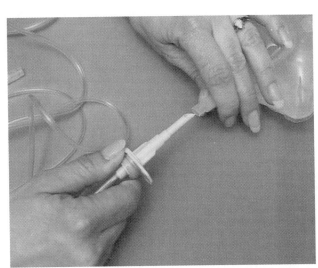

Step 8

9. Fill drip chamber of tubing until half full by gently squeezing and releasing.

Creates vacuum, allowing fluid to enter drip chamber.

10. Open rate-controlling clamp and fill remainder of tubing (see illustration). Invert Y connector sites to displace air. Most tubings can be fully filled or primed without removing the cover on the end of the IV tubing.

Tubing must be fully filled with fluid before connecting to client to avoid air embolus.

11. Close rate-controlling clamp on tubing.

12. Perform venipuncture (see Skill 30.1) and attach catheter to end of IV tubing, maintaining sterility.

13. With IV fluid bag a minimum of 36 inches (90 cm) above IV insertion site, adjust rate-controlling clamp to deliver drops per minute.

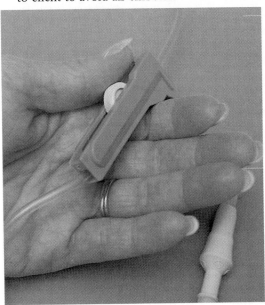

Step 10

Steps

Rationale

14. *Option:* Attach to electronic infusion device or rate controller.

   a. Place electronic eye on half-filled drip chamber above fluid line if required (see illustration). NOTE: Some devices do not use electronic eye.

   b. Insert IV tubing into chamber of control mechanism (see illustration). (Consult manufacturer's instructions for use of pump.)

Positioning necessary for accurate drip count.

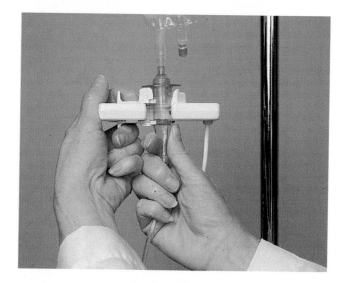

Step 14a

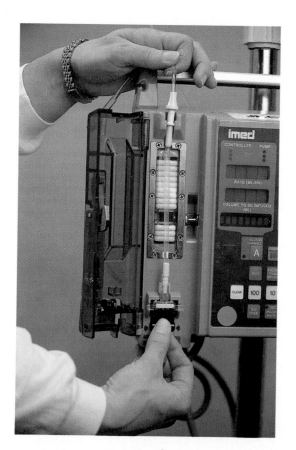

Step 14b

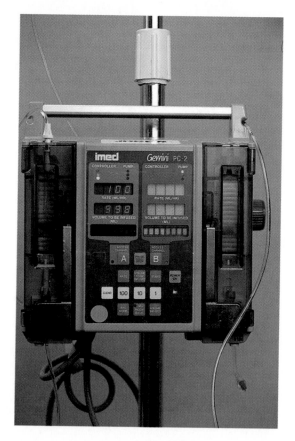

Step 14e

Steps	Rationale

   c. Secure portion of IV tubing through "air in line" alarm system.

   d. Turn on pump, and select rate per hour and total volume to be infused (VTBI).

   e. Open rate-controlling clamp if closed and press start (see illustration).

   f. Monitor infusion hourly to assess patency of system when in alarm mode and monitor for proper infusion rate and infiltration.

15. *Option.* Attach IV tubing to volume control device.

   a. Place volume control device between IV bag and insertion spike of infusion set using sterile technique (see illustration).

   b. Fill IV tubing with fluid by opening regulator clamp.

   c. Place 2 hours of fluid allotment in chamber device.

16. Instruct client about the following:

   a. To avoid raising hand or arm to a position that will affect flow rate.

   b. To avoid manipulation of rate control clamp.

   c. Purpose and significance of alarms.

17. See Completion Protocol (inside front cover).

Allows for detection of air in tubing, which can enter vascular system, causing an embolus.

This prevents infusion from running dry if 60 minutes elapses before nurse returns. Should infusion rate accidentally increase, will only allow 2 hours of fluids to infuse.

• • •

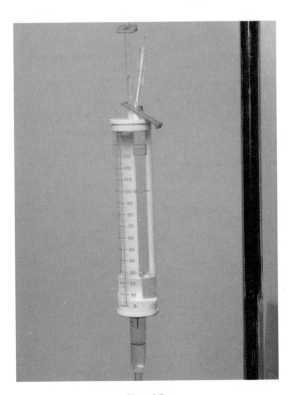

Step 15a

EVALUATION

1. Monitor client's IV infusion hourly for proper rate of infusion.
2. Observe client for therapeutic response to medication(s).
3. Observe client and client's laboratory values for signs and symptoms of overhydration or dehydration during infusion, observing for restoration of fluid and electrolyte balance and therapeutic response.
4. Evaluate client during ADLs for proper positioning of extremity and care of infusion tubing during activity.

Unexpected Outcomes and Related Interventions

1. During hourly check, infusion is found to be behind.
   a. Evaluate reason for delay in fluids.
   b. Recalculate remainder of infusion and confer with physician before reregulating.
2. Client experiences sudden onset of shortness of breath, tachycardia, restlessness, and confusion. Assessment of lung sounds reveals inspiratory crackles. Client has received more than prescribed infusion volume.
   a. Evaluate for proper function of IV access device.
   b. Slow rate to keep vein open (KVO).
   c. Place client in high Fowler's position and notify physician.

Recording and Reporting

- Record rate of infusion, drops/min, and ml/hr in nurses' notes every 4 hours or according to agency policy.
- Immediately record in nurses' notes any new IV fluid rates.
- Document use of any electronic infusion device or controlling device and number on that device.
- At change of shift or when leaving on break, report rate of infusion to nurse in charge or next nurse assigned to care for client.

Sample Documentation

Routine documentation is included on the IV Maintenance Record (see Figure 30-2, p. 694).

1700   Client complaining of SOB. Lungs auscultated with inspiratory crackles in rt lower lobe. Dr. Lee notified. Order noted to decrease IV to 25 ml/hr. Positive blood return noted via 20-gauge IV right cephalic vein. Changed to IMED Gemini infusion at 25 ml/hr via pump. Purpose of fluid restriction and symptoms of pulmonary edema reviewed with client and wife with verbalized understanding.

Geriatric Considerations

- Changes in cardiac and renal function related to the aging process or chronic conditions indicate the need for extreme accuracy in flow control, requiring electronic infusion devices.
- Fragility of veins in older adult client increases risk of infiltration. The infusion device may continue to infuse fluid into sites where infiltration is occurring. Monitor infusion site carefully and frequently.

Home Care and Long-Term Care Considerations

- Ensure that client is able and willing to operate the electronic infusion device (if applicable) and administer IV therapy, or ensure that there is a reliable caregiver or nursing support personnel at home to provide this IV therapy care. Closely assess any visual or physical limitations.
- Make sure nurse is in the home when IV pump is delivered. This enables nurse to determine that equipment works properly.
- Teach client and primary caregiver to time drops per minute using watch with second hand.
- Ensure that client's electrical outlets are properly grounded.

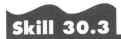

Skill 30.3

MAINTENANCE OF IV SITE

Peripheral IV catheters and the therapy being infused are frequently associated with complications such as local or systemic infections, phlebitis, and infiltration. Appropriate management of IV sites will prevent or minimize these complications.

The skin is one of the primary sources of catheter-related infection. Therefore catheter dressings must be securely applied and be changed when loose, wet, or soiled. Sterile gauze secured with tape or transparent membrane dressings is used to cover the site. Peripheral catheter dressings are applied when the catheter is inserted or when the site is changed. Peripheral IV sites are usually changed between 48 and 72 hours and the dressing changed at that time (INS, 1998; Pearson, 1996). Routine dressing changes on midline catheters vary from one to three times per week and immediately if they become wet, dirty, or loose. The procedure for changing the midline catheter dressing is the same as for central venous catheter dressing change (see Chapter 39). Check agency policy.

Fluid containers include plastic bags, plastic bottles, and glass bottles. These containers may be changed frequently depending on the rate of infusion and the volume in the container. The CDC (1996) does not make a recommendation for the hang time of IV fluids, but the INS recommends that each container be changed within 24 hours after the administration set is added (INS, 1998). Fluid containers on ambulatory infusion devices may remain longer than 24 hours if aseptic technique is used, the system remains closed without injection ports or add-on tubing, and the medication is stable for the anticipated infusion time (INS, 1998; Pearson, 1996). The nurse must allow adequate time for this procedure, follow proper technique to prevent infection, and adhere to the specific agency policy.

Changing infusion tubing is much simpler and more efficient if changed when hanging a new fluid container. The CDC (1996) recommends changing tubing no more frequently than every 72 hours. The INS (1998) recommends 48-hour intervals for tubing changes, adding that 72-hour tubing changes may be considered if the rate of phlebitis and infection are low. INS also states that tubing used for intermittent infusion through an injection/access port should be changed every 24 hours. Both ends of this tubing are manipulated more frequently than tubing used for continuous infusion.

An injection cap or prn adapter on a peripheral catheter is changed when the catheter is changed. A short extension tubing or loop may be placed between the catheter hub and injection cap. This allows manipulation of the injection cap without movement of the catheter. This tubing remains attached to the peripheral catheter and is changed when the catheter is changed. For midline

and central venous catheters, these caps should be changed at least every 7 days (INS, 1998). The fluid pathway and capped ends on all infusion tubing, stopcocks, extension tubing, and injection caps are sterile. The nurse must exercise caution to prevent contamination of these surfaces during changes.

The nurse must be prepared to assist the client with many aspects of hygiene, such as gown changes, while the client is receiving IV therapy (see Chapter 7). Gowns with snaps across the shoulders are best, especially for multiple infusions. When using a regular gown or the client's clothing, the nurse must thread the fluid container and tubing through the sleeve of the gown in the same manner as the client's arm. Infusion tubing should not be disconnected to change a gown or any article of clothing. Care can be coordinated so that bathing or hygiene activities are done after removal of an old infusion site and before another venipuncture is made.

Equipment

Changing a peripheral IV dressing
  Alcohol swabsticks
  Povidone-iodine swabsticks
  Skin protectant solution
  Adhesive remover (optional)
  Strips of sterile, precut tape (or 36-inch roll tape)
  Clean gloves
  Sterile 2 × 2 gauze pad and tape or transparent membrane dressing
  Arm board or housing device
Changing infusion tubing
  Continuous infusion:
    Microdrip or macrodrip infusion tubing, as appropriate for rate
    0.22-μ filter and extension tubing if necessary
    Tubing label
  Intermittent saline/heparin lock:
    Injection cap or prn adapter
    Loop or short extension tubing (if necessary)
    Sterile 2 × 2 gauze pads
    Saline-filled flush syringe and heparin-filled flush syringe (check agency policy)
    Clean gloves
    If a new IV dressing must be applied, assemble additional equipment (see Skill 30.2)
Changing infusion container
  Bottle/bag of IV solution as ordered by physician or appropriate prescriber
  Time tape
  Pen
Discontinuing IV medications
  Clean gloves

Sterile cap or cover for infusion tubing
Saline-filled syringe
Heparin-filled syringe for intermittent lock
Alcohol swabs
Injection cap replacement, if necessary
Discontinuing peripheral IV access
Clean gloves
Sterile 2 × 2 or 4 × 4 gauze pad
Tape

ASSESSMENT

1. *Changing a peripheral IV dressing:*
   a. Determine when the dressing was last changed by checking the dressing label. **Rationale: This labeling provides instant identification for assessing and determining status of the site (INS, 1998).**
   b. Observe present dressing for moisture and occlusiveness. Determine if moisture is from leakage from the puncture site or from an external source.
   c. Observe IV system for proper functioning or complications (tubing or catheter kinks). Palpate the catheter site through the intact dressing for inflammation; drainage; or complaints of tenderness, pain, or burning.
   d. Inspect exposed catheter site for swelling, redness, or blanching.
   e. Monitor body temperature.
   f. Determine client's understanding of the need for continued IV infusion.

2. *Changing infusion tubing:*
   a. Determine when new infusion set is needed (e.g., according to agency policy, or after contamination or puncture of infusion tubing).
   b. Observe for occlusions in tubing such as kinking, drug or mineral precipitate and blood. **Rationale: Infusion of incompatible medications can lead to precipitate formation. Blood may flow retrograde from vein and adhere to tubing. Infusion of viscous blood components may adhere to tubing.**
   c. Determine client's understanding of the need for continued IV infusions.

3. *Changing fluid container:*
   a. Check physician's orders. **Rationale: Ensures that correct solution will be used and that the order is complete.**
   b. If order is written for keep vein open (KVO), contact physician for clarification of the rate of infusion. Note date and time when solution was last changed. **Rationale: Orders for KVO do not provide complete information and can result in fluid overload or deficit and electrolyte imbalance (INS, 1998). Refer to agency policy.**
   c. Determine the compatibility of all IV fluids and additives by consulting appropriate literature or the pharmacy. **Rationale: Incompatibilities can cause physical or chemical changes in the admixture, such as precipitation or gas formation and changes in color or clarity. These changes increase the risk of catheter obstruction and decrease the therapeutic effect of the solution (Trissel, 1997).**
   d. Determine client's understanding of need for continuing IV therapy.
   e. Assess patency of current IV access site.

4. *Discontinuing IV medications:*
   a. Observe fluid container for complete infusion of all medication.
   b. Review care plan for any blood samples required after medication infusion. **Rationale: Monitoring of serum concentrations of some IV medications is required to avoid reaching toxic levels. Dosage adjustments or alterations of timing for next dose may be required. Check agency policy.**

5. *Discontinuing peripheral IV access:*
   a. Observe IV site for signs and symptoms of infection, infiltration, or phlebitis.
   b. Review physician order for discontinuation of IV therapy. **Rationale: Physician's order is required to discontinue IV therapy. The specific wording may not include removal of the catheter, but this is implied.**
   c. Determine client's understanding of the need for removal of peripheral IV catheter.

PLANNING

Expected outcomes focus on reducing the risk of infection and phlebitis, minimizing client discomfort, reducing risk of overhydration, and maintaining a patent IV catheter.

Expected Outcomes

1. Client will have IV that flows freely without infiltration, phlebitis, or clot.
2. Client's temperature will remain normal.
3. Client will continue to receive the prescribed fluid infusion and/or medication as ordered.
4. Client's serum electrolyte levels remain or return to normal.

DELEGATION CONSIDERATIONS

These skills require problem solving and knowledge application unique to a professional nurse. In many states, these skills are included within the scope of practice for licensed practical (vocational) nurses. AP may be delegated the task of collecting supplies, assisting with comfort measures, and distracting the client during the procedure.

IMPLEMENTATION

Steps	Rationale

1. See Standard Protocol (inside front cover).

2. 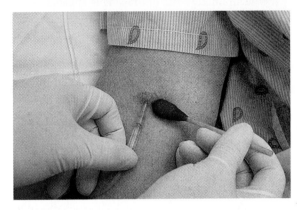 *Changing peripheral IV dressing:*

    a. Remove tape and gauze from old dressing one layer at a time by pulling toward the insertion site. Leave tape securing catheter to skin. Transparent membrane dressings may be removed by pulling each side laterally while holding catheter hub. Check agency procedure.

    b. Observe insertion site for redness, swelling, drainage, pallor, or pain. If present, discontinue infusion (see step 6).

    c. If IV is infusing properly, gently remove tape securing catheter. Stabilize catheter with one finger. Remove adhesive residue with adhesive remover, if necessary.

    d. Using circular motion, cleanse peripheral insertion site with alcohol, then povidone-iodine solution (see illustration), starting at insertion site and working outward creating concentric circles. Allow povidone-iodine solution to dry for 2 minutes.

    e. OPTION: Apply skin protectant solution (SkinPrep or No Sting Barrier Film) to the area where the tape or dressing will be applied. Allow to dry.

    f. Gauze dressing:

    (1) Place single strip of sterile ½-inch nonallergenic tape under peripheral catheter with sticky side up to anchor catheter to skin. Fold tape ends around catheter hub or wings. Place a second piece of sterile tape across catheter at hub.

    (2) Place a 2 × 2 gauze over venipuncture site and secure with tape on all edges. Do not cover the catheter hub/tubing junction with the dressing.

    g. Transparent dressing: Place transparent dressing over venipuncture site using the application method recommended by the dressing manufacturer. Do not cover the catheter hub/tubing junction with the dressing (see Skill 3.1, Step 20a(1)).

    h. Fold a 2 × 2 gauze in half and cover with 1-inch-wide tape extending about an inch from each side of gauze. Place under the tubing/catheter hub junction. Curl a loop of tubing to the outside of the arm and place a second piece of tape directly over the padded 2 × 2, securing the tubing in two places.

    i. Label the dressing with date and time of insertion, date and time of dressing change, gauge and length of catheter, and identification of nurse.

Step 2d

Drying allows time to effectively reduce microbial counts (INS, 1998).

Coats the skin with protective solution to maintain skin integrity, prevent irritation from the adhesive, and promote adhesion of the dressing.

Securing the tubing at two places prevents catheter movement and dislodgement that increase the risk of phlebitis and infiltration. Placing tape on tape makes tubing removal easier and decreases the skin irritation.

Steps	**Rationale**

    j. Apply hand board or commercial housing device if venipuncture site or dressing is affected by the motion of the wrist.

Reduces the risk of phlebitis and infiltration from motion of the joint.

    k. Discard used supplies, remove gloves, and wash hands.

3. *Changing infusion tubing:*

    a. Open new infusion set and connect add-on pieces such as filters or extension tubing. Keep protective covering over spike and distal needle adapter. Secure all junctions with Luer-loks, clasping devices, or threaded devices. Avoid the use of tape.

Separation of infusion tubing increases the risk of air emboli, hemorrhage, and infection.

    b. If needle or catheter hub is visible, remove IV dressing as directed in Step 2a. Do not remove tape securing catheter to skin (if gauze dressing was used). If transparent dressing is removed, place small piece of tape to temporarily anchor catheter.

    c. For continuous infusion:

      (1) Close roller clamp on new tubing.

      (2) Slow rate of infusion to KVO on existing IV by regulating roller clamp on old tubing.

      (3) Compress and fill drip chamber of old tubing.

      (4) Remove old tubing from solution and hang or tape drip chamber on IV pole 36 inches above IV site.

      (5) Place insertion spike of new tubing into old fluid container opening, compress and release drip chamber on new tubing, and fill drip chamber one-third to one-half full (see illustration). Hang container on IV pole.

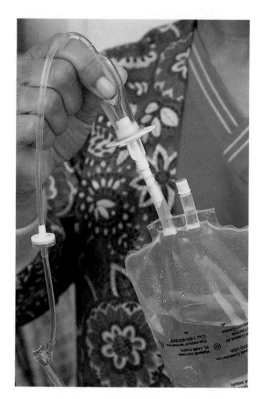

Step 3c(5)

      (6) Slowly open roller clamp, remove protective cap from needle adapter (if necessary), and flush new tubing with solution. Stop infusion and replace cap.

      (7) Turn roller clamp on old tubing to "off" position.

    d. OPTION: Place 2 × 2 gauze under catheter hub.

Prevents tubing from accidentally contacting skin and collects blood that may leak from catheter hub.

    e. Stabilize hub of catheter and apply pressure over vein just above catheter tip (at least 1½ inches above insertion site). Gently disconnect old tubing from catheter hub and quickly insert needle adapter of new tubing into catheter hub (see illustrations).

    f. Open roller clamp on new tubing, allowing solution to run rapidly for 30 to 60 seconds, then regulate IV drip according to physician's orders and monitor rate hourly (see illustration).

    g. Remove and discard 2 × 2 gauze (if used). If necessary, apply new dressing (see Step 2).

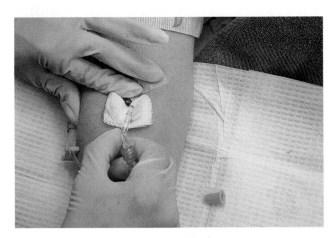

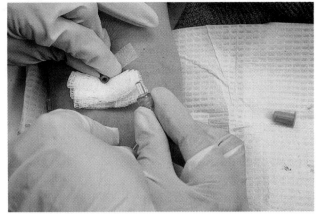

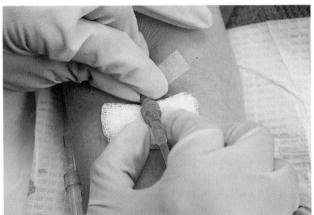

Step 3e

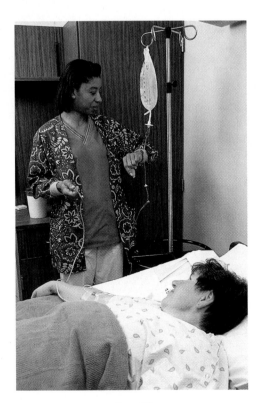

Step 3f

Steps	Rationale

4. *Changing fluid container:*

   a. Prepare next solution at least 1 hour before needed. If prepared in pharmacy, be sure it has been delivered to the client's location. Check that the solution is correct and properly labeled. Check solution expiration date.

   b. Change solution when fluid remains only in neck of container.

   c. Move roller clamp to stop flow rate, and remove old IV fluid container from IV pole.

   d. Quickly remove spike from old container. Without touching tip, insert spike into new bag or bottle.

   e. Hang new bag or bottle of solution on IV pole.

   f. Check for air in tubing. If bubbles form, they can be removed by closing the roller clamp, stretching the tubing downward, and tapping the tubing with the finger (the bubbles rise in the tubing to the drip chamber) (see illustration). For larger amounts of air, connect a syringe to an injection port below the air and aspirate the air into the syringe.

COMMUNICATION TIP

Tell client the "champagne-type bubbles" inside the tubing are not a problem. They will be removed by the filter in the line.

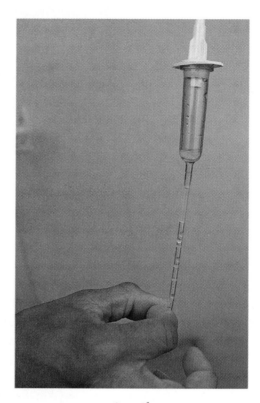

Step 4f

   g. Make sure drip chamber is one-third to one-half full. If drip chamber is too full, pinch off tubing below the drip chamber, invert the container, squeeze the drip chamber, hang container, and release the tubing.

   h. Regulate flow to prescribed rate.

   i. Place time label on the side of container and label with the time hung, the time of completion, and appropriate interval. If using plastic bags, mark only on the label and not the container.

5. *Discontinuing IV medications:*

   a. Move roller clamp on infusion tubing to the "off" position.

   b. Remove any clasping devices and disconnect medication delivery tubing from injection port.

   c. Remove the needle or needleless adapter on the infusion tubing; discard appropriately in receptacle and replace with a sterile cap or cover.

   d. Swab injection port or prn adapter on main IV tubing with alcohol (see illustration, p. 709).

   e. For intermittent medication "piggybacked" into a continuous infusion, attach saline-filled syringe to injection port and flush the line gently. Regulate fluid flow of the continuous infusion as ordered.

NURSE ALERT

If the tubing spike, connector end, fluid pathway, or fluid container is contaminated, a new tubing set or fluid container is required.

Saline flush prevents incompatible medications from coming into contact in the infusion tubing.

Steps	Rationale

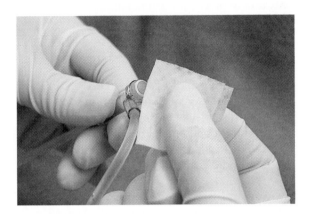

Step 5d

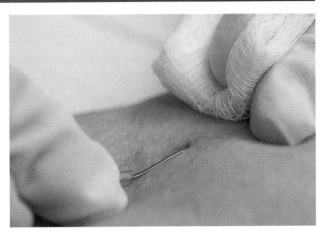

Step 6d

  f. For intermittent medications through a saline or heparin lock, attach saline-filled syringe to injection port and flush catheter gently, or attach heparin-filled syringe to injection port and flush gently, if necessary. Check agency policy. Attach sterile injection port cover, if necessary.

  g. Remove gloves, discard used supplies, and wash hands.

  h. Prepare client for obtaining blood samples after medication infusion, if necessary.

6. *Discontinuing peripheral IV access:*

  a. Explain procedure to client. Explain that affected extremity must be held still and how long procedure will take.

  b. Turn IV tubing roller clamp to "off" position.

  c. 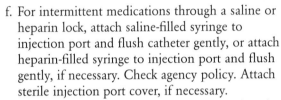 Remove IV site dressing and tape while stabilizing catheter.

NURSE ALERT

Never use scissors to remove the tape or dressing, because the catheter could accidentally be cut.

  d. With dry gauze or alcohol swab held over site, withdraw the catheter using a slow steady movement, keeping the hub parallel to the skin (see illustration).

  e. Apply pressure to the site for 2 to 3 minutes, using a dry, sterile gauze pad. Secure with tape.

  f. Inspect the catheter for intactness, noting tip integrity and length.

  g. Discard used supplies.

  h. Remove and discard gloves and wash hands.

  i. Instruct client to report any redness, pain, drainage, or swelling that may occur after catheter removal.

NURSE ALERT

Gentle technique is required when flushing all IV catheters. If resistance is encountered, do not forcefully flush the line. Investigate the cause of the resistance (e.g., kinked tubing, catheter position, position of extremity, drug precipitate, blood clot) and resolve the problem. Forceful flushing could cause catheter damage, vein trauma, or emboli. If in doubt, restart IV.

Changing the angle of the catheter inside the vein could cause additional vein irritation, increasing the risk of postinfusion phlebitis.

Dry pad controls bleeding and causes less irritation to the puncture site.

Postinfusion phlebitis may occur within 48 to 96 hours after catheter removal (Perdue, 1995).

EVALUATION

Changing Peripheral IV Dressing:
1. Observe functioning and patency of IV system after changing dressing.
2. Inspect condition of IV site, noting color. Palpate for skin temperature, edema, and tenderness.
3. Monitor client's body temperature.

Changing Infusion Tubing:
1. Evaluate flow rate of flush, and observe connection site for leakage.

Changing Fluid Container:
1. Observe client for signs of fluid volume excess or deficit to determine response to IV fluid therapy.
2. Monitor IV infusion for correct solution and additives.

Discontinuing IV Medications:
1. Observe site for redness, pain, drainage, or swelling.
2. Observe continuous infusion for correct rate.
3. Observe tubing for leaking.

Discontinuing Peripheral IV Access:
1. Observe site for evidence of bleeding.
2. Observe site for redness, pain, drainage, or swelling.

Unexpected Outcomes and Related Interventions

Changing Peripheral IV Dressing:
1. IV catheter is infiltrated, as evidenced by edema, pallor, leakage from puncture site, or decreased skin temperature around insertion site.
2. Phlebitis is present, as evidenced by redness and tenderness along vein pathway.
3. IV catheter is accidentally dislodged.
4. Catheter is infected, as evidenced by redness, swelling, pain, and/or exudate.
   NOTE: For all of the above, temporarily discontinue infusion and remove catheter. Insert another catheter, preferably on the opposite extremity. Check agency policy for complication management.
5. Client has an elevated temperature, but the insertion site is free of signs and symptoms of infection.
   Assess all vital signs and inform the physician of the client's condition.

Changing Infusion Tubing:
1. Decreased or absent flow of IV fluid indicated by a slowed or obstructed flow.
   a. Open roller clamp, slide clamps, and recalibrate drip rate.
   b. Evaluate any pain or discomfort at the site for infiltration or temporary venous spasm.

Changing Fluid Container:
1. Flow rate is incorrect; client receives too little or too much fluid.
   a. Regulate to the correct rate.
   b. Determine and correct the cause of the incorrect flow rate (e.g., change in client position, change in catheter position, kinked tubing).
   c. Use electronic infusion device when accurate flow rate is critical.

Discontinuing IV Medications:
1. Solution in tubing below piggyback site turns cloudy because of precipitate formation, indicating medication incompatibility.
   a. Stop all infusions.
   b. Change tubing on continuous infusion.

Discontinuing Peripheral IV Access:
1. Hematoma formation.
   a. Apply a pressure dressing to the site.
   b. Apply ice to slow or stop bleeding.
   c. Monitor for additional bleeding.
   d. Assess circulatory, motor, and neurological function of the extremity.

Recording and Reporting

- Record time peripheral dressing was changed, reason for dressing change, type of dressing material used, patency of system, and observation of venipuncture site.
- Record changing tubing on client's record, including the rate of infusion. A special IV flow sheet may be used.
- Attach a piece of tape or preprinted label with date and time of tubing change below the drip chamber.
- Record amount and type of fluid infused and amount and type of new fluid according to agency policy. A special flow sheet may be used for parenteral fluids.
- Record time of discontinuing medication and flushing infusion tubing/catheter, including amount and type of flush solution and condition of site.
- Report the time to obtain blood sample to the laboratory, if necessary.
- Record time peripheral IV was discontinued. Include site assessment information and gauge and length of catheter removed.
- Report to nurse in charge or oncoming nurse that the dressing was changed, any significant information about IV site or IV system, the time the medication or IV was discontinued, and the time of obtaining any blood samples.

Sample Documentation

1300 IV dressing became wet during shower; applied transparent membrane dressing; insertion site without redness, edema, or drainage. Infusing at 125 ml/hr. Client states there is no discomfort or tenderness in the hand or extremity.

1700 Gentamicin infusion complete; line flushed with 3 ml NS and 5% dextrose and water with multivitamins infusing at 125 ml/hr. IV site without redness or edema; client states there is no pain or discomfort at the site. Lab notified to obtain blood sample at 1745.

2100 20-g IV catheter removed from right hand. Site without redness or swelling. Client states, "My hand feels good with the IV out." Removed catheter length is 1 inch; catheter tip intact.

Geriatric Considerations

- Fragile skin requires the use of nonporous tapes and skin protectant solutions.
- Older adults are more prone to fluid imbalances and require careful monitoring of all infusions.
- Visual and hearing deficits can lead to challenges in client education. Face the client while speaking clearly and calmly.
- Short-term memory loss, depression, and confusion may lead to clients removing the IV catheter or a change in their attitude or decision about care.

Home Care and Long-Term Care Considerations

- Ensure that the client or caregiver is able and willing to provide the care needed for the IV site.
- If the client is unable to provide the needed care because of loss of vision, explore alterations in the delivery methods used. Medications can be admixed for multiple doses to be delivered through an ambulatory infusion pump, decreasing the need for repeated flushing and tubing changes.
- Assess support from caregiver to assist with providing care.
- Ensure that the client has adequate facilities for storing supplies and medications that need refrigeration.
- Ensure that the long-term care facility is capable of managing a client with peripheral IV therapy.

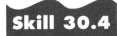

Skill 30.4

ADMINISTERING IV MEDICATIONS

Technological advances have resulted in the increase of drug delivery by the IV route. IV administration of medications is often preferred to oral or intramuscular (IM) administration because of efficacy of concentration, absorption, and rapid onset. The IV route is often required if the client is unable to take oral medications. Some drugs can be administered only by the IV route. Because of the principles that make IV administration the preferred route (rapid onset, improved serum drug concentrations), it also requires greater knowledge and skill by the nurse to prevent potentially dangerous complications when administering any IV medication. Parenteral administration of any drug is invasive and poses greater risk to the client.

When administering IV medications, the principles associated with delivery of any medication remain the same. The nurse should ensure it is the right client, right drug, right dose, right time, and right route. Drugs are documented immediately after administration. In addition to these basic rights, the nurse must also apply principles of IV therapy. Physical incompatibilities of IV medications, osmolality of drug admixtures, and potential for IV therapy–related complications must be considered before administering any medication intravenously.

A variety of methods are available for IV medication delivery. Because drugs given by the IV route are delivered directly into the vascular system, dosages are usually lower than for those given orally (LaRocca and Otto, 1994). Dosages and admixtures vary and are usually calculated based on the client's weight, drug distribution and absorption, safety of administration, excretion, and solubility in solution. IV medications can be mixed in large admixture volumes (e.g., addition of 40 mEq KCL to 1000 ml IV fluid), by "piggyback" infusion (e.g., administration of an antibiotic concurrently with an IV infusion), or by bolus injection (delivery of a small-volume admixture through an existing IV access device). In all three methods of IV medication administration, the client is required to have an IV access device.

The nurse also must know the absorption, metabolism, and excretion rate and route of IV medications. Because the liver and kidneys metabolize and excrete byproducts of the IV drug, systemic diseases such as liver and renal impairment affect absorption. Older adults usually have diminished renal and liver function and are more likely to experience toxicity related to IV drug administration than individuals with normal liver and kidney function. Clients with lower plasma proteins have more adverse effects when receiving IV medications, because therapeutic response to the drug is related to the amount of drug not bound to a plasma protein or tissue. Drug binding influences both the effectiveness of the drug given and the duration of the effect (LaRocca and Otto, 1994).

Some drugs such as heparin are required to be given by continuous infusion to maintain a therapeutic action. The efficacy of other drugs (e.g., antibiotics) and their therapeutic response are determined by therapeutic drug monitoring. Serum drug levels such as peak and trough levels of aminoglycosides (e.g., gentamicin, tobramycin, amikacin) and vancomycin are performed at specific intervals during IV medication therapy to monitor response and to protect the client from adverse effects if excretion of the metabolized drug is reduced. Serum drug levels reveal if drug doses are too high or low. Dosages are adjusted by increasing or decreasing the time between administration or by increasing or decreasing the drug amount to provide therapeutic levels within a narrow range. Monitoring therapeutic drug levels is an additional responsibility of the nurse when administering IV medications and is crucial in safe and effective delivery of care to the client.

When giving IV medications, the nurse also assesses clients for hypersensitivity (allergic) reactions. The rapid absorption of IV medications, if the client has an allergic response or delayed hypersensitivity, occurs quickly and can be exhibited by reactions ranging from a mild skin rash to anaphylaxis. The extent of the reaction is related to the hypersensitivity to the drug and the amount actually infused. If an allergic reaction occurs, the nurse should stop the medication, keep the IV line open with a plain fluid infusion, monitor the client for respiratory distress and changes in vital signs, notify the physician, and be prepared to administer emergency medications and resuscitative measures if necessary.

The CDC and the Occupational Safety and Health Administration (OSHA) have made recommendations that all intermittent infusions be administered via a needleless system. This can be achieved by the use of a manufactured needleless system. Needleless infusion lines allow a direct connection with the IV line via a recessed connection port or a blunt-ended cannula or shielded needle device (Figure 30-4). The risk of exposure to an IV needle is eliminated when using these devices.

Equipment

IV medication
  Vial or ampule of prescribed medication
  Small-volume admixture (Normal saline, Dextrose and water, or sterile water) in either syringe or 50- to 250-ml IV fluid bag
Container for admixture diluent (Volutrol)
Sterile 19- to 21-gauge needle, 1 to 1½ inches (20-gauge, 1-inch needle typically used) if system is not needleless
Label, if needed (Many small-volume admixtures are premixed and dispensed from pharmacy.)
Syringe pump, if applicable
Secondary administration set, if needed
Disposable gloves
Two 3-ml syringes filled with NS 0.9%
One 3-ml syringe filled with dilute heparin (10 U/ml) (optional)
Antiseptic swabs
Tape (optional)
IV pole
Medication administration record or computer printout

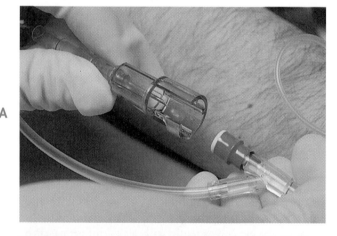
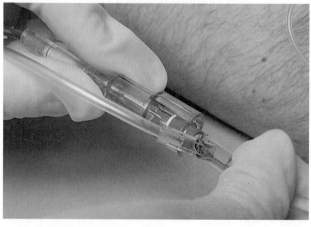

Figure 30-4 A, Needleless infusion system. **B,** Connection into an injection port.

ASSESSMENT

1. Check physician's orders to determine type of IV solution, medication, dose, and route and frequency of administration.
2. Review information about drug, including action, purpose, peak onset, normal dose, side effects, and nursing implications. Note appropriate time for infusion (e.g., mg/min).
3. Assess appropriate laboratory values (e.g., creatinine, peak and trough levels). **Rationale: Determines drug efficacy and toxicity.**

4. Assess existing IV line for patency (see Skill 30.3), and note rate of main IV line.
5. Assess IV insertion site for signs of infiltration or phlebitis (pain, tenderness, redness, swelling, heat on palpation). **Rationale: Administration of hyperosmolar drugs by IV route increases risk of phlebitis.**
6. Assess client's history of drug allergies. **Rationale: Ensures a contraindicated medication is not administered.**
7. Assess client's understanding of purpose for drug therapy.

PLANNING

Expected outcomes of IV medication administration focus on ensuring therapeutic response of drug with minimum adverse reactions.

Expected outcomes
1. Drug infuses within desired period.

2. Client's IV site remains free of phlebitis or infiltration.
3. Client's laboratory values of therapeutic drug monitoring reveal desired response without renal toxicity.
4. Client does not show evidence of hypersensitivity or allergic reaction to IV medication.
5. Client or family is able to explain drug's purpose, action, side effects, and dosage.

DELEGATION CONSIDERATIONS

This skill requires problem solving and knowledge application unique to a professional nurse. In many states, the administration of certain IV medications is included within the scope of practice for licensed practical (vocational) nurses. Follow agency policy for the specific medications that may be administered by LPN/LVN. Delegation of this skill to AP is inappropriate.

IMPLEMENTATION

Steps	Rationale
1. See Standard Protocol (inside front cover).	
2. Assemble medications in medication room using aseptic technique (see Chapter 3).	
3. Check client identification, look at armband, and ask client to state name.	Identification of client is required before any medication administration.
4. Explain procedure, and encourage client to report any symptoms of discomfort at IV site during infusion.	
5. IV push (bolus) (through existing line)	
a. ▨ Select injection port closest to client. If add-on 0.22-μ filter is used, give IV push medications below the filter next to client, preventing medication from being absorbed in filter.	Ensures small-volume bolus enters vein quickly and directly.
b. Prepare injection site or cleanse connection port with antiseptic swab. Allow to dry.	
c. Connect syringe to IV line.	
(1) Needleless system Remove cap of needleless injection port. Connect tip of syringe directly.	
or	
Insert blunt cannula through appropriate injection cap (see illustration, p. 714).	
(2) Needle system Insert short, small-gauge needle through center of injection port.	
d. Occlude IV system by pinching tubing above injection port (see illustration, p. 714).	Prevents reflux of medication up tubing and inadvertent bolus when infusion is resumed.
e. Aspirate gently on syringe plunger, observing for blood return.	Ensures drug will be delivered intravascularly.

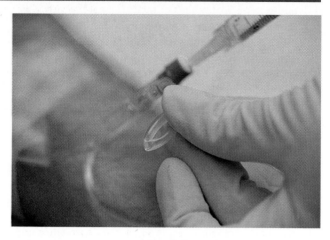

Step 5d

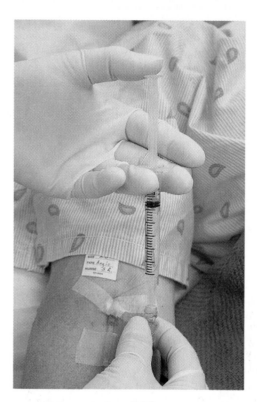

Step 5c(1)

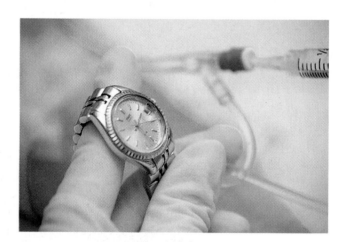

Step 5f

    f. After observing for blood return, continue to occlude IV tubing and inject medication slowly over appropriate time. Use watch to time administration (see illustration).

    g. Release tubing, withdraw syringe, and recheck fluid infusion rate.   Fluid infusion may need to be readjusted if injection changed drip rate.

    h. If using a needleless system, replace injection port cap with new sterile cap.

    i. Remove gloves and wash hands.

    j. Dispose of needles and syringes in appropriate container. *Do not* recap needles.   Prevents contamination from needle-stick injury.

6. IV push (through IV lock)

    a. 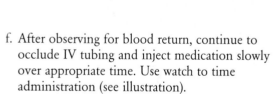 Fill two 3-ml syringes with NS 0.9%. Attach blunt cannula or remove needle from syringe as indicated by the type of needleless system.   Flush will be used to clear lock before medication administration.

    b. Cleanse injection port of IV lock with antiseptic swab, or remove cap.

Steps	Rationale

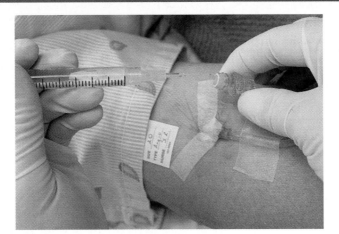

Step 6c

c. Insert syringe of NS 0.9% through injection port of IV lock (see illustration).

d. Aspirate gently and observe for blood return.

e. Flush gently with NS while assessing for resistance. If resistance is felt, never continue to apply force. Stop and evaluate cause.

Ensures IV catheter is correctly positioned in vein.
Ensures catheter patency and prevents dislodging blood clot or drug precipitate into blood stream.

f. Detach NS syringe, reprepare with antiseptic swab, and attach syringe filled with medication (see Step 6c).

g. Inject medication slowly over appropriate time, using a watch to ensure proper time of delivery.

h. Remove medication syringe.

i. Reclease cap or port with antiseptic swab and attach syringe with 1 ml 0.9% NS. Inject NS flush.

Irrigation with NS prevents occlusion of IV access device.

j. OPTION (if agency protocol): Inject 1 ml dilute heparin, maintaining positive pressure in IV access device.
   Using SASH:
      Saline
      Administration
      Saline
      Heparin

Prevents incompatibility of heparin with drug administered because 0.9% NS is isotonic.

k. Remove gloves and wash hands.

l. Dispose of all needles and syringes in proper container. *Do not* recap needle.

Prevents accidental needle-stick injury with contaminated needle.

NURSE ALERT

NS effectively maintains patency of peripheral IV lines (Perucca, 1995). To maintain positive pressure in IV access device when flushing, clamp extension tubing if present or withdraw syringe during the final 0.2 to 0.4 ml of injection, creating a splash of NS *(or dilute heparin if used) on the gloved hand when withdrawing syringe. This prevents reflux of blood in the IV catheter and prolongs patency of the access device. Some needleless system injection ports have an antireflux valve in injection port.*

Steps	Rationale

7. IV piggyback (IVPB) through existing line

a. 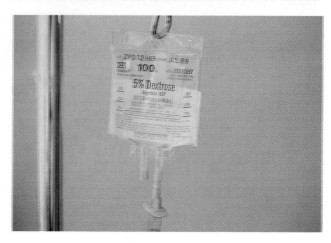 Attach tubing of administration set to prepared admixture container.

   (1) *Tandem (piggyback) infusion:* Small-volume admixture (50 to 100 ml) in a minibag that dilutes and administers drug. Insert spike of tubing into port of minibag (see illustration).

   (2) *Syringe pump:* Small-volume admixture in a syringe (10 to 60 ml) to dilute and administer drug. Attach tubing to end of syringe.

Step 7a(1)

b. Fill tubing with IV fluid.

   (1) *Tandem (piggyback) infusion:* Close roller clamp, squeeze chamber, and fill half full. Open roller clamp and prime remaining tubing.

   (2) *Syringe pump:* Gently push plunger of syringe to fill tubing completely.

Infusion tubing should be fluid filled and free of air bubbles to prevent air embolism.

COMMUNICATION TIP

If client complains during infusion of hyperosmolar drugs (e.g., erythromycin, vancomycin), assess IV site for symptoms of chemical phlebitis. IV infusion of drug greater than 650 mOsm/L is known to cause chemical phlebitis. If client is symptom free, slow infusion and decrease rate to infuse over maximum time allowed.

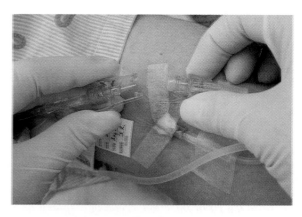

Step 7c

Steps	Rationale

c. Administer IVPB (tandem infusion). Attach needle to end of IV minibag tubing and insert into injection port farthest away from client after cleansing port with antiseptic swab. For needleless system, attach tubing to recessed connection port above backcheck valve (see illustration).

Use of injection port closest to drip chamber of primary IV line allows piggyback to infuse while stopping the flow of primary IV line through backcheck valve.

  (1) Lower primary IV line. (Hook may be used to lower primary IV line.)

Allows infusion of minibag and prevents infusion of primary line.

  (2) Open regulator or clamp on minibag infusion.

  (3) Regulate flow rate of infusion with roller clamp on primary tubing to deliver medication over 20 to 90 minutes (see agency policy or pharmacy instruction).

  (4) After medication has infused, check flow rate of primary infusion.

Backcheck valve prevents infusion of primary line while medication is infusing. Primary infusion will automatically begin to flow when tandem (piggyback) infusion is empty.

  (5) Reregulate primary infusion to desired IV rate.

Prevents infusion of excess fluid.

  (6) Leave secondary bag and tubing in place for future drug administration or discard in appropriate container. Discard needle in sharps container.

Establishment of secondary line produces route for microorganisms to enter main line. Repeated changes in tubing increase risk of infection. Check agency policy and procedure for frequency of administration set tubing change.

  (7) Remove gloves and wash hands.

8. Mini-infusion or syringe pump

a. Place prefilled syringe with primed tubing into mini-infusor pump (follow manufacturer's directions) (see illustration).

b. Attach end of tubing to designated port *or* insert sterile needle into injection port of existing IV line after cleansing injection port with antiseptic swab.

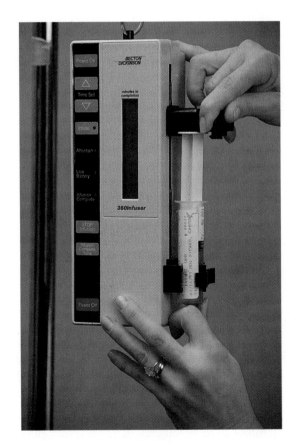

Step 8a

Steps	Rationale

c. Hang mini-infusor pump with syringe on IV pole with primary IV line. Press button to "on" position. The infusion-complete alarm in "on" position should be used if available and if infusing via saline/heparin lock.

Prevents delay in flushing after completion of infusion, maintaining patency of access device.

d. After medication infuses, turn off pump. Check flow rate of primary IV infusion and regulate to desired rate. (If stopcock is used, turn to "off" position after infusion is complete, and cap.)

Prevents infusion of excess fluid.

Maintains sterility of system.

e. Leave infuser tubing attached to primary line. Disconnect and cover end with sterile cap, or disconnect and discard in appropriate container.

9. IVPB: saline or heparin lock (see illustration).

a. Take minidrip (60 gtt/ml) IV tubing and insert spike into minibag.

Minidrip used to regulate small-volume infusion.

b. Close roller clamp and squeeze drip chamber to fill half full.

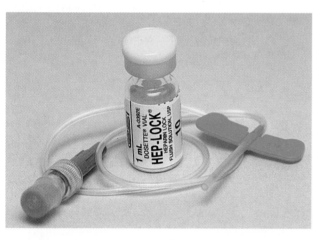

Step 9

c. Open roller clamp and fill remaining tubing.

Flushes air from tubing.

d. Attach sterile needle (e.g., 20 gauge, 1 inch) to tubing. Attach sterile cap to end of primed tubing if using needleless system.

Needle should be changed with each administration.

e. Prepare injection port of needleless system or heparin stopper with antiseptic swab.

f. Insert 3-ml syringe filled with 1 ml NS 0.9% and gently aspirate. Check for blood return, then flush NS slowly. Note any pain, swelling, or burning at IV site.

Ensures placement of IV in vein. Symptoms may suggest phlebitis or infiltration and the need to restart peripheral IV line.

g. Reprepare port or stopper with antiseptic swab. Attach end of tubing to port, or insert sterile needle.

h. Open flow clamp and regulate IV medication to infuse 20 to 90 minutes. (Refer to agency policy or pharmacy instructions.)

Steps	Rationale

i. Continue to observe infusion periodically until complete. When complete, disconnect, maintaining aseptic technique.

j. Prepare injection port with antiseptic swab, insert syringe with 1 ml NS, and gently flush, maintaining positive pressure in IV access device.

Always use SASH technique to flush port and prevent drug incompatibilities (see Step 6j).

k. Reprepare and inject dilute heparin concentration (per agency and procedure), repeating procedure and using positive pressure.

l. Apply new sterile needle and cap to minibag tubing and retain for next administration.

Maintains sterility of IV tubing for future reuse.

m. Dispose of syringe and needles in appropriate container.

10. See Completion Protocol (inside front cover).

NURSE ALERT

Prompt flushing after IVPB via saline/heparin lock prevents clotting inside catheter lumen when infusion is completed. Should IV access device clot after IVPB administration, do not forcefully flush. INS standards prohibit declotting of peripheral IV access

(INS, 1998). If blood collects in IV tubing, clear tubing with remaining solution or change tubing. Blood retained in IV tubing promotes bacterial growth and predisposes client to risk of infection.

• • •

EVALUATION

1. Observe client's infusion for proper rate of administration, and note time of completion.
2. Inspect client's IV site and tubing for symptoms of IV complications (e.g., swelling, pain, tenderness, redness at site).
3. Monitor therapeutic drug levels (e.g., aminoglycosides, vancomycin, aminophylline, phenytoin).
4. Monitor client during infusion for allergic response or adverse reaction (e.g., urticaria, respiratory distress, tachycardia, hypotension).
5. Ask client to name IV medication, purpose, side effects, dosage, and frequency.

Unexpected Outcomes and Related Interventions

1. Client experiences burning, irritation, redness, or pain during infusion.
   a. Reinspect site and check for blood return.
   b. If phlebitis is present, discontinue infusion and reinsert another catheter, preferably in the opposite extremity, if IV therapy is still necessary.
2. Client experiences adverse reaction or allergic reaction during infusion of drug.
   a. Stop the infusion.
   b. Maintain existing IV line with NS 0.9% or ordered solution.
   c. Notify physician.
   d. Monitor vital signs and respiratory status.
   e. Administer medications as ordered.
   f. Be prepared to perform cardiac or respiratory resuscitation.
   g. After acute episode subsides, advise client of allergy and necessity for future reporting to health care personnel; advise client of significance of allergy; advise client as to the availability of Medic Alert identification tags.
3. Client is unable to state purpose of drug, significance to treatment of current illness, side effects, or health management related to drug.
   a. Reinforce information, giving simple instructions, written if necessary.
   b. Communicate to other health personnel, particularly if client is to continue IV therapy in home setting.
   c. Include family or care provider during instruction.

Recording and Reporting

• Record drug dose, route, amount and type of diluent (e.g., 1 g in 50 ml D_5W), and time of administration on medication administration record or computer printout. (See Medication Administration Record, Appendix A).

- Record volume of fluid on client's I&O record. (See Intake and Output Summary.)

Sample Documentation

0810   During first 5 minutes of infusion of 100 ml NS and 1 g Ampicillin, client complained of sudden onset of "can't catch my breath," clutching at throat; high-pitched inspiratory stridor noted. Macular rash generalized over face and upper extremities noted. Ampicillin stopped immediately and IV fluids maintained at 125 ml/hr. VS 98/60, 120, 26. M.D. notified. Epinephrine 0.5 mg IVP given, with inspiratory distress subsiding within 30 seconds of administration. Allergy band applied.

0830   VS 120/84, 96, 18. Client states breathing is normal. Expressing some fear over "how fast it came on." Significance of allergy, implications for future administration, and notification of dentists, physicians, and other health care providers discussed. Aware that vital signs will continue to be monitored and to notify immediately for any signs of respiratory distress.

Geriatric Considerations

- Because of fragility of veins, use extra care in injecting bolus of medications.

Skill 30.5

TRANSFUSIONS WITH BLOOD PRODUCTS

Technological advances in transfusion therapy now allow administration of various blood components specifically needed by the client. These technological advances also create an increased responsibility for nurses to have expanded knowledge of transfusion therapy, allowing for safe administration.

Blood and blood component transfusion is a major factor in restoring and maintaining quality of life for the client with hematological disorders, cancer, injury, or surgical intervention (LaRocca and Otto, 1994). Caring for the client receiving blood or blood components may be a routine nursing responsibility, but overlooking a minor detail could be dangerous to the client.

Transfusions of blood and blood products are closely regulated and monitored. Standards of operations for all blood bank centers are set by the American Association of Blood Banks (AABB), OSHA, Food and Drug Administration (FDA), and the American Red Cross. These standards include the collection of donor blood, distribution of the product, and standards for transfusion. Always verify specific agency or institutional policy as to specific procedural requirements before any transfusion.

Blood and blood component therapies treat and restore hemodynamic homeostasis. A written physician's order to transfuse should always include which component to transfuse and the duration of the transfusion. A single unit of whole blood or red blood cells should be infused within a 4-hour period (INS, 1998; Vengelen-Tyler, 1996). If more than one blood product is to be given, the sequence or order of transfusion should be specified. Any additional medications, such as antihistamine (given when

history shows previous allergic response), antipyretics (given when history shows previous febrile nonhemolytic response), or diuretics (given when history shows potential for CHF or pulmonary edema), or any other special treatment of the components should also be prescribed by the physician when ordering the transfusion (Vengelen-Tyler, 1996).

Three blood typing systems, ABO, Rh, and most recently HLA typing, are used to ensure transfusion products match the recipient's blood as closely as possible (Table 30-5). Before transfusion in nonemergent situations, the client's blood type and Rh factor *must always* be verified to be compatible with the donor transfusion.

There is increasing public awareness of the possible transmission of infectious diseases through transfusion of blood products. Because of improved testing of donor blood, the risk of the blood recipient developing an infectious disease is lower than ever before. However, viral, bacterial, and parasitic diseases can still be transmitted through blood. Screening of blood donors is one of the most important steps to identify persons with a medical history, behavior, or events that put them at risk of transmissible disease. All donor blood is tested for syphilis, hepatitis B, and the presence of antibodies to hepatitis C, HIV 1 and 2, human T-cell lymphotropic virus I, and cytomegalovirus. Liver enzymes are also measured to determine the possibility of liver disease from other types of hepatitis (Vengelen-Tyler, 1996).

Nurses and physicians must be prepared to inform the client thoroughly about the options, benefits, and risks of transfusion and must reassure the client that every effort

Table 30-5

Blood Type Identification

Client	Compatible Transfusion
Type A	A or AB plasma A or O RBCs
Type B	B or AB plasma B or O RBCs
Type AB	AB plasma A, B, AB, or O RBCs
Type O	A, B, AB, or O plasma O RBCs
Rh^-	Must receive Rh^- blood
Rh^+	Can receive Rh^- or Rh^+ blood
O^-	Universal donor for RBCs
AB^-	Universal donor for plasma

RBCs, red blood cells.

has been taken to ensure a safe blood supply. Clients should know that there is never a completely risk-free transfusion.

One avenue for preventing the transmission of infectious diseases during blood transfusion is the use of autologous blood (i.e., the client's own blood). This can be done in several ways; however, the most frequent method is preoperative collection from the client. AABB standards establish the process for determining client eligibility, collecting, testing, and labeling the unit. Before transfusion, ABO and Rh typing of the client are performed. Autologous units must be used before units from the general blood supply. Identification and checking processes and methods of administration for autologous units are the same as those used for other units of blood. If unused, autologous units are not added to the general blood supply (Vengelen-Tyler, 1996).

The skill of transfusing blood or blood products requires the nurse to know thoroughly the policy and procedure of the agency or institution. The nurse must ensure the safe administration of the product and closely monitor before, during, and after the transfusion.

Equipment
Blood administration set with standard 170-μ filter
Ordered blood product
IV solution: NS 0.9%
Disposable gloves
Tape
Optional equipment
Infusion pump (Verify that infusion pump can be used to deliver blood or blood products.)
Leukocyte-depleting filter
Blood warmer (used mainly when massive transfusion is needed)
Pressure bag (used for rapid infusion in acute blood loss)

ASSESSMENT
1. Assess physician's order for type of blood product, length of transfusion (up to 4 hours for whole blood or red blood cells), and pretransfusion or posttransfusion medications to be given.
2. Assess client's transfusion history, including previous transfusion reaction. Verify that type and crossmatch has been completed within 72 hours of transfusion and, if applicable, that consent for transfusion is signed. **Rationale: Clients with recent transfusion, pregnancy (within 3 months), or uncertain history are at high risk because of potential antibody response.**
3. Establish that client has a patent large-bore IV catheter with positive blood return. **Rationale: Catheters used for blood transfusion should be large enough to accommodate the appropriate flow rate, but not large enough to damage the vein. Small-gauge catheters (e.g., 22 gauge) may be used in clients whose larger veins are inaccessible (Vengelen-Tyler, 1996).**
4. Assess pretransfusion, baseline vital signs (blood pressure, pulse, respiration, temperature). If client is febrile (greater than 100° F or 37.8° C), notify physician before initiating transfusion (check agency policy). **Rationale: This provides comparison to detect change in client's condition during transfusion.**
5. Assess client's medication schedule.

PLANNING
Expected outcomes focus on safe, complication-free transfusion therapy, restoration of normal cell count, and improvement in oxygenation and tissue perfusion.

Expected Outcomes
1. Client is free of signs and symptoms of transfusion reaction or fluid volume overload, evidenced by normal temperature and blood pressure and absence of chest pain, dyspnea, dizziness, or tachydysrhythmias.
2. Client demonstrates normal fluid balance, evidenced by normal urine output, improved hemoglobin (Hgb) and hematocrit (Hct), and normal red blood cell indices.
3. Client does not experience signs and symptoms of blood or blood product infiltrate or phlebitis.
4. Client lists two benefits and risks of transfusion therapy.
5. Client experiences lessened stress or fear, evidenced by verbalized understanding and acceptance of transfusion therapy.

DELEGATION CONSIDERATIONS

This skill requires problem solving and knowledge application unique to a professional nurse. In many states, the administration of blood and blood components is included within the scope of practice for licensed practical (vocational) nurses. Follow agency policy. Delegation to AP may include obtaining vital signs, collecting equipment, transporting units from the blood bank, and instituting client comfort measures. However, the primary responsibility for donor and recipient identification, infusing the unit within the required time, and assessing outcomes remains with the nurse-transfusionist.

IMPLEMENTATION

Steps	Rationale

1. See Standard Protocol (inside front cover).
2. Obtain blood bag from laboratory following agency protocol. Blood transfusions must be initiated 15 to 30 minutes after release from laboratory.

3. Open blood administration set and prime the tubing with NS 0.9% (see illustration), completely filling filter with saline. Maintain sterility of system and close lower clamp.

Agencies differ as to personnel who can release a blood bag from a blood bank, but they always require two witnesses and some form of client identification. Only one unit is usually released at a time.

If filter is not completely primed with saline, transfusion will slow because of collection of debris in partially primed filter. Saline is used to wet the filter, dilute red blood cells to reduce their viscosity if necessary, and flush blood components from the tubing. If a reaction occurs, a separate bag of saline with a separate infusion tubing must be hung to decrease the amount of blood given to the client.

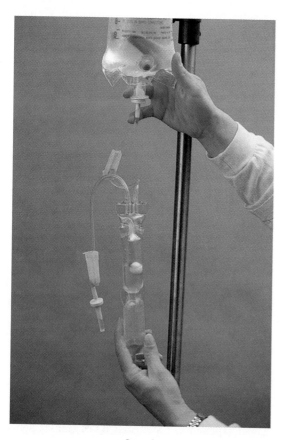

Step 3

NURSE ALERT

IV medications cannot be added to a blood bag or infused through a transfusion administration set. An additional IV site may be required if IV medications cannot be delayed or adjusted during blood transfusion(s).

COMMUNICATION TIP

While preparing for blood administration, explain to client, "I will be staying with you for the first few minutes of the transfusion. We will be checking with you frequently while the blood is infusing, and taking your blood pressure and temperature frequently. If you feel discomfort of any type while the blood is infusing, please let me know immediately."

Steps	Rationale

4. Have client void or empty urinary drainage collection container.

    If transfusion reaction occurs, urine specimen obtained must be recent and preferably taken after transfusion is initiated to assess for presence of red blood cells from a hemolytic reaction.

5. With another registered nurse or licensed nurse, correctly verify blood product and identify client (check agency policy):
   a. Client's name and identification number
   b. Client's name and identification number with forms from blood bank and with physician's order in client's record
   c. Client's blood group and Rh type
   d. Crossmatch compatibility
   e. Donor's blood group and Rh type
   f. Unit and hospital number
   g. Expiration date and time on blood unit
   h. Type of blood component is correct component ordered by physician

    If possible, have client identify self. Correct product must be administered to right client to avoid transfusion reaction.

NURSE ALERT

Because most severe transfusion reactions occur from identification error (Vengelen-Tyler, 1996), verification of client, product, product type, and crossmatch may be the most important step of the entire procedure.

6. Inspect blood product for signs of leakage or unusual appearance, including clots, bubbles, or purplish color.

    If signs of contamination are present, return blood product to laboratory.

7. Attach blood product by inserting spike of Y tubing located next to NS 0.9% tubing (see illustration). Close NS clamp above filter and open clamp above filter to blood product.

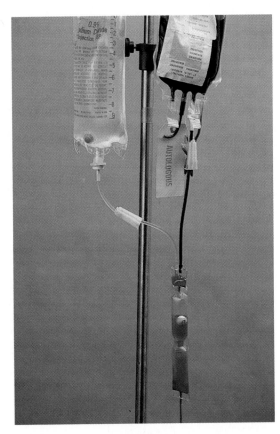

Step 7

Steps	Rationale

8. Review with client the purpose of transfusion. Ask client to report immediately any signs and symptoms (during or after transfusion), including chills, low back pain, shortness of breath, nausea, excessive perspiration, rash, or even a vague sense of uneasiness.

Once transfusion reaction occurs, staff must respond immediately with treatment.

9. Connect NS-primed blood administration set directly to client's IV site. Remove and discard gloves and wash hands.

NURSE ALERT

A transfusion reaction is an emergency.

10. Open lower clamp and regulate blood infusion to allow only 10 to 24 ml to infuse in the first 15 minutes. Remain with client.

If a reaction occurs, infusion of this amount minimizes the amount of incompatible blood transfused.

11. Obtain vital signs (temperature, pulse, respiration, blood pressure) 15 minutes after initiation of transfusion.

Change from baseline vital signs may indicate transfusion reaction.

12. Reregulate flow clamp if there is no transfusion reaction, and infuse the remaining volume of blood as ordered by physician. Packed red blood cells are usually infused over 2 hours and whole blood over 3 to 4 hours. Check blood tubing package for correct drop factor.

Careful regulation prevents adverse response. Client's condition and physician's orders dictate rate of blood infusion.

NURSE ALERT

Blood must be transfused within 4 hours of spiking the blood bag. Even if infusion is not complete, blood must be discontinued. This reduces the potential for exposure to bacterial infection from blood. Blood bank can split blood units if client is at risk for fluid overload.

13. Continue to monitor vital signs per agency/agency procedure and procedure during transfusion.

Ensures early identification of adverse response.

14. After blood has infused, close roller clamp above filter to blood and open NS.

15. Infuse NS until blood administration is completely clear.

Ensures all blood cells infused.

16. Discontinue transfusion and blood administration set.

17. Follow standard precautions and agency protocol for disposal of old blood bags and tubing. Remove and discard gloves and wash hands.

18. Blood transfusion increases risk of phlebitis. Apply injection cap and flush existing IV line or restart IV fluids as ordered only after assessing IV site for patency and signs and symptoms of phlebitis. If transfusing more than one unit of blood or blood product, maintain NS via blood administration set at KVO rate until second unit is started. Because of the risk of bacterial growth, blood administration sets should be changed after each unit or at the end of 4 hours (INS 1998; Vengelen-Tyler, 1996).

19. See Completion Protocol (inside front cover).

EVALUATION

1. Observe for chills, flushing, itching, hives, dyspnea, tachycardia, drop in blood pressure, or any sign of transfusion reaction.
2. Monitor I&O and laboratory values (Hgb, Hct, prothrombin time [PT], partial thromboplastin time [PTT], platelet count) after transfusion. (In the hematologically stable adult, one unit of PRBCs should increase the Hgb by 1 g/dl and Hct by 3%. A unit of platelet concentrate prepared from a single unit of whole blood should increase the client's platelet count by 5000 to 10,000/mL (Vengelen-Tyler, 1996).
3. Observe that client's behavior or appearance does not demonstrate signs of physical or emotional stress during the transfusion and that client can verbalize understanding of the need for transfusion.
4. Monitor IV site and status of infusion every time vital signs are taken.
5. Ask client to describe purpose, benefit, and risk of transfusion.

Unexpected Outcomes and Related Interventions

1. Client experiences pain, swelling, or discoloration at the IV site.
   a. Stop the transfusion and discontinue the IV infusion.
   b. Restart the IV infusion in another site.
2. Client complains of pain at infusion site when blood is first initiated, but IV site is patent and not infiltrated.
   Apply warm pack to arm to prevent venous spasm from infusion of cold blood products.
3. Transfusion slows and client is not receiving proper volume.
   a. Check patency of set.
   b. Ensure blood bag is elevated to proper height.
   c. Verify that all clamps and stopcocks are open.
   d. Ensure filter is completely primed.
   e. Gently agitate blood bag.
   f. Close primary clamp (below the filter). Lower blood bag and open NS roller clamp. Dilute blood with 25 to 50 ml NS to facilitate infusion.
   g. Place unit to be infused in an electronic infusion device that permits blood transfusion.
   h. Apply pressure bag and inflate to a maximum of 300 mm Hg.
   i. Restart IV infusion with a large-gauge catheter.
4. Client has sudden temperature spike (greater than 100° F or 38.7° C), tachycardia, fall in blood pressure, low back pain, or dyspnea during transfusion.
   a. Stop the transfusion.
   b. Keep the IV open with NS 0.9% via a new infusion set.
   c. Notify physician and blood bank immediately.
   d. Follow agency protocol for reporting and intervention.

5. Client's laboratory values fail to normalize after transfusion.
   Notify physician and continue to monitor client for active bleeding.

Recording and Reporting

- Record pretransfusion medications, vital signs, and location and condition of IV catheter.
- Record type of blood component, recipient and unit identification, compatibility, and expiration date according to agency policy.
- Record volume of NS and blood component infused.
- Record vital signs taken during transfusion.
- Report signs and symptoms of a transfusion reaction immediately.

Sample Documentation

1000   Early AM CBC noted. MD aware of Hct 22. Type & cross match drawn with two witnesses per phlebotomy.

1230   Voided 320 ml clear, amber urine. 18 angiocath inserted left cephalic vein. NS 0.9% initiated at KVO. 1 unit PRBCs started at 40 ml/hr, after witnessed by J. Doe, RN.

Geriatric Considerations

- If the client cannot tolerate the volume of 1 unit of whole blood or red blood cells to be infused in 4 hours, request the blood bank to split the unit into two bags, and leave the second bag under the appropriate refrigeration during the infusion of the first.
- If accurate rate control with an electronic infusion device is required, check agency policy for information about use of the specific brand for blood infusor.

Home Care and Long-Term Care Considerations

- Pretransfusion client assessment and identification are the same as in the hospital.
- Blood and blood products must be transported in a container with an appropriate coolant. Check and record the temperature at the time of delivery. Nurses or blood bank personnel may transport blood.
- Easy access to emergency medical services and the primary physician are required during transfusion outside the hospital.

CRITICAL THINKING EXERCISES

1. You have received information about Mr. Smith, a 75-year-old client with a preliminary diagnosis of fever of unknown origin, being admitted to your unit. The physician's orders include 1000 ml 5% dextrose in 0.45% sodium chloride at 80 ml/hr.
   a. What other information do you need to learn about Mr. Smith before starting the IV infusion?
   b. What factors should be considered in determining the gauge of catheter to use?
   c. What factors must be considered for a safe infusion?

2. What is the most appropriate action to take for each of the following situations?
   a. The IV site is located slightly above the client's wrist in the cephalic vein. When the client moves his arm, the infusion rate slows down dramatically.
   b. The client complains of pain at the site of the IV catheter. On examination, no redness, edema, or skin temperature changes are found.
   c. While flushing an intermittent IV lock after a dose of medication has been infused, you notice clear liquid leaking from under the transparent dressing.

3. You have returned from the blood bank with a unit of red blood cells for Mrs. Jones. While checking the identification of the client and blood with another nurse, you find that the identification number on the client's armband is not the same as the number on the unit of blood. What is the appropriate action to take?

4. You have hung a dose of vancomycin to the client's intermittent IV lock. After 15 minutes of infusion, you learn that the client is complaining of feeling flushed and itching.
   a. What is the first action to take?
   b. What other signs or symptoms should be assessed?
   c. What information should be conveyed to the physician?

REFERENCES

Camp-Sorrell D: *Access device guidelines: recommendations for nursing practice and education,* Pittsburgh, 1996, Oncology Nursing Society.

Fabian B: Intravenous therapy in the older adult. In Terry LBJ, Lonsway RA, Hedrick C, editors: *Intravenous therapy: clinical principles and practice,* Philadelphia, 1995, WB Saunders.

Centers for Disease Control: Guidelines for prevention of intravascular device-related infections. Infection Control & Hospital Epidemiology, 17(7):438–472, 1996.

Intravenous Nurses Society: Intravenous nursing standards of practice, *J Intraven Nurs* 21(1S):35–36, 1998.

Ippolito G et al: *Prevention, management and chemoprophylaxis of occupational exposure to HIV,* Charlottesville, 1997, International Health Care Worker Safety Center, University of Virginia.

LaRocca J, Otto S: *Pocket guide to intravenous therapy,* St Louis, 1994, Mosby.

Pavlin DJ et al: Vasovagal reactions in an ambulatory surgery center, *Anesth Analg* 76(5):931–935, 1993.

Pearson ML: Guideline for prevention of intravascular device related infections, *Infect Control Hosp Epidemiol* 17(7): 438–473, 1996.

Perdue M: Intravenous complications. In Terry LBJ, Lonsway RA, Hedrick C, editors: *Intravenous therapy: clinical principles and practice,* Philadelphia, 1995, WB Saunders.

Perucca R: Obtaining vascular access. In Terry LBJ, Lonsway RA, Hedrick C, editors: *Intravenous therapy: clinical principles and practice,* Philadelphia, 1995, WB Saunders.

Perucca R, editor: Intravenous monitoring and catheter care. In Terry LBJ, Lonsway RA, Hedrick C, editors: *Intravenous therapy: clinical principles and practice,* Philadelphia, 1995, WB Saunders.

Rapp SE et al: Effect of patient position on the incidence of vasovagal response to venous cannulation, *Arch Intern Med* 153(7):1698–1704, 1993.

Trissel LA: *Handbook on injectable drugs,* ed 9, Bethesda, Md, 1996, American Society of Health-System Pharmacists.

Vengelen-Tyler V, editor: *Technical manual,* ed 12, Bethesda, Md, 1996, American Association of Blood Banks.

CHAPTER 31

Promoting Oxygenation

Skill 31.1
Oxygen Administration, 728

Skill 31.2
**Airway Management: Noninvasive
Interventions, 735**

Skill 31.3
Airway Management: Suctioning, 739

Skill 31.4
**Airway Management: Endotracheal Tube
and Tracheostomy Care, 747**

Skill 31.5
**Managing Closed Chest Drainage
Systems (Including Managing Postoperative
Autotransfusions), 754**

Physiological needs, such as food, water, and air, are the primary stimulus for behavior according to Maslow's hierarchy of human needs. It is only when these needs are met that humans may attempt to reach higher levels of needs, such as safety, intimacy, and the need for knowledge and understanding.

Respirations are effective when sufficient oxygenation is obtained at the cellular level and when cellular waste and carbon dioxide are adequately removed via the bloodstream and lungs. When this system is interrupted, such as by lung tissue damage, obstruction of airways by inflammation and excess mucus, or impairment of the mechanics of ventilation, intervention is required to support the client or death may occur.

NURSING DIAGNOSES

A variety of nursing diagnoses may apply to clients requiring promotion of oxygenation. Nursing diagnoses directly related to promoting optimum oxygenation include **Ineffective Airway Clearance** resulting from an ineffective cough or excessive secretions, **Ineffective Breathing Pattern** exhibited by clients with respiratory muscle weakness and fatigue or abnormal breathing pattern, **Impaired Gas Exchange** resulting from altered oxygen supply or alveolar hypoventilation, **Inability to Sustain Spontaneous Ventilation** for those clients who exhibit an imbalance between ventilatory capacity and demand because of decreased ventilatory capacity and increased ventilatory demand, and **Dysfunctional Ventilatory Weaning Response (DVWR)** for those clients who are physically or psychologically unable to wean from mechanical ventilation.

Clients with breathing problems may be at risk for **Altered Thought Processes** from inadequate oxygenation and carbon dioxide retention. **Activity Intolerance** related to imbalance between oxygen supply and demand may lead to a **Self-Care Deficit** and **Risk for Infection** a result of the damaged defense systems of the lungs. Psychosocial factors such as **Anxiety, Fear,** and **Hopelessness** may be related to dyspnea and feelings of suffocation, as well as the fear of dying. **Ineffective Coping** may be related to the chronicity of many pulmonary diseases. **Impaired Verbal Communication** when the client receives a tracheostomy or is intubated may also be appropriate.

Skill 31.1

OXYGEN ADMINISTRATION

Oxygen therapy refers to the administration of oxygen to a client to prevent or relieve hypoxia. *Hypoxia* is a condition in which insufficient oxygen is available to meet the metabolic needs of tissues and cells. Hypoxia results from *hypoxemia*, which is a deficiency of oxygen in the arterial blood. Supplemental oxygen for the relief of hypoxemia may be temporary, until the cause of the problem is corrected, or long term, when it is required for a chronic condition. The delivery method used depends on the amount of supplemental oxygen required (Table 31-1), hospital or home use, and the portability desired (see Chapter 40).

Equipment

Delivery device ordered by physician
Oxygen tubing (consider extension tubing)
Humidifier
Sterile water
Oxygen source
Flow meter
"Oxygen In Use" sign

ASSESSMENT

1. Perform a complete assessment of the respiratory system (see Chapter 14). Assess for hypoxia including:
   a. Behavioral changes, apprehension, anxiety, decreased ability to concentrate, decreased level of consciousness, fatigue and dizziness.
   b. Changes in vital signs of increased depth and rate of respirations, dyspnea and use of accessory muscles of respiration, decreased oxygen saturation, tachycardia, and cardiac dysrhythmias.

Table 31-1

Oxygen Delivery Systems

Delivery system	F_iO_2* Delivered	Advantages	Disadvantages
Nasal cannula	1–6 L/min: 24%–44%	Safe and simple Easily tolerated Effective for low concentrations Does not impede eating or talking Inexpensive, disposable	Unable to use with nasal obstruction Drying to mucous membranes Can dislodge easily May cause skin irritation or breakdown Client's breathing pattern will affect exact F_iO_2
Oxymizer	1–15 L/min: 24%–60%	Higher concentrations without mask Releases O_2 only on inhalation Conserves O_2, increased portability Does not require humidification	Interferes with drinking from cup May be cosmetically unappealing Potential reservoir membrane failure Client's breathing pattern will affect exact F_iO_2
Venturi mask	4–10 L/min: 24%–50%	Delivers exact preset F_iO_2 despite client's breathing pattern Does not dry mucous membranes Can be used to deliver humidity	Hot and confining, mask may irritate skin F_iO_2 may be lowered if mask does not fit snugly Interferes with eating and talking
Partial rebreather	6–15 L/min: 35%–60%	Delivers increased F_iO_2 Easily humidifies O_2 Does not dry mucous membranes	Hot and confining, may irritate skin, tight seal necessary Interferes with eating and talking Bag may twist or kink; should not totally deflate
Nonrebreather	6–15 L/min: 60%–100%	Delivers highest possible F_iO_2 without intubation Does not dry mucous membranes	Requires tight seal, difficult to maintain and uncomfortable May irritate skin Bag should not totally deflate

*FiO_2, Fraction of inspired oxygen concentration.

c. Changes in color: pallor or cyanosis.
Rationale: Early detection of hypoxia will result in prompt treatment. Untreated hypoxia is life-threatening.

2. Check arterial blood gas (ABG) results. **Rationale: Objectively quantifies changes in oxygen and carbon dioxide changes that affect acid-base balance (see Chapter 37).**

periences of anxiety, fatigue, and decreased oxygenation status return to normal by discharge.

3. Client is able to state the indications for supplemental oxygen by discharge.
4. Client follows safety guidelines for supplemental oxygen therapy by discharge.
5. Client uses supplemental oxygen as prescribed by discharge.

PLANNING

Expected outcomes focus on optimum oxygenation, safe application of oxygen therapy, and an understanding of and compliance with the oxygen prescription.

Expected Outcomes

1. Client's oxygen saturation and ABGs return to or remain within normal limits or baseline levels.
2. Client's pulse; respirations; color; and subjective ex-

DELEGATION CONSIDERATIONS

The skill of oxygen administration by nasal cannula or mask can be delegated to appropriately trained assistive personnel (AP). The nurse assesses for correct administration and client response.

- Care provider should demonstrate correct technique for the application of oxygen: the correct setup, device, and flow rate.
- Instruct the care provider on possible unexpected outcomes associated with oxygen delivery and the need to report these to the nurse if they occur.

IMPLEMENTATION

Steps	Rationale

1. See Standard Protocol (inside front cover).

COMMUNICATION TIP

Explain to client the purpose of oxygen administration and safety precautions (Table 31-2).

Client may continue to have dyspnea while receiving oxygen because of other etiology (e.g., narrowed airways). Understanding of purpose and safety guidelines increases compliance and safety.

2. Attach delivery device to oxygen tubing. Consider extension tubing for clients who are not confined to bed.

Avoids complications of bed rest.

3. Attach appropriate flow meter to oxygen source.

Flow meters with smaller calibrations may be safer for clients requiring low-dose oxygen when larger doses may be harmful, as in client with chronic obstructive pulmonary disease (COPD).

4. Attach tubing to flow meter.
5. Adjust oxygen flow rate to prescribed dosage. If humidifier is used, verify that water is bubbling (see illustration, p. 730).

Humidifier prevents drying of mucosa and airway secretions but may not be necessary for flow rates less than 3 L/min. Presence of bubbling indicates that oxygen is humidified before delivery to client.

Table 31-2

Oxygen Safety Guidelines

Guideline	Explanation
Make sure oxygen is set at prescribed rate.	Oxygen is a medication and should not be adjusted without a physician's order.
Smoking is not permitted. Avoid electrical equipment that may result in sparks.	Oxygen supports combustion. Delivery systems must be kept 10 feet from open flames and at least 5 feet from electrical equipment.
Store oxygen cylinders upright.	Secure with chain or holder to prevent tipping and falling while stationary or when client is being transported.
Check oxygen available in portable cylinders before transporting or ambulating clients.	Gauge on cylinder should register in green range, indicating oxygen is available for transport and ambulation. Have back-up supply available if level is low.

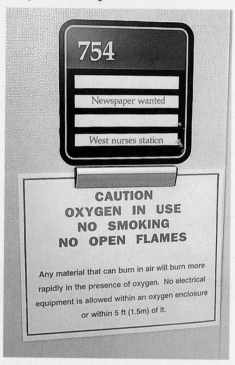

Figure 31-1

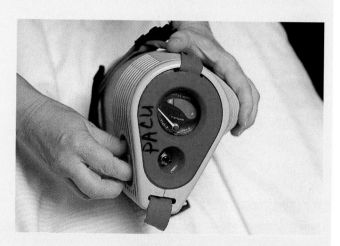

Figure 31-2

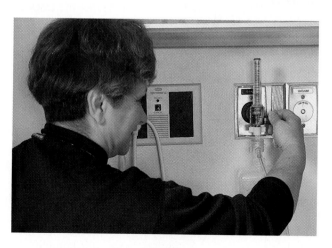

Step 5

Steps	Rationale

6. Observe for proper fit and function of delivery device (Lewis and Collier, 1992).

a. Nasal cannula

Place tips of cannula into client's nares and adjust headband or plastic slide until cannula fits snugly and comfortably (see illustration).

Effective mechanism of oxygen delivery up to 6 L/min.

b. Reservoir nasal cannula

Fit as for nasal cannula. Reservoir is located under nose or as a pendant (see illustration).

Able to deliver higher flow of oxygen than cannula without changing to a mask, which is claustrophobic for some clients. Delivers a 2:1 ratio (e.g., 6-L nasal cannula is approximately equivalent to 3-L reservoir device or Oxymizer).

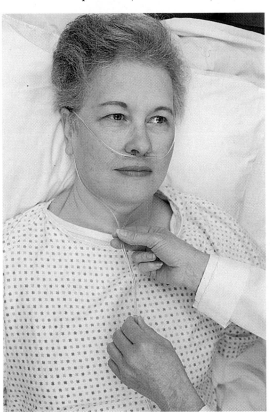

Step 6a

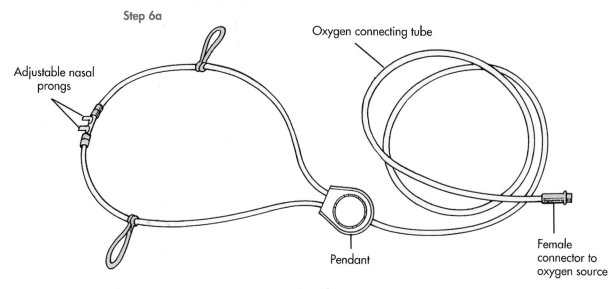

Step 6b

Steps	Rationale

c. Venturi mask

Rate set on flow meter will determine fraction of inspired oxygen concentration (F_iO_2). Low- and high-concentration adapters are available. Setting should correlate with prescribed dosage (see illustration).

Delivers exact oxygen concentration despite respiratory pattern.

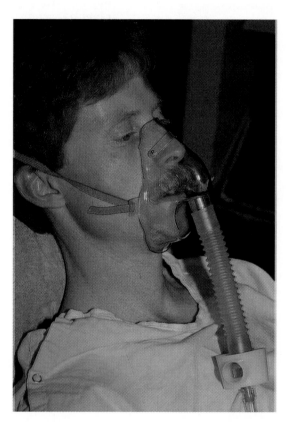

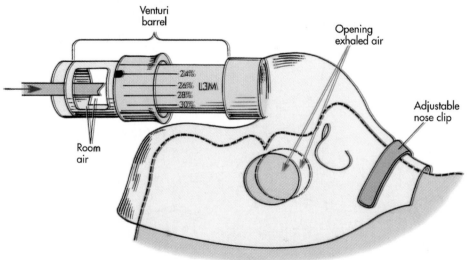

Step 6c

Steps	Rationale

d. Partial rebreather mask
Reservoir should fill on exhalation and almost collapse on inhalation (see illustration).

Effectively delivers higher oxygen concentrations.

e. Nonbreathing mask
Reservoir should fill on exhalation and should never totally collapse on inhalation.

Delivers highest possible oxygen concentration for nonintubated clients.

f. Simple face mask
Place securely over client's nose and mouth (see illustration).

NURSE ALERT

To ensure the client's inspiratory demands are being met, observe the reservoir bag; it should not completely collapse on inspiration.

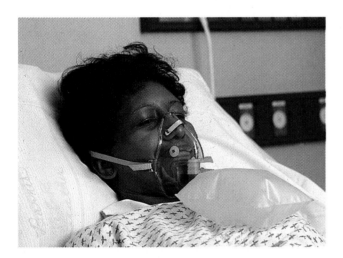

Step 6d

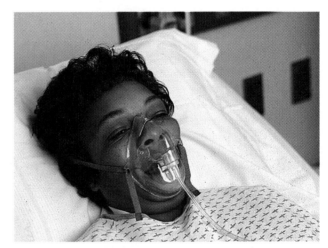

Step 6f

7. Obtain an order for ABGs 10 to 15 minutes after initiation of therapy or change in oxygen concentration.

ABGs provide objective data regarding blood oxygenation and acid-base status (see Chapter 37).

8. Consult with physician regarding the need for pulse oximetry if client's oxygen level may be unstable.

Oximetry provides objective data regarding blood oxygenation and is used for trending (see Chapter 12).

9. See Completion Protocol (inside front cover).

• • •

EVALUATION

1. Observe repeat ABGs and/or pulse oximetry for objective measurement of improvement.
2. Observe client for improved oxygen saturation, as demonstrated by decreased anxiety, improved level of consciousness and cognitive abilities, decreased fatigue, and absence of dizziness.
3. Assess pulse and respirations, decreased pulse with regular rhythm, decreased respiratory rate, and improved color. These are signs that oxygenation is improving.

4. Ask client to verbalize indications for supplemental oxygen.
5. Observe if client follows safety guidelines in present setting, and ask client to verbalize safety guidelines for home use.
6. Observe for compliance to oxygen prescription.

Unexpected Outcomes and Related Interventions

1. Client experiences nasal irritation, drying of nasal mucosa, sinus pain, or epistaxis.
   a. Apply a water-soluble lubricant to areas of irritation around nares.
   b. Recommend use of an isotonic saline nasal spray.
   c. Determine if a reservoir cannula is appropriate; obtain order.
2. Client develops irritation of the face or posterior surfaces of the ear.

   Apply ear protectors or reposition nasal cannula so that it does not come into contact with irritated areas.
3. Client has continued hypoxia.
   a. Monitor ABGs and/or pulse oximetry.
   b. Perform a complete respiratory assessment.
   c. Notify physician.
   d. Identify methods to decrease oxygen demand (e.g., total bed rest).
4. Client develops carbon dioxide retention, as demonstrated by confusion, headache, decreased level of consciousness, flushing, somnolence, carbon dioxide narcosis, or respiratory arrest.
   a. Monitor ABGs.
   b. Notify physician.
   c. Assist in maintaining oxygen pressure (PO_2) at 55 mm Hg. (Hypoxia must be treated, but PO_2 levels that exceed 60 to 70 mm Hg may worsen hypoventilation.)

Recording and Reporting

- Record the respiratory assessment findings, method of oxygen delivery, flow rate, client's response, any adverse reactions, and change in physician's order.

Sample Documentation

0800   Client alert and oriented. Respirations even and easy. Color pink. O_2 4-L nasal cannula. Productive cough of yellow sputum. Fluids encouraged.

1000   Reddened areas are noted behind right ear, without breakdown. Foam ear protector added to nasal cannula tubing.

1200   No further redness noted behind ears. Client denies discomfort from cannula.

Geriatric Considerations

- Normal arterial oxygen levels may decrease with age. A 70 year old may have a normal arterial PO_2 between 75 and 80.
- The drive to breathe in clients who have chronically increased CO_2 levels is based on their oxygen status. Oxygen flow rates greater than 2 L are given with great caution in these individuals.
- The older adult may be at increased risk for skin breakdown. Frequent monitoring for redness is necessary. Early interventions such as loosening the straps, repositioning, or adding padding may prevent breakdown.

Home Care and Long-Term Care Considerations

- The client and family must be taught how to correctly administer oxygen based on which system is used and the safety measures to be followed. These considerations are discussed more fully in Chapter 40.
- The dangers of changing the oxygen flow rate from the prescribed flow should be stressed. Emphasize that the client may be short of breath because of reasons other than hypoxemia and to contact the physician if increased shortness of breath occurs.
- The client and family must be taught the signs and symptoms for which to call the physician.

Skill 31.2

AIRWAY MANAGEMENT: NONINVASIVE INTERVENTIONS

The respiratory system is comprised of a system of airways that must remain open and free of obstruction to decrease resistance of airflow to and from the lung. Interventions to maintain the airways depend on the pathophysiology responsible. Positioning, controlled cough, medications, hydration, and suctioning may be considered.

Positioning and coughing are two noninvasive techniques that may assist in improving airway patency. Positioning to enhance airway patency should be considered with all clients. The goal is to position the client to allow the greatest chest expansion with the least amount of effort. Generally, if a client is short of breath, this position will be semi-Fowler's or Fowler's position. The supine position may be preferred for clients with increased abdominal girth. Controlled coughing is used to clear secretions that may obstruct the airway. Repeated coughing that does not mobilize secretions is tiring and ineffective and should be prevented.

Medications such as bronchodilators can be used to dilate airways with some disease processes of the respiratory system. The purpose of hydration, through the oral route if possible, is to thin pulmonary secretions so that they can be expectorated more easily. Suctioning is discussed in Skill 31.3.

Clients with certain disorders such as obstructive sleep apnea (OSA) may be unable to maintain a patent airway. In OSA, nasopharyngeal abnormalities that cause narrowing of the upper airway produce repetitive airway obstruction during sleep with the potential for periods of apnea and hypoxemia. Treatment of OSA can be a challenge for the client and nurse or health care provider. Pressure can be delivered during the inspiratory and expiratory phases of the respiratory cycle by mask to maintain airway patency during sleep, but the process requires consideration of each individual's needs to obtain compliance. Pressure applied during the expiratory phase alone is administered by continuous positive airway pressure (CPAP) and during both inspiration and expiration by bilevel positive airway pressure (BiPAP).

For clients who have measurable changes in the flow of their airways, such as clients with asthma or reactive airways disease, peak expiratory flow rate (PEFR) measurements may be useful. The PEFR is the maximum flow that a client can force out during one quick forced expiration, measured in liters. The client or nurse can use these measurements as an objective indicator of the client's current status and effectiveness of treatment. Decreased peak flow rates may indicate the need for further treatment such as bronchodilators or antiinflammatory medications.

Equipment

Application of CPAP or BiPAP (Figure 31-3)
Mask with straps (face or nasal)
Valve (CPAP or BiPAP)
Oxygen source
Generator (CPAP or BiPAP)
Appropriate signs
PEFR measurements (Figure 31-4)
Peak flow meter
Client diary, if appropriate

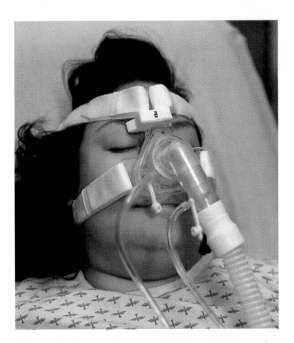

Figure 31-3   Application of CPAP or BiPAP mask.

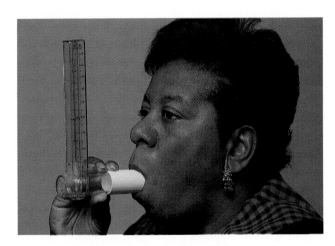

Figure 31-4   PEFR measurement.

ASSESSMENT

1. Assess for possible impairment of airway clearance: increased work of breathing or inability to clear copious or tenacious secretions by coughing.
2. Observe for signs of airway obstruction; shortness of breath, wheezing, use of accessory muscles of respiration, pallor or cyanosis, nasal flaring, snoring respirations, or sleep apnea.
3. Assess client's baseline knowledge of positioning, CPAP/BiPAP, and PEFR.
4. Review physician's order for CPAP/BiPAP and predicted values for PEFR.

PLANNING

Expected outcomes focus on client's airway patency, comfort, and ability for self-care.

Expected Outcomes

1. Client maintains a position that promotes maximum lung expansion and comfort.

2. Client's airways are cleared of retained secretions.
3. Client's periods of sleep apnea are reduced to fewer than two episodes in 6 hours.
4. Client's objective measures of oxygenation improve or remain normal (ABGs, pulse oximetry).
5. Client expresses comfort while CPAP/BiPAP is in place by discharge.
6. Client and family demonstrate correct use of CPAP/BiPAP or PEFR by discharge.
7. Client and family verbalize an appropriate action plan based on PEFR values obtained by discharge.
8. Client verbalizes the benefits of positioning, CPAP, and/or PEFR by discharge.

DELEGATION CONSIDERATIONS

The skills of positioning, therapeutic coughing, CPAP/BiPAP mask application, and PEFR measurements can be delegated to appropriately trained AP. The nurse assesses for correct administration and client response.

IMPLEMENTATION

Steps	Rationale
1. See Standard Protocol (inside front cover).	

COMMUNICATION TIP

Explain to client that you are aware of the discomfort he or she is experiencing (i.e., breathlessness, pain) and that correct positioning will aid in the relief of this discomfort.

2. **Correct positioning of client**
   a. **Sitting**
   Semi-Fowler's or high Fowler's, sitting on side of bed, or in chair with elbows resting on knees. Clients with COPD may benefit from leaning over table with arms propped up (see illustrations).

   Promotes optimum lung expansion and maximizes use of accessory muscles.

   b. **Standing**
   When client who is ambulating experiences shortness of breath or the need to cough, encourage a position that supports client (see illustrations).

   c. **Supine**
   Most clients are more comfortable supported by two pillows or head of bed up at least 30°. Turn at least every 2 hours to encourage secretion drainage. Consider maneuvers to drain areas of lungs with retained secretions by gravity if tolerated by client. If unilateral reexpansion is needed (e.g., after surgery), have client lie with side requiring expansion up: "good side down, affected lung up."

   Decreases orthopnea. Obese clients may experience decreased abdominal interference of full lung expansion when lying flat.

   Promotes lung expansion on the affected side. Exchange of respiratory gases is improved.

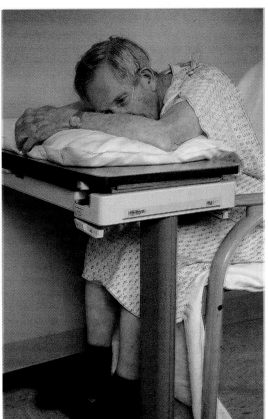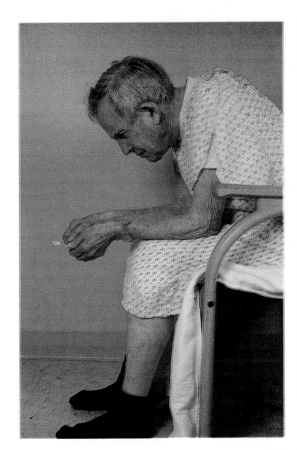

Step 2a

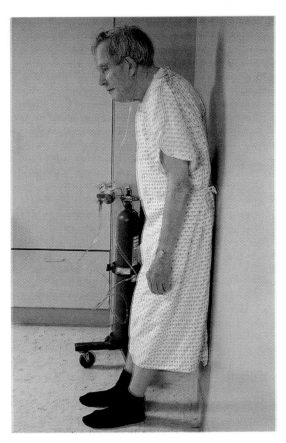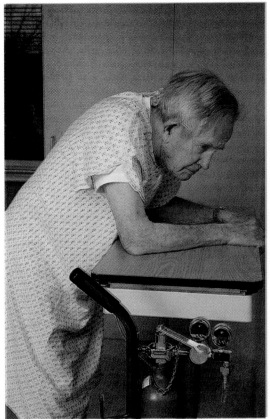

Step 2b

Steps	Rationale

3. Controlled coughing
   a. Place client in upright position. High Fowler's, leaning forward, or with knees bent and a small pillow or hand to support the abdomen may augment expiratory pressure.
   b. Instruct client to take two slow, deep breaths, inhaling through the nose and exhaling out the mouth.
   c. Instruct client to inhale deeply a third time, hold this breath, and count to three; then cough deeply for two or three consecutive coughs without inhaling between coughs. Instruct the client to push air forcefully out of the lungs.

COMMUNICATION TIP

Explain to client that controlled coughing clears secretions that may obstruct the airway by allowing air behind the mucus to move during the cough.

COMMUNICATION TIP

Explain that tight seal around face is needed to improve symptoms

4. **Apply CPAP/BiPAP**
   a. Position client.
   b. Position face mask or nasal mask tightly and adjust head strap until seal is maintained and client is able to tolerate (see Figure 31-3).

Client may experience claustrophobic sensations and feelings of discomfort from continuous pressure. Support and education help client develop tolerance. Promotes optimum lung expansion. Several types of masks are available because of the difficulties in achieving a comfortable fit.

   c. Instruct client to breath normally.
   d. Apply at ordered setting for prescribed length of time.

Reduces hyperventilation and fatigue.

5. **Obtain PEFR measurements**
   a. Instruct client about purpose and rationale.
   b. Place client in an upright position.
   c. Slide indicator to base of the numbered scale.
   d. Instruct client to take a deep breath.
   e. Have client place meter mouthpiece in the mouth and close lips, making a firm seal (see Figure 31-4).
   f. Have client blow out as hard and fast as possible through the mouth only.

Promotes optimum lung expansion.

Tight seal ensures all expired breath will be measured for accurate reading.

Maximum effort is required for an accurate reading. Air expelled through nares will not be measured and will decrease PEFR readings.

   g. This maneuver should be repeated two additional times, with the highest number recorded.
   h. If client is to record PEFR at home, have client demonstrate PEFR technique independently and assess ability to record PEFR accurately in a diary.
6. See Completion Protocol (inside front cover).

COMMUNICATION TIP

Help client implement an appropriate action plan as prescribed by physician. Explain that PEFR is just one objective measure that can be used to judge symptom severity.

EVALUATION

1. Observe client's body alignment and position whenever in visual contact with client. Reposition as needed, at least every 2 hours.
2. Auscultate and examine chest at least every 8 hours.
3. Assess client's respiratory status during sleep to determine response to CPAP. Ask if client subjectively feels more rested after arising.
4. Observe repeat ABGs and/or pulse oximetry for objective measure of improvement.

5. Assess client's tolerance of CPAP/BiPAP mask and compliance to therapy.
6. Observe a return demonstration by client/family to determine if correct technique is being used with CPAP/BiPAP or PEFR.
7. Ask client to explain the appropriate response to different PEFR values he or she may obtain.
8. Ask client to explain purpose and benefits of positioning, controlled coughing, CPAP/BiPAP, and PEFR.

Unexpected Outcomes and Related Interventions

1. Client is unable to maintain a patent airway.
   a. Evaluate positioning. Consider suctioning.
   b. Monitor ABGs/pulse oximetry.
   c. An artificial airway may be considered, if not present.
2. Client experiences worsening dyspnea with bronchospasm and hypoxemia.
   a. Notify physician.
   b. Monitor ABGs/pulse oximetry.
   c. Medicate as ordered.
   d. Evaluate for methods to decrease oxygen demand.
3. Client is unable to tolerate CPAP/BiPAP because of feeling of suffocation, shortness of breath, and discomfort related to pressure applied during CPAP/BiPAP.
   a. Check fit of delivery device. Consider alternative if difficulties continue.
   b. Provide client with encouragement, support, and education.
4. Client is unable or unwilling to give maximum effort for PEFR.
   a. Provide client with encouragement and education.
   b. If unable to achieve adequate readings, contact physician immediately, medicate as ordered, and give support.

Recording and Reporting

- Record activity level, including assistance with positioning, if needed. Record cough effectiveness and respiratory assessment.
- For CPAP/BiPAP, record client compliance and tolerance, mask fit and skin assessment beneath mask, effectiveness of therapy, witnessed periods of apnea, and status of daytime hypersomnolence.
- For PEFR record measurement before and after therapy and client's ability and effort to perform PEFR.

Sample Documentation

Positioning

0300 Dyspneic at rest, O_2 saturations 88%–90%. Respiratory rate 26 and shallow with use of accessory muscles. States he is unable to tolerate supine position. Assisted to chair, leaning forward with head and shoulders resting on pillow on stationary table. Pursed-lip breathing encouraged.

0315 States he is breathing easier. Color pink. O_2 saturations 90%–92%. Respiratory rate 28 with good pursed-lip breathing technique. Remains in chair.

CPAP

2400 Appears to sleep restfully. Respirations even and easy without snoring. No jerking movements noted. CPAP continues per face mask with good seal at 7.5 cm H_2O.

0800 No change noted in assessment during night. CPAP applied for 10 hours. No areas of irritation noted from mask. States he slept well without awakening.

Home Care and Long-Term Care Considerations

- Frequent follow-up may be necessary to enhance CPAP/BiPAP compliance and address unexpected outcomes promptly.
- PEFR may be incorporated into an "action plan" for the client at home as an objective measure of when a change in therapy is required.

Skill 31.3

AIRWAY MANAGEMENT: SUCTIONING

For some clients, use of noninvasive techniques, along with medications, is not sufficient to maintain a patent airway. In these cases, suctioning is considered. The method of suctioning used depends on the level of the secretions to be removed, the presence of an artificial airway, and the client's condition. Oropharyngeal (Yankauer) suctioning is performed by using a rigid plastic catheter with one large and several small eyelets (Figure 31-5) through which mu-

cus enters when suction is applied. Alert clients can easily be taught this suction method to control the secretions in the oral cavity.

Nasotracheal suctioning is used to clear secretions from the trachea. This type of suctioning is used when secretions cannot be expectorated from the lower airway, thus requiring sterile technique.

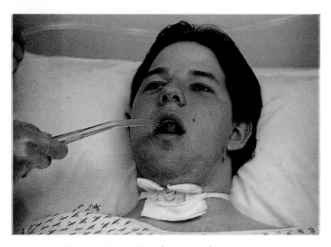

Figure 31-5 Oropharyngeal suctioning.

Endotracheal (ET; Figure 31-6) and tracheostomy (trach; Figure 31-7) tubes allow direct access to the lower airways for suctioning. These artificial airways may be inserted to create a route for mechanical ventilation, allow easy access of suctioning, relieve mechanical airway obstruction, or protect the airway from aspiration because of impaired cough or gag reflexes.

Figure 31-6 **A,** Endotracheal (ET) tube with inflated cuff. **B,** ET tubes with uninflated and inflated cuffs and syringe for inflation. Client is unable to speak while tube is in place because air cannot flow through the vocal cords.

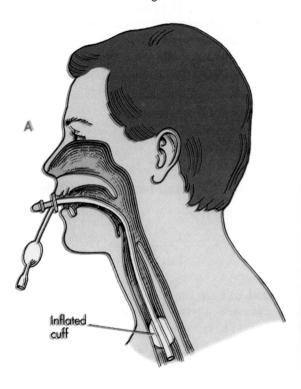

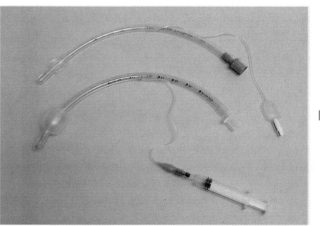

Equipment

Oropharyngeal suctioning

Oropharyngeal suction catheter or Yankauer suction tip

Nonsterile gloves

Nonsterile basin (e.g., disposable cup)

Water (about 100 ml)

Portable or wall suction machine

Connecting tubing (6 feet)

Face shield, if indicated

Nasotracheal suctioning

12 to 16 French suction catheter (adult)

Water-soluble lubricant

Two sterile gloves or one sterile and one nonsterile glove

Sterile basin

Sterile normal saline (NS) (about 100 ml)

Clean towel or paper drape

Portable or wall suction

Connecting tubing (6 feet)

Face shield, if indicated

Endotracheal or tracheostomy suctioning

12 to 16 French catheter (adult)

Bedside table

Two sterile gloves or one sterile and one nonsterile glove

Sterile basin

Sterile NS (about 100 ml)

Clean towel or sterile drape

Portable or wall suction machine

Connecting tubing (6 feet)

Face shield, if indicated

Closed-system or in-line suctioning

Closed-system or in-line suction catheter

5 to 10 ml NS in syringe or vials

Portable or wall suction apparatus

Connecting tubing (6 feet)

Two clean gloves (optional)

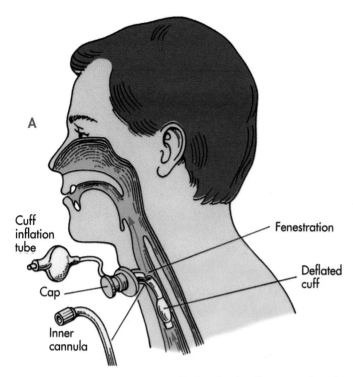

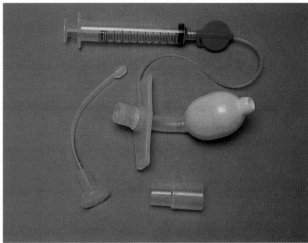

Figure 31-7   A, Trach tube (fenestrated) with inner cannula removed and cap in place to allow speech (Lewis and Collier, 1992). Tubes without opening interfere with speech. **B,** Trach tube with obturator for insertion and syringe for inflation of cuff.

ASSESSMENT

1. Observe for signs and symptoms of excess secretions.
    a. Assess oral cavity: gurgling on inspiration or expiration; obvious oral secretions, drooling, gastric secretions or vomitus in mouth, and productive cough without expectorating secretions from the oral cavity.
    b. Assess for lower airway obstruction: coughing, secretions in the airway, labored breathing, restlessness or irritability, unilateral breath sounds, cyanosis, decreased oxygen saturations or level of consciousness, or ineffective cough before deflation of ET tube or trach cuff.
2. Assess lung sounds.
3. Assess client's understanding of procedure and feeling of congestion to indicate that the oral cavity or lower airway needs suctioning.

PLANNING

Expected outcomes focus on airway patency, avoidance of infection, and client's comfort and understanding.

Expected Outcomes

1. Client's airways are cleared of secretions. No sounds of congestion can be detected, and lung sounds are improved.
2. Client indicates easier breathing and decreased congestion.
3. Client performs correct oropharyngeal suctioning technique.

DELEGATION CONSIDERATIONS

The skill of suctioning, other than oropharyngeal suctioning (Yankauer), requires problem solving and knowledge application unique to a professional nurse or other licensed health care professional. Oropharyngeal suctioning may be delegated to AP, including the client and family when appropriate.

   In special situations, the skill of performing a permanent tracheostomy tube suctioning can be delegated to AP. These situations include stable clients with permanent tracheostomy tubes after head and neck surgery and clients receiving mechanical ventilation at home.

IMPLEMENTATION

Steps	Rationale

1. See Standard Protocol (inside front cover).
2. **Preparation for all types of suctioning**
   a. Fill basin or cup with approximately 100 ml of water.
   b. Connect one end of connecting tubing to suction machine. Check that equipment is functioning properly by suctioning a small amount of water from basin.
   c. Turn on suction device. Set regulator to appropriate negative pressure: wall suction, 80 to 120 mm Hg; portable suction, 7 to 15 mm Hg for adults.

   Elevated pressure settings increase risk of trauma to mucosa.

3. **Oropharyngeal suctioning**
   a. Consider applying mask or face shield. Attach suction catheter to connecting tubing. Remove oxygen mask if present.
   b. Insert catheter into client's mouth. With suction applied, move catheter around mouth, including pharynx and gum line, until secretions are cleared.

   If catheter does not have a suction control to apply intermittent suction, take care not to allow suction tip to invaginate oral mucosal surfaces with continuous suction.

   c. Encourage client to cough, and repeat suctioning if needed. Replace oxygen mask if used.

   Coughing moves secretions from lower and upper airways into mouth.

   d. Suction water from basin through catheter until catheter is cleared of secretions.

   Clearing secretions before they dry reduces probability of transmission of microorganisms and enhances delivery of preset suction pressures.

   e. Place catheter in a clean, dry area for reuse with suction turned off or within client's reach, with suction on, if client is capable of suctioning self.
   f. Discard water if not used by client. Clean basin or dispose of cup. Remove gloves and dispose.
4. Nasotracheal suctioning
   a. Prepare suction catheter.
      (1) Open suction kit or catheter using aseptic technique. If sterile drape is available, place it across client's chest. Do not allow suction catheter to touch any nonsterile surfaces.

      Prepares catheter and prevents transmission of microorganisms.

      (2) Unwrap or open sterile basin and place on bedside table. Be careful not to touch inside of sterile basin. Fill with about 100 ml sterile NS (see illustration).

      NS is used to rinse catheter after suctioning.

   b. Apply one sterile glove to each hand, or apply nonsterile glove to nondominant hand and sterile glove to dominant hand. Attach nonsterile suction tubing to sterile catheter, keeping hand holding catheter sterile (see illustration).

      Reduces transmission of microorganisms and allows nurse to maintain sterility of suction catheter.

   c. Secure catheter to tubing aseptically. Coat distal 6 to 8 cm (2 to 3 inches) of catheter with water-soluble lubricant.

Steps	Rationale

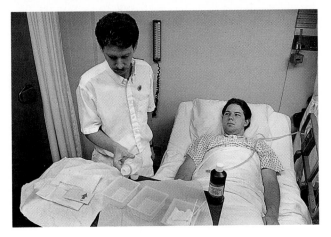

Step 4a(2)

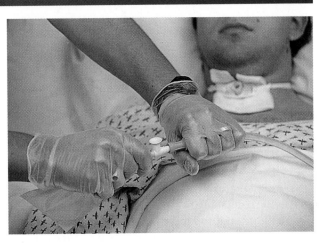

Step 4b

d. Remove oxygen delivery device, if present, with nondominant hand. Use dominant hand to insert catheter into nares during inspiration without applying suction. Do not force catheter.

e. Insert catheter approximately 16 cm (6½ inches) in adults. One method of approximating the correct length of catheter to insert is to use the distance from the client's nose to the base of the earlobe as a guide.

f. Apply intermittent suction by placing and releasing nondominant thumb over vent of catheter. Slowly withdraw catheter while rotating it back and forth with suction on for as long as 10 to 15 seconds. Replace oxygen device, if applicable.

g. Rinse catheter and connecting tubing by suctioning normal saline from the basin until tubing is clear. Dispose of catheter, gloves, and remaining saline in basin. Turn off suction device.

5. **Endotracheal or tracheostomy tube suctioning**

a. Prepare suction catheter.

(1) Aseptically open suction kit or catheter. If sterile drape is available, place it across client's chest. Do not allow suction catheter to touch any nonsterile surfaces.

(2) Unwrap or open sterile basin and place on bedside table. Be careful not to touch inside of sterile basin. Fill with about 100 ml sterile NS (see Step 4a(2)).

b. Apply one sterile glove to each hand, or apply nonsterile glove to nondominant hand and sterile glove to dominant hand. Attach nonsterile suction tubing to sterile catheter, keeping hand holding catheter sterile (see Step 4b).

NURSE ALERT

Keep oxygen delivery device readily available in case the client exhibits symptoms of hypoxemia.

Prepares catheter and prevents transmission of microorganisms.

NS is used to rinse catheter after suctioning.

Reduces transmission of microorganisms and allows nurse to maintain sterility of suction catheter.

Steps	Rationale
c. Check that equipment is functioning properly by suctioning small amounts of saline from basin.	Lubricates catheter and tubing.
d. Hyperinflate and/or hyperoxygenate client before suctioning, using manual resuscitation bag or sigh mechanism on mechanical ventilator.	Hyperinflation decreases atelectasis caused by negative pressure. Preoxygenation converts large proportion of resident lung gas to 100% oxygen to offset amount used in metabolic consumption while ventilator or oxygenation is interrupted, as well as to offset volume lost out of suction catheter.
e. Open swivel adapter, or if necessary, remove oxygen or humidity delivery device with nondominant hand.	Exposes artificial airway.
f. Without applying suction and using dominant thumb and forefinger, gently but quickly insert catheter into artificial airway (best to time catheter insertion with inspiration) until resistance is met or client coughs, then pull back 1 cm (see illustration).	Application of suction pressure while introducing catheter into trachea increases risk of damage to tracheal mucosa. Stimulates cough and removes catheter from mucosal wall.

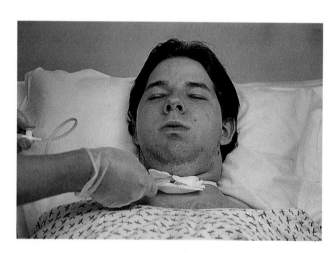

Step 5f

Steps	Rationale
g. Apply intermittent suction by placing and releasing nondominant thumb over vent of catheter, and slowly withdraw catheter while rotating it back and forth between dominant thumb and forefinger. The maximum time catheter may remain in airway is 10 seconds. Encourage client to cough.	Intermittent suction and rotation of catheter prevent injury to tracheal mucosal lining. If catheter "grabs" mucosa, remove thumb to release suction. Increased hypoxia related to removal of oxygen in airways and blockage of airways will occur during suctioning procedure.
h. Close swivel adapter or replace oxygen delivery device. Encourage client to deep breathe. Some clients respond well to several manual breaths from the mechanical ventilator or resuscitation bag.	Reoxygenates and reexpands alveoli. Suctioning can cause hypoxemia and atelectasis.
i. Rinse catheter and connecting tube with NS until clear. Use continuous suction.	Removes catheter secretions. Secretions left in tubing decrease suction and provide environment for growth of microorganisms.

Steps	Rationale

j. Assess client's cardiopulmonary status for secretion clearance and complications. Repeat Steps d through i once or twice more to clear secretions. Allow adequate time (at least 1 full minute) between suction passes for ventilation and reoxygenation.

Suctioning can induce dysrhythmias, hypoxia, and bronchospasms. Repeated passes with suction catheter clear airway of excessive secretions and promote improved oxygenation.

k. Perform nasopharyngeal and oropharyngeal suctioning to clear upper airway of secretions. After these suctionings are performed, catheter is contaminated; do not reinsert into ET or trach tube.

Removes upper airway secretions. Upper airway is considered "clean," whereas lower airway is considered "sterile." Therefore same catheter can be used to suction from sterile to clean areas, but not from clean to sterile areas.

l. Disconnect catheter from connecting tube. Roll catheter around fingers of dominant hand. Pull glove off inside out so that catheter remains in glove. Pull off other glove in same way. Discard into appropriate receptacle. Turn off suction device.

Reduces transmission of microorganisms. Clean equipment should not be touched with contaminated gloves.

m. Place unopened suction kit on suction machine or at head of bed.

Provides immediate access to suction catheter.

6. **Endotracheal or tracheostomy tube suctioning with a closed-system (in-line) catheter**

a. Attach suction.

(1) In many institutions, catheter is attached to mechanical ventilator circuit by personnel from respiratory therapy (see illustration, *A*). If not already in place, open suction catheter package using aseptic technique, attach closed-suction catheter (see illustration, *B*) to ventilator circuit by removing swivel adapter and placing closed-suction catheter apparatus on ET or tracheostomy tube, and connect **Y** on mechanical ventilator circuit to closed-suction catheter with flex tubing.

Catheter becomes part of the circuit and is often changed by respiratory therapist with each circuit change or every 24 hours.

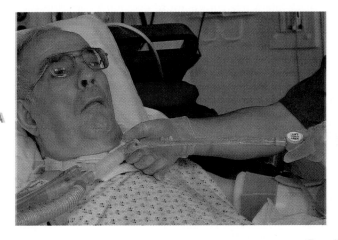

A

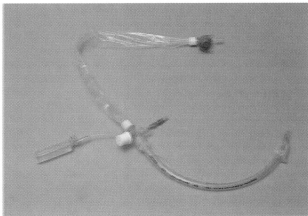

B

Step 6a(1)

Steps	Rationale
(2) Connect one end of connecting tube to suction machine and connect other to end of closed-system or in-line suction catheter if not already done. Turn suction device on and set vacuum regulator to appropriate negative pressure (80 to 120 mm Hg for adults).	Prepares suction apparatus. Excessive negative pressure damages tracheal mucosa and can induce greater hypoxia.
b. Hyperinflate and/or hyperoxygenate client using resuscitation bag or manual breathing mechanism on mechanical ventilator according to institution protocol and clinical status (usually 100% oxygen).	Decreases atelectasis caused by negative pressure and increases oxygen available to tissues during suctioning.
c. Unlock suction control mechanism if required by manufacturer. Open saline port and attach saline syringe or vial.	
d. Pick up suction catheter enclosed in plastic sleeve with dominant hand. From 2 to 3 ml NS may be instilled to attached port to stimulate cough if secretions are thick and tenacious.	Saline travels down suction catheter and into airway. Timing NS with inhalation allows it to be delivered into lung rather than blown into ventilatory circuit.
e. Wait until client inhales NS or mechanical ventilator delivers a breath to dispense NS, then quickly but gently insert catheter on next inhalation. To insert catheter, use a repeating maneuver of pushing catheter and sliding (or pulling) plastic back between thumb and forefinger until resistance is felt or client coughs. (NOTE: Some catheters contain depth markings that are useful in positioning catheter.)	Catheter sterility and secretion containment are provided by plastic sheath. Mechanical ventilator breaths, oxygen, and positive end-expiratory pressure (PEEP) are not interrupted during suctioning. Catheter slides within plastic sheath. Coughing occurs or resistance is felt when catheter touches carina.
f. Encourage client to cough and apply suction by squeezing on mechanism while withdrawing. Be sure to withdraw catheter completely into plastic sheath so it does not obstruct airflow.	Removes secretions from airway. Catheter left in ET or trach tube limits airflow.
g. Reassess cardiopulmonary status, including pulse oximetry, to determine need for subsequent suctioning or complications. Repeat Steps c through f 1 or 2 more times to clear secretions. Allow adequate time (at least 1 full minute) between suction passes for ventilation and reoxygenation.	Repeated passes clear airway of secretions to promote ventilation and oxygenation. Suctioning can cause complications such as dysrhythmias, hypoxia, and bronchospasm.
h. When airway is clear, withdraw catheter completely into sheath. Be sure black line on catheter is visible in sheath. Squeeze vial or push syringe while applying suction to rinse inner lumen of catheter. Use at least 5 to 10 ml of NS. Lock suction mechanism, if applicable, and turn off suction.	Black line is reference point to determine correct position of catheter when not in use. Inability to see black line suggests catheter is in airway and may be impeding airflow. Interior of catheter must be rinsed to prevent bacterial growth. Failure to lock mechanism can result in inadvertent continuous suction and serious complications.
i. Client may require suctioning of oral cavity.	Catheter is continuously connected to ET or trach tube. Separate suction catheter is necessary for oral cavity.

7. See Completion Protocol (inside front cover).

EVALUATION

1. Compare client's respiratory assessments before and after suctioning.
2. Ask client if breathing is easier and if congestion is decreased.
3. Observe client's technique and compliance with suctioning procedures.

Unexpected Outcomes and Related Interventions

1. Client becomes cyanotic or restless or develops tachycardia, bradycardia, or other dysrhythmia.
   a. Discontinue attempt at suctioning until stabilized, unless client's condition is deteriorating because of secretions in airway.
   b. Monitor vital signs and pulse oximetry.
   c. Preoxygenate for repeated attempts.
2. Bloody secretions are returned, which may indicate trauma.
   a. Evaluate technique and frequency of suctioning.
   b. If bleeding continues, notify physician of potential hemorrhage and monitor vital signs.
3. Client has paroxysms of coughing.
   a. Reassure client.
   b. Instruct client about relaxation techniques. Medicate as needed.
4. No secretions are obtained.
   a. Reassess respiratory system for presence of secretions.
   b. Stimulate client's cough.
   c. Check that suction system is functioning.
5. Thick secretions are present and difficult to suction.
   a. Stimulate client's cough.
   b. Notify physician if signs and symptoms of infection are present.
   c. Provide increased fluids if not contraindicated. Inadequately hydrated clients may have thick secretions.

Recording and Reporting

- Record respiratory assessments before and after suctioning; size of catheter used; route; amount, consistency, and color of secretions obtained; frequency of suctioning; and the client's tolerance.

Sample Documentation

1200 Occasional productive cough. Client requires hourly suctioning per ET tube of moderate amount (5 ml or less) of thick yellow sputum. Able to use Yankauer catheter to suction mouth with good technique. Lungs clear after cough and suctioning. O$_2$ 92% to 94%. Respirations nonlabored.

Geriatric Considerations

- Older adults with ischemic cardiac or obstructive pulmonary disease may benefit from maintenance of oxygen supply during suctioning.

Home Care and Long-Term Care Considerations

- In the home, it is necessary to adhere to best practices for infection control while weighing the necessity of cost-effectiveness in a chronic situation. For example, clean suctioning techniques may be acceptable and the secretion collection container may be cleaned and disinfected every 24 hours.
- Assess the knowledge level of the client and caregivers to determine the amount of instruction and frequency of visits required for safe, effective practices.
- For portable suction machines, as the secretion jar fills, efficiency of the suction decreases.

Skill 31.4

AIRWAY MANAGEMENT: ENDOTRACHEAL TUBE AND TRACHEOSTOMY CARE

The presence of an artificial airway places the client at high risk for infection. Correct care of the artificial airway will help to prevent infection from occurring. Artificial airways also make the client susceptible to airway injury. When artificial airways are used, it is essential that they be maintained in the correct position, or damage may occur.

Endotracheal tubes are used as short-term artificial airways to administer mechanical ventilation, relieve upper airway obstruction, protect against aspiration, or clear secretions (see Figure 31-6, p. 740). ET tubes are generally removed within 14 days. If the client requires continued assistance from an artificial airway, a tracheostomy is considered for long-term use. A surgical incision is made into the trachea, and a short artificial airway (a trach) is inserted (see Figure 31-7, *A,* p. 741).

Equipment

Endotracheal tube care
Towel
ET and oropharyngeal suction equipment
1 to 1½-inch adhesive or waterproof tape (not paper tape) or commercial ET holder (follow manufacturer's instructions for securing)
Two pairs of nonsterile gloves
Adhesive remover swab or acetone on a cottonball
Mouth care supplies (e.g., toothbrush, toothpaste, mouth swabs)
Face cleanser (e.g., wet washcloth, towel, soap, shaving supplies)
Clean 2 × 2 gauze
Tincture of benzoin or liquid adhesive
Face shield (if indicated)
Tracheostomy care
Bedside table
Towel
Tracheostomy suction supplies
Sterile tracheostomy care kit, if available, *or*
   Three sterile 4 × 4 gauze pads
   Sterile cotton-tipped applicators
   Sterile trach dressing
   Sterile basin
   Small sterile brush (or disposable cannula)
   Tracheostomy ties (e.g., twill tape, manufactured trach ties, Velcro trach ties)
Hydrogen peroxide
Normal saline (NS)
Scissors
Two sterile gloves
Face shield, if indicated

ASSESSMENT

1. Assess client for ineffective cough, secretions, decreased oxygen saturations, restlessness or irritability, and decreased or adventitious breath sounds.

2. Identify factors that increase risk of complications from ET tubes: type and size of tube, movement of tube up and down trachea, duration of placement.
3. Assess client's knowledge and comfort with procedure.
4. If applicable, assess client's understanding of and ability to perform own tracheostomy care.

PLANNING

Expected outcomes focus on the prevention of infection and breakdown around the artificial airway.

Expected Outcomes

1. Client's artificial airway/tube is in correct position and properly secured.
2. Client remains afebrile without signs and symptoms of infection.
3. Client's oral mucous membrane/stoma remains free of breakdown or accumulation of secretions.
4. Client's artificial airway is intact without persistent dried secretions.
5. Client understands purpose and is cooperative with care.
6. Client is able to demonstrate correct technique of tracheostomy care when appropriate.

DELEGATION CONSIDERATIONS

The skill of ET tube care requires problem solving and knowledge application unique to a professional nurse. The skill of trach care can be delegated to AP when a permanent or long-term trach is in place. In critically ill clients receiving mechanical ventilation this skill should not be delegated. Teach care provider emergency procedures in case the trach tube inadvertently becomes dislodged when ties are changed.

IMPLEMENTATION

Steps	Rationale

1. See Standard Protocol (inside front cover).
2. **Endotracheal tube care**
   a. Initiate endotracheal suction.

Removes secretions. Diminishes client's need to cough during procedure.

   b. Leave Yankauer suction catheter connected to suction source.

Prepares for oropharyngeal suctioning.

   c. Prepare tape. Cut piece of tape long enough to go completely around client's head from naris to naris plus 15 cm (6 inches): adult, about 30 to 60 cm (1 to 2 feet). Lay adhesive side up on bedside table. Cut and lay 8 to 16 cm (3 to 6 inches) of tape, adhesive side down, in center of long strip to prevent tape from sticking to hair.

Adhesive tape must be placed around head from cheek to cheek below ears.

   d. Have an assistant apply a pair of gloves and hold ET tube firmly so that tube does not move.

Reduces transmission of microorganisms. Maintains proper tube position and prevents accidental extubation.

   e. Carefully remove tape from ET tube and client's face. If tape is difficult to remove, moisten with water or adhesive tape remover. Discard tape in appropriate receptacle if nearby. If not, place soiled tape on bedside table or on distant end of towel.

Provides nurse with access to skin under tape for assessment and hygiene. Reduces transmission of microorganisms.

   f. Use adhesive remover swab to remove excess adhesive left on face after tape removal.

Promotes hygiene. Unremoved adhesive can cause damage to skin and prevent poor adhesion of new tape.

   g. Remove oral airway or bite block if present.

Provides access and complete observation of client's oral cavity.

   h. Clean mouth, gums, and teeth opposite ET tube with mouthwash solution and 4 × 4 gauze, sponge-tipped applicators, or saline swabs. Brush teeth as indicated. If necessary, administer oropharyngeal suctioning with Yankauer catheter.

   i. Oral ET tube only: Note "cm" ET tube marking at lips or gums. With help of assistant, move ET tube to opposite side or center of mouth. Do not change tube depth.

Prevents pressure sore formation at sides of client's mouth. Ensures correct position of tube.

   j. Repeat oral cleaning as in Step h on opposite side of mouth.

Removes secretions from mouth and oropharynx.

   k. Clean face and neck with soapy washcloth; rinse and dry. Shave male client as necessary.

Moisture and beard growth prevent adhesive tape adherence.

   l. Pour small amount of tincture of benzoin on clean 2 × 2 gauze and dot on upper lip (oral ET tube) or across nose (nasal ET tube) and cheeks to ear. Allow to dry completely.

Protects and makes skin more receptive to tape.

Steps	Rationale

m. Slip tape under client's head and neck, adhesive side down. Take care not to twist tape or catch hair. Do not allow tape to stick to itself. It helps to stick tape gently to tongue blade, which serves as a guide. Then slide tongue blade under client's neck. Center tape so that double-faced tape extends around back of neck from ear to ear.

Positions tape to secure ET tube in proper position.

n. On one side of face, secure tape from ear to naris (nasal ET tube) or edge of mouth (oral ET tube). Tear remaining tape in half lengthwise, forming two pieces that are ½ to ¾ inch wide. Secure bottom half of tape across upper lip (oral ET tube) or across top of nose (nasal ET tube) (see illustration, *A*). Wrap top half of tape around tube (see illustration, *B*).

Secures tape to face. Using top tape to wrap prevents downward drag on ET tube.

o. Gently pull other side of tape firmly to pick up slack and secure to remaining side of face (see illustration). Assistant can release hold when tube is secure. Nurse may want assistant to help reinsert oral airway.

Secures tape to face and tube. ET tube should be at same depth at the lips. Check earlier assessment for verification of tube depth in centimeters.

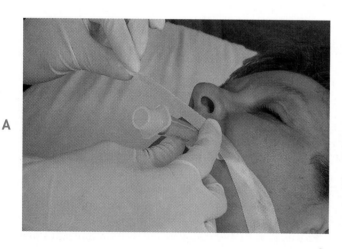

A

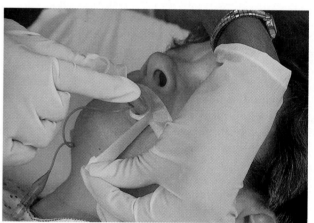

B

Step 2n

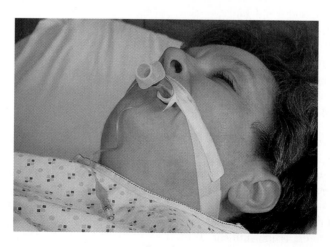

Step 2o

Steps	**Rationale**

p. Clean oral airway in warm soapy water and rinse well. Hydrogen peroxide can aid in removal of crusted secretions. Shake excess water from oral airway.

Promotes hygiene. Reduces transmission of microorganisms.

q. Reinsert oral airway without pushing tongue into oropharynx.

Prevents client from biting ET tube and allows access for oropharyngeal suctioning.

3. **Tracheostomy care**

a. Suction trach (see Skill 31.3). Before removing gloves, remove soiled trach dressing and discard in glove with coiled catheter.

Removes secretions so as not to occlude outer cannula while inner cannula is removed. Reduces need for client to cough.

b. While client is replenishing oxygen stores, prepare equipment on bedside table. Open sterile trach kit. Open three 4 × 4 gauze packages using aseptic technique and pour NS on one package and hydrogen peroxide on another. Leave third package dry.

Allows for smooth, organized completion of trach care.

c. Open two packages of cotton-tipped swabs and pour NS on one package and hydrogen peroxide on the other.

d. Open sterile trach package. Unwrap sterile basin and pour about 2 cm (¾ inch) hydrogen peroxide into it (see illustration). Open small sterile brush package and place aseptically into sterile basin.

e. If using large roll of twill tape, cut appropriate length of tape (see Step 2c) and lay aside in dry area. Do not recap hydrogen peroxide and NS.

COMMUNICATION TIP

Explain the importance of routine trach care to prevent infections or crusting and blockage. Explain that the procedure is not painful but that movement of the trach may promote coughing.

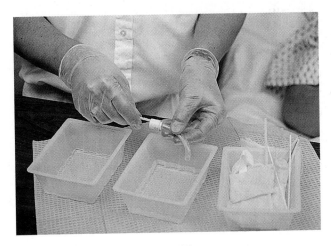

Step 3g(3)

f. Apply gloves. Keep dominant hand sterile throughout procedure. Remove oxygen source.

Reduces transmission of microorganisms.

g. If a nondisposable inner cannula is used:
   (1) Remove with nondominant hand. Drop inner cannula into hydrogen peroxide basin.
   (2) Place trach collar or T tube and ventilator oxygen source over or near outer cannula. (NOTE: T tube and ventilator oxygen devices cannot be attached to all outer cannulas when inner cannula is removed.)
   (3) To prevent oxygen desaturation in affected clients, quickly pick up inner cannula and use small brush to remove secretions inside and outside cannula (see illustration).

Removes inner cannula for cleaning. Hydrogen peroxide loosens secretions from inner cannula.

Maintains supply of oxygen to client.

Trach brush provides mechanical force to remove thick or dried secretions.

Steps	Rationale
(4) Hold inner cannula over basin and rinse with NS, using nondominant hand to pour.	Removes secretions and hydrogen peroxide from inner cannula.
(5) Replace inner cannula and secure "locking" mechanism (see illustration). Reapply ventilator or oxygen sources.	

h. If a disposable inner cannula is used:
   (1) Remove cannula from manufacturer's packaging.
   (2) Withdraw inner cannula and replace with new cannula. Lock into position.
   (3) Dispose of contaminated cannula in appropriate receptacle.

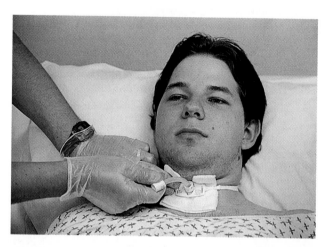

Step 3g(5)

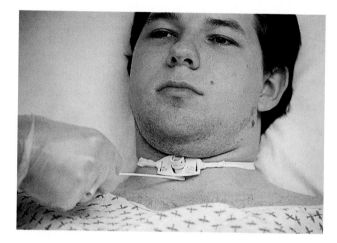

Step 3i

i. Using hydrogen peroxide–prepared cotton-tipped swabs and 4 × 4 gauze, clean exposed outer cannula surfaces and stoma under faceplate, extending 5 to 10 cm (2 to 4 inches) in all directions from stoma (see illustration). Clean in circular motion from stoma site outward, using dominant hand to handle sterile supplies.	Aseptically removes secretions from stoma site.
j. Using NS-prepared cotton-tipped swabs and 4 × 4 gauze, rinse hydrogen peroxide from trach tube and skin surfaces.	Rinses hydrogen peroxide from surfaces, preventing possible irritation.
k. Using dry 4 × 4 gauze, pat lightly at skin and exposed outer cannula surfaces.	Dry surfaces prohibit formation of moist environment from growth of microorganisms and skin excoriation.
l. Instruct assistant, if available, to hold trach tube securely in place while ties are cut.	Promotes hygiene, reduces transmission of microorganisms, and secures trach tube.

NURSE ALERT

Assistant must not release hold on trach tube until new ties are firmly tied to reduce risk of accidental extubation. If no assistant is present, do not cut old ties until new ties are in place and securely tied. (Follow manufacturer's guidelines for Velcro ties.)

Steps	Rationale
(1) Cut length of twill tape long enough to go around client's neck 2 times, about 60 to 75 cm (24 to 30 inches) for an adult. Cut ends on a diagonal.	Cutting ends of tie on a diagonal aids in inserting tie through eyelet.

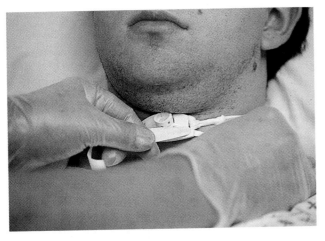

Step 3l(2)

(2) Insert one end of tie through faceplate eyelet and pull ends even (see illustration).	
(3) Slide both ends of tie behind head and around neck to other eyelet, and insert one tie through second eyelet.	
(4) Pull snugly.	
(5) Tie ends securely in double square knot, allowing space for only one finger in tie.	One-finger slack prevents ties from being too tight when trach dressing is in place.
m. Insert fresh trach dressing under clean ties and faceplate (see illustration).	Absorbs drainage. Dressing prevents pressure on clavicle heads.
n. Position client comfortably and assess respiratory status.	Promotes comfort. Some clients may require post–trach care suctioning.
4. See Completion Protocol (inside front cover).	

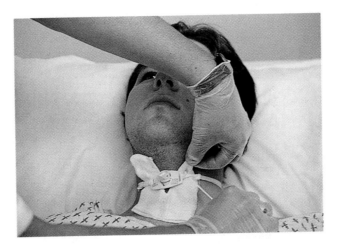

Step 3m

EVALUATION

1. Observe that airway is in proper position with tape/ties secure and comfortable for client. ET tube should be at the same depth as before care (as per physician order), with the same centimeter marking at lips and equal bilateral breath sounds.
2. Measure client's temperature; observe stoma for signs of infection.
3. Observe client's oral mucosa.
4. Compare assessments before and after artificial airway care. Observe for signs of tissue breakdown or persistent dried secretions.
5. Observe client's actions to determine compliance with the procedure.
6. Have client indicate when trach care is required and independently demonstrate the technique for trach tube care.

Unexpected Outcomes and Related Interventions

1. Tube is not secure, and artificial airway moves in or out or is coughed out by client.
2. Breath sounds are unequal with ET tube.
   a. Evaluate ET tube for proper depth. If incorrect, arrange for ET tube to be repositioned as allowed by institution.
   b. Obtain order for chest x-ray study to verify placement if applicable.
   c. Evaluate for mucus plugs.
3. Breakdown or pressure areas are observed.
   a. Increase frequency of tube care.
   b. Make sure skin areas are clean and dry.
4. Hard, reddened areas with or without excessive or foul-smelling secretions are observed.
   a. Indicates infection. Notify physician.
   b. Increase frequency of tube care.
5. Respiratory distress is caused by mucus plug. Remove inner cannula, if applicable, for cleaning and suctioning.

Recording and Reporting

- Record respiratory assessments before and after care.
- Record ET tube care: depth of ET tube, frequency and extent of care, client tolerance, and any complications related to presence of the tube.
- Record trach care: type and size of trach tube, frequency and extent of care, client tolerance, and any complications related to presence of the tube.

Sample Documentation

0800　Routine ET tube care done. Size 7.5-cm tube remains with 22-cm marking at lips. No irritation or skin breakdown noted. Mouth care given. Respirations even and easy at a rate of 16/min. Clear breath sounds bilaterally.

◆ Geriatric Considerations

- Older adult skin may be more fragile and prone to breakdown from secretions or pressure or to tearing when tape is removed.

◆◆ Home Care and Long-Term Care Considerations

- Trach care may be performed in the home and is discussed more fully in Chapter 40.

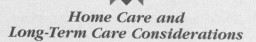

Skill 31.5

MANAGING CLOSED CHEST DRAINAGE SYSTEMS (INCLUDING MANAGING POSTOPERATIVE AUTOTRANSFUSIONS)

Trauma, disease, or surgery can interrupt the closed negative-pressure system of the lungs, causing lung collapse. Air (pneumothorax) or fluid (hemothorax) may leak into the pleural cavity. A chest tube is inserted and a closed chest drainage system is attached to promote drainage of air and fluid (Figure 31-8). Suction may be added to assist gravity in draining the lung. Lung reexpan-

sion and improved oxygenation occurs as the fluid or air is removed.

The location of the chest tube indicates the type of drainage expected. Because air rises, apical and anterior chest tube placement (Figure 31-9, *A*) promotes removal of air. Chest tubes are placed low and posterior or lateral (Figure 31-9, *B*) to drain fluid. A mediastinal chest tube is

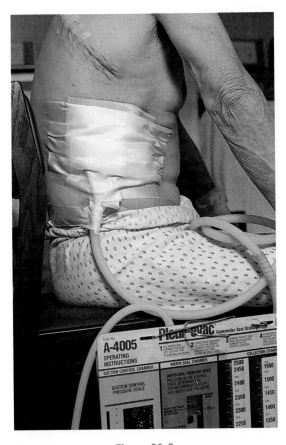

Figure 31-8

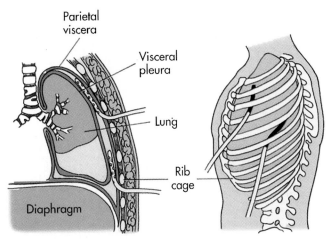

Figure 31-9

placed just below the sternum (Figure 31-10) and drains blood or fluid, preventing its accumulation around the heart (e.g., after open heart surgery).

Although single-bottle systems are available, single-unit water-seal or waterless systems are most often used. The water-seal system is composed of two or three compartments or chambers (Figure 31-11, p. 756). Fluid is drained into the first chamber. The second chamber contains the water seal, which allows air to escape because of the force of expiration but not to reenter on inspiration. If suction is to be used, a third chamber is used. The amount of suction depends on the amount of sterile water in the suction chamber.

The waterless system (Figure 31-12, p. 756) follows the same principles, except sterile water is not required for setup. The water seal is replaced by a one-way valve located near the top of the system. Most of the single unit is the drainage chamber. The suction chamber contains a suction control float ball that is set by a suction control dial after the suction source is turned on.

Autotransfusion can be linked with chest drainage after open heart surgery or thoracic surgery to replace mediastinal blood lost and allow lung reexpansion (Figure 31-13, p. 757). Autotransfusion enables the client to avoid

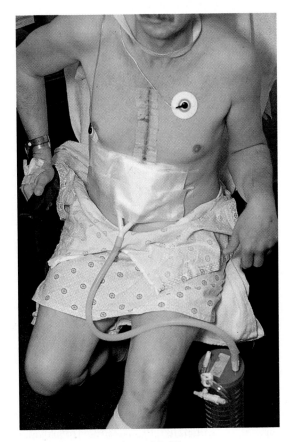

Figure 31-10

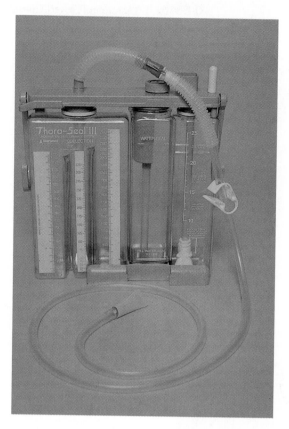

Figure 31-11

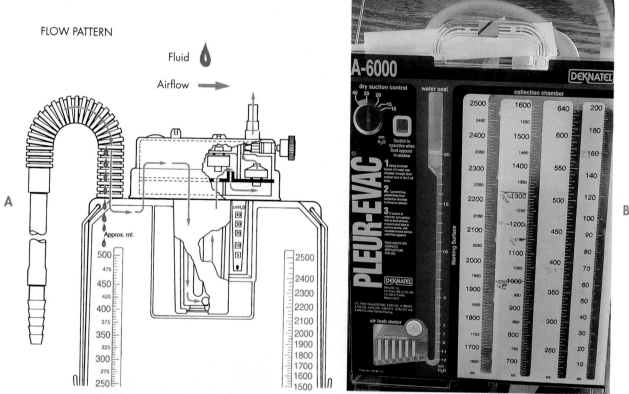

Figure 31-12 A, Suction-regulating device. **B,** Collection chamber is marked at specified intervals to monitor amount of drainage.

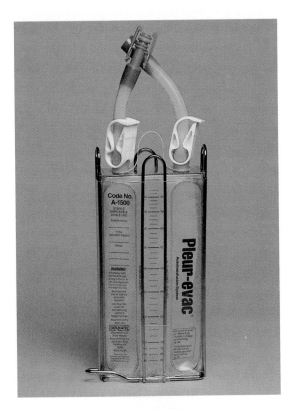

Figure 31-13

other donor blood transfusion. The client's own blood is drained from the chest and reinfused.

Equipment
Prescribed drainage system
Water-seal system
Sterile water or NS to fill 2.5 cm (1 inch) of water-seal U tube
Suction control chamber, if used
Waterless system
30-ml vial of injectable sodium chloride (NaCl) or water
20-ml syringe
21-gauge needle

Two shodded hemostats for each chest tube
1-inch adhesive tape for taping connections

ASSESSMENT
1. Perform a complete respiratory assessment (Chapter 14).
2. Obtain vital signs.
3. Assess client's breathing pattern.
4. Ask if client is able to breathe deeply and comfortably. **Rationale: Detects early signs and symptoms of complications. Promotes reexpansion of the lung.**

PLANNING
Expected outcomes should focus on removal of air and fluid from the pleural space and reexpansion of the lung with maximum client comfort.

Expected Outcomes
1. Client's respirations are nonlabored.
2. Client's breath sounds are present in all lobes, and lung expansion is symmetrical.
3. Client's vital signs, hemoglobin, and hematocrit are within normal ranges by discharge.
4. Client uses breathing exercises and remains comfortable.
5. Chest tube remains in place, and chest drainage system remains airtight and functioning properly.
6. Client's oxygen saturation is within client's normal range.

DELEGATION CONSIDERATIONS

The skill of chest tube management requires problem solving and knowledge application unique to a professional nurse. Delegation is inappropriate.

IMPLEMENTATION

Steps	Rationale
1. See Standard Protocol (inside front cover).	
2. **Set up water-seal system**	
a. Obtain a chest drainage system. Remove wrappers and prepare to set up as a two- or three-chamber system.	Maintains sterility of system for use under sterile operating room conditions.
b. While maintaining sterility of the drainage tubing, stand system upright and add sterile water or NS to appropriate compartments.	Reduces possibility of contamination.

Steps	Rationale

c. For a two-chamber system (without suction), add sterile solution to water-seal chamber (second chamber), bringing fluid to the required level as indicated.

Maintains water seal.

d. For a three-chamber system (without suction), add sterile solution to the water-seal chamber (second chamber). Add amount of sterile solution prescribed by physician to the suction control (third) chamber, usually 20 cm (8 inches). Connect tubing from suction control chamber to suction source.

Depth of rod below fluid level dictates highest amount of negative pressure that can be present within system. For example, 20 cm of water is approximately −20 cm of water pressure. Any additional negative pressure applied to system is vented into atmosphere through suction control vent. This safety device prevents damage to pleural tissues from an unexpected surge of negative pressure from suction source.

3. Set up waterless system

a. Remove sterile wrappers and prepare to set up.

Maintains sterility of system for use under sterile operating room conditions.

b. For a two-chamber system (without suction), nothing is added or needs to be done to system.

Waterless two-chamber system is ready for connecting to client's chest tube after opening wrappers.

c. For a three-chamber waterless system with suction, connect tubing from suction control chamber to suction source.

Suction source provides additional negative pressure to system.

d. Instill 15 ml sterile water or NS into diagnostic indicator injection port located on top of system.

This is not necessary for mediastinal drainage because there will be no tidaling. Also, in an emergency, this is not necessary because system does not require water for setup.

4. Tape all connections in a spiral fashion using 1-inch adhesive tape. Then check both systems for patency by:

Prevents atmospheric air from leaking into system and client's intrapleural space. Provides chance to ensure airtight system before connecting it to client. Allows correction or replacement of system if it is defective before connecting it to the client.

a. Clamping the drainage tubing that will connect client to system.

b. Connecting tubing from the float ball chamber to suction source.

c. Turning on suction to prescribed level.

> **NURSE ALERT**
>
> *Bubbling will be seen at first because there is air in tubing and system initially. This should stop after a few minutes unless other sources of air are entering system. If bubbling continues, check connections and locate source of air leak as described in Table 31-3.*

5. Turn off suction source and unclamp drainage tubing before connecting client to system.

Having client connected to suction when it is initiated could damage pleural tissues from sudden increase in negative pressure. Suction source is turned on again after client is connected to three-chamber system.

6. Position the client

During tube insertion, position client so the side in which the tube will be placed is accessible to physician. After tube placement client is positioned:

a. Using semi-Fowler's to high Fowler's position to evacuate air (pneumothorax).

Permits optimum drainage of fluid and/or air.
Air rises to highest point in the chest.

b. Using high Fowler's position to drain fluid (hemothorax).

Permits optimum drainage of fluid.

Steps	Rationale

7. Assist physician with chest tube insertion by providing needed equipment, analgesic, and offering support and instruction to the client.

8. ▨ Help physician attach drainage tube to chest tube.

Connects drainage system and suction (if ordered) to chest tube.

9. Tape tube connection between chest and drainage tubes. One method: one long strip of tape on each side with an overlapping tape wrapped spirally enables connections to be observed and remain secure.

Secures chest tube to drainage system and reduces risk of air leaks causing breaks in airtight system.

10. Check patency of air vents in system.
a. Water-seal vent must have no occlusion.
b. Suction control chamber vent must have no occlusion when using suction.
c. Waterless systems have relief valves without caps.

Permits displaced air to pass into atmosphere.
Provides safety factor of releasing excess negative pressure into atmosphere.

11. Coil excess tubing on mattress next to client. Secure with a rubber band and safety pin or system's clamp.

Prevents excess tubing from hanging over edge of mattress in a dependent loop. Drainage could collect in loop and occlude drainage system.

12. Adjust tubing to hang in a straight line from top of mattress to drainage chamber.

Promotes drainage.

13. Provide two shodded hemostats for each chest tube. Shodded hemostats are usually attached to top of client's bed with adhesive tape or clamped to client's clothing during ambulation.

Chest tubes are double-clamped under specific circumstances: (1) to assess for an air leak (see Table 31-3, p. 761), and (2) to empty or change collection bottle or chamber or disposable systems.
Have new system ready to be connected before clamping tube so that transfer can be rapid and drainage system reestablished.

14. Care for client with chest tubes
a. Assess vital signs, oxygen saturation, skin color, breath sounds, and rate, depth and ease of respirations.

Provides baseline and information about procedure related complications.

b. Monitor color, consistency and amount of drainage every 15 minutes for the first 2 hours indicating level of drainage fluid, date and time on chamber's write on surface (see illustration).
(1) From mediastinal tube less than 100 ml/hr is expected and a total of approximately 500 ml in first 24 hrs.
(2) From a posterior chest tube between 100 and 300 ml is expected during first 2 hours after insertion which decreases and a total of 500 to 1000 ml can be expected in first 24 hrs.
(3) From an anterior chest tube which primarily removes air, much less drainage is expected.

Provides baseline for continuous assessment of type and quantity of drainage. Ensures early detection of complications.

Sudden gush of drainage may result from coughing or changing client's position releasing blood rather than indicating active bleeding (Carroll, 1995).

COMMUNICATION TIP

Discuss client's continued participation in care, as appropriate. Medicate as needed.

c. Observe chest dressing for drainage.

Increase in drainage may indicate blockage in chest tube.

d. Palpate around the tube for swelling and crepitus as evidenced by crackling.

Indicates presence of air trapping in subcutaneous tissues. Large areas that travels to neck or face can result in respiratory distress (O'Hanlon-Nichols, 1996).

Steps	Rationale
e. Check tubing to ensure it is free of kinks and dependent loops. Excess tubing should be coiled on bed or chair.	Promotes drainage.
f. Observe for fluctuation of drainage in the tubing during inspiration and expiration. Observe for clots or debris in tubing.	If fluctuation, or tidaling stops it means either the lung is fully expnded or the system is obstructed.
g. Keep drainage system upright and below level of the client's chest.	Promotes gravity drainage and presents backflow of fluid and air into the pleural space.
h. Check for air leaks by monitoring the bubbling in the water seal chamber: Intermittent bubbling is normal during expiration when air is being evacuated from the pleural cavity, but continuous bubbling during both inspiration and expiration indicates a leak in the system.	Absence of bubbling may indicate that the lung has expanded sealing the opening.
15. Obtain specimen	
a. Cleanse resealing diaphragm or tubing with an antiseptic.	Reduces transmission of microorganisms.
b. Insert needle with bevel in the fresh drainage.	
c. Gently aspirate appropriate amount of fluid and place into properly labeled container.	
d. Recleanse diaphragm with antiseptic swab.	
16. Assist in chest tube removal	
a. Administer prescribed medication for pain relief about 30 minutes before procedure.	Reduces discomfort and relaxes client.
b. Assist client to sit on edge of bed or to lie on side without chest tubes.	Physician prescribes client's position to facilitate tube removal.
c. Physician prepares an occlusive dressing of petroleum gauze on a pressure dressing and sets it aside on a sterile field.	Essential to prepare in advance for quick application to wound during tube withdrawal.
d. Physician asks client to take a deep breath and hold it or exhale completely and hold it.	Prevents air from being sucked into chest as tube is removed.

COMMUNICATION TIP

Support client physically and emotionally while physician removes dressing and clips sutures.

Table 31-3

Problem Solving with Chest Tubes

Assessment	Intervention
Air leak can occur at insertion site, connection between tube and drainage, or within drainage device itself. Continuous bubbling is noted in water-seal chamber and water seal. Leaks are corrected when constant bubbling stops.	Locate leak by clamping tube at different intervals along the tube.
Assess for location of leak by clamping chest tube with 2 rubber shod or toothless clamps close to the chest wall. If bubbling stops, air leak is inside client's thorax or at chest insertions site.	NURSE ALERT: Unclamp tube, reinforce chest dressing, and notify physician immediately. **Rationale: Leaving chest tube clamped can cause collapse of lung, mediastinal shift, and eventual collapse of other lung from build up of air pressure within the pleural cavity.**
If bubbling continues with the clamps near the chest wall, gradually move one clamp at a time down drainage tubing away from client and toward suction control chamber. When bubbling stops, leak is in section of tubing or connection between the clamps.	Replace tubing or secure connection and release clamps.
If bubbling still continues, this indicates the leak is in the drainage system.	Change the drainage system.
Assess for tension pneumothorax: • Severe respiratory distress • Low oxygen saturation • Chest pain • Absence of breath sounds on affected side • Tracheal shift to unaffected side • Hypotension and signs of shock • Tachycardia	Make sure chest tubes are patent: remove clamps, eliminate kinks, or eliminate occlusion. **Rationale: Obstructed chest tubes trap air in intrapleural space when air leak originates within the thorax. Notify Physician immediately and prepare for another chest tube insertion.** A flutter (Heimlich) valve or large-gauge needle may be used for short term emergency release of pressure in the intrapleural space. Have emergency equipment, oxygen, and code card available since condition is life-threatening.
Water seal tube is no longer submerged in sterile fluid due to evaporation.	Add sterile water to water-seal chamber until distal tip is 2 cm under surface level.

Steps	Rationale

e. Physician quickly pulls out chest tube.

f. Physician quickly applies prepared dressing over wound and firmly secures it in position with elastic bandage (Elastoplast) or wide tape. Physician sometimes uses skin clips or draws purse string sutures together before applying dressing.

Prevents entry of air through chest wound.

Keeps wound aseptic. Prevents entry of air into chest. Wound closure occurs spontaneously. Clips or sutures aid in skin closure.

17. Perform postoperative autotransfusion

a. Set up the Pleur-evac autotransfusion system (ATS) using technique that maintains the sterility of unit and following three steps printed on front of unit (Deknatel, Inc.) (see Figure 31-13).

Contamination of unit provides a ready source of infection to client.

b. Make sure all connections are tight and all clamps are open.

Tight connections ensure an airtight system, and open clamps allow chest drainage to enter the ATS bag.

c. A 200-μ double-sided mesh filter is located in the ATS bag to filter drainage.

Filtering drainage removes extraneous materials and microemboli.

d. ATS collection bag has a capacity of 1000 ml, marked in increments of 25 ml, and an area for marking times and amounts.

e. Continue collection.

(1) Open Pleur-evac A-1500 replacement bag using proper technique and close two white clamps.

Contamination of unit provides a ready source of contamination to client. Closed clamps maintain a closed system during replacement.

(2) Use high-negativity relief valve to reduce excessive negativity.

Eases removal of initial collection bag from metal support stand.

(3) Perform bag transfer.

(a) Close clamp on chest drainage tubing.

Prevents air from entering chest cavity through tube and collapsing lung.

(b) Close two white clamps on top of initial ATS collection bag.

Maintains a closed system for reinfusion, preventing contamination of blood.

(c) Connect chest drainage tube to new ATS bag using red containers.
Make certain that all connections are tight.

(d) Open all clamps on chest drainage tube and replacement bag.

Reestablishes an autotransfusion collection system.

f. Connect red and blue connectors on top of initial collection bag, and remove it by lifting it from side hook and then from foot hook.

Maintains a closed system within bag and removes it for use in autotransfusion.

g. Secure replacement bag by connecting foot hook, replacing metal frame into side hook of Pleur-evac unit, and pushing down to secure frame into hook.

h. Replacement bag is removed by placing the thumbs on top of metal frame and pushing up with fingers to slide bag out.

i. Initiate Pleur-evac autotransfusion reinfusion.

(1) Use a new microaggregate filter to reinfuse each autotransfusion bag.

Prevents infusion of microemboli and provides maximum filtration for each bag.

(2) Access bag by inverting it, spiking it through spike port with microaggregate filter, and twisting.

Connects autotransfusion bag to transfusion tubing.

(3) With bag upside down, gently squeeze it to remove the air and prime the filter with blood.

Gentle pressure is used to prevent hemolysis.

Steps	**Rationale**

(4) Hang bag on an intravenous (IV) pole and continue to prime tubing until all air is gone. Clamp tubing, attach it to client's IV access, and adjust clamp to deliver the reinfusion at the appropriate rate.

Removes all air from transfusion tubing and establishes the reinfusion. Gravity, a blood cuff (not to exceed 150 mm Hg pressure), or a blood-compatible IV pump may be used.

(5) If ordered, anticoagulants (i.e., heparin) can be added to the reinfusion through self-sealing port in autotransfusion connector.

Prevents clotting in the autotransfusion.

NURSE ALERT

Stripping or milking the chest tube is controversial and should be performed according to hospital policy. Stripping creates a high degree of negative pressure and potentially may pull lung tissue or pleura into drainage holes of chest tube.

j. Discontinue autotransfusion.
   (1) Clamp chest drainage tube and connect it directly to Pleur-evac unit using red and blue connectors.

Prevents air from entering chest cavity through tube and collapsing lung.

   (2) Open chest drainage tube clamp.

All drainage will be collected directly in Pleur-evac unit and must be appropriately discarded.

18. See Completion Protocol (inside front cover).

• • • •

EVALUATION

1. Assess client for decreased respiratory distress and chest pain.
2. Auscultate client's lungs and observe chest expansion.
3. Monitor vital signs, hematocrit, and hemoglobin.
4. Evaluate client's ability to use deep-breathing exercises while maintaining comfort.
5. Monitor continued functioning of system, as indicated by reduction in the amount of drainage, resolution of the air leak, and complete reexpansion of the lung.
6. Monitor client's oxygen saturation.

Unexpected Outcomes and Related Interventions

1. Air leak is unrelated to client's respiration.
   See Table 31-3, on p. 761 for determining the source of an air leak and problem solving.
2. Chest tubes become obstructed by a clot or kinked tube.
   a. Observe client for mediastinal shift or respiratory distress, which may constitute a medical emergency.
   b. Determine source of obstruction, as noted by lack of flow through tube or clot detected in system. If kinked, straighten tubing and adjust to prevent continued problems.
   c. If clot is identified, notify physician. (Duncan, Erickson, and Weigel, 1987.)

3. Chest tube becomes dislodged.
   a. Immediately apply pressure over chest tube site with anything that is within immediate reach (e.g., several layers of client's hospital gown, bed sheet, or towel).
   b. Have assistant obtain a sterile petroleum dressing. Apply as client exhales. Secure dressing with a tight seal.
   c. Notify physician.
4. Substantial increase in bright-red drainage is observed.
   a. Observe for tachycardia and hypotension.
   b. Report to physician, because this may indicate that client is actively bleeding.
5. Drainage system is knocked on side or damaged.
   a. Observe for signs of increasing pneumothorax, which would indicate that water seal is not being maintained. Notify physician.
   b. Obtain a second unit and change system after following setup guidelines.

Recording and Reporting

• Record respiratory assessment; amount of suction, if used; amount of drainage since the previous assessment; type of drainage in chest tubing; presence or absence of an air leak, including amount if present; status of dressing; and client tolerance.

Sample Documentation

0800   Client resting comfortably, denies complaint. Respirations even and easy. Lungs clear with breath sounds heard over all lung fields. Posterior chest tube and dressing remain intact with oscillation present in water-seal chamber. No air leak noted. 50 ml serous drainage collected in past 8 hours. Continues to take deep breaths without complaints of discomfort as instructed.

CRITICAL THINKING EXERCISES

1. In report you are informed by the previous nurse that a client you are to care for is complaining of being unable to breathe. The client was admitted for an exacerbation of her asthma. The nurse states that the client is "just faking it." What would you include in your assessment to determine if this evaluation is correct?

2. CPAP was started on a client you are seeing in his home. On arrival for a follow-up visit you find that the client has been noncompliant with the CPAP. He states that he is unable to tolerate the CPAP.
   a. What parameters do you assess?
   b. What suggestions/interventions can you suggest to increase compliance?

3. While you are caring for a client with a trach tube, the client develops respiratory distress during the suction procedure. What should you do?

4. You have just received a client with a chest tube from the recovery room. The client is not completely alert, but he is exhibiting signs and symptoms of poor pain control. Knowing the effect of analgesics on respiration, what should you do?

REFERENCES

Carroll PF: *Nurs 86* 16(12):26, 1986.

Chulay M: Arterial blood gas changes with a hyperinflation and hyperoxygenation suctioning intervention in critically ill patients, *Heart Lung* 17(6): 654–661, 1988.

Dettenmeier PA: *Pulmonary nursing care,* St Louis, 1992, Mosby.

Duncan C, Erickson R, Weigel RM: Effect of chest tube management on drainage after cardiac surgery, *Heart Lung* 16(1):1, 1987.

Kryger M, Roth T, Dement W: *Principles and practice of sleep medicine,* Philadelphia, 1994, Saunders.

Lewis SM, Collier IC: *Medical-surgical nursing: assessment and management of clinical problems,* ed 3, St Louis, 1992, Mosby.

NIH Publication: *Guidelines for the diagnosis and management of asthma, expert panel report 2,* 1997, National Institutes of Health.

O'Hanlon-Nichols T: Commonly asked questions about chest tubes, *AJN* 96(5):1, May 1996.

Perry AG, Potter PA: *Clinical nursing skills and techniques,* ed 4, St Louis, 1998, Mosby.

Shapiro BA et al: *Clinical application of respiratory care,* ed 4, St Louis, 1991, Mosby.

Weilitz PB: *A pocket guide to respiratory care,* St Louis, 1991, Mosby.

CHAPTER 32

Gastric Intubation

Skill 32.1
Inserting Nasogastric Tube, (Includes Checking Placement of Nasal Tube), 766

Skill 32.2
Irrigating Nasogastric Tube, 770

Skill 32.3
Removing Nasogastric Tube, 773

NURSING DIAGNOSES

Nursing diagnoses for clients who may undergo nasogastric intubation include **Risk for Aspiration,** in which clients are at risk of aspiration related to nausea and vomiting or delayed gastric emptying, and this risk is a primary reason for placement of the tube. The presence of an NG tube can lead to the diagnosis of **Altered Oral Mucous Membranes** because NG tubes typically cause irritation, drying, and crusting of secretions. Removal of gastric secretions can produce **Fluid Volume Deficit** associated with altered electrolyte imbalance (see Chapter 37).

Intubation of the stomach with a flexible tube passed through the client's nares, nasopharynx, and esophagus and into the stomach (Figure 32-1) is sometimes performed after surgical procedures, when vomiting and gastric distention occur, and for irrigation of the stomach. Decompression of the stomach with removal of fluids and gas promotes abdominal comfort, decreases the risk of aspiration, and allows surgical anastomoses to heal without distention. When used for decompression, the tube is usually attached to low intermittent suction to facilitate the removal of secretions. For clients who are unable to swallow, the nasogastric (NG) tube is frequently used for the administration of medications. The tube can also be used to irrigate the stomach and to remove toxic substances, such as in poisoning.

NG tubes are typically of a larger diameter (12 to 18 Fr) than feeding tubes to enhance the removal of thick secretions or to instill fluids rapidly. Their stiffer composition and larger diameter make these tubes more uncomfortable for the client, and these tubes cause more irritation of the sensitive nasopharyngeal mucosa. NG tubes are constructed of a single lumen (Levin tube) or a central lumen and a separate air vent lumen (Salem sump tube). Important nursing measures for the client with an NG tube include measures to maintain patency of the tube, such as irrigation, and measures to promote comfort, such as positioning the tube to prevent pressure on the nares, cleansing around the nares, and lubrication of the oral and nasal membranes.

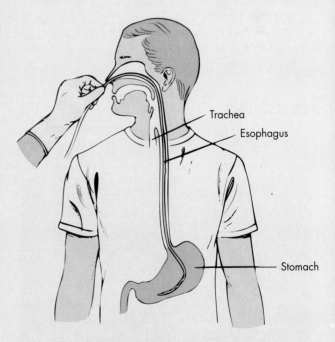

Figure 32-1 Placement of NG tube.

Skill 32.1

INSERTING NASOGASTRIC TUBE (INCLUDES CHECKING PLACEMENT OF NASAL TUBE)

This skill includes insertion of a large-bore flexible tube into the client's nares, nasopharynx, esophagus, and stomach. Placement of an NG tube requires a physician's order. The tube can be accidentally displaced into the pulmonary system, lie in the distal esophagus or gastric antrum rather than well into the stomach, or kink on itself in the stomach. In addition to displacement, other complications of NG tubes include impaired skin integrity of nares and nasal mucosa, sinusitis, earache, esophagitis, gastric or esophageal ulceration and bleeding, and pulmonary aspiration.

Care must be taken to reduce the discomfort related to an NG tube and to ensure that it remains correctly positioned and patent.

Equipment (Figure 32-2)
Nasogastric tube
Water-soluble lubricant
60-ml catheter tip syringe
Emesis basin
Towel
Clean gloves
Stethoscope
Cup of water and straw
Tongue blade
Tissues
Safety pin and rubber band
pH test strip
Indelible marker
Hypoallergenic tape and tincture of benzoin (or tube fixation device)
Suction source

ASSESSMENT
1. Assess client's nares and oral cavity for deviated nasal septum, nasal surgery, inability to breathe well when either nasal opening is occluded, and nasal or oral irritation or bleeding. **Rationale: This information determines which naris the tube should be inserted through and the need for special measures for oral hygiene or comfort after the tube is inserted.**
2. Assess client's ability and willingness to cooperate or assist with the procedure and the need for special positioning during insertion.
3. Palpate client's abdomen for distention or pain and auscultate for bowel sounds. **Rationale: No abdominal pain/distention do not confirm need for tube. Provides baseline data regarding abdominal or intestinal functioning prior to intubation.**
4. Assess client's need for specialized nutrition support. **Rationale: Clients who take nothing by mouth for more than 7 days may require specialized nutritional support.**
5. Check medical record for surgeon's order, type of NG tube to be placed, and whether tube is to attach to suction or drainage bag.

PLANNING
Expected outcomes focus on decompression of the stomach, comfort, adequacy of fluid volume, adequacy of nutrition, and prevention of complications related to nasogastric intubation.

Expected Outcomes
1. Client has no abdominal distention or pain.
2. Client's NG tube remains patent.
3. Client verbalizes enhanced comfort after nursing measures to promote oral and nasal hygiene and after lubrication of mucous membranes.
4. Client maintains good skin turgor, adequate urine output, and normal electrolyte balance.
5. Client's nasal membranes remain clear of abrasions, excoriation, or erosion, and membranes remain moist.

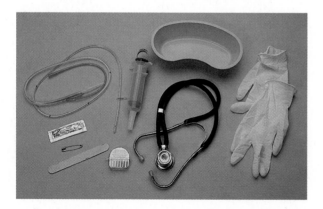

Figure 32-2   Nasogastric tube insertion equipment.

DELEGATION CONSIDERATIONS

This skill requires problem solving and knowledge application unique to a professional nurse. Assistive personnel (AP) may measure and record the drainage from the NG tube and provide oral and nasal hygiene. For this reason, this skill is usually not delegated.

IMPLEMENTATION

Steps	Rationale

1. See Standard Protocol (inside front cover).
2. 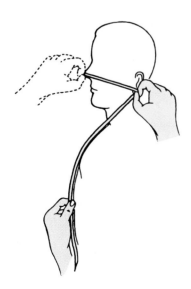 Stand on client's right side if right-handed, left side if left-handed.

NURSE ALERT

Client should be sitting upright in bed if possible. Have suction equipment and emesis basin within reach in case of vomiting.

3. Measure estimated length of tube to reach well into stomach: measure distance from tip of nose to earlobe to xiphoid process of sternum (see illustration).

    Approximates distance from nares to stomach.

4. Mark this distance on tube with a removable piece of tape or an indelible marker.
5. Cut a piece of tape about 4 inches (10 cm) long, and split one half of it into two pieces to form a Y.
6. Curve 10 to 15 cm (4 to 6 inches) of end of tube tightly around index finger and then release.

    Curving tube tip aids insertion and decreases tube stiffness.

7. Lubricate about 4 inches (10 cm) of the distal end of the tube with a water-soluble lubricant.
8. Tell client that insertion is about to begin, and ask client to extend neck back against pillow (see illustration).

    Promotes comfort and reduces friction during insertion.

9. Insert tube slowly through naris with curved end pointing downward. Continue to insert tube along floor of nasal passage aiming down toward ear. If resistance is met, apply gentle downward pressure to advance tube. (Do not force past resistance.)

    Promotes comfort and reduces friction during insertion.

10. With continued resistance, withdraw tube, allow client to rest, lubricate it again, and attempt insertion in opposite nostril.

NURSE ALERT

Do not force tube past point of resistance, because force may cause trauma to nasal mucosa.

Step 3

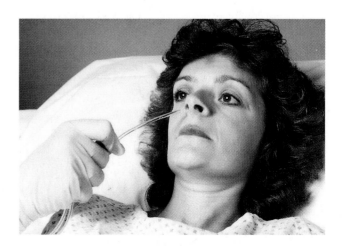

Step 8

Steps	Rationale
11. Insert tube to nasopharynx, rotate it toward the opposite nostril, then pass just above oropharynx.	Helps prevent coiling of tube in oropharynx.
12. Stop and allow client to relax. Provide tissues as needed to remove tears or excess lubrication around nares.	Mucosal irritation and discomfort can produce tearing.
13. Ask client to bend head forward and swallow small sips of water if allowed or to swallow without water as tube is advanced.	
14. Advance tube 1 to 2 inches (2.5 to 5 cm) with each swallow. If coughing or gagging occurs, withdraw tube a bit and allow client to relax and breathe easily.	Tube may be displaced into larynx and produce coughing.
15. Ask client if tube feels as though it is coiling in back of throat, and check back of oropharynx using tongue blade to compress client's tongue. If tube has coiled, withdraw it until the tip is back in the oropharynx. Then reinsert with client swallowing.	
16. Continue to advance tube with swallowing until tape or mark is reached.	Tip of tube must be well within stomach for adequate decompression.
17. Temporarily anchor tube to cheek with a piece of tape until placement is checked.	
18. Ask client to speak.	Inability to speak can indicate that tube is through vocal cords into the lungs.
19. Check the placement.	
a. Inspect posterior pharynx for presence of coiled tube.	Tube is pliable and can coil up in back of pharynx instead of advancing into esophagus.
b. Attach catheter-tipped syringe to end of tube, then aspirate gently back on syringe to obtain gastric contents, observing color. Measure pH of aspirate with color-coded pH paper with range of whole numbers at least 0 to 10 (see illustration).	Gastric secretions are usually highly acidic. A pH reading between 0 to 6 is a reasonable value to indicate gastric versus respiratory, or intestinal, placement. Gastric fluid is usually grass green, tan, bloody, or brown. A higher pH means it is in the small intestine or respiratory tract (Metheny et al, 1998).
20. If pH of aspirate is not 4 or less, advance tube by about 2 inches (5 cm) and repeat Steps 17 and 18.	

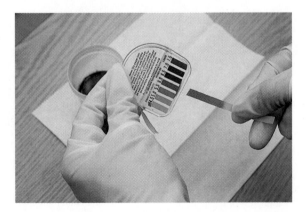

Step 19b

NURSE ALERT

Traditionally, nurses checked tube placement by injecting air into the tube and listening for a "whooshing" sound with a stethoscope. Sounds may be transmitted from the pleural space and are not reliable in testing placement (Metheny, 1998).

Steps	Rationale

21. When gastric aspirates are obtained, anchor tube to nose and avoid pressure on nares. Remove and discard gloves and wash hands.
    a. Apply tincture of benzoin sparingly to nose and allow it to become "tacky."
    b. Apply tube fixation device using shaped adhesive patch (see illustration)
    c. Alternative: Apply tape to client's nose. Wrap two ends of tape around tube (see illustration).
22. Fasten rubber band to end of NG tube in a slip knot, and pin rubber band to client's gown, allowing enough slack for movement of head.

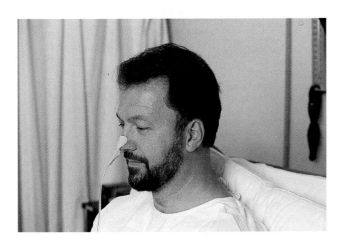

Step 21b

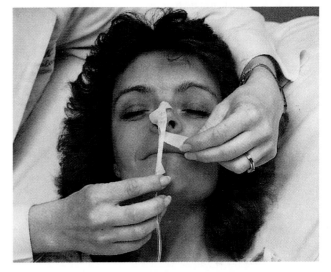

Step 21c

23. Keep head of bed elevated at least 30 degrees unless physician orders otherwise.
24. Attach NG tube to drainage bag or suction source.
25. Provide regular oral hygiene (see Chapter 7) every 2 to 3 hours.
26. See Completion Protocol (inside front cover).

Presence of NG tube renders the pyloric sphincter incompetent and increases the risk of gastroesophageal reflux.

• • •

EVALUATION

1. Palpate client's abdomen for distention and pain. Auscultate for bowel sounds.
2. Observe color of gastric secretions and patency of NG tube.
3. Ask client if oral and nasal hygiene measures have increased comfort.
4. Assess client's skin turgor. Measure urine output and specific gravity, and monitor client's laboratory studies.
5. Observe integrity or condition of nasal and oral mucosa.

Unexpected Outcomes and Related Interventions

1. Client develops abdominal distention, vomiting, or absence of drainage from tube.
    Assess patency of tube and irrigate tube as needed.
2. Client complains of sore throat from dry irritated mucous membranes.
    a. Perform oral hygiene more frequently.
    b. Ask physician whether client can suck on ice chips or throat lozenges or chew gum.
3. Client develops signs of fluid volume deficit (see Chapter 37).
    Report decreased urine output, poor skin turgor, or excessive loss of secretions to physician.

4. Client develops signs and symptoms of pulmonary aspiration: fever, shortness of breath, pulmonary congestion.
   a. Contact physician to report symptoms.

Recording and Reporting
- Record length, size, and type of gastric tube inserted and through which nostril it was inserted.
- Record the client's response to tube insertion, any symptoms that could indicate malposition, and the client's status after the tube was inserted.
- Record the pH readings that were obtained to indicate correct placement and the color of secretions withdrawn from the tube.

Sample Documentation
1000   Inserted 16 Fr Salem sump tube into left nares and advanced it to 50-cm mark. Client assisted with insertion by swallowing and states he is comfortable following procedure. 50 ml of light-green gastric secretions were aspirated from tube with a measured pH of 3. Tube secured with tape and attached to low intermittent suction.

1200   Client given moistened swabs to lubricate oral mucosa. Stated increased comfort after use of.

Geriatric Considerations

- Geriatric clients may have sensory deficits that affect their ability to assist with NG tube insertion. If the client has hearing impairment, make sure that the client's hearing aid is in place and adjusted appropriately so that the client will be able to hear instructions.
- Check for ill-fitting dentures and remove them for the client's safety and comfort during the insertion.
- Oral and nasal mucosal drying may be present. Be sure that the tube is adequately lubricated for insertion.

Home Care and Long-Term Care Considerations

- Clients are seldom sent home with NG suction. If long-term decompression of the stomach is required, such as when the bowel is obstructed, a permanent decompression tube, such as a gastrostomy tube, is surgically inserted. Clients and caregivers should be taught how to take care of the gastrostomy tube and suction device. A portable, intermittent suction device is usually used in the home.

Skill 32.2

IRRIGATING NASOGASTRIC TUBE

This skill involves irrigation of the NG tube with an isotonic saline solution to maintain patency of the tube. Irrigation should be performed when the tube's patency is in question, such as when the volume of gastric secretions has decreased or the client is experiencing symptoms such as abdominal pain or nausea, or if the client's abdomen is distended. The NG tube should also be irrigated before and after its use for the administration of medications.

Equipment (Figure 32-3)
   60-ml catheter tip syringe
   Normal saline solution for irrigation
   Towel
   Disposable gloves

ASSESSMENT
1. Assess the volume, color, and character of gastric secretions. **Rationale: Thick secretions and a reduced volume of secretions may indicate the need to irrigate the NG tube.**
2. Assess client's abdomen for distention or pain.
3. Assess bowel sounds and passage of flatus.

PLANNING
Expected outcomes focus on maintenance of tube patency to ensure adequate decompression of the stomach.

Expected Outcomes
1. Client's NG tube remains patent.
2. Client denies abdominal discomfort or nausea.

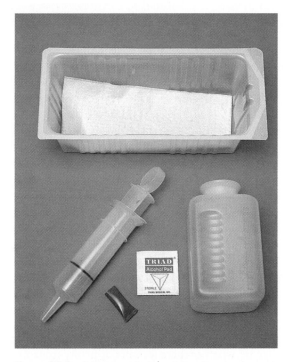

Figure 32-3   Nasogastric tube irrigation equipment.

DELEGATION CONSIDERATIONS

The skill of irrigating a nasogastric tube requires problem solving and knowledge application unique to a professional nurse.

IMPLEMENTATION

Steps	Rationale

1. See Standard Protocol (inside front cover).
2. Determine that NG tube is properly placed (see Skill 32.1, Steps 17 to 19). Inject saline solution steadily; do not force.
3. Draw up 30 ml of normal saline solution into large syringe.
4. Kink NG tube and remove from suction source. Lay end of suction tubing on towel.
5. Insert tip of irrigation syringe into end of NG tube and unkink tubing (see illustration).

Prevents soiling of client's gown and bed by drainage of gastric secretions.
Avoid use of pigtail vent on Salem Sump for irrigation.

NURSE ALERT

Client should be sitting upright in bed if possible.

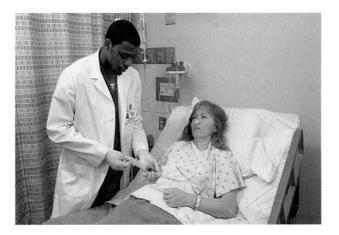

Step 5

Steps	Rationale
6. If unable to instill fluid, reposition client on left side and try again.	Tip of tube may be against stomach wall. Notify physician if unable to instill fluid.
7. When saline solution has been instilled, withdraw fluid by pulling back gently on syringe.	
8. Reconnect NG tube to suction. Remove and discard gloves and wash hands.	
9 Record difference in volume instilled and volume withdrawn. If equal, no documentation is required.	Maintains accurate intake and output records.
10. See Completion Protocol (inside front cover).	

• • •

EVALUATION

1. Measure client's abdominal girth and inspect the color, volume, and character of NG secretions.
2. Assess client for abdominal pain, nausea, or bloating.

Unexpected Outcomes and Related Interventions

1. Client's NG tube cannot be irrigated and is no longer patent.
   Contact physician. The buildup of secretions poses a risk for aspiration.
2. Client's NG tube can be irrigated, but irrigation fluid cannot be withdrawn and the tube continues to drain poorly.
   Contact physician. Position of tube may need to be confirmed.

Recording and Reporting

- Record volume and color of drainage from the NG tube before irrigation of the tube and any symptoms of discomfort that the client is having.
- Record the amount and type of irrigation solution.
- Record whether there was any difficulty irrigating the tube and the volume of secretions withdrawn after irrigation.
- Record the client's response to irrigation, including any discomfort or relief of symptoms.

Sample Documentation (See Intake and Output Summary, Chapter 9)

0800   NG tube draining scant amounts. Irrigated with 30 ml normal saline. Initially, NG tube irrigated sluggishly, but became easier to irrigate. Withdrew 20 ml light-green fluid at end of irrigation. Client stated he had been feeling mild nausea.

1000   Increased volume of light-green gastric secretions draining from NG tube. Client states he no longer feels nauseated.

Skill 32.3

REMOVING NASOGASTRIC TUBE

This skill involves removal of the NG tube when it is no longer needed for decompression of the stomach. A physician's order is required for this procedure. Generally, an NG tube is no longer required when gastric secretions empty normally into the duodenum through the pyloric sphincter and when intestinal motility returns. The client's ability to handle gastric secretions is sometimes evaluated by removing the NG tube from suction and putting it to gravity drainage, or by clamping the NG tube for a specified number of hours per day. If the client has not had a return of gastric or intestinal motility, the symptoms of abdominal distention, discomfort, or nausea will return.

Equipment

Tissues
Towel
Disposable gloves
60-ml catheter tip syringe

ASSESSMENT

1. Assess client for abdominal distention and symptoms such as nausea or abdominal pain.
2. Assess client for signs of returning bowel function, such as bowel movements, flatus, and presence of bowel sounds. **Rationale: Return of peristalsis confirms that tube can be removed.**

PLANNING

The expected outcome focuses on minimizing the discomfort caused by removal of the tube.

Expected Outcome

Client remains comfortable after removal of the tube.

DELEGATION CONSIDERATIONS

The skill of removing a nasogastric tube requires problem solving and knowledge application unique to a professional nurse.

IMPLEMENTATION

Steps	Rationale
1. See Standard Protocol (inside front cover).	
2. Place towel over client's chest to protect gown and cover tube.	
3. Turn off suction and disconnect NG tube from drainage bag or suction.	Avoids trauma to mucosa during removal.
4. Attach large syringe to tube and flush with 20 ml of air.	Clears gastric fluids from tube that could irritate esophagus and mouth during tube removal.
5. Remove tape from client's nose and unpin tube from gown.	
6. Tell client that removal of tube is about to begin and will not be as uncomfortable as insertion.	Reduces anxiety and enhances cooperation.
7. Hand the client facial tissue and ask client to take a deep breath and hold it as tube is removed.	Airway is partially occluded during removal of tube. Minimizes risk of aspirating gastric contents if spilled from tube during removal.
8. Kink tube securely and pull tube out quickly and steadily onto towel.	Kinked tube is less likely to expel gastric contents (if present) into throat or trachea.
9. Give tissues to client to clean nares or assist client as needed.	
10. Measure volume of drainage and note character of content. Record on Intake and Output Summary (see Chapter 9). Dispose of NG tube, remove and discard gloves, and wash hands.	Maintains accurate intake and output.
11. Clean nares and provide mouth care.	Promotes comfort.
12. See Completion Protocol (inside front cover).	

EVALUATION

Ask client about level of comfort after removal of the tube and after provision of mouth care.

Unexpected Outcomes and Related Interventions

Client complains of pain after removal of the NG tube.
   a. Consult with physician about the use of topical anesthetics to reduce pain from irritated nasal mucosa.
   b. Encourage client to ingest warm, soothing liquids if able. Be alert for any swallowing problems that may indicate erosion of the esophagus.

Recording and Reporting

- Record whether there was any difficulty removing the NG tube.
- Record the client's level of comfort and any symptoms after removal of the tube.
- Record any nursing interventions for client's discomfort or relief of other symptoms.

Sample Documentation

1300   Removed NG tube without difficulty. Mouth care provided after the removal. Client stated throat was sore but mouth care provided some relief.

CRITICAL THINKING EXERCISES

1. While inserting an NG tube, the client initially complains of burning and then begins to swallow as the tube reaches the back of the throat. The client requires some effort to swallow continuously. Should the nurse be concerned with this response?

2. The nurse irrigates Mrs. Alvera's NG tube with 20 ml of saline solution and senses a sudden release of pressure. When withdrawing the fluid, the nurse obtains 150 ml of light green fluid. Is this normal? What could explain these findings?

3. Ms. Olivera has an NG tube placed during surgery to prevent fluid build-up around her surgical anastomosis. On the first postoperative day, Ms. Olivera complains of stomach distention and the nurse notices that her abdomen appears distended. The drainage from her tube has decreased over the last 4 hours, and Ms. Olivera states that she accidentally pulled on the tube when trying to reach for her glasses. The tube appears to be the same length as before. What actions should the nurse consider?

REFERENCES

American Society for Parenteral and Enteral Nutrition Board of Directors: *Clinical pathways and algorithms for delivery of parenteral and enteral nutrition support in adults,* Silver Springs, Md, 1998, American Society for Parenteral and Enteral Nutrition.

Barnie DC, Currier J: What's that GI tube being used for? *RN* 58(8):45–48, 1995.

Metheny NA, Smith L, Wehrle M, Wiersma L, and Clark J: pH, color and feeding tubes, *RN* Jan, 1998, p 25-27.

Metheny N, Smith L, Aud MA Ignatavicius, DD: *Detection of improperly positioned feeding tubes, J Healthcare Risk Manage* 98:37–48, 1998.

Surratt S: Trouble shooting a sump tube, *Am J Nurs* 93(1):42–47, 1993.

Viall C: When your patient has an NG tube, what's the most important thing?–Location, location, location, *Nursing* 26(9):43–45, 1996.

CHAPTER 33

Enteral Nutrition

Skill 33-1
Intubating the Client with a Small-Bore Nasogastric or Nasointestinal Feeding Tube, 776

Skill 33-2
Administering Tube Feedings, 781

Skill 33-3
Administering Medication Through a Feeding Tube, 787

When clients have an intact and functional gastrointestinal (GI) tract but are unable to consume food or fluids orally, enteral nutrition is the preferred technique for nourishment. Enteral nutrition involves the provision of nutrients to the GI tract for digestion and absorption.

Tube feedings may be used for short-term management of nutritional problems during acute illness and recovery. The primary reason that clients receive tube feedings is to prevent or treat malnutrition related to diminished intake. Also, clients may require tube feeding because of ineffective swallowing or a weakened gag reflex causing aspiration. Some clients are "hypermetabolic" as a result of sepsis or burns and are unable to ingest enough calories to meet their bodies' needs. After the feeding tube is placed, all clients remain at risk for aspiration and need careful nursing management to avoid this complication.

For short-term nutritional support, 4 weeks or less, soft, small-diameter enteral feeding tubes are usually placed nasally into the stomach, duodenum, or jejunum (Eisenberg, 1994). Clients in acute care facilities also often have firm, large-diameter nasogastric-tubes placed for multiple purposes such as medication administration, gastric suction, or short-term feeding (Metheny et al, 1998b). Tube feedings may also be used to provide long-term nu-

tritional support for clients who cannot swallow safely or those who are unable to eat enough to sustain daily function. These groups may include clients with brain injury or an altered or reduced level of consciousness and clients with neuromuscular diseases who have a high incidence of aspiration, such as those with amyotrophic lateral sclerosis (ALS) and muscular dystrophy (MD). In these clients, tubes may be placed endoscopically or surgically through the abdominal wall gastrostomy (into the stomach) or jejunostomy (into the small intestine) (Figure 33-1).

Tube feeding formulas may consist of blended table food; commercial preparations that are of varying osmolarity and caloric, fat, protein, and lactose content; or ele-

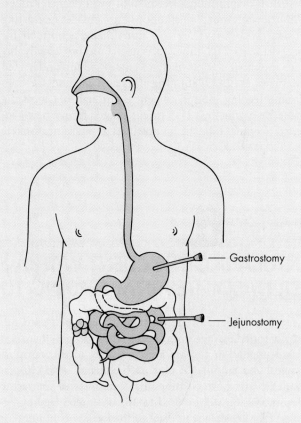

Figure 33-1 Placement for gastrostomy and jejunostomy enteral feeding tubes.

mental formulas that require no digestion to absorb. Some tube feedings are also designed for specific diseases, such as renal, respiratory, or hepatic failure. The choice of tube feeding depends on the client's clinical condition (Bockus, 1993).

Tube feedings may be administered in several ways. They can be given as a bolus amount via gravity, several times a day through a large-bore syringe; as a continuous gravity drip for ½ to 1 hour several times per day using a pouch to hang the feeding; or as a continuous drip per infusion pump, on whatever schedule best meets the client's needs: 8 or 12 or 24 hours per day.

Checking for placement of a feeding tube before administering medication or tube feeding is critical to safe client care. A feeding tube is improperly positioned when it is accidentally placed in the lung, esophagus, or even the stomach when it should be in the small bowel (Metheny et al, 1998a, b). Tubes can easily be misplaced or migrate into the esophagus and lung. Complications such as aspiration, pneumonia, pneumothorax, and peritonitis can develop if the tube becomes misplaced and feedings are subsequently administered.

The most dependable means for checking tube placement is through radiologic confirmation (Fater, 1995). Chest x-ray films are considered the standard of care, especially for confirming placement of small-diameter tubes. Unfortunately, not all institutions have policies mandating this method. X-rays are also not usually performed for large-diameter NG tubes, because clinicians usually believe the tubes are less likely to enter the lung undetected (Metheny et al, 1998b). The next best method for confirming feeding tube placement is through pH measurement. By testing the pH of fluid aspirated from a newly inserted feeding tube, it is possible to make reasonable assumptions about the tube's location (Metheny et al, 1998a). Traditionally, the auscultatory method has been used to determine NG tube placement. The use of a syringe to insufflate air through a tube and then using a stethoscope to listen for a gurgling sound over the epigastric region was long thought to indicate proper tube placement. Studies have shown that the reliability of this method is highly questionable, and it should not be used as the sole method to rule out inadvertent respiratory positioning of feeding tubes (Metheny et al, 1990b; 1998b).

Many potential complications may arise from tube feeding administration. The cost of managing the ensuing complications and infections is expensive. Complications may be related to the tube itself, such as placement of the tube in the lung, frequent tube clogging, or the tube inadvertently being pulled out. Complications may also occur when the administered tube feeding causes delayed gastric emptying, bloating, diarrhea, or aspiration pneumonia (Bowers, 1996).

NURSING DIAGNOSES

Altered Nutrition: Less Than Body Requirements related to insufficient intake is appropriate when there is evidence of weight loss and/or inability to ingest food. **Impaired Swallowing** related to neuromuscular impairment makes a client a likely candidate for feeding tube placement. **Risk for Aspiration** is another indication for use of tube feedings. Clients may experience **Diarrhea** or **Constipation** related to altered intake associated with tube feedings.

Skill 33.1

INTUBATING THE CLIENT WITH A SMALL-BORE NASOGASTRIC OR NASOINTESTINAL FEEDING TUBE

Large-bore NG tubes are contraindicated when used primarily for enteral feedings because they carry an increased risk of aspiration and are more irritating to the nasopharyngeal and esophageal mucosa (Lehmann, 1992). Occasionally, large-bore GI tubes that were inserted for gastric decompression will be used to initiate enteral feeding because they are already in place. If the feeding continues for more than a few days, the nurse should consult with the physician about placement of a small-bore enteral feeding tube (Figure 33-2). Small-bore feeding tubes are available in weighted (tungsten) or unweighted designs. Weighted tubes were thought to pass more easily into the duodenum or jejunum via peristalsis; however, research has not demonstrated an advantage of the weight in promoting intestinal passage (Lord et al, 1993). Because the tubes are flexible, a guidewire or stylet is used to provide rigidity and to facilitate positioning, and then they are removed once correct placement is verified. Small-bore tubes can be left in place for an extended period with less irritation to the nasopharyngeal, esophageal, and gastric mucosa. Placing an **NG** or **nasointestinal** (NI) **feeding tube** requires a physician's order.

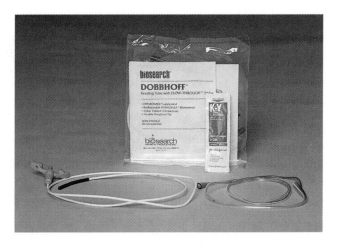

Figure 33-2 Small-bore feeding tubes.

Equipment

NG or NI tube (8 to 12 Fr) with guidewire or stylet
60-ml or larger Luer-Lok or catheter-tipped syringe
Stethoscope
Hypoallergenic tape or tube fixation device
Tincture of benzoin and cotton-tipped applicator
pH Indicator strip (scale 0.0 to 10.0)
Glass of water and straw
Emesis basin
Safety pin
Rubber band
Towel
Facial tissues
Clean gloves
Suction equipment in case of aspiration
Penlight
Tongue blade

Assessment

1. Review client's history and current health status for presence of impaired swallowing, head or neck surgery, decreased level of consciousness, surgeries involving upper alimentary tract, or facial trauma. **Rationale: Indications suggest need for tube feeding; order to be obtained after consultation with physician.**

2. Assess weight for client's height, hydration status, electrolyte balance, and organ function. **Rationale: Enteral feeding preserves function and mass of the gut, promotes wound healing, and may decrease the incidence of infection in the critically ill (Zaloga, 1994).**

3. Have client close each nostril alternately and breathe. Examine each naris for patency and skin breakdown. **Rationale: Assessment determines most patent naris for tube insertion.**

4. Assess client's history for nosebleeds, nasal surgery, deviated septum, anticoagulant therapy, and coagulopathy. **Rationale: Factors may require nurse to seek physician's order to change route of nutritional support.**

5. Assess client for gag reflex. Place tongue blade in client's mouth, touching uvula. **Rationale: Identifies client's ability to swallow and determines if risk for aspiration exists.**

6. Assess client's mental status. **Rationale: An alert client is better able to cooperate with procedure.**

7. Assess for bowel sounds (notify physician if sounds are absent). **Rationale: Absence of bowel sounds may indicate decreased or absent peristalsis and increased risk of aspiration or abdominal distention.**

PLANNING

Expected outcomes focus on safe insertion of feeding tube with placement in stomach, duodenum, or jejunum.

Expected Outcomes

1. Feeding tube will remain patent in appropriate location of stomach or intestine.
2. Client does not experience aspiration.
3. Bowel sounds will be normoactive.
4. Client has no complaints or signs of discomfort or nasal trauma.

DELEGATION CONSIDERATIONS

This skill requires problem solving and knowledge unique to a professional nurse. For this skill, delegation is inappropriate.

IMPLEMENTATION

Steps	Rationale
1. See Standard Protocol (inside front cover).	
2. Position client in sitting or high Fowler's position. If client is comatose, place in semi-Fowler's position	Reduces risk of pulmonary aspiration in event client should vomit.
3. Check feeding tube for flaws: rough or sharp edges on distal end and closed or clogged outlet holes.	Flaws in feeding tube hamper tube intubation and can injure client.
4. Determine length of tube to be inserted and mark with tape or indelible ink (see illustration).	Determines approximate depth of insertion.

COMMUNICATION TIP

Explain to client how to try to relax and communicate during tube insertion. "Now I will explain each step as we go along. The tube will cause a burning pain as it passes through your nose. I want you to raise one finger to tell me when it really hurts so that I can be gentle and at the same time get this done as quickly as possible."

NURSE ALERT

Tip of tube must reach stomach. Measure distance from tip of nose to earlobe to xyphoid process of sternum (see illustration). Add additional 20 to 30 cm (8 to 12 in) for NI tube (Welch, 1996; Lord et al, 1993; Hanson, 1979).

Steps	Rationale
5. Prepare NG or NI tube for intubation:	
a. Plastic tubes should not be iced.	Tubes will become stiff and inflexible, causing trauma to mucous membranes.
b. Wash hands.	
c. Inject 10 ml of water from 30-ml or larger Luer-Lok or catheter-tipped syringe into the tube.	Aids in guidewire or stylet insertion.
d. Make certain that guidewire is securely positioned against weighted tip and that both Luer-Lok connections are snugly fitted together.	Promotes smooth passage of tube into GI tract. Improperly positioned stylet can induce serious trauma.
6. Cut tape 10 cm (4 in) long.	
7. ▨ Inspect nares for any irritation or obstruction.	

COMMUNICATION TIP

Explain that you are now about to insert the feeding tube. Let client know how he or she can assist. "I will insert the tube through your nose toward the back of your throat. Once the tip is in the back of your throat, I will ask you to begin to swallow. The water (ice chips) are something we may use if you find it hard to swallow. I will tell you when to stop swallowing"

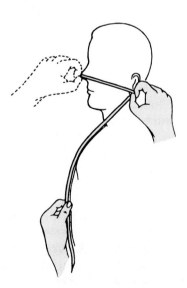

Step 4

Steps	Rationale
8. Dip tube with surface lubricant into a glass of water.	Activates lubricant to facilitate passage of tube into naris to GI tract.
9. Hand client a glass of water with straw or glass with crushed ice.	
10. Gently insert tube through nostril to back of throat (posterior nasopharynx). Aim back and down toward ear.	Natural contour facilitates passage of tube into GI tract.
11. Have client flex head toward chest after tube has passed through nasopharynx.	Closes off glottis and reduces risk of tube entering trachea.

NURSE ALERT

Encourage client now to swallow by giving small sips of water or ice chips when possible. Advance tube as client swallows. Rotate tube 180 degrees while inserting.

NURSE ALERT

Do not force tube. If resistance is met or client starts to cough, choke, or become cyanotic, stop advancing the tube and pull tube back.

12. Emphasize need to mouth breathe and swallow as tube continues to be inserted.	Swallowing facilitates passage of tube past oropharynx. Rotating tube decreases friction.
13. Advance tube each time client swallows until desired length has been passed.	Reduces discomfort and trauma to client.
14. Check for position of tube in back of throat with penlight and tongue blade.	Tube may be coiled, kinked, or entering trachea.
15. Check placement of tube (see Skill 33.2).	Proper position is essential before starting feedings.
16. When gastric aspirates are obtained, anchor tube to nose and avoid pressure on nares.	A properly secured tube allows client more mobility and prevents trauma to nasal mucosa.
a. Apply tincture of benzoin sparingly to nose and allow it to become "tacky."	
b. Apply tube fixation device using shaped adhesive patch (see illustrations). Remove and discard gloves and wash hands.	
c. *Option:* split one end of a 2-inch-long piece of hypoallergenic tape lengthwise about halfway down tape. Place intact end over bridge of client's nose. Wrap each of the strips around tube as it exists nose.	

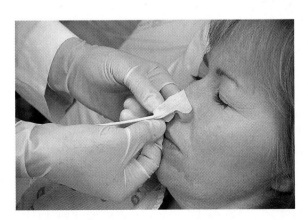

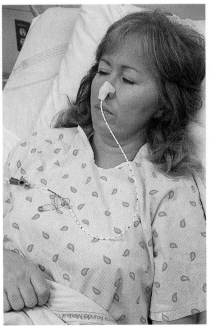

Step 16b

Steps	Rationale
17. Fasten end of NG tube to client's gown by looping rubber band around tube in slip knot. Pin rubber band to gown. Allow slack for movement of head.	Reduces traction on naris when tube is moved.
18. For intestinal placement, position client on right side when possible until radiologic confirmation of correct placement has been verified. Otherwise, assist client to a comfortable position.	Promotes passage of the tube into the small intestine (duodenum or jejunum).

NURSE ALERT

Leave guidewire or stylet in place until correct position is ensured by x-ray film. Never attempt to reinsert partially or fully removed guidewire or stylet while feeding tube is in place.

Guidewire or stylet may perforate GI tract, especially esophagus or nearby tissue, and seriously injure the client.

Steps	Rationale
19. Obtain x-ray film of abdomen.	Placement of tube is verified by x-ray examination (Metheny, 1988).
20. Apply gloves and administer oral hygiene. Cleanse tubing at nostril.	Promotes client comfort and integrity of oral mucous membranes.
21. See Completion Protocol (inside front cover).	

• • •

EVALUATION

1. Placement is verified by x-ray examination.
2. Observe client for persistent gagging or paroxysmal coughing.
3. Routinely reassess client's bowel sounds every 4 hours.
4. Reinspect condition of nasal mucosa at least every 8 hours.

Unexpected Outcomes and Related Interventions

1. Persistent gagging leads to vomiting with aspiration of GI contents.
   a. Position client on side, remove feeding tube if gagging continues and suction airway as needed (see Skill 31.1)
   b. Contact physician and consider need for immediate chest x-ray film.
2. Bowel sounds become absent or decreased.
   a. Notify physician.
   b. Consider need to temporarily discontinue or reduce size of feedings.
   c. Monitor for gastric distention.
3. Nasal mucosa becomes inflamed, tender, and/or eroded.
   a. Retape tube to relieve pressure on mucosa.
   b. Consider removal of tube and reinsert in opposite naris (physician order required).

Recording and Reporting

- Record in nurse's notes type and size of tube placed, length of tube insertion, client's tolerance of procedure, confirmation of tube position by x-ray film, and pH and appearance of aspirate.
- Report to physician any incidence of aspiration or suspected change in tube position

Sample Documentation

1000   Number 10 Fr small-bore feeding tube inserted into right naris, advanced approximately 60 cm. Client experienced usual discomfort without gagging or vomiting. Chest x-ray confirmed duodenal placement. Intestinal aspirate tested at pH 7.0, bile colored in appearance.

Geriatric Considerations

- Ensure adequate lubrication of tube to decrease discomfort for the older adult, who may have decreased oral or nasopharyngeal secretions.

Home Care and Long-Term Care Considerations

- Assess environmental safety and sanitation of client's home to determine potential for infection or injury if tube is to be inserted for ongoing nutritional support.
- See home care considerations from Skill 33.2.

Skill 33.2

ADMINISTERING TUBE FEEDINGS

This skill includes the administration of tube feeding via bolus, and continuous drip via gravity or infusion pump. It is very important to check placement of NG and NI tubes before initiating feedings. Using good handwashing technique and clean equipment and hanging formula only for the recommended time to prevent spoiling are critically important for avoiding contamination of the system and subsequent infection in the client.

Equipment (Figure 33-3)

Formula (Figure 33-4)
50- to 60-ml syringe
  Catheter tip for large-bore tubes
  Luer-lock tip for small-bore tubes
pH test strip (range 0.0 to 10.0)
Graduate container
Administration set
  Bolus: 60 ml bulb or plunger syringe *or*
  Gavage/intermittent infusion: plastic feeding bag with drip chamber and tubing *or*
  Infusion pump: pump, plastic feeding bag with appropriate drip chamber and tubing for pumps
Tap water

ASSESSMENT

1. Identify signs and symptoms of malnutrition, including baseline weight and laboratory values (albumin, protein, lymphocyte, etc.). **Rationale: Determine client's need for enteral nutrition: depressed level of consciousness, surgery, swallowing disorders, or trauma.**
2. Verify physician orders for tube feeding formula, rate, and frequency. Laboratory data and bedside assessments, such as finger-stick blood glucose measurements, are also ordered by the physician. **Rationale: Tube feedings, laboratory tests, and bedside tests must be ordered by the physician.**
3. Assess for food allergies. **Rationale: Prevents client from developing localized or systemic allergic reactions.**
4. Assess abdomen for distention or tenderness. Auscultate for active bowel sounds before each feeding. **Rationale: Absent bowel sounds indicate inability of the GI tract to digest or absorb nutrients.**

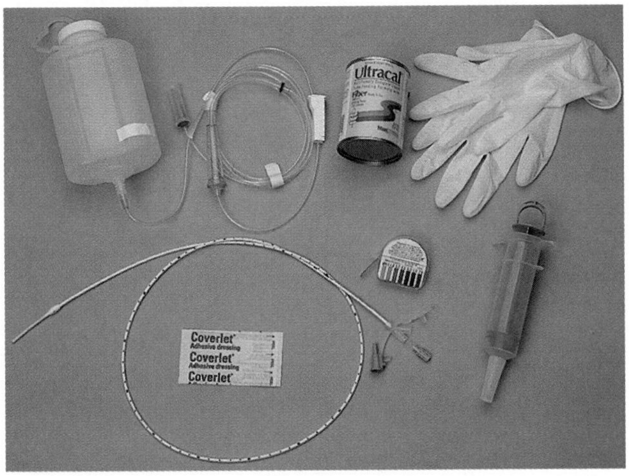

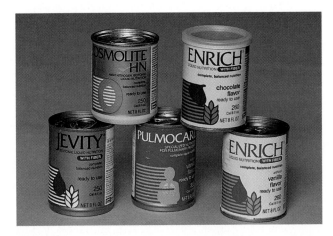

Figure 33-3 Graduate feeding container with tubing, 50-60 ml syringe with catheter tip, pH test strip, formula, gloves, feeding tube with guide wire, and fixation device.

Figure 33-4 A variety of formula preparations for tube feedings.

PLANNING

Expected outcomes focus on safe administration of tube feeding formula, client tolerance of the formula, and avoidance of complications related to tube feeding administration.

Expected Outcomes

1. Client's nutritional monitoring parameters (laboratory values, weight status, wound healing) trend toward normal by discharge.
2. Client maintains body weight or trends toward IBW.
3. Client verbalizes no complaints of abdominal discomfort.
4. Client experiences no aspiration by discharge.
5. Client has residual volume less than 150 ml before tube feeding.

DELEGATION CONSIDERATIONS

Administration of enteral tube feeding via syringe is a procedure that can be delegated to assistive personnel (AP).

- The professional nurse should verify tube placement before the feeding and establish patency of the tube by flushing it with water.
- The nurse should also ensure that the client is sitting upright in a chair or in bed and instruct the assistive personnel to infuse the feeding slowly.
- AP should be instructed to report any difficulty infusing the feeding or any discomfort voiced by the client.

IMPLEMENTATION

Steps	Rationale
1. See Standard Protocol (inside front cover).	
2. Elevate head of bed to high Fowler's, at least 30 degrees, or reverse Trendelenburg if spinal injury present.	Reduces risk of aspiration during feeding with head higher than stomach.
3. Check placement of feeding tube.	Radiographic evidence of placement is the most accurate, but cost and radiation exposure prohibit frequent checks many times per day (Metheny, 1993).
a. Aspirate gastric or intestinal contents with appropriate cone-tipped syringe inserted into end of tube (see illustration).	Gastric secretions are usually green, brown, or tan, to off-white.; intestinal fluid is medium to deep golden brown or bile stained. Pleural fluid is pale, clear yellow, and watery (Metheny et al, 1998a).
b. Place drop of GI contents on pH test paper for measurement (see illustration).	Gastric contents should have a pH range of 0–4; tracheobronchial and pleural secretions should have a pH >6 and intestinal contents usually have a pH of 7 or greater (Metheny et al, 1998a; 1998b). Visual inspection of fluid helps differentiate gastric from intestinal.

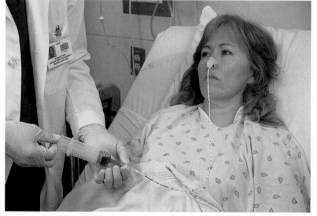

Step 3a

COMMUNICATION TIP

Let client know the purpose of your testing: "I'm checking the fluid from your stomach to make sure that the tube is in the right place. I put a drop on this paper strip and the value tells me the tube is where it belongs."

Steps	Rationale

c. Auscultate over left upper quadrant with stethoscope. Do not insufflate air.

Determines presence of peristalsis. Auscultation is no longer considered a reliable method for verification of placement of tube because air in tube inadvertently placed in lungs, pharynx, or esophagus can transmit sound similar to that of air entering stomach (Metheny et al, 1998a).

d. If tube is nasally inserted, inspect oral cavity for tube kinking or curling in back of the throat.

Indicates that tube may no longer be correctly positioned in the GI tract.

e. If unable to aspirate, consider that tube is clogged or kinked, and attempt to flush with 30 ml of warm water.

Using a small syringe (3 to 6 ml) generates a large force and may rupture small-bore feeding tubes.

4. Aspirate GI contents for residual volume; if client has a small-bore feeding tube, aspirate slowly to avoid collapse. Determine volume with graduate container if necessary.

Evaluates absorption and tolerance of last feeding, or may indicate delayed gastric emptying. Small-bore feeding tubes in the intestine may not have residual volumes.

NURSE ALERT

If residual amount is greater than last hour's infusion or 150 ml, hold feeding 1 hour and recheck residual (Bockus, 1993).

5. Readminister residual volume to client by allowing it to flow from syringe into tubing. If large volume of residual, administer slowly.

Avoids fluid and electrolyte imbalance. Slow administration minimizes nausea.

6. Prepare formula for administration.
   a. If pouring directly from a can, check expiration date and wipe off top of can (see illustration).
   b. If using premixed bags, check date and time of mixing, as well as correct strength (full, half strength, etc.).

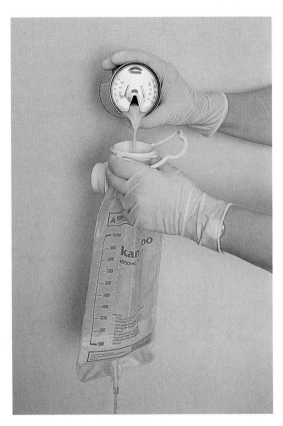

Step 6a

Steps	Rationale

7. Bolus or intermittent feedings
  a. Administer the tube feeding with 60-ml bulb or plunger syringe.
  b. Remove cap or plug from end of feeding tube and pinch closed to prevent leakage.
  c. Attach syringe by removing bulb or plunger and inserting tip into end of tube. Elevate to no more than 18 inches (45 cm) above insertion site (see illustration).

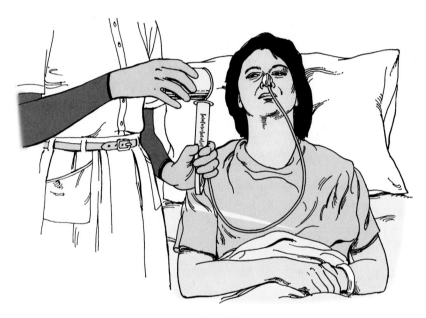

Step 7c

  d. Fill syringe with formula, release tube, and allow syringe to empty gradually, refilling until prescribed ordered amount has been administered.

  Slow delivery of tube feeding (50 to 100 ml/min) is better tolerated. Continuous draining from syringe avoids air entry and gas production.

  e. Flush tube with 30 to 60 ml tap water (or ordered amount) when feeding complete.

  Prevents tube clogging with thicker feeding.

  f. Recap/plug tube.

8. Continuous drip method
  a. Administer the tube feeding with gavage bag (see illustration).

  Easily tolerated in the stomach. Allows periods for client to be unattached to a feeding system.

  b. Prepare administration set: clamp tubing, prepare gavage bag with prescribed type and amount of formula, unclamp and prime tubing to remove air, then reclamp tubing.
  c. Label bag with tube feeding type, strength, and amount. Include date, time, and initials.
  d. Pinch end of feeding tube. Remove plug/cap.

  Prevents air from entering stomach.

  e. Securely attach gavage tubing to end of feeding tube.
  f. Set rate by adjusting roller clamp on tubing. Usually this type of tube feeding infuses for 30 to 60 minutes 3 to 6 times per day.

Steps	**Rationale**

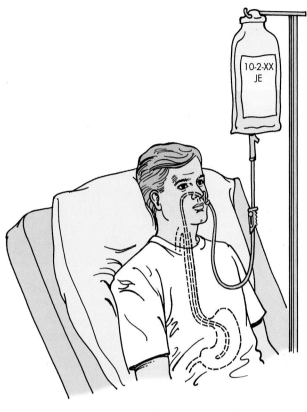

Step 8a

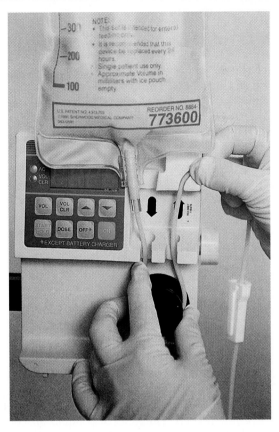

Step 9a

---

   g. Flush tube with 30 to 60 ml tap water (or ordered amount) when feeding complete.

Prevents tube clogging.

   h. Recap/plug tube.

9. **Feeding via infusion pump**

   a. Administer the tube feeding as a continuous drip via infusion pump (see illustration).

Allows a smaller volume of feeding to be delivered continuously. There is less risk of aspiration or missed feedings.

   b. Prepare administration set, with type and amount of formula to last no more than 8 hours. Clamp tubing, spike bag, and unclamp and prime tubing. Reclamp tubing.

Avoids spoilage. Prefilled vacuum packages are available from the manufacturer and are less likely to spoil.

   c. Label bag with tube feeding type, strength, and amount. Include date, time, and initials.

   d. Hang tube feeding set on intravenous (IV) pole with infusion pump. Connect tubing to pump and set rate.

   e. Pinch end of feeding tube. Remove plug/cap. Connect infusion tubing to client feeding tube.

   f. Open roller clamp on infusion tubing. Turn infusion pump on.

   g. Check residual volumes every 4 hours by aspirating with 60 ml syringe.

Ensures that tube feeding is continuing to infuse through the GI system.

Steps	Rationale
10. Fill 60 ml syringe with ordered volume of water (generally 30 to 50 ml). Inject into feeding tube to flush after bolus, or as ordered with continuous drip.	Aids in avoiding a clogged tube. Water replacement is vital to help client maintain adequate fluid and electrolyte balance.
11. Flush tube with water every 4 to 8 hours as in Step 8g, and clamp end when no feedings are infusing.	
12. Rinse syringe or bag and tubing with warm water after all bolus and gavage feedings. Remove and discard gloves and wash hands.	Rinsing removes formula left in equipment, reduces potential for bacterial growth, and allows for reuse of equipment. Most institutions require replacement with new equipment every 24 hours.
13. Ask if client is comfortable while the infusion is continuing.	Complaints of cramping may indicate tube feeding is too cold or is infusing too fast. Diarrhea should be reported to the physician. Client may need antidiarrheal agents (e.g., Kaopectate, Lomotil).
14. See Completion Protocol (inside front cover).	

• • •

EVALUATION

1. Monitor weight and laboratory values daily.
2. Assess client's level of comfort with each tube feeding or at each shift if a continuous drip is given. Nausea or vomiting may indicate need for change in rate of administration.
3. Observe and assess client for shortness of breath, low oxygen saturation, and presence of liquid the color of feeding from airway. Blue dye may be added to feeding to confirm presence of feeding in lungs. (check agency policy.)
4. Monitor the amount of residual tube feeding aspirated to evaluate for absorption vs. decreased gastric motility.

Unexpected Outcomes and Related Interventions

1. Client's feeding tube is unable to be aspirated or injected with air or water.
   a. For a newly inserted tube, notify physician and obtain x-ray confirmation of positioning (Metheny et al, 1998b).
   b. Attempt to flush with large-bore syringe and warm water. (Avoid using a small-bore syringe because this exerts large amounts of pressure and may rupture tube.)
   c. Notify physician if unable to clear feeding tube.
   d. If tube cleared, keep tube patent by flushing every 4 hours, before clamping off each time, and before and after each feeding and medication infusion.

2. Aspirated residual appears straw colored with a pH of 7.0.
   a. Hold tube feeding.
   b. Contact physician. Consider chest x-ray film to evaluate tube placement.
3. Client vomits. Heart rate and respiratory rate are elevated, and client is coughing.
   a. Hold tube feeding; assess lungs.
   b. Notify physician of probable aspiration.
4. Client receiving a continuous-infusion tube feeding appears ashen. Respirations are rapid and shallow. Breath sounds are full of rhonchi. Client coughs up secretions that are very similar to the tube feeding.
   a. Turn off tube feeding.
   b. Notify physician. Prepare for supplemental oxygen, chest x-ray film, and probable tube removal.

Recording and Reporting

- Record amount of feeding.
- Record client's response to tube feeding, patency of tube, and any side effects.
- Record and report type of feeding, status of feeding tube, client's tolerance, and adverse effects.

Sample Documentation

0900 NG feeding tube placement confirmed, aspirant pH 3.0. Bowel sounds normoactive. Abdomen soft and nondistended. Full-strength Osmolyte hung per infusion pump at 60 ml/hr. Head of bed elevated 30 degrees. Denies discomfort.

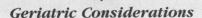

Geriatric Considerations

- Assess the client for hyperglycemia, because older adults may be more susceptible to the high glucose concentration in enteral formulas.
- Assess the client frequently for gastric residual, because older adults may have decreased transit time so that formula remains in the stomach longer.
- The use of intestinal feeding tubes may reduce the risk of aspiration of tube feeding for the older adult.

Home Care and Long-Term Care Considerations

- Teach the client or primary caregiver to check placement of tube before administering formula.
- Instruct the client or primary caregiver in the method of GI fluid pH measurement and expected range.
- Instruct the client or primary caregiver not to administer a feeding if there is any doubt concerning the placement of the tube.
- Instruct the client or primary caregiver that feedings should be administered at room temperature.

Skill 33.3

ADMINISTERING MEDICATION THROUGH A FEEDING TUBE

This skill involves the safe administration of oral medications through a feeding tube. Specific attention must be paid to proper placement of the tube and whether the medication can be crushed for administration through the tube. Liquid medication and elixirs are the best choice to administer through a feeding tube, but some medicines only come in tablet form. Most tablets may be crushed; however, those that are sublingual, enteric coated, or sustained release should not be given by tube, because their absorption, metabolism, and effectiveness will be unpredictable. Capsules (except sustained-release preparations) may be emptied of powder or aspirated of gelatin, dissolved, and given through the feeding tube (Lehmann, 1992). A pharmacist should be consulted before pills are crushed or before capsules are opened and dissolved for tube feeding administration.

Medications should not be mixed in with tube feedings because of potential interruptions in tube feeding flow (e.g., turning feeding off while client in radiology department), spillage, delayed absorption of the medication, or possible drug precipitation. It is always best to consult with a pharmacist before administering medications through a feeding tube.

Equipment

50- to 60-ml syringe
   Catheter tip for large-bore tubes
   Luer-lock tip for small-bore tubes
pH test strip
Graduate container
Medication to be administered
Pill crusher if medication in tablet form

Syringe with needle if medication in gelatin form
Warm water (to dissolve dry/gelatin medication)
Tap water
Tongue blade or straw to stir dissolved medication

ASSESSMENT

1. Assess for any contraindications to client receiving oral medication: Has the client been diagnosed as having bowel inflammation or reduced peristalsis? Has client had recent gastrointestinal surgery? Does client have gastric suction? **Rationale: Alterations in GI function interfere with drug distribution, absorption, and excretion. Clients with GI suction might not receive benefit from the medication because it may be suctioned from GI tract before it can be absorbed.**

2. Assess client's medical history, history of allergies, medication history, and diet history. **Rationale: These factors can influence how certain drugs act. Information also reflects client's need for medications.**

3. Gather and review assessment and laboratory data that may influence drug administration. **Rationale: Physical examination or laboratory data may contraindicate drug administration.**

4. Before the administration of medication, verify placement of the gastric tube (see Skill 33.1).

PLANNING

Expected outcomes focus on administration of appropriate medication via the tube feeding route and avoidance of tube clogging from medication administration.

Expected Outcomes

1. Client experiences desired medication effect within period of onset of medication.
2. Client's feeding tube remains patent after medication administration.

IMPLEMENTATION

Steps	Rationale

1. See Standard Protocol (inside front cover).
2. Elevate head of bed to high Fowler's, at least 30 degrees, or in reverse Trendelenburg if spinal injury present.

    Reduces risk of aspiration.

3. Prepare medication for instillation in feeding tube.
   a. Review five "rights" for administration of medication (see Chapter 16).

NURSE ALERT

Verify that medications to be administered do not include any sublingual, enteric-coated, or sustained-release medications.

   b. *Tablets:* Crush pill (in its package if possible) with pill crusher (see illustration). Dissolve the powder in 15 to 30 ml warm water.

    Crushing medication in its package prevents some from being lost.

   c. *Capsules:* Open and dissolve the powder in 15 to 30 ml warm water.
   d. *Gelatin capsules:* Aspirate with a syringe, or capsule may be dissolved in warm water (see illustration) over several minutes. After capsule dissolves, remove its gelatin outer layer.

    Less medication is wasted if capsule is dissolved in warm water, but this may require 15 to 20 minutes before administration.

4. Check placement of feeding tube (see Skill 33.1).

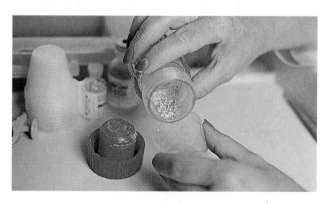

Step 3b

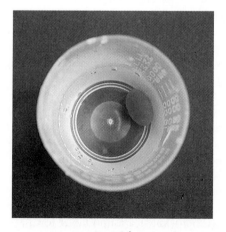

Step 3d

Steps	Rationale

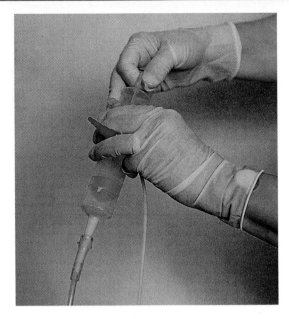

Step 5

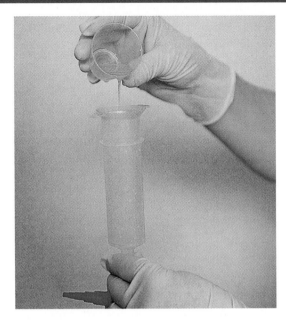

Step 6

5. Aspirate stomach contents for residual volume, determine volume with graduate container if necessary and reinstill to client (see illustration).

6. Pour dissolved medication into syringe and allow to flow by gravity into feeding tube (see illustration). Flush with 10 ml water after each medication.

7. Follow medication with 30 to 60 ml of water to flush tube of medications.

8. See Completion Protocol (inside front cover).

If residual remains greater than 100 ml, hold medication and contact physician for further orders.

If a problem develops during medication administration (e.g., spillage, coughing, tube clogging), nurse can tell which medications have been lost and which are still available for later administration.

Avoids tube clogging with medication and ensures medication enters stomach, where it can be absorbed.

• • •

EVALUATION

1. Observe for desired effects within appropriate time frame depending on medication administered.

2. Observe tube patency before and after medication administration.

Unexpected Outcomes and Related Interventions

1. Client has Theo-Dur 300 mg ordered bid per tube.
   a. Note that Theo-Dur is a sustained-release medication intended to break down and be absorbed slowly over 8 to 12 hours.
   b. Contact physician for orders to have client receive theophylline elixir every 4 to 6 hours for better tolerance.

2. Client is unable to receive medication because of blockage in tube.
   a. Attempt to flush tube with warm water to clear clog.
   b. If unable to flush clog, contact physician for replacement of tube and potential need to reroute medication if dose cannot be skipped or delayed until a new feeding tube is placed.

Recording and Reporting

• Record in nurses' notes method used to check placement of NG tube, volume of stomach aspirate, and, if indicated, pH of stomach aspirate.

• Record time each drug was administered on the

MAR or computer printout. Include initials or signature.

- If drug is withheld, record reason in nurses' notes. Circle time the drug normally would have been given on the MAR or computer printout.
- Report adverse effects/client response to nurse in charge or M.D.

Sample Documentation

NOTE: Documentation for medications via feeding tube is usually done on the medication sheet, the same as for any other medication. Other documentation occurs only if a problem is noted.

1300   Unable to administer medication because of clogged tube, despite efforts to unclog. Physician notified, medications held pending placement of new tube.

Geriatric Considerations

Assess the client for use of medications that may affect the pH of gastric secretions, such as histamine-receptor antagonists or antacids.

Home Care and Long-Term Care Considerations

- Teach the client or primary caregiver to check placement of tube before administering any medication.
- Instruct the client or primary caregiver not to administer medication if there is any doubt concerning the placement of the tube.
- Instruct the client or primary caregiver that medications, especially elixirs, may clog feeding tubes. Be sure to administer water before and after giving the medications.
- Instruct the client or primary caregiver that sublingual, enteric-coated, or sustained-release pills can not be given through the tube.

CRITICAL THINKING EXERCISES

1. Your client has an NG tube in place. You need to administer two medications via the tube. One medication is an elixir; the other is a gelatin capsule. Describe your nursing actions related to the medication administration.

2. You have just checked the placement of your client's NG tube. You obtain a pH reading of 7.0. Discuss the implications of this value and what nursing actions you would take.

3. Mr. H. is on continuous tube feedings. During your initial assessment you discover that his respirations are 30 per minute and that he has bilateral rales at the bases of his lungs. What are your nursing actions based on these data?

REFERENCES

Bockus S: When your patient needs tube feedings: making the right decision, *Nursing '93* 23(7):34, 1993.

Bowers S: Tubes: a nurses guide to enteral feeding devices, *Med Surg Nursing* 5(5):315, 1996.

Chang J et al: Inadvertent endobronchial intubation with nasogastric tube, *Arch Otolaryngol* 108:528, 1982.

Eisenberg PG: Nasoenteral tubes: a nurse's guide to tube feeding, *RN* 57(10):62, 1994.

Fater KH: Determining nasoenteral tube placement, *Med Surg Nursing* 4(1):29, 1995.

Goff KL: The nuts and bolts of enteral infusion pumps, *Med Surg Nursing* 6(1):9–15, 1997.

Hanson RL: Predictive criteria for length of nasogastric tube insertion for tube feeding, *JPEN* 3:(6), 1979.

Lehmann S: Parenteral and enteral access devices. In Teasley-Strausberg KM, editor: *Nutrition support handbook*, Cincinnati, 1992, Harvey Whitney Books.

Lord L et al: Comparison of weighted vs unweighted enteral feeding tubes for efficacy of transpyloric intubation, *JPEN* 17(3):271, 1993.

Metheny N: Measures to test placement of nasogastric and enteral feeding tubes: a review, *Nurs Res* 37(6): 323, 1988.

Metheny N et al: Detection of inadvertent respiratory placement of small bore feeding tubes: a report of 10 cases, *Heart Lung* 19(6):631, 1990a.

Metheny N et al: Effectiveness of the auscultatory method in predicting feeding tube location, *Nurs Res* 39(5):262, 1990b.

Metheny N: Minimizing respiratory complications of nasoenteric tube feedings: state of the science, *Heart Lung* 22(3):213, 1993.

Metheny N et al: pH, color, and feeding tubes, *RN* 61(1):25–27, 1998a.

Metheny N et al: Detection of improperly positioned feeding tubes, *J Healthcare Risk Management* Summer pp 37–47, 1998b.

Welsch SK: Certification of staff nurses to insert enteral feeding tubes using a research-based procedure, *NCP* 11(1):21, 1996.

Zaloga G: Timing and route of nutritional support. In Zaloga G, editor: *Nutrition in critical care*, St Louis, 1994, Mosby.

CHAPTER 34

Altered Bowel Elimination

Skill 34.1
Removing Impactions, 792

Skill 34.2
Pouching an Enterostomy, 794

Skill 34.3
Irrigating a Colostomy, 803

Disorders of the bowel may be caused by various factors. Those requiring direct nursing intervention commonly result from constipation or surgical removal of various portions of bowel. Left unrecognized, constipation can progress to fecal impaction, in which stool may block the intestinal lumen. Stasis of bowel contents produces abdominal distention and pain. In some cases, liquid stool passes around the obstruction, which can be misinterpreted as diarrhea. If enemas and suppositories do not facilitate passage of stool, the impaction may need to be removed manually.

An ostomy is an opening made to allow passage of feces. The piece of intestine brought out onto the client's abdomen is called a stoma. An enterostomy is any surgical procedure that produces an artificial stoma in a portion of intestine through the abdominal wall. Depending on the reason for the surgery, an ostomy can be permanent or temporary. There are two types of ostomies in the gastrointestinal (GI) tract (Figure 34-1). The most common type is a *colostomy,* which is a stoma made from the large intestine or colon. The other, an *ileostomy,* is found in the small intestine (Fazio and Tjandra, 1992; Hampton and Bryant, 1992; Nadler, 1992). The drainage from the stoma is often called *effluent.* Ostomies of the genitourinary (GU) tract are addressed in Chapter 35.

Care of a client with an ostomy involves many dimensions. These include providing the physical care of the stoma, containing the ostomy output or effluent, protecting the skin around the stoma (peristomal skin), preventing peristomal irritation, and preventing fecal contamination of the surgical wound (Hampton and Bryant, 1992). Teaching the client self-ostomy care is critical. This includes pouch change techniques, colostomy irrigation, and diet management.

Regardless of the type of ostomy, a threat to body image may be perceived (Kluka and Kristijanson, 1996; Piper and Mikols, 1996; Piper, Mikols, Grant, 1996; Quayle, 1994; Walsh et al., 1995). The client with a new ostomy

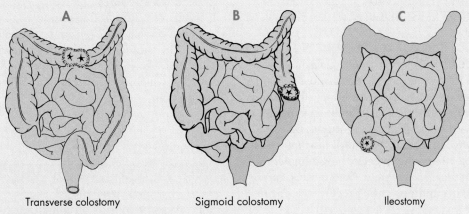

Transverse colostomy   Sigmoid colostomy   Ileostomy

Figure 34-1 Types of colostomies. **A,** Transverse (double barrel) colostomy. **B,** Sigmoid colostomy. **C,** Ileostomy.

has undergone a significant body image disturbance. It is of primary importance when caring for a client with a new ostomy to use neutral, nonjudgmental verbal and nonverbal communication. Researchers have shown that clients with ostomies not only have body image concerns but also concerns about stool leakage and odor, self-care, and surgical complication management. Education and counseling of clients with ostomies are major interventions for the nurse (Piper and Mikols, 1996).

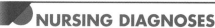

NURSING DIAGNOSES

Nursing diagnoses associated with clients who have an impaction include **Constipation** related to dehydration, decreased activity, postsurgical ileus, or inadequate dietary fiber; and **Pain** related to bowel distention. Those common diagnoses associated with clients who have ostomies include **Knowledge Deficit** related to ostomy self-care or irrigation management, **Body Image Disturbance** related to presence of the ostomy, **Risk for Impaired Skin Integrity** related to irritation of peristomal skin, **Anxiety** related to bowel function or rejection by friends, and **Ineffective Individual Coping** related to daily ostomy care requirements.

Skill 34.1

REMOVING IMPACTIONS

This skill is usually performed when the administration of enemas or suppositories have been unsuccessful at removing hard or large stools. Digital removal of an impaction may be embarrassing and uncomfortable for the client. Excessive rectal manipulation may cause irritation to the mucosa and subsequent bleeding or vagus nerve stimulation, which can produce a reflex slowing of the heart rate (Wright and Staats, 1986).

Equipment

Clean gloves
Water-soluble lubricant
Waterproof pad
Toilet tissue/Wipettes
Bedpan
Bedpan cover
Basin, washcloth, towel, and soap
Bath blanket

ASSESSMENT

1. Assess client's normal and current bowel elimination pattern as to frequency, characteristics of stool, use of laxatives and other medications; urge to defecate but inability to do so, and abdominal discomfort, especially when attempting to defecate. **Rationale: This information is valuable in determining contributing factors and preventing recurrence of this problem.**
2. Assess client's abdomen for distention, auscultate for the presence of bowel sounds, and palpate the abdomen for masses. **Rationale: Distention may con-**

tribute to constipation. **Hyperactive bowel sounds may result from partial obstruction of GI tract.**
3. Measure client's current vital signs to establish a baseline. **Rationale: Vagus nerve stimulation may slow the heart rate.**
4. Check client's record for physician's order for digital removal of impaction. **Rationale: A physician's order is necessary because of possible vagus nerve stimulation.**

PLANNING

Expected outcomes focus on removal of the impaction and prevention of further occurrences.

Expected Outcomes

1. Client's rectum is free of stool.
2. Client's vital signs remain normal after procedure.
3. Client resumes normal defecation within 2 to 3 days.
4. Client experiences minimal discomfort.
5. Client/family verbalize ways to prevent fecal impaction.

DELEGATION CONSIDERATIONS

The skill of removing an impaction requires problem solving and knowledge application unique to a professional nurse.

IMPLEMENTATION

Steps	Rationale

1. See Standard Protocol (inside front cover).
2. Assist client to a left side-lying position with knees flexed.

Provides access to the rectum.

3. Drape client's trunk and lower extremities with bath blanket and place waterproof pad under buttocks.

Prevents unnecessary exposure of body parts.

4. Place bedpan next to client.

COMMUNICATION TIP

At this time, instruct client to take slow, deep breaths during procedure. Breathe slowly with client.

5. Lubricate gloved index finger with lubricating jelly.
6. Insert index finger into rectum and advance finger slowly along rectal wall toward umbilicus.

Permits smooth insertion of finger into anus and rectum. Allows nurse to reach impacted stool high in rectum.

7. Gently loosen fecal mass by massaging around it. Work finger into hardened mass.

Loosening and penetrating mass allows nurse to remove it in small pieces, resulting in less discomfort to client.

8. Work stool downward toward end of rectum. Remove small sections of feces.

Prevents need to force finger up into rectum and minimizes trauma to mucosa.

9. Periodically assess heart rate and look for signs of fatigue.

Vagal stimulation slows heart rate and may cause dysrhythmia. Procedure may exhaust client.

NURSE ALERT

Stop procedure if heart rate drops or rhythm changes, or if bleeding occurs.

10. Continue to clear rectum of feces and allow client to rest at intervals.

Rest improves client's tolerance of procedure.

11. After removal of impaction, provide washcloth and towel to wash buttocks and anal area.
12. Remove bedpan and dispose of feces. Remove gloves by turning inside out and discarding in proper receptacle.

Reduces transmission of microorganisms.

13. Assist client to toilet or clean bedpan. (Procedure may be followed by enema or cathartic.)

Disimpaction may stimulate defecation reflex.

14. See Completion Protocol (inside front cover).

• • •

EVALUATION

1. Perform rectal examination for stool.
2. Reassess vital signs and compare to baseline values.
3. Monitor bowel elimination pattern.
4. Palpate abdomen to determine if it is soft and non-tender.
5. Have client identify ways to prevent fecal impaction.

Unexpected Outcomes and Related Interventions

1. Client has seepage of liquid fecal material after removal of impaction.
   a. Contact physician. An enema may be needed to remove hardened feces higher in the rectum.
   b. Increasing fluids, fiber in the diet, and activity level may aid peristaltic activity.

2. Client experiences bradycardia, decrease in blood pressure, and decrease in level of consciousness as a result of vagus nerve stimulation.
   a. Stop procedure.
   b. Notify physician immediately.
   c. Monitor the client's vital signs and level of consciousness.
   d. Be prepared for potential emergency intervention.
3. Client has trauma to the rectal mucosa, as evidenced by blood on the gloved finger.
   a. Assess rectal area every hour for bleeding.
   b. If bleeding continues, contact physician for further treatment measures.

Recording and Reporting
- Record and report any changes in vital signs, character of pain, presence of bleeding, client's comments, amount and consistency of stool removed, and adverse effects.

Sample Documentation
1600   Moderate amount of hard, dark brown stool removed from rectum. Pulse ranged 86 to 94 beats/min. Procedure tolerated without rectal bleeding, pain, or fatigue.

Home Care and Long-Term Care Considerations
- Consider having client or family member keep a week's diary of meals and fluid intake. Determine if dietary pattern contributes to constipation. Recommend a diet adequate in fiber.
- In long-term care, maintenance of activity can be very important in maintaining peristalsis.

Geriatric Considerations
- Many older adult clients are especially prone to dysrhythmia and other problems related to vagal stimulation; monitor heart rate and rhythm closely.
- At least 28% of older adults are constipated as a result of insufficient dietary bulk, inadequate fluid intake, laxative abuse, diminished muscle tone and motor function, decreased defecation reflex, mental or physical illness, and presence of tumors or structures (Ebersole and Hess, 1994).
- For the elderly, instituting a diet adequate in dietary fiber (6 to 10 g/day) adds bulk, weight, and form to stool and improves defecation (Ebersole and Hess, 1994).
- Consider development of a regular toileting routine that includes responding to the urge to defecate (Lueckenotte, 1996).

Skill 34.2

POUCHING AN ENTEROSTOMY

Immediately after surgical diversion or removal of a portion of bowel, it is necessary to place a pouch over the newly created stoma because in noncontinent ostomies effluent may begin immediately. The pouch collects all effluent and protects the skin from irritating drainage. A pouch with its skin barrier should fit comfortably, cover the skin surface around the stoma, not cut the stoma, and create a good seal. The postoperative pouch should allow visibility of the stoma.

Pouching a newly formed stoma differs from techniques used to pouch a stoma several days or weeks old. The new stoma is edematous during the postoperative healing process. An incision line from the bowel resection may lie close to the stoma. The stoma itself often has a series of small stitches around its perimeter. A pouch and its skin barrier must be applied so that they do not constrict the stoma or traumatize healing tissues. Initially, the pouch over a postoperative colostomy may not need to be emptied frequently because drainage is diminished or lacking. Several days may pass before a client's normal elimination pattern returns. In the case of an ileostomy, the client will have frequent loose or watery stools when peristalsis returns.

Many types of pouches and skin barriers are available. Some pouches are one piece and have skin barriers directly preattached. Some of these one-piece pouches already are precut to size by the manufacturer, and others must be custom cut to fit the client's stoma. Other systems are two separate pieces. The pouch can be applied to the skin barrier by attaching it to the flange (a plastic ring) on the barrier. Often the skin barrier must be custom cut to the client's specific stoma size. For two-piece systems, the skin barrier with flange must be used with the corresponding size pouch that fits that flange *from the same manufacturer.* Nurses should understand how to use each of these different pouching systems.

Equipment

Pouch, clear drainable colostomy/ileostomy in correct size for two-piece system or custom cut-to-fit one-piece type with attached skin barrier (Figure 34-2)
Pouch closure device, such as a clamp
Ostomy measuring guide
Adhesive remover (optional)
Clean disposable gloves
Deodorant
Gauze pads or wash cloth
Towel or disposable waterproof barrier
Basin with warm tap water
Scissors
Skin barrier such as sealant wipes or wafer
Tape or ostomy belt
Skin cleanser

ASSESSMENT

1. Identify the type of ostomy (e.g., colostomy or ileostomy) the client has (see Figure 34-1, p. 791). **Rationale: Type of client ostomy is important when deciding on type of pouching system to use. Pouch type will vary as to amount and consistency of drainage and client's stoma characteristics.**

2. Auscultate for bowel sounds. **Rationale: Validates the presence of peristalsis.**

3. Observe skin barrier and pouch for leakage and length of time in place. Depending on type of pouching system used (such as an opaque pouch), the nurse may have to remove the pouch to fully observe the stoma. **Rationale: Extended exposure of the skin to effluent can cause maceration.**

4. Assess client's stoma for the following characteristics:
   a. *Size:* Use a measuring card to determine the correct size of the client's stoma (Figure 34-3). **Rationale: Accurate stoma size is critical for planning and selecting ostomy pouch size.**
   b. *Shape:* If the stoma is round, use the precut, presized pouches as an option. **Rationale: Irregularly shaped stomas require a custom-cut shape made on the skin barrier to match the shape of the stoma (Figure 34-4, p. 796).**
   c. *Type:* Determine whether the stoma is flush to the skin or protruding (Figure 34-5, p. 796). **Rationale: Type of stoma is important when selecting skin barrier and pouch.**
   d. *Color:* Stoma should be pink-red in color. **Rationale: Dark-colored stoma can indicate stoma necrosis.**
   e. *Effluent:* Determine amount and consistency of the fecal drainage from the stoma (Table 34-1, p. 797). **Rationale: Differences in drainage in the type of ostomies should be considered when selecting the ostomy pouch. Only a pouch designed for stool should be used.**

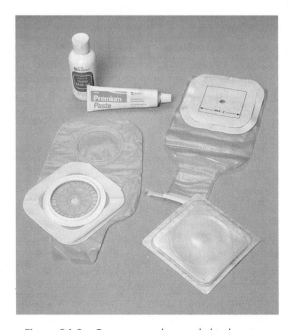

Figure 34-2 Ostomy pouches and skin barriers.

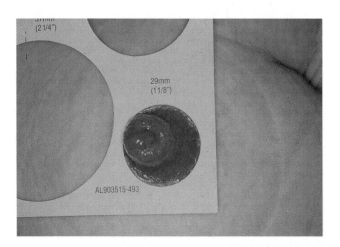

Figure 34-3 Measuring an ostomy using a measuring card.

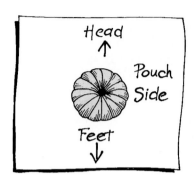
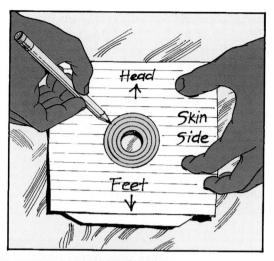

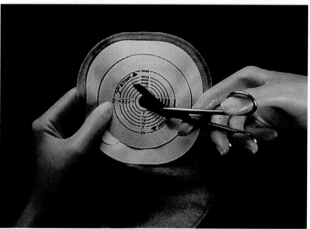

Figure 34-4   Steps for preparing skin barrier and pouch.   *Courtesy Hollister, Inc., Libertyville, Ill.*

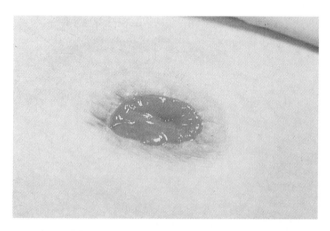

Figure 34-5   *Courtesy Hollister, Inc., Libertyville, Ill.*

PLANNING

Expected outcomes focus on helping client adjust to life with an ostomy emotionally as well as physically when performing self-ostomy care, preventing peristomal skin breakdown, and containing effluent.

Expected Outcomes

1. Client denies discomfort.
2. Stoma is moist and reddish pink. Skin is intact and free of irritation; sutures are intact.
3. Stoma is functioning with moderate amount of liquid or soft stool and flatus in pouch. Bowel sounds are present. (Flatus is noted by bulging of pouch in absence of drainage; flatus initially indicates return of peristalsis after surgery.)
4. Client observes stoma and steps of procedure carefully. Reveals acknowledgment of body alterations.
5. Client indicates readiness to learn and to begin self-care.

Table 34-1

Characteristic Output of GI Stomas

Type	Amount (ml)	Consistency	pH
Esophagostomy	1000–1500	Saliva	Slightly alkaline
Gastrostomy	2000–2500	Liquid	0.5–1.5
Jejunostomy	1000–3000	Liquid	Slightly acid
Ileostomy	750–1000	Toothpaste	Alkaline
Cecostomy and ascending colostomy	500–750	Toothpaste	Alkaline
Transverse colostomy		Mushy to semiformed	Alkaline
Descending and sigmoid colostomy		Semiformed to formed	Alkaline

DELEGATION CONSIDERATIONS

The skill of pouching a stoma requires problem solving and knowledge application unique to a professional nurse. In some agencies the pouching of an established ostomy may be delegated. In this case the Assistive personnel (AP) must report any changes in the appearance of the stoma or peristomal skin that the nurse has not assessed.

IMPLEMENTATION

Steps	Rationale

1. See Standard Protocol (inside front cover).
2. Inspect pouch periodically to see if it has to be emptied.

Minimizing leaking fosters a positive body image.

Empty ostomy pouch when pouch is ⅓ to ½ full.

A full, heavy ostomy pouch will break the seal and cause leakage.

3. For one-piece system
   a. Open end of drainable pouch and empty contents into bedpan or toilet.

   Do not let effluent splash on client when emptying pouch. Observe effluent.

   b. Rinse inside of pouch with a cup of warm water. Wipe and dry end of pouch.

   Empties pouch of effluent and cleans the inside.

   c. Close end of pouch by applying the pouch closure device (or rubber band) according to manufacturer's instruction (fold end of pouch over one time only).

   Lessens chance of pouch accidentally opening and stool coming out on client.

4. For two-piece system
   a. Hold one hand on skin barrier, and with other hand on pouch pull tab, remove pouch from skin barrier.

   Avoid unnecessary removal of skin barrier.

   b. Empty contents of pouch into toilet and observe effluent.

Steps	Rationale

c. Rinse pouch, clean, dry, and reattach to flange of skin barrier. Avoid excessive pressure to abdomen.

Some two-piece pouches can be reused. Others are disposable.

d. Close end of pouch by applying pouch closure device (or rubber band) according to manufacturer's instruction.

Lessens chance of pouch accidentally opening and stool coming out on the client.

Apply/Change ostomy pouch.

Only replace if pouch is leaking. Disposable pouches should not be routinely changed daily.

5. Remove pouch (one-piece system) or pouch and skin barrier (two-piece system) and discard according to hospital policy for standard precautions.

6. Wash gently around stoma with warm water and washcloth. Gently pat dry.

Stoma may bleed slightly; this is normal.

7. Inspect stoma daily and peristomal skin for color (redness) and any trauma, such as ulceration, cuts, or necrosis (Table 34-2).

COMMUNICATION TIP

While caring for the stoma, talk in a pleasant tone and use normal facial gestures to convey acceptance. Encourage the client by saying "the stoma appears to be healing well," for example.

NURSE ALERT

The stoma should be measured at each pouching system change to determine the correct size of equipment needed. Follow each ostomy pouch manufacturer's directions and measuring guide as to which size ostomy pouch to use based on the client's actual stoma measurement size.

8. Remeasure stoma using measuring card at each pouch change.

Stoma will shrink postoperatively. Client's weight gain or loss can affect pouching needs.

9. Select appropriate pouch for client based on assessment. With a custom cut-to-fit pouch, use an ostomy guide to cut opening on the pouch $\frac{1}{16}$ to $\frac{1}{8}$ inch larger than stoma before removing backing. Prepare pouch by removing backing from barrier and adhesive (see illustration). With ileostomy, apply thin circle of barrier paste around opening in pouch; allow to dry.

Paste facilitates seal and protects skin. Size of pouch opening keeps drainage off skin and lessens risk of damage to stoma during peristalsis or activity. Stool is alkaline, and this irritates the skin; fecal bacteria can colonize on the skin and increase risk of infection.

NURSE ALERT

When applying a skin barrier to a stoma that is close to a client's abdominal incision, the skin barrier may have to be trimmed for it to fit.

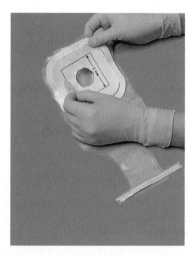

Step 9

Table 34-2

Peristomal Skin Damage

Type or Cause of Damage	Appearance	Treatment Principles
CHEMICAL DAMAGE Effluent in contact with skin Incorrect use of adhesives or solvents	Erythematous and denuded areas corresponding to leakage of effluent *or* areas of product use (adhesives, solvents)	Eliminate effluent contact with skin; allow adhesives to dry and remove solvents from skin. *Topical:* Skin barrier powder; sealants if needed

MECHANICAL DAMAGE (Figure 34-6, *A*)
Inappropriate skin care
  (scrubbing or "picking")
Incorrect tape removal or fragile
  skin, resulting in "stripping"
  of epidermis
	Patchy areas of erythema or denudation corresponding with areas subjected to trauma or "taped" areas	Eliminate cause; teach atraumatic skin care, appropriate tape removal, and use of sealants when indicated.
		Topical: Skin barriers (powder; with sealant as indicated; solid barriers until area has healed)

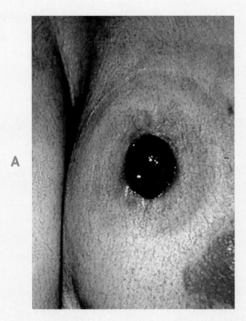 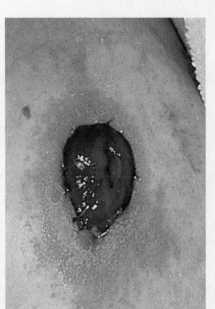

Figure 34-6   **A,** Mechanical injury. **B,** Candidiasis.   *Courtesy Hollister, Inc., Libertyville, Ill.*

Type or Cause of Damage	Appearance	Treatment Principles
FUNGAL RASH *(CANDIDA)* (Figure 34-6, *B*) Antibiotics resulting in fungal overgrowth Persistent skin moisture	Maculopapular rash with satellite lesions	Keep skin dry; eliminate pooled urine; restore normal flora. *Topical:* Antifungal powder and sealant as indicated
ALLERGIC REACTION Can be caused by any product	Areas of erythema or pruritus corresponding to area of skin exposed to allergen	Use patch test if needed to determine allergen; eliminate contact with allergen. *Topical:* Corticosteroid agent if needed for control of pruritus (cream or spray, not ointment, which would interfere with pouch adherence)

From Hampton BG, Bryant RA: *Ostomies and continent diversions: nursing management,* St Louis, 1992, Mosby.

Steps	Rationale
10. Place skin barrier around stoma as single unit.	Enhances sticking of skin barrier to peristomal skin.
a. For one-piece pouching system:	
(1) Use skin sealant wipes on part of skin directly under adhesive skin barrier or pouch; allow to dry. Press the adhesive backing of the pouch and/or skin barrier smoothly against the skin, starting from the bottom and working up and around the sides.	
(2) Hold pouch by barrier, center over stoma, and press down gently on barrier; bottom of pouch should point toward client's knees.	**NURSE ALERT** *Excessive pressure may cause the client pain.*
(3) Maintain gentle finger pressure around the barrier for 1 to 2 minutes.	Enhances the sticking of skin barrier to peristomal skin.
b. If using a two-piece pouching system:	
(1) Apply flange (barrier with adhesive) as in steps above for one-piece system. Then snap on pouch and maintain finger pressure.	Creates wrinkle-free, secure seal; decreases irritation from the adhesive on skin.
11. *Option:* Apply nonallergeric paper tape around the pectin skin barrier in a "picture frame" method. Half of the tape should be on the skin barrier and half on the client's skin. Some clients may prefer a belt attached to the pouch for extra security rather than tape.	"Picture framing" the pectin skin barrier keeps the pouch system attached securely.
12. Make sure a client who chooses to wear an ostomy belt does not have the belt too tight. To check for appropriate tightness, two fingers should be able to be placed between belt and skin.	
13. Although many ostomy pouches are odor-proof, some nurses and clients like to add a small amount of ostomy deodorant into the pouch. Do not use "home remedies," which can harm the stoma, to control ostomy odor.	**NURSE ALERT** *Aspirin should never be added to the ostomy pouch. It can cause stomal bleeding.*
14. Fold bottom of drainable open-ended pouches up once and close using a closure device such as a clamp (or follow manufacturers' instructions for closure).	Maintains secure seal to prevent leaking.
15. Properly dispose of old pouch and soiled equipment. Remove and discard gloves and wash hands. Consider using room deodorant if needed.	
16. Change pouch every 3 to 7 days unless leaking; pouch can remain in place for tub bath or shower; after bath, pat adhesive dry.	Avoids unnecessary trauma to skin from too frequent changes. Dryness ensures adhesion of pouch.
17. See Completion Protocol (inside front cover).	

• • • •

EVALUATION

1. Observe client for nonverbal indication of pain.
2. Inspect peristomal skin for signs of skin breakdown and assess stoma status.
3. Monitor amount, color, consistency, and frequency of fecal elimination from the stoma. Check bag for leakage. Check for odor and seepage under the skin barrier. Auscultate bowel sounds.
4. Observe client perform self-care of ostomy pouching.
5. Observe client's behavior when looking at stoma and handling equipment. Note whether client talks about stoma.

Unexpected Outcomes and Related Interventions

1. Client's peristomal skin breaks down.
   a. Assess for causes of the skin breakdown.
   b. Remeasure the stoma size.
   c. Check if the selected pouch is correct for client's stoma size.
   d. Use a skin barrier for subsequent pouch changes.
2. Client's skin barrier and pouch leak.
   a. Assess if client is waiting too long (e.g., if pouch more than half full of stool) to empty pouch.
   b. Remeasure stoma and reevaluate pouch and skin barrier size.
   c. Determine if client is cutting out the correct size on the skin barrier.
   d. Evaluate if stoma is in a skin fold or whether other irregularities exist (Figure 34-7).
   e. Assess for peristomal hernia (Figure 34-8).
   f. Determine whether a convex disk, skin barrier paste, or other measures are needed to prevent leakage (Young, 1992).
3. Client cannot do self-ostomy pouching change.
   a. Determine if client lacks the physical or mental ability to do self-ostomy care.
   b. Eliminate distractions and other factors (e.g., pain) that might interfere with client's performance of self-ostomy care.

   c. Reevaluate client's understanding of self-ostomy care.
   d. Reevaluate client's problems with self-image, coping skills, and support systems (Salter, 1992).

Recording and Reporting

- Chart type of pouch and skin barrier applied.
- Record amount and appearance of stool or drainage in pouch, size, color, and shape of stoma, condition of peristomal skin, and sutures.
- Report any of the following to the charge nurse and/or physician:
   a. Abnormal appearance of stoma, suture line, peristomal skin, character of output, absence of bowel sounds.
   b. No flatus in 24 to 36 hours and no stool by third day.
- Document abdominal distention and excessive tenderness, nature of bowel sounds.
- Record client's level of participation and need for teaching.

Sample Documentation

1600   Bud colostomy stoma is 1½ in diameter, round, slightly swollen, and red in color. Peristomal skin is intact. Stoma is functioning × 3300 ml of dark brownish liquid stool. Normal bowel sounds present. Two-piece ostomy pouching system with hydrocolloid skin barrier in place without odor or other signs of leaks. Client has not yet looked at stoma. ET nurse began instruction of client's self-ostomy care technique.

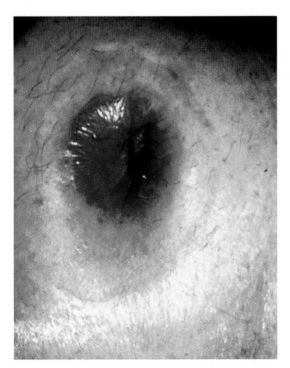

Figure 34-7   Irregular stoma (flush on right side, raised on left with skin irritation).

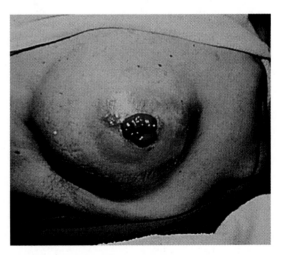

Figure 34-8   Peristomal hernia. *Courtesy Hollister, Inc., Libertyville, Ill.*

Geriatric Considerations

- Evaluate the older adult's cognitive status for understanding ostomy self-care instructions.
- Evaluate the older adult's motor and visual ability to prepare ostomy equipment. For clients who are unable to custom cut the size of their skin barriers, consider having barriers precut by the ostomy equipment supplier or using a precut two-piece system.
- Avoid hot water and harsh soaps when washing the peristomal skin.
- Teach older clients about the change in the number of eliminations (from an incontinent ostomy) that would be normal on a daily status.
- Financial concerns about the cost of ostomy supplies and reimbursement may be an important issue for clients on Medicare (Halvorson and Kertz, 1996).

Home Care and Long-Term Care Considerations

- Evaluate the client's home toileting facilities. This includes:
  - The presence of adequate functioning and accessible toileting facilities.
  - Number and location of toileting facilities.
  - Number of other people living with the client who must share the toileting facilities.
  - Identification of the toileting facilities pattern of use as to time of day and amount of time spent in bathroom by the other people living with the client.
- Evaluate the client's ostomy routine in relationship to usual lifestyle after discharge.
- Caution the client that most ostomy pouches and barriers cannot be flushed down the toilet; they clog the system. Dispose of used ostomy pouch according to local sanitation regulations.
- Client should understand that it is *not* necessary to use sterile gauze to cleanse the stoma. A washcloth or any soft material can be used.
- Review the client's dietary pattern. Help client and family members learn the types of foods to avoid so as to prevent problems with effluent or odor (Box 34-1).

Box 34-1 Effects of Food on Stoma Output

Foods that Thicken Stool		**Foods that Cause Stool Odor**	
Bananas	Cheese	Fish	Turnips
Rice	Tapioca	Eggs	Cabbage
Bread	Yogurt	Asparagus	Onions
Potatoes	Pasta	Garlic	Brussel sprouts
Creamy peanut butter	Pretzels	Some spices	Broccoli
Applesauce	Marshmallows	Beans	Cauliflower

Foods that Loosen Stool		**Foods that Cause Gas**	
Dried or string beans	Fried foods	Dried and string beans	Broccoli
Chocolate	Greasy foods	Beer	Cauliflower
Raw fruits	Prune or grape juice	Carbonated beverages	Dairy products
Raw vegetables	Leafy green vegetables	Cucumbers	Spinach
Highly spiced foods	(lettuce, broccoli, spinach)	Cabbage	Corn
		Onions	Radishes
		Brussel sprouts	

Foods that Color Stool	
Beef	
Red jello	

From Hampton BG, Bryant RA: *Ostomies and continent diversions: nursing management,* St Louis, 1992, Mosby.

Skill 34.3

IRRIGATING A COLOSTOMY

The purpose of a colostomy irrigation is to establish a pattern of regular bowel elimination after ostomy surgery, to cleanse the bowel of feces before tests or surgical procedures, and to relieve constipation. Irrigation of a colostomy is a simple procedure that clients can learn. The muscular quality of the colon allows it to be safely irrigated with a relatively large amount of fluid. Clients who perform irrigations at home learn to establish an irrigation routine so that regular evacuation of the bowel occurs without stomal discharge between irrigations. Irrigations for achieving regular bowel evacuation can be achieved only with descending and sigmoid end colostomies and are not usually done for pediatric clients.

Irrigating an ileostomy is rarely necessary, except in cases of food blockage near the stomal outlet. Then a gentle lavage may be performed, but only by a qualified person such as an ET nurse. An ileostomy produces a liquid drainage containing a high concentration of electrolytes such as sodium, chloride, potassium, magnesium, and bicarbonate. Because excessive lavage could lead to a serious fluid and electrolyte imbalance, normal saline solution is used. Smaller amounts of solution are used on pediatric clients. Volume is determined by the physician.

Equipment

Ostomy irrigation set that consists of an irrigation solution bag and tubing with a fluid control clamp and cone tip (Figures 34-9 and 34-10)
Irrigation sleeve (with belt tabs or stick-on ring and end-closure device)
Water-soluble lubricant
Ostomy pouch and skin barrier or stoma cap cover
Clean disposable gloves
Toilet facilities that include
A flushable toilet
A hook or some device to hold the irrigation container
Toilet tissue
Running water (that is suitable for use)
For clients who are bedridden
Bedpan
Towels
Waterproof pad

ASSESSMENT

1. Assess frequency of defecation, character of stool, and placement of stoma, as well as client's regular nutritional pattern. **Rationale: May indicate a need to irrigate to stimulate elimination function; consistency of stool varies along length of GI tract.**

2. Assess time when client normally irrigates colostomy. In the case of a new ostomy, confer with physician about whether and when irrigations can begin. Obtain written order. Confer with client for best time to irrigate. **Rationale: Irrigation helps to establish regular bowel emptying. Bowel must be totally healed so irrigation fluid will not cause perforation. This usually occurs 3 to 7 days after surgery. Irrigation can be planned to coincide with other hygiene activities.**

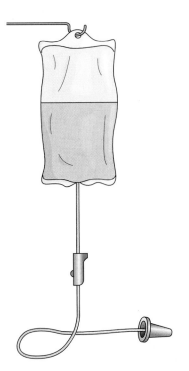

Figure 34-9   Irrigation bag with tubing and control clamp.

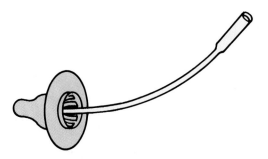

Figure 34-10   Cone tip.

3. Assess client's understanding of procedure and ability to perform techniques. **Rationale: Determines level of participation to expect from client, level of explanations nurse should provide, and if irrigation is appropriate for client.**

PLANNING
Expected outcomes focus on regular bowel evacuation and client learning to perform the colostomy irrigation.

Expected Outcomes
1. Client achieves regular bowel movements from the stoma with no leakage between irrigations.
2. Client independently does the colostomy irrigation procedure.

IMPLEMENTATION

Steps	Rationale
1. See Standard Protocol (inside front cover).	
2. Summarize for client how procedure will be performed. Encourage questions as you proceed.	Helps client anticipate steps in procedure. Active dialogue during procedure can enhance learning.
3. ![] Position client either: (NOTE: Gloves are optional for client.) a. On toilet or in chair in front of toilet, if ambulatory b. On side, with head slightly elevated, if unable to be out of bed	Allows for placement of irrigation sleeve into toilet or bedpan.
4. For adult clients, fill irrigation bag with 500 to 1000 ml warm irrigation solution (tap water or saline solution) (see illustration); clear tubing of air by opening flow control clamp and allow solution to run through tubing. Close clamp.	Volume will adequately distend colon and cause evacuation. Cold solution can cause syncope; hot solution could injure mucosa. Air entering colon can cause cramping.

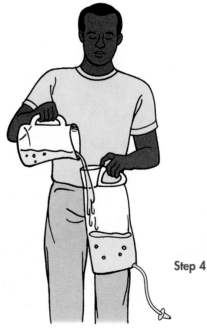

Step 4

Steps	Rationale
5. Hang the irrigation solution container on a hook so that the lower end of the bag is no higher than client's shoulder height when sitting or 18 to 20 inches (45 to 50 cm) above stoma.	This position prevents too high a water pressure and reduces possibility of bowel damage.
6. Remove client's pouch by gently pushing skin from adhesive and barrier; dispose of according to hospital policy for standard precautions. (save clamp if attached to pouch)	
7. Lubricate client's little finger and gently guide it into stoma for about 1 inch to learn the direction or angle of bowel from stoma. Have client hold finger in stoma for about 1 minute.	Teaches client the direction of the colon and helps dilate stoma. If bright-red blood is noted when client removes finger, reassure client that this will occasionally happen because mucosa bleeds readily as a result of higher vascularity in this area.
8. Place irrigation sleeve over client's stoma. Angle sleeve for appropriate flow of fecal returns (e.g., if client is using bedpan at 45 degrees). Angle of irrigation sleeve facilitates flow of fecal returns. Know particular use of the selected irrigation equipment. Some irrigation sleeves attach to flange of the two-piece skin barrier. Some sleeves require use of a belt. If so, adjust belt so it fits comfortably and is not too tight or too loose (Beare and Myers, 1994).	Make sure irrigation sleeve is correctly attached. End of sleeve *must* be in toilet or bedpan to prevent spillage of feces.

9. Lubricate tip of irrigating cone. Reach through the top of the irrigation sleeve and insert the cone gently into the stoma (see illustrations).	Prevents tearing, bleeding, and rupturing of stoma.

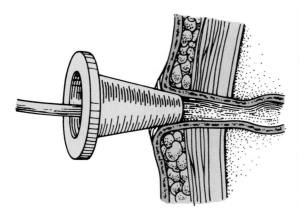 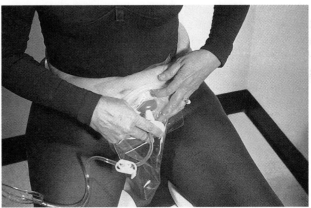

Step 9

10. With client holding cone, have client open flow control clamp and allow solution to flow. Start with 500 ml; this should take 5 to 10 minutes. Adjust direction of cone to facilitate inflow of solution as needed.	Too rapid instillation of irrigation solution can cause cramping and risk bowel perforation.

Steps	Rationale
11. If cramping occurs, reduce or stop flow of irrigation fluid.	Client's complaint of abdominal cramps indicates need to stop irrigating and wait until cramps subside.
12. When all the irrigation fluid has been instilled into client's stoma, close flow control clamp and wait 15 seconds before removing irrigation cone from stoma. Close top of irrigation sleeve using appropriate closure method (e.g., Zip-loc top, clothes pins). Discard gloves.	
13. Allow 15 to 20 minutes for initial evacuation of stool. Keep end of sleeve in toilet or bedpan.	Keeps the device balanced and prevents injury from bumping against objects.

COMMUNICATION TIP

Now is a good time to review with client importance of instilling fluid slowly. Reinforce positive performance. "You did very well. Remember, it helps to hold the cone *so that fluid runs easily. Next time, you can show me how you would insert it."*

14. [glove icon] Use gloves when assisting client. After initial evacuation of stool is over, dry tip of irrigation sleeve and close end with the clip or closure device. Leave in place 30 to 45 minutes while waiting for the secondary evacuation. Client may get off toilet and walk around at this time. Discard gloves.	Client may walk around, shower, or shave. Exercise stimulates bowel.
15. [glove icon] Use gloves. Unclamp sleeve and empty any fecal contents into toilet or bedpan. Rinse sleeve by pouring a small amount of water through the top, then remove sleeve. Rinse with liquid cleanser and cool water. Hang sleeve to dry.	Maintains sleeve in clean condition for future use.
16. Wipe stoma with toilet tissue to remove any stool. Put an appropriate colostomy pouch over stoma. If client is using a two-piece pouching system, place a new flange cap or closed-end pouch onto skin barrier (see Skill 34.2).	An appropriate pouch or cap may be worn to contain feces in case of elimination between irrigations.
17. See Completion Protocol (inside front cover).	

• • •

EVALUATION

1. Observe amount and character of fecal material and fluid that is returned after the irrigation.
2. Evaluate degree to which regularity of bowel movements is being achieved.
3. Determine if client has fecal drainage between irrigations.
4. Observe client's response to the irrigation procedure.
5. Evaluate client's knowledge and ability to do the irrigation procedure correctly.

Unexpected Outcomes and Related Interventions

1. Client has feces from the colostomy stoma between irrigations.
   a. Reassess if client is an appropriate candidate for this management option.
   b. Evaluate whether anything has changed in client's treatment plan or life-style that could account for this finding.
   c. Evaluate whether client understands to follow the schedule for irrigation at the same time each day.

d. Evaluate if sufficient time has occurred since beginning the irrigation routine (6 to 8 weeks) to allow the bowel time to react to the irrigation stimulus.

2. Client cannot independently perform the irrigation procedure correctly.
   a. Instruct primary caregivers in this technique.
   b. Reassess client's self-irrigation technique for accuracy.
   c. Observe client perform the irrigation technique, and monitor for errors in technique that could account for this finding.

3. Client has no fecal returns after the irrigation.
   a. Evaluate client for possible absence of bowel sounds, abdominal pain, or distention. More often, lack of fecal returns may indicate that client is dehydrated.
   b. Encourage client to increase fluid intake, to alter diet intake if constipated, and to wear a pouch that can contain the expected fecal output until the next scheduled irrigation.

Recording and Reporting

- Record procedure, time of irrigation, volume and type of solution, amount and type of return, and client's tolerance.
- Record reapplication of skin barrier and pouch and condition of stoma and skin.
- Report symptoms of extreme discomfort, onset of severe diarrhea, poor results, or excessive bleeding to nurse in charge or physician.

Sample Documentation

0800   Second colostomy irrigation done in bathroom by client with minimal nurse assistance. 500 ml lukewarm water instilled easily into stoma using cone applicator. Effective for large amount of brownish fluid and semisoft stool. Tolerated procedure without cramping or complaints. Correctly replaced ostomy pouch onto ostomy skin barrier at end of irrigation procedure. States, "Feels like I'm beginning to do this right."

Geriatric Considerations

- Assess the client's willingness to do ostomy self-irrigations. This takes a time commitment to be able to perform the skill correctly.
- Assess the client's physical ability to do ostomy self-irrigations. Motor and/or visual limitations may make it difficult but not impossible for client to do the procedure. Some adaptions in the irrigation technique may need to be made to enable older clients with motor and/or visual limitations to successfully do self-irrigation.
- Some older adults become upset if they do not have a daily bowel movement. With some irrigation routines, irrigation is not done daily, therefore the client will not have a daily bowel movement. Client needs to understand and accept this.

Home Care and Long-Term Care Considerations

- Evaluate the client's home toileting facilities. This includes:
  - The presence of functional and accessible toileting facilities in the client's home.
  - Number and location of toileting facilities.
  - Number of other people living with the client who must share the toileting facilities.
  - Identification of the toileting facilities pattern of use as to time of day and amount of time spent in bathroom by the other people living with the client.
- Establish scheduled time (approximately 1 hour) for uninterrupted ostomy care.
- Assess bathroom for towel rack, hook, or other device from which irrigation device may be hung; end of irrigation solution bag should hang at shoulder level when client is sitting on the toilet.
- Irrigation sleeve may be attached by a belt, by a stick on, or by snapping directly onto the flange of the skin barrier. For home care, two-piece system is easier to use and more cost-effective; it allows client to remove pouch from flange and then attach irrigation sleeve, then snap on a clean pouch or stoma cap when evacuation is completed.
- Tell clients if they travel in a foreign country that if they cannot drink the water, they should not irrigate with it.

CRITICAL THINKING EXERCISES

1. An 80-year-old client was admitted yesterday with a diagnosis of weakness and dehydration. The history indicates no bowel movement for the past 3 days, and the client is having episodes of diarrhea today. How would you proceed and what are your rationales?

2. You just started irrigating your client's colostomy and the client begins to complain of cramping. What should you do and why?

3. You have an elderly client using a two-piece pouching system who tells you she is having difficulty changing the pouch. What nursing assessments are important to make at this time?

REFERENCES

Beare PG, Myers JL: *Principles and practice of adult health nursing,* ed 2, St Louis, 1994, Mosby.

Ebersol P, Hess P: *Toward healthy aging: human needs and nursing response,* ed 3, St Louis, 1994, Mosby.

Fazio VW, Tjandra JJ: Prevention and management of ileostomy complications, *J ET Nurs* 19(2):48, 1992.

Halvorson ML, Kertz JM: Changes in Medicare reimbursement for ostomy supplies: an overview, *Journal of WOCN* 23(1): 26-32, 1996.

Hampton BG, Bryant RA: *Ostomies and continent diversions: nursing management,* St Louis, 1992, Mosby.

Kluka S, Kristijanson LJ: Development and testing of the ostomy concerns scale: measuring ostomy-related concerns of cancer patients and their partners, *JWOCN* 23(3):166, 1996.

Lueckenotte AG: *Gerontologic nursing,* St Louis, 1996, Mosby.

Nadler LH: General considerations and complications of the ileostomy, *Ostomy Wound Manage* 38(4):18, 1992.

Piper B, Mikols C, Grant TRD: Comparing adjustment to an ostomy for three groups, *JWOCN* 23(4): 197, 1996.

Piper B, Mikols C: Predischarge and postdischarge concerns of persons with an ostomy, *JWOCN* 23(2):105, 1996.

Quayle BK: Making positive choices: body image and the new ostomy patient, *Ostomy Wound Manage* 40(4):16, 1994.

Salter MJ: Aspects of sexuality for patients with stomas and continent pouches, *J ET Nurs* 19(4):126, 1992.

Thelan LA, Davie JK, Urden LD: *Textbook of critical care nursing: diagnosis and management,* ed 2, St Louis, 1994, Mosby.

Walsh BA et al.: Multidisciplinary management of altered body image in the patient with an ostomy, *JWOCN* 22(5):227, 1995.

Wright BA, Staats DO: The geriatric implications of fecal impaction, *Nurs Pract* 11(10):53, 1986.

Young MJ: Convexity in the management of problem stomas, *Ostomy Wound Manage* 38(4):53, 1992.

CHAPTER 35

Altered Urinary Elimination

Skill 35.1
Urinary Catheterization: Male and Female, 810

Skill 35.2
Urinary Diversions (Continent and Incontinent, 818

Skill 35.3
Continuous Bladder Irrigation, 825

Skill 35.4
Suprapubic Catheters, 828

Urinary elimination, micturition, is a necessary natural process in clients. Clients normally urinate or void through the genitourinary system. When the urinary system fails to function properly, virtually all body systems can be affected. Normal urine output is at least 30 ml per hour or a total of 1 to 2 L per day.

The urinary system consists of two kidneys, where wastes are removed from blood to form urine. Urine passes through the two ureters and on into the bladder. Once the bladder has accumulated 250 to 300 ml of urine, a signal is sent to the central nervous system indicating fullness and the need to void. Once the bladder contracts, urine passes through the urethra to the urinary meatus.

If urine flow is altered, the client may have a catheter, either indwelling or suprapubic, to assist in correcting the body's inability to empty the bladder. At other times, urine must be redirected to another outlet, a urinary diversion. Urinary diversions are ostomies, or openings, coming from the bladder, ureters, or kidneys to the outer wall of the abdomen. Another intervention to correct altered urine flow may be irrigating catheters to prevent obstruction of urine outflow.

Clients may have altered body images with urinary system dysfunctions. The genitourinary system is a very private body part and one that is not seen or freely discussed. When an external device, such as a urinary diversion or an indwelling catheter, is used, the client's body image may be further altered. Privacy, confidentiality, and explanations are necessary interventions when dealing with altered urinary elimination.

 NURSING DIAGNOSES

Altered Urinary Elimination is a diagnosis that applies when clients have sensory, neuromuscular, or traumatic alterations affecting normal voiding. Clients may have a nursing diagnosis of **Risk for Infection** related to urinary retention, inadequate perineal hygiene, or lack of knowledge of care for a urinary catheter or stoma. **Urinary Retention** may result from obstructions, paralysis, or inadequate muscle tone of the bladder. Clients with urinary obstruction may also experience **Pain** related to a distended bladder. Several diagnoses pertaining to **Incontinence** (e.g., **Functional, Reflex, Stress, Total,** and **Urge**) are appropriate depending on whether the client has neurological deficits or bladder dysfunction. **Impaired Skin Integrity** related to inadequate knowledge of stoma care or to irritation from incontinence or adhesive around the stoma may also apply.

Another possible nursing diagnosis is **Sexual Dysfunction** related to presence of a catheter for a prolonged time or to altered body image. **Social Isolation** may be appropriate when a client believes that limited involvement with other people is imposed by physical changes or by anxiety related to altered body image. **Ineffective Family Coping** may be appropriate when family members are unable to support adaptation to artificial urinary devices. **Alteration in Body Image** may also be appropriate when clients have urinary diversions.

Skill 35.1

URINARY CATHETERIZATION: MALE AND FEMALE

Catheterization of the bladder involves introducing a rubber or plastic tube through the urethra and into the bladder to provide a continuous flow of urine. Aseptic technique must be used when inserting a catheter into the urinary meatus because the urinary system is sterile. An indwelling or a straight catheter may be used to relieve the bladder of urine either because obstructions are present (e.g., from cancer or trauma) or normal emptying is impaired (e.g., from neurologic impairment). In addition, catheterization may be indicated to obtain sterile urine specimens, to prevent leakage of urine when performing a surgical procedure (e.g., a hysterectomy), to relieve postoperative urinary retention, or as a last resort for clients who are incontinent of urine. Intermittent catheterization is preferable to indwelling catheterization (Davey, 1994) because the likelihood of a urinary tract infection is reduced.

Equipment

Catheter kit with appropriate catheter (size and type)
   (Figure 35-1, *A* and *B*)
Urinary drainage device (for indwelling catheter)
Extra sterile gloves and catheter
Clean gloves
Bath cloth, towel, soap, and basin for water
Flashlight and gooseneck lamp
Flat sheet or bath blanket
Measuring container for urine

ASSESSMENT

1. Assess client's weight, age, level of consciousness, ability to cooperate, and mobility of lower extremities. **Rationale: This determines how much assistance is needed holding client's legs in correct position.**
2. Assess client's knowledge and prior experience with catheterization. **Rationales: This reveals need for client instruction and likelihood of client cooperation.**
3. Palpate for bladder over symphysis pubis. **Rationale: This indicates distended bladder and the need to insert catheter if client is unable to void independently.**
4. Inspect perineal region, observing for perineal landmarks, erythema, drainage, or discharge. **Rationale: This determines condition of the perineum.**

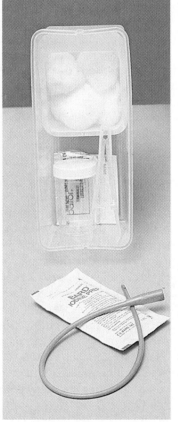

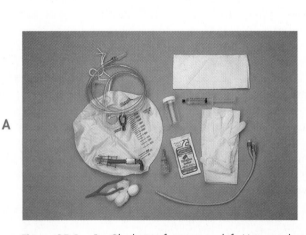

Figure 35-1 A, *Clockwise from upper left:* Urinary drainage device, sterile specimen cup, sterile drape, sterile gloves, indwelling catheter, sterile cleanser, sterile saline, and sterile cotton balls with forceps. **B,** Catheter kit with straight catheter and iodine cleanser.

5. Ask client the time of last voiding and to describe urine (if nurse did not observe). Check I&O flow sheet. **Rationale: This determines if urinary retention is likely.**

6. Ask client and check chart for allergies. **Rationale: This determines allergy to antiseptic, tape, latex, and lubricant. Povidone iodine allergies are common; if client is unaware of allergy, ask instead if allergic to shellfish.**

7. Assess any pathological condition that may impair passage of catheter (e.g., enlarged prostate gland in men).

8. Review client's medical record, including physician's order and nurse's notes. Note previous catheterization, including catheter size, response of client, and time of last catheterization. **Rationale: This determines purpose of inserting catheter and can indicate potential difficulty with new catheter insertion.**

PLANNING

Expected outcomes focus on emptying the bladder and on client comfort.

Expected Outcomes

1. Client's bladder is not distended.
2. Client will verbalize relief of discomfort in bladder after catheter insertion.
3. Client has a urine output of at least 30 ml per hour.

DELEGATION CONSIDERATIONS

The skill of urinary catheterization may be delegated to assistive personnel (AP) in some settings (see agency policy). First-time catheterizations or catheterization of clients with urethral trauma may best be performed by an RN. The nurse should be sure the care provider is properly instructed on client positioning, aseptic technique, proper insertion, and balloon inflation.

IMPLEMENTATION

Steps	Rationale

1. See Standard Protocol (inside front cover).
2. Explain procedure to client. Describe how client can participate.
3. Arrange for extra nursing personnel to assist with positioning as needed.
4. Option: Apply disposable gloves. Cleanse clients' perineal area with soap and water, rinse off soap and dry.
5. **Position and drape client.**
   a. *Female client*
      (1) Assist client into dorsal recumbent position (on back with knees flexed) (see illustration).

Female clients often have difficulty maintaining dorsal recumbent position.

COMMUNICATION TIP

"First we will position you as comfortably as we can. I want you to be able to lie still so that you do not accidentally contaminate the sterile equipment. I will let you know before I actually begin to insert the catheter."

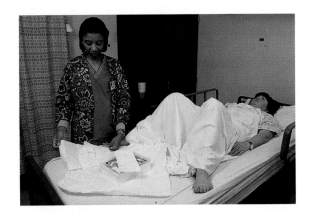

Step 5a(1)

Steps	Rationale

(2) If client cannot lie supine, then position client in side-lying (Sim's) position with upper leg flexed at knee and hip. The nurse must take extra precautions to cover rectal area with the drape during the procedure to reduce risk of cross-contamination.

(3) Drape with bath blanket so that only perineum is exposed (see illustration).

b. *Male client*

(1) Assist client to lie flat, with legs abducted.

(2) Drape upper body with small sheet or towel, and cover legs with sheet so that only genital area is exposed (see illustration).

This alternate position is used if client cannot abduct leg at the hip joint (e.g., if client has arthritic joints or contractions). This position may also be more comfortable for the client. Support client with pillows if necessary to maintain position (Perry and Potter, 1998).

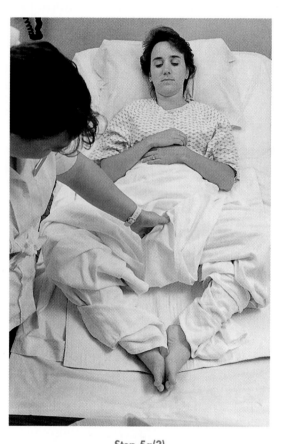

Step 5a(3)

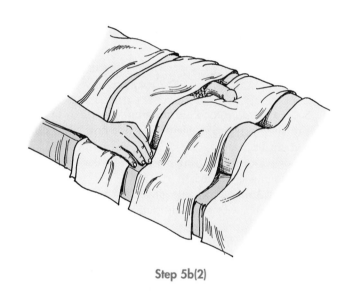

Step 5b(2)

6. Position light to illuminate perineum.

7. Place catheter kit on overbed table and open outer wrap using sterile technique. Then open package containing drainage system: place drainage bag over edge of bottom bed frame and bring drainage tube up between side rail.

Outer wrap serves as sterile work field.

8. Put on sterile gloves (see Chapter 4).

9. Organize supplies on sterile field, maintaining sterility of gloves.

Steps	Rationale

10. Prepare equipment.
  a. Check bag clamp.
  b. Test balloon of retention catheter by injecting saline solution into balloon port (see illustration). Withdraw if no leakage.
  c. Lubricate catheter with water-soluble gel 2.5 cm to 5 cm (1 to 2 inches) for women and 12.5 to 17.5 cm (5 to 7 inches) for men.
  d. Open specimen container if needed.
  e. Pour antiseptic solution over all but one cotton ball.

Will prevent urine leakage from bag.
Ensures proper inflation and deflation.

Makes insertion easier.

Dry cotton ball is used to remove excess antiseptic solution from meatus.

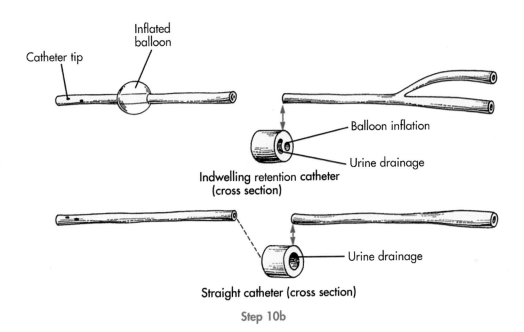

Catheter tip   Inflated balloon

Indwelling retention catheter (cross section)

Balloon inflation

Urine drainage

Straight catheter (cross section)

Urine drainage

Step 10b

11. Cleansing and catheter insertion: female
  a. Allow top edge of sterile drape to form cuff over both hands. Place drape down on bed between client's thighs and slip drape under buttocks. Client's knees remain flexed.
  b. Place sterile tray and contents on sterile drape between thighs.
  c. Separate labia with fingers of nondominant hand (now contaminated). This hand remains in this position for remainder of the procedure.
  d. Cleanse labia and meatus.
    (1) With dominant hand (sterile), use forceps to hold cotton balls.
    (2) Use each cotton ball for one stroke, then discard.
    (3) Cleanse from anterior to posterior.
    (4) First stroke is on farthest side from nurse and closest to meatus.

Prevents contamination of catheter by having it close to perineum.
Prevents labia from contaminating area being cleansed.

COMMUNICATION TIP

Tell the client "you will feel cold and wet" as you prepare to cleanse the area.

Steps	Rationale

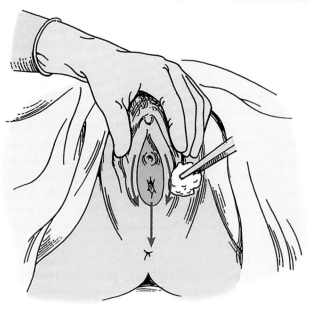

Step 11d(5)

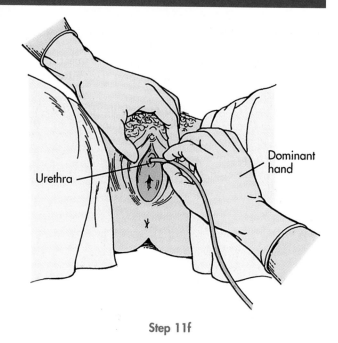

Urethra

Dominant hand

Step 11f

(5) Second stroke is on side of meatus closest to nurse (see illustration).

(6) Third stroke is down center of meatus.

Cleans from clean area to dirty area.

e. If meatus is difficult to visualize, have a second person hold a flashlight or direct lamp.

f. Holding catheter near tip, slowly insert catheter until urine flows, then advance another 1 to 2 inches (2.5 to 5 cm) for a total of 2 to 3 inches (5 to 7.5 cm) (see illustration). Place end of catheter in urine tray.

Female urethra is short. Appearance of urine indicates that catheter tip is in bladder or lower urethra. Advancement of catheter ensures bladder placement.

COMMUNICATION TIP

Tell the client "I want you to bear down gently as if you were passing urine. This will burn and you may feel pressure."

NURSE ALERT

Do not force catheter against resistance.

12. Cleansing and catheter insertion: male

a. Touching only corners, place sterile drape with hole centered over penis.

b. Place sterile tray and contents on sterile drape between client's thighs.

c. Hold shaft of penis at right angle to body with nondominant hand while retracting foreskin (if present). This hand remains in this position for remainder of the procedure. Retract urethral meatus between thumb and forefinger.

Provides sterile field.

Keeps equipment accessible.

Proper angle ensures that urethra is straight and ready for catheter insertion. Prevents contamination of glove.

Steps	Rationale

d. Use forceps to hold cotton balls and cleanse penis and meatus with dominant hand (sterile).
  (1) Use forceps to hold cotton balls.
  (2) Use each cotton ball for one stroke, then discard.
  (3) Use circular strokes from meatus outward and downward with three cotton balls (see illustration).

Cleans from clean area to dirty area.

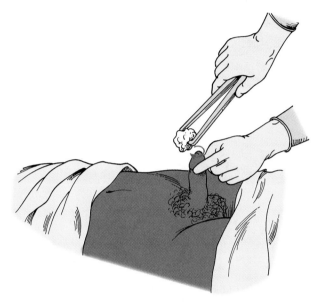

Step 12d(3)   Urinary diversions.

e. Pick up catheter with gloved dominant hand. Gently apply traction to penis and insert catheter 6 to 7 inches (15 to 17.5 cm) in adult or until urine flows out catheter end. If resistance is met with catheter, do not force it through urethra. When urine appears, advance catheter another 1 to 2 inches (2.5 to 5 cm).

Adult male urethra is long. It is normal to meet resistance at the prostatic sphincter. When resistance is met, nurse should hold catheter firmly against sphincter without forcing catheter. After a few seconds, sphincter relaxes and catheter is advanced. Appearance of urine indicates catheter tip is in bladder or urethra. Further advancement of catheter ensures proper placement (Perry and Potter, 1998).

13. a. *Retention catheter:* hold catheter securely in place with nondominant hand until bladder is empty or urine specimen obtained (volume depends on test ordered).
  b. *Indwelling catheter:* Urine specimen can be collected. Then, while holding catheter securely in place with nondominant hand, use dominant hand to insert syringe into port and inflate catheter balloon (see illustration, p. 816) (Box 35-1).

Retention catheter is removed once urine is drained or collected.

Allows catheter to settle against neck of bladder.

Steps	Rationale

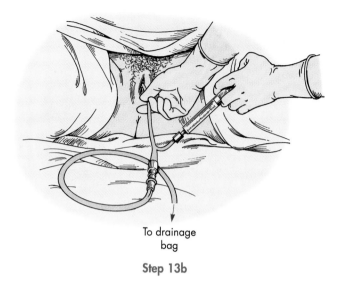

To drainage bag

Step 13b

Box 35-1 Inflation of Balloon for Indwelling Catheter

Inflate indwelling catheter with amount of fluid recommended by the manufacturer.

a. While holding catheter with thumb and little finger of nondominant hand at urethral meatus, take end of catheter and place it between first two fingers of nondominant hand.
b. With free dominant hand, attach syringe to injection port at end of catheter.
c. Slowly inject total amount of solution. If client complains with sudden pain, aspirate solution and advance catheter farther.
d. Release catheter and pull gently to feel resistance. Then move catheter slightly back into bladder.

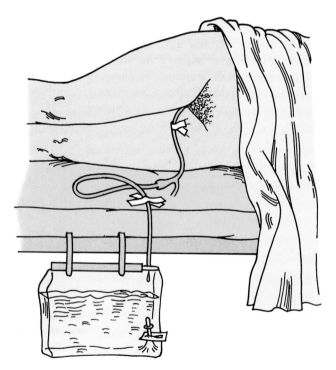

Step 15a

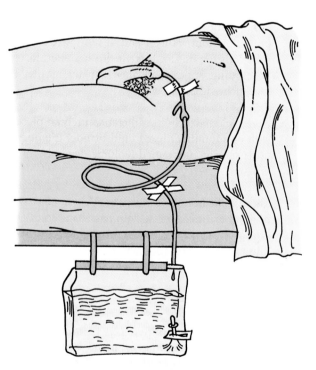

Step 15b

Steps	Rationale
14. Remove straight catheter, pulling slowly but evenly.	Reduces trauma to urethra.
15. Secure indwelling catheter and attach to drainage bag.	Proper taping prevents pulling on catheter and possible trauma to urethra.
a. **Female:** Secure to inner thigh with nonallergenic tape or catheter strap (see illustration, *A*). Allow for slack so movement of thigh does not create tension on catheter.	
b. **Male:** Secure to top of thigh or lower abdomen with tape or catheter strap (see illustration, *B*). Replace foreskin if present.	
16. Position drainage bag lower than bladder and coil tubing on bed.	Prevents reflux of urine. Catheter drains by gravity.
17. Cleanse and dry perineal area. Position client for comfort.	Povidone iodine is irritating to skin.
18. Measure urine.	Monitors output as baseline assessment.
19. See Completion Protocol (inside front cover).	

• • •

EVALUATION

1. Palpate bladder and observe urine in catheter bag for amount, color, and clarity.
2. Ask client if comfortable.
3. Measure intake and output per routine.

Unexpected Outcomes and Related Interventions

1. Client complains of discomfort during inflation of balloon.
   a. Stop immediately—if not advanced far enough in urethra, could cause serious trauma to urethra.
   b. Advance another 1 inch (2.5 cm) and reattempt inflation.
   c. If client sill complains of pain, remove catheter and report to physician.
2. Catheter does not insert easily into urethra.
   a. For male, reposition penis toward head of client and retract (pull) gently and attempt reinsertion.
   b. For male and female, have client take deep breaths to relax and attempt reinsertion.
   c. Never force if still unable to advance. Remove and report to physician.
3. Catheter goes into vagina.
   a. Leave catheter in vagina.
   b. Reclean urinary meatus. With another sterile catheter, insert catheter into meatus.
   c. Remove catheter in vagina after inserting second catheter in bladder.
4. Sterility is broken during catheterization by nurse or client.
   a. Replace gloves if contaminated and start over.
   b. If client places foot or body part in sterile field, but not on equipment, do not use that part of the sterile field.
   c. If client touches equipment, nurse *must* replace with sterile items or replace with new kit and start over.

Recording and Reporting

• Report and record type and size of catheter inserted, amount of fluid used to inflate balloon, characteristics of urine, amount of urine, reasons for catheterization, specimen collection, and, if appropriate, client's response to procedure and teaching concepts.
• Initiate I&O records.

Sample Documentation

0800 Bladder distended 4 cm above symphysis pubis. C/O full sensation but unable to void. #18 Fr catheter inserted. 700 ml of clear yellow urine returned. Tolerated with "mild discomfort." Bladder nondistended, lower abdomen soft. Catheter to bedside drainage with client on rt. side.

Geriatric Considerations

- A client with a catheter is especially vulnerable to UTI. The frail older adult client who is physically compromised runs the additional risk of developing septicemia, a life-threatening infection that has spread to the blood. The client who is incontinent should not be routinely catheterized.
- An adequate oral fluid intake of 2000 ml/day and assisting the older adult to toilet on a regular timed basis will help bladder retraining and minimize the need for excessive catheterization.
- Attached equipment such as a catheter may make it more likely that the older adult will not be fully ambulatory, thereby increasing the risks associated with decreased mobility. When catheters are required, they should be removed as soon as the client's condition allows.

Home and Long-Term Care Considerations

- Clients who are at home may use a leg bag during the day and switch to a large-volume bag at night so that sleep can remain uninterrupted.
- Clients may catheterize themselves at home on an intermittent basis using clean technique. Self-catheterization has been shown to be successful in maintaining continence and results in fewer infections than with the use of indwelling catheters.

Skill 35.2

URINARY DIVERSIONS (CONTINENT AND INCONTINENT)

Urinary diversions are surgical procedures performed on clients who have partial or complete excision of the bladder (cystectomies) because of malignancies or trauma to the bladder. Urinary diversions are ostomies, or openings, coming from the bladder, ureters, or kidneys to the outer wall of the abdomen (Figure 35-2). Urine is rerouted through the urinary diversion instead of the bladder.

There are two types of urinary diversions. The first type or continent diversion consists of an internal pouch or reservoir for urine, surgically created from a segment of the bowel. The stoma has a muscular closure or nipple valve similar to the meatus sphincter so urine does not leak involuntarily. The client will need to self-catheterize or intubate every 4 to 6 hours but will not need to wear an external appliance. Irrigation of the reservoir will also be necessary because mucus is always secreted from pouches constructed from the bowel. When the catheter is not in use, a small gauze pad covers the stoma to protect the client's clothes from mucus drainage.

Examples of continent diversions are the Kock, Mainz, Indiana, and Florida pouches. The main difference between the various diversions are the segments of bowel used (Lewis and Collier, 1996). If the urethra is not diseased, a "neobladder" may be created by attaching a portion of the large bowel to the urethra. The result is closer to normal anatomy (Bradley and Pupiales, 1997). Conti-

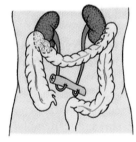

Ileal loop

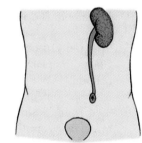

Single ureterostomy

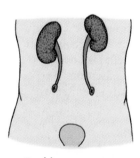

Double ureterostomy

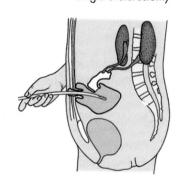

Continent urinary diversion

Figure 35-2 Types of urinary diversions.

nence can be a problem with this procedure, and the client may have to be taught how to self-catheterize. Despite this difficulty there is a greater acceptance rate among clients because normal anatomy is maintained.

During the immediate postoperative period, ureteral stents extend from the renal pelves through the ureters and through the reservoir, conduit, or neobladder. They exit through the stoma and are usually contained in the pouch. A catheter is also placed to keep the internal reservoir drained for 2 to 3 weeks. Both stents and catheter are removed once adequate healing has occurred. With reservoirs, clients must learn to drain and irrigate the reservoir at regular intervals before discharge from the hospital (Black and Matassarin-Jacobs, 1997).

The second type of urinary diversion is an *incontinent* urinary diversion, such as the ileal conduit (ureter transplanted into a closed-off portion of the ileum, which has one opening going to the outer wall of the abdomen) and ureterostomy (opening from the ureter to the abdomen's outer wall). The diversions require pouching continuously. The pouch must be emptied frequently, and the adhesive holding the pouch may cause skin irritation. Numerous products on the market are available for pouching and skin barrier protection. Check your agency's protocol and client preference.

Incontinent and continent urinary diversions affect the body image of clients. The nurse may have to help the client deal with psychological problems as well as care of the stoma. Clients should be informed that the stoma will continue to shrink for approximately 1 year.

Equipment (see Figure 34-2, p. 795)
   Clean gloves
   Washcloth, towel, nonmoisturizing soap, and water
   Underpad
For incontinent diversions
   Scissors with pointed end
   Measuring guide
   Tissue or toilet paper
   Gauze pad or tampon
   New pouch and adhesive if required
For continent diversions, varies with recovery phase, postoperative care to 3 weeks
- Sterile normal saline solution (NS)
- Sterile catheter-tipped irrigating syringe
- Sterile gauze pads
- Sterile gloves
- Povidone-iodine swabs
- Sterile specimen cup
- Sterile water
- Towels
Postoperative care 4 to 6 weeks:
- Sterile NS
- Sterile catheter-tipped irrigating syringe
- Sterile gauze pads
- Sterile gloves

- Povidone-iodine swabs
- Sterile basin
- Sterile 14 to 16 Fr red rubber catheter
- Water-soluble lubricant
- Stoma cover (commercial or Band-Aid or nonstick dressing)
- Liquid antimicrobial soap
- Towels

ASSESSMENT

1. Observe location of stoma and type of appliance in use. (If first time and no pouch selected, consider location and size of stoma, client's age and weight, activity level, and financial situation.)
2. Observe stoma site for color (pink with no erythema or necrotic tissue), moistness, or irritation, and check peristomal skin for maceration. Inspect all external suture lines for healing progress.
3. Observe and palpate skin around stoma for erythema, excoriation, edema, and drainage. **Rationale:** Determines need for skin barrier.
4. Assess client's ability and willingness to learn self-care. **Rationale: The nurse must ensure that client or significant other can comprehend and follow directions and that he or she understands the importance of following protocol for care of urinary diversions to prevent infections, irritation of peristomal skin and stoma, and obstruction of urine flow.**

PLANNING

Expected outcomes focus on maintaining urine flow and stoma and skin integrity.

Expected Outcomes
1. Client's urine output is maintained at 30 ml per hour.
2. Client's stoma remains red, shiny, moist, and free of erythema and purulent drainage.
3. Client's peristoma skin and suture line are intact.
4. Client and/or primary caregiver correctly cares for stoma, skin, and pouch by discharge.

DELEGATION CONSIDERATIONS

Delegation of this skill is inappropriate because it requires knowledge and problem solving unique to a professional nurse. One exception in some agencies is pouching of established ostomies. AP should be instructed to report any leakage of urine and/or breakdown of skin integrity to the professional nurse.

IMPLEMENTATION

Steps	Rationale

1. See Standard Protocol (inside front cover).
2. Position client to allow for easy access to stoma so that abdomen is as smooth or flat as possible. Be sure client can view procedure.
   For continent diversion, client should be supine or sitting.
3. Continent urinary diversion (postoperative care up to 3 weeks)
   a. Set up sterile supplies on work surface and put on sterile gloves.
   b. Note presence or absence of ureteral stents.

> **NURSE ALERT**
>
> *Pouch should be changed every 3 to 7 days and emptied when ⅓ to ½ full. Apply protective barrier to healthy skin only, if used (contains alcohol).*

> **NURSE ALERT**
>
> *Hospital protocols vary; generally, immediately after surgery, continent diversions are irrigated every 2 to 4 hours to maintain patency of the stomal catheter, allowing urine to drain freely. Stomal catheter is usually removed the third week.*

c. Draw 20 to 30 ml sterile NS into syringe. Cleanse connection of indwelling stoma catheter and drainage to be with povidone-iodine swabs using a circular motion; use each swab once.

    This prevents nosocomial infections.

d. Disconnect catheter, insert syringe, and gently irrigate stomal catheter; do not contaminate tip of drainage tubing.

    Internal anastomotic sites require strict asepsis during postoperative phase (Perry and Potter, 1998).

e. Reconnect drainage system. Record volume used for irrigation, and subtract this from total urine output at the end of each shift.

    This computes actual urine output.

4. **Continent urinary diversion** (postoperative care of 4 to 6 weeks)
   a. Set up sterile supplies and apply sterile gloves. Draw 30 to 60 ml of sterile NS into syringe. Cleanse "face" of stoma with povidone-iodine swab starting from center and using circular movements to outer edge; wait 30 seconds.

    This reduces risk of nosocomial infection and removes any accumulation of mucus (Perry and Potter, 1998).

   b. Lubricate catheter well with water-soluble lubricant. Insert into stoma by gently rotating during insertion; insert until urine starts to drain. Some resistance to insertion is normal, client may need to change position or take slow, deep breaths to facilitate insertion (Perry and Potter, 1998).

    This reduces trauma to continence mechanism (valve) during insertion.

   c. If this is a scheduled time for irrigation, proceed after urine has drained by irrigating with 30 to 60 ml of sterile NS; allow to drain.

    Continent diversions must be irrigated at scheduled times because mucus is always produced (Perry and Potter, 1998).

   d. Before withdrawing catheter, have the client cough 3 or 4 times, then slowly remove.

    Positive pressure inside the abdomen clears residual urine from the pouch and continence valve (Perry and Potter, 1998).

   e. Gently cleanse the peristomal skin with gauze pads and liquid antimicrobial soap; rinse; pat dry.

    This reduces bacterial colonization and removes any dry mucus to maintain skin integrity (Perry and Potter, 1998).

   f. Cover stoma with gauze dressing.

    Until full recovery from surgery, some leakage will occur; mucus will always be produced.

   g. Record output and amount used for irrigation.

    This keeps accurate output record.

Steps	Rationale

5. Continent urinary diversion, (fully recovered client)
   a. Intubate (or be intubated if unable to do so) every 4 to 6 hours and prn at night; irrigate bid and prn. Physician's protocols may vary.

Regular intubation times allow for gradual expansion of the pouch. Pouches or reservoirs vary as to maximum amount of urine they can hold after complete recovery; the amount may range from 150 to 600 ml. Routine irrigations are necessary because reservoirs constructed from bowel always secrete mucus (Perry and Potter, 1998).

   b. Keep schedule of intubation and irrigation times at bedside. A time card at the bedside will facilitate this.

Client, family, and all caregivers should be aware of scheduled times.

COMMUNICATION TIP

This is a good time to review home care measures. Tell client that uric acid crystals may collect on skin. Explain, "Use a washcloth with a vinegar soak (⅓ white vinegar and ⅔ water) to the skin around the stoma.

Rinse with warm tap water." Also reinforce importance of reporting fever, chills, back or flank pain, or cloudy, foul-smelling urine to the physician as soon as possible.

6. Incontinent urinary diversion
   a. Prepare new pouch.
      (1) It may be possible to measure stoma size without removing pouch. If not, apply clean gloves and follow steps 6b(1–5).

Accurate stoma measurement for appliance ring is necessary to prevent leakage and damage to stoma.

      (2) Use measuring guide to cut appliance ring so margin around stoma and pouch is ¹/₁₆ to ⅛ inch (Perry and Potter, 1998). Do not leave a tight margin that might cut stoma.

Protect skin.

      (3) Check drainage valve on pouch.
      (4) Remove protective covering over adhesive ring (see illustration).

Prevents leakage.

      (5) Have all equipment ready to decrease leakage of urine when removing old pouch and applying new one.

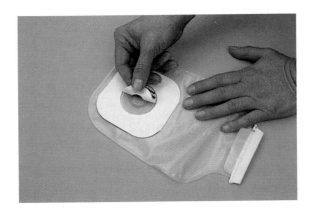

Step 6a(4)

Steps	Rationale

b. Replace pouch.
   (1) 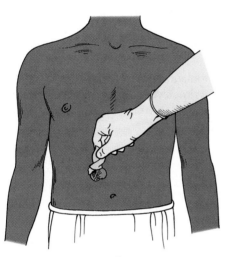 Place towel or disposable waterproof barrier under client.
   (2) Remove old pouch and place in plastic bag.
   (3) Remove any drainage and/or urine on stoma or around catheter (if in use) with tissue.

   Prevents skin irritation.

   (4) Apply a rolled gauze pad or tampon over stoma while cleaning around stoma (see illustration).

   Wicking collects urine and prevents leakage on skin and bed linens.

   (5) Cleanse area around stoma with nonmoisturizing soap and water, and pat dry.

   For better pouch adherence (Bradley and Pupiales, 1997).

   (6) Apply prepared pouch over stoma or catheter and hold pressure for 5 minutes.

   Helps to adhere pouch to skin. Skin barriers help protect peristomal skin from breakdown.

   (7) If skin barriers or additional adhesives are used, apply before pouch placement. Remove and dispose of gloves and wash hands.

Step 6b(4)

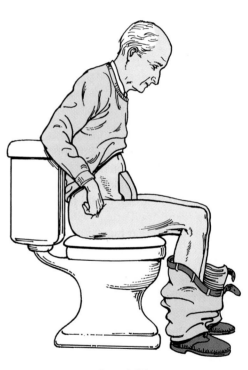

Step 6c(1)

c. Empty pouch.
   (1) 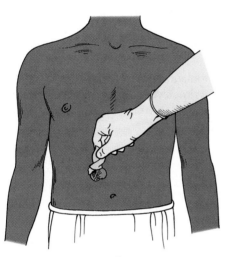 Place client on toilet or commode and put pouch valve end between legs or hold container under valve and empty (see illustration).
   (2) Rinse pouch with tepid tap water (may use perineal bottle) (see illustration).
   (3) After rinsing, pat valve dry and close. Remove and dispose of gloves and wash hands.
7. Allow client time to ask questions regarding procedure.
8. See Completion Protocol (inside front cover).

• • •

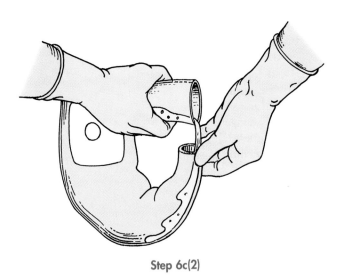

Step 6c(2)

EVALUATION

1. Observe urine output through stoma: urine is free flowing and greater than 240 ml every 8 hours.
2. Inspect and palpate stoma for color, shine, moistness, erythema, edema, or tenderness.
3. Observe peristomal skin for excoriation or erythema. If suture line present, inspect for approximation and signs of inflammation.
4. Observe client demonstrating pouch care during next change.

Unexpected Outcomes and Related Interventions

1. Output from pouch is less than anticipated.
   a. Use problem-solving method below (Figure 35-3) (Perry and Potter, 1998):
2. Skin irritation around stoma: itching and burning (usually from improperly fitted pouch).
   a. Remove pouch immediately.
   b. Cleanse area with nonmoisturizing soap and water and pat dry.
   c. If lotion or moisturizer used to ease irritation, use a dissolving base so adhesive will adhere.
   d. Apply new pouch.
3. Odors are coming from pouch.
   a. If pouch is leaking, change complete pouch.
   b. Increase intake of cranberry juice, ascorbic acid, protein, grains, and cereals. (This will acidify the urine and decrease odor and potential for infection.)
4. Client will not participate in care of stoma.
   a. Give psychological support to client's feelings.
   b. Contact local support group with physician's approval.
   c. Guard against displaying disapproval or disgust while caring for client.
5. Continence valve leaks excessively and continuously after stomal catheter is removed. Dysfunction of

valve is major complication that may result from stricture of stoma, incomplete healing, anastomotic leaks, failure to empty reservoir at scheduled times (overdistention), and damage from improper catheter insertion (perforation).
   a. Notify charge nurse and physician.
   b. Protect skin from excoriation while seeking help.

Recording and Reporting

- Record type of pouch, time of change, condition and appearance of stoma and peristomal skin, character of urine, time of irrigation and/or intubation, and client response.
- Record actual urinary output (subtract irrigation from volume measured to obtain amount). Note characteristics of urine.
- Document client's, family's, or significant other's verbal and nonverbal reaction to stoma and level of participation.
- Report abnormalities in stoma or peristomal structures and absence or decrease in urinary output to nurse in charge or physician.

Sample Documentation

0800 Pouch changed on ileal conduit, client assisted with handling supplies. Stoma is shiny, moist, and beefy red. Peristomal skin has no excoriation, erythema, or drainage. 250 ml of clear yellow urine. Cleansed with soap and water. Client correctly reapplied pouch.

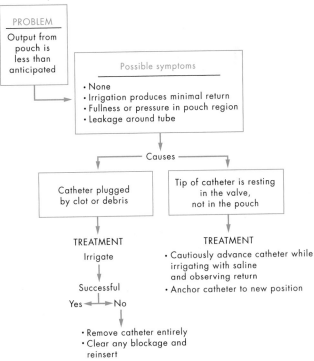

Figure 35-3 Problem solving when output from the pouch is less than anticipated. *Modified from Hull, Erwin-Toth* Journal of WOCN, 1996, Mosby.

Geriatric Considerations

- Some older clients feel that they can cope with the continuous flow of urine from the stoma by decreasing the amount of fluid they drink so they will have less output. This can be very dangerous because older adults are more susceptible to fluid imbalance. Client needs appropriate teaching to change this misconception.
- Limitations in physical and visual ability may require adjustments in self-ostomy routine.

Home Care and Long-Term Care Considerations

1. Care of continent diversions
   - Teach clients to *not* use petroleum-based products for lubricating the catheter, because this increases the risk of infection; client may use plain warm tap water or water-soluble lubricant (preferred). May use plain warm tap water to irrigate after week 6 (this may vary with physician's protocol).
   - Taking deep breaths facilitates intubation, because it helps to relax abdominal muscles; massaging the lower abdomen aids emptying; coughing periodically while draining effluent helps clear mucus from catheter because of increasing positive pressure.
   - Keeping a small card in pocket or purse with time schedule for intubation and irrigation is a helpful reminder.
   - Client may use moist towel or nonalcohol towelette to cleanse face of stoma before intubation; may use catheter-tipped syringe or bulb syringe for irrigation.
   - Client can sit on stool or stand next to a sink to perform irrigation and intubation. Teach client to not let end of catheter come in contact with fixtures or water in toilet or sink.
   - Teach clients proper care of intubation catheters: After use, rinse inside to clear any mucus and wash with warm, soapy water; rinse well inside and out; suspend catheter so that it hangs to dry. Dry completely and keep in a clean plastic bag or toothbrush holder container.

   - Clients must always carry their catheter with them.
   - Discard catheter after 1 month's use.
2. Care of incontinent diversions
   - At home, pouch spout should be opened and connected to straight drainage at night. Make sure client understands that using the wrong adaptor piece causes leakage.
   - Many different types of one-piece and two-piece pouching systems are available. All disposable pouches are odor proof, and most have an anti-reflux valve. Clients should be encouraged to find a pouch that they can apply easily and that satisfies them.
   - Clients should avoid placing pouches in extremely hot or cold locations, because temperature may affect the barrier and adhesive materials.
   - Pouch covers are available or can be easily made. Special underwear and sleep garments are also available.
   - Advise clients when they travel to always keep spare ostomy supplies with them in case luggage gets lost.
   - While swimming, clients may find that applying waterproof tape to the skin barrier and/or wearing an ostomy belt prevents the pouch and skin barrier from becoming dislodged.
3. All diversions
   - Client must always wear Medic-Alert bracelet or necklace.

Skill 35.3

CONTINUOUS BLADDER IRRIGATION

Continuous bladder irrigation (CBI) requires a physician's order and must be performed using sterile technique. CBI is a continuous infusion of a sterile solution into the bladder, usually using a three-way irrigation set and a triple-lumen catheter, which has three ports (Figure 35-4). One port goes to the client to drain urine, one goes to the irrigation solution, and one is used to inflate the catheter balloon (Figure 35-5). The primary use of CBI is to keep an indwelling catheter patent and free of blood clots or sediment. CBI is frequently ordered after bladder surgeries.

The physician must order the solution, strength, and flow rate. If the physician only specifies solution, check your agency's protocol for strength and rate. The irrigation solution infuses continuously through one port while the second port drains the urine and irrigation solution.

Equipment
Clean gloves
Irrigation solution and tubing
IV pole
Antiseptic swab

ASSESSMENT
1. Assess client's level of consciousness and ability to cooperate.
2. Palpate bladder for distention and tenderness. **Rationale: This indicates flow of urine may be blocked from draining (Perry & Potter, 1998).**
3. Ask client about the presence of bladder pain or spasms. **Rationale: Blood clots will cause bladder spasms and may be too large to come through the irrigation catheter lumen. This is one way to determine whether the irrigation solution's rate should be increased.**

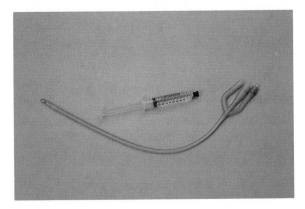

Figure 35-4 *From bottom:* Triple lumen catheter with sterile syringe to inflate catheter balloon.

4. Observe urine for color, amount, clarity, and presence of mucus, clots, or sediment. **Rationale: This indicates if client is bleeding or sloughing tissue and determines necessity for increasing irrigation rate (Perry and Potter, 1998).**
5. Compare amount of irrigation solution infused with urine output. **Rationale: A blood clot may obstruct the catheter and not allow urine and the irrigation solution to flow from the bladder. If irrigation solution still infuses into the bladder, the bladder may become overdistended and rupture.**
6. Review I&O record. **Rationale: This determines baseline for prior output measures.**
7. Assess client's knowledge regarding purpose of performing catheter irrigation. **Rationale: This reveals need for client instruction.**

PLANNING
Expected outcomes focus on continuous urine flow and client comfort.

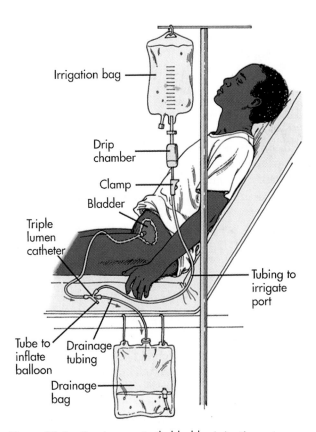

Figure 35-5 Continuous sterile bladder irrigation setup.

Irrigation bag

Drip chamber

Clamp

Bladder

Triple lumen catheter

Tubing to irrigate port

Tube to inflate balloon

Drainage tubing

Drainage bag

Expected Outcomes

1. Client's urine drains freely (at least 30 ml/hr). (NOTE: Urine will be bloody following bladder/urethral surgery, gradually becoming lighter and blood tinged in 2 to 3 days.)
2. Client's urine output has decreased blood clots and sediment.
3. Client does not complain of bladder pain or spasms.
4. Client is free from infection.

IMPLEMENTATION

Steps	Rationale
1. See Standard Protocol (inside front cover).	
2. Place label on irrigation solution bag with client's name, room number, date, and time. Mark bag for GU IRRIGATION ONLY in red, type of solution, and any additives.	Indicates fluid is not to be infused intravenously.
3. Prepare the solution (must maintain sterility).	
a. Close clamp on tubing and spike the bag with the tubing.	
b. Place bag on an IV pole.	
c. Fill the drip chamber one-half full by squeezing the chamber.	
d. Open the clamp to completely fill tubing and remove air.	Air will cause bladder fullness and spasms.
e. Close the clamp and maintain sterility.	
4. Wipe off irrigation port of triple-lumen catheter with antiseptic swab and connect to irrigation tubing aseptically.	
5. Remove gloves.	
6. Adjust rate at roller clamp (according to physician's orders or agency protocol).	
7. If urine is bright red or has clots, increase irrigation rate until clears.	Assists with clotting active bleeding in bladder and flushes clots out of bladder.
8. Change irrigation solution as needed.	
9. Using gloves, empty catheter bag as needed.	Bag will fill rapidly and may need to be emptied every 1-2 hrs.
10. Compare urine output with irrigation solution's infusion every hour.	May overdistend bladder if irrigant and urine do not flow from bladder.
11. See Completion Protocol (inside front cover).	

NURSE ALERT

Irrigation solution and tubing should be changed every 24 hours to decrease potential for infection.

• • • •

EVALUATION

1. Measure client's *urine* output by subtracting total irrigating solution used from total drainage in bag.
2. Observe client's urine for blood clots and sediment.
3. Ask if client is experiencing pain and assess for fever.
4. Monitor for fever. Inspect urine for cloudiness or foul odor.

Unexpected Outcomes and Related Interventions

1. Irrigation solution will not infuse or is slower than previous set.
   a. Check for kinks in the tubing.
   b. Assess for clots or sediment obstruction (may need to irrigate manually; follow agency protocol).
   c. Readjust height of IV pole and readjust clamp.

2. Irrigant going in but not being returned.
   a. Assess for clots and manually irrigate with 50 ml sterile NS "using gentle pressure" (or follow agency protocol).
   b. Assess client for bladder spasms and distended bladder (may need antispasmodics).
   c. Notify physician or charge nurse.
3. Signs of fever or cloudy, foul urine.
   a. Send urinalysis and urine for culture and sensitivity to laboratory.
   b. Notify physician or charge nurse.
4. Bright-red bleeding occurs even with irrigation drip wide open.
   a. Assess for hypovolemic shock (vital signs, color and moisture on skin, anxiety level).
   b. Leave irrigation drip wide open and call physician or charge nurse.
5. Client has bladder spasms.
   a. Reassure and try methods to relax: apply warm cloth to lower abdomen, use heating pad (with order), flex knees to 45 degrees, and reposition catheter. Ensure catheter and tubing are not kinked and tubing is coiled on the bed to facilitate drainage by gravity.
   b. Administer ordered urinary antispasmodics.
   c. If unrelieved, call physician.

Recording and Reporting
- Record amount and type of solution used as irrigant, amount returned as drainage, characteristics of output, and urine output of drainage in nurses' notes and I&O sheet.
- Report catheter occlusion, sudden bleeding, infection, or increased pain to physician.
  Bleeding is common after transurethral prostatectomy. Nurse should expect bright red–tinged urine during first 48 hours postoperatively followed by pink-tinged to clear urine by fifth postoperative day.

Sample Documentation
0800   Lower abdomen soft and flat, catheter to bedside drainage with 225 ml of bright-red urine with moderate-size dark bloody clots passing 3000 ml of NS to irrigation port infusing at 60 gtt per minute. Client rates spasms at a 5 on a 0 to 10 scale (with 10 the worst). Lying on lt. side, knees flexed.

Geriatric Considerations

- Benign prostatic hypertrophy is common as men age, and surgical intervention on the prostate gland may be required. After surgery, continuous and rapid irrigation of the bladder with a three-way Foley catheter is often necessary to prevent clotting and obstruction of the catheter.

Home Care and Long-Term Care Considerations

- Assess the client and primary caregiver for ability and motivation to perform catheter irrigation.
- Assess client's environment for appropriate storage space for materials needed for procedure.
- Observe client and primary caregiver while they perform procedure.
- Refer client to home care agency for in-home follow-up.
- Instruct client and primary caregiver to observe urine daily for changes in color, presence of mucus or blood, and changes in consistency and odor.
- Instruct client to maintain adequate oral intake of 2 L per day (unless contraindicated).

Skill 35.4

SUPRAPUBIC CATHETERS

Suprapubic catheters are inserted by physicians either at the bedside with the client under local anesthesia or while in surgery under general anesthesia. An incision is made through the abdominal wall above the symphysis pubis (Figure 35-6). Benefits of suprapubic catheters are (1) lower incidence of urinary infection, (2) client is able to void naturally when suprapubic catheter is clamped, and (3) client experiences more comfort when ambulating and can handle catheter easier.

Disadvantages of suprapubic catheters include (1) they require physician to insert through abdominal wall and (2) they must be cleansed each day using sterile technique and supplies.

The nurse is responsible for maintaining the suprapubic catheter and teaching the client about the catheter before discharge. Numerous suprapubic catheters and appliances are available. They may be attached to the skin with sutures or adhesive material.

Equipment

Clean gloves	Antiseptic swabs
Sterile gloves	Split gauze
Gauze	Nonallergenic tape
Antiseptic solution	Plastic bag

ASSESSMENT

1. Assess client's level of consciousness and ability to cooperate.
2. Assess old dressing for drainage (color, odor, amount). **Rationale: Drainage indicates potential complication of infection.**

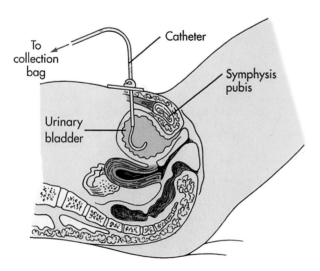

Figure 35-6 Suprapubic catheter.

3. Assess catheter insertion site for erythema, edema, drainage, and odor. **Rationale: This may indicate potential infection. If insertion site is new, slight inflammation may be expected as part of wound healing.**
4. Assess urine in catheter or bag for color, clarity, and odor. **Rationale: Abnormal findings may indicate potential complications like urinary tract infection, decreased urinary output, and blockage.**
5. Assess for increase in body temperature. **Rationale: Infection at the suprapubic catheter site or of the urinary tract may cause an elevated body temperature.**
6. Assess how catheter is held in place. **Rationale: Catheter may be sutured or retained by a commercial body seal.**
7. Assess tape site for signs of irritation. **Rationale: Client may be sensitive to tape or antiseptic solution.**

PLANNING

Expected outcomes focus on prevention of infection, maintaining the integrity of the client's urinary system, and maintaining client's level of comfort.

Expected Outcomes

1. Client's urine is free from odor, sediment, and bacteria.
2. Client's urine culture remains free of bacterial infection by discharge.
3. Client remains afebrile.
4. Client's catheter site is free of erythema, edema, discharge, or tenderness.
5. Client's catheter is patent, and output is 30 ml or greater per hour.
6. Client verbalizes signs and symptoms of urinary tract infection and insertion site infection by discharge.
7. Client correctly demonstrates care for insertion site by discharge.
8. Client's level of discomfort is 4 or less (scale of 0 to 10).

DELEGATION CONSIDERATIONS

The skill of caring for a suprapubic catheter requires the knowledge and decision-making skills unique to the professional nurse and is not usually delegated to AP.

IMPLEMENTATION

Steps	Rationale

1. See Standard Protocol (inside front cover).
2. 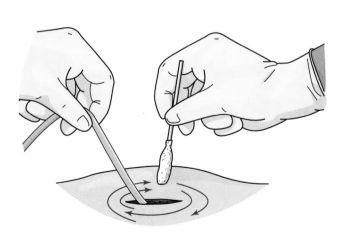 Position client so that catheter site can be seen easily.
3. Remove old dressing and place dressing and gloves in bag.
4. Put on sterile gloves.
5. Assess insertion site and patency of catheter (see assessment).

6. Maintaining sterility, clean site by swabbing in circular motion starting closest to the catheter site and continuing in outward widening circles for approximately 2 inches (5 cm) (see illustration). If necessary, use nondominant sterile gloved hand to hold catheter erect while cleaning.

   Follows principle of sterile technique to move from area of least contamination to area of most contamination. (Perry and Potter, 1998).

7. Perform Step 6 as many times as needed to cleanse site.

COMMUNICATION TIP

During cleansing routine, caution client about risk for infection. Explain, "It is important to drink at least 6 glasses of fluids daily." Also show client how to keep drainage bag below level of bladder.

8. Take one gauze pad moistened in antiseptic solution and cleanse catheter from proximal to distal.

   Cleanses organisms off catheter that could migrate to site.

9. With sterile gloved hand, apply split gauze around catheter and tape in place.
10. Secure catheter to abdomen with tape or Velcro multipurpose tube holder to reduce tension on insertion site.

    Secures catheter and reduces risk of excessive tension on suture and/or body seal (Perry and Potter, 1998).

11. Ensure bag and catheter junctions are securely in place.

    Prevents leakage of urine or organisms from entering bladder.

12. Ask client if there are any questions about catheter care.
13. See Completion Protocol (inside front cover).

• • •

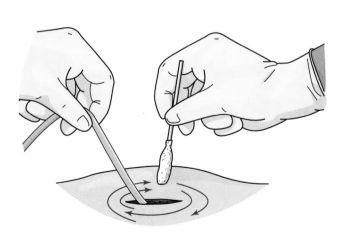

Step 6

EVALUATION

1. Observe client's urine for sediment or unusual odor.
2. Review laboratory urine culture and sensitivity for presence of bacteria.
3. Monitor body temperature and elevated white blood cell count.
4. Observe catheter insertion site.
5. Monitor suprapubic catheter output.
6. Ask client to state signs and symptoms of urinary tract infection and insertion site infection.
7. Observe client demonstrate care of insertion site.
8. Ask client to rate discomfort (scale of 0 to 10).

Unexpected Outcomes and Related Interventions

1. Urine through catheter is obstructed (may be caused by blood clots, catheter tip against wall of bladder, or sediment collection).
   a. Call physician for irrigation orders.
   b. Increase fluids (if not contraindicated) to at least 1500 ml/day.
2. Client has urinary tract infection or catheter site infection.
   a. Increase fluids to at least 1500 ml/day (if not contraindicated).
   b. Increase protein, cereal, and grain foods to increase acidity of urine, and increase intake of cranberry juice.
   c. Perform good handwashing and use sterile technique for catheter care.
   d. Monitor body temperature and notify physician for temperatures greater than 101° F (38.3° C).
   e. Follow agency or CDC protocol and culture drainage at site of catheter.
3. Catheter becomes dislodged.
   a. Apply sterile gauze to site.
   b. Apply pressure if bleeding.
   c. Reassure client.
   d. Notify physician.
4. When catheter clamped, client complaints of distended bladder before time to release clamp.
   a. Release clamp and drain no more than 1000 ml of urine at one time.
   b. Recalculate time for clamping, if off schedule.

Recording and Reporting

- Report and record dressing replacement including assessments of wound and tolerance of client to dressing.
- Report any unexpected outcomes.

Sample Documentation

0800 Client alert and awake, old dressing removed from suprapubic catheter site with small amount of dark-brown drainage on gauze with no unusual odor. Site has no redness, edema, or drainage. Cleaned with povidone-iodine swabs around site. Redressed with split gauze. Tolerated without complaints of discomfort. Side rails up × 4, in supine position.

Home Care and Long-Term Care Considerations

- With shortened hospital stays it is common for the postsurgery client to go home with a suprapubic catheter.
- Teach client or caregiver how to clean and dress the suprapubic site.
- Teach client or caregiver how to empty a catheter bag and assess urine for color, odor, clarity, and amount.

CRITICAL THINKING EXERCISES

1. Mrs. Smith is 1 day postpartum and has been having difficulty voiding. She was catheterized 8 hours ago for 750 ml of urine. She currently is complaining of not being able to pass her urine, and she has abdominal pain. The physician's order states that the client can be catheterized every 8 hours if unable to void and to insert an indwelling catheter for a volume of urine greater than 200 ml. What assessments would you make to determine the client's bladder status? What information would you need before proceeding with the procedure?

2. Mr. Jones is undergoing continuous bladder irrigation following prostate surgery, 6 hours ago. What assessments are important at this time? What color would you expect the urine to be at this time and 3 days from now? How would the nurse plan for the client's discharge?

3. While cleansing around a client's incontinent urinary diversion stoma, the nurse notes the peristomal skin to be inflamed and macerated. What might be the cause? What actions might the nurse take to relieve skin impairment?

REFERENCES

Black I, Matassarin-Jacobs E: *Medical-surgical nursing: clinical management for continuity of care,* ed 3, Philadelphia, 1997, WB Saunders.

Bradley M, Pupiales M: Essential elements of ostomy care, *Am J Nurs* 97(7):38–45, 1997.

Davey F: Myths surrounding use of urinary catheters: a summary of key beliefs that inhibit acute care nurses from altering their use of indwelling catheters, *Can J Infect Control* 9(2):39, 1994.

Hull TL, Erwin-Toth P: The pelvic pouch procedure and continent ostomies: overview and controversies, *JWOCN* 23(3):156, 1996.

Hutchinson M: Caring for a patient with ileal or colon conduit, *J Urol Nurs* 14(2):1009–1014, 1995.

Lewis S, Collier I: *Medical-surgical nursing: assessment and management of clinical problems,* ed 4, St Louis, 1996, Mosby.

Mekresh M et al: Double folded rectosigmoid bladder with a new ureterocolic antireflux technique, *J Urol* 157:2085–2089, 1997.

Perry P, Potter P: *Clinical nursing skills & techniques,* ed 4, St Louis, 1998, Mosby.

CHAPTER 36

Altered Sensory Perception

Skill 36.1
Caring for Clients with Contact Lenses, 833

Skill 36.2
Caring for an Eye Prosthesis, 839

Skill 36.3
Eye Irrigations, 842

Skill 36.4
Caring for Clients with Hearing Aids, 845

Skill 36.5
Ear Irrigations, 848

Meaningful sensory stimuli allow a person to learn about the environment and are necessary for healthy functioning and normal development. Many clients seeking health care have preexisting sensory alterations, whereas others might develop alterations after medical treatment. The nurse plays an important role in helping clients care for sensory aids such as contact lenses, hearing aids, and eye prosthetics. In addition, the nurse provides care, such as eye or ear irrigations, that promotes the integrity of sensory organs.

Whenever you care for clients with sensory alterations, safety is a priority. The nurse must be able to anticipate how the client's sensory alteration places the client at risk for injury. Orientation to any new environment, arranging an existing living environment to minimize safety hazards, and educating family and friends about ways to help clients adapt to sensory loss are just some of the interventions nurses may use.

In an acute care environment the nurse may need to provide clients more direct supervision. When assisting ambulation for a visually impaired client, the nurse should stand on the client's nondominant side approximately one step ahead, with the client lightly holding the nurse's arm. Items such as the call light, overbed table, and telephone should be placed within the client's reach and their locations described to the client. If a client has a hearing deficit, the nurse may need to ensure the client can understand caregivers' communication. Face the client before beginning to speak and to make sure there is enough light for the client to see the nurse's lips. By eliminating external noises; speaking in a slow, clear, normal tone of voice; and accentuating facial gestures, the nurse helps the client to hear correctly. Sign language, lipreading, writing with pad and pencil, or use of communication boards may be necessary for hearing-impaired clients. Family or friends should be taught these same techniques so that they can become a source of support.

Clients may be very sensitive about lens or prosthetic care. Accidental breakage or malfunction may seriously impair sensory function and threaten self-esteem if the client becomes dependent on others for assistance. Most clients have established routines for cleaning contact lenses or eye prostheses. Nurses should adapt to these routines as much as possible when administering care to clients. Likewise, clients should be encouraged to participate in care of sensory aids as much as possible. Careful handling of these devices is vital to avoid damage or injury.

A visual or hearing impairment may be caused by the presence of foreign bodies, irritants, or secretions. In the older adult or in clients who wear hearing aids, cerumen impaction can cause discomfort and further hearing loss. Inflammation or infection of the eyes may produce drainage or secretions that reduce vision. Irrigation of the eye or ear may help restore or maintain existing function. The presence of a foreign body or irritant in the eye or ear requires immediate intervention to restore function and prevent possible permanent sensory loss.

◗ NURSING DIAGNOSES

An appropriate nursing diagnosis associated with a visual or hearing impairment is **Sensory/Perceptual Alterations. (Visual/Auditory),** in which clients experience a change in how they perceive and respond to environmental stimuli. Clients with a hearing loss may also have **Impaired Verbal Communication,** depending on their ability to use and understand language. Clients requiring irrigations of the eye or assistance with contact lenses or prostheses may be at **Risk for Infection** if the client does not use the proper technique. A client with a sensory impairment in an unfa- miliar environment, such as a hospital room, is especially at **Risk for Injury.** A nursing diagnosis of **Pain** may also apply when injury or infection involves the eye or ear. Clients who are unable to demonstrate proper care tech- niques may have a **Knowledge Deficit.** Visual or hearing impairments can also affect psychosocial status, resulting in **Impaired Social Interaction** or **Social Isolation.**

Skill 36.1

CARING FOR CLIENTS WITH CONTACT LENSES

For vision to occur, light must reach and stimulate the cells in the retina. A refractive error in the eye that results in light not falling directly on the retina indicates that a corrective lens is necessary for improving acuity. The con- tact lens provides the eye with a double cornea (Lake, 1996). As long as the contact lens is the correct size, shape, and fit it will bend the rays of light, allowing a clear pic- ture to be focused on the retina. The four types of contact lenses include rigid or hard, hard gas-permeable, soft, and disposable. Contact lenses are also available as daily wear and extended wear. Because an artificial surface is placed over the cornea, the risks of oxygen deprivation to corneal tissues and trauma are great. Selection of an appropriate lens should minimize these complications (Box 36-1).

Many contact lens–related complications have been linked to inappropriate lens care (Martin and Barr, 1997; Turner et al., 1993) or excessive wear. Conjunctivitis and corneal abrasions tend to be the most common problems for contact lens wearers (Lake, 1996). Proteins present in tears may build up on the surface of a lens. Unless re- moved by effective cleansing, these proteins will act as a culture medium for bacteria development (Elder and Daniel, 1993). Sight-threatening corneal keratitis (corneal infection) is the most severe complication caused by

Box 36-1 Types of Contact Lenses

Rigid Hard Lenses
- Impervious to oxygen; rely on pumping of tears into the space between lens and cornea during blinking to give oxygen to the cornea.
- Good vision correction
- Can be uncomfortable

Hard Gas-Permeable Lenses
- Durable and inexpensive
- Oxygen transmission lower than in soft lenses but higher than in rigid lenses
- Prone to deposit formation

Soft Contact Lenses
- Good oxygen transmission
- Water content and thickness of lenses affect refrac- tion, requiring appropriate fitting

Disposable Lenses
- Discarded after 1 day (daily) to 1 week (extended wear) of wear
- Less likely to build up deposits; reduce risk of aller- gies and infection
- If problems occur, user may change lens rather than seek medical advice

Data from Lake A: Prevention of complications related to contact lens wear, *Nurs Times* 92:36–38, 1996.

Box 36-2 Guidelines for Care and Wear of Contact Lenses

- Do not wear lenses beyond prescribed interval (daily removed overnight, should not be worn more than 10 to 14 hours; extended wear, should not be worn more than 6 consecutive nights).
- Before handling lenses, thoroughly wash and rinse hands. Shake hands dry or dry on lint-free towel.
- Be sure eye makeup does not come in contact with lens.
- When wearing soft lenses, never sleep in them or ex- ceed recommended wearing time.
- Do not swim or use a whirlpool bath while wearing lenses.
- Do not place lenses in your mouth to clean them.
- Do not use salt tablets.
- Disinfect daily wear lenses daily. Disinfect extended wear lenses when removed for cleaning.

Data from Lake A: Prevention of complications related to contact lens wear, *Nurs Times* 92:36–38, 1996.

Pseudomonas aeruginosa or the difficult-to-treat *Acanthamoeba*, which is found in common tap water. Box 36-2 on p. 833 lists guidelines for proper wear and care of contact lenses.

Nurses need to assess whether dependent clients wear contact lenses, especially those admitted to a hospital in an unresponsive or confused state. If a seriously ill client is wearing lenses that go undetected, severe corneal injury can result. Upon removal of any lens, labeling should include the client's name, room number, and the eye from which the lens was removed. Sterile saline can be used to soak the lens until the correct solution can be found.

Equipment

    Clean lens storage container
    Bath towel
    Small lens suction cup (optional)
    Sterile lens cleaning disinfectant solution (surfactant agents, 3% hydrogen peroxide preservative free)
    Sterile lens rinsing solution (sterile saline)
    Sterile enzyme solution (depends on care regimen)
    Sterile rewetting solution (depends on care regimen)
    Cotton ball or cotton-tipped applicator
    Emesis basin
    Disposable gloves

ASSESSMENT

1. Inspect the eye or ask client if contact lens is in place. **Rationale: Lenses are generally comfortable to wear, and client may forget they are in place.**
2. Ask client the following questions:
   How long do you normally wear your lenses on an average day?
   Do you wear the lenses overnight?
   What method of lens care do you use?
   How frequently do you clean and disinfect the lenses?
   When did you last clean and disinfect them? **Rationale: Determines client's compliance with lens care.**
3. Observe client's ability to manipulate and hold contact lens. **Rationale: Determines level of assistance required in care.**

4. Wearing gloves, inspect the eye and note presence of redness, tearing or watering, discharge, or swelling of eyelids or conjunctivae. Ask if client notices pain, burning, itching, reduced visual acuity, or blurred vision. **Rationale: Indicates signs and symptoms of infection, overwear of lenses, corneal abrasion, or sensitivity to lens care solutions** (Cohen and Krachmer, 1992; Martin and Barr, 1997).

PLANNING

Expected outcomes focus on maintaining vision, preventing ocular complications, and improving client's knowledge of lens care.

Expected Outcomes

1. Client verbalizes comfort after removal and reinsertion of lenses.
2. Client's eye shows no signs of ocular infection, injury, or overwear.
3. Client verbalizes improved visual perception after lens cleaning.
4. Client demonstrates no signs of eye injury, as evidenced by irritation, pain, foreign body sensation, redness, and tearing.
5. Client shows no signs of overwear such as blurred vision or severe ocular pain.
6. Client demonstrates the proper technique for removing, cleaning, and reinserting lenses.

DELEGATION CONSIDERATIONS

The skills of removal, cleansing, and insertion of contact lenses can be delegated to assistive personnel (AP).

- Confirm that care provider knows proper way to care for lenses.
- Stress to care provider that careful handling of lenses is necessary to prevent loss or damage.
- Inform care provider of types of findings to report (e.g., eye pain, drainage).

IMPLEMENTATION

Steps	Rationale
1. See Standard Protocol (inside front cover).	Be sure to wash hands with nonoily soap, rinse thoroughly, and dry with a lint-free towel (Lewis, Collier, and Heitkemper, 1996).
2. With client in sitting position, place towel just below client's face.	

Steps	Rationale

3.   **Removing soft lenses for a dependent client**
   a. Add a few drops of sterile saline to client's eye.

   b. Tell client to look straight ahead. Using gloved middle finger, retract lower eyelid to expose lower edge of lens.

   c. With pad of index finger of same hand, slide lens off cornea onto white of eye.

   d. Pull upper eyelid down gently with thumb of other hand and compress lens slightly between thumb and index finger.

   e. Gently pinch lens and lift out without allowing lens edges to stick together.

   f. If lens edges stick together, place lens in palm and soak thoroughly with sterile saline. Gently roll lens with index finger in back-and-forth motion. If gentle rubbing does not separate edges, soak lens in sterile solution.

   g. Place lens in storage case; **R** for right lens; **L** for left.

   h. Follow procedure for cleansing and disinfecting.

   i. Repeat Steps a to g for other lens.

   j. Remove and discard gloves and wash hands.

Lubricates eye to facilitate lens removal.

Use of finger pads prevents injury to cornea and damage to lens.

> **NURSE ALERT**
>
> *Handle lens with care. Soft lenses are prone to damage from fingernails during care.*

4.   **Removing rigid lenses for a dependent client**
   a. Be sure lens is positioned directly over cornea. If it is not, have client close eyelids, place index and middle fingers of one hand beside the lens, and gently but firmly massage lens back into place.

   b. Place index finger on outer corner of client's eye and draw skin gently back toward ear (see illustration).

   c. Ask client to blink. Do not release pressure on lids until blink is completed.

   d. If lens fails to pop out, gently retract eyelid beyond edges of lens. Press lower eyelid gently against lower edge of lens.

Maneuver should cause lens to dislodge and pop out. Lid margins must clear top and bottom of lens until the blink.

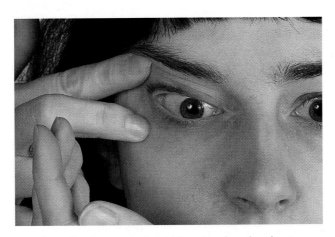

Step 4b   Removal of rigid lens (as done by client).

Steps	Rationale
e. Allow both eyelids to close slightly and grasp lens as it rises from eye. Cup lens in hand. A lens suction cup can be used for confused or unconscious clients. Gently apply suction cup to lens surface and lift lens out.	Lens suction cup helps reduce the risk of scratching the eye as lens is removed.
f. Place lens in storage case (see illustration): **R** for right lens; **L** for left.	
g. Follow procedure for cleansing and disinfecting.	
h. Repeat Steps a to g for other lens.	
i. Remove and discard gloves and wash hands.	

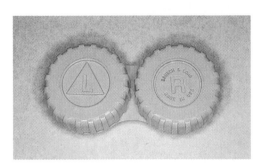

Step 4f

NURSE ALERT

Always perform procedure with the same lens first. Remove, clean, and insert one lens before the other lens is handled (Lake, 1996).

5. **Cleansing and disinfecting**
   a. Open lens storage case. Check expiration dates of solutions.
   b. After removal of one lens from case, apply 1 or 2 drops of cleaning solution to lens in palm of hand (use cleaning solution recommended by lens manufacturer or eye care practitioner).

   Removes tear components, including mucus, lipids, and proteins that collect on lens. Cleaning solutions incorporating a surfactant agent can remove 90% to 95% of all microorganisms (Rakow, 1993).

   c. Rub lens gently but thoroughly on both sides for 20 to 30 seconds. Use index finger (soft lenses) or little finger or cotton-tipped applicator soaked with cleaning solution (rigid lenses) to clean inside lens. Be careful not to touch or scratch lens with fingernail.

COMMUNICATION TIP

With the lens out and the client observing your cleansing technique, explain why cleansing is important in the prevention of infection. For example, "Notice how I want to make sure both surfaces are completely cleaned and then rinsed thoroughly. Bacteria can easily grow on the lens over a period of time. A serious infection can cause loss of sight."

   d. Holding lens over a small clean emesis basin, rinse thoroughly with manufacturer-recommended rinsing solution (soft lenses) or normal saline (rigid lenses). Reinsert (Step 6) or store (Step 5e).

   Lenses may be different prescriptions.

   e. Place lens in proper clean storage case compartment: **R** for right lens and **L** for left lens. Center lens in storage case, convex side down. Fill with recommended disinfecting solution. Label case with client's name and room number.

NURSE ALERT

Do not clean lens over open sink or drain. Do not use tap water.

Steps	Rationale

6. Inserting soft lenses

   a. Remove right lens from storage case and rinse with recommended rinsing solution; inspect lens for foreign materials, tears, or other damage.

   b. Check that lens is not inverted (inside out). Apply wetting agent (sterile saline).

                                                          Soft lens is inverted if the edge has a lip; it is in proper position if curve is even from base to rim.

   c. Using middle or index finger of opposite hand, retract upper lid until iris is exposed.

   d. Use middle finger of the hand holding lens to pull down lower lid.

   e. Tell client to look straight ahead; gently place lens directly on cornea; release lids slowly, starting with lower lid.

   f. Tell client to close eyes slowly and roll them toward lens if not on the cornea.

   g. Tell client to blink a few times.

   h. Ask client to open eyes. Check for blurred vision or discomfort.

   i. Repeat Steps a to h for left eye.

   j. Discard used solution in the storage case.

   k. Wash lens case with soap and a scrubber. Rinse case in sterile saline or a known disinfectant. Store dry.

7. Inserting rigid lenses

   a. Remove right lens from storage case; attempt to lift lens straight up (see illustration).

NURSE ALERT

Follow instructions of manufacturer or eye care practitioner regarding the time and procedure for disinfection/neutralization, because they vary among products. Some disinfecting solutions can harm the eyes if used improperly.

Ensures lens is centered, free of trapped air, and comfortable.

Prevents multiplication of amoeba and bacteria (Martin and Barr, 1997).

Sliding lens out of case can cause scratches on the surface.

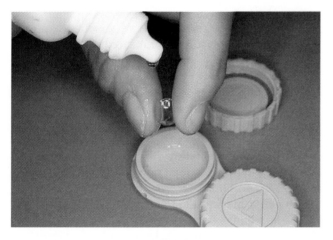

Step 7a

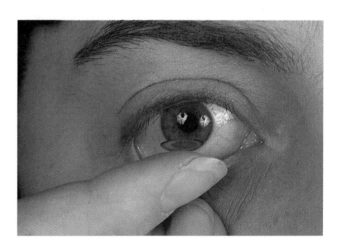

Step 7d

   b. Rinse with recommended rinsing solution; inspect lens for foreign material or chips.

   c. Wet lens on both sides, using prescribed wetting solution.

   d. Place right lens concave side up on tip of index finger of dominant hand (see illustration).

Hot water causes lens to warp.

Inner surface of lens should face up so that it is applied against cornea.

Steps	Rationale

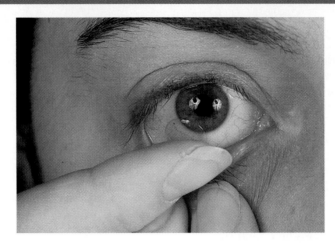

Step 7e

e. Instruct client to look straight ahead while retracting both upper and lower lids; place lens gently over center of cornea (see illustration).

f. Ask client to close eyes briefly and avoid blinking. Helps to secure position of lens.

g. Ask client to open eyes. Check for blurred vision or discomfort.

h. Repeat Steps a to g for left eye.

i. Discard used solution. See Step 6; for case cleansing.

8. See Completion Protocol (inside front cover).

• • •

EVALUATION

1. Ask client about comfort after removal and reinsertion of lenses.
2. Inspect eye for signs of ocular infection, over wear, and abrasion.
3. Ask client about visual perception after lens cleaning.
4. Ask if client is experiencing eye irritation or tearing.
5. Ask if client is having blurred vision or eye pain.
6. Observe client demonstrating technique for lens care.

Unexpected Outcomes and Related Interventions

1. Client complains of burning, pain, or foreign body sensation.
   a. Remove lenses.
   b. If symptoms persist, notify physician.
2. Client complains of blurred vision.
   a. Retract eyelids and locate position of lens. Ask client to look in direction opposite of lens and, with index finger, apply pressure to lower eyelid margin and position lens over cornea.
   b. If lenses feel dry, apply a wetting solution (if recommended) according to instructions.
   c. If symptoms persist, remove lenses and notify physician.

3. Client develops inflammation of conjunctiva, pain, discharge, excess tearing, or reduced vision.
   a. Remove lenses and notify physician.
4. Client is unable to perform lens care correctly.
   a. Demonstrate correct lens care.
   b. Observe return demonstration until correctly performed.

Recording and Reporting

• Record in progress notes or report to physician any signs or symptoms of visual alterations or corneal irritation/inflammation noted during procedure.

• Record on nursing care plan or Kardex times of lens insertion and removal if client is going to surgery or special procedure.

Sample Documentation

2000 Client complaining of eye discomfort. Slight redness of conjunctivae noted bilaterally. Contact lenses removed by client. Cleansing and disinfecting performed according to instructions. Client wearing glasses.

2200 No complaints of eye discomfort. Conjunctivae pink, no redness noted.

Geriatric Considerations

Some older adults experience dry eyes as a result of inadequate tear production. Itching, burning, and reduced vision can result (Lueckenotte, 1996). These reactions may contraindicate use of contact lenses.

Home Care and Long-Term Care Considerations

- Freshly boiled and cooled tap water may be used for rinsing off disinfecting solutions from hard lenses (Larkin, Kilvington, and Easty, 1990).
- The use of cold tap water and homemade saline for rinsing lenses between the use of solutions and in storage cases is not recommended (Larkin, Kilvington, and Easty, 1990; Martin and Barr, 1997).

Skill 36.2

CARING FOR AN EYE PROSTHESIS

As a result of tumor, infection, congenital blindness, or severe trauma to the eye, clients may have to undergo an enucleation, a procedure involving the complete removal of the eyeball. All that remains is the socket and eyelids. For obvious cosmetic purposes, clients who have had an enucleation are often fitted with an artificial eye, or prosthesis.

Artificial eyes are made of glass and plastic and fit just behind the client's eyelids. Each prosthesis is designed to take on the appearance of the client's natural iris, pupil, and sclera. Prostheses are relatively easy to remove and insert and can be worn day and night. Cleansing with soap and water can be done daily or any time up to several months based on client preference.

Equipment (Figure 36-1)

 Soft washcloth or cotton gauze square
 Wash basin with warm water or saline
 4 × 4 gauze pads
 Mild soap
 Facial tissues
 Bath towel
 Suction device (e.g., rubber bulb syringe, medicine dropper bulb) (OPTIONAL: Syringe removes prosthesis by suction if manual removal is not successful.)
 Disposable gloves
 Covered plastic storage case

ASSESSMENT

1. Determine which eye is artificial (no movement or pupillary reaction to light).

2. Inspect surrounding tissues of eyelid and eye socket for inflammation, tenderness, swelling, or drainage after prosthesis removal. Wear gloves if drainage is suspected or present.

3. Assess client's routines for prosthetic care: frequency and methods of cleaning. **Rationale: Determines compliance with and knowledge of self-care.**

4. Assess client's ability to remove, clean, and reinsert prosthesis.

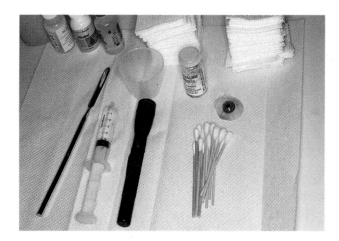

Figure 36-1

PLANNING

Expected outcomes focus on client's comfort and prevention of infection.

Expected Outcomes

1. Client verbalizes feelings regarding prosthesis removal.
2. Client's eyelid margins and eye socket are clean and of normal pink color, with lashes turned away from prosthesis.
3. Client demonstrates no signs of infection, such as redness, tenderness, swelling, or discharge of socket or eyelid margins.
4. Client verbalizes that prosthetic eye fits comfortably.
5. Client demonstrates the proper technique for removing, cleaning, and reinserting prosthesis.

DELEGATION CONSIDERATIONS

The skills of removal, cleansing, and insertion of an eye prosthesis can be delegated to AP.

- Confirm that care provider knows proper way to remove and reinsert prosthesis.
- Stress to care provider the importance of maintaining client's dignity and privacy during procedure.
- Inform care provider of types of findings to report (e.g., inflammation, drainage).

IMPLEMENTATION

Steps	Rationale
1. See Standard Protocol (inside front cover).	
2. With thumb, gently retract lower eyelid against lower orbital ridge (see illustration).	
3. Exert slight pressure below eyelid (see illustration). If prosthesis does not slide out, use bulb syringe or medicine dropper bulb to apply direct suction to prosthesis.	Maneuver breaks suction, causing prosthesis to rise and slide out of socket (Bocking et al., 1990).

4. Place prosthesis in palm of hand and clean with mild soap and water or plain saline by rubbing between thumb and index finger.
5. Rinse well under running tap water and dry with soft washcloth or facial tissue (see illustration, p. 841).
6. If client is not to have prosthesis reinserted, store in sterile saline or water in plastic storage case. Label with client's name and room number.

COMMUNICATION TIP

During this time make client feel at ease by using a calm, gentle approach

- *Avoid any facial expressions that might suggest discomfort or aversion toward handling the prosthesis. Now is a good time to ask, "Tell me how often you find it necessary to clean your artificial eye. Have you ever had difficulty with that?"*

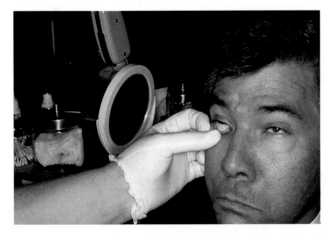

Step 2

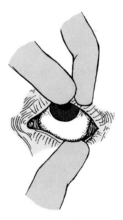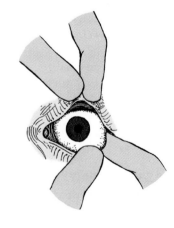

Step 3

Steps	Rationale

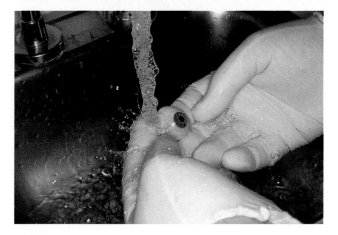

Step 5

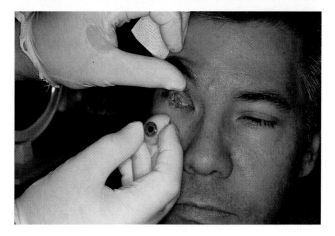

Step 9

7. Clean eyelid margins and socket.
   a. Retract upper and lower eyelids with thumb and index finger. (Inspection can be done at this time.)
   b. Wash socket with washcloth or gauze square moistened in warm water or saline.
   c. Dry socket well with gauze pads.
   d. Wash eyelids with mild soap and water, wiping from inner to outer canthus, using a clean part of cloth with each wipe. Dry eyelids using the same method.
8. Moisten prosthesis with water or saline.

9. Retract client's upper eyelid with index finger or thumb of nondominant hand (see illustration).
10. With dominant hand, hold prosthesis so that notched or pointed edge is positioned toward nose. Iris faces outward.
11. Slide prosthesis up under upper eyelid as far as possible. Then push down lower lid to allow prosthesis to slip into place.
12. Gently wipe away excess fluid if necessary. Remove and discard gloves and wash hands.
13. See Completion Protocol (inside front cover).

Rationale:

Removes moisture that can harbor microorganisms.

Makes insertion easier because dry plastic would rub against tissue surfaces.

Correct positioning of prosthesis ensures proper fit (Bocking et al., 1990).

Wipe toward nose to prevent dislodgement.

• • •

EVALUATION
1. Ask client about feelings regarding prosthesis removal.
2. Inspect eyelids and eye socket for cleanliness, color, and position of eyelashes.
3. Inspect eyelids and socket for signs of infection.
4. Ask client if prosthesis fits comfortably.

5. Observe client demonstrating technique for prosthesis care.

Unexpected Outcomes and Related Interventions
1. Client states prosthesis feels uncomfortable.
   a. Reposition prosthesis.
   b. Remove prosthesis. Inspect for any rough areas.

2. Client develops signs of inflammation in socket or eyelid.
   a. Remove prosthesis for a few days if necessary. Clean eyelid and socket.
   b. Provide client with an eye patch if desired.
3. Client develops excessive, purulent, or foul drainage.
   a. Remove prosthesis and clean area. Provide eye patch if desired.
   b. Evaluate temperature every 4 hours and as necessary.
   c. Notify physician of assessment findings.
4. Client is unable to perform prosthesis care correctly.
   a. Demonstrate correct prosthesis care.
   b. Observe return demonstration until correctly performed.

Recording and Reporting

- Record appearance and condition of eye socket in nurses' notes.
- Record and report any signs and symptoms of infection involving eye socket.

Sample Documentation

1400 *Client complaining of tenderness at left artificial eye. Prosthesis removed. No scratches or rough edges noted. Slight redness and edema noted at outer canthus. Socket and eyelids cleaned with normal saline. Client agrees not to wear prosthesis until symptoms improve. Prosthesis cleaned and stored. Eye patch provided.*

Geriatric Considerations

- Older adults normally experience a reduction in visual function. With only one eye, the older adult may require greater assistance with respect to safety precautions.

Home Health and Long-Term Care Considerations

- If a client becomes disabled and suffers an inability to perform self-care measures on a regular basis, be sure the prosthesis is cleaned regularly to prevent possible infection.

Skill 36.3

EYE IRRIGATIONS

Eye irrigation is performed to flush out exudate or irritating solutions. It is a procedure typically used in emergency situations when a foreign object or some other substance has entered the eye (Perry and Potter, 1998). When a chemical or irritating substance contaminates the eyes, irrigate *immediately* with copious amounts of water for at least 15 minutes to prevent corneal burning (McConnell, 1991).

Equipment

Prescribed irrigating solution: volume usually varies from 30 to 180 ml at 98.6° F (37° C). (For chemical flushing, use tap water or prescribed IV fluid in volume to provide continuous irrigation over 15 minutes.)
Sterile basin for solution
Curved emesis basin
Waterproof pad or towel
Cotton balls
Soft bulb syringe, eyedropper, or IV tubing
Disposable gloves

ASSESSMENT

1. Assess reason for eye irrigation. **Rationale: This information determines the amount and type of solution and the immediacy of treatment.**
2. Assess the eye for redness, excessive tearing, and discharge. Assess the eyelids and lacrimal glands for edema. Ask client about itching, burning, pain, blurred vision, or photophobia (McConnell, 1991). **Rationale: Provides baseline for condition of eye.**
3. Assess client's ability to cooperate. **Rationale: Extra assistance may be needed.**

PLANNING

Expected outcomes focus on client's physical and psychological comfort and improving vision.

Expected Outcomes

1. Client verbalizes reduced burning/itching after eye irrigation.
2. Client demonstrates minimal anxiety during irrigation.
3. Client verbalizes improved visual acuity after eye irrigation.
4. Client maintains normal pupillary reaction and eye movement after irrigation.

IMPLEMENTATION

Steps	Rationale
1. See Standard Protocol (Inside front cover).	
2. Remove contact lenses (if possible) before beginning irrigation.	Relieves client's anxiety.
3. Assist client to side-lying position on the same side as the affected eye. Turn head toward affected eye.	Irrigation solution will flow from inner to outer canthus, preventing contamination of unaffected eye and nasolacrimal duct.

COMMUNICATION TIP

Reassure client that eye can be closed periodically and that no object will touch eye.

NURSE ALERT

Remove contact lenses (if possible) before beginning irrigation.

Steps	Rationale
4. Place waterproof pad under client's face.	
5. With cotton ball moistened in prescribed solution (or normal saline), gently clean eyelid margins and eyelashes from inner to outer canthus.	Minimizes transfer of debris from lids or lashes into eye during irrigation.
6. Place curved emesis basin just below client's cheek on side of affected eye.	
7. With gloved finger, gently retract upper and lower eyelids to expose the conjunctival sacs. To hold lids open, apply pressure to lower bony orbit and bony prominence beneath eyebrow. Do not apply pressure over eye.	Retraction minimizes blinking and allows irrigation of conjunctiva.
8. Hold irrigating syringe, dropper or IV tubing approximately 1 inch (2.5 cm) from the inner canthus.	If irrigator touches the eye, there is risk of injury.

COMMUNICATION TIP

Use a calm, confident, soft voice when talking with client and reinforcing the importance of the procedure. For example, "You are doing great; just relax; that's it, we need to flush this out of your eye as completely as possible to lessen the chance of an eye injury."

Steps	Rationale

9. Ask client to look up. Gently irrigate with a steady stream toward the lower conjunctival sac to the outer canthus (see illustration).
10. Allow client to close the eye periodically.

11. Continue irrigation until all solution is used or secretions have been cleared. (NOTE: A 15-minute irrigation is needed to flush chemicals.)
12. Dry eyelids and facial area with sterile cotton ball. Remove and discard gloves and wash hands.
13. See Completion Protocol (inside front cover).

Lid closure moves secretions from upper to lower conjunctival sac.

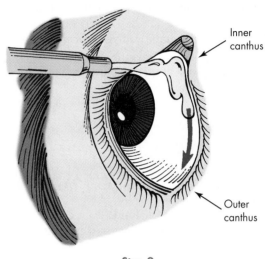

Step 9

• • •

EVALUATION
1. Assess client's comfort level after eye irrigation.
2. Observe for verbal and nonverbal signs of anxiety during irrigation.
3. Ask client if vision is blurred after irrigation.
4. Observe pupillary reaction (to light and accommodation) and extraocular eye movement (see Skill 14.3).

Unexpected Outcomes and Related Interventions
1. Client demonstrates extreme anxiety during irrigation.
   a. Reinforce the rationale for irrigation.
   b. Allow client to close eye periodically during irrigation.
   c. Instruct client to take slow, deep breaths.
   d. Seek extra assistance if needed to prevent injury.
2. Client complains of pain and foreign body sensation in the eye after irrigation. Excessive tearing and photophobia noted.
   a. Advise client to close the eye and avoid eye movement.
   b. Notify physician or eye care practitioner of findings.

Recording and Reporting
• Record in nurses' notes condition of eye, type and amount of solution used for irrigation, length of time for irrigation, and client's report of pain and visual status.

• Report continued symptoms of pain and visual blurring to physician.

Sample Documentation
0800 Client complaining of blurred vision and tenderness in left eye. Yellow, crusty drainage noted on eyelids with slight edema and redness of conjunctiva. Eyelids cleaned and eye irrigated with 30 ml warm, sterile, normal saline for 10 minutes. Bacitracin ophthalmic ointment applied. Client had no complaint of discomfort.
0900 Client states that eye "feels better." Vision clearer. PERRLA. Normal eye movements noted. Conjunctiva remains red with slight edema.

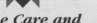

Home Care and Long-Term Care Considerations

• If client suffered injury in the home, instruct on ways to minimize chemical injuries in the future. Have client wear eye goggles when working with chemicals.
• Instruct client and family on how to perform emergency irrigation of the eye.

Skill 36.4

CARING FOR CLIENTS WITH HEARING AIDS

Hearing is vital for normal communication and orientation to sounds in the environment. For people with hearing loss, hearing aids improve the ability to hear and understand spoken words. Hearing aids amplify so that sound is heard at a more effective level. All aids have four basic components:

1. A microphone, which receives and converts sound into electrical signals.
2. An amplifier, which increases the strength of the electrical signal.
3. A receiver, which converts the strengthened signal back into sound.
4. A power source (batteries).

In addition, programmable hearing aids are now available. These aids input signals rather than just amplifying the sounds. They are programmed by an audiologist with the use of a computer specific to a client's hearing impairment.

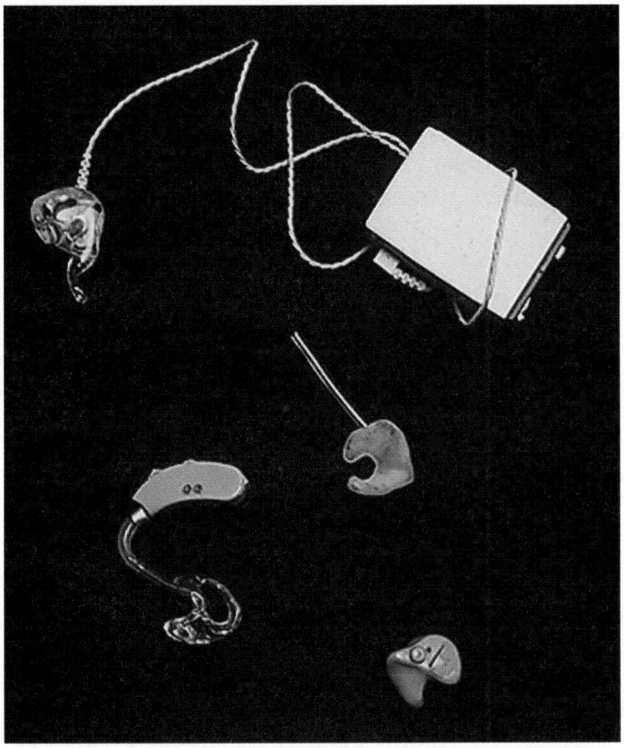

These aids are adjusted to accommodate the range of the client's residual hearing. Programmable aids independently amplify high-frequency (soft-spoken consonants) from low-frequency (loudly spoken vowels) sounds; this process occurs rapidly and continuously. (ReSound Corporation, 1994; 1995). Several styles of hearing aids are available to clients today (Figure 36-2).

1. An in-the-canal (ITC) aid fits entirely in the ear canal. It has cosmetic appeal, is easy to manipulate and place in the ear, does not interfere with the wearing of eyeglasses or use of the telephone, and can be worn during most physical exercise. However, obtaining a proper fit is more difficult, and cerumen tends to plug this model more than others.
2. An in-the-ear (ITE) or intraaural aid, fits into the external auditory ear and allows more fine-tuning (Figure 36-3). It is more powerful and therefore is useful for a wider range of hearing loss than the ITC aid. It is easy to position and adjust and does not interfere with eyeglass wearing. It is slightly more noticeable than the ITC aid and is not recommended for persons with moisture or skin problems in the ear canal. It is the most common type worn.
3. A behind-the-ear, (BTE) or postaural aid, hooks around and behind the ear and is connected by a short, clear, hollow plastic tube to an ear mold inserted into the external auditory canal. It is used for clients with rapidly progressive hearing loss or manual dexterity difficulties and those who find partial ear occlusion intolerable. Disad-

Figure 36-2 Types of hearing aids. **A,** Older aid with a battery pack worn on the body and a wire connected to the ear mold. **B,** Behind-the-ear (BTE) battery with ear mold. **C,** In-the-ear (ITE) mold with battery. **D,** Small in-the-canal (ITC) mold. *Courtesy CLG Photographics, Inc.*

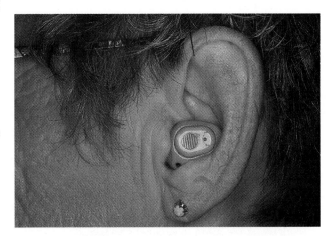

Figure 36-3 Small canal type hearing aid.

vantages are that it is more visible, may interfere with eyeglasses and telephone use, and is more difficult to keep in place during physical exercise.

4. The eyeglass aid is a hearing aid that fits in the ear canal and attaches to a battery located on the arm of the eyeglass frame. The frame must be bulky to accommodate the equipment; therefore style selection is limited.

5. The body aid is a bulky instrument used for severe hearing loss. A fitted ear mold attaches to a round receiver that connects to a transmitter the size of a cigarette case. The devices can be tailored to a client's specific amplification need.

Equipment
Overbed table
Soft towel and washcloth
Brush or wax loop
Storage case
Disposable gloves (if drainage is present)

ASSESSMENT
1. Assess client's knowledge of and routines for cleansing and caring for hearing aid. **Rationale: Determines compliance with and knowledge of self-care.**
2. Observe whether client can hear clearly with use of aid by talking slowly and clearly in normal tone of voice.
3. Assess if hearing aid is working by removing from client's ear. Close battery case and turn volume slowly to high. Cup hand over hearing aid. If squealing sound (feedback) is heard, it is working. If no sound is heard, replace batteries and test again.

4. Inspect ear mold for cracked or rough edges.
5. Inspect for accumulation of cerumen around aid and plugging of opening in aid. **Rationale: Cerumen can block sound reception.**

PLANNING
Expected outcomes focus on facilitating communication and promoting comfort and appropriate self-care.

Expected Outcomes
1. Client hears conversation spoken in normal tone of voice and responds appropriately.
2. Client responds appropriately to environmental sounds.
3. Client demonstrates proper care of the hearing aid.
4. Client verbalizes that the aid fits comfortably.

DELEGATION CONSIDERATIONS

The skill of caring for a hearing aid can be delegated to AP.

- Confirm that care provider knows proper way to care for prosthetic device.
- Clarify communication tips to use for individual client while aid is being cleaned.
- Have care provider report presence of any drainage to RN.

IMPLEMENTATION

Steps	Rationale
1. See Standard Protocol (inside front cover).	
2. Have equipment at bedside for client to see.	
3. **Cleaning hearing aid**	
a. Wipe aid with soft washcloth. Use wax loop or brush (supplied with aid) or tip of syringe needle to clean the holes in the aid; do not jam wax deeper into holes.	Impaction of wax blocks normal sound transmission (Meador, 1995).

NURSE ALERT

Caring for a hearing aid should protect the device from moisture, heat, breakage, and loss.

COMMUNICATION TIP

Ask client to share at this time any tips for care of the aid. Use the time to discuss whether the client is having any difficulty hearing or using the aid at home, at work, or in social situations. When children are clients, involve parents.

Steps	Rationale
b. Open battery door and allow it to air dry.	Increases battery life and allows moisture to evaporate (Olson, 1995).
c. Wash ear canal with washcloth moistened in soap and water. Rinse and dry.	Removes cerumen from ear canal.
d. If hearing aid is to be stored, place in dry storage case with dessicant material. Label case with client's name and room number. If more than one aid, note right or left. Turn off hearing aid when not in use.	
4. Inserting hearing aid	
a. Check batteries (see Assessment).	
b. Turn aid off and volume control down.	Protects client from sudden exposure to feedback sounds.
c. Hold aid so that the bore–the long portion with the hole(s)–is at the bottom.	
d. Insert bore into the canal first. Use other hand to pull up and back on outer ear. Gently twist and push aid into ear until it is in place and fits snugly in the midline.	
e. Adjust volume gradually to comfortable level for talking to client in regular voice 3 to 4 feet away. Rotate volume control toward nose to increase volume and away from nose to decrease volume. Note that some ITC hearing aids have preset sound levels that require a special instrument to adjust. Most clients leave setting at an acceptable level.	For most people, hearing aids work best at lower volume settings.
5. See Completion Protocol (inside front cover).	

• • •

EVALUATION
1. Converse with client in a normal tone of voice and observe response.
2. Observe client's response to environmental sounds.
3. Observe client perform hearing aid care.
4. Ask client about comfort after hearing aid insertion.

Unexpected Outcomes and Related Interventions
1. Client is unable to hear conversations or environmental sounds clearly. Client's verbal responses are inappropriate.
   a. Remove hearing aid and check battery for power and correct placement.
   b. Inspect ear mold for cerumen blockage.
   c. Change volume setting as needed.
   d. If problems persist, contact audiologist or hearing aid specialist.
2. Client is unable to perform care of hearing aid.
   a. Demonstrate correct aid care.
   b. Observe return demonstration until correctly performed.

3. Client complains of ear discomfort and may complain of whistling sound.
   a. Remove aid and reinsert.
   b. Assess external ear for signs of inflammation.
   c. If problems persist, contact audiologist or hearing aid specialist.

Recording and Reporting
- Record that hearing aid is removed and stored if client is going for surgery or special procedure.
- Report to nursing staff and document on plan of care tips that promote communication with client.

Sample Documentation
1000   Client responding inappropriately to questions. Unable to hear normal conversation tone. Complains of hearing an "echo." Volume turned down on ITE aid in right ear. Daughter states that client frequently turns the volume up so he can "hear better." Reviewed proper volume settings and improved listening techniques with client and daughter.

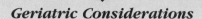

Geriatric Considerations

* The small size of hearing aids may make it difficult for older adults to handle and manipulate the devices. Clients who have this difficulty should contact their hearing aid specialist for assistance. Family members may be able to assist with care of device.

Home Care and Long-Term Care Considerations

* Initial use of a hearing aid should be restricted to quiet situations in the home. Clients need to adjust gradually to voices and household sounds (Lewis, Collier, and Heitkemper, 1996).
* Avoid exposure of aid to extreme heat or cold. Do not leave in case near stove, heater, or sunny window. Do not use with hair dryer on hot settings or with sunlamp.
* Remove aid for bathing and when at hair stylist.
* Hair spray tends to clog the aid.

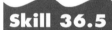

EAR IRRIGATIONS

The common indications for irrigation of the external ear are presence of certain foreign bodies and accumulation of cerumen. The procedure is not without potential hazards. Damage to the external auditory meatus may occur by scratching the lining of the canal if the client suddenly moves or if there is inadequate control of the irrigating syringe (Meador, 1995). Improperly drying the ear may lead to an episode of acute otitis externa. If the client moves suddenly during irrigation, the tympanic membrane can be perforated. Water pressure can also cause perforation. Never irrigate the ear if vegetable matter is occluded in the canal; the tympanic membrane is ruptured; or the client has otitis externa, myringotomy tubes, or a mastoid cavity (McConnell, 1992; Zivic and King, 1993).

In addition to irrigation, cerumen can be removed by use of a currette, which is performed by a physician or advanced nurse practitioner. Instillation of ceruminolytic agents that soften and loosen the matter for cleaning is another alternative.

Equipment
Otoscope
Prescribed sterile irrigating solution warmed to 98.6° F (37° C)
Otological syringe (20 to 50 ml) with needle replaced by an angiocath or dental irrigation device set at low setting (Zivic and King, 1993)
Sterile basin for solution
Curved emesis basin
Towel or waterproof pad
Cotton-tipped applicators
Antiseptic otic solution (e.g., VoSol Otic Solution or 70% isopropyl alcohol)

ASSESSMENT
1. Review medical history for ruptured tympanic membrane, myringotomy tubes, or surgery of auditory canal. **Rationale: These factors contraindicate ear irrigation.**
2. Assess client's comfort level. **Rationale: Provides baseline to evaluate changes in client's condition.**
3. Assess client's hearing ability in the affected ear.
4. Assess client's knowledge of proper ear care.
5. Inspect the pinna and external auditory meatus for redness, swelling, drainage, abrasions, and presence of cerumen or foreign objects. (If indicated, use an otoscope to inspect deeper portions of the auditory canal.

PLANNING
Expected outcomes focus on client comfort and improved auditory perception.

Expected Outcomes
1. Client denies increased pain during instillation.
2. Client verbalizes increased comfort, using a scale of 0-10, after irrigation.
3. Client demonstrates minimal anxiety during irrigation.
4. Client's ear canal is clear of discharge, cerumen, or foreign material after irrigation.
5. Client demonstrates improved hearing acuity in the affected ear after irrigation.

DELEGATION CONSIDERATIONS

The skill of irrigating the external ear requires knowledge application and decision making unique to a professional nurse. Delegation is inappropriate.

IMPLEMENTATION

Steps	Rationale
1. See Standard Protocol (inside front cover).	
2. ![icon] Assist client to a sitting or lying position with head turned toward the affected ear. Place towel or waterproof pad under client's head and shoulder. Have client help hold basin under affected ear (see illustration).	Solution will flow from ear canal to basin.
3. Pour prescribed irrigating solution into sterile basin. Check the temperature of the solution (98.6° F or 37° C) by pouring a small drop on your inner forearm.	Solution that is too hot or too cold can cause nausea, vertigo, and vomiting.
4. Gently clean auricle and outer ear canal with moistened cotton applicator. Do not force drainage or cerumen into ear canal.	

NURSE ALERT

Advise client to not make any sudden moves, to prevent trauma to the ear.

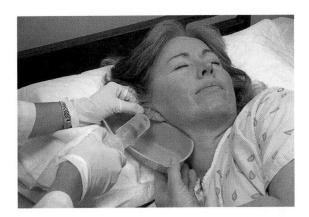

Step 2

5. Fill syringe and expel air. If using dental irrigating device, use low setting.	Prevents sudden expulsion of fluid.
6. Place the tip of the irrigating device just inside the external meatus. Leave a space around the irrigating tip and canal. With nondominant hand, straighten the auditory meatus by gently drawing the pinna up and back (for adult) or down and back (for young child).	Prevents obstruction of canal with device, which can lead to increased pressure on tympanic membrane. Pulling of pinna straightens external ear canal.
7. Direct the fluid gently toward the posterior wall of the ear canal. Compare the perimeter of the ear to that of a clock face. Direct the fluid toward 1 o'clock in the left ear and toward 11 o'clock in the right ear (Zivic and King, 1993).	Fluid is directed back behind impacted cerumen.
8. Maintain the flow of the irrigation in a steady stream until you see small to large pieces of cerumen flow from the canal.	

COMMUNICATION TIP

Talk in a confident, calm voice to help the client relax. As you begin the irrigation, say, "Now you are going to feel the warm water. I am going to be sure to do this gently. If you feel any discomfort at all, let me know."

Steps	Rationale
9. Periodically ask if the client is experiencing pain, nausea, or vertigo.	Symptoms indicate irrigating solution is too hot or too cold.
10. Periodically examine the canal during the irrigation for patency or cerumen plug.	Determines if cerumen is being removed.
11. Drain excessive fluid from the ear by having client tilt the head toward the affected side.	
12. Dry the canal gently with a cotton-tipped applicator and then chemically dry with an antiseptic otic solution such as VoSol Otic Solution or 70% isopropyl alcohol (Meador, 1995). Remove and discard gloves and wash hands.	Drying prevents buildup of moisture that can lead to otitis externa.
13. See Completion Protocol (inside front cover).	

• • •

EVALUATION

1. Ask client about pain level during irrigation.
2. Ask client about comfort level after irrigation.
3. Observe for verbal and nonverbal signs of anxiety during irrigation.
4. Inspect condition of external meatus and ear canal.
5. Assess hearing acuity in the affected ear after irrigation.

Unexpected Outcomes and Related Interventions

1. Client complains of increased ear pain during irrigation.
    Discontinue irrigation and notify physician.
2. Client's ear canal remains occluded. Client's hearing acuity has not improved in the affected ear.
    a. Repeat irrigation if prescribed.
    b. If condition persists, notify physician.

Recording and Reporting

• Record type of solution and amount, ear irrigated, appearance of irrigant, and condition of external ear canal.
• Report if client complains of sudden pain or if irrigation results in drainage of purulent-looking fluid.

Sample Documentation

1000 Client complaining of difficulty hearing in right ear. Cerumen plug noted in canal. Irrigated right ear with 50 ml warm normal saline. Return fluid clear with brown particles. No complaints of pain or discomfort. States that hearing "is fine." Responding appropriately to normal conversation tone. Right ear canal clear.

Geriatric Considerations

• Older adults often require ongoing ear care for cerumen removal. Use of a softening agent, such as slightly warmed mineral oil (0.5 to 1 ml), twice daily for several days before irrigation is helpful.
• Older adults with higher risk of cerumen impaction include those with large amounts of ear canal hair, those with benign growths that narrow the ear canal, and those who habitually wear hearing aids (Ebersole and Hess, 1994).

Home Care and Long-Term Care Considerations

• Instruct client to clean ears with a damp washcloth wrapped around a finger. Do not use a cotton-tipped applicator.
• If client uses a ceruminolytic agent, instruct that these are softening products and that they will not remove the impaction (Meador, 1995).
• Severe cerumen impactions may cause a decrease in hearing, pain, ringing, or a crackling noise in the ear. This requires referral to a physician.

CRITICAL THINKING EXERCISES

1. Ms. Sorenstam comes to the clinic with a complaint of eye pain during the past 24 hours. She appears to have inflammation of the conjunctiva. Your assessment reveals that she wears soft contact lenses. Ms. Sorenstam reports that she cleans her lenses daily, using a prescribed disinfectant from her ophthalmologist and tap water for rinsing. What might be the source of Ms. Sorenstam's eye discomfort?

2. What do clients in need of prosthetic care have in common?

3. Mr. Zisk is a 74-year-old client who wears an ITE hearing aid. He has noted a decrease in hearing over the past 2 weeks despite use of the hearing aid, which functions normally. What nursing intervention might Mr. Zisk require, and why?

REFERENCES

Bocking H et al: Artificial eyes, *Nurs Times* 86(18):40, 1990.

Cohen E, Krachmer J: Red eyes and contact lenses, *Patient Care* 26(9):143, 1992.

Ebersole P, Hess P: *Toward healthy aging,* St Louis, 1994, Mosby.

Elder M, Daniel R: Contact lenses and their implications, *Practitioner* 237:509–512, 1993.

Lake A: Prevention of complications related to contact lens wear, *Nurs Times* 92:36–38, 1996.

Larkin DFP et al: Contamination of contact lens storage cases by *Acanthamoeba* and bacteria, *Br J Ophthalmol* 74(1):133–135, 1990.

Lewis SM, Collier I, Heitkemper M: *Medical-surgical nursing: assessment and management of clinical problems,* St Louis, 1996, Mosby.

Lueckenotte A: *Gerontologic nursing,* St Louis, 1996, Mosby.

Martin S, Barr O: Preventing complications in people who wear contact lenses, *Br J Nurs* 6(11):614–619, 1997.

McConnell E: How to irrigate the eye, *Nurs '91* 21(3):28, 1991.

McConnell E: How to irrigate the ear, *Nurs '92* 22(1):66, 1992.

Meador JA: Cerumen impaction in the elderly, *J Gerontol Nurs* 21(12):43–45, 1995.

Olson R: Now hear this! *RN* 58(8):43, 1995.

Perry A, Potter P: *Pocket guide to basic skills and procedures,* ed 4, St Louis, 1998, Mosby.

Rakow PL: Managing contact lens non-compliance, *J Ophthal Nurs Technol* 12(1):47–48, 1993.

ReSound Corporation: *Hear what you've been missing,* Redwood City, Calif, 1994, ReSound Corporation.

ReSound Corporation: ReSound hearing health care, *Hearing J* 48(7):53, 1995.

Turner FD et al: Compliance and contact lens care: a new assessment method, *Optom Vision Sci* 70(12):998–1004, 1993.

Zivic RC, King S: Cerumen impaction management for clients of all ages, *Nurs Pract* 18(3):29–37, 1993.

CHAPTER 37

Fluid, Electrolyte, and Acid-Base Balance

Skill 37.1
Monitoring Fluid Imbalance, 856

Skill 37.2
Monitoring Electrolyte Imbalance, 859

Skill 37.3
Monitoring Acid-Base Imbalance, 864

Fluid, electrolyte, and acid-base imbalances occur to some degree in most clients with a major illness or injury. A variety of factors increase the risk for fluid, electrolyte, and acid-base imbalances, and several imbalances in the same client are common (Boxes 37-1 and 37-2). Many fluid, electrolyte, and acid-base imbalances are directly related to illness or disease such as with diabetes, burns, renal failure, or congestive heart failure (CHF). In other situations, therapeutic measures such as major surgery, intravenous (IV) fluid therapy, diuretics, or mechanical ventilation indirectly influence fluid, electrolyte, and acid-base balance (Lewis, Collier, and Heitkemper, 1996).

◢ DISTRIBUTION AND COMPOSITION OF BODY FLUIDS

Body fluids are distributed in two distinct compartments: intracellular fluids and extracellular fluids. The fluid environment inside the cells (intracellular fluid, or ICF) must remain stable to maintain healthy cellular function. The fluid environment outside the cells (extracellular fluid, or ECF) includes both intravascular fluid (within the blood vessels) and interstitial fluid (between the cells and the blood vessels). Fluids in these compartments interact with the outside environment to provide the cells with the steady delivery of nutrients and removal of metabolic wastes. Body fluids are composed of water, nonelectrolytes (e.g., glucose, bilirubin, minerals, urea), and electrolytes. Homeostasis requires that the intake of water and electrolytes is equal to their elimination.

◢ Movement of Body Fluids

Because the cell membranes that separate the body fluid compartments are selectively permeable, water can pass through them easily. However, most ions and molecules

---

Box 37-1 Risk Factors for Fluid Imbalances

Fluid Volume Deficit (FVD)
Losses from the gastrointestinal system such as from diarrhea, vomiting, or drainage from fistulas or tubes
Loss of plasma or whole blood, such as with burns or hemorrhage
Excessive perspiration
Fever
Decreased oral intake of fluids
Use of diuretics

Fluid Volume Excess (FVE)
Congestive heart failure (CHF)
Renal failure
Cirrhosis
Increased serum aldosterone and steroid levels
Excessive sodium intake

Third-Space Syndrome
Portal hypertension
Small bowel obstruction
Peritonitis
Burns
Nephrosis (nephrotic syndrome)

Box 37-2 Risk Factors for Electrolyte Imbalances

Hyponatremia
  Renal disease
  Adrenal insufficiency
  Gastrointestinal losses
  Excessive sweating
  Use of diuretics (especially along with low-sodium diet)
  Interruption of sodium-potassium pump with decreased cell potassium and decreased serum sodium
  Metabolic acidosis

Hypernatremia
  Ingestion of large amounts of concentrated salt solution
  Iatrogenic administration of hypertonic saline IV solution
  Excess aldosterone secretion

Hypokalemia
  Use of potassium-wasting diuretics
  Diarrhea, vomiting, or other gastrointestinal losses
  Alkalosis
  Cushing's syndrome or adrenal hormone–producing tumors
  Polyuria
  Excessive sweating
  Excessive use of potassium-free IVs

Hyperkalemia
  Renal failure
  Hypertonic dehydration
  Massive cellular damage such as from burns and trauma
  Iatrogenic administration of large amounts of potassium IV

  Adrenal insufficiency
  Acidosis
  Rapid infusion of stored blood
  Use of potassium-retaining diuretics

Hypocalcemia
  Rapid administration of blood containing citrate
  Hypoalbuminemia
  Hypoparathyroidism
  Vitamin D deficiency
  Neoplastic diseases
  Pancreatitis

Hypercalcemia
  Hyperparathyroidism
  Metastatic bone tumors
  Paget's disease
  Osteoporosis
  Prolonged immobilization

Hypomagnesemia
  Inadequate intake: malnutrition and alcoholism
  Inadequate absorption: diarrhea, vomiting, nasogastric drainage, fistulas, excessive dietary calcium (competes with magnesium for transport sites) small intestine diseases
  Hypoparathyroidism
  Excessive loss resulting from thiazide diuretics
  Aldosterone excess
  Polyuria

Hypermagnesemia
  Renal failure
  Excessive parenteral administration of magnesium

---

pass through them more slowly (Tate, Seeley, and Stephens, 1994). Fluids and solutes move across these membranes by means of four processes: osmosis, diffusion, filtration, and active transport. Osmosis involves the movement of water from areas of lesser concentration to areas of greater concentration (Figure 37-1, p. 854). Changes in ECF osmolarity (number of solutes in solution) produce changes in ICF volume because of water movement toward the greater concentration of particles. Osmolality of serum refers to its osmotic pressure, which is normally 280 to 295 mOsm/kg.

Diffusion is the movement of dissolved substances across a semipermeable membrane from an area of higher concentration to an area of lower concentration (Figure 37-2, p. 854). An example of diffusion is the movement of oxygen and carbon dioxide between the alveoli and the blood vessels in the lungs.

Filtration is the process by which water and diffusable substances move together in response to fluid pressure. This process is active in capillary beds, where hydrostatic pressure differences determine the movement of water (Figure 37-3, p. 854). When there is increased hydrostatic pressure on the venous side of the capillary bed, as occurs in the presence of congestive heart failure (CHF), the normal movement of water from the interstitial space into the intravascular space by filtration is reversed, resulting in an accumulation of excess fluid in the interstitial space, known as *edema*.

Active transport uses energy (adenosine triphosphate [ATP]) to move sodium and potassium molecules against the gradient across a semipermeable membrane from an area of lesser concentration to an area of greater concentration (Figure 37-4, p. 854). This process makes it possible to keep a higher concentration of potassium in the ICF and a higher concentration of sodium in the ECF. Normally movement of water and solutes occurs to maintain homeostasis.

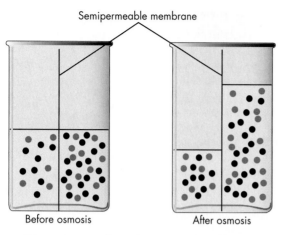

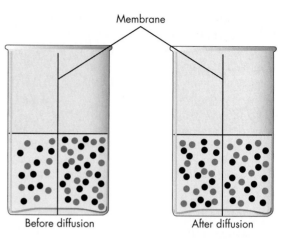

Figure 37-1 Osmosis through a semipermeable membrane; water moves from area of low solute concentration to an area of high solute concentration. *From Lewis SM, Collier IC, Heitkemper M: Medical-surgical nursing: assessment and management of clinical problems, ed 4, St Louis, 1996, Mosby.*

Figure 37-2 Diffusion is the movement of molecules from an area of high concentration to an area of low concentration. *From Lewis SM, Collier IC, Heitkemper M: Medical-surgical nursing: assessment and management of clinical problems, ed 4, St Louis, 1996, Mosby.*

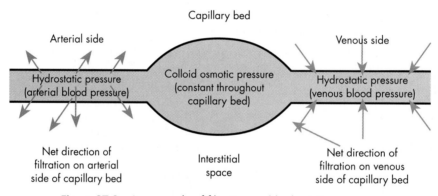

Figure 37-3 An example of filtration and hydrostatic pressure.

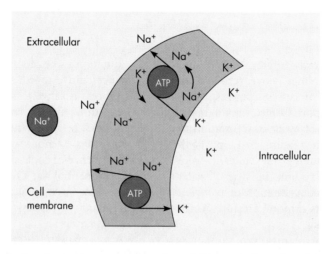

Figure 37-4 Sodium-potassium pump. As sodium diffuses into the cell and potassium out of the cell, an active transport system supplied with energy delivers sodium back to the extracellular compartment and potassium to the intracellular compartment. *ATP,* Adenosine triphosphate. *From Lewis SM, Collier IC, Heitkemper M: Medical-surgical nursing: assessment and management of clinical problems, ed 4, St Louis, 1996, Mosby.*

When illness or injury results in fluid and electrolyte imbalances, treatment may involve administration of IV fluids. An isotonic IV solution such as 0.9% normal saline (NS) has the same osmolality as blood plasma and will increase intravascular fluid volume without a fluid shift to other compartments. A hypotonic IV solution such as 0.45% saline has a lesser concentration of solutes than plasma and will move water into the cells. Hypertonic solutions such as those containing 3% saline have a greater concentration of solutes than plasma and will move water out of the cells and into the blood vessels.

Regulation of Body Fluids

Fluid intake is regulated primarily through the thirst mechanism, controlled by the hypothalamus in the brain. The thirst mechanism is affected by increased plasma osmolality, decreased plasma volume, dry mucous membranes, and other factors (Potter and Perry, 1998). Clients who are unable to perceive or respond to the thirst mechanism are at risk for dehydration. This includes infants, clients with neurological impairment or who are unconscious for any reason, and clients who are immobilized or restrained.

Fluid output is primarily regulated by the kidneys. In adults the kidneys produce about 60 ml per hour and about 1.5 L of urine per day. Water loss from the skin oc-

Table 37-1

Adult Average Daily Fluid Gains and Losses

Fluid Gains		Fluid Losses	
Oral fluids	1100–1400 ml	Kidneys	1200–1500 ml
Solid foods	800–1000 ml	Skin	500–600 ml
Metabolism	300 ml	Lungs	400 ml
		Gastrointestinal	100–200 ml
TOTAL GAINS	2200–2700 ml	TOTAL LOSSES	2200–2700 ml

curs in the form of sweat, which is increased with exercise; exposure to a warm environment, and fever. Excessive perspiration or diaphoresis may result in losses of 1000 ml or more in 24 hours.

Other insensible water losses are not perceptible to the person, include about 400 ml per day, and are increased substantially with an increased respiratory rate and depth, as well as fever. Normal loss via the gastrointestinal tract is 100 ml per day. Vomiting or diarrhea increases fluid loss substantially. The average daily fluid gains and losses in adults are 2200 to 2700 ml (Table 37-1).

Box 37-3 Clinical Applications of Alterations in Fluid Balance

Surgery

Because of the stress response to surgical trauma, 24 to 48 hours after surgery aldosterone and glucocorticoid hormones are increased, resulting in sodium, chloride, and fluid retention and potassium excretion. An increase in ADH secretion results in decreased urinary output, which helps maintain blood volume and blood pressure. After the second postoperative day, a diuretic phase begins as hormone levels return to normal and excess sodium and water are excreted.

Burns

In clients with severe burns, the body loses fluids in several ways. The greater the body surface burned, the greater the fluid loss. Plasma leaves the intravascular space and enters the interstitial fluid as trapped edema. This phenomena is also called "third-spacing." Plasma and fluids are lost as burn exudate (weeping tissues). Sodium and water shift into the cells, depleting ECF volume.

CHF

In CHF, decreased cardiac output results in less perfusion to the kidneys and decreased urine output. The client retains sodium and water, resulting in circulatory overload that may lead to pulmonary edema.

COPD

Alterations in respiratory function may interfere with the elimination of carbon dioxide to the extent that exceeds the buffers' ability to manage, resulting in a chronic acidosis and decreased pH. In chronic conditions the kidneys conserve bicarbonate to achieve compensation. When assessing arterial blood gases (ABGs) with chronic obstructive pulmonary disease (COPD), it is important to compare present values with a previous baseline reflection of what is normal for the client.

Kidney Failure

Kidney failure results in abnormal retention of sodium, chloride, potassium, and water in the ECF and increased plasma levels of waste products such as blood urea nitrogen (BUN) and creatinine. Hydrogen ions are retained, resulting in metabolic acidosis. Because of the disease process, compensation by bicarbonate reabsorption in the kidneys is not possible.

Infants and small children are at greater risk for fluid volume deficit (FVD) because body water losses are proportionately greater per kilogram of body weight. Children frequently respond to illness with fevers of higher temperature or longer duration than adults, resulting in increased insensible water losses.

Hormone Regulation

Antidiuretic hormone (ADH) is released by the posterior pituitary gland and decreases the production of urine by reabsorption of water by the kidney tubules. In the presence of FVD, as with vomiting and diarrhea, ADH levels increase, resulting in conservation of water. Aldosterone is a hormone produced by the adrenal cortex that regulates sodium and thus potassium and water balance. In response to aldosterone, the kidneys excrete potassium and reabsorb sodium, and as a result water is also retained. Fluid deficits such as those produced by hemorrhage or gastrointestinal losses can increase aldosterone levels. Glucocorticosteroids are hormones that increase in response to stress and result in retention of sodium and water. Clients taking steroid medication such as prednisone for its anti-inflammatory effects tend to retain sodium and water also. Box 37-3 on p. 855 gives examples of changes in fluid balance related to several clinical situations.

 NURSING DIAGNOSES

Nursing diagnoses relating to fluid and electrolyte imbalance include two major categories: **Fluid Volume Deficit (FVD)** and **Fluid Volume Excess (FVE).** FVD may be related to excessive fluid losses, decreased intake, or both. **Hyperthermia** (associated with systemic infection, septicemia, or draining wounds) and **Impaired Skin Integrity** (associated with burns) also contribute to fluid loss and electrolyte imbalance. FVE may be related to excessive intake of fluids, especially rapid IV infusion and excess sodium intake. FVE may also occur from retention of fluids as a result of decreased circulation and/or redistribution within the compartments and compromised regulatory mechanisms as occurs with CHF and renal failure.

Skill 37.1

MONITORING FLUID IMBALANCE

Fluid balance is neither a static nor simple physiological entity. Many variables can change the distribution of fluids in the body. During assessment the nurse considers variables influencing the fluid status and whether the change is normal and adaptive or the result of a pathological process. Certain conditions such as burns require frequent, in-depth assessment. Postoperative clients and clients recovering from gastroenteritis also require careful routine monitoring.

ASSESSMENT
1. Consult the medical record, or complete a nursing history with the client and family to identify risk factors for fluid volume imbalances (see Box 37-2).
2. Assess client's and family's understanding of fluid imbalances and the importance of accurate assessment data.

PLANNING

Expected outcomes focus on identifying fluid imbalances. Treatment often needs to begin quickly to avoid potentially life-threatening complications.

Expected Outcomes
1. Client will achieve or maintain normal fluid balance.
2. Causes of imbalance are identified and corrected.
3. Complications will be prevented or detected and managed promptly.

DELEGATION CONSIDERATIONS

Monitoring fluid balance requires the problem solving and knowledge application unique to a professional nurse. Assistive personnel (AP) may monitor assessment data (e.g., daily weight, I&O, vital signs) and report a client's subjective symptoms. All monitoring data must be reported to an RN.

IMPLEMENTATION

Steps	Rationale
1. See Standard Protocol (inside front cover).	
2. Monitoring FVD	
a. Monitor cardiovascular status for the following changes at least every 4 hours:	Assessments indicating hypovolemia (decreased circulating volume) are related to FVD.
(1) Falling blood pressure, especially orthostatic hypotension. Compare blood pressure lying, sitting, and standing.	
(2) Increased pulse rate, weak pulse, and capillary filling time longer than 3 sec.	
(3) Flat neck veins when supine.	
(4) Slow venous filling of dependent hands longer than 3 to 4 seconds.	
b. Check daily weights for losses (see Skill 8.3).	Daily weight is the most effective way to evaluate fluid balance. Rapid weight loss of 5% to 10% of body weight suggests moderate FVD; greater than 10% loss suggests severe FVD. Each kg of loss equals 1 L fluid loss (Potter and Perry, 1998).
c. Compare fluid intake and output (I&O) over 24 to 48 hours (see Skill 9.1).	
(1) Intake includes all liquids taken by mouth, fluids given through nasogastric or jejunostomy feeding tubes, IV fluids, IV piggyback medications, and blood or blood components.	
(2) Output includes urine, diarrhea, vomitus, gastric suction, and drainage from surgical tubes. Observe urine for oliguria, dark, concentrated (tea-colored) appearance.	Output greater than intake over time results in FVD. In the presence of FVD the body conserves water, resulting in more concentrated urine.
d. Inspect oral mucous membranes.	Sticky, dry membranes; dry, cracked lips; and decreased saliva production suggest dehydration.
e. Provide oral hygiene every 2 to 4 hours and keep lips moist with petrolatum jelly (see Skill 6.3).	
f. If oral intake is not restricted, encourage fluids. If client is NPO or unable to tolerate oral fluids, parenteral fluid administration is indicated (see Chapter 30).	
g. Inspect skin for temperature and moisture.	Dryness and flushed appearance suggest dehydration. Cool, clammy skin suggests hypovolemia.
h. Palpate skin for inelastic turgor (tenting) over the sternum in adults or the abdomen in infants.	Tenting indicates significant FVD related to dehydration. The back of the hand is not a reliable place to test skin turgor because of loose, thin skin, especially in older adults.

Steps	Rationale
i. Assess mental status and level of consciousness (LOC).	Dizziness, restlessness, confusion, lethargy, and coma may be related to dehydration or decreased cardiac output with hypovolemia.
j. In infants, inspection will reveal depressed or sunken fontanels in the presence of FVD.	
k. Monitor laboratory values: (1) Hematocrit (Hct): increased (2) BUN: increased (3) Urine specific gravity: increased	Increased Hct suggests hemoconcentration caused by fluid loss. Increased BUN suggests hemoconcentration in the presence of normal kidney function. Increased urine specific gravity indicates concentrated urine.
3. Monitoring FVE a. Monitor vital signs for: (1) Bounding pulse. (2) Increased respiratory rate, orthopnea, shortness of breath, or cough	
b. Inspect for jugular venous distention (JVD) when client is sitting upright (see Chapter 14).	Indicates increased venous pressure and compromised ability of the right atrium to receive blood and pump it throughout the circulatory system.
c. Auscultate lungs for crackles (rales) and rhonchi.	Indicates fluid buildup in the lung interstitial tissue (pulmonary edema), which requires immediate medical intervention.
d. Assess for peripheral or central edema. (1) Rapid weight gain (greater than 5% is significant).	
(2) Palpate dependent body parts such as feet/ankles for pitting edema (1+ to 4+). Clients on bedrest develop edema in sacral area when supine. Edema may shift from side to side as the client is turned (see Skill 13.5).	Pitting edema indicates fluid excess of 10 pounds (20 L) or more.
(3) Inspect for periorbital edema and blurred vision.	
(4) Monitor for intake greater than output.	In the presence of normal kidney function, urine will be pale and dilute and output will be increased. In the presence of kidney failure, oliguria intensifies the accumulation of fluids in the body.
(5) Monitor laboratory values: (a) Hct: decreased (b) Urine specific gravity: decreased in the presence of diuresis	Decreased Hct suggests hemodilution casued by fluid retention. Decreased urine specific gravity indicates dilute urine.
(6) Palpate the abdomen for ascites, an accumulation of fluid in the abdomen. Measure abdominal girth every 12 to 24 hours.	
(7) Infants may exhibit bulging fontanels in the presence of FVE.	
(8) See Completion Protocol (inside front cover).	

• • •

EVALUATION

1. Conduct ongoing assessment to determine whether the fluid imbalance has been corrected.
2. Evaluate effectiveness of corrective action based on identified cause(s).
3. Evaluate for possible complications of overcorrection of the original problem. For example, if the client is treated for FVD, observe for FVE.

Unexpected Outcomes and Related Interventions

1. After treatment for FVD, client remains either hypovolemic or dehydrated.
   a. Analyze the data supporting the persistent fluid imbalance (excess loss or inadequate intake).
   b. In collaboration with other health team members, increase volume or rate of ordered fluids either orally or intravenously, or identify medications such as antiemetics that decrease losses.
2. After treatment for FVD, client has evidence of FVE.
   a. Analyze the data to determine extent of overload.
   b. Decrease the infusion rate of parenteral fluids, and administer diuretics as ordered.

Recording and Reporting

- Describe assessment data that indicate the extent of FVD.
- Report significant alterations in vital signs, oliguria, laboratory results, and mental status to the physician promptly.
- Record independent and collaborative nursing interventions implemented, including oral or IV fluids, medications, and comfort measures.

Sample Documentation

1000   States nausea, vomiting × 3 days at home. Vital signs: T 98.4, P 100, R 12, supine BP 118/80, standing BP 90/60. Alert; oriented to person, place, time. Complains of dizziness, thirst, nausea. Oral mucous membranes dry, jugular veins flat with head of bed flat, inelastic skin turgor, capillary refill longer than 3 seconds. IV infusing at 125 ml/hr via infusion pump. Antiemetic given as ordered.

Geriatric Considerations

- The amount of fluid in the body decreases with age. As much as 80% of an infant's body weight is water, whereas a person over 70 years of age may have as little as 45% to 50%.
- Older adults tend to have decreased thirst sensation or may have altered ability to request or obtain needed fluids.
- After age 65, the kidneys lose nephrons and therefore the ability to concentrate urine.
- Atrophy of adrenal glands results in altered regulation of sodium and potassium and predisposes the client to fluid and electrolyte imbalance.

Home Care and Long-Term Care Considerations

If client or family is required to monitor I&O, have them use household measures and calculate totals accordingly.

Skill 37.2

MONITORING ELECTROLYTE IMBALANCE

Disturbances in electrolyte balance seldom occur alone and often are related to fluid imbalances. The basic types of electrolyte imbalances include sodium, potassium, calcium, and magnesium imbalances. A variety of risk factors are associated with these imbalances (see Box 37-2, p. 852). Electrolytes are substances that separate in solution into negatively charged ions (anions) and positively charged ions (cations) that conduct electrical currents. The numbers of positive and negative charges must be equal in body fluids. Electrolytes are vital to many body functions, including neuromuscular function, cardiac rhythm and contractility, mental processes, and gastrointestinal function. Major electrolytes are sodium, potassium, calcium, and magnesium. Most serum electrolytes are measured in milliequivalents (mEq) per liter.

Sodium is the most abundant cation in the ECF. Water follows sodium so that when sodium is excreted by the kidneys, water is also excreted. (This is the mechanism of action for some diuretics.) Hyponatremia is a low serum sodium level, associated with kidney disease, gastrointestinal losses, increased sweating, and certain diuretics. Severe hyponatremia can result in vascular collapse and shock.

Dilutional hyponatremia occurs in the presence of water excess. Hypernatremia is caused by extreme water loss or overall sodium excess.

Potassium is the predominant intracellular cation, which regulates neuromuscular excitability and muscle contraction and is primarily regulated by the kidneys. Relatively small deviations from normal can be very serious because only 3% of potassium is in the blood. Any condition that decreases urine output also decreases potassium excretion. Hyperkalemia is an elevated serum potassium, which may be caused by altered kidney function, massive cell damage such as from burns, myocardial infarction, crushing injuries, and cell destruction after chemotherapy and radiation therapy. Hypokalemia (low serum potassium) can result from prolonged malnutrition; gastrointestinal losses with vomiting, diarrhea, or gastric suctioning; kidney disease; diabetic ketoacidosis; and the use of potassium-wasting diuretics.

The functions of calcium include transmission of nerve impulses, cardiac contractions, blood clotting, and formation of teeth and bone (Lewis, Collier, and Heitkemper, 1996). Hypocalcemia represents a low serum calcium and causes altered blood clotting and a tendency toward tetany. Hypocalcemia is associated with surgical removal of the parathyroid glands, acute pancreatitis, renal failure, decreased dietary intake, and excess loss with laxative abuse. Hypercalcemia is an increase in the total serum calcium level and frequently is a symptom of an underlying disease resulting in excess bone resorption with release of calcium (Potter and Perry, 1998). The most common cause of hypercalcemia is malignancy. Other causes include parathyroid disease, vitamin D overdose, and prolonged immobilization.

Magnesium imbalances directly influence neuromuscular function. Hypomagnesemia increases neuromuscular and central nervous system (CNS) activity. Hypermagnesemia diminishes the excitability of muscle cells and contributes to hypertension, cardiac dysrhythmias, ischemic heart disease, and sudden cardiac death. Magnesium deficit may be caused by excess losses via vomiting and diarrhea; large urine output; nasogastric suction; and decreased dietary intake because of chronic alcoholism, malnutrition, or inadequate absorption. Elevated magnesium levels are associated with renal failure, adrenal insufficiency, and overdose associated with IV administration for the prevention of seizures in toxemia of pregnancy.

ASSESSMENT

1. Consult the medical record, or complete a nursing history with the client and family to identify risk factors for electrolyte imbalances (see Box 37-2).
2. Check laboratory results to identify abnormal electrolyte levels.
3. Assess client and family's understanding of the risk for electrolyte imbalances.

PLANNING

Expected outcomes focus on identifying a high risk for or actual electrolyte imbalance. Treatment should begin quickly because complications can be life threatening.

Expected Outcomes

1. Client will have normal serum electrolyte levels.
2. There will be no evidence of complications of electrolyte imbalance.

DELEGATION CONSIDERATIONS

Monitoring electrolyte balance requires complex problem solving and knowledge application unique to a professional nurse. AP may monitor assessment data (e.g., daily weight, I&O, vital signs) and report a client's mental status (sudden confusion), changes in strength (weakness or muscle rigidity), and subjective symptoms. All monitoring data must be reported to an RN.

IMPLEMENTATION

Steps	Rationale
1. See Standard Protocol (inside front cover).	
2. Assess for sodium imbalance: Identify conditions that contribute to sodium imbalance, including loss of sodium-containing fluids or water excess (see Box 37-2, p. 853).	Hyponatremia causes hypoosmolality with a shift of water into cells (Lewis, Collier, and Heitkemper, 1996).
a. *Hyponatremia:* Assess for evidence of hyponatremia (serum sodium level less than 137 mEq/L):	

Steps	Rationale

(1) Assess mental status for personality change, irritability, apprehension, anxiety, convulsions, or coma.

Neurological symptoms are caused by fluid shift into brain cells (Lewis, Collier, and Heitkemper, 1996). Severe hyponatremia (less than 120 mEq/L) can result in neurological changes and irreversible neurological alterations or death at 110 mEq/L (Potter and Perry, 1998).

(2) Monitor vital signs for weak, rapid pulse and hypotension.

(3) Assess for abdominal cramps, nausea, and vomiting.

b. *Hypernatremia:* Assess for evidence of hypernatremia (serum sodium level less than 145 mEq/L):

Hypernatremia causes hyperosmolality with a shift of water out of the cells.

(1) Assess vital signs for low-grade fever and postural hypotension.

(2) Inspect mouth for dry tongue and mucous membranes.

(3) Assess for dry, flushed skin and thirst.

(4) Assess for agitation, restlessness, hyperreflexia, excitability, or convulsions.

(5) Monitor urine output for oliguria or anuria.

c. Provide comfort and safety measures, including preparation for potential convulsions in severe cases (see Skill 5.2).

d. If a low-sodium diet is prescribed, teach the client ways to consume less salt and sodium.

NURSE ALERT

IV fluids rates should be carefully monitored. When clients require rapid rates of infusion they must be assessed frequently for FVE, especially in the presence of cardiac, renal, or neurological problems.

(1) Read the nutrition labels and minimize the use of processed foods containing high levels of sodium. Look for canned foods with reduced or no sodium.

(2) Use fresh and plain frozen vegetables.

(3) Request no added salt when eating out or traveling.

(4) Use spices and herbs rather than salt to enhance the flavor of food.

(5) Avoid condiments such as pickles, olives, soy sauces, and other sauces high in sodium.

(6) Choose fresh fruits and vegetables as snacks rather than salted chips, nuts, or popcorn.

(7) Avoid over-the-counter medications that contain sodium (Na).

3. Assess for potassium imbalance: Identify conditions that contribute to potassium imbalance.

a. *Hypokalemia:* Assess for evidence of hypokalemia (serum potassium level less than 3.5 mEq/L):

The most common cause of hypokalemia is the use of potassium-wasting diuretics such as thiazides and loop diuretics.

(1) Assess vital signs for a weak, irregular pulse; shallow respirations; and hypotension.

(2) Assess electrocardiogram (ECG) changes (depressed ST, T wave inversion or flattening, and U waves).

(3) Assess for generalized weakness, decreased muscle tone, decreased reflexes, or fatigue.

(4) Assess abdomen for decreased bowel sounds and abdominal distention.

Steps	Rationale

    (5) Assess extremities for muscle cramps and paresthesias.

  b. Maintain adequate dietary intake of potassium (potatoes, spinach, broccoli, winter squash, dates, bananas, cantaloupes, dried apricots, orange and grapefruit juice, dry beans, milk, and yogurt).

  c. Administer IV fluids with KCl as ordered.

NURSE ALERT

The rate of administration of IV fluids containing KCl should not exceed 20 mEq of potassium per hour.

  d. *Hyperkalemia:* Assess for evidence of hyperkalemia (serum potassium greater than 5.5 mEq/L):

    (1) Assess ECG changes, including peaked T waves, prolonged PR interval, widening of QRS, complete heart block, ectopic beats, and ventricular fibrillation leading to cardiac arrest.

    (2) Assess for nausea, vomiting, diarrhea, and cramping pain.

    (3) Assess for muscle twitching, paresthesias or paralysis, or seizures.

  e. In the presence of hyperkalemia, collaborate with the physician to prescribe Kayexalate (exchanges Na for K, and K is excreted in stool), and/or promote the excretion of potassium with dialysis.

4. Calcium Imbalance: Identify conditions that contribute to calcium imbalance.

  a. *Hypercalcemia:* Assess laboratory reports for hypercalcemia (total serum calcium greater than 11 mg/dl):

    (1) Assess for lethargy, fatigue, malaise, confusion, impaired memory, sudden psychosis, or coma.

    (2) Monitor for weight loss, dehydration, and increased thirst.

    (3) Assess for hypertension or ECG changes.

    (4) Assess for decreased muscle strength, hypoventilation, and depressed reflexes.

    (5) Assess for anorexia, nausea, or constipation.

    (6) Assess abdomen for hypoactive bowel sounds or paralytic ileus.

  b. Promote the excretion of calcium in urine by increasing fluid intake to 3000 to 4000 ml of fluid daily or administration of a loop diuretic as ordered.

  c. *Hypocalcemia:* Monitor laboratory reports for hypocalcemia (total serum calcium less than 8.5 mg/dl):

    (1) Assess for personality changes, depression, irritability, anxiety, or confusion.

    (2) Assess for ECG changes, laryngeal spasm, or respiratory arrest.

    (3) Assess for colicky discomfort or diarrhea.

    (4) Assess for muscle cramps, numbness, and tingling in extremities.

Hyperkalemia is caused by renal failure, massive tissue damage, and rapid IV administration.

NURSE ALERT

Severe hypocalcemia is a medical emergency, particularly if laryngeal spasms and respiratory arrest are imminent. It is treated with IV calcium gluconate.

Steps	**Rationale**

(5) Assess for Chvostek's sign, a contraction of facial muscles in response to a light tap over the facial nerve in front of the ear (see illustration).

(6) Assess for Trousseau's sign, carpal spasm induced by inflating a blood pressure cuff above the systolic pressure for as long as 3 minutes (see illustration).

(7) Prepare for possible seizures and tetany (see Skill 5.2).

5. **Magnesium Imbalance:.** Identify factors that contribute to magnesium imbalance.

   a. *Hypomagnesemia:* Assess for evidence of magnesium deficit:

     (1) Assess mental status for sudden changes, including confusion.

     (2) Assess for hyperactive deep tendon reflexes (DTR), tremors, and convulsions.

     (3) Monitor for cardiac dysrythmias.

   b. *Hypermagnesemia:* Assess for evidence of magnesium excess:

     (1) Assess for lethargy and drowsiness.

     (2) Assess for hyporeflexia.

     (3) Assess for nausea and vomiting.

     (4) Promote urinary excretion in the presence of normal kidney function.

6. See Completion Protocol (inside front cover).

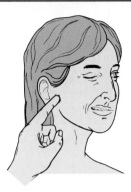

Step 4c(5) *From Lewis SM, Collier I, Heitkemper MM: Medical-surgical nursing: assessment and management of clinical problems, ed 4, St Louis, 1996, Mosby.*

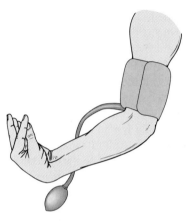

Step 4c(6) *From Lewis SM, Collier I, Heitkemper MM: Medical-surgical nursing: assessment and management of clinical problems, ed 4, St Louis, 1996, Mosby.*

• • •

EVALUATION

1. Check laboratory values and physical signs to identify trends in response to medical treatment.
2. Monitor for evidence of complications related to treatment resulting in the opposite imbalance (i.e., treatment for hypokalemia may result in hyperkalemia).

Unexpected Outcomes and Related Interventions

1. After treatment, client has a persistent electrolyte imbalance.
   a. Analyze the available data supporting the imbalance.
   b. In collaboration with other health team members, administer appropriate therapies to restore electrolyte balance.

Recording and Reporting

- Laboratory tests may be done frequently to monitor response to therapy. Report should include when electrolytes were drawn and abnormal results. When significantly abnormal, results should be called to the physician immediately for appropriate management.
- Documentation should include positive and negative assessment data related to abnormal electrolyte laboratory results and action taken, including notification of the physician.

Sample Documentation

1100   Serum Na 135 and K 3.2. Pulse 110, weak and irregular, respirations 28. Client reports weakness, fatigue, nausea, and anorexia. Dozing and arouses easily. States, "My legs have been aching since yesterday." Dr. Johnson notified. Orders received.

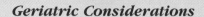

Geriatric Considerations

*   Atrophy of adrenal glands results in altered regulation of sodium and potassium and predisposes the client to fluid and electrolyte imbalance.

Home Care and Long-Term Care Considerations

*   Management of fluid and electrolyte problems in the home involves teaching caregivers of high-risk clients how to monitor for developing problems by recognizing risk factors.

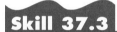

MONITORING ACID-BASE IMBALANCE

The body's metabolic processes constantly produce acids, which must be neutralized and excreted to maintain acid-base balance. Normally the body maintains an arterial pH between 7.35 and 7.45 by three regulatory mechanisms (Figure 37-5). These are buffer systems, the respiratory system, and the renal system. The buffer system reacts immediately to absorb or release hydrogen ions to maintain acid-base balance. The respiratory system responds within minutes, and the renal system takes 2 to 3 days to respond.

The lungs excrete carbon dioxide (CO_2) and water. The amount of CO_2 in the blood is directly related to the carbonic acid concentration. With increased respirations, more CO_2 is eliminated, which results in less carbonic acid. With decreased respirations, more CO_2 remains in the blood, which results in more carbonic acid.

Under normal conditions the kidneys reabsorb and conserve bicarbonate, which is the alkaline portion of the balance. The kidneys can generate additional bicarbonate and eliminate excess hydrogen ions as compensation for acidosis. The body normally excretes an acidic urine to help maintain acid-base balance. An acid-base imbalance is produced when the ratio between acid and base content of the blood is altered.

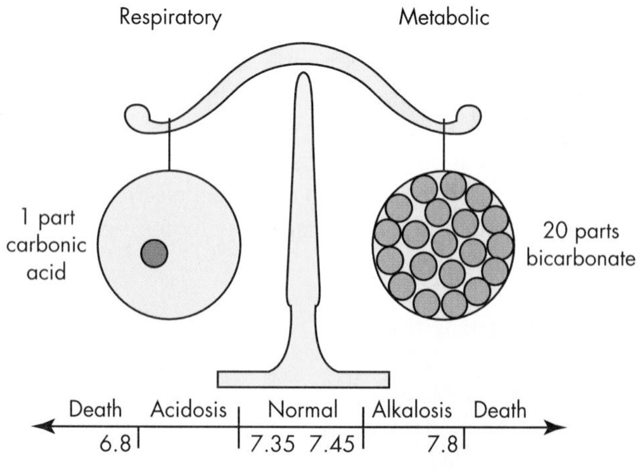

The primary types of acid-base imbalance are respiratory acidosis, respiratory alkalosis, metabolic acidosis, and metabolic alkalosis. To assess acid-base balance, a specimen of arterial blood is analyzed to determine the pH, amount of oxygen, amount of carbon dioxide, and amount of bicarbonate. This test, called an *arterial blood gas (ABG),* gives information about the cause of acid-base imbalances (respiratory or metabolic) and whether the imbalance is being compensated for by the respiratory or renal system. Normal ABG values are listed in Appendix D.

ASSESSMENT

1. Assess client's risk factors for acid-base imbalances (Box 37-4).
2. Identify potential complications.

PLANNING

Expected outcomes focus on identifying risks for or actual acid-base imbalance. Treatment should begin quickly to avoid any life-threatening complications.

Expected Outcomes

1. Client will maintain or achieve normal acid-base balance.
2. Complications will be prevented or minimized.

Death   Acidosis   Normal   Alkalosis   Death
6.8   7.35 7.45   7.8

Figure 37-5   Carbonic acid bicarbonate ratio and pH.

DELEGATION CONSIDERATIONS

Monitoring acid base balance requires the complex problem solving and knowledge unique to a professional nurse. AP may monitor assessment data (including vital signs) and report a client's subjective symptoms. All monitoring data must be reported to an RN.

Box 37-4 Risk Factors for Acid-Base Imbalances

Respiratory Acidosis
Pneumonia
Respiratory failure
Atelectasis
Drug overdose
Paralysis of respiratory muscles
Traumatic injury
Obesity
Airway obstruction
Head injuries
Stroke
Drowning
Cystic fibrosis

Respiratory Alkalosis
Anxiety
Fear
Anemia
Hypermetabolic states
CNS injuries or infections
Asthma
Inappropriate mechanical ventilator settings

Metabolic Acidosis
Starvation
Diabetic ketoacidosis
Renal failure
Shock
Diarrhea
Drug use (methanol, ethanol, formic acid, paraldehyde, aspirin)
Renal tubular acidosis

Metabolic Alkalosis
Excessive vomiting
Prolonged gastric suctioning
Hypokalemia
Hypercalcemia
Cushing's syndrome
Drug use (steroids, diuretics, sodium bicarbonate)

IMPLEMENTATION

Steps	Rationale

1. See Standard Protocol (inside front cover).
2. Check the pH to determine if it is alkalotic (greater than 7.45) or acidotic (less than 7.35).
3. Check the PaO_2 (norm is 80 to 100 mm Hg) and the SaO_2 (norm is 95% to 100%). NOTE: PaO_2 has no bearing on acid-base balance. Laboratory report includes whether supplementary oxygen was being administered when blood sample was drawn.

   Hypoxemia refers to low levels of oxygen in the arterial blood, whereas *hypoxia* refers to low tissue oxygenation. Hypoxia can exist with normal ABGs when the oxygen-carrying capacity of the blood is compromised (low hemoglobin) or there is low cardiac output and inadequate perfusion.

4. Determine the primary cause of the change in the pH. Check the $PaCO_2$ to determine if it is high, within normal limits (WNL) or low (normal is 35 to 45 mm Hg).
   a. If the $PaCO_2$ is high, the client is hypoventilating and retaining carbonic acid, resulting in *respiratory acidosis* (see illustration, p. 866). In collaboration with other health team members, determine ways to improve the client's ventilation to eliminate excess CO_2 (e.g., deep breathing, pursed-lip breathing, bronchodilators). Administer sodium bicarbonate intravenously as ordered.

Steps	**Rationale**

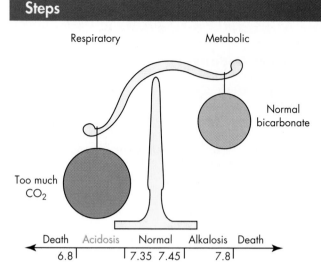

Step 4a

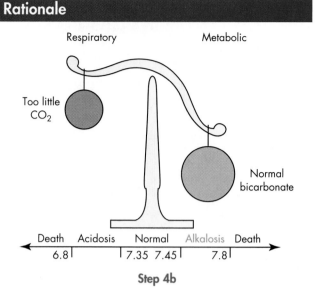

Step 4b

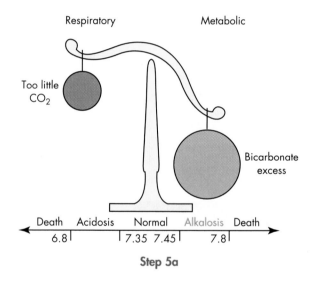

Step 5a

b. If the PaCO₂ is low, the client is hyperventilating and too much CO_2 is eliminated, resulting in *respiratory alkalosis* (see illustration). In collaboration with other health team members, determine ways to promote retention of CO_2 (e.g., minimize anxiety, slow rate of breathing and breathe less deeply, breathe into a paper bag).

c. If the PaCO₂ is WNL, the client is ventilating adequately.

5. Check the HCO₃ to determine if it is high, WNL, or low (normal is 22 to 26 mEq/L).

a. If the HCO₃ is high, there is a bicarbonate excess, which can result from retention of bicarbonate or a *metabolic loss* of acids; for example, with prolonged vomiting or gastric suction (see illustration). In collaboration with other health team members, determine ways to minimize the metabolic loss of acids.

b. If the HCO₃ is low and the CO_2 is normal, there is most likely a *bicarbonate deficit* from an accumulation of acids caused by a metabolic process such as diabetic ketoacidosis or lactic acid resulting from shock (see illustration). In collaboration with health team members, you may give sodium bicarbonate intravenously to treat the condition causing abnormal production of acids, thereby decreasing acid production. NOTE: Acidosis can be caused by carbon dioxide excess or by a bicarbonate deficit, and alkalosis can be caused by a carbon dioxide deficit or bicarbonate excess.

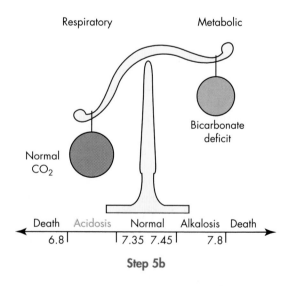

Step 5b

Steps	Rationale

6. Determine if there is evidence of the body attempting to compensate for the pH change.

   a. If the primary problem is respiratory acidosis (pH less than 7.4 with an elevated PCO_2), the kidneys may compensate by retaining bicarbonate, which will cause the pH to trend toward the normal range (7.35 to 7.39). This process may take hours or days (see illustration).

   b. If the primary problem is metabolic acidosis (pH less than 7.4 with a bicarbonate deficit), the body may compensate by hyperventilating immediately and eliminating carbon dioxide, causing the pH to trend toward the normal range (7.35 to 7.39) (see illustration).

   c. If the primary problem is respiratory alkalosis (pH greater than 7.4 with low CO_2), the body may compensate by decreasing renal absorption of bicarbonate. The pH trends toward the normal range (less than 7.45). This begins in 8 hours and is maximal in 3 to 5 days (see illustration).

   d. If the primary problem is metabolic alkalosis (pH greater than 7.4 with bicarbonate excess), the body may compensate immediately with hypoventilation to promote retention of carbonic acid. The pH trends toward the normal range (less than 7.45) (see illustration).

7. See Completion Protocol (inside front cover).

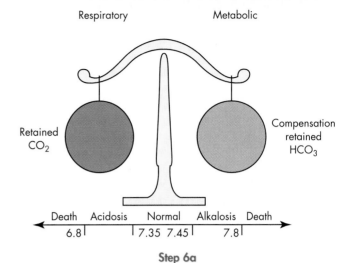

Step 6a

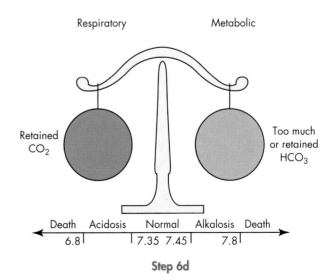

Step 6b

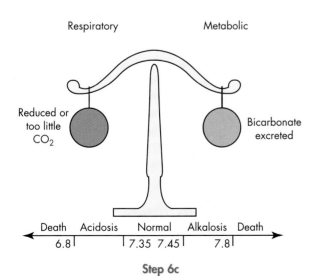

Step 6c

Step 6d

EVALUATION

1. Analyze the ABG to determine if acid-base imbalance has been corrected as a result of medical and nursing interventions. (Correction is evident by pH, CO_2, and HCO_2 all WNL.)
2. Assess for evidence of complications.

Unexpected Outcomes and Related Interventions

1. After treatment, the client continues to have persistent acid-base imbalance.
   a. Analyze the available data to determine confounding factors.
   b. In collaboration with other health team members, identify ways to correct imbalance.

Recording and Reporting

- Clients with acid-base imbalances are usually critically ill and may require frequent ABG analysis and prompt medical and nursing interventions.
- Often blood samples are drawn in emergency situations and sent to the laboratory STAT. Results must be reported to the physician as soon as available.
- Documentation should include assessments related to client status, interventions utilized, and evaluation of client response.

Sample Documentation

2300   Admitted in acute respiratory distress. Vital signs: P 112, R 36, BP 148/84. Reports dyspnea at rest and speech interrupted to breathe. Alert and oriented X 3. Lung sounds reveal coarse crackles and wheezing throughout. Oxygen at 2 L per nasal cannula. HOB elevated. ABGs PaO_2 68, pH 7.32, $PaCO_2$ 50, and HCO_3 24. Dr. Lindsay notified. Orders received.

CRITICAL THINKING EXERCISES

1. A client is extremely anxious after an automobile accident. The client complains of neck pain. Respirations are very rapid and the pulse rate is 110. Would the acid-base balance most likely to develop be acidosis or alkalosis, and would the cause be respiratory or metabolic? Explain.

2. A client has several days of severe vomiting and diarrhea. ABGs reveal a pH of 7.3, pCO_2 of 35, and HCO_3 of 20. What acid-base imbalance is present? What assessments could you make to detect compensation efforts by the body?

3. An older adult client has been living alone in an apartment. During your home health visit, the client demonstrates the following: weight loss of 5 pounds in 3 days; weak pulse; blood pressure 90/50 (baseline 115/80); oliguria with dark, tea-colored urine; weakness; and dry lips and mucous membranes. What additional data would you need to determine if the condition is caused by decreased intake, excessive losses, or both?

REFERENCES

Lewis SM, Collier IC, Heitkemper M: *Medical-surgical nursing: assessment and management of clinical problems,* ed 4, St Louis, 1996, Mosby.

Perry AG, Potter PA: *Clinical nursing skills and techniques,* ed 4, St Louis, 1998, Mosby.

Potter PA, Perry AG: *Fundamentals of nursing,* ed 4, St Louis, 1998, Mosby.

Tate P, Seeley RR, Stephens TD: *Understanding the human body,* St Louis, 1994, Mosby.

CHAPTER 38

Emergency Measures for Life Support in the Hospital Setting

Skill 38.1
Resuscitation, 870

Skill 38.2
Code Management, 877

Skill 38.3
Care of the Body after Death, 882

The cardiovascular and pulmonary systems work together to transport oxygen to the tissues and remove carbon dioxide and other waste products of metabolism. The amount of oxygen delivered to the tissues depends on several physiological components. These components include ventilation (the amount of oxygen entering the blood), perfusion (the circulation of blood to lungs and tissues), and diffusion (the transference of oxygen and carbon dioxide to and from the tissues during inspiration and exhalation). Diffusion occurs at the alveolar level. Critical to the transport of oxygen to the tissues is the ability of the heart to pump blood between the lungs and the periphery. Other components to be considered are the oxygen-carrying capacity of the blood and oxygen requirements of the tissues. The oxygen-carrying capacity of blood depends on the presence of adequate numbers of hemoglobin molecules and an environment conducive to the attachment of oxygen and carbon dioxide to the hemoglobin molecule.

Respiratory arrest and cardiac arrest are emergency situations that the nurse must be prepared to handle at any time. Respiratory arrest, or absence of breathing, results in the absence of oxygen delivery to the alveoli. This in turns leads to no oxygen or carbon dioxide exchange, which creates a buildup of waste products in the tissues. Cardiac arrest is the cessation of circulating blood, which in turn eliminates oxygen transport.

Predisposing factors to a cardiac or pulmonary arrest may include illnesses involving the cardiopulmonary system, presence of an airway obstruction, fluid and electrolyte imbalances, and ingestion of toxic substances. Unless otherwise indicated, such as a client having a do not resuscitate (DNR) status, all clients receive cardiopulmonary resuscitation (CPR) in the event of arrest. Individual hospital policy and procedures define methods of identification of a client's resuscitation status.

Advance directives offer valuable information concerning resuscitation status and individual client decisions regarding resuscitation efforts. Although advance directives may be addressed before or during the client's hospital admission, the nurse can play an important role in encouraging clients to complete the document. Nurses, because of their unique relationship with clients and the associated high level of trust, are the ideal facilitators for the initiation of advance directives (Johns, 1996). Clients want to discuss end-of-life care, and they expect providers to initiate these conversations (Bettrell, Mezey, and Ramsey, 1996). Advance directives may be used as a tool to minimize disagreements among family members regarding resuscitation status determination when the client is physically unable to make decisions. Many hospitals have a mechanism to assist the client/family regarding this issue. Social services and an ethics committee may be of assistance to the client and family.

NURSING DIAGNOSES

Nursing diagnoses that apply to clients who receive CPR include **Ineffective Breathing Pattern,** in which a client who is not breathing (respiratory arrest) is unable to achieve adequate gas exchange of oxygen and carbon dioxide. This may be related to injury, paralysis affecting the diaphragm or phrenic nerve, a collapsed lung (pneumothorax), chest trauma with blood accumulation in the chest (hemothorax), or drug overdose. **Ineffective Airway**

Clearance related to copious secretions associated with pneumonia or airway obstruction can also result in respiratory distress. **Impaired Gas Exchange** can be associated with cardiac and pulmonary disorders that interfere with the body's ability to exchange carbon dioxide and oxygen at the cellular level. **Decreased Cardiac Output** occurs when there is a cardiac arrest and/or cardiac disorders such as dysrhythmias, blockage of coronary arteries, or conges-tive heart failure (CHF). Finally, **Altered Tissue Perfusion** of vital organs (e.g., brain, kidney, heart) occurs if cardiopulmonary function is not maintained or restored.

After death, the following nursing diagnoses may apply: **Risk for Impaired Skin Integrity** associated with the decomposition of tissue and **Grieving** related to family members or friends facing difficulty with loss or **Dysfunctional grieving** in which there is prolonged grief.

Skill 38.1

RESUSCITATION

Cardiopulmonary arrest is identified by the absence of pulse or respiration. Once this is assessed, the nurse must immediately begin CPR. CPR is an emergency procedure that combines artificial breathing techniques with external cardiac massage. This technique is accomplished in an established and orderly pattern known as the *ABCs*. Resuscitation efforts include establishing the *Airway*, initiating *Breathing*, and maintaining *Circulation*. This can be expanded to include *Defibrillation*. Defibrillation involves delivery of a direct electrical current, through the heart, that is sufficient to depolarize cells of the myocardium. The intent of defibrillation is that subsequent repolarization of the heart will allow the sinoatrial (SA) mode to resume the role of pacemaker. The heart will then resume more normal conduction. Early CPR followed by immediate electrical defibrillation of the heart (when indicated) and advanced cardiac life support (ACLS) can improve the survival of cardiopulmonary arrest victims. ACLS training and certification combines cognitive and psychomotor skills with systematic critical thinking skills in the management of the client experiencing cardiopulmonary arrest. ACLS teaches the support of ventilation, establishment of intravenous (IV) access, recognition of dysrythmias, administration of drugs, and delivery of electrical shock. Early ABCD is crucial for a favorable client outcome. Without oxygen delivery, brain damage begins within 4 minutes of arrest, brain damage almost always occurs at 6 minutes, and brain death is certain at 10 minutes (Chandra and Hazinski, 1997).

Being prepared for a cardiopulmonary arrest is important. The ability of non–ACLS-trained nurses to initiate a code contributes significantly to the code team's ability to function effectively (Brown et al., 1995). Equipment may be readily available at the bedside or in a designated area of the hospital unit. It is the nurse's responsibility to know the location of emergency equipment, including the resuscitation cart. It is also the nurse's responsibility to know the contents of the resuscitation cart (Figure 38-1).

Equipment

Air-mask-bag-unit (Ambu bag), if available (Figure 38-2)
CPR pocket mask or barrier device, if available (Figure 38-3)
Clean gloves, face shield, and gown if available
Suction apparatus

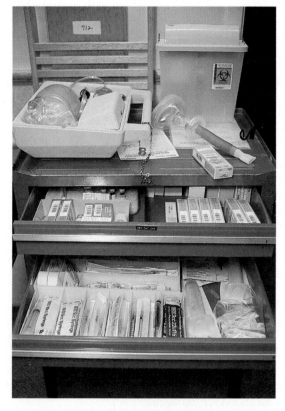

Figure 38-1 Emergency resuscitation cart.

Resuscitation cart with
    Cardiac monitor with defibrillator and pads
    Emergency medications
    Endotracheal intubation equipment
    IV catheters (sizes 16 and 18), tubing, and fluids
        (0.9% normal saline [NS])
Pulse oxymetry monitoring equipment

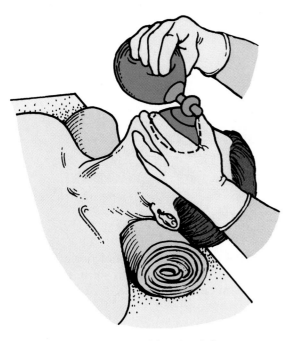

Figure 38-2 Ambu bag and face mask for resuscitation.

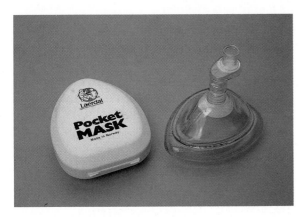

Figure 38-3 Pocket mask.

ASSESSMENT

1. Assess the client's unresponsivenenss by shaking the client and shouting, "Are you OK?" **Rationale: Assists the nurse in determining if the client is unconscious rather than intoxicated, sleeping, or hearing impaired.**
2. Activate the emergency medical services according to hospital policy and procedure (e.g., call a code 99). **Rationale: The majority of adult victims are in ventricular fibrillation and need defibrillation and antidysrhythmic drugs as soon as possible. Early access to emergency cardiac care systems improves client outcome.**

PLANNING

Expected outcomes focus on the establishment and maintenance of artificial breathing and circulation.

Expected Outcomes

1. Adequate oxygenation and tissue perfusion are maintained during artificial resuscitation.
2. Client regains spontaneous respirations during resuscitation.
3. Client regains adequate cardiac output as a result of resuscitation.

DELEGATION CONSIDERATIONS

The skill of cardiopulmonary resuscitation can be performed by assistive personnel (AP).

- Caution the care provider to make certain the client is indeed pulseless before initiating chest compressions.
- Review the procedures for opening the airway if the client is at risk for cervical neck trauma.
- Caution the AP regarding the differences in technique between infants, children, and adults.
- Ensure that the care provider is using correct hand and body positioning for CPR and is cycling breathing and compressions correctly.

IMPLEMENTATION

Steps	Rationale
1. Observe for chest movement; listen and feel for breaths.	Indicates client has spontaneous respirations.
2. If client is breathing and no trauma is present, place client in the recovery position (see illustration).	In the recovery position, the airway is more likely to remain open and unrecognized airway obstruction (the tongue) is less likely to occur (Chandra and Hazinski, 1997).

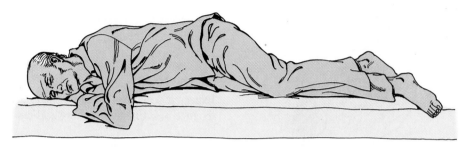

Step 2

Steps	Rationale
3. If no respirations are detected, call for assistance.	Effective CPR cannot be continuously maintained by one person. The helper can also obtain the resuscitation cart or equipment.

> **NURSE ALERT**
>
> *This skill requires application of the basic principles of CPR to maintain tissue perfusion until additional assistance of the cardiac arrest or code team arrives.*

Steps	Rationale
4. Place victim on hard surface, such as floor or ground, or use the backboard found on the resuscitation cart or the headboard of the hospital bed. If the client must be moved to the supine position, use the log-rolling technique to maintain spinal integrity.	External cardiac compressions are most effective when the heart is compressed between the sternum and a hard surface (Chandra and Hazinski, 1997).
5. Correctly position for resuscitative efforts.	
a. *One-person rescue:* face client while kneeling parallel to the client's sternum.	Allows rescuer to move quickly between head and sternum.
b. *Two-person rescue:* one person faces client while kneeling parallel to the client's head. Second person is on the opposite side parallel to the client's sternum.	Allows one rescuer to perform artificial respirations while the second rescuer performs chest compressions.
6. Open the airway.	
a. If no head or neck trauma is suspected, use the head-tilt, chin-lift method (see illustration).	The head-tilt, chin-lift maneuver prevents the tongue from obstructing the airway of the unconscious client. The tongue is the most common obstruction.
b. If head or neck trauma is suspected, use the jaw-thrust maneuver only. Grasp angles of client's lower jaw and lift with both hands, displacing the mandible forward (see illustration).	This maneuver allows opening of airway without disrupting head and neck alignment, therefore preventing any further damage.

Steps	Rationale

NURSE ALERT

The nurse must be aware if the client has a DNR status.

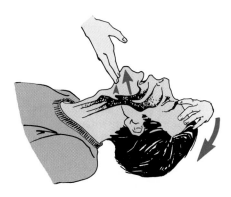

Step 6a

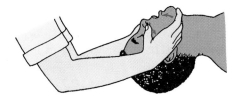

Step 6b

7. Mouth-to-mouth artificial respirations:
   a. *Adult:*
      (1) Pinch client's nose with thumb and index finger and occlude mouth with rescuer's mouth or use CPR pocket mask (see illustration). Attempt two slow breaths, 1½ to 2 seconds per breath.
      (2) The rescuer should take a breath after each ventilation.

      (3) Allow the client to exhale between breaths.
      (4) Continue with 12 breaths per minute.

Forms an airtight seal around the client's mouth and prevents air from escaping through the nose. Give breaths with only enough force to make the chest rise. Slow breaths deliver air at a low pressure to reduce the risk of gastric distention.

Taking a breath ensures the client is receiving an adequate volume of oxygenated air with each ventilation.

An excess of air may result in gastric distention.

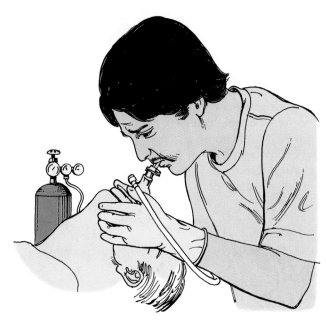

Step 7a(1)

Steps	Rationale

b. *Child* (1 to 8 years of age):
   (1) Pinch the victim's nose tightly with thumb and forefinger. Place rescuer's mouth or CPR pocket mask over client's mouth, forming an airtight seal. Give two slow breaths, 1 to 1½ seconds per breath.

Forms an airtight seal around the client's mouth and prevents air from escaping through the nose. Give breaths with only enough force to make the chest rise. Slow breaths deliver air at a low pressure to reduce the risk of gastric distention.

   (2) Pause after the first breath to take a breath.

Taking a breath ensures the client is receiving an adequate volume of oxygenated air with each ventilation.

   (3) Continue with 20 breaths per minute.

c. *Infant:*
   (1) Place the rescuer's mouth over the infant's nose and mouth, forming an airtight seal.

Rescue breaths are the single most important maneuver in assisting a nonbreathing infant or child.

   (2) Give two breaths slowly at 1 to 1½ seconds per breath.

Infants and children have small airways that provide high resistance to airflow. To minimize the resistance and to prevent gastric distention, give breaths slowly.

The correct volume for each breath is the volume that makes the chest rise (Chandra and Hazinski, 1997).

   (3) Continue with 20 breaths per minute.

8. Ambu bag artificial respirations:
  a. *All ages:*
   (1) Connect oxygen supply tubing to Ambu bag and oxygen flowmeter. Adjust oxygen to 100% F_iO_2 or ordered rate.

Provides supplemental oxygen.

   (2) Insert oropharyngeal airway.

Prevents tongue from obstructing the airway and provides patent airway.

   (3) Position the face mask of the Ambu bag over the client's mouth and nose.

Selection of the proper size face mask is essential in achieving an airtight seal.

   (4) Give slow breaths by squeezing the bag.

As the bag is compressed, oxygen enters the client.

   (5) Allow time for client to exhale.

Exhalation prevents overinflation of the lungs and gastric distention.

9. If ventilation attempt is unsuccessful, reposition the client's head and reattempt rescue breathing again. If ventilation attempt remains unsuccessful, the airway may be obstructed by a foreign body that will need to be removed.

Patent airway and oxygen delivery must be ensured before beginning compressions.

  a. *Adult:* Foreign body removal may be facilitated by blind finger sweeps and the Heimlich maneuver (see illustration). For finger sweep, keep victim's head up. Open victim's mouth by grasping both the tongue and lower jaw between the thumb and fingers and lifting. This draws the tongue from the back of the throat and away from foreign body. Maneuver object into mouth for removal (see illustration).

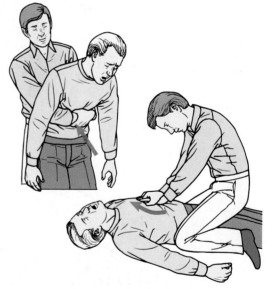

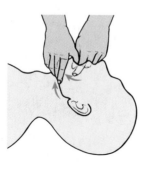

Step 9a   *From Lewis SM, Collier I, Heitkemper MM: Medical-surgical nursing: assessment and management of clinical problems, ed 4, St Louis, 1996, Mosby.*

Steps	Rationale

b. *Child:* Heimlich maneuver and back blows and chest thrusts are recommended.

c. *Infant:* Back blows and chest thrusts are recommended.

Finger sweep may push foreign body back into the airway.

Serious complications related to the use of the Heimlich maneuver on infants include rupture of the stomach, diaphragm, esophagus, and jejunum (Chandra and Hazinski, 1997).

10. Suction secretions as needed or turn client's head to the side if no trauma is suspected.

Suctioning secretions assists in preventing airway obstruction. Turning the head to one side allows the secretions to drain to gravity.

11. Check for the presence of carotid pulse in adult and child or brachial pulse in infant. Feel for 3 to 5 seconds.

Carotid pulse is present when other peripheral pulses are not. The neck of an infant is usually fat and chubby, so the carotid pulse is difficult to locate. Delivering cardiac compressions in the presence of a pulse contraindicated.

12. If no pulse, initiate chest compressions.

a. *Adult:* Place heel of hands, one atop the other, on lower third of the sternum. Lock elbows and maintain shoulders in line sternum (see illustrations).

b. *Child:* Place the heel of one hand on the lower half of the sternum (see illustration).

c. *Infant:* Place two or three fingers on the lower half of the sternum just below the level of the infant's nipples (see illustration).

Correct positioning of the hands decreases chance of injury.

NURSE ALERT

Ensure fingers are off the ribs and the lowermost part of the xiphoid process. This minimizes the chance of rib fracture.

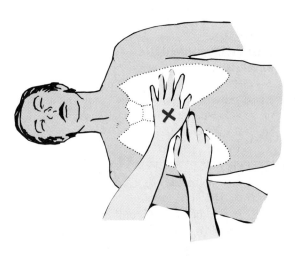

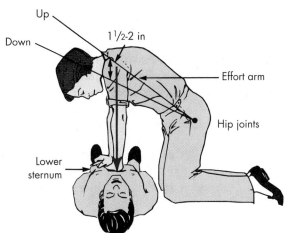

Step 12a

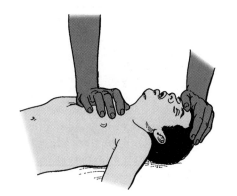

Step 12b

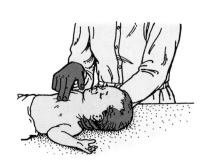

Step 12c

Steps	Rationale

13. Compress chest downward to proper depth and then release. Maintain constant contact with skin.
   a. *Adult:* 1½ to 2 inches (4 to 5 cm)
   b. *Child:* 1 to 1½ inches (2.5 to 4 cm)
   c. *Infant:* ½ to 1 inch (1 to 2.5 cm)
	Compression of the sternum provides circulation as a result of direct compression of the heart and increase in intrathoracic pressure (Chandra and Hazinski, 1997).

14. Maintain correct ratio proportionate to number of rescuers:
     One rescuer: 15 compression, 2 breaths
     Two rescuers: 5 compressions, 1 breath
   a. *Adult:* minimum of 80 to 100 compressions per minute
   b. *Child:* minimum of 100 compressions per minute
   c. *Infant:* minimum of 100 compressions per minute (Chandra and Hazinski, 1997)
	Number of effective compressions per minute determines the cardiac output.

15. Continue artificial respiration.	Maintains oxygen concentration during compressions.
16. Monitor the adequacy of the compressions during two-rescuer CPR with palpation of the carotid (adult, child) or brachial (infant) pulse during compressions. Have the rescuer performing the breathing palpate the pulse during compression. Do not delay compression.	If the pulse is not palpable, compressions may not be strong enough or hand position on the sternum may be incorrect. CPR cannot be interrupted for more than 5 seconds. Interruption of CPR for intubation should be closely monitored to avoid prolonged cessation of life-support measures.
17. Continue CPR until the rescuer is relieved, client regains cardiopulmonary function independently, or physician directs that CPR be discontinued.	Artificial respiration and cardiac function are provided as long as necessary.
18. See Completion Protocol (inside front cover).	

• • • •

EVALUATION

1. Inspect client's chest wall for rise and fall during administration of artificial breathing. Monitor for adequate seal over client's mouth.
2. Palpate for presence of pulse after four cycles of compressions and breaths. Assess every few minutes thereafter.
3. Observe for return of respirations and pulse.

Unexpected Outcomes and Related Interventions

1. Client develops a fractured rib or sternum or a laceration of an internal organ such as a lung or the liver.
   a. Monitor correct hand placement during the administration of CPR.
   b. Assess client for predisposing factors that make the client susceptible to injury during CPR. *Note:* CPR takes precedence over predisposing factors for injury.

Recording and Reporting

- Immediately report arrest, indicating the exact location of the arrest (follow hospital policy).
- Record in nurses' notes onset of arrest; actions taken, including all medications and treatments; and client's response. A special resuscitation sheet is available in most acute care settings.

Sample Documentation

2230 Client found lying in bed and unresponsive. No breathing noted. Code called, CPR begun.

2342 Client resuscitated by Code 99 team and transferred to the medical intensive care unit with team in attendance.

Geriatric Considerations

- In the older adult, compressions often result in rib and cartilage fractures. Cardiopulmonary resuscitation should be continued.

Home Care and Long-Term Care Considerations

For clients with implanted cardioverter-defibrillators, families should know how to administer CPR. CPR should be delayed until the device fires unsuccessfully 4 to 7 times or fails to fire after 30 seconds (Lewis et al., 1996).

CODE MANAGEMENT

This skill includes the initial response and management of cardiopulmonary arrest. Care must be taken to perform the basic skills of CPR immediately after discovery of an unresponsive client. In many hospital settings, a code team or cardiac arrest team is available to respond and assist in resuscitation of a client with cardiac arrest.

The team usually includes a physician, intensive care nurse, respiratory therapy personnel, radiology and laboratory technologists, and other personnel. A representative from pastoral care may be available to be with the family. Family and visitors have traditionally been asked to wait in a nearby area. The Emergency Nurses Association (ENA) has issued a statement regarding the family's presence during the resuscitative phase of a client's care. The ENA asserts the family should be given the choice of staying with the client or waiting in another area. Continued research is necessary to determine the impact on family members, clients, and health care personnel (Lenehan, 1995). If the client is in a two-bed room and the roommate can be assisted to leave, this is appropriate. If the roommate cannot leave, it is appropriate for someone to remain with the person. Excess furniture is moved out of the way and resuscitation equipment is brought into the room.

CPR is initiated and maintained by the discovering staff until the code team arrives. As soon as possible, the client's cardiac rhythm is determined and the client is defibrillated if warranted. The client may also be intubated, and an Ambu bag is used for ventilatory support. Usually specially trained staff from the code team initiate defibrillation. When code teams are not used, nurses should be proficient with defibrillation. A code team should have access to a defibrillator immediately or within 1 to 2 minutes of cardiac arrest (Cummins, 1997).

Automatic external defibrillators (AEDs) are available. The advantage of the AED is that basic life support (BLS) personnel who have less training than ACLS personnel can defibrillate. AEDs eliminate the training in rhythm interpretation and make early defibrillation practical and achievable. The AED is an external defibrillator that incorporates a rhythm analysis system. The device attaches to a client by two adhesive pads and connecting cables. The pads can relay the rhythm for interpretation and deliver the electric shock. A fully automatic defibrillator requires only that the operator attach the pads and turn on the device.

A cardiopulmonary arrest is approached in a systematic and organized fashion to ensure the most expedient care. The goal is to restore cardiopulmonary function as soon as possible and decrease the likelihood of an adverse outcome. The Committee on Emergency Cardiac Care (1992) continues to research cardiac arrest treatment and outcomes and has created guidelines for the initial care of these special specific recommendations for emergency cardiac drugs, electrical defibrillation, and supportive measures are included in the Advanced Cardiac Life Support Guidelines (Cummings, 1997).

ASSESSMENT

1. Assess client's unresponsiveness. **Rationale: This information assists the nurse in determining if the client is unconscious rather than asleep, intoxicated, or hearing impaired.**
2. Activate the emergency medical service in accordance with hospital policy and procedure (e.g., call a code 99 or 555). **Rationale: The majority of adult victims are in ventricular fibrillation and need defibrillation and antidysrhythmic drugs as soon as possible. Early access to emergency cardiac care systems improves client outcomes (Cummings, 1997).**
3. Begin CPR efforts (see Skill 38.1). **Rationale: Without oxygen delivery, brain damage begins within 4 minutes. Brain damage almost always occurs at 6 minutes, and brain death is certain at 10 minutes (Chandra and Hazinski, 1997).**

PLANNING

Expected outcomes focus on the goals of care, which are restoration of cardiac and pulmonary function before irreversible organ damage occurs.

Expected Outcomes

1. Client regains cardiopulmonary function without adverse effects.

DELEGATION CONSIDERATIONS

The skill of cardiopulmonary resuscitation can be performed by AP. The administration of emergency drugs and treatment is the responsibility of the RN and physician. An ACLS-certified RN is responsible for coordinating nursing and some ancillary department activities in a code situation.

IMPLEMENTATION

Steps	Rationale

1. Follow Skill 38.1.
Establish absence of respirations, begin artificial respirations, establish absence of pulse, and begin compressions (ABC).

NURSE ALERT

This skill requires that CPR be performed immediately after discovery of the client with cardiopulmonary arrest and that electrical defibrillation equipment be obtained as soon as possible.

NURSE ALERT

Know the client's code status.

2. First available person brings the resuscitation cart with emergency drugs, intubation equipment, IV access supplies, and other equipment.

Positive client outcome is directly related to the timeliness of administration of ACLS.

3. If an AED is available, attach to client and deliver shock.

   a. Turn on the power.

Turning on the power allows the machine to warm up while the defibrillator pads are being applied.

   b. Attach the device. One pad to the right of the sternum just below the clavicle and the other to the left of the precordium.

Maximizes current flow through the cardiac chambers (Cummins, 1997).

   c. Initiate analysis of the rhythm. Each brand of AED is different, so familiarity with the model is important.

The AED automatically interprets the rhythm upon operator's command.

   d. Deliver the shock in a series of three as indicated by the AED. The AED has a pause time of 10 to 15 seconds for rhythm analysis.

Series of three repeated shocks decreases intrathoracic pressure to the electrical current (Cummins, 1997). This pause time is the exception to American Heart Association (AHA) guidelines, which recommend that CPR not be stopped for more than 5 seconds.

   e. Check for pulse after three shocks. If no pulse, resume CPR for 1 minute, then begin the shock sequence again.

The purpose of defibrillation is to return the heart to a rhythm that produces a pulse.

4. Have someone assist the victim's roommate away from the code scene.

The victim's privacy must be protected. The code scene is intense and has the potential to create emotional distress for the roommate.

5. The client's nurse must relay information about the client to the team. This information includes events occurring immediately before the arrest, vital signs, laboratory results, radiology findings, and medications. The code leader may want information about the location of family members.

This information is critical in the selection of appropriate treatment for the client.

6. If respirations are absent but pulse is present, assist the code team to:

   a. Administer oxygen at high flow rate by mask or Ambu bag (see illustration).

Increases the oxygen concentration in the blood circulating to the tissues.

   b. Monitor vital signs, including cardiac rhythm via resuscitation monitor (see illustration).

A cardiac dysrhythmia resulting in hypotension requires immediate intervention.

   c. Prepare for endotracheal intubation.

Intubation provides a patent airway and increases pulmonary ventilation.

Steps

Rationale

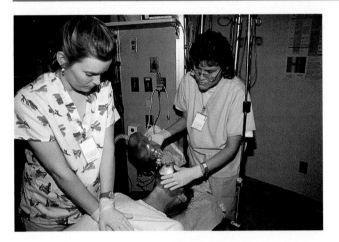

Step 6a

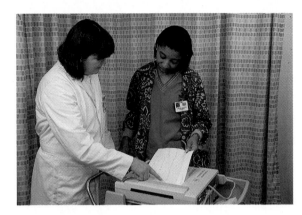

Step 6b

d. Establish IV access with large-bore needle and begin infusion of 0.9% NS.

Provides a route for rapid drug administration, access for blood samples, and fluid administration. Physiological saline is isotonic.

e. Assist ancillary team to obtain blood samples, including arterial blood gases (ABGs).

Provides valuable information regarding electrolytes, oxygenation, and ventilation.

f. Review history for suspected causes of cardiac arrest.

Hypotension, shock, pulmonary edema, and dysrhythmias are possible causes of a respiratory arrest. Treatment depends on the cause.

7. If respirations and pulse are absent and no AED is available, assist the code team to:

a. Prepare for defibrillation and defibrillate. NOTE: **Defibrillation is performed only by personnel trained and certified to do so.**

b. Defibrillator is turned on and proper energy level is selected.

Output in joules or watts per second. Shock may be delivered at 200j and increased as necessary.

c. Conductive materials (electrode gel or defibrillator gel pads) are applied to client's chest where defibrillator paddles will be placed.

Decreases electrical opposition and helps minimize burns (Cummings, 1997).

d. Paddles are charged and placed on the client's chest wall with one to the right of the sternum just below the clavicle and the other to the left of the precordium (see illustration, p. 880).

e. Operator applies a firm pressure to the paddles, announces intent to shock the client, and makes sure no personnel are directly or indirectly in contact with the client.

Firm pressure lowers transthoracic impedance of the electrical current (Cummings, 1997). Anyone in direct or indirect contact with the client during the shock will also receive the shock.

f. Operator depresses the buttons on the defibrillator paddles at the same time to discharge the electrical current.

g. The first defibrillation activity is performed as a rapidly repeated series of three if the monitor displays persistent ventricular fibrillation or ventricular tachycardia without a pulse.

The series of three repeated shocks decreases the intrathoracic impedance to the electrical current (Cummings, 1997).

Steps	Rationale

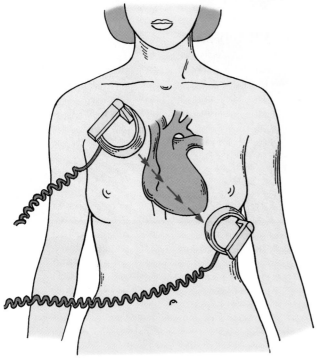

Step 7d

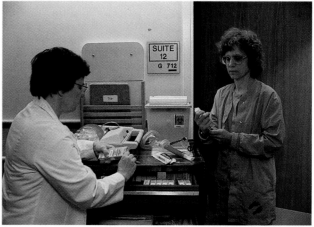

Step 9

8. If three shocks fail or a different dysrhythmia is present:
   a. Continue CPR.
   b. Establish IV access.
   c. Administer medications.
   d. Establish ventilation (intubation).
   e. Repeat shocks if warranted.

The code team is trained to interpret dysrhythmias and intervene with appropriate treatment.

9. If not involved in the performance of CPR, nurse should obtain supplies and drugs as requested (see illustration).

The code team is specially trained in advanced life support techniques. Rapid location of supplies assists the team in providing care to clients.

10. Anticipate the types of vasoactive medications that will likely be used (Box 38-1). Double-check dosages to be given (Box 38-2).

Ensures prompt and accurate administration of medications.

11. Remain in the room during the resuscitative phase.

Nurse caring for the client is the person most familiar with the client's medical history, which aids in diagnosis and treatment by the code team.

12. Keep unnecessary personnel out of the room during the resuscitative phase.

Cardiopulmonary arrest situations attract many hospital personnel. Too many people may interfere with the expeditious delivery of care.

13. Ensure all interventions, medication administration, and client responses are being recorded.

At the onset of a code, designation of a recorder is important. Several medical personnel are performing different interventions in a rapid sequence. Accurate recording of the events assists the code team in planning the next intervention.

14. Continue resuscitative efforts until the client regains pulse or until the physician determines cessation of efforts.

15. See Completion Protocol (inside front cover).

• • • •

Box 38-1 Critical Care Calculations

Basic Formula

$$\frac{\text{Concentration}}{60} = \frac{\text{Total minute dose}}{\text{Rate}}$$

Present Rate

$$\text{Rate} = \frac{60 \times \text{Total minute dose}}{\text{Concentration}}$$

Desired Dose

$$\text{Total minute dose} = \frac{\text{Concentration} \times \text{Rate}}{60}$$

Reminders

1. Rates in cc/hr = microdrops/minute (μgtt/min)
2. Concentration of solution is in mg/ml or μg/ml.

$$\text{Concentration} = \frac{\text{Drug in solution (mg)}}{\text{Volume of solution (ml)}}$$

To convert mg/ml to μg/ml, multiply by 1000.
EXAMPLE: 0.2 mg/ml = 200 μg/ml
3. Total minute dose is in mg/min or μg/min, depending on solution strength. When prescribed as μg/kg/min, multiply by client weight.
EXAMPLE: Desired dose = 3 μg/kg/min for 50-kg person
Total minute dose = 3 μg/kg/min $\times$ 50 kg = 150 μg/min
4. Client's lean body weight is suggested reference weight for titration of potent medications. To convert lbs to kg, divide by 2.2.

Modified from Keen JH, Baird MS, Allen JH: *Mosby's critical care and emergency drug reference*, St Louis, 1994, Mosby.

Box 38-2 Common Vasoactive Infusions

dobutamine (Dobutrex)
Concentration: 250 mg/250 D$_5$W (1000 μg/ml)
   Usual dose: 2.5–20 μg/kg/min
   Initial dose: 60 kg: 9 ml/hr is 2.5 μg/kg/min
                80 kg: 12 ml/hr is 2.5 μg/kg/min
               100 kg: 15 ml/hr is 2.5 μg/kg/min

dopamine (Intropin)
Concentration: 400 mg/250 D$_5$W (1600 μg/ml)
   Usual dose: 2.5–20 μg/kg/min
   Initial dose: 60 kg: 6 ml/hr is 2.5 μg/kg/min
                80 kg: 8 ml/hr is 2.5 μg/kg/min
               100 kg: 9 ml/hr is 2.5 μg/kg/min

epinephrine (Adrenalin)
Concentration: 1 mg/250 D$_5$W (4 μg/ml)
   Usual dose: 2–10 μg/min
   Initial dose: 30 ml/hr is 2 μg/min

nitroglycerin (Tridil)
Concentration: 50 mg/250 D$_5$W (200 μg/ml)
   Usual dose: 10–200 μg/min
   Initial dose: 3 ml/hr is 10 μg/min

nitroprusside (Nipride)
Concentration: 50 mg/250 D$_5$W (200 μg/ml)
   Usual dose: 0.5–10 μg/kg/min
   Initial dose: 60 kg: 9 ml/hr is 0.5 μg/kg/min
                80 kg: 12 ml/hr is 0.5 μg/kg/min
               100 kg: 15 ml/hr is 0.5 μg/kg/min

norepinephrine (Levophed)
Concentration: 4 mg/250 D$_5$W (16 μg/ml)
   Usual dose: 0.5–30 μg/min
   Initial dose: 4 ml/hr is 1 μg/min
               15 ml/hr is 4 μg/min

From Keen JH, Baird MS, Allen JH: *Mosby's critical care and emergency drug reference*, St Louis, 1994, Mosby.

COMMUNICATION TIP

When assisting a client from a room during a code situation, remain calm. Use words that convey a sense of urgency and also portray a sense of competency and assurance. "There will be many people in the room soon to help your roommate. I will help you to a less busy area/room." If the client must stay in the room because it is impossible to leave, stay with the client. "A team of professionals is going to help your roommate. It will be a very busy area and may be noisy. I will be with you to answer questions." Remember the issue of confidentiality when answering questions. If the family is at the bedside, assist them away from the area. "Your brother is in an emergency situation. We need to give the emergency team time and space to work to help your brother. I will keep you informed of his condition frequently."

EVALUATION

1. Inspect the client's chest wall for rise and fall during administration of artificial respiration.
2. Assess pulse during compressions to determine the adequacy of compressions.

   NOTE: CPR is not interrupted for more than 5 seconds. CPR is resumed between all interventions.
3. Assess client for predisposing factors for injury such as osteoporosis or other medical problems. Remember CPR takes precedence over all predisposing factors.

Unexpected Outcomes and Related Interventions

1. Client experiences injury as a result of cardiac compressions, such as rib or sternum fracture or lacerated lung or liver.

   Monitor correct hand placement before cardiac compressions.
2. Client converts back to life-threatening dysrhythmia of ventricular fibrillation or pulseless ventricular tachycardia.
   a. Continuously monitor cardiac rhythm and vital signs after resuscitation phase.
   b. Reinitiate or continue CPR.
3. Client is pronounced dead by physician member of the code team after all emergency life-support interventions are unsuccessful.
   a. Support family/significant others during initiation of grieving process.
   b. Perform postmortem care (see Skill 38.3).
   c. Review resuscitation efforts with team members and evaluate effectiveness of interventions.
   d. Discuss personal feeling regarding client's death and resuscitative efforts with team members, supervisor, or other professional as needed.

Recording and Reporting

- Cardiopulmonary arrest requires precise documentation. Most hospitals use a form designed specifically for in-hospital arrests. These forms are reviewed by a committee to ensure the code was performed according to ACLS recommendations.
- Information included in the form are time of the arrest, initiation, continuation, and cessation of CPR; cardiac rhythm; pulse; defibrillation attempts; medication administration; procedures performed; and the client's response.

Sample Documentation without Code Sheet

0734   Client found unresponsive in bed. Code 99 called. Compression board under client. CPR begun.

0736   Code 99 team arrives. Cardiac monitor shows ventricular fibrillation. CPR continues.

0738   Client defibrillated at 200, 300, and 360j with monitor showing continued ventricular fibrillation. No pulse. Continue CPR.

0740   18-gauge IV inserted in right and left antecubital site. Blood sent to lab for electrolytes and complete blood count. NS wide open via right antecubital site. ABG drawn via right femoral site by M.D.

0741   Intubated with #8 endotracheal tube, left side of mouth at 26 cm. Securely taped. CPR continues. Epinephrine 1 mg IV given left antecubital site.

0742   Repeat defibrillation at 360j. Monitor shows sinus tachycardia. Carotid pulse felt. BP 96/46.

0745   Prepare for transport to cardiac care unit with M.D, RN, and respiratory therapist. Client remains intubated with monitor showing sinus tachycardia.

Skill 38.3

CARE OF THE BODY AFTER DEATH

When death occurs, the traditional clinical signs are cessation of pulse and respirations. When the physician pronounces the client dead, the time of death is documented. The RN can pronounce "absence of life" in some states. The physician may request permission from the family for an autopsy. An autopsy, or postmortem examination, is performed to confirm or determine the cause of death, gather data regarding the nature and progress of a disease, study the effects of therapies on body tissue, and provide statistical data for epidemiology and research purposes. A consent form must be signed by the appropriate family member and the physician. Autopsies are required in circumstances of unusual death (e.g., violent trauma, unexpected death in the home) and death occurring within a set time after hospitalization. Each state has guidelines for when autopsies are requested. Autopsies normally do not affect the client's appearance or delay burial. In some cases, removal of invasive tubes and appliances is prohibited, especially in coroners' cases or cases requiring autopsies.

The topic of organ/tissue donation can be introduced by the nurse. One research study has concluded that physicians, nurses, and social workers are not the most suitable individuals to present the option of donation to ensure the family's right to make the decision without the pressure of consent (Von Pohle, 1996). The nurse can also contact a representative from an organ procurement agency who is trained to deal with issues surrounding organ donation and may be best suited to request organ donation (Edwards, Hasz, and Menendez, 1997; Von Pohle, 1996). The success of organ donation depends on the joint involvement of nursing, medical, and organ procurement organization staff (Edwards, Hasz, and Menendez, 1997).

Equipment

Disposable gloves, gown, and other protective clothing

Plastic bag for hazardous waste disposal

Wash basin, washcloth, warm water, and bath towel

Clean gown or disposable gown for body (consult agency policy)

Absorbent pads

Body bag or shroud kit (consult agency policy)

Paper tape and gauze dressing

Paper bag, plastic bag, or other suitable receptacle for client's clothing, belongings, and other items to be returned to family

Valuables envelope

Identification tags as specified by agency policy

ASSESSMENT

1. Assess for presence of family members or significant others and their knowledge of client's death. Take to a private location and allow time for family to ask questions. **Rationale: Physician usually informs the family of client's death, depending on the circumstances. Nurse provides emotional support and guidance. Appropriate communication skills such as active listening, acknowledgment of feelings and emotions, or silence can assist the family during the grieving process (Wheeler, 1996).**

2. Determine who is legally able to give permission for organ/tissue donation. This person could be the next of kin or someone appointed by the client or the court to make these types of decisions. The nurse

may desire the expertise of specially trained personnel from an organ/tissue bank to make the request. **Rationale: Organ/tissue donation options and implications need to be explained completely to the appropriate party.**

3. Complete necessary organ/tissue donation request form. **Rationale: Federal guidelines require documentation that request has been made. Some hospitals pose the question of organ/tissue donation upon admission into the hospital.**

4. Determine if autopsy is planned. **Rationale: If autopsy is planned, some procedures such as removal of tubes and lines may be altered or prohibited.**

PLANNING

Expected outcomes focus on preventing injury to the deceased's body tissue and facilitating grieving of family and friends.

Expected Outcomes

1. Deceased's body will be free of skin damage.
2. Significant others will express grief.

DELEGATION CONSIDERATIONS

Most hospitals and long-term care facilities allow AP to prepare the body for viewing and for transport to the morgue. When delegating to personnel, the nurse should do the following:

- Review any instruction and reinforce the importance of handling the body with respect.
- Reinforce to staff the importance of following infection-control guidelines.
- Inform the staff of any special needs the family might have regarding the preparation of the body.

IMPLEMENTATION

Steps	Rationale
1. See Standard Protocol (inside front cover).	
2. Check with significant others about notifying other significant people.	Significant others may have trouble dealing with the concrete details surrounding the death and may need assistance.
3. Discuss procedure of preparing the body with significant others. Inquire if there are particular cultural or spiritual practices that are significant for the deceased or significant others.	Having some ability to direct what is happening can increase the significant others' sense of control. Discussing these aspects of care with the significant others can convey your caring and concern.

Steps	Rationale
4. If tissue donation has been made, consult policy for specific guidelines in care of the body.	Retrieval of tissues (e.g., eyes, bone, skin) may require certain preparation measures.
5. Apply gown or protective barriers as applicable.	Body excretions may harbor infectious microorganisms. Withdrawal of IV tubing or other tubing may cause temporary bleeding.
6. Identify the body according to agency policy. Leave identification in place as directed in agency policy.	Ensures proper identification of the body.
7. If in keeping with agency procedures, remove all indwelling catheters, IV, oxygen, and other tubes. (If an autopsy is to be performed, policy may direct to leave these devices in place.) Dress puncture wounds with a small dressing and paper tape.	Creates a normal appearance. Paper tape minimizes skin trauma.
8. If the person wore dentures, insert them. If mouth fails to close, place a rolled up towel under the chin.	It is difficult to insert dentures after rigor mortis occurs. Dentures maintain natural facial expression.
9. Position client as outlined in agency procedures. In general, do not place one hand on top of the other.	Client appears natural and comfortable. Placing one hand on top of another can lead to skin discoloration.
10. Place small pillow or folded towel under the head or elevate head of bed 10 to 15 degrees.	Prevents pooling of blood in the face and subsequent discoloration.
11. Close eyes gently by grasping the eyelashes.	Closed eyes present a more natural appearance. Pressure on the lids can lead to discoloration.
12. Wash body parts soiled by blood, urine, feces, or other drainage. (A mortician will provide a complete bath.) Place an absorbent pad under the client's buttocks.	Prepares body for viewing and reduces odors. Relaxation of sphincter muscles after death may cause release of urine or feces.
13. Remove soiled dressings and replace with clean gauze dressings. Use paper tape.	Paper tape minimizes skin trauma. Changing dressings helps to control odors caused by microorganisms and to create a more acceptable appearance.
14. Place a clean gown on the client (agency policy may require removal before body is wrapped).	Prepares body for viewing.
15. Brush and comb client's hair. Remove any clips, hairpins, or rubber bands.	During viewing, the client should appear well-groomed. Hard objects such as pins can damage or discolor the face and scalp.

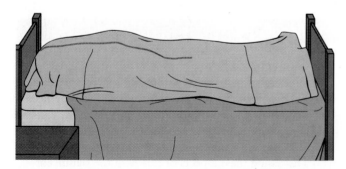
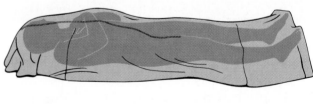

Step 18

Steps	**Rationale**
16. Remove all jewelry and give to family member. EXCEPTION: Family may request wedding band be left in place. Place a small strip of tape around client's finger over the ring.	Prevents loss of client's valuables.
17. If significant others request viewing, place a sheet or light blanket over the body with only the head and upper shoulders exposed. Remove unneeded equipment from the room. Provide soft lighting and offer chairs.	Maintains dignity and respect for the client and significant others. Prevents exposure of body parts.
18. After the significant others have left the room, remove all linen and the client's gown (refer to agency policy). Place body in body bag or apply the shroud as required by the agency (see illustration).	
19. Label the body as directed by agency policy.	Ensures proper identification of the body.
20. Arrange transportation of the body to the morgue or mortuary.	If delay is anticipated before the mortician arrives, the body should be cooled in the morgue to prevent further tissue damage.

• • •

EVALUATION

1. Observe significant others' response to the loss.
2. Provide significant others with the opportunity to express feelings.
3. Note appearance and condition of client's skin during preparation of the body.

Unexpected Outcomes and Related Interventions

1. Significant others become immobilized by their grief and have difficulty functioning.
   a. Consider pastoral care or social work consult.
   b. Do not rush family. Give them time to ask questions. Assist in contacting physician.
2. Lacerations, bruises, or abrasions are noted on skin surfaces of deceased.
   a. Cleanse areas thoroughly before family viewing.
   b. Inform family of any bruises or lacerations that they may see.

Recording and Reporting

- Record date and time of death, time physician notified, name of physician pronouncing death, delivery of postmortem care, identification of body, consent form signed by significant other, disposition of the body, and information provided to significant others (Figure 38-4, p. 886).
- Document any marks, bruises, wounds on body before death or those observed during care of the body.
- Document how valuables and personal belongings were handled and who received them. Secure signatures as required by agency policy.

Sample Documentation

0245   David Knight pronounced dead by Dr. J. White at
0213.   Wife and family members aware. Organ and tissue donation declined. Two bruises, approximately 1 cm diameter each, on left forearm noted. Body prepared for mortuary, Allen and Son Funeral Home in New Castle. Mortuary aware of death. Teeth, glasses, hearing aid, and clothes with body to morgue with security personnel.

CRITICAL THINKING EXERCISES

1. The code team, physical therapist, and dietitian arrive. What action do you take, and why?

2. A code is called in Room 211, bed 2. Your client is in Room 211, bed 1. Upon entering the room, what should you assess? What would you do after making your assessment?

3. You find your client on the floor without respirations or pulse. You know the client has terminal illness but has been unable to make a resuscitation decision. What do you do?

4. The nurse discovers the client, a nursing home resident with severe Alzheimer's disease and contractures, unresponsive in bed. The nurse calls a code 99 and begins cardiac compressions. Assistive personnel arrive to assume CPR, and the nurse leaves the room to get the client's chart. Critique this nurse's critical thinking and activities.

Expiration Flow Sheet

Time of death _____   Pronounced dead by _____

Family notified: Name & Relationship _____

Family member responsible for funeral arrangements   Name: _____

_____   Relationship: _____   Time available: _____

Address: _____   # can be reached at _____

Physicians notified: _____

_____   Time _____

Hospital chaplain/family pastor notified _____   Time _____
Funeral home _____   Time notified _____
     Isolation Information: Infection Hazard?   YES   NO
Autopsy requested   YES   NO   Requested by: _____
Permission obtained for autopsy   YES   NO
Permission Experienced: Fall _____   Fracture _____
Security notified   Time: _____
Coroner notified (M-F [tel. no.] evening & weekends [tel. no.]) (if applicable)
     I. Time notified: _____
     II. Information the Coronary needs:
          Name of patient, time of death, age, address, physician, next of kin, autopsy (yes or no), procedure _____

ORGAN/TISSUE DONATION **(PLEASE COMPLETE I A&B, & II A BEFORE APPROACHING FAMILY)**
I.   A. Is the patient 70 years old or older?   YES   NO
     B. Is the patient currently positive for HIV, Hepatitis A or B?   YES   NO
II. A. If you have answered "NO" TO THOSE TWO QUESTIONS, this patient may be a candidate for organ and/or tissue dona-
         tion. Please contact the ROBI Coordinator who is "On Call" at (tel. no.) (24 hours/day) to verify eligibility of patient to do-
         nate.
     B. Name of ROBI Coordinator: _____
     C. Patient is a candidate for donation.   YES   NO
         If yes, family permission obtained.   YES   NO
         Patient is not a candidate due to: _____

Disposition of chart   _____   To Laboratory (if autopsy)
                        _____   To medical records (if no autopsy)

Disposition of body   _____   Morgue   Time _____
                       _____   Funeral home
                       _____   Pathology

Disposition of valuables _____

DATE _____

SIGNATURE _____

Courtesy Memorial Medical Center, Springfield, Ill.

Figure 38-4 Expiration flow sheet.   *Courtesy Memorial Medical Center, Springfield, Ill.*

REFERENCES

Betrell M, Mezey M, Ramsey G: Advance directives protocol: nurses helping protect the patient's rights, *Geriatr Nurs* 17(5):204, 1996.

Brown J et al: The first 3 minutes: code preparation for the staff nurse, *Orthop Nurs* 14(3):35, 1995.

Chandra NC, Hazinski MF, editors: *Basic life support for healthcare providers*, Dallas, 1997, American Heart Association.

Committee on Emergency Cardiac Care: Guidelines for cardiopulmonary resuscitation and emergency cardiac care, *JAMA* 268:16, 1992.

Cummins R, editor: *Textbook of advanced cardiac life support*, Dallas, 1997, American Heart Association.

Edwards J, Hasz R, Menendez J: Organ donors: your care is critical, *RN* 60(6):46, 1997.

Johns J: Advance directives and opportunities for nurses, *Image J Nurs Sch* 28(2):149, 1996.

Keen JH, Baird MS, Allen JH: *Mosby's critical care and emergency drug reference*, St Louis, 1994, Mosby.

Lenehan GP, editor: Emergency Nurses Association position statement, *J Emerg Nurs* (21)(2):26A, 1995.

Lewis et al: *Medical-surgical nursing: assessment and management of clinical problems*, ed 4, St Louis, 1996, Mosby.

Von Pohle W: Obtaining organ donation: who should ask? *Heart Lung* 25(4):304, 1996.

Wheeler SR: Helping families cope with death and dying, *Nurs 96* 7:25, 1996.

CHAPTER 39

Care of the Client with Special Needs

Skill 39.1
Managing Central Venous Lines, 889

Skill 39.2
Administration of Total Parenteral Nutrition, 898

Skill 39.3
Mechanical Ventilation, 901

Skill 39.4
Care of Client Receiving Hemodialysis, 907

Skill 39.5
Peritoneal Dialysis, 911

The client with special needs includes the population with complex medical and nursing diagnoses, who require nursing interventions that are more elaborate than those of basic nursing care. These interventions require a higher level of problem solving and coordination. Many of the interventions required by these clients are performed in cooperation with physicians or allied health professionals, which means that communication skills are also a part of these processes. It is common for facilities to have in-service or certification programs that are required before implementation of these skills; the nurse should be familiar with the facility's expectations and standards of performance in the clinical area.

The role of assessment on the part of the nurse takes on special importance in these skills. Because of more frequent and more prolonged contact with the client in most instances, the nurse has a unique perspective on the progress toward goals and the factors that might affect that progress. This includes positive factors such as family support and adequate resources, as well as factors that might have a negative impact on the outcome, such as the development of complications or the presence of family stressors. The observation and interpretation of all facts will be critical in the ongoing process of client care, and the foundation of this must be assessment. Systematic and objective assessments on the part of the nurse ensure the highest-quality, individualized client care.

 NURSING DIAGNOSES

The following nursing diagnoses apply to multiple skills in this chapter (Kim, McFarland, and McLane, 1997):

- **Noncompliance** and/or **Ineffective Individual Coping** related to possible side effects of treatment, knowledge deficit or poor relationships with the health care team.
- **Body Image Disturbance** related to physical changes brought on by illness or side effects of treatment.
- **Anxiety** related to possible outcomes of both treatment and disease process.
- **Risk for injury** and/or **Impaired Skin Integrity** related to disease process, invasive treatment procedures, and altered fluid/nutritional balance.
- **Knowledge Deficit** related to inexperience with procedures.
- **Fluid Volume Deficit** and/or **Fluid Volume Excess** related to disease process and/or side effects of medication or treatment.
- **Risk for Infection** related to disease process and/or invasive treatment procedures.

Additional nursing diagnoses may be applicable as a result of the unique implications for each skill. The nurse must use critical thinking in selecting nursing diagnoses that are appropriate.

Skill 39.1

MANAGING CENTRAL VENOUS LINES

Long-term central venous access devices are indicated for some clients who will receive IV therapy for longer than 7 days and up to 3 years. The lines are used to administer IV fluids, medications, blood products, and parenteral nutrition fluids. They may be single-, double-, or triple-lumen catheters. The use of intravascular devices is frequently complicated, including instances of septic thrombophlebitis, endocarditis, bloodstream infection, and metastatic infection (e.g., osteomyelitis, arthritis). Catheter-related infections are associated with increased morbidity and mortality rates, prolonged hospitalization, and increased medical costs.

Central venous catheters are inserted by physicians through the subclavian or jugular veins. These sites are preferred in providing a flat, relatively immobile area on the chest and blood flows at a high rate. Peripherally inserted central catheters (PICCs) are inserted by specially trained nurses or physicians, with the insertion from the antecubital site, and the distal end of the catheter resting in the central circulation. These catheters may be inserted at the client's bedside, in the outclient department, or in the client's home. Other long-term devices may be divided into two categories: surgically tunneled catheters, which are designed to have a portion lie within an SQ passage before exiting the body (e.g., Broviac, Hickman, Groshong); and surgically implanted infusion ports, which are placed in a vessel, body cavity, or organ and are attached to a reservoir placed under the skin (e.g., Port-A-Cath).

Equipment

Insertion
Central line insertion kit
Underpad
Masks
Gowns
Head coverings
Towels
Extra drapes
Extra local anesthetic
Sterile and nonsterile gloves
Heparin flush solution (10 u/ml)
10 ml syringe
Clear occlusive or gauze dressing
Label
Tape
Povidone-iodine or chlorhexidine (if client is allergic to povidone-iodine)
Goggles
100-mg lidocaine syringe
Sterile and unsterile tape measure (for PICC line insertion)

Removal
Nonsterile gloves
Povidone-iodine swabs (or chlorhexidine if client is allergic to povidone-iodine)
Suture removal set
4 × 4s
Tape
Site care and dressing change
Gloves (sterile and nonsterile)
Alcohol and povidone-iodine swabs or combination swabs (chlorhexidine if client is allergic to povidone-iodine)
Clear occlusive or gauze dressing
Label
Blood drawing through insertion cap
Gloves
Povidone-iodine swabs (chlorhexidine if client is allergic to povidone-iodine)
Three 5-ml Luer-lok syringes
Two 10-ml Luer-lok syringes
Saline flush
Heparin flush (10 u/ml)
Blood tubes
Injection cap

ASSESSMENT

1. Assess client for indications for long-term device.
   a. IV therapy anticipated for longer than 7 days, including transfusions, total parenteral nutrition administration, or continuous infusions such as narcotics.
   b. Infusion of vesicants or irritants, such as in chemotherapy.
   c. Poor peripheral venous circulation.
   d. Frequent long-term phlebotomy.
2. Assess for indications for particular type of long-term device, such as PICC line for client with chest injury or central line for client with peripheral vein thrombosis.
3. Consider client's preference for long-term device.
4. Assess baseline for vital signs and I&O.

PLANNING

Expected outcomes focus on maintaining a patent channel of venous access, maintaining fluid and electrolyte balance, and preventing complications related to insertion and maintenance of access devices.

Expected Outcomes

1. Intake and output remains in balance with electrolytes within normal limits.
2. IV setup is intact and functioning properly with infusion flowing freely.
3. Client has no evidence of complications: clotting, local inflammation or phlebitis, systemic infection, venous thrombosis, air embolus, extravasation (leaking of medication into the tissues around the site), or migration of catheter.

DELEGATION CONSIDERATIONS

The skill of insertion and maintenance of venous access devices requires problem solving and knowledge application unique to a professional nurse. Delegation is inappropriate for this skill.

IMPLEMENTATION

Steps	Rationale
1. See Standard Protocol (inside front cover).	
2. Provide client education with respect to insertion and maintenance of catheter.	Allays client's fears and ensures cooperation.
3. Review facility's guidelines on personnel who are authorized to implement insertion.	Procedure may be limited to physicians or certified nurses only.
4. Witness/obtain consent.	Needed for invasive procedure; increases client's level of commitment and cooperation for procedure.
5. Place client in supine or Trendelenberg position (NOTE: If client is dyspneic, wait until after skin preparation).	Decreases risk of air embolus during insertion.
6. Place moisture-proof underpad beneath client's shoulder on side of insertion.	Maintains hygiene during procedure and protects linens from soiling.
7. Clip heavy hair growth at and around insertion site.	Decreases risk of infection, increases adherence of dressing, and avoids impairment of skin integrity possible with shaving.

NURSE ALERT

Be sure that emergency equipment and medications are on hand before beginning procedure.

Steps	Rationale
8. If assisting physician in procedures, help with donning sterile garb.	
9. Put on mask and gown.	
10. Open sterile packages.	
11. Monitor heart rate, respiratory rate and rhythm, and client's comments and reactions.	
12. [image] Prepare tubing:	Prevents air from entering system.
a. Attach injection cap to extension tubing (one set for each lumen).	
b. Draw up enough NS for 2 ml per lumen, and flush each cap.	
c. Inspect catheter equipment for defects.	Cracks or kinks render equipment unusable; must ensure function after insertion.
d. Verify patency of introducer.	
13. Assist with insertion of catheter (PICC or subclavian):	
a. Prepare site by placing drapes; hand sterile equipment to physician; discard contaminated supplies.	

COMMUNICATION TIP

Review steps and rationale with client by saying, "Can you tell me in your own words why this procedure is important for you to have?" Explain each step of procedure as it is performed if client desires.

Steps	Rationale
b. Assist with injection of local anesthetic as directed; if transdermal analgesic creme (EMLA) is used, apply 60 minutes before procedure and cover site with occlusive dressing (see illustration).	Allows time for analgesic creme to take effect (Intravenous Nurses Society [INS], 1998).
c. Assist with venipuncture as directed.	

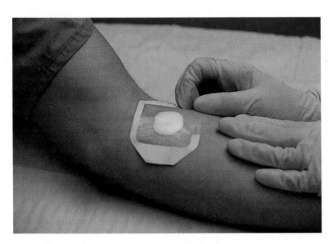

Step 13b

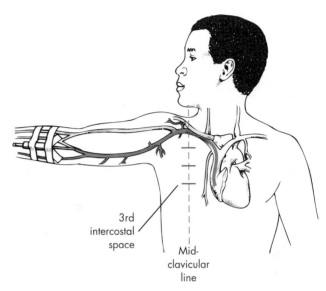

3rd intercostal space

Mid-clavicular line

Step 14d

Steps	Rationale
14. Insertion of PICC line:	
a. If using EMLA anesthetic, see Step 13b.	
b. Identify appropriate vein in antecubital fossa; place tourniquet on upper arm to identify vein, then release to prevent venous engorgement.	Basilic vein preferred over cephalic because of less tortuosity (Camp-Sorrell, 1996).
c. Position client in supine position with arm at 45- to 90-degree angle to trunk.	Provides straighter course for advancing catheter to large veins in the chest.
d. Measure distance from insertion site to proposed site for catheter tip using unsterile tape measure (see illustration). Subclavian placement: from insertion site up the arm to the shoulder and across to the midclavicular line. Superior vena cava placement: continue to the sternal notch and down to the third intercostal space on the right of the sternum.	Landmarks correspond to venous structures underneath.
e. Apply mask, gown, and goggles; client may also wear mask.	Reduces transmission of microorganisms.
f. Open sterile supplies/kit. Arrange supplies using kit's wrap as a sterile field. Cleanse top of NS, heparin, and lidocaine vials; set aside.	
g. Apply sterile gloves.	
h. With assistance from nurse, draw up NS, heparin, and lidocaine (optional).	
i. Measure catheter with sterile tape measure to the length previously determined, plus 1 inch.	
j. Cut catheter to desired measurement using sterile scissors.	

Steps	Rationale

k. Prepare insertion site by placing sterile drape under arm. Prepare with each of three alcohol swab sticks and each of three povidone-iodine swab sticks, allowing skin to dry between scrubbings. Using concentric circular motion, prepare a site 6 inches in diameter around the insertion site (see illustration).

Alcohol swabs defat the skin; povidone-iodine reduces the skin surface bacteria. Circular scrubbing motions move bacteria on the skin away from the insertion site. Allowing scrubs to dry completely promotes maximum bacteriocidal effectiveness.

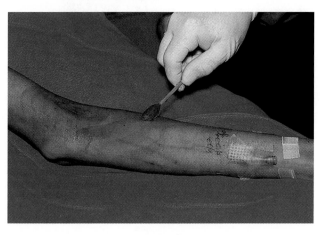

Step 14k

NURSE ALERT

Review facility policy with regard to use of guidewire or stylet. Make sure catheter remains on sterile field during procedure. Guidewires provide more rigidity to the catheter, thus aiding in insertion. Catheters contaminated in any way must be discarded.

l. Remove gloves and reapply new pair of sterile, powder-free latex gloves.

Powder might adhere to catheter.

m. Apply sterile tourniquet or place sterile gauze 4 × 4s over nonsterile tourniquet.

n. Place fenestrated drape over insertion site. Administer lidocaine if transdermal analgesic has not been used.

Local anesthetic reduces discomfort of procedure.

o. Insert introducer at 20- to 30-degree angle and look for brisk blood return (see illustration).

Angular approach reduces risk of puncturing posterior wall of vein with large-bore introducer.

p. Advance introducer (parallel to skin) 0.5 to 1 cm further into vein.

Ensures that vein is securely cannulated.

q. Advance the plastic cannula that fits over the introducer forward slightly to cover the needle tip. Release tourniquet.

Slow advancement of catheter prevents trauma to intima of vein.

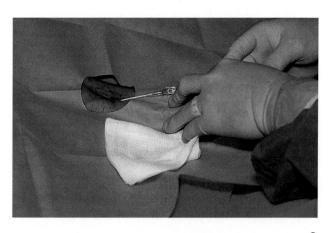
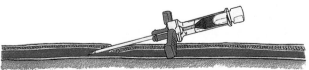

Step 14o

Steps	Rationale

r. Withdraw needle of introducer from the plastic cannula while holding plastic cannula in place. Then apply mild pressure near tip of plastic cannula (see illustration).

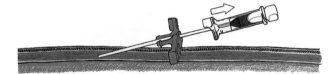

Step 14r

s. Thread the catheter slowly through the plastic cannula (see illustration) 2 to 3 inches (5 to 7.5 cm) using nontoothed forceps, or fingers of gloved hand.

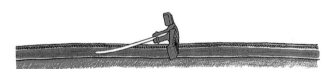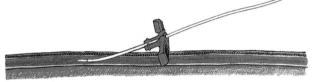

Step 14s

t. Advance catheter until tip is at shoulder (6 inches or more, depending on client's size).

Catheter is marked at 10-cm intervals to allow for identification of catheter tip location.

NURSE ALERT

Observe cardiac monitor or palpate peripheral pulse during advancement of catheter. Prepare to bolus IV lidocaine if ordered. Client is at risk of cardiac dysrhythmia because of irritation during procedure.

u. Instruct client to turn head toward side of venous access and drop chin to chest.

v. Continue to slowly advance catheter until predetermined length is reached.

w. Apply pressure to the vein just distal to the tip of the plastic cannula. Withdraw the plastic cannula with a firm steady motion out of the vein (see illustration) 2 inches above insertion site during withdrawal.

Closes internal jugular vein and prevents it from being accidentally cannulated.

Premeasuring aids in proper placement of tip.

Introducer might accidentally puncture vein if left in place. Stabilizing ensures against accidental removal of catheter during step.

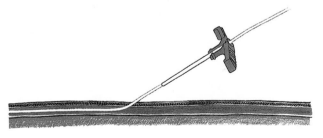

COMMUNICATION TIP

Explain to client that snapping sound is about to be heard. Prevents anxiety when sound occurs.

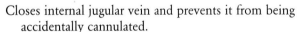

Step 14w

Steps

Rationale

x. When cannula is out, press or peel wings out together until they snap, then peel the cannula from around the catheter (see illustration).

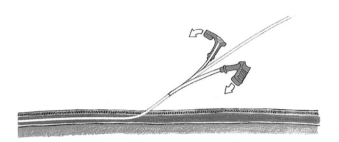

Step 14x

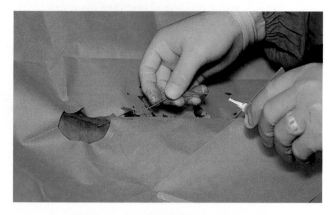

Step 14z

y. Attach syringe with 10 ml NS to lumen tip of catheter, aspirate for blood return, and flush the catheter.

z. Remove syringe from lumen and attach extension tubing and cap (see illustration).

15. Prepare PICC site for dressing application.
   a. Cleanse insertion site with antiseptic swab to remove blood, then allow site to dry.
   b. Anchor hub of catheter to skin with Steristrips (see illustration).
   c. Assist physician with suturing of catheter. (Some State Boards allow nurses to suture.)
   d. Apply sterile dressing (see Chapter 30). Place 2 × 2 gauze pads over insertion site. Cover with transparent dressing (see illustration); mark date, time, and initials on label.
   e. Coil extension tubing and tape securely to client's arm. Do not pull catheter or apply undue pressure during manipulation.
   f. Flush each lumen with 10 ml heparin solution.

Makes lumen of catheter available for use; prevents damage to catheter and vein. Verifies patency of lumen; prevents clotting.

Prevents blood loss; maintains closed system.

Helps maintain catheter's position for long-term use.

Catheter is at risk of migration if not secured.

Provides pressure to control oozing caused by large-gauge introducer.

Prevents accidental dislodgement and catheter breakage.

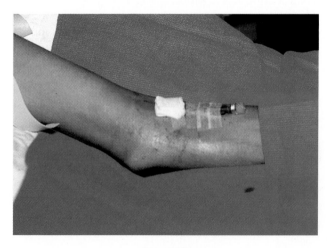

Step 15b

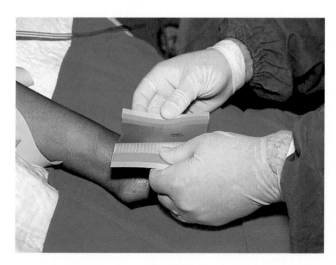

Step 15d

Steps	Rationale
g. Obtain portable chest xray.	Verifies location of catheter.
h. See Completion Protocol (inside front cover).	
16. Removal of Central venous Catheter.	
a. See Standard Protocol (inside front cover).	
b. Explain procedure to client.	
c. Place client in supine or Trendelenberg position.	
d. Place moisture-proof underpad beneath site.	
e. Remove old dressing and tape.	
f. Cleans site using povidone-iodine swabs, starting at site and working outward in a circular motion. Allow to air dry.	
g. Open suture removal set.	
h. With nondominant hand, grasp suture with forceps. Using dominant hand, cut suture carefully with sterile scissors, making sure to avoid damage to skin or catheter. Lift suture out and discard.	
i. Using nondominant hand, apply sterile 4 × 4 to site. Instruct client to take deep breath as catheter is withdrawn.	Reduce risk of air embolus by decreasing negative pressure in respiratory system.
j. With dominant hand, remove catheter in a smooth, continuous motion. Apply pressure to site immediately and continue for 5 to 10 minutes. Observe for bleeding.	Client is at risk for bleeding and needs direct pressure on site to prevent hematoma or hemorrhage.
k. Apply sterile dressing to site. Write the date and time and initials on the dressing.	
l. Inspect catheter integrity and discard.	
m. See Completion Protocol (inside front cover).	
17. Site Care and Dressing Change	
a. See Standard Protocol (inside front cover).	
b. Explain procedure to client. (Provide care every 24 to 48 hours and prn)	
c. Don mask.	
d. Remove old dressing and tape. Discard in receptacle.	
e. Inspect the catheter, insertion site, suture, and surrounding skin.	
f. Remove and discard nonsterile gloves; apply sterile gloves.	
g. Using combination antiseptic swab, cleanse catheter and site, working outward in a circular motion, or follow steps h and i.	
h. Using alcohol swab, cleanse catheter and site, working outward in a circular motion. Repeat × 2; allow to dry completely. Use chlorhexidine if client is allergic to alcohol.	
i. Using povidone-iodine swab, cleanse catheter and site, working outward in a circular motion. Use chlorhexidine if client is allergic to povidone-iodine. Repeat × 2. Allow povidone-iodine to dry completely.	

NURSE ALERT

If catheter is removed because of suspected infection, send to laboratory for culturing.

Steps	Rationale
j. Apply sterile gauze or clear occlusive dressing.	
k. Tape dressing in "window-frame" fashion as needed.	Permits visual inspection while securing dressing.
l. Write the date and time and your initials on the label.	
m. Clamp lumens one at a time and remove injection caps.	
n. Cleanse ports with povidone-iodine and allow to dry completely.	
o. Put new caps in place. Open clamps for infusion.	
p. See Completion Protocol (inside front cover).	
18. Blood drawing through insertion cap	
a. See Standard Protocol (inside front cover).	
b. Explain procedure to client.	
c. Cleanse injection cap with povidone-iodine and allow to dry completely.	
d. Stop IV infusion. NOTE: If infusion is critical for client's well-being, draw blood peripherally.	
e. Flush catheter port with 5 ml NS.	
f. Aspirate 5 ml blood and discard.	Specimen is diluted with saline solution.
g. Aspirate specimen and place in appropriate laboratory tube/s.	Multiple specimens can be removed at one time and placed in various different tubes.
h. Flush catheter with 10 ml NS solution. Reduces risk of clotting in tube after procedure.	
i. Flush catheter port with 3 ml heparin solution.	
j. Clamp lumen and remove cap.	
k. Cleanse port with povidone-iodine and allow to dry completely.	
l. Put on new cap/s. Open clamps for infusion and resume.	
m. See Completion Protocol (inside front cover).	

• • •

EVALUATION

1. Evaluate for signs of clot formation in catheter including difficulty flushing, sluggish infusion, absent or sluggish blood return.
2. Inspect IV setup and catheter/port every 8 hours for leaks or tears, secure connections, integrity of dressing, tubing free of obstruction or kinks, correct solution, tubing labeled, and electronic infusion pump functioning properly.
3. Monitor I&O every 8 hours for fluid balance and monitor laboratory values for electrolyte balance as ordered.
4. Evaluate for complications:
   a. Inspect insertion site every 4 hours for the first 48 hours, then every 8 hours for warmth, tenderness, swelling, drainage, or bruising or bleeding. Observe skin around the site for cellulitis.
   b. Monitor for systemic infection every 12 hours including fever, hypotension, tachycardia, increased WBC's, confusion or change in level of conciousness and decreased urinary output.
   c. Observe for thrombosis every 8 hours including pain, tenderness, or numbness in the neck, shoulder, or arm on affected side of the body.
   d. Observe for air embolism every 8 hours including dyspnea, respiratory distress, or cyanosis.
   e. Observe for extravasation during infusions including burning or swelling around insertion site or port (Port-A-Cath).
   f. Observe for migration of catheter or port every 12 hours:

All:
a. Irregular heart rate or dysrhythmia
PICC
b. Frequent nausea and emesis
c. Frequent, severe episodes of coughing
d. Client manipulation of site
Hickman/Groshong:
e. Swelling
f. S. burning sensation

Unexpected Outcomes and Related Interventions
1. Client has broken or leaking catheter.
   a. Hickman/Broviac:
      (1) Cease use of catheter.
      (2) Clamp with nonserrated instrument between the broken area and the exit site.
      (3) Cover the broken part with sterile gauze and tape securely.
   b. PICC:
      (1) Cease use of catheter.
      (2) Cover the broken part with sterile gauze and tape securely.
2. Client has extravasation.
   a. Stop infusion immediately.
   b. Consult clinical pharmacist for antidote.
3. Client has air embolus.
   a. Close off open end of catheter.
   b. Place client in Trendelenberg position on left side.
   c. Obtain immediate emergency assistance.

Recording and Reporting
- Notify physician immediately for signs/symptoms of the following: local or systemic infection; thrombosis/thrombophlebitis; air embolus; extravasation; suspected catheter or port occlusion or migration; dysrhythmias; or leaks, tears, or breaks in catheter.
- Notify nurse who inserted PICC immediately for phlebitis/cellulitis of affected arm; suspected catheter occlusion/migration; or leaks, tears, or breaks in catheter.
- Document for insertion: site and length of catheter in centimeters, client's tolerance of procedure, complications of procedure, heart rate and respiratory rate during and after insertion, chest x-ray done, and confirmation of line placement.
- Document for catheter removal: appearance of site, integrity of catheter on removal, client's tolerance of procedure, and presence/absence of bleeding every 15 minutes × 4.
- Document for changing injection caps: appearance of site, catheter, and suture; date and time of dressing change; injection caps changed.
- Document for drawing blood via injection cap: date, time, sample drawn.
- Document site care and dressing/tubing cap changes on IV record.

- Document unexpected outcomes, physician notification, and interventions in nurses' notes.

Sample Documentation
1030   Informed consent was obtained after discussion with client about risks and benefits of PICC line insertion. PT and PTT values were WNL. Measured for determination of insertion length. Skin cleaned with alcohol and povidone-iodine. Vein in the inside of the left arm chosen for cannulation with a 4 Fr Groshong PICC. Catheter flushed with NS. Brisk return of venous blood noted upon venipuncture. Cannula threaded without difficulty to the 44-cm mark. A portable chest x-ray done, with confirmation of placement in the SVC. Catheter sutured in place, and occlusive dressing applied over the site.

The client instructed to return to the office tomorrow for dressing change and inspection of the site. Instructed to notify the office immediately if there is sign of bleeding or excessive bruising at site. Weekly checks and dressing changes will be done thereafter.

Geriatric Considerations

- The older adult client is at greater risk for alterations in skin integrity, nutritional imbalance, and fluid and electrolyte imbalance.
- Cardiac complications are more likely to arise in a client who may already have underlying cardiac disease.
- During insertion, monitor the older adult client's progress carefully.

Home Care and Long-Term Care Considerations

- Instruct client/significant other to notify the nurse/physician immediately for pain, swelling, burning, or numbness at site, affected arm, or side of body; bleeding or leaking; difficulty breathing; any perceived change in well-being; or pump alarming.
- Instruct client/significant other in flushing technique, site care and dressing change, and emergency interventions.

Skill 39.2

ADMINISTRATION OF TOTAL PARENTERAL NUTRITION

Total parenteral nutrition (TPN) is the administration through a vein of a nutritionally complete formula including amino acids, glucose, lipids, electrolytes, vitamins, and trace elements. The purpose of the administration of TPN is to promote wound healing and avoid malnutrition. Hyperalimentation solutions that have very high osmolarities (i.e., containing 15% to 30% dextrose) are infused into a wide-diameter, high-flow central vein to reduce the risk of chemical phlebitis. The commonly accepted sites for vascular access of the central venous system are the subclavian and internal jugular veins. The catheter-tip location is usually the superior vena cava, although other sites may be the innominate vein, the intrathoracic subclavian vein, and the right atrium (for silastic catheters only).

TPN is typically used for clients with severe burns, sepsis, cardiac conditions, trauma, liver failure, gastrointestinal conditions impairing absorption, or anorexia nervosa. The regimen is individually designed for a client; the prescription should be ordered by the physician and reviewed daily, with special consideration given to the electrolyte, fluid, and nitrogen balance. The choice of solution varies with the client's condition and nutritional needs. Lipid infusions are commonly given on a scheduled basis alongside TPN (Perry and Potter, 1998).

Equipment

Glucometer kit
IV tubing
IV solution of TPN
IV infusion pump
IV filter (OPTIONAL: 0.22 μ for dextrose/amino acids, 1.2 μ for three-in-one solutions)
Alcohol swabs
Sterile needles

ASSESSMENT

1. Assess indications of and risks for protein/calorie malnutrition: weight loss from baseline or ideal, muscle atrophy/wasting/weakness, edema, lethargy,

failure to wean from ventilatory support, chronic illness, allergy to foods (especially eggs), and NPO more than 6 days.
2. Assess serum albumin, total protein, transferrin, prealbumin, triglycerides, glucose, and urine nitrogen balance as ordered by physician. **Rationale: Provides baseline measure of nutritional status and blood sugar level.**
3. Consult with physician and dietitian on calculation of calorie, protein, and fluid requirements for client. **Rationale: Provides multidisciplinary plan for client's nutritional support.**
4. Assess baseline vital signs and weight. **Rationale: Subsequent measures will evaluate effectiveness of nutritional support.**
5. Verify physician's order for nutrients, vitamins, minerals, trace elements, electrolytes, and flow rate.

PLANNING

Expected outcomes focus on adequacy of nutrition, adequacy of fluid volume, and prevention of complications related to TPN therapy.

Expected Outcomes

1. Client will achieve/maintain ideal body weight.
2. Client will achieve/maintain fluid and electrolyte balance.
3. Client will maintain serum glucose levels at less than 200mg/dl.
4. Client will remain free of local and systemic infection.

DELEGATION CONSIDERATIONS

The skill of TPN management requires problem solving and knowledge application unique to a professional nurse. Delegation is inappropriate.

IMPLEMENTATION

Steps	Rationale

1. See Standard Protocol (inside front cover).
2. Initiate central line management protocol (see Skill 39.1).
3. Explain purpose of TPN.

COMMUNICATION TIP

Describe for client the nutrients contained in the solution. Also explain, "We will be checking your blood often to be sure your blood sugar is just right and that other blood values are where we want them."

Steps	Rationale
4. Inspect TPN solution for particulate matter or separation of fat into a layer.	Presence of matter or lipid separation requires solution to be discarded.
5. Connect TPN solution to appropriate IV tubing and fill; then connect to dedicated port of multilumen central catheter, and label port.	
6. Use IV pump or volume controller (see illustration) to infuse solution.	
7. Assess appearance of central line site routinely (see agency policy).	
8. Change tubing every 24 hours or anytime contamination is suspected or integrity of product may have been compromised.	Client is at increased risk of infection because of impaired nutritional status. High concentration of glucose in infusion also increases risk of infection.
9. Do not add medications to parenteral nutrition solution.	In rare circumstances, medications may be added if verified as compatible by pharmacy and no other ports are available.
10. Make sure adequate solution is available to ensure continuous infusion if ordered.	Blood glucose levels must be maintained to avoid complications of hypoglycemia. Patency of line must be maintained to ensure continued use.

NURSE ALERT

Have backup fluids available if new TPN solution cannot be obtained on time.

11. See Completion Protocol (inside front covers).

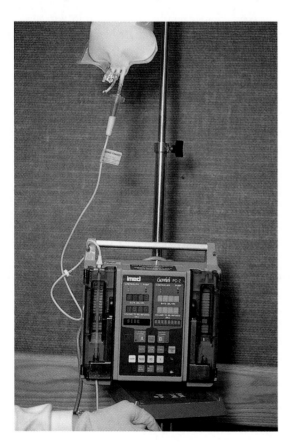

Step 6

• • •

EVALUATION

1. Monitor daily weights for trend toward normal.
2. Monitor I&O and evaluate for fluid overload or dehydration (see Chapter 9).
3. Monitor finger stick blood sugar every 6 hours or as ordered.
4. Monitor for signs and symptoms of infection at infusion site including redness, swelling, tenderness or drainage; monitor for systemic signs of infection including fever, elevated WBC, and malaise.

Unexpected Outcomes and Related Interventions

1. Client develops hypoglycemia or hyperglycemia.
   a. Client may need gradual adjustment of concentration of glucose in TPN solution.
   b. Insulin may be necessary to maintain proper blood glucose.
2. Client has sharp chest pain, dyspnea, decreased breath sounds on one side, crepitus, cyanosis, or resonance to percussion. These indicate pneumothorax, hydrothorax, or hemothorax.
   a. Stop infusion.
   b. Get chest x-ray as ordered by physician.
   c. Monitor vital signs.
   d. Provide emotional support.
   e. Assist with aspiration or insertion of chest tube.
   f. Assist with removal of catheter and insertion of replacement.
3. Client has bright red blood filling syringe, or tracheal compression with respiratory distress, indicating arterial laceration.
   a. Notify physician.
   b. Apply direct pressure to artery for 15 minutes.

Recording and Reporting

- Report to physician deviation from baseline assessment or laboratory parameters and signs/symptoms of dehydration or fluid overload.
- Document assessment of physical condition, capillary blood glucose values, and IV solution on applicable flow sheet.
- Document I&O and weight on graphic sheet.
- Document unexpected outcomes, notification of physician, and interventions on nurses' notes/plan of care.

Sample Documentation

0700 Weight maintained at 58 KG for 1 week. Central line insertion site free of infection. Vital signs stable. Client denies discomfort from catheter. Daily infusions continued with 2000 ml/day as ordered. 150 g dextrose, 42.5 m amino acids, 200 ml fat emulsion, 50 mEq Na, 30 mEq K, 4.5 mEq Ca, 5 mEq Mg, 50 mEq Cl, 12 mEq PO$_4$, 10 ml multivitamins, 1 ml trace minerals, and 100 units heparin.

Geriatric Considerations

TPN is appropriate treatment for older adults with the following conditions:

- Cachexia (chronic protein colorie malnutrition), is more common in older adults with cancer, hepatic disease, or chronic neurological disease. Manifestations of cachexia include emaciation, loss of subcutaneous fat and lean body mass, brittle hair, and banded nails.
- Older adults may also have protein malnutrition. Malnutrition is primarily the result of protein losses (not reduced intake), as with burns, pemphigus, or albuminuria.

Older adults are at higher risk for complications related to TPN therapy

Home Care and Long-Term Care Considerations

- Assess client's/family member's ability to manage enteral feedings. Also assess environmental conditions: sanitation, equipment storage, power source.
- For long-term management of TPN administration, the client and significant others must be taught to monitor the results as outlined above and should be instructed to report the following immediately: perceived change in physical condition, weight change, altered glucose values, or change in skin turgor or integrity; pain, redness, or swelling at infusion site; infusion pump alarm that cannot be corrected.
- Instruct client/family member on proper steps used to obtain capillary blood sample and measure glucose level.

Skill 39.3

MECHANICAL VENTILATION

Mechanical ventilation controls or assists the client's respirations when the client is unable to provide an adequate gas exchange to body tissues because of respiratory or ventilatory failure (Table 39-1, p. 902). The treatment takes over the physical work of moving air in and out of the lungs, but it does not replace nor alter the physiological function of the lung. Mechanical ventilation is used to maintain or improve ventilation, oxygenation, and breathing pattern. It corrects profoundly impaired ventilation that may be evidenced by hypercapnia and symptoms of breathing difficulty. Mechanical ventilation typically requires the use of an endotracheal or tracheostomy tube (see Chapter 31) and delivers room air under positive pressure or oxygen-enriched air in concentrations of up to 100%. The ultimate goal of timely and successful discontinuation of mechanical ventilation is achieved differently with every client. In general, clients will remain on mechanical ventilation only as long as necessary and will not require reintubation within 24 to 48 hours of discontinuation of treatment. Management of the client receiving mechanical ventilation is a continual challenge. Strong interdisciplinary collaboration among physicians, nurses, respiratory therapists, pharmacists, nutritionists, pastoral care personnel, and rehabilitation services is essential to manage and eventually terminate mechanical ventilatory assistance. Nursing care for the client requiring mechanical ventilation includes provision of emotional support, prevention of equipment failure, prevention of complications (e.g., pneumothorax, atelectasis, decreased cardiac output, pulmonary barotrauma, stress ulcer, infection), and promotion of optimum gas exchange.

Equipment

 Inline suction catheter
 Suction unit
 Nonsterile latex gloves
 10-ml syringe
 Stethoscope
 Ambu bag with oxygen tubing
 Adhesive tape
 Roll of 1-inch gauze
 Scissors
 Bite block
 Oral airway

ASSESSMENT

1. Assess the client's ability and willingness to cooperate or assist with the procedure and the need for special positioning during the intubation procedure.

Rationale: Combative behavior on the part of the client not only makes the procedure more difficult but also requires greater respiratory effort for the client.
2. Assess the client's ability (e.g. use of notepad or alphabet board or hand signals) and willingness to communicate, and establish an appropriate means to do so. **Rationale: Decreasing apprehension and facilitating communication will allow the client to remain calmer and more cooperative during mechanical ventilation.**
3. Assess the client's need for specialized nutrition support. **Rationale: Client will not be able to have any oral intake and will have increased nutritional needs from the stress related to the condition.**
4. Assess the client's baseline vital signs and laboratory values (e.g., electrolytes, arterial blood gases [ABGs], hemoglobin [Hg]/hematocrit [Hct]) ordered by the physician. After initiation of treatment, monitor and evaluate client's SaO_2 continuously, and monitor ABGs as ordered and prn with respiratory distress.

PLANNING

Expected outcomes focus on establishing and maintaining a patent airway; facilitating effective gas exchange, adequacy of fluid volume, and adequacy of nutrition; and preventing complications related to intubation and mechanical ventilation.

Expected Outcomes

1. Client's airway remains clear of secretions.
2. Client's PaO_2, respiratory pattern, and SaO_2 remain within desired parameters.
3. Client's oral and nasal mucous membranes and lips remain moist and clear of abrasions, excoriations, or erosions.
4. Client maintains fluid and electrolyte balance.
5. Client maintains mental status and level of conciousness.
6. Client remains free of lung infection.

DELEGATION CONSIDERATIONS

The skill of maintenance of mechanical ventilation requires problem solving and knowledge application unique to professional nurses. Delegation is inappropriate.

Table 39-1

Overview of Mechanical Ventilation Types

Types	Description	Nursing Considerations
POSITIVE PRESSURE		
Continuous Positive–Airway Pressure (CPAP)	Applies positive pressure during entire respiratory cycle	Used for clients who breathe spontaneously but have hypoxemic respiratory failure; also useful during weaning
Positive End-Expiratory Pressure (PEEP)	Applies positive pressure during expiration	Used for treating hypoxemic respiratory failure, usually at 5 to 20 cwp
Volume-cycled	Delivers a preset volume to client	Useful when excessive inspiratory pressure could damage lungs, as in neonates; tidal volume varies with airway resistance and lung compliance
HIGH FREQUENCY		
High-Frequency Jet Ventilation (HFJV)	Delivers gas rapidly under low pressure via special injector cannula	
	Delivers 100 to 200 breaths/min with tidal volume of 50 to 400 ml	Most common of high-frequency types; maintains alveolar ventilation with low airway pressure; useful for treating esophageal or bronchopleural fistulas or pneumothorax; may avert barotrauma in high-risk clients if used early in treatment
High-Frequency Oscillatory Ventilation (HFOV)	Delivers over 200 breaths/min or 900 to 3000 vibrations, with tidal volume of 50 to 80 ml	
High-Frequency Positive-Pressure Ventilation (HFPPV)	Delivers 60 to 100 breaths/min, with tidal volume of 3 to 6 ml/kg	Tidal volume is less than the normal 5 to 7 ml/kg
MODE OF USE		
Control	Fully regulates ventilation in client with paralysis or in arrest	
	Delivers set tidal volume at prescribed rate, using predetermined inspiratory/expiratory times	
Assist	Client initiates inspiration and receives preset tidal volume that augments ventilatory effort	
Assist-control	Client initiates breathing, but backup control delivers a preset number of breaths at a set volume	
Synchronized Intermittent Mandatory Ventilation (SIMV)	Ventilator delivers set number of breaths at specified volume; client may breathe spontaneously between SIMV breaths at volumes differing from those set on machine; used for weaning	

IMPLEMENTATION

Steps	Rationale

1. See Standard Protocol (inside front cover).
2. Explain the system to the client, using descriptions of anticipated experiences and benefits.
3. Set up a communication system and reassure the client that assistance will always be nearby.

Presence of endotracheal tube prevents client from being able to talk.

NURSE ALERT

Be sure that communication device/system is always within reach and available to client.

4. If client does not have an endotracheal or tracheostomy tube, assist physician with insertion; then order chest x-ray.

X-ray evaluates tube placement.

5. Implement safety and infection-control measures:
   a. Check ventilator and cardiac alarm at beginning of each shift and after visits to bedside by others.
   b. Check for endotracheal tube position in centimeters every shift, and secure stabilization of artificial airway with every client contact.
   c. Keep airway, face mask, and Ambu bag at bedside.
   d. Ensure availability of emergency supplies on unit (e.g. extra endotracheal [ET] tubes, chest tubes).
   e. Check endotracheal tube cuff using minimal leak technique every shift and after any change in tube position.
   f. Verify tube position after every chest x-ray.
   g. Using inline catheter, suction prn; suction oro/nasopharynx after endotracheal suctioning and before any cuff manipulation.
   h. Use swivel adaptor between endotracheal tube and ventilator.
   i. Rotate oral endotracheal tube from one side of mouth to the other every 24 hours; retape endotracheal tube every 24 hours and prn, using skin prep pads.
   j. Perform oral hygiene every 2 hours with oral suction close at hand.
   k. Monitor inline temperature continuously.
   l. Keep ventilator tubing clear of condensation and secretions.
   m. Place bite block or airway if client is biting tube.
   n. Administer sedatives or neuromuscular blocking agents as ordered if client is fighting ventilator and ineffective ventilation occurs; observe carefully after administration.
   o. Troubleshoot high-pressure alarms within 15 sec.

Prevents accidental migration of tube into right or left bronchus.

Necessary to ventilate client if endotracheal tube is inadvertently removed

Ensures stable position of tube.

Maintains patency of airway

Helps to minimize oral mucosa irritation and erosion.

Prevents accidental spillage into client's airway.

Establishes more relaxed breathing pattern.

6. When possible place client in semi-Fowler's position.

Promotes lung expansion and prevents aspiration if client is on enteral feedings.

7. If client becomes confused or combative, consult physician on use of soft restraints to prevent the client from extubating self.

COMMUNICATION TIP

Reassure the client, "This is a way of helping you remember not to pull out the tube that you need to help you breathe."

Steps	Rationale

8. Monitor ABGs regularly to detect possible overventilation or inadequate alveolar ventilation or atelectasis
   a. Check oxygen saturation every 8 hours.
   b. Check ABGs whenever ventilator settings are changed.

NURSE ALERT

Overventilation causes respiratory alkalosis from decreased carbon dioxide. Inadequate ventilation may cause respiratory acidosis.

---

   c. Pulse oximetry may be used for continuous monitoring of blood gases in addition to periodic laboratory analysis of blood specimens.
9. Perform the following at least hourly:
   a. Make sure that the client can reach the call light if able to use it.   Ensures mode of communication for client.
   b. Check all connections between the client and the ventilator, making sure that the alarms are turned on, including both high- and low-pressure alarms and volume alarms.   Maintains pressure within system.
   c. Verify that the ventilator settings are correct and that the ventilator is operating at those settings. Compare the client's respiratory rate with the setting. Make sure that the spirometer reaches the correct volume for volume-cycled machines; for pressure-cycled machines, use a respirometer to determine exhaled tidal volume.   Maintains integrity of system and ensures that settings are consistent with current physician's orders.

NURSE ALERT

Do not assume that ventilator settings are correct, because they may be altered accidentally or intentionally by other personnel such as respiratory therapists or physicians. Do not assume that the machine is operating correctly, because loose connections or obstructions in tubings can cause altered function despite ventilator settings.

---

   d. Check the humidifier and refill if necessary. Check the corrugated tubing for condensation, and drain any accumulation to be discarded.   Do *not* return condensation to humidifier, because of possible bacterial contamination.
   e. Check temperature gauges and make sure that gas is being delivered at the correct temperature. The desired range of temperatures is between 89.6° F (32° C) and 98.6° F (37° C).   Maintain client's body temperature.
   f. If ordered, give the client several deep breaths every hour by setting the sigh mechanism on the ventilator or by using the Ambu bag.
10. At least every 4 hours, assess client for:
   a. Confusion, anxiety/restlessness, agitation/lethargy, headache.   Sign of inadequate ventilation/gas exchange.

Steps	Rationale

   b. Adventitious breath sounds, dyspnea, tachypnea, inability to move secretions.

   c. Decreased urine.

Sign of inadequate renal perfusion.

11. Assess client at least every 4 hours for:

   a. Nasal flaring, tracheal tug, intractable cough, fremitus, use of accessory muscles.

Signs of ineffective breathing patterns, possibly related to problem with equipment.

   b. Changes in respiratory depth, prolonged expiratory phase, or altered chest excursion during spontaneous breaths.

12. Auscultate for decreased breath sounds on the left side. Arrange for chest x-rays as ordered.

Determines whether the tube has slipped into the right mainstem bronchus.

13. Auscultate over trachea for presence of air leaks.

Excessive pressure causes tissue necrosis.

   a. Using minimal occlusive pressure, inflate cuff with 10-ml syringe.

   b. Leave syringe attached to cuff of tubing.

14. Monitor fluid I&O and electrolyte balance. Weigh client as ordered.

Fluid retention can signal early pulmonary edema.

15. Using aseptic technique, change the tubing every 48 hours, including the humidifier, the nebulizer, and the ventilator. During the tubing change the client should be manually ventilated.

16. Change the client's position frequently to avoid impaired circulation of both air and blood.

17. Perform chest physiotherapy (see Chapter 14) as necessary, including percussion and postural drainage as appropriate.

18. Monitor gastrointestinal function to prevent complications.

Inactivity and stress can produce decreased bowel function.

   a. Administer antacids and other medications as ordered to reduce gastric acid production.

   b. Auscultate for decreased bowel sounds and check for abdominal distention, which may signal paralytic ileus.

Nasogastric tube may be needed to provide decompression.

   c. Check nasogastric secretions for blood using Hemoccult or other agency-approved reagent.

Stress ulcer is a common complication of mechanical ventilation.

19. Provide emotional support to minimize stress. Apprehension and anxiety can increase client's respiratory rate and respiratory effort.

   a. Ensure that means of communication is intact.

   b. Explain procedures and events to client.

20. Maintain activity level at toleration.

   a. Do passive/active range-of-motion (ROM) exercises.

   b. Change position every 2 hours and prn.

   c. Evaluate for rotational therapy.

   d. Assist client to chair 3 times daily if tolerated.

   e. Assist client to stand and walk in place at bedside if tolerated.

COMMUNICATION TIP

Explain procedures even to clients who are unresponsive, because they may still be able to hear and understand. "I am going to suction you now so that you can breathe better."

21. Initiate interdisciplinary consults as indicated.

Potential needs for nutritional support, spiritual support, physical therapy support, or other needs.

22. See Completion Protocol (inside front cover).

• • •

EVALUATION

1. Assess respiratory pattern, vital signs, and arterial blood gases and oxygen saturation at least every 2 hours for acutely ill clients and at least every 4 hours in stable chronically ill clients.
2. Inspect oral/nasal mucosa and lips for integrity and adequate moisture.
3. Monitor daily weights, I&O, and related laboratory values.
4. Use Glasgow Coma Scale to evaluate mental status and level of conciousness.
5. Monitor for signs and symptoms of infection including fever, and WBC.

Unexpected Outcomes and Related Interventions

1. Client develops signs/symptoms of inadequate ventilation/gas exchange/ineffective breathing pattern:
   a. Remove from ventilator and ventilate with bag/mask device at 100% O_2.
   b. Search for reversible cause.
   c. Call code blue if indicated.
2. Client develops signs of inadvertent extubation/ malposition of endotracheal tube or leak in cuff, characterized by vocalization/gurgling sounds, activated low-pressure alarm, decreased/absent breath sounds, gastric distention, asymmetrical chest expansion, increased/decreased peak inspiratory pressure (PIP), air leak around mouth/nose, loss of tidal volume, radiographical evidence of malposition.
   a. Notify physician.
   b. Manually ventilate client with Ambu bag until reintubation or repositioning of tube is achieved.
3. Client develops extubation/malposition of endotracheal tube.
   a. Deflate cuff if still in airway and remove endotracheal tube.
   b. Ventilate with bag/mask device at 100% O_2.
   c. Prepare for reintubation.
4. Client develops signs/symptoms of pneumothorax: absent/diminished breath sounds on the affected side, acute chest pain, and possibly tracheal deviation or submucosal or mediastinal emphysema.
   a. Remove from ventilator and ventilate with bag/mask device at 100% O_2.
   b. Prepare for chest tube insertion (see Chapter 39).
5. Client develops signs of atelectasis, characterized by decreased or bronchial breath sounds, increased breathing effort, tracheal deviation toward side of abnormal findings, increased peak inspiratory pressure, decreased lung compliance, decreased PaO_2, SaO_2 in the presence of constant ventilator parameters, or localized consolidation on chest x-ray.
   Notify physician.
6. Client develops oxygen toxicity (clients receiving high concentrations of oxygen are especially at risk), characterized by substernal chest pain, increased coughing, tachypnea, decreased lung compliance and vital capacity, and decreased PaO_2 without a change in oxygen concentration.
   Notify physician and prepare to reduce oxygen concentration.
7. Client develops signs of nosocomial lung infection, characterized by purulent secretions or change in consistency/color of secretions, decreased bronchial breath sounds, coarse rales/rhonchi/wheezes, positive sputum Gram stain, positive sputum and/or blood cultures, progressive/persistent infiltrate on chest x-ray.
   a. Notify physician.
8. Client develops signs of nutritional deficiencies as characterized by progressive weight loss, decreased serum plasma proteins (albumin, prealbumin, transferrin), decreased lymphocyte count, slow wound healing, lethargy.
   a. Notify physician.
   b. Initiate dietary consult as ordered.

Recording and Reporting

Document the following on appropriate forms in client record:

- Date/time ventilatory support initiated, size of endotracheal tube, and position in centimeters.
- Ventilator settings and client mechanics, including FiO_2 delivered/exhaled tidal volume, mode of ventilation, breaths per minute, Positive end expiratory pressure (PEEP), inspiration/expiration ratio or inspiratory time, PIP, compliance, date/time of changes in ventilator parameters.
- Physical assessment findings, weight, vital signs, lung sounds, and hemodynamic parameters and waveforms.
- ABG results and other laboratory work.
- Interventions/comfort measures and client's response.

Sample Documentation

0930   Intubated with 7 Fr endotracheal tube; insertion depth marked at 22 cm. Cuff inflated to minimal occlusive pressure as verified by auscultation for air leaks. 10-ml syringe left in place at bedside; cuff tubing clamped. FiO_2 at 100%; will titrate down to maintain SaO_2 at or above 92%. Ventilator set on assist control, with respiratory rate at 12 and tidal volume at 700 ml. Client was sedated with 1 mg lorazepam IV push; will sedate prn if client is combative or fighting ventilator. Tube placement verified with chest x-ray; no epigastric gurgling noted, bilateral breath sounds auscultated. Client tolerated procedure without adverse effects.

Geriatric Considerations

- Older adult clients are at risk for complications with greater frequency and intensity than younger clients.
- Because of alterations in sensory capabilities, the older adult client has special considerations in communication techniques and emotional support.
- Alterations in electrolyte balance, nutritional status, or cardiovascular function can produce sudden changes in the client's condition.
- Underlying medical conditions and the presence of multiple medications can have significant effects on the client's progress.
- The older adult client is at greater risk for infection because of diminished immune function.
- The nurse must exercise diligence in monitoring the older adult client's condition on an ongoing basis and perform interventions to limit or control complications quickly and aggressively.

Home Care and Long-Term Care Considerations

- Family/significant others must accept responsibility for performing all procedures related to mechanical ventilation support, as allowed by available equipment.
- Backup supplies must be present, including airways, oxygen supply, Ambu bags, and endotracheal tubes or tracheostomy tubes.
- The preparation for transition to the home must begin as soon as possible to allow maximum time to instruct family members and evaluate their return demonstrations.
- Emergency interventions should be clearly outlined to prevent life-threatening complications of treatment.

Skill 39.4

CARE OF CLIENT RECEIVING HEMODIALYSIS

The purpose of hemodialysis is to remove toxic wastes and other impurities from the blood in a client with renal failure. The blood is removed from the body through a surgically created access site, pumped though a dialyzing unit to filter out toxins, and returned to the body (Figure 39-1, p. 908). The procedure may be performed in an emergency in acute renal failure, or it may be performed as a long-term therapy in end-stage renal disease. The frequency and duration of dialysis are determined by the client's condition; a client in chronic renal failure may need treatments up to 3 hours in length, several times a week. The goals of hemodialysis are to help restore or maintain acid-base balance, help restore or maintain electrolyte balance, prevent complications associated with uremia, and help restore or maintain fluid balance. These goals are accomplished by extracting by-products of protein metabolism (especially urea and uric acid), creatinine, excess water, and other unmeasured toxins. This is done by allowing the client's blood to flow between surfaces of semipermeable membranes. At the same time the dialysis solution (called *dialysate)* is pumped around the other side of the apparatus using hydrostatic pressure. The dialysate is an aqueous fluid usually containing isotonic concentrations of sodium and chloride ions; low concentrations of potas-

sium, calcium, and magnesium ions; and high concentrations of bicarbonate and glucose. The toxic wastes and excess water are removed as a result of the differing pressure and concentration gradients between the blood and the dialysis solution.

Because the blood has greater concentrations of hydrogen ions and other electrolytes than the dialysate, the solutes diffuse across the semipermeable membrane into the solution. In the other direction, glucose and acetate are more highly concentrated in the dialysate, so they diffuse across the semipermeable membrane into the blood.

Vascular access with high blood flow is required for hemodialysis. For chronic, long-term dialysis, an arteriovenous fistula or graft is created. In the case of an external shunt (Figure 39-2, *A*, p. 909), a cannula is implanted in both the artery and vein and is connected to a silicone rubber tubing that exits from the skin (Lewis, Collier, and Heitkemper, 1996). The two ends are connected with a U-shaped shunt. In the center of the shunt is a connector, accessed for attaching the client to the dialysis machine.

Internal arteriovenous fistulas and vein or synthetic grafts (39-3, *B* and *C*, p. 912) are created in the forearm or thigh. The increased pressure of the arterial bloodflow through the vein causes the vein to dilate and toughen, al-

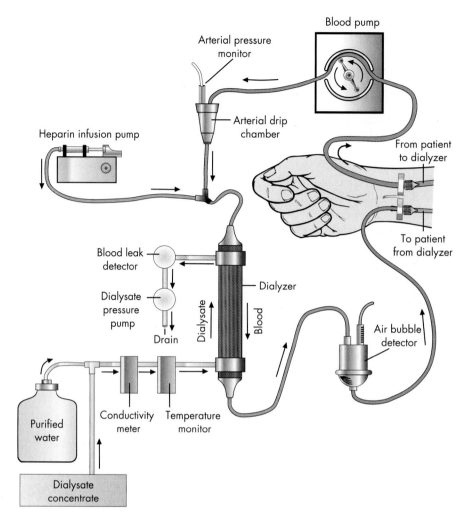

Figure 39-1 Components of a hemodialysis system. *From Thelan LA, Davie JK, Urden LD: Textbook of critical care nursing: diagnosis and management,* ed 3, 1998, Mosby.

lowing easy access for venipuncture. The fistula or graft is accessed using two large-gauge steel needles. For temporary dialysis, dual-lumen dialysis catheters can be placed in the subclavian, internal jugular, or femoral veins.

Nurses who work in outpatient dialysis centers receive specialized training to administer dialysis. Clients visit these centers usually 3 times per week with treatment lasting 3 to 4 hours. When these clients become acutely ill and hospitalized, nursing staff must know how to monitor their status and provide appropriate supportive care.

Equipment
 Stethoscope
 Antiseptic swabs
 4 × 4 gauze squares or 2-inch gauze roll
 Nonallergenic tape (optional)

ASSESSMENT

1. Assess client's weight and compare to weight from end of previous dialysis and dry weight. **Rationale: Fluid retention can be quickly assessed by weight gain.**
2. Assess client's vital signs with blood pressure taken in both supine and standing positions.
3. Assess client for changes in mentation, speech, and thought processes. **Rationale: Change in cognition can reveal fluid and electrolyte imbalance.**
4. Assess client's peripheral pulses with special attention to extremity where shunt is located. **Rationale: Determines adequacy of peripheral circulation.**
5. Assess client's heart rate and rhythm. **Rationale: Determines adequacy of systemic circulation and establishes baseline for assessments after dialysis.**

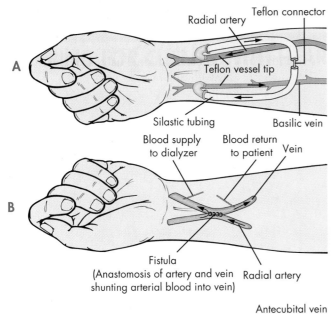

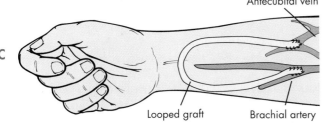

Figure 39-2 Methods of vascular access for hemodialysis. **A,** External cannula or shunt. **B,** Internal arteriovenous fistula. **C,** Looped graft in forearm. *From Lewis SL, Collier IC, Heitkemper MM: Medical-surgical nursing: assessment and management of clinical problems, ed 4, St Louis, 1996, Mosby.*

6. Assess client's respiratory rate, rhythm, and quality and character of lung sounds. **Rationale: Determines baseline for assessing client's respiratory status after dialysis, because of potential changes related to fluid overload.**

7. Inspect condition of skin around vascular access. If external device is present, inspect insertion/exit sites.

PLANNING

Expected outcomes focus on relieving client's anxiety; maintaining comfort; maintaining adequacy of fluid volume, electrolyte balance, and nutrition; and preventing complications related to the dialysis process.

Expected Outcomes

1. Excess fluid and solute wastes are removed from the blood and lymph as evidenced by decreased weight, blood pressure WNL, and electrolyte balance.
2. Client relates a feeling of improved well-being.
3. Client has no complications as evidenced by absence of nausea, vomiting, cardiovascular complications, or alteration in sensorium.
4. Arteriovenous shunt is patent and intact.
5. Client verbalizes understanding of dialysis purpose and procedure.

DELEGATION CONSIDERATIONS

The skill of administering hemodialysis treatment requires problem solving and knowledge application unique to a professional nurse. Delegation is inappropriate.

IMPLEMENTATION

Steps	Rationale
1. See Standard Protocol (inside front cover).	
2. Thoroughly review steps of procedure with client and family member if new to procedure. If client has received dialysis in the past, ask if there are any questions or if client wants to discuss the experience.	
3. Restrict fluids to 1 to 1.5 L/day.	Reduced renal function limits volume of fluid that can be filtered by body.
4. Develop adequate diet plan in collaboration with dietitian and client. Encourage compliance on the part of the client.	Reduced renal function limits type and quantity of nutrients that can be metabolized/excreted by the body.

COMMUNICATION TIP

Review with client the role diet plays in disease management by asking questions such as, "Have you no- *ticed a difference in the way you feel when you go off your prescribed diet?"*

Steps	Rationale

5. Before dialysis, provide light meals.

Large meals cause shunting of blood to gut. Hemodynamics are altered during dialysis and hypotension, and vomiting may develop.

6. Routine administration of medications must be altered to avoid complications of dialysis.
   a. Antihypertensives must be withheld in vast majority of clients until after treatment.
   b. For IV fluids, lactated Ringer's solution must not be used because of potassium load.
   c. Calcium for use as a phosphate binder must be given *with* meal, not just "around mealtime."

If client is normotensive before dialysis and medication is given, the client might become hypotensive.

7. For care of access:
   a. Palpate for thrill and auscultate for bruit. Client should learn to assess bruit/thrill daily.

COMMUNICATION TIP

Be sure that client knows how to properly assess patency of access site by asking for return demonstration. "Please show me where you feel your shunt and listen to it to be sure that it is not clotted."

   b. If clotting is suspected or confirmed, declotting is usually performed in radiology.
   c. Use dual-lumen catheters for blood draws and IV fluids *only* with approval of nephrologist.
   d. Post a warning sign in prominent location and instruct client to observe by refusing to allow others to perform venipuncture or blood pressure measurements on affected extremity.

Risk of damage to access site; risk of clotting. Goal is to avoid stagnation of flow to decrease clotting and reduce risk of infection.

NURSE ALERT

No blood pressures, needle sticks, or any constricting procedure on access arm.

   e. If access device is external and newly placed, clean around insertion site with antiseptic swab. Using sterile gloves, apply sterile gauze squares or gauze roll (see agency policy).
8. See Completion Protocol (inside front cover).

• • •

EVALUATION

1. Compare weight and blood pressure to preprocedure parameters. A weight change of 1 kg is equivalent to 1 L of fluid.
2. Ask client to describe general feeling of well-being.
3. Observe for nausea, vomiting, change in vital signs, or altered level of consciousness. NOTE: Temperature may rise because BUN is an antipyretic and is decreased with dialysis. Hypotension may indicate hypovolemia or a drop in Hct. Rapid respirations may indicate hypoxemia.
4. Palpate arteriovenous shunt for thrill and auscultate for bruit.
5. Ask client to describe the purpose and process of hemodialysis.

Unexpected Outcomes and Related Interventions

1. Client develops internal bleeding, which may be manifested by apprehension; restlessness; pale, cold, clammy skin; excessive thirst; hypotension; rapid, weak, thready pulse; increased respirations; or decreased body temperature.
   a. Report to physician immediately.

b. Prepare to transfuse if ordered.

2. Client develops excessive site bleeding.
   a. Maintain pressure on site and notify physician.

3. Client develops fever.
   a. Assess for sources and signs of infection.
   b. Culture blood as ordered.
   c. Administer antipyretics and antibiotics as ordered.

4. Client develops hypotension, which may be related to antihypertensive medications, inadequate sodium in diet, unstable cardiovascular disease, hypoalbuminemia, or hypovolemia from excessive fluid and sodium removal during dialysis.
   a. Place client in Trendelenberg position.
   b. Administer 100 to 500 ml NS boluses as ordered by physician.
   c. Measure blood pressure frequently during episode.
   d. Administer colloid osmotic agent as ordered.

Recording and Reporting

After dialysis, record the following in the client's record:

- Client education given and client's ability to discuss.
- All vital signs measured, all laboratory data, and client's weight before and after treatment.
- All food and fluid intake before treament.
- Assessment of venous access before treatment, including site inspection and appreciation of thrill and bruit.

Sample Documentation

1045   Client scheduled for hemodialysis. Discussed wife's concerns about patency of fistula. Arteriovenous shunt in left forearm has palpable thrill; able to auscultate bruit. Dry weight before treatment 91.2 Kg. BP 170/102 (sitting); 155/97 (standing).

Geriatric Considerations

- Older adults are at greater risk for complications including systemic or peripheral circulatory problems such as hypotension and hypoxia that can be life threatening.

Home Care and Long-Term Care Considerations

- The client must be taught to care for the vascular access site, which includes keeping incision clean and dry to prevent infections and cleaning site with hydrogen peroxide daily until healing is complete and sutures are removed; notifying health care team of pain, swelling, redness, or drainage in accessed arm; use of stethoscope to auscultate bruit daily and palpation technique to appreciate thrill daily; free use of arm after site has healed, with care not to exert excessive pressure on it; avoiding any treatments or procedures on the access arm; and use of exercises for access arm to promote vascular dilation and enhance bloodflow.
- The client who will be performing hemodialysis at home must thoroughly understand all aspects of the procedure. The client should be given the phone number for contacting the health care team for any questions or to report any problems. The client should be encouraged to have another person present during the home dialysis sessions in case problems develop.

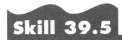

PERITONEAL DIALYSIS

Peritoneal dialysis removes toxins from the blood of a client with acute or chronic renal failure who does not respond to other treatments. It uses the body's peritoneal membrane as the semipermeable dialyzing membrane (Figure 39-3, p. 912). A hypertonic dialysate is instilled through a catheter inserted into the peritoneal cavity; then diffusion moves the excessive concentrations of electrolytes and uremic toxins across the membrane into the dialysate. Excessive water is removed in the same way by osmosis. After an appropriate dwell time, the dialysate so-lution is removed, to be replaced by fresh solution. The procedure may be performed manually or by a cycler machine (Figure 39-4, p. 913). Table 39-2, p. 912 summarizes the types of peritoneal dialysis.

Equipment

Peritoneal dialysis administration set
Mask
Graduated containers for measuring I&O
Stethoscope

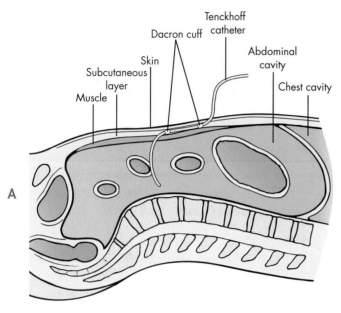
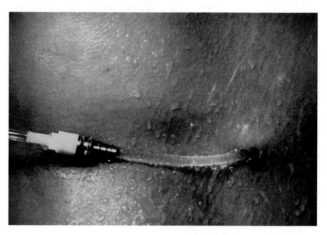

Figure 39-3   A, Tenckhoff catheter used in peritoneal dialysis. **B,** Placement of peritoneal catheter.   **A,** *From Lewis SL, Collier IC, Heitkemper MM: Medical-surgical nursing: assessment and management of clinical problems, ed 4, St Louis, 1996, Mosby.* **B,** *Courtesy Baxter Healthcare.*

Table 39-2

Methods of Peritoneal Dialysis

Type	Description
Continuous ambulatory peritoneal dialysis (CAPD)	Manual; three to five exchanges daily; last batch of solution remains in abdomen overnight
Continuous cycling peritoneal dialysis (CCPD)	Cycler machine changes solution 3 to 5 times overnight; last batch of solution remains in abdomen during daytime
Intermittent peritoneal dialysis (IPD)	Manual or automated; connected for about 10 hours, with cycle changing every 30 to 60 minutes; abdomen left "dry" between sessions
ADDITIONAL PROCEDURES	
Continuous arteriovenous hemofiltration (CAVH)	Treats clients who have fluid overload but do not need dialysis; mechanically filters toxic wastes and infuses a replacement fluid such as Ringer's lactate; blood may be accessed by femoral catheters, internal arteriovenous graft, or arteriovenous shunt
Continuous arteriovenous ultrafiltration (CAVU)	Similar to CAVH, but slower (2 to 6 L/day); blood accessed by femoral catheters or by large-bore percutaneous catheters

ASSESSMENT

1. Assess client's weight and vital signs for baseline. Blood pressure should be measured with the client standing and supine.
2. Assess client's serum electrolytes, especially potassium. **Rationale: Determines amount of potassium to be added to dialysate, ordered by physician.**
3. Assess client's knowledge and compliance with diet plan. Review sources of high sodium that often require restriction.

PLANNING

Expected outcomes focus on successful filtering of toxic wastes from the client's blood, adequacy of fluid volume and of nutrition, and prevention of complications related to the dialysis treatment.

Expected Outcomes

1. Excess fluid and solute wastes are removed from the blood and lymph as evidenced by decreased weight, blood pressure WNL, electrolyte balance (especially potassium).
2. Client relates a feeling of improved well-being.

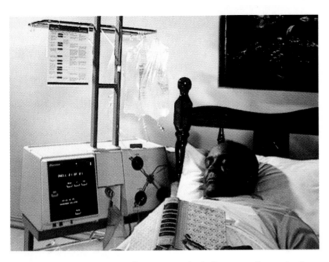

Figure 39-4 Automated peritoneal dialysis cycler, which is used while the client is sleeping at night. *Courtesy Baxter Healthcare.*

3. Client has no complications as evidenced by absence of nausea, vomiting, cardiovascular complications, or alteration in sensorium.
4. Client's catheter remains patent and intact.
5. Client verbalizes understanding of peritoneal dialysis purpose and procedure.

DELEGATION CONSIDERATIONS

The skill of performing peritoneal dialysis requires problem solving and knowledge application unique to professional nurses. Supportive comfort or assistive measures may be performed by other members of the health care team or by family members.

IMPLEMENTATION

Steps	Rationale

1. See Standard Protocol (inside front cover).
2. Review client's understanding of treatment (Khanna, Nolph, and Oreopoulus, 1993) and provide emotional support.

COMMUNICATION TIP

Client often is fatigued and may experience other symptoms because of blood toxins. Keep discussion simple and focused on client needs.

3. Ask client to void before procedure of catheter insertion.

Reduces risk of bladder perforation and increases comfort during catheter insertion.

4. Warm dialysate solution to body temperature according to agency procedure.

Avoids hypothermia and shock during procedure.

5. Add any prescribed medications to dialysate.
6. Prepare dialysis administration set, wearing mask.

Avoids introducing pathogens into peritoneal cavity.

   a. Place drainage bag below client.
   b. Connect outflow tubing to drainage bag.

Facilitates drainage by gravity.

7. Connect dialysis infusion lines to the bags/bottles of dialysate and hang at client's bedside.
8. Place client in supine position when the equipment and solutions are ready.

Promotes comfort and relaxation. Abdominal distention from fluid instillation may make breathing difficult in Fowler's or semi-Fowler's position.

9. Prime tubing by allowing solution to fill tubes. Keeping clamps closed, connect one infusion line to the abdominal catheter.

Maintains integrity of system and prevents air from entering line.

NURSE ALERT

Avoid introducing air into peritoneal cavity.

Steps	Rationale
10. Check patency of catheter:	Ensures that catheter is ready for use and that client will tolerate initiation of treatment.
a. Rapidly instill 500 ml of dialysate into client's peritoneal cavity.	
b. Immediately unclamp the outflow line and let fluid drain into the collection bag.	
11. Open the clamps on the infusion lines and infuse the prescribed amount of dialysate over 5 to 10 minutes; allow solution to dwell for prescribed interval (10 minutes to 4 hours). Remove and discard gloves and wash hands.	
12. When dwell time is completed, open the outflow clamps and allow the solution to drain into the collection bag.	
13. Repeat the cycles of infusion-dwell-drainage (using new batches of solution each cycle) until the prescribed amount of dialysate and the prescribed number of cycles have been achieved.	
14. When the dialysis treatment is completed, put on sterile gloves and clamp the catheter.	
15. After carefully disconnecting the inflow line from the catheter, place a sterile tip over the catheter end.	Avoid introducing pathogens into the peritoneal cavity.
16. Apply sterile povidone-iodine solution to the site using a sterile gauze sponge.	
17. Apply two split-drain sponges around the site and tape securely in place.	
18. Monitor vital signs every 10 minutes until stable, then every 2 to 4 hours as ordered.	Client is at risk for respiratory distress from fluid overload.
19. During treatment, have client change positions frequently, do ROM exercises, and do deep breathing.	Improves client comfort, reduces risk of skin integrity impairment, reduces risk of respiratory complications, and enhances dialysate drainage.
20. Maintain adequate nutrition, adhering to any prescribed diet.	Protein needed to replace that lost during dialysis.
21. Maintain standard precautions when emptying collection bag and measuring solution.	Fluid is contaminated and may carry transferable diseases such as hepatitis.
22. See Completion Protocol (inside front cover).	

• • • •

EVALUATION

1. Compare weight and blood pressure to preprocedure parameters. A weight change of 1 kg is equivalent to 1 L of fluid. Monitor electrolytes (especially potassium).
2. Ask client to describe general feeling of comfort.
3. Observe for respiratory distress indicating fluid overload or leakage of dialysate into pleural cavity. Watch for abdominal pain and fever, which can indicate peritonitis.
4. Observe catheter that there are no kinks and observe outflow for cloudiness, blood, or blood clots. Clear fluid drainage should be present after a few fluid changes. Observe the site for signs of infection.
5. Ask client to describe the purpose and process of peritoneal dialysis.

Unexpected Outcomes and Related Interventions

1. Client develops peritonitis, which may be manifested by abdominal pain and elevated temperature.
   a. Culture all sites to determine portal of entry: transluminal, periluminal, hematogenous, or through bowel wall.
   b. Administer prescribed antibiotics.
   c. Consult with physician for possible removal of catheter.
2. Client develops exit site infection, which may be manifested by redness, swelling, heat, and pain.
   a. Assess response to cleansing agents.
   b. Continue thorough daily site care.
   c. Administer antibiotics as ordered.

3. Client develops abdominal pain.

    If related to rapid inflow, decrease rate of infusion during initial exchanges.

4. Client develops shoulder pain, which may be related to abdominal distention secondary to air in the peritoneal cavity.

    Prime new tubing carefully and do not use vented systems.

5. Client develops increased body temperature, abdominal pain, or cardiac dysrhythmias related to receiving overheated dialysate.

    a. Drain solution.

    b. Treat for hyperthermia.

    c. Evaluate warming procedure.

6. Client develops hypothermia, which may be related to receiving inadequately warmed dialysate.

    a. Drain solution.

    b. Treat hypothermia.

    c. Evaluate warming procedure.

7. Client develops fluid overload, which may be manifested by dyspnea, altered mental status, and alteration in breath sounds.

    a. Calculate fluid balance accurately.

    b. Use a more hypertonic dialysate as ordered by physician.

    c. Limit fluid intake.

    d. Shorten dwell time.

    e. Correct any catheter malfunction.

    f. Monitor weight, vital signs, and cardiorespiratory status frequently.

8. Client develops fluid deficit, which may be manifested by alteration in fluid and electrolyte balances.

    a. Calculate fluid balance accurately.

    b. Discontinue use of hypertonic solution.

    c. Replace fluid and sodium losses.

    d. Monitor vital signs and weight closely.

    e. Lengthen dwell time.

9. Client develops hypokalemia, which is manifested by decreased levels of serum potassium.

    a. Monitor serum potassium.

    b. Add potassium to dialysate for clients with normal levels.

    c. Instruct clients with chronic problems to increase dietary intake of potassium.

Recording and Reporting

- Document the client's vital signs, weight, laboratory results, type of solution, number of cycles, and volume of infusion and return.

- Document any unexpected outcomes and interventions performed.

- Report any significant changes to physician.

Sample Documentation

1015   Weight after peritoneal dialysis is 70 Kg. Abdominal girth is 94 cm. Electrolytes are WNL. Vital signs: BP 159/82, Pulse 94, resp. 20. Temperature 37° C. Catheter patent. Drainage clear pale yellow. Site nontender without redness or drainage. Client reports feeling much better. Denies questions or concerns about the procedure.

Geriatric Considerations

- The older adult client is at risk for complications related to alterations in metabolic and nutritional changes, as well as related to difficulty in following through with instructions because of alterations in sensory perceptions and judgment.

- The client must be monitored carefully to ensure that complications are prevented or minimized.

Home Care and Long-Term Care Considerations

- The client who will perform CAPD or CCPD at home will usually undergo a 2-week training program before performing the treatment independently.

- The client must be able to understand and perform all the necessary steps of the procedure, in addition to reporting any untoward effects of treatment such as infection and fluid imbalance.

- A support group can be helpful in facilitating adjustment to the client's new regimen.

- Home care nursing can provide periodic supervision and assessment of the client's performance of the treatment.

- The client should carry emergency medical information and identification at all times, including the phone number of the dialysis center.

- The client should record vital signs and response to each treatment.

- The nurse stresses the importance of follow-up visits with the dialysis team to evaluate the effectiveness of the treatment and detect any problems that may arise.

CRITICAL THINKING EXERCISES

1. A client who is receiving TPN infusions begins to complain of sharp chest pain and shortness of breath. His symptoms progress quickly, and you note on assessment of his chest that there are decreased breath sounds on the side where the central venous catheter is inserted. What are the most likely complications developing in this client, and what are the appropriate interventions to correct the problem?

2. During a home visit to a peritoneal dialysis client, you note bags of chips, bottles of carbonated beverages, and cans of salted nuts in the kitchen. What nutritional intervention might be indicated for this client, and why? How will you assess to determine your instructions to the client?

3. Three days after insertion of a Port-A-Cath, the client develops symptoms of fever, hypotension, tachycardia, decreased urine output, and elevated white blood cell count. What do these symptoms indicate, and what interventions are appropriate to correct the problem?

REFERENCES

Alspach J: *Core curriculum for critical care nursing,* Philadelphia, 1998, WB Saunders.

Boggs R, Wooldridge-King M: *AACN procedure manual for critical care.* ed 3, Philadelphia, 1997, WB Saunders.

Camp-Sorrell D, editor: *Access device guidelines: recommendations for nursing practice and education,* Pittsburg, 1996, Oncology Nursing Press.

Cancer chemotherapy guidelines and recommendations for practice, Pittsburgh, 1996, Oncology Nursing Press.

Flynn JB, Hackel R: *Technological foundations in nursing,* East Norwalk, Conn, 1990, Appleton-Lang.

Huddleston S, Ferguson S: *Critical care and emergency nursing,* Bethleham Pike, Pa, 1997, Springhouse.

Illustrated manual of nursing practice, Bethlehem Pike, Pa, 1993, Springhouse.

Intravenous Nurses Society: Intravenous nursing standards of practice, *J Intraven Nurs* 21(15):51–85, 1998.

Khanna R, Nolph K, Oreopoulos D: *The essentials of peritoneal dialysis,* Dordrecht, The Netherlands, 1993, Kluwer Academic Publishers.

Kim M, McFarland G, McLane A: *Pocket guide to nursing diagnoses,* St Louis, 1997, Mosby.

Lancaster L, editor: *Core curriculum for nephrology nursing,* Pitman, NJ, 1995, Jannetti.

Lewis SL, Collier IC, Heitkemper MM: *Medical-surgical nursing: assessment and management of clinical problems,* ed 4, St Louis, 1996, Mosby.

Macklin D: How to manage PICCs, *Am J Nurs* 97(9):21–33, 1997.

Mostellar RD: Simplified calculation of body surface area, *N Engl J Med* 317:1078, 1987.

Perry A, Potter P: *Clinical nursing skills and techniques,* ed 4, St Louis, 1998, Mosby.

Peterson M: Guideline for prevention of intravascular device-related infections, *Am J Infect Control* 24(4):262–293, 1996.

Phipps W et al: *Medical-surgical nursing: concepts and clinical practice,* ed 5, St Louis, 1995, Mosby.

Tucker S et al: *Client care standards: collaborative practice planning guides,* St Louis, 1996, Mosby.

CHAPTER 40

Discharge Teaching and Home Health Management

Skill 40.1
Risk Assessment and Accident Prevention, 918

Skill 40.2
Teaching Self-Administration of Non-Parenteral Medications, 922

Skill 40.3
Teaching Self-Injections, 926

Skill 40.4
Teaching Home Self-Catheterization, 932

Skill 40.5
Using Home Oxygen Equipment, 936

Skill 40.6
Teaching Home Tracheostomy Care, 941

Clients must have the necessary knowledge, skill, and resources to meet self-care needs at home before discharge from a health care facility. Therefore, discharge teaching and planning are of utmost importance. Discharge planning is an organized, coordinated, interdisciplinary process that provides a plan of care for the client leaving the health care setting. The goal of discharge planning is to provide continuity of care, thereby ensuring a smooth transition for the client from the health care setting to the home environment.

The nurse's role in discharge planning follows the nursing process. The nurse must assess the biophysical, psychosocial, educational, self-care, environmental, and discharge needs of the client. The discharge needs are determined from the analysis of the total assessment, and nursing diagnoses are then identified.

In the planning phase, the nurse and client jointly identify goals and expected outcomes. Achievement of these goals is based on selection of appropriate therapies and therapeutic services available. The nurse must know what family and community resources are available, the referral process, and the client's financial support. Because of shortened length of stays, heavy client case loads, and quick discharge decisions, a discharge planning department may be needed to assist the nurse in preparing the client for discharge.

Teaching is the major intervention in the implementation phase. Teaching strategies are based on assessment of the client's physical and emotional readiness to learn, educational level, and learning needs. Teaching is integrated throughout the client's stay in a health care facility and must be followed up in the home setting. For example, teaching clients how to self-administer medications or modify risk factors are teaching actions that may begin in the health care facility but need to continuously be evaluated and reinforced at home. Written and/or visual guidelines reinforce verbal instructions and should be provided to the client on discharge home.

When clients become actively engaged in the learning process, teaching/learning effectiveness is enhanced.

Therefore the best way for the nurse to evaluate a client's understanding of the material presented is to ask clients about the treatment regimen or to demonstrate a procedure that will be done by the client, family member, or significant other. Discharge instructions should reflect nursing actions of teaching, counseling, and appropriate referrals. Clear, concise, accurate documentation of the client's needs and abilities on the discharge plan improves the continuity of care. The nurse should also document the client's and family's knowledge of and ability to comply with discharge instructions.

Finally, the discharge plan is confirmed with the client and family. The nurse can follow up several days after discharge by telephone to answer questions or may secure a follow-through from a referral agency such as home health care.

NURSING DIAGNOSES

Health-Seeking Behaviors is appropriate when the client is in stable health and is actively seeking to alter personal habits to achieve better health.

Altered Health Maintenance is appropriate when a client or family is unable to identify, manage, or seek help to maintain health.

Health beliefs, cultural influences, spiritual values, financial constraints, and the client-provider relationship may result in **Noncompliance** with self-care therapies. In the case of noncompliance, the nurse tries to help the client adhere to self-administered therapies. **Ineffective Individual Management of Therapeutic Regimen** may apply when the client has difficulty meeting health goals. Complexity of treatments, knowledge deficit, and per-

ceived susceptibility cause the client to integrate treatments ineffectively in their daily lives.

Knowledge Deficit is appropriate when the client has not been exposed to a new procedure, lacks recall, or verbalizes misinterpretation of previously learned information. **Anxiety** results from the client's concern about how illness may change lifestyle or the client may be unsure about learning a new behavior and performing it correctly in the home environment.

The aging process and chronic illnesses such as diabetes mellitus and cataracts may elicit the **Sensory/Perceptual Alterations** diagnosis. With these conditions, the client's sensory acuity is decreased and adaptations to the home environment may be needed. **Impaired Physical Mobility** from activity intolerance, perceptual or cognitive impairment, disabilities, or age-related changes may limit the client's ability to take medications or perform self-care skills. Impaired physical mobility can also lead to **Risk for Injury,** which can occur as a result of potentially unsafe environmental conditions (e.g., physical setup of the home). Clients who have sensory, cognitive, or motor disabilities are at highest risk.

Risk for Infection is appropriate when clients are initiating an invasive procedure such as performing a self-catheterization. This diagnosis may also exist if the home is not environmentally clean and the client does not follow aseptic technique when necessary. All clients after discharge may be at risk for **Impaired Home Maintenance Management.** This may be associated with client's disease or disability, motor skills, inadequate support systems, decreased knowledge of available resources and ways to initiate contact, communication skills, and impaired cognitive or emotional functioning (Kim, McFarland, and McLane, 1997).

Skill 40.1

RISK ASSESSMENT AND ACCIDENT PREVENTION

This skill focuses on preparing the client to go home to a risk-free, safe environment. Discharge from an agency can be stressful if a client and family feel unprepared to resume normal activities or unable to adapt therapeutic regimens to living at home. Before the client is discharged, the client and family must know how to manage care in the home and what to expect regarding any continuing physical problems. Without the necessary equipment and professional resources to care for continuing health problems, the client risks loss of any rehabilitation gains made before discharge. Failure to understand

restrictions or implications of health problems may cause a client to develop complications after leaving the health care setting. Inadequate discharge planning overlooks the client's needs within the home and increases the chance of the client reentering the health care system prematurely.

Unintentional injuries can occur at all ages of the life span. Many of these injuries result from hazards that are easy to overlook but easy to fix. Knowledge of specific motor and cognitive developmental changes enables the nurse to assess for potential injury for each client. After the area of risk is identified, the nurse designs interventions to eliminate or reduce the threat to the client's safety.

Equipment

Assessment form(s)

Home safety checklist

ASSESSMENT

1. Assess client's physical and mental status before discharge and determine the type of adaptions necessary in the home. **Rationale: The nature of physical and cognitive limitations determines the type of adjustments to be made in the home.**

2. Assess client's attitudes toward returning home and following health care provider recommendations. Determine the perceived susceptibility to harm, perceived seriousness of any physical condition, perceived benefit in changing behavior, and perceived barriers related to changing the behavior. **Rationale: The health-belief model (HBM) addresses attitudinal components of health behaviors. If attitudes related to health behaviors can be identified, nursing interventions for attitude change can be developed (Becker, 1974; Champion, 1984).**

3. Review risk factors from nursing history in relation to lifestyle patterns: smoking, stress, drug use, alcohol use, unplanned exercise habits, and personal hygiene. **Rationale: Lifestyle habits frequently increase the risk for developing illnesses or disabilities during middle or older years.**

4. Obtain client's employment history to determine risks within the work setting. **Rationale: Occupational inhalants such as asbestos, plastics, dusts, and gases have potential for causing chronic lung diseases or cancer.**

5. Assess client's and family's understanding of home therapies, restrictions resulting from health alterations, and possible complications. **Rationale: Determines level and extent of health education needed by client.**

6. Determine client's actual or potential limitations resulting from sensory, motor, cognitive, or physical changes. **Rationale: This provides the opportunity to identify factors that increase client's risk of injury.**

7. Consult other health team members about needs after discharge (e.g., dietitian, social worker, home health care nurse). Make appropriate referrals. **Rationale: Members of all health care disciplines should collaborate to determine client's needs and functional abilities.**

PLANNING

Expected outcomes focus on improving client's knowledge level, and motivation to learn, identification of risk factors, provision of a safe environment, and ability to perform self-care in the home environment.

Expected Outcomes

1. Client explains how health care is to continue at home, including what treatments and medications are needed and when to seek medical attention for problems.

2. Client demonstrates self-care activities.

3. Client identifies safety risks in the home.

4. Client maintains a home environment that is adapted to client's motor, sensory, and cognitive developmental needs.

5. Client identifies community resources available and how to initiate contact.

DELEGATION CONSIDERATIONS

Some of the principles that are involved in changing the home environment are both practical and common sense in approach. Assistive personnel (AP) such as home health aides often interact with clients and make suggestions for ways to make the home safer. However, an RN is best qualified to conduct a thorough home safety assessment and to determine what alterations or revisions are preferred on the basis of the client's physical and/or cognitive limitations. The RN should provide supervision to any unlicensed personnel who suggest changes.

IMPLEMENTATION

Steps	Rationale
1. See Standard Protocol (inside front cover).	
2. Assemble teaching materials and provide a comfortable and quiet setting, free of distractions.	Comfortable environment enhances learning. Interruptions interfere with concentration.

Steps	Rationale
3. Begin teaching sessions with client and family as soon as possible during hospitalization (use time when giving a bath, passing medications, ambulating, or feeding client). Pamphlets or books may be given to client and family.	Gives client opportunity to practice new skills, ask questions, and obtain necessary feedback to ensure learning. Incorporating teaching during care activities maximizes use of available time.
4. Set up equipment and show skill to client. Utilize supplies and equipment that client will use at home. Employ teaching techniques of repetition, rephrasing, and summarizing. Have client demonstrate skill. Provide client with positive feedback.	Facilitates transfer of learning.
5. Teach health promotional activities in areas of nutrition, exercise, relaxation, and smoking cessation (if applicable). Review risks for cancer and teach warning signs.	Reduces risk of certain diseases (e.g., cardiopulmonary disease, cancer, obesity). There is supportive evidence that with certain disorders, exercise and nutrition enable wellness (Grimby et al., 1992).
6. Teach client how to recognize stress and measures to deal effectively with psychophysiological effects.	Prolonged stress response can increase client's risk of stress-related illnesses.
7. With the client and family as active participants, conduct a home safety assessment using a checklist or flow sheet (Kravitz et al., 1994). NOTE: The assessment may need to be validated later with client in the home.	
8. Suggest ways to make home environment safe.	Client's level of independence and ability to retain function can be maintained within safe environment.
a. Involve client and family in all decisions if possible.	
b. Explain benefits of all recommendations.	
9. Disposal of in-home medical supplies:	
a. Instruct client to place needles, syringes, lancets, or other sharp objects in a hard plastic or metal container such as soda bottles or laundry detergent containers with screw-on or tightly secured lid.	Prevents injury to self or others and prevents pollution.
b. Soiled bandages, disposable sheets, and medical gloves are placed in securely fastened plastic bag before being placed in garbage can.	
10. Physical arrangements that can reduce predisposition to falls:	
a. *Stairs*	
(1) Install treads with uniform depth of 9 inches (23 cm) and 9-inch risers (vertical face of steps).	If stairs are of uniform size, older adult client need not continually adjust vision.
(2) Install uniform-textured or plain-colored surfaces on each tread, and mark edge of tread with contrasting color (e.g., orange, yellow).	Uniform texture or color helps to decrease vertigo. Marking edge of tread provides obvious visual target for client to see edge of stairs more clearly.
(3) Ensure proper lighting of each tread. Block sun or light bulb glare with translucent shades or screens, or use lower-wattage bulbs. Do not use fluorescent lighting.	Older adult's eyes are unable to adjust quickly to changes in lighting and are more sensitive to glare.

Steps	Rationale

(4) Ensure adequate head room so that client does not have to duck to use stairs.

Sudden changes in head position may result in dizziness.

(5) Remove protruding objects from staircase walls.

Decreased peripheral vision may prevent client from seeing objects.

(6) Keep outdoor walkways and stairs in good condition (free of holes, cracks, and splinters) and well lighted.

Decreased visual acuity can prevent client from seeing structural defect.

b. *Handrails*

(1) Install smooth but slip-resistant handrails at least 2 inches (5 cm) from wall.

Distance allows client to grasp handrail firmly for support.

(2) Secure handrail firmly so that client's weight can be supported, especially at bottom and top of stairway.

Older client has greatest risk of falling at top and bottom of stairs because center of gravity is being shifted and balance is unstable.

(3) Install guardrails in bathroom near toilet and bathtub.

Enables clients to have support while rising from sitting to standing position.

c. *Floor coverings*

(1) Secure all carpeting, mats, and tile; place skid backing under area rugs.

Sudden slip may cause dizziness and inability of client to regain balance. Decrease in muscle strength may decrease client's ability to adjust to slip and prevent fall.

(2) Provide unobstructed pathways.

11. Prevention of fires and burns

a. Install smoke detectors on each floor of the house.

Prevents injury.

b. Have client select a fire extinguisher that is easy to handle and manipulate.

Older adults or clients with disabilities may have difficulty gripping mechanisms on certain extinguishers.

c. Keep hot water temperature 120° F (48.8° C) or lower by adjusting water heater setting.

d. Discourage smoking when client is sleepy or in bed (if applicable).

e. Keep flammable objects away from stove when cooking.

f. Provide client and family with information about community health care resources.

Community resources may offer services that client or family cannot provide.

12. See Completion Protocol (inside front cover).

• • •

EVALUATION

1. Ask client and family to describe treatment regimens and physical signs and symptoms to be reported to physician.
2. Have client or family perform treatments and procedures to be continued at home.
3. Ask client to identify safety risks.
4. Ensure that family or a home health nurse inspects home environment so that it is free of obstacles and risks.
5. Ask client and family to identify resources available for a particular problem and how to initiate contact with that resource.

Unexpected Outcomes and Related Interventions

1. Client is unable to identify safety risks.
   a. Reevaluate home environment with client and family members.
   b. Teach client the rationale for preventing and removing potential hazards from home environment.
2. Client demonstrates procedure incorrectly.
   a. Reassess client's knowledge level.
   b. Teach procedure, and reinforce areas of learning deficit.
   c. Demonstrate procedure, and have client return demonstration.
   d. Provide praise throughout learning session.

Recording and Reporting

- Retain copy of the home safety assessment in the client's home health record.
- Record assessment of the client's cognitive and mental status, recommended interventions, and client's and caregiver's response in progress notes.
- Record any instruction provided, client's response, and changes made to the environment in progress notes.

Sample Documentation

0900 Safety risks and hazards found in home environment discussed with client and family. Checklist completed with client and family members. Instructed to correct potential hazards of throw rugs and to install handrails in bathroom. Heartland Home Health Care Agency referral made with physician's order and discussed with client and family members.

1115 Client states family members will make necessary changes in home environment before discharge. Client able to correctly identify benefits of receiving home health nursing care to meet his needs.

Geriatric Considerations

- Physiological changes and mental status alterations that accompany aging, such as a slower reaction time, muscular weakness, reduced pain and temperature perception, reduced depth perception and color discrimination, reduced visual acuity, confusion, memory loss, and poor orientation, place older adults at risk for injury in the home environment.
- Older adults learn to negotiate their environments relatively well and are usually more aware of potential dangers (Ebersole and Hess, 1994).

Home Care and Long-Term Care Considerations

- Any changes in the client's home environment should be made to retain as much of the client's independence as possible.
- Before making any revisions to a client's home, know the client's financial resources and wherever possible let the client be the final decision maker in the types of alterations to be made.
- Caregivers must learn the importance of preserving client autonomy, and any modifications to the home environment should consider the client's physical strengths and remaining functional abilities, not just the client's disabilities.

Skill 40.2

TEACHING SELF-ADMINISTRATION OF NON-PARENTERAL MEDICATIONS

This skill focuses on teaching techniques and strategies to ensure client safety and compliance with home medication regimens. It is very important to use every opportunity that the nurse has in the hospital setting to teach clients about how their medications are to be taken.

Noncompliance with medication regimen is a common problem. Some clients tend to "forget" to take their medications, whereas others refuse to do so. Some individuals may have sensory or motor impairments and/or financial constraints that may make them unable to comply correctly with medication administration, and others fail to understand the necessity of taking their medications. Noncompliance may be aggravated in older adults by the lack of family support systems and because multiple chronic conditions are often treated with multiple med-

ications, sometimes prescribed by more than one physician (Esposito, 1995). In many instances, noncompliance accompanies clients' lack of understanding about their own illness or injury; therefore follow-up treatment with medications may be adversely affected. The nurse teaches and counsels clients to enhance their knowledge, safety, and compliance with their medication regimen. Teaching individualized for each client because each person has unique characteristics and capabilities. Make sure that a client who has a sensory impairment is equipped with the appropriate appliances (e.g., hearing aid, glasses).

Review the discharge order and clarify any misinformation with the physician. Also, arrange a time that the client's significant other may participate in the teaching session(s).

Equipment

Medication

Liquid to take with medication

Measuring devices (teaspoon, measuring cups, syringe)

Medication chart/record

Special containers for daily or weekly preparation

ASSESSMENT

1. Assess client's cognitive, sensory, and motor function; level of consciousness; sight; hearing; touch; reading ability and comprehension; ability to swallow; ability to ambulate and tolerate activity; and willingness to cooperate. **Rationale: Cognitive sensory, and motor deficits may influence client's ability to take or prepare prescribed medication correctly and to participate in instruction.**

2. Assess the client's resources to obtain medications when needed. **Rationale: Lack of financial resources or transportation will negatively affect compliance with a medication regimen.**

3. Assess client's and significant other's knowledge related to medication therapy: names of drugs, action or purpose, daily dosages and time taken, potential side effects, and what to do if problems arise. **Rationale: This determines how much teaching will be needed, providing the nurse with baseline information. Family members (or caregivers) are important resources to help clients comply with therapy.**

4. Assess client's belief in the need for drug-therapy. Consider cultural values, religious beliefs, personal experiences with medications, and significant others' values about drugs. **Rationale: These factors influence client's compliance with drug therapy.**

5. Check client's prescribed drugs. Has more than one physician prescribed medications? Are medications obviously inappropriate? Are labels clearly marked? Are time schedules confusing? Do different drugs look alike? Does client store medications together? **Rationale: This assists nurse in determining sources of confusion affecting client's compliance.**

PLANNING

Expected outcomes focus on improving client's and caregiver's knowledge level, self-care, motivation to learn, and ability to comply with medication regimen.

Expected Outcomes

1. Client or significant other explains the purpose, action, and common side effects of each medication by discharge.

2. Client or significant other identifies by discharge whom to contact for questions or problems and what to do if a dose is missed.

3. Client or significant other explains how to self-administer medication.

4. Client or significant other reads and interprets the drug label properly.

5. Client or significant other prepares proper drug doses.

6. Client or significant other demonstrates self-administration of medications by the prescribed route before discharge.

DELEGATION CONSIDERATIONS

This skill requires problem solving and knowledge application unique to a professional nurse. Delegation is inappropriate.

IMPLEMENTATION

Steps	Rationale
1. See Standard Protocol (inside front cover).	
2. Assemble teaching materials and provide a comfortable, quiet, well-lit setting, free of distractions at a time when family members may participate in teaching.	Comfortable environment enhances learning. Interruptions interfere with concentration. Family can serve as a positive resource to client.
3. Be sure that hearing aids and/or glasses are worn during the teaching.	Increases client's sensory perception and likelihood of attending to teaching session and understanding content.
4. Present the information clearly and concisely in understandable terms in accordance with client's educational level and age.	

Steps	Rationale
5. Provide frequent pauses to allow client and caregiver to ask questions.	Increases client's participation in learning process. Ongoing feedback ensures nurse that client is acquiring information.
6. Discuss the following information in relation to medication regimen: purpose, action, common side effects, significance of taking, dosage schedules, what to do if experiencing side effects, when and whom to call for/with problems/concerns, drug safety guidelines, and implications when medications are not taken.	Content learned improves client's ability to self-medicate and comply with medication regimen.
7. Discuss additional information related to medication therapy as appropriate: always take the drug as prescribed for duration of course; consult physician before switching medications; follow the pharmacy directions on medication label; examine labels of other over-the-counter (OTC) drugs to prevent possible adverse reactions when drugs are inadvertently mixed; advise on storing medications.	Minimizes chances of adverse or undesirable side effects.
8. Provide frequent, short teaching sessions.	Improves attention and retention of information discussed.
9. Provide learning aids, special charts, and devices to increase compliance (e.g., calendars, pill box with color-coded compartments) (see illustration).	
10. Demonstrate preparation of medication.	

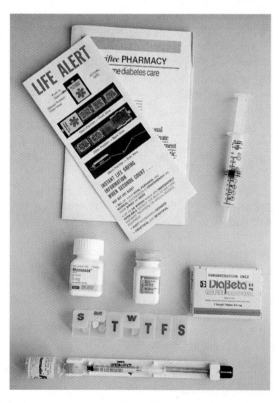

Step 9

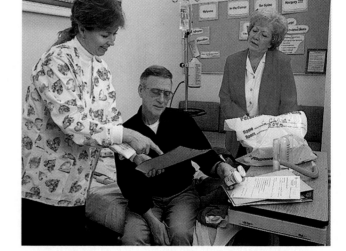

Step 13

Steps	Rationale
11. Have client practice preparing medication(s). Offer assistance by having the pharmacy provide flip-top or screw-top containers and larger labels on medication containers when necessary.	Nurse can observe client's ability to read labels correctly and prepare all medications for prescribed times. Visual alterations or weakened grasp can cause inaccurate medication preparation.
12. Have client demonstrate steps in medication administration. Be sure to assess technique of swallowing.	Some clients do not drink enough water to swallow properly; the tablet could become lodged in the esophagus and cause esophageal lesions.
13. Provide client and family written instructions to take home (see illustration).	While hospitalized, client may be anxious and easily distracted during teaching sessions. Written instructions help ensure compliance.
14. Arrange for regular visits by home health nurse as deemed necessary.	Provides health care provider with knowledge of client's compliance with medication administration in the home; early intervention is then possible.
15. See Completion Protocol (inside front cover).	

• • •

EVALUATION
1. Ask client and significant other to explain purpose, action, and side effects of the prescribed medications, as well as foods or OTC drugs to avoid.
2. Ask client and significant other to identify whom to contact with concerns and what to do if a dose is missed.
3. Have client and significant other read and interpret the pharmacy label.
4. Have client and significant other verbalize the steps in preparing the medication.
5. Have client and significant other prepare proper drug dosages.
6. Observe client and/or significant other prepare and self-administer the medications.

Unexpected Outcomes and Related Interventions
1. Client is unable to recall or explain information discussed in teaching session.
   a. Determine what information client does have.
   b. Determine what remaining information is essential for client safety and compliance, and provide additional teaching.
2. Client is unable to prepare medications as prescribed.
   a. Reassess client's sensory and motor abilities to ensure safety and compliance.
   b. Identify areas of concern in administering drugs. Provide emotional (positive) support of client's ability.
   c. Have client demonstrate preparation of medications until successful.
   d. Have family member prepare medications.
3. Client fails to comprehend the importance of information provided in the teaching session.

a. Observe client's emotional status and acceptance of the need for medication.
b. Enlist support of significant others to verify importance of medication regimen.

Recording and Reporting
• Document instruction provided and learning outcomes achieved by client on progress notes.
• Develop a client recording mechanism of dosage schedules and self-monitoring regimen for the home.

Sample Documentation
1000   Teaching regarding self-medication administration completed. Verbalized need to follow written instructions regarding medications while at home.
1200   Client correctly administered own medications following appropriate guidelines.

Geriatric Considerations

• Older adults often have reduced visual and hearing acuity and difficulty understanding language because of high-frequency tones being less perceptible. Therefore, speak in a slow, low-pitched voice when teaching the older adult.
• The capacity for learning new information remains as we age, in the absence of dementia (Lueckenotte, 1996). Allow adequate time and number of teaching sessions to support successful learning.

Home Care and Long-Term Care Considerations

- Pill counts and visual check of the medication delivery system (e.g., weekly pill dispensing system) may help to assess learning follow-through, especially if memory loss is a concern.
- Written instructions should be at the reader's level of understanding. Client education materials are of-

ten too complex or contain confusing medical jargon (Wilson, 1996).

- If difficulties arise regarding the schedule of medicines, frequency of dosing, or cost, the nurse must notify the prescribing physician of the factors negatively affecting an accurate self-medication plan in the home setting.

Skill 40.3

TEACHING SELF-INJECTIONS

Many drugs may be administered subcutaneously (e.g., narcotics, vaccines, insulin, heparin). Insulin and heparin are the medications most likely to be self-administered in the home environment. These medications must be administered subcutaneously because they are not absorbed by the oral route. It is recommended that heparin be injected into the subcutaneous tissue of the abdomen, and the client should be instructed to observe for signs of bleeding such as bruising, bleeding gums, or bloody stools. The client is instructed not to aspirate or rub the injection site after heparin or insulin administration with heparin. These actions could result in tissue damage and severe bruising. Also, massaging an insulin injection site could lead to increased absorption of the medication (Haire-Joshu, 1996).

This skill focuses on teaching clients how to administer insulin self-injections. Almost 3 million diabetic clients may require daily subcutaneous injections of insulin (ADA, 1993). The nurse is responsible for teaching clients how to give injections for the first time, as well as for evaluating the injection techniques of clients administering their own insulin. Some clients with diabetes are still trying to learn proper technique, and others do not realize they have been doing it incorrectly.

The ability of a client with diabetes to learn how to administer injections depends in part on the progress of the disease. Diabetes is a chronic condition that can cause loss of vision and peripheral nerve damage. The nurse may need to adapt the equipment available to the client or educate a significant other. Special syringes with plunger locks ensure that only a specific dose is prepared. Syringe magnifiers, insulin pens, needle guides, and vial stabilizers are available for clients with visual or motor impairments to aid in insulin administration (Figure 40-1).

Equipment

Vial of insulin in correct concentration (U-100)
Two or three insulin syringes (0.25 ml, 0.3 ml, 0.5 ml, or 1 ml, calibrated in units)
Bottle of sterile water or normal saline
Antiseptic/alcohol swabs
2 × 2 gauze pads
Rotation chart

ASSESSMENT

1. Assess client's readiness and ability to learn: Does client ask questions about disease, treatment, or injections or request to learn how to give injections? Is client mentally alert? Does client participate in own care? Determine client's ability to read and see clearly. **Rationale: This reflects client's ability to**

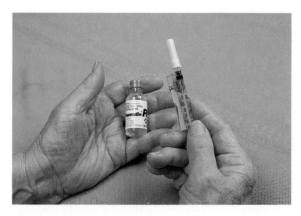

Figure 40-1 A syringe magnifier aids clients with visual or motor impairments.

understand explanations and actively participate in teaching process. Mental or physical limitations affect client's ability to learn and alter nurse's method of instruction.

2. Assess client's ability to hold and manipulate a syringe and hold insulin vial. **Rationale: Peripheral neuropathy can alter diabetic client's sensation of touch and affect ability to handle syringe and vial safely.**

3. Assess client's visual ability by having client read numbers on insulin syringe or directions on a vial. If acuity is reduced, ask client to use syringe magnifier. **Rationale: Clients with diabetes often experience swelling of the lens because of elevated blood glucose levels, causing a transient reduction in visual acuity. It may be necessary to educate family members or significant others.**

4. Assess client's knowledge and understanding of diabetes; purpose, action, and side effects of insulin; and reason insulin is required. **Rationale: Client must know implications of too much or too little insulin, which can be fatal.**

5. Assess significant others' interest in and ability to provide injections. **Rationale: Significant other may be principal administrator of injections; even if client can administer own injections, significant other should be available as resource if client becomes ill.**

6. Assess drug dosage and schedule client is ordered to receive at home.

7. If client administers own injections, assess client's techniques in preparation and administration of injection. **Rationale: Nurse's instruction may require only simple reinforcement, depending on client's level of skill.**

PLANNING

Expected outcomes focus on improving client and caregiver's knowledge level and motivation to learn, and ability to self-administer injection.

Expected Outcomes

1. Client or significant other identifies the parts of the needle and syringe.
2. Client or significant other correctly manipulates the syringe and needle using aseptic technique.
3. Client or significant other uses aseptic technique throughout the procedure.
4. Client or significant other states which insulin is to be administered, as well as the correct dosage.
5. Client or significant other correctly draws up the ordered insulin dose in corresponding insulin syringe.
6. Client or significant other selects injection sites recommended for insulin administration.
7. Client or significant other discusses the rationale for rotating sites.
8. Client or significant other correctly demonstrates an insulin self-injection.
9. Client and significant other describe signs of low blood sugar and how to treat.
10. Client or significant other identifies proper disposal of used needles.

DELEGATION CONSIDERATIONS

This skill requires problem solving and knowledge application unique to a professional nurse. The RN is best equipped to identify the adaptations needed within the home based on the client's limitations. However, (AP), such as home health aides, will frequently be in a situation to be able to see how clients use these adaptations. AP can learn how to make suggestions that further ensure client safety:

- Use of basic infection-control practices
- How to dispose of sharps and needles
- How to dispose of contaminated supplies

IMPLEMENTATION

Steps	Rationale
1. See Standard Protocol (inside front cover).	
2. Assemble teaching materials and equipment needed. Provide a comfortable, quiet, well-lit setting, free of distractions. Have client sit at table where all equipment is displayed; make sure equipment is within easy reach and organized logically.	Comfortable environment enhances learning. Interruptions interfere with concentration. Enables client to visualize entire procedure.
3. Have client wash hands. Explain importance of handwashing.	

Steps	Rationale
4. Have client manipulate syringe. Explain which parts must remain sterile and which can be touched.	Familiarity with aseptic technique in handling syringe ensures safe drug administration.
5. Have client compare syringe scale with insulin label concentration on insulin vial.	Concentration of insulin in units and number of units marked on syringe should match; for example, 100-unit syringe is used only with U-100 insulin.
6. Discuss client's ordered dose.	
7. Have client check the vial label indicating the type of insulin and expiration date of insulin, and examine solution for color change, clumping, or frosting of the vial. If insulin has been refrigerated, allow to warm to room temperature.	Client should not take expired medication. Regular and lispro insulin should be clear. All other insulin types (intermediate-acting, long-acting, and premixed) should be uniformly cloudy. A cold insulin injection can be painful and less effective than one at room temperature.

NURSE ALERT

It is not necessary that insulin be stored in the refrigerator. A cool place at room temperature will keep the insulin from losing potency for as long as 30 days. Any *unused insulin vials should be kept refrigerated. If a client must use prefilled syringes, they must be refrigerated and used within 30 days (ADA, 1998).*

Steps	Rationale
8. Demonstrate technique for mixing cloudy insulin vial by gently rolling bottle between the hands; then allow client to mix the vial. *Never* shake the vial.	After sitting, insulin forms crystal on bottom of vial. Mixing produces uniform solution. Shaking creates air bubbles.
Drawing up insulin	
9. Demonstrate and explain steps used to prepare syringe.	Demonstration is the most effective technique for teaching motor skill.
a. Wipe off top of vial with alcohol and remove needle cover.	
b. Pull plunger out to same number of units to be removed from vial. This pulls air into syringe.	
c. With vial still on table, push needle slowly into rubber on top of vial while holding syringe barrel carefully. Do not bend needle (see illustration).	

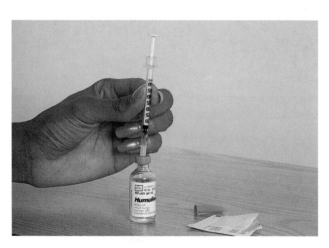

Step 9c

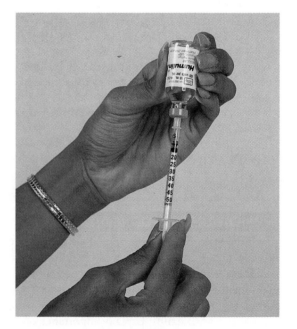

Step 9e

Steps	Rationale

d. Push in plunger to push air into bottle; this prevents vacuum.

e. Hold vial and syringe together; turn both upside down. Hold vial between thumb and forefinger, supporting syringe with other hand (see illustration).

f. With the other hand, slowly pull back on plunger to number of units of insulin to be given. Be sure needle stays under fluid in vial.   Explanation includes basic principles for syringe preparation (see Chapter 18).

g. Do not touch inside of plunger.

h. Check for clear air bubbles inside syringe.   With bubbles present, correct amount of insulin may not be prepared.

i. If bubbles can be seen, use the plunger to push the insulin back into the vial and then slowly pull the insulin into the syringe again, stopping at the correct dose of insulin. Repeat this procedure until there are no large air bubbles in the syringe.

j. Check to be sure correct amount of insulin is in syringe and no air bubbles are present.

k. Remove syringe from vial by pulling it straight out.

l. Put cap or sheath back without touching needle.

10. Show chart of injection sites and find each accessible site on client's body (see illustration).   Comparing body parts allows nurse to point out areas to be avoided, such as scars and bruises.

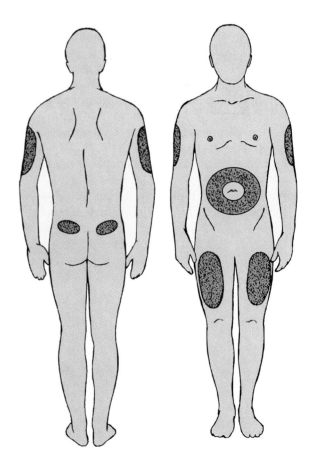

Step 10

Steps	Rationale
11. Discuss importance of rotating sites systematically, using all the sites in one area before changing to another. If client takes more than one shot each day, a different area should be used for each shot (e.g., the morning shot may be given in the outer thigh and the evening shot in the inner thigh).	Insulin is absorbed differently in different parts of the body. Insulin is absorbed most predictably and completely in the abdomen (Haire-Joshu, 1996). Using the same area at the same time every day provides client with more consistent dosing and smoother control of diabetes.
12. Have client choose injection site in abdomen or thigh where nurse can easily demonstrate injection.	
13. Administer injection while explaining each step slowly, using simple terms.	Nurse's instructions during demonstration should include principles for minimizing pain, injecting needle correctly, maintaining asepsis, and checking for insulin leakage.
a. Wipe off site with alcohol swab to clean area; let dry.	
b. Take cover or sheath off needle.	
c. Hold syringe as you would a pencil.	
d. Grasp (or pinch up skin fold) injection site between thumb and fingers of free hand. To self-inject arm, press back of upper arm against wall or back of chair. "Roll" arm down to push up skin.	
e. With a quick jab, insert needle into cleansed area at a 90-degree angle. (A 45-degree angle may be used for children or thin adults.)	
f. Insert needle all the way to hub. Hold onto syringe.	
g. Let go of skin, push plunger in to administer insulin. Be sure to inject all the insulin.	
h. Put 2 ×2 gauze over needle gently, and pull needle out quickly at same angle it was inserted. Check for insulin leakage at site.	
i. Briefly hold dry 2 ×2 over site.	
j. Discard uncapped needle or needle enclosed in safety shield and attached syringe in a plastic receptacle.	Prevents needle sticks.
k. Have client indicate on record chart where injection was given.	Facilitates rotation of injection sites.
14. Encourage client to ask questions about procedure.	Allows clarification of any misunderstanding and facilitates recall.
15. Provide client with written and visual guidelines.	
16. See Completion Protocol (inside front cover).	

NURSE ALERT

Clients who exercise should avoid injecting into the subcutaneous tissue adjacent to the muscles to be exercised, because this can lead to more rapid insulin absorption and subsequent hypoglycemia.

NURSE ALERT

Routine aspiration (drawing back on the syringe to check for blood) is no longer recommended, even for children and thin adults (ADA, 1998).

COMMUNICATION TIP

Reinforce key points for client to remember; for example, take your insulin every day. Never skip a shot. "Do not hesitate or jab when inserting the needle, just apply smooth even pressure and the injection will be more comfortable. You may feel a slight stinging sensation when you inject the medication."

EVALUATION

1. Ask client or significant other to identify the parts of the syringe and needle.
2. Observe client or significant other manipulating syringe.
3. Ask client or significant other to explain what is meant by *aseptic technique*. Observe client's or significant other's ability to follow through with aseptic technique throughout procedure.
4. Have client or significant other verify physician orders for insulin type and insulin dosage. Have client or significant other explain which insulin to administer and the amount to give.
5. Observe client or significant other preparing insulin injection.
6. Have client or significant other point out on self the areas for site rotations.
7. Ask client or significant other why it is important to rotate sites.
8. Observe client's or significant other's technique for self-administering an insulin injection in the proper location.
9. Ask client or significant other signs of low blood sugar and how to treat.
10. Ask client or significant other how to dispose of used needles.

Unexpected Outcomes and Related Interventions

1. Client or significant other is unable to meet one or more of the expected outcomes.
   a. Reassess readiness and ability to learn.
   b. Reassess sensory and motor capabilities and provide adaptive devices such as a syringe magnifier if needed.
   c. Determine if client is in pain or has other symptoms that can detract from learning and demonstrating.
   d. Identify areas of deficiencies.
   e. Reteach those areas where there are deficiencies.
   f. Provide teaching booklet.
   g. Have client or significant other explain and demonstrate the self-injection technique several times in nurse's presence following procedural guidelines.

Recording and Reporting

- Document instruction provided and learning outcomes achieved by client on progress notes and in care plan.
- Develop an at-home recording system to be used by the client/significant other to provide information on injection site, time, and dosage of insulin injection.

Sample Documentation

0900   Teaching self-injection of insulin started; client able to identify correct parts of syringe and basic principles of aseptic technique. Encouraged client to manipulate syringe and ask questions.

1000   Teaching continued; discussion and demonstration of drawing up insulin and injection technique completed. Chart shown of available injection sites; rationale provided for rotation of sites. Practiced drawing up normal saline in syringe.

0700   Administered own insulin injection following proper procedure with verbal cues only from RN.

Geriatric Considerations

- Older adults frequently suffer from chronic diseases that leave deficits, making syringe visualization and manipulation difficult and place them at risk for unsafe parenteral medication administration. The nurse must assess any special needs of the older adult and adapt the teaching strategy accordingly by providing assistive devices such as a syringe magnifier or enlisting the help of the client's significant other.

Home Care and Long-Term Care Considerations

- Note the temperature of medication storage area. Medications should not be stored in extreme heat or cold.
- If there are small children in the home, with easy access to the medication storage area, be sure medications and equipment are stored in a secure place.

Skill 40.4

TEACHING HOME SELF-CATHETERIZATION

This skill addresses the proper way to teach a client to perform clean, intermittent self-catheterization. Many clients in the home environment use self-catheterization to manage acute or chronic bladder dysfunctions. Self-catheterization can be taught to clients with paraplegia, hemiplegia, or other illnesses that limit voluntary bladder control. When teaching self-catheterization to a client, the nurse must also teach a family member or significant other to complete the procedure.

Clients performing self-catheterization can choose to use either clean or sterile technique (see Chapter 4). Clients who are prone to infection should use sterile technique, whereas others can use medical asepsis (clean technique) without the risk of infection. For these clients, the bladder's natural resistance to microorganisms normally found in the home environment makes it unnecessary to use sterile technique.

Self-catheterization is an important component of a client's rehabilitation and return to a maximal level of functioning. Therefore, instruction is integrated into the rehabilitation program at an early stage and not merely tacked onto the end of the hospital stay.

Equipment

Catheter(s) (one or two, red rubber), size 14 to 16 Fr for an adult, or size 8 to 10 Fr for a child
Zephrin towelettes, "baby wipes," soap and water
Surgical lubricant that is water soluble (K-Y jelly or Surgilube)
Container with a cover to store catheter
Germicide solution
Toilet/container for draining urine
Mirror

ASSESSMENT

1. Assess client's and significant other's knowledge base related to self-catheterization. Does client know why self-catheterization is the best technique? **Rationale: This determines if client is ready and motivated to learn. Highly motivated people perform more successfully.**
2. Assess client's developmental, cognitive, and physical able to do the procedure? Can client assume the position for self-catheterization? Can client manipulate the catheter? Is client able to care for the equipment used for the procedure? **Rationale: The procedure may have to be adapted to individual needs.**
3. Assess client's present knowledge base? **Rationale: This aids in developing appropriate teaching strategies.**

PLANNING

Expected outcomes focus on improving client's and caregiver's knowledge level, ability to perform self-catheterization, motivation to learn the technique, and ability to comply with procedure guidelines.

Expected Outcomes

1. Client and significant other provide reasons why self-catheterization is the best technique for managing bladder dysfunction.
2. Client correctly demonstrates self-catheterization before discharge.
3. Urine is clear, dilute, and odor free after self-catheterization.
4. Client verbalizes satisfaction with procedural technique.
5. Client demonstrates care of equipment after self-catheterization according to institutional recommendations.

DELEGATION CONSIDERATIONS

This skill requires problem solving and knowledge application unique to a professional nurse. Delegation is inappropriate.

IMPLEMENTATION

Steps	Rationale

1. See Standard Protocol (inside front cover).
2. Before demonstrating actual procedure, review and summarize all steps with client. Allow client to ask questions and inspect equipment.

   a. A reduction of microorganisms

     (1) Teach and demonstrate handwashing and its significance.

     (2) Explain and demonstrate opening catheter package, manipulating supplies, and handling catheter.

     (3) Explain and demonstrate cleansing of urethral meatus.

Starting with simple concepts and working toward more complex ones facilitates learning. Return demonstration actively involves client in performing procedure on self, or client may need to start on model and work up to performing procedure on self with nurse's supervision.

   b. Insertion of catheter into bladder

     (1) Identify possible positions for client to assume: sitting on toilet or frog leg (lying on bed with legs bent and knees apart).

     (2) Review anatomical landmarks. Female may need mirror to view urinary meatus.

     (3) Explain insertion of catheter: how to hold penis or separate labia and distance to insert catheter.

Practicing psychomotor skills after cognitive learning allows client to apply and practice principles learned.

   c. Care of equipment

     (1) Discuss and demonstrate principles of medical asepsis.

     (2) Explain that the following changes must be reported to health care provider:

       (a) Urine changes: color changes such as dark or cloudy appearance, bleeding or sediment, odor changes, or decrease in urine volume

       (b) Pain or discomfort: In bladder area while performing procedure or at any time in bladder area with accompanying fever

       (c) Inability to perform procedure, inability to pass catheter

Proper care of equipment prevents spread of infection.

Indicates possible urinary tract infection. Antibiotic treatment may be required.

3. Gather equipment: catheter, towelettes or soap and water, wet washcloth for rinsing, lubricant, container for urine collection if toilet unavailable, and container to store catheter.
4. Wash hands with soap and water.
5. Have client assume comfortable position of choice.
6. **Coach client in performing female self-catheterization.**

(Reinforce with written instructions and visual guidelines.)

   a. Client may wish to use a mirror while in bed to aid in visualizing the urinary meatus (Haas, 1997).

   b. Wash urinary meatus (opening) with towelette or soapy washcloth. Spread vaginal folds with nondominant hand to expose urinary meatus, and cleanse with front-to-back motion (see illustration). Rinse with damp washcloth.

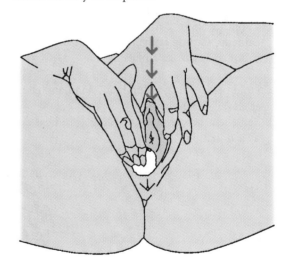

Step 6b *Courtesy Methodist Medical Center of Illinois, Peoria, Ill.*

Front-to-back motion decreases chance of contamination.

Steps	Rationale

    c. Lubricate 1 to 3 inches (2.5 to 7.5 cm) of catheter, starting at the tip. Do not allow catheter to touch any other surfaces (see illustration).

    d. Separate labia with nondominant hand.

COMMUNICATION TIP

Tell client just before inserting catheter to bear down gently as if urinating. Explain that this helps the catheter be inserted more easily. Also warn that a slight burning sensation or pressure might be felt.

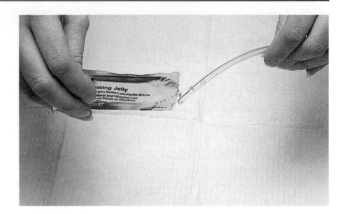

Step 6c

    e. Hold catheter in dominant hand, and use mirror to visualize meatus. slowly insert it into urinary meatus about 3 inches (7.5 cm) or until urine flows through (see illustration).

    f. While holding catheter in place, place other end into the container or toilet; allow all the urine to drain. Then press on abdomen to be sure bladder is empty.

    g. Slowly remove catheter after all urine has been drained.

7. **Coach client in performing male self-catheterization.**

    (Reinforce with written instructions and visual guidelines.)

    a. Wash urinary meatus (end of penis) with towelette or warm soapy water (see illustration).

    b. Lubricate about 2 to 3 inches (2.5 to 7.5 cm) of catheter, starting at the tip. Do not allow catheter to touch any other surfaces.

    c. Hold penis with nondominant hand and at an angle "J" position.

    d. Tell client before inserting catheter to bear down as if urinating.

Ensures catheter tip enters bladder.

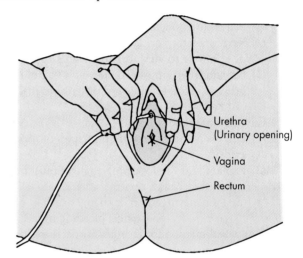

Step 6e *Courtesy Methodist Medical Center of Illinois, Peoria, Ill.*

Straightens urethra for easier catheter passage.

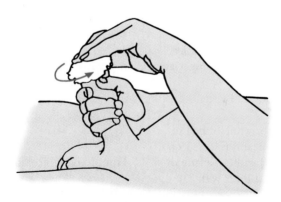

Step 7a *Courtesy Methodist Medical Center of Illinois, Peoria, Ill.*

Steps	Rationale

e. Insert catheter into urinary opening about 8 inches (20 cm) into bladder (see illustration).

f. Let penis return to natural position after urine starts to flow. Allow urine to drain, making sure to hold catheter at all times; then slowly withdraw catheter after urine flow ceases.

8. Rinse catheter in cold water inside and out and place in covered container with a germicide solution (e.g., Detergicide, Sporiciden), or wash it in warm soapy water and allow to air dry. (Refer to agency policy.)

9. Discard catheter if it becomes difficult to clean. Catheters may be used for 7 to 30 days depending on cleansing of equipment and agency policy.

10. See Completion Protocol (inside front cover).

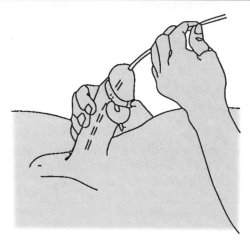

Step 7e   *Courtesy Methodist Medical Center of Illinois, Peoria, Ill.*

• • •

EVALUATION

1. Ask client to state reasons self-catheterization is an appropriate choice for controlling bladder dysfunction.

2. Observe client performing catheterization on "like" model independently. Then observe client's ability to perform self-catheterization using procedural guidelines.

3. Observe client's urine after self-catheterization.

4. Ask client for any questions or concerns about the procedure.

5. Have client explain proper care of the equipment, and evaluate ability to follow guidelines after self-catheterization.

Unexpected Outcomes and Related Interventions

1. Client is unable to complete procedure.
   a. Reassess knowledge base.
   b. Assess for changes in cognition or psychomotor skill.
   c. Try different position for catheterization.
   d. Assess client's personal feelings about performing procedure.
   e. Reteach areas in which client is deficient.

2. Client develops a urinary tract infection (Signs and symptoms include fever, cloudy foul-smelling urine, and back or flank pain.)
   a. Reevaluate client's technique for performing procedure and cleaning equipment.

b. Assess home environment.
   c. Assess fluid intake. Encourage client to drink plenty of fluids.
   d. Instruct client to switch from clean to sterile catheter technique.

Recording and Reporting

• Record and report the type and size of catheter used.

• Record and report the amount and characteristics of the urine.

• Record and report instructions provided and the client's ability to perform the procedure.

Sample Documentation

1400   Instructions regarding home self-catheterization given to client. Use of equipment, medical asepsis, and reasons for self-catheterization discussed. Catheterization demonstrated on model by nurse. Encouraged client to practice on model and ask questions.

1700   Client demonstrated procedure on model. Written and visual guidelines for self-catheterization given and explained to client.

Next day

1300   Client performed self-catheterization using aseptic technique in nurse's presence. 400 ml clear, yellow, odorless urine returned. Client praised on performance.

- A frail older adult is especially vulnerable to urinary tract infections and runs the additional risk of developing septicemia, an infection that has spread to the blood. Self-catheterization with sterile technique may be most appropriate for these clients.
- Failing vision or deficits from other chronic diseases such as arthritis may necessitate assistance from a family member or significant other when performing self-catheterization.

- Assess the client's home environment for appropriate clean storage space for equipment needed for self-catheterization.
- Refer client to home care agency for in-home follow-up.

Skill 40.5

USING HOME OXYGEN EQUIPMENT

Clients with alterations in oxygenation often require continuous oxygen therapy. The duration of therapy may be several weeks or months as clients recover for an acute lung injury or continuously for the remainder of their lives. Oxygen is a drug and is administered and monitored with the same care as any other medication. Box 40-1 lists oxygen safety measures to be followed.

Oxygen therapy is covered by Medicare and other third-party payors. Medicare has specific guidelines for reimbursement of oxygen therapy in the home e.g. serious reduction in PaO$_2$ during sleep or following exercise.

Three types of oxygen are available for home use: compressed oxygen, liquid oxygen and oxygen concentrators. Liquid oxygen systems have smaller portable units that are filled from a larger stationary unit in the home. When at home, the client uses the stationary unit. The reservoir unit is refilled weekly or more often depending on the client's use. Liquid oxygen is the most portable and the most expensive. Table 40-1 lists the length of time a liquid oxygen system will last depending on the liter flow. Oxygen concentrators are moderate-sized units that extract oxygen from the room air, concentrate it, and deliver the prescribed liter flow to the client. Oxygen concentrators (Figure 40-2) are the most economical but do not provide portability. Clients with an oxygen concentrator usually have small E cylinder tanks available for trips outside the home (Figure 40-3). Compressed oxygen is usually available in large H cylinders and in the small E cylinder tanks on carts, which are easily pulled along as the client walks. The large H cylinder tank will last approximately 50 hours at 2 L/min.

The type of oxygen delivery is based on a thorough assessment of the client's needs. Criteria for determining the right oxygen delivery for the client include the client's activity level, the amount of oxygen prescribed for the client, the client's physical ability, the availability of assistance for activities such as refilling a liquid tank, and where the client lives. A client who is very mobile and active would benefit from a liquid oxygen system to encourage continuation of activities. A client who is homebound is best served with an oxygen concentrator and smaller E cylinder for infrequent trips outside the home. The nurse, physician, client, and home health company can determine the right system to meet a client's needs.

Box 40-1 Oxygen Safety Guidelines

- Oxygen is a medication and should not be adjusted without a physician's order.
- No smoking should be allowed in the client's room.
- A "No Smoking" sign is placed in a spot visible to visitors.
- Oxygen delivery systems must be kept 10 feet from any open flames.
- Oxygen supports combustion; however, it will not explode.
- When oxygen cylinders are used, they must be secured so that they will not fall over. Oxygen cylinders are stored upright and chained or in appropriate holders.

Table 40-1

Liquid Oxygen Timetable (in Hours)

L/min	Stationary Reservoirs		Portable Units	
	17,000 L	25,000 L	800 L	1000 L
1	248	396	7	14
2	124	198	3	7
3	83	134	2	4½
4	61	99	1½	3½
5	40	80	–	–
6	–	–	1	2

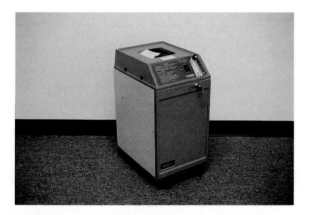

Figure 40-2   Oxygen concentrator.   *From Sorrentino SA: Assisting with patient care, St Louis, 1999, Mosby.*

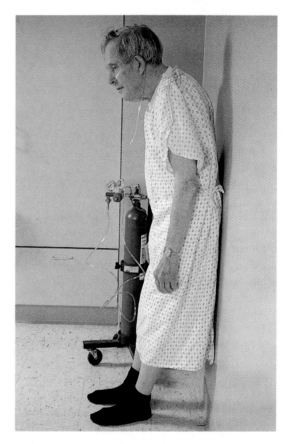

Figure 40-3   Portable compressed oxygen.

The client receiving home oxygen usually has the oxygen delivered via nasal cannula. More recently, oxygen is administered through a reservoir nasal cannula, which stores oxygen in a chamber during the expiratory phase of respirations (Rice, 1996), or through a Venturi mask. Transtracheal oxygen is delivered directly into the trachea via a catheter (Figure 40-4, p. 938). A T tube with reservoir or tracheostomy collar is used for clients with a permanent tracheostomy.

Nasal cannulas are changed weekly and cleaned with mild soap and water. Face masks, T tubes, and tracheostomy collars are cleaned daily with mild soap and water and allowed to air dry. Clients should have more than one delivery device so they can clean one and hang it to air dry while using the other.

This skill involves setting up and administering oxygen therapy to the client requiring oxygen administration in the home.

Equipment

Oxygen delivery device   Oxygen source
  Nasal cannula   Oxygen cylinders
  Simple mask   Liquid system
  Tracheostomy collar   Concentrator
Oxygen tubing

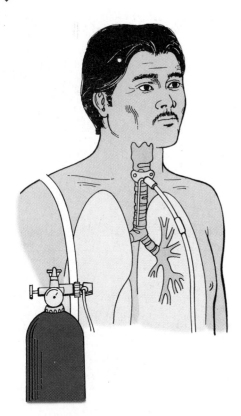

Figure 40-4 Transtracheal oxygen delivery via a catheter placed directly into the trachea.

ASSESSMENT

1. Assess client's and family's ability to apply and manipulate oxygen equipment while in the hospital or in the home. **Rationale: Physical or mental impairment may indicate a need for assistance in the home.**

2. Assess client's and family's ability to determine the signs and symptoms of hypoxia. **Rationale: Hypoxia can occur at home when client uses oxygen and can be caused by worsening of the client's physical problem or an underlying change in respiratory status.**

3. Assess the availability of community resources for home oxygen therapy. **Rationale: Ensures repair service and purchasing service availability.**

4. Determine appropriate backup system, if compressor is used, in event of power failure.

PLANNING

Expected outcomes focus on correct and safe use of the home oxygen equipment.

Expected Outcomes

1. Client receives oxygen at prescribed rate.
2. Client and family verbalize the purpose and correct use of home oxygen by discharge.
3. Client and family demonstrate how to set up the oxygen system.
4. Client and family are able to verbalize safety guidelines for oxygen use.
5. Client and family are able to verbalize emergency plan of care.

DELEGATION CONSIDERATIONS

This skill requires problem solving and knowledge application unique to the professional nurse. The nurse assumes accountability for appropriate assessment and implementation of home oxygen therapy by the client or appropriate caregiver after the teaching has occurred.

IMPLEMENTATION

Steps	Rationale
1. See Standard Protocol (inside front cover).	
2. Place oxygen system in a clutter-free environment.	Keeps the device balanced and prevents injury from bumping against objects
3. Check oxygen level remaining.	Ensures adequate oxygen supply.
a. Check liquid system by depressing button at lower right corner and reading the dial on the Liberator or Stroller (see illustration).	
b. Check cylinders by reading amount on pressure gauge.	
4. Connect oxygen delivery device (e.g., nasal cannula) to oxygen system.	

Steps	Rationale

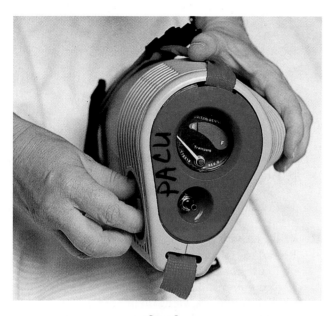

Step 3a

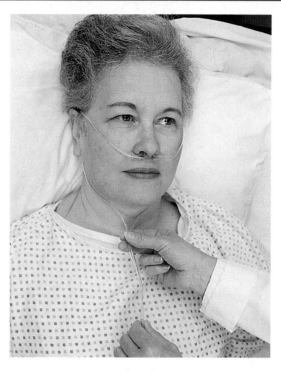

Step 6

5. Determine and set correct liter flow rate.
   Ensures delivery of prescribed amount of oxygen.
6. Place oxygen delivery device on client (see illustration).
7. When client is leaving the home and needs portability, the following steps are needed to prepare the portable units:

Liquid system
   a. Refill Stroller by turning bayonet coupling lock on Stroller 45 degrees.
   b. Insert female adaptor on Stroller onto male adaptor on Liberator.
   c. Refill Stroller until indicator reaches full.
   d. Disconnect from Liberator.
   e. Return bayonet coupling lock to original position.
   f. Set prescribed flow rate and lock flow meter.

   g. Connect appropriate oxygen delivery device and oxygen tubing to Stroller.
   h. Place Stroller on cart.

E tank oxygen source
   a. Place unused E tank in portable carrier.
   b. Turn valve at top of tank on for 1 second.
   c. Attach regulator to E tank.
   d. Using oxygen key, open E tank.

NURSE ALERT

Equipment vendor and nurse should instruct client how frequently Liberator and Stroller must be filled. Small Liberator (Sprint) has 4-hour capacity, whereas 9½-lb Stroller has 8-hour capacity. Refilling occurs automatically and takes a few seconds to a minute, depending on amounts of oxygen required to fill Stroller.

Allows secure connection to prevent leakage of liquid oxygen into the room.

Ensures delivery of prescribed amount of oxygen and prevents client from changing oxygen flow rate.

Removes dust particles and metal filings from fittings.

Steps	Rationale

    e. Determine level of oxygen in tank by reading gauge on regulator.

    f. Set prescribed flow rate.

    g. Connect appropriate oxygen delivery device and oxygen tubing to E tank.

8. See Completion Protocol (inside front cover).

• • •

EVALUATION

1. Observe client's respiratory pattern and breathlessness to determine if client is receiving oxygen as prescribed.
2. Ask client and family to describe reasons for and correct setup for home oxygen use.
3. Observe client and family use of home oxygen system to determine ability to set up equipment correctly.
4. Ask client and family to describe safety and emergency guidelines for home oxygen use.
5. Ask client/family to describe emergency plan.

Unexpected Outcomes and Related Interventions

1. Client develops signs and symptoms associated with hypoxemia.
   a. Determine if oxygen delivery device and source are delivering oxygen properly.
   b. Determine if prescribed oxygen flow rate is set correctly.
   c. Assess client for change in respiratory status, such as airway plugging, respiratory infection, or bronchospasm.
2. Client uses unsafe practices with oxygen therapy, such as using oxygen near fire or cigarette smoking or setting incorrect flow rate.
   a. Discuss with client risks created through unsafe behavior.
   b. Attempt to identify reason client is unable to use oxygen correctly (e.g., health beliefs, incorrect information).

Recording and Reporting

- Record teaching plan for instructing client and family to use home oxygen on nursing care plan.
- Record information given to client and family and any validation of learning on progress notes.
- Communicate client's or family's learning progress to other health care providers involved.

Sample Documentation

1600   Client and family able to return demonstrate appropriate use of liquid oxygen system, including refilling Stroller and monitoring oxygen level. Correctly stated signs and symptoms of hypoxemia and safety precautions for home oxygen use.

Home Care and Long-Term Care Considerations

- Oxygen desaturation and decreased oxygen delivery to the brain can impair the client's ability to remember previous learning. Thus, written or pictorial instructions should be provided for the home setting.
- Some clients are able to manage portable oxygen system but are unable to fill portable system.
- Assess the home for availability of a three-pronged outlet for the compressor to prevent electric shock.
- Equipment must be kept out of reach of children in the home, because manipulation of dials or flow meters could have disastrous effects on the oxygen-delivery process.

Geriatric Considerations

- Older adults have less efficient respiratory systems and less surface area for gas exchange, so their response to decreased oxygen and infection may cause cerebral anoxia and lead to confusion. They may be unable to recognize respiratory problems or problems with the delivery system; therefore, they must have frequent contact with a designated caregiver.
- Older adults are prone to skin breakdown; therefore it is important to keep skin dry under the mask, and wash with mild soap and water.

Skill 40.6

TEACHING HOME TRACHEOSTOMY CARE

The indications and procedure for performing tracheostomy care and suctioning in the home are similar to the care in the hospital except for the use of principles of medical asepsis or clean technique rather than surgical asepsis. In the hospital, principles of surgical asepsis are used because the client is more susceptible to infection from the pathogenic microorganisms present. In the home setting the risk to the client is greatly reduced, and clean technique provides safe care for most clients.

Immunocompromised clients, clients with active infections, and clients living in unclean home environments are not appropriate candidates for clean technique. In these instances, surgical asepsis is indicated to reduce the client's risk of infection.

Home tracheostomy care actually begins in the hospital as the nurse teaches the client and family how to care for the tracheostomy. The client usually learns more easily when less invasive techniques such as stoma care precede more invasive techniques such as inner cannula care and suctioning.

Suctioning is done when the client feels resistance in the airways or coughs up mucus that cannot be expectorated. The client and family are taught how to assess for the need to suction based on the client's need to clear the airways. Tracheostomy care is performed at least daily but may be necessary as often as every 4 hours for clients with copious secretions. Hydration helps keep secretions thin and makes them easier to cough up and expectorate or suction.

This skill involves use of clean technique for suctioning and cleaning the tracheostomy tube in the home care setting. Care must be taken to provide safe and effective airway care with minimal disruption of the client's breathing pattern.

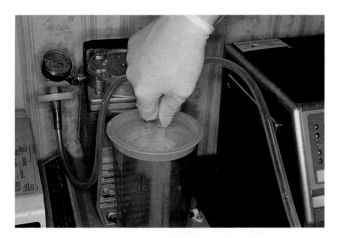

Figure 40-5

Equipment

Suction machine with connecting tube (Figure 40-5)
Nonsterile gloves
3 small basins
Hydrogen peroxide, water (boiled preferred over tap)
Normal saline
Clean 4 × 4 gauze pads (nonshredding)
Appropriate size of sterile or clean and disinfected catheter (diameter should be no greater than half the diameter of the tracheostomy tube)
Tracheostomy care kit *or*
   Clean 4 × 4 gauze pads (nonshredding)
   Water-soluble lubricant
   Small nylon bottle brush or pipe cleaners
   Cotton-tipped applicators
   Trach ties (twill 3/8-inch preferably)
Mirror
Wet washcloth or paper towel
Dry cloth, towel, or paper towel
Protective eyewear (optional)
Trash bag (plastic, nonleaking preferred)
Disposable apron (optional)

ASSESSMENT

1. Assess client's and family's ability to perform tracheostomy care and suctioning properly while in the hospital. **Rationale: Physical and cognitive impairment or an emergency may necessitate a family member or significant other performing tracheostomy care or suctioning.**

2. Assess client's and family's knowledge and ability to observe for signs and symptoms of need to perform suctioning and tracheostomy care. Prompt response to airway obstruction is necessary.

3. Observe client and family member performing complete tracheostomy tube care and suctioning. **Rationale: Allows nurse to determine which specific components of skill client and family member can easily complete and which are more difficult.**

PLANNING

Expected outcomes focus on client learning correct assessment of need for suctioning, proper suction procedure, and proper tracheostomy care.

Expected Outcomes

1. Client/family identifies signs and symptoms indicating need for tracheostomy care and suctioning.

2. Client/family can identify signs and symptoms of stoma inflammation, respiratory tract infection, and when to notify physician.
3. Lower and upper airways are free of secretions.
4. Stoma site is clean and free of infection.

5. Inner cannula of tracheostomy tube and dressings are free of secretions.
6. Client/family demonstrates clean technique for tracheostomy care and suctioning.

IMPLEMENTATION

Steps	Rationale

1. See Standard Protocol (inside front cover).
2. Instruct client on signs and symptoms indicating need for suctioning (e.g. difficulty breathing, productive cough, sensed airway congestion) and tracheostomy care (e.g. build up of secretions on faceplate, soiled dressing and tie).

3. ![] **Tracheostomy suctioning**

COMMUNICATION TIP

While preparing client, explain: "Suctioning will help to clear your secretions and make you more comfortable. Try to cough deeply. Take two to three deep breaths after I suction you and replace your oxygen."

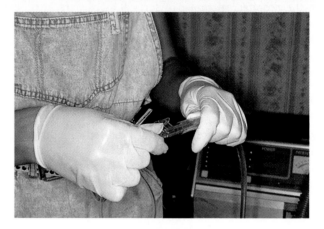

Step 3c

    a. Have client sit in chair or sit up in bed.
    b. Fill basin with ½ cup water or normal saline.
    c. Connect suction catheter to suction apparatus and check that equipment is functioning (see illustration).
    d. Remove oxygen or humidity source from client.
    e. Insert catheter 6 to 8 inches (15 to 20 cm) without applying suction. If resistance is met, pull back catheter ½ inch (1 cm) (see illustration).
    f. Apply intermittent suction, for 5 to 10 seconds, by placing and releasing thumb over catheter vent and slowly withdrawing catheter while rotating it between thumb and forefinger. Explain that catheter will cause client to cough.

Provides easier access to airway.

NURSE ALERT

Before continuing suction, allow client to rest and encourage to take two to three deep breaths to reduce oxygen loss and prevent hypoxia.

Intermittent suction and rotation of catheter prevent injury to tracheal mucosal lining.

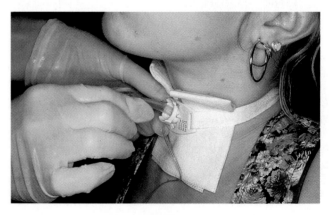

Step 3e

Steps	Rationale

g. Reapply oxygen or humidity source.

h. Repeat Steps e through g as needed to remove secretions.

i. Suction nasal and oral pharynx if needed.

NURSE ALERT

Do not reinsert catheter into trachea after oral or nasal suction.

j. After suctioning is completed, rinse catheter with water in basin until clean.

Removes secretions from catheter and reduces transmission of microorganisms.

k. Disconnect suction catheter and coil around gloved hand.

(1) If catheter is to be cleaned and disinfected, set aside.

(2) If catheter needs to be discarded, pull glove over coiled catheter and discard.

NURSE ALERT

With pediatric clients, many physicians order the client to receive 10% to 15% higher oxygen before tracheostomy tube changes.

4. **Tracheostomy care**

a. To clean inner cannula, place impervious trash bag near work site and create a clean field for equipment; place the three basins on the field.

Ensures maintenance of standard precautions.

b. Pour hydrogen peroxide in one container and water or normal saline in second container. Pour hydrogen peroxide or normal saline in third container with 4 × 4 gauze pads.

c. Remove old tracheostomy bib or dressing and discard using standard precautions.

Reduces transmission of microorganisms.

d. Remove and discard contaminated gloves.

e. Put on clean gloves.

Reduces transmission of microorganisms.

f. Using presoaked 4 × 4 gauze sponges and damp applicators, gently wash skin around stoma, under trach ties and flanges (see illustration).

Removes secretions that predispose client to localized infection.

g. Dry exposed outer cannula and skin with dry tracheostomy gauze/towel.

Prevents moist environment for organism growth.

h. Unlock safety lock and remove inner cannula of tracheostomy tube by pulling it out following the curve of the tube (see illustration) and place in hydrogen peroxide solution to soak.

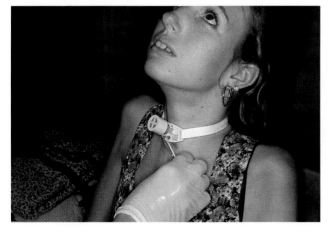

Step 4f

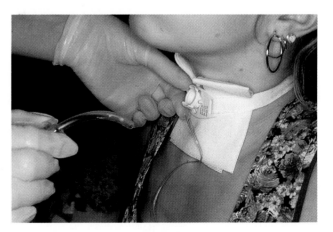

Step 4h

Steps	Rationale

i. Using nylon brush or pipe cleaners, gently scrub inner cannula.

j. Rinse inner cannula with water or NS for at least 15 seconds.

Removes remaining hydrogen peroxide from inner cannula that could cause airway or stoma irritation.

k. Replace inner cannula and lock into position.

l. Change tracheostomy ties. Have client hold face plate of tracheostomy tube while removing old ties and applying new ones (see illustration). Secure ties in a knot along the side of client's neck, but be sure that one finger can fit under the ties so they are not too tight.

m. Gently slip edge of clean gauze under tie and around one side of tracheostomy tube. Repeat for other side (see illustration).

n. Clean reusable supplies in warm soapy water. Rinse thoroughly and air dry.

o. Store clean, dry supplies in loosely closed plastic bag.

p. Place "button" on tracheostomy to facilitate speech (see illustration).

q. Remove and discard gloves.

NURSE ALERT

Client is at risk for tube coming out as ties are changed. Another tube may be needed, including a stylet for insertion.

Air must circulate, or humidity in bag can promote growth of microorganisms.

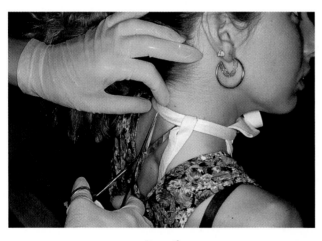

Step 4l

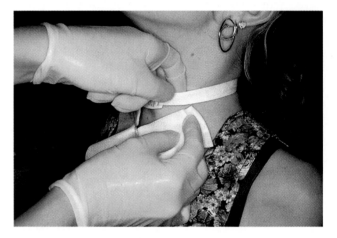

Step 4m

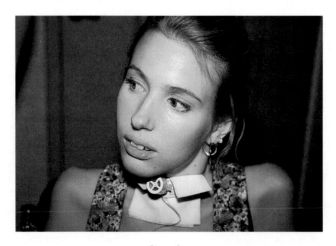

Step 4p

Steps	Rationale

5. **Disinfecting supplies**
   a. Reusable supplies should be disinfected at least weekly by one of the following methods:
   Method 1
   (1) Boil reusable supplies for 15 minutes.
   (2) Allow to cool, air dry, and store.
   Method 2
   (1) Soak reusable supplies in equal parts of vinegar and water for 30 minutes.
   (2) Remove and rinse thoroughly.
   (3) Air dry and store.
   Method 3
   (1) Soak reusable supplies in prepared disinfectant solution (quaternary ammonium chloride compounds) according to manufacturer's recommendations.
   (2) Rinse thoroughly.
   (3) Air dry and store.

Rationale: Home environment is less likely to have pathogens to which the client is susceptible; therefore sterilization is not necessary.

   b. Discuss signs and symptoms of stomal infection (redness, tenderness, drainage) and respiratory tract infection (fever, increased sputum, sputum color change, foul sputum odor, increased cough, chills, night sweats).

Rationale: Client must be able to recognize onset of inflammation or infections.

6. See Completion Protocol (inside front cover).

• • •

EVALUATION

1. Ask client to list signs and symptoms that indicate the need for suctioning, including difficulty breathing and continued coughing of secretions.
2. Observe for signs of stomal or respiratory tract infections.
3. Inspect tracheostomy tube and dressings for secretions or crusting.
4. Ask client to demonstrate technique for tracheostomy care and suctioning.

Unexpected Outcomes and Related Interventions

1. Client develops reddened or hard stoma site with or without drainage.
   a. Report finding to physician.
   b. Monitor for fever, malaise, or sputum color changes.
2. Client has copious colored secretions around stoma site or when suctioned.
   a. Notify physician.
   b. Increase suction frequency.
   c. Increase fluid intake to thin secretions.

3. Client is unable to perform skill.
   a. Review procedures with client and family.
   b. Assess need for home health nurse or aide to assist with care.
4. Tracheostomy tube comes out.
   a. Instruct client to remain calm and breathe slowly.
   b. Replace tube with new, clean tube, using stylet. Remove stylet and replace with inner cannula.
   c. Lock inner cannula into place.
   d. If unable to replace, notify physician immediately and support respirations as necessary.
5. Skin breakdown is present at stoma site.
   a. Clean around stoma site more frequently, and make sure area is kept clean and dry.
   b. Change tracheostomy dressing and ties when they become moist.

Recording and Reporting

• Record in client record the teaching done and accuracy of care delivered by client or family member.
• Develop a system of recording to be used by the client/caregiver to provide information that compliance is achieved or maintained.

Sample Documentation

0800 Client able to suction adequately and performs tracheostomy care without difficulty. Secretions are white and thin. Stoma site is clean and dry without redness or evidence of infection.

Geriatric Considerations

- Loss of upper airway functions with tracheostomy can predispose client to greater secretions. Older adults have lost some properties of elastic recoil and gas exchange.
- Manual dexterity may be limited because of arthritic changes of the upper extremities.
- Skin integrity may be compromised and at risk for breakdown from secretions and/or tape.

Home Care and Long-Term Care Considerations

- Suctioning should be performed at least daily in the home setting and more frequently as needed if secretions are copious. Secretions are likely to be greater in the morning when the client awakes.
- Most clients benefit from a room humidifier.
- Clients with impaired or absent cough or gag reflex, decreased level of consciousness, neuromuscular diseases, pneumonia, chronic obstructive pulmonary disease, congestive heart failure, and pulmonary edema are at great risk. Families of tracheostomy clients must learn how to obtain emergency assistance within their community.

REFERENCES

American Diabetes Association: Position statement: implications of the diabetes control and complications trial, *Diabetes Spectrum* 6(4):225, 1993.

American Diabetes Association: 1998 Buyer's guide to diabetes products, *Diabetes Forecast* 50(10):68–71, 1997.

American Diabetes Association: Clinical practice recommendations, *Diabetes Care* 21(51):51, 1998.

Beare P, Myers J: *Principles and practices of adult health nursing,* ed 2, St Louis, 1994, Mosby.

Becker MH, editor: *The health belief model and personal health behavior,* Thorofare, NJ, 1974, Charles B Slack.

Champion VL: Instrument development for health belief model constructs, *Adv Nurs Sci* 7:73–85, 1984.

Ebersole P, Hess P: *Toward healthy aging: human needs and nursing response,* ed 4, St Louis, 1994, Mosby.

Esposito L: The effects of medication education on adherence to medication regimens in an elderly population, 21:935, 1995.

Grimby G et al: Training can improve muscle strength and endurance in 78- to 84-year-old men, *J Appl Physiol* 73(6):2517, 1992.

Haas M: The long way to self-catheterization with a zip, *Urol Nurs* 17(1):35, 1997.

Haire-Joshu D: *Management of diabetes mellitus: perspectives across the life span,* ed 2, St Louis, 1996, Mosby.

Kim M, McFarland G, McLane A: *Pocket guide to nursing diagnoses,* ed 7, St Louis, 1997, Mosby.

Kravitz R et al: Geriatric home assessment after hospital discharge, *J Am Geriatr Soc* 42(12):1232, 1994.

Lueckenotte A: *Gerontologic nursing,* St Louis, 1996, Mosby.

Occupational Safety and Health Administration (OSHA): *Occupational Safety and Health Act: blood-borne pathogens, Fed Register* 56(235):64, 1991.

Rice R: *Home health nursing practice,* ed 2, St Louis, 1996, Mosby.

Sorrentino SA: *Assisting with patient care,* St Louis, 1999, Mosby.

Wilson F: Patient education materials nurses use in community health, *West J Nurs Res* 18(2):204, 1996.

CRITICAL THINKING EXERCISES

1. You are a home health nurse who has been assigned to care for Mr. and Mrs. Reynolds. Mr. Reynolds is recuperating from left hip replacement surgery and needs the assistance of a walker to ambulate. Mrs. Reynolds is scheduled to have cataract surgery in the next month. They live alone in a two-bedroom, one-bathroom home that has no stairs. Your first visit to the home reveals numerous sidewalk cracks on the walkway to the home. The doorbell does not work, and there is not a working porch light. The kitchen cabinets are low, and the counters are cluttered with mail and newspapers. The bathroom has a tub with a grab bar and a loose bath mat. There are several area rugs scattered throughout the home. Other than a neighbor who checks on them weekly, the couple has no other family or significant others. From this case study, what safety hazards do Mr. and Mrs. Reynolds need to be made aware of, and what other areas should you investigate?

2. You observe Mrs. Shaw (age 72) preparing and administering her insulin. She is to take NPH 20 units in the morning before breakfast. Describe what parameters you would assess to be certain that she can perform the procedure independently and accurately.

3. You have been instructed to teach Mandy how to perform sterile self-catheterization. Previously, Mandy was allowed to do clean catheterization. What conclusion can be drawn about the need to teach Mandy the new procedure?

APPENDIXES

Appendix A
Sample Forms

Appendix B
Abbreviations and Equivalents

Appendix C
Nursing Diagnoses (1999-2000 NANDA) Classification of Nursing Diagnoses by Functional Health Patterns

Appendix D
Norms for Common Laboratory Tests

Appendix E
Height and Weight Tables

APPENDIX A

Sample Forms

Admission Patient Profiles, 949

Diabetic Management Record, 954

Patient/Visitor Incident Report, 955

Routine Nursing Assessment, 956

Vital Signs, 958

Critical Care Path, 959

ST. JOHN'S HOSPITAL
Springfield, Illinois

ADMISSION PATIENT PROFILE

*Asterisk markings identify those areas that have more detailed assessment forms that may be appropriate for this patient.

HEALTH PATTERNS ASSESSMENT (May be completed by RN or LPN)

Information Obtained From: ☐ Patient   ☐ Family   ☐ Friend   ☐ Old Chart   ☐ Transfer Sheet   ☐ ER Record

Reason for Admission (as stated by patient): _____

_____

Previous Surgery(ies)/Hospitalizations: _____

_____

_____

Previous Transfusion(s)?   ☐ No   ☐ Yes   Date _____

Known Food, Drug, Contact Allergies   ☐ None   *If yes, list and state reaction:* _____

_____

_____

_____

Latex Allergy: ☐ No   ☐ Yes   *(describe)* _____

MEDICATIONS: Patient is currently taking (include over-the-counter medications)				
Name	**Dose**	**Dosing Time**	**Day/Time of Last Dose**	**Brought to Hospital**
				☐ No ☐ Yes Disposition:
				☐ No ☐ Yes Disposition:
				☐ No ☐ Yes Disposition:
				☐ No ☐ Yes Disposition:
				☐ No ☐ Yes Disposition:
				☐ No ☐ Yes Disposition:
				☐ No ☐ Yes Disposition:
				☐ No ☐ Yes Disposition:
				☐ No ☐ Yes Disposition:
				☐ No ☐ Yes Disposition:
				☐ No ☐ Yes Disposition:
				☐ No ☐ Yes Disposition:
				☐ No ☐ Yes Disposition:
				☐ No ☐ Yes Disposition:

#4678   (R 04/95)
(1 OF 5)

ADMISSION PATIENT PROFILE

(Courtesy St. John's Hospital, Springfield, Ill.)

SYSTEMS ASSESSMENT (May be completed by RN or LPN)

NEURO/SENSORY

Additional Comments   **Nursing Diagnosis Cues**

☐ CVA ☐ Side affected: ☐ Rt ☐ Lt   ☐ Head injury _____

☐ Headache _____   ☐ Hx of Seizures _____   ☐ Stiff Neck

☐ Alert ☐ Oriented ☐ Confused ☐ Comatose ☐ Cooperative ☐ Withdrawn

☐ Anxious ☐ Hearing Difficulty ☐ P.E.R.L. ☐ Unsteady Gait

☐ Vision Difficulty Cataracts: ☐ Rt ☐ Lt Blind: ☐ Rt ☐ Lt Glaucoma: ☐ Rt ☐ Lt

☐ Syncope _____   ☐ Speech impairment (describe)

*Pain/Discomfort   ☐ Yes ☐ No   Describe _____

　　How is pain controlled? _____

☐ All above areas addressed

Sensory/Perceptual Alterations

Impaired Communication

Altered Thought Processes

Potential for Injury

Pain

Pain, chronic

PERFUSION

Additional Comments   **Nursing Diagnosis Cues**

☐ Congenital Heart defects (describe) _____ ☐ CHF ☐ Anemia

☐ Heart Attack _____ ☐ Hypertension ☐ Perpheral Vascular Disease

☐ Pacemaker   Check pt. I.D. Card for Model # _____ Manufacturer _____

☐ Automatic Implantable Cardioverter Defibrillator (AICD) Model # _____ Manufacturer _____

☐ Angina (describe) _____

☐ Stent (describe) _____   Apical Pulse: ☐ Reg. ☐ Irreg.

KEY:　P = Pulse Present by Palpation　　Pulses:　Radial 　___ Rt. ___ Lt.

　　　D = Pulse Audible with Doppler　　　　Posterior Tibial 　___ Rt. ___ Lt.

　　　A = Absent　　　　　　　　　　　　　Pedal 　___ Rt. ___ Lt.

☐ All above areas addressed

Decreased Cardiac Output

Fluid Volume Deficit

Fluid Volume Excess

Altered Tissue Perfusion

Pain

OXYGENATION

Additional Comments   **Nursing Diagnosis Cues**

Respiration history: ☐ Asthma ☐ COPD ☐ Pneumonia ☐ TB ☐ Other _____

Smoking History: Do you smoke? ☐ Yes ☐ No Packs/day: ___ # of years ___

Have you ever smoked? ☐ Yes ☐ No Packs/day: ___ # of years ___

When did you quit? _____

Oxygen Therapy/Resp. Therapy used at home? ☐ Yes ☐ No Describe: _____

Breathing: ☐ Deep and regular ☐ Shallow ☐ Irregular ☐ SOB (describe) _____

Breath Sounds: ☐ Clear bilaterally ☐ Abnormal (describe) _____

Describe Cough: _____   Describe Sputum: _____

☐ All above areas addressed

Impaired Gas Exchange

Ineffective Airway Clearance

Ineffective Breathing Pattern

Activity Intolerance

*SKIN CONDITION

Additional Comments   **Nursing Diagnosis Cues**

Indicate locations of any of the following by number:

1. Abrasion   5. Bruise
2. Burn   6. Laceration
3. Contusion   7. Rash
4. Decubitis   8. Scars
　　　　　　　　9. Sutures

Skin color _____

Skin temperature _____

Skin moisture _____

☐ Edema _____

☐ All above areas addressed

Impaired Skin Integrity

Altered Oral Mucous Membrane

MUSCULO-SKELETAL/PHYSICAL MOBILITY

Additional Comments   **Nursing Diagnosis Cues**

☐ Arthritis ☐ Gout ☐ Fracture _____ ☐ Deformity noted (describe)

☐ Contractures: ☐ Rt. Arm ☐ Lt. Arm ☐ Rt. Leg ☐ Lt. Leg

☐ Previous limitations in mobility (specify)* _____

☐ Wheelchair**   ☐ Bed Bound**

☐ History of falls (indicate frequency and reason) _____

Gait: ☐ Steady ☐ Unsteady ☐ Independent ☐ Needs ___ # of persons assist

Ambulatory devices: ☐ Cane ☐ Crutches ☐ Walker ☐ Other _____

☐ Assistance needed with bathing   ☐ Assistance needed with dressing

☐ Amputations _____   ☐ Prosthesis _____

*☐ Pain Location _____   Describe _____

☐ All above areas addressed

Activity Intolerance

Self-care Deficit

Impaired Physical Mobility

Potential for Injury

Pain

** (NOTE: IF patient in wheelchair or bed bound complete "Pressure Ulcer Therapy" form)

ST. JOHN'S HOSPITAL
Springfield, Illinois

ADMISSION PATIENT PROFILE

SYSTEMS ASSESSMENT (continued)   (May be completed by RN or LPN)

IMMUNE FUNCTION

	Additional Comments	Nursing Diagnosis Cues
☐ Fever in last 48° ☐ Transplant history _____	_____	Potential for Infection
☐ Radiation therapy (date) _____ ☐ Chemotherapy (date)_____	_____	
☐ Venous access device _____ Site:_____	_____	
☐ Central Catheter_____ Site:_____	_____	
Malignancy history_____	_____	
☐ All above areas addressed	_____	

NUTRITIONAL/METABOLIC

	Additional Comments	Nursing Diagnosis Cues
☐ Home Diet _____ ☐ Assistance with eating needed (describe) _____	_____	Altered Nutrition
☐ Recent Weight Changes ☐ Increase ☐ Decrease (reason)_____	_____	Noncompliance
Time Frame _____ Amount _____ ☐ Intentional ☐ Unintentional	_____	
☐ Nausea and vomiting ☐ Heartburn ☐ *Abdominal pain (describe)_____	_____	Self-Care Deficit, Feeding
☐ Diabetes: ☐ Insulin Dependent ☐ Diet Controlled ☐ Oral Meds_____	_____	Pain
☐ Thyroid problems ☐ Hepatitis ☐ Alcohol use (Avg. number drinks/week)_____	_____	
☐ All above areas are addressed.	_____	

ELIMINATION

	Additional Comments	Nursing Diagnosis Cues
BOWEL: ☐ GI Bleed ☐ Colitis ☐ Diverticulitis ☐ Hemorrhoids Date of last BM_____	_____	Constipation
Bowel pattern (describe)_____ ☐ Stool changes (describe)_____	_____	Diarrhea
☐ Constipation ☐ Diarrhea Frequency_____ x/day ☐ Involuntary	_____	
Bowel Sounds: ☐ Present ☐ Absent ☐ Abdominal Distention	_____	Bowel Incontinence
URINE: ☐ Burning ☐ Hematuria ☐ Urgency ☐ Retention ☐ Renal disease	_____	Urinary Incontinence
☐ Dysuria ☐ Incontinence (describe)_____	_____	Urinary Retention
☐ Nocturia (_____ x/night) ☐ Stream initiation difficulty	_____	Altered Patterns of Urinary
☐ Foley in place Date inserted/changed _____	_____	Elimination
☐ Stent	_____	
☐ All above areas addressed.	_____	

REPRODUCTIVE

	Additional Comments	Nursing Diagnosis Cues
MALE: ☐ Prostate Problem (describe)_____	_____	Sexual Dysfunction
☐ History of Sexually Transmitted Disease:_____	_____	Body Image Disturbance
FEMALE: ☐ Menstrual changes/problems (describe)_____	_____	
☐ History of Sexually Transmitted Disease:_____	_____	
☐ Breast changes/problems (describe)_____	_____	
☐ LMP_____ ☐ Pregnant_____ — EDD _____	_____	
For female over age 20, date of last pap smear:_____	_____	
☐ All above areas addressed	_____	

ADMISSION PATIENT PROFILE

SYSTEMS ASSESSMENT (continued)   (May be completed by RN or LPN)

PSYCHO-SOCIAL/SPIRITUAL/CULTURAL	Additional Comments	Nursing Diagnosis Cues
☐ Lives with spouse ☐ Lives alone ☐ Lives with family	_____	Ineffective Coping
☐ Lives with friend ☐ Nursing Home ☐ Other _____	_____	
Do you plan to return to the same living arrangement? ☐ No ☐ Yes	_____	Altered Family Process
Do you have close family members or significant others that are supportive to you if you	_____	Altered Health Maintenance
need help? ☐ No ☐ Yes Name _____	_____	
Relationship _____	_____	Spiritual Distress
☐ Are you the primary caregiver for someone at home? ☐ No ☐ Yes		

Do you have special religious/spiritual requests during this hospitalization?   ☐ No ☐ Yes
Describe _____
_____
_____
_____
_____

What concerns you most about your hospitalization?
Describe _____
_____
_____
_____
_____

What concerns you most about your illness?
Describe _____
_____
_____
_____
_____

From an ethnic or cultural perspective, please describe any special habits, customs, beliefs or values that we
need to honor while you are a patient at St. John's Hospital. (For Example: Special food/dietary needs that
are based on your religion/culture.)
Describe _____
_____
_____
_____
_____

Signature of Data Collector: _____   Date: _____   Time: _____

ST. JOHN'S HOSPITAL
Springfield, Illinois

ADMISSION PATIENT PROFILE

ADVANCED DIRECTIVES

1. Do you want further information regarding advanced directives?   ☐ Yes   ☐ No
    - Patient received a copy of the patient handbook and was shown the advanced directive brochure.   ☐ Yes   ☐ No
      If no, (explain) _____

    - Notify Social Service as needed.   ☐ Yes   ☐ No
      If no, (explain) _____

2. If completed, do we have your current copy?
    ☐ Yes *(Nursing: Place in patient's chart and mark the front of the chart.)*
    ☐ Yes, placed in my record at a previous admission.
       (Nursing: Obtain copy from Medical Records and place copy in patient's current chart and mark the front of the chart.)
    ☐ No, Please advise patient to bring a copy to the hospital.
       (Nursing: Make a reminder note on the Patient Care Summary to follow-up.)

INITIAL TEACHING/DISCHARGE PLANNING / REFERRALS (*MUST* be completed by RN)

1. Patient/family teaching needs identified at this time:
    ☐ Medication _____   ☐ Pre-op _____   ☐ Other (specify) _____
    ☐ Dietary _____   ☐ Pre-Procedure _____
    ☐ Wound Care _____   ☐ Diabetic _____
    ☐ Ostomy Care _____   ☐ Pressure Ulcer Prevention _____

2. Does anyone from a community agency visit you at home?   ☐ Yes   ☐ No
    If yes, specify _____

3. Based on this Admission Patient Profile do you anticipate the patient needing any assistance when they are discharged from the hospital?   ☐ No   ☐ Yes
    If yes, specify _____
    _____

4. Screening Referrals to: Date/Time
    ☐ Cardiac Rehabilitation (ext. 4448 - order required)   _____
    ☐ Clinical Dietitian (ext. 4880)   _____
    ☐ Home Health Services (ext. 5641)   _____
    ☐ Oncology Clinical Nurse Specialist (ext. 4547)   _____
    ☐ Oncology Pain Management Service (ext. 4547)   _____
    ☐ Pastoral Care (ext. 4500)   _____
    ☐ Rehabilitation Department (ext. 4800 - order required)   _____
    ☐ Social Worker (ext. 4480)   _____
    ☐ Stoma Nurse (ext. 4035)   _____
    ☐ Other   _____

Signature _____ R.N.   Date _____   Time: _____

*Asterisk markings identify those areas that have "more detailed" assessment forms that may be appropriate for this patient.

ADMISSION PATIENT PROFILE

St. John's
Hospital
Springfield, Illinois

DIABETIC MANAGEMENT RECORD

DATE:	Time									
	Blood Glucose									
	Ketones									
	Medication Dosage									
	Comments									
	Initials									
DATE:	Time									
	Blood Glucose									
	Ketones									
	Medication Dosage									
	Comments									
	Initials									
DATE:	Time									
	Blood Glucose									
	Ketones									
	Medication Dosage									
	Comments									
	Initials									

INITIALS	SIGNATURE	INITIALS	SIGNATURE	INITIALS	SIGNATURE

#700 (R 11/93)

DIABETIC MANAGEMENT RECORD

(Courtesy St. John's Hospital, Springfield, Ill.)

An Affiliate of Hospital Sisters Health System

This report is not a part of a patient's medical record. It is a Risk Management/Quality Improvement Tool.

"An incident is any happening which is not consistent with the routine operation of the hospital or routine care of a particular patient. It may be any situation, condition or event which could adversely affect the patient, visitor or the hospital."

HS HS HS
Hospital Sisters
Health System

Patient / Visitor
Incident Report
C O N F I D E N T I A L

A) If patient, use addressograph; B) If no plate, give name/age/patient # and medical record #; C) If visitor, give name/age/address/phone #.

Procedure:
A. Complete all applicable sections with facts
B. Do not complete shaded areas
C. Route according to hospital directive
D. Retain property and physical evidence involved

Facility/City/State

Incident Number:

Diagnosis

Incident Identification:

I ☐ Inpatient   O ☐ Outpatient   V ☐ Visitor

Type of incident: (check one only)				
AM ☐ Against Medical Advice/Elopement	CN ☐ Consent	IV ☐ Intravascular		
AD ☐ Adverse Reaction	CT ☐ Count	ME ☐ Medication		
BE ☐ Behavioral	DE ☐ Delay	PP ☐ Policy/Procedure		
BN ☐ Burn	EQ ☐ Equipment Related	PR ☐ Property		
CO ☐ Complaint	FL ☐ Fall	TT ☐ Test/Treatment		
	IN ☐ Infection	OT ☐ Other - Explain _____		

Location of incident, be specific (eg., 5 North hallway, Radiology exam room, grounds, etc.):

Date of incident: /   /

Time of incident: ☐ A.M. ☐ P.M.

Describe exactly what happened; why it happened; what causes were; use additional sheet of paper if needed.

_____

_____

_____

_____

_____

_____

_____

_____

_____

☐ Property or equipment involved — describe:

Category:

☐ No apparent injury   If injury, state nature and part of body affected:

Injury:

Patient Factor:

Condition	Activity Orders	Bed Rails (Circle)	Bed Position	Restraints
A ☐ Alert	A ☐ Ambulatory with assistance	1 2 3 4 Raised	A ☐ Up	A ☐ YES
B ☐ Sedated	B ☐ Ambulatory w/o assistance	1 2 3 4 Lowered	B ☐ Down	B ☐ NO
C ☐ Confused	C ☐ Bed rest	**Call button within reach:**	**Floor condition:**	
D ☐ Sleeping	D ☐ _____	A ☐ Yes	A ☐ Wet	
		B ☐ No	B ☐ Dry	

Referred for Treatment:	Was Physician Notified:	☐ A.M.	Physician's Name:
☐ YES ☐ NO ☐ Refused	☐ YES ☐ NO Date: Time:	☐ P.M.	

Was person seen by: ☐ Emergency Dept.

☐ Physician/Name_____   ☐ Other _____

Employee Involved:

Witness (Name/Address/Phone):

Person Completing Report: Date:

Witness (Name/Address/Phone):

Supervisor Signature: Date:

RM-1 9/92

(Courtesy Hospital Sisters Health System, Springfield, Ill.)

ST. JOHN'S HOSPITAL
Springfield, Illinois
ROUTINE NURSING ASSESSMENT
Medical/Surgical

EDEMA: +1 = 0″ - ¼″
         +2 = ¼″ - ½″
         +3 = ½″ - 1″
    ∅ = Negative/No
    √ = observed or positive response
Blank = no assessment at this time
   NN = see nurses notes
   LE = lower extremity
   UE = upper extremity
  OTA = open to air

PU = purulent
SS = serosanguinous
 B = brown
 R = red
 Y = yellow
 G = green
 P = pink
 A = amber
 C = clear
CL = cloudy

Date									
Time									
MENTAL STATUS	Alert								
	Oriented/Disoriented								
	Lethargic								
	Unresponsive								
BEHAVIOR	Agitated								
	Anxious								
	Restless								
MOTOR/SENSORY FUNCTION	Moves all extremities								
	Weakness UE LT / RT								
	LE LT / RT								
	Paralysis UE LT / RT								
	LE LT / RT								
	Numbness/Tingling								
	location								
SKIN/MUCOUS MEMBRANE	Temperature: warm/cool								
	Moisture: dry/moist								
	Skin: pink/pale								
	flushed/cyanotic								
	jaundiced								
	Mucous Membrane: pink/pale								
	flushed cyanotic								
	Edema:								
	location								
CARDIO-VASCULAR	Apical rate: reg./irreg.								
	Dorsalis pedis LT / RT								
	Posterior tibial LT / RT								

#4747 (R 10/91)
(1 of 2)

ROUTINE NURSING ASSESSMENT — Medical/Surgical

(Courtesy St. John's Hospital, Springfield, Ill.)

		Date								
		Time								
RESPIRATORY		Quality: unlabored/labored								
		deep/shallow								
		O₂ Therapy:								
		Sounds: clear LT / RT								
		diminished LT / RT								
		rales (crackles) LT / RT								
		rhonchi LT / RT								
		wheeze LT / RT								
		Cough: productive/nonproductive								
		Sputum: Color								
GASTROINTESTINAL/ ABDOMEN		Nondistended / Distended								
		Sounds: present/absent								
		Firm / Soft								
		Hyperactive / Hypoactive								
		Expelling flatus								
		Nausea								
WOUND		Location (✓ = no redness or edema)								
		#1								
		#2								
		#3								
DRESSING		Location (✓ = clean & dry)								
		#1								
		#2								
		#3								
DRAINAGE		Device and location:	description	description	description	description	description	description	description	description
		#1								
		#2								
		#3								
PAIN		Absent/Present								
		Location:								
		#1								
		#2								
		Severity scale (0-10) #1 / #2								
		Intervention								
PATIENT TEACHING		Description								
		#1								
		#2								
		#3								
		Signature								

#4747   (R 10/91)
(2 of 2)

ST. JOHN'S HOSPITAL
Springfield, Illinois

VITAL SIGNS RECORD

KEY:

V = systolic	• = temperature	RA = right arm
∧ = diastolic	A = axillary	LA = left arm
LY = lying	O = oral	RL = right leg
ST = standing	R = rectal	LL = left leg
SIT = sitting	S = skin	
D = Doppler	P = temperature probe	

Date																						
Time																						
Weight (kg)																						
Temp site																						
B/P site																						

43.0 - 240	
42.5 - 230	
42.0 - 220	
41.5 - 210	
41.0 - 200	
40.5 - 190	
40.0 - 180	
39.5 - 170	
39.0 - 160	
38.5 - 150	
38.0 - 140	
37.5 - 130	
37.0 - 120	
36.5 - 110	
36.0 - 100	
35.5 - 90	
35.0 - 80	
34.5 - 70	
34.0 - 60	
33.5 - 50	
33.0 - 40	

Pulse																						
Respiration																						

#284   (R 09/88)   **VITAL SIGNS RECORD**

(Courtesy St. John's Hospital, Springfield, Ill.)

1

BARNES

CARE PATH®
501
LUNG TRANSPLANT EVALUATION

SERVICE		PHYSICIAN	
PRIMARY NURSE		PRIMARY NURSE	
DC DATE	ADM DATE	DATE OF SURGERY	A-8

Problem Number	PATIENT PROBLEMS / NURSING DIAGNOSES
#1	LACK OF KNOWLEDGE R/T LUNG TRANSPLANT EVALUATION EXPERIENCE
#2	DECREASE IN EXERCISE CAPACITY R/T IMPAIRED OXYGENATION/VENTILATION/DECONDITIONING
#3	POTENTIAL FOR ALTERATION IN COPING R/T SITUATIONAL CRISIS/TRANSITION
#4	POTENTIAL FOR ALTERATION IN FAMILY PROCESSES R/T SITUATIONAL CRISIS/TRANSITION
#5	POTENTIAL FOR ALTERATION IN NUTRITION R/T INAPPROPRIATE INTAKE/DYSPNEA
#6	IMPAIRED GAS EXCHANGE R/T ALVEOLAR-CAPILLARY MEMBRANE CHANGE/ALTERED BLOOD FLOW *IF APPROPRIATE

#	1 - 12	1 - 12	1 - 2, 6 - 8, 12	2, 10, 12	1
	ASSESSMENT / MONITORING	CONSULTS	PROCEDURES / TEST	TREATMENT	ACTIVITY
PRE ADMIT		Transplant office to preschedule following as needed for pt.: 2-D Echo, Quant. V-Q, Resting RVG, PFTs, MRI, Cardiac Cath, Chest CT, Transesophageal echocardiogram			
DAY 1	Braden scale Respiratory status Fall prevention Assess/individualize pt. problem list	Notify consults as per orders. Check with transplant P.A. for additional tests which may be needed. SMA 6 and 12, CBC, CMV, HSV, EBV, Vz titers, HbsAq, HbsAb, HIV, Hep. A, Hep. C titers, T & S, PT, PTT HLA (A,B,C,DR) Typing, incl. cytotoxic screen, u/a - routine & micro, CXR-AP & lat EKG	Apply skin tests 07 } Nursing, Pulm. Rehab., 08 } & H.O. 09 10 11 12 } Psychologist 13 14 } CDL 15 16 } PFTs 17 } Chaplain 18 19 Cardiology Consult 20	Appropriate bed surface for Braden scale O₂ • At rest _____ • Activity _____ CPT x1 x2 x3 x4 by Nursing, Physical Therapy, family Aerosols x1 x2 x3 x4 (Self)	Continue activity as done at home

SIGNATURE	INIT.	SIGNATURE	INIT.	SIGNATURE	INIT.

3100-45 (REV. 10/93)

501

Unn Fig A-6 Portion of critical pathway.   Courtesy Barnes-Jewish Hospital, St. Louis

APPENDIX B
Abbreviations and Equivalents

ABBREVIATIONS AND CONVERSION FROM APOTHECARY TO METRIC

1 grain (gr) = 60 milligram (mg)
15 gr = 1 gram (g, gm)
15 minims = 1 milliter (ml, mL)
1 dram (dr) = 4 ml
1 ounce (oz) = 30 cubic centimeters (cc, ml)

ABBREVIATIONS FOR CONVERSION USING HOUSEHOLD MEASURES

1 drop (gtt) = 1 minim
1 teaspoon (1 tsp) = 5 ml
3 tsp = 1 tablespoon (tbsp)
1 cup = 8 oz
16 oz = 1 pound (lb)

STANDARD EQUIVALENTS, ABBREVIATIONS, AND CONVERSIONS

1000 mg = 1 g
1000 ml = 1 liter (L)
2.2 lb = 1 kilogram (kg) = 1000 g
1 tsp = 5 ml (cc)
1 dr = 4 ml (cc)
mEq: millequivalent
mcg (μg): microgram

SYMBOLS

/	Per
<	Less than
>	More than
≤	Equal to or less than
≥	Equal to or more than
≅	Approximately equal to
+ / −, ±	Plus or minus
♂	Male
♀	Female
1°	Primary; first degree
2°	Secondary; second degree
3°	Tertiary; third degree
↑	Up; increase
↓	Down; decrease
μ	Micron

ABBREVIATIONS RELATED TO TYPES OF INTRAVENOUS (IV) FLUIDS

D5W, D_5W: 5% dextrose and water
NS: normal saline
LR: lactated Ringer's solution
D5NS, D_5NS: 5% dextrose in 0.9% (normal) saline
D5 ½ NS, D_5½ NS: 5% dextrose in 0.45% saline
D5 ⅓ NS, D_5⅓ NS: 5% dextrose in 0.33% saline

ABBREVIATIONS

$\bar{a}$: before
abd: abdomen
ABGs: arterial blood gases
ac: before meals
ab lib: as desired
ADH: antidiuretic hormone
ADLs: activities of daily living
AFB: acid-fast bacillus (related to tuberculosis)
AIDS: acquired immunodeficiency syndrome
ALL: acute lymphoblastic leukemia
AMB: ambulatory
AP (and lateral chest): anterior and posterior
ASA: aspirin
ASHD: arteriosclerotic heart disease
ax: axillary
BE: barium enema
bid: twice a day
BM: bowel movement
BP: blood pressure
BPH: benign prostatic hypertrophy
BR: bed rest
BRP: bathroom privileges
BSE: breast self-examination
BSI: body substance isolation
BUN: blood urea nitrogen
bx: biopsy
$\bar{c}$: with
C&S: culture and sensitivity
CA: cancer
CABG: coronary artery bypass graft
CAD: coronary artery disease
cap: capsule

CBC: complete blood count
CBI: continuous bladder irrigation
CBR: complete bed rest
CC: chief complaint
CDC: Centers for Disease Control
CHF: congestive heart failure
Cl: chloride
CN: cranial nerve
CNS: central nervous system
c/o: complains of
CO_2: carbon dioxide
COPD: chronic obstructive pulmonary disease
CPM: continuous passive motion
CPR: cardiopulmonary resuscitation
CSF: cerebrospinal fluid
CT: computed tomography
CVA: cerebrovascular accident (stroke)
CVP: central venous pressure
D/C: discontinue
DM: diabetes mellitus
DNR: do not resuscitate
DSD: dry sterile dressing
DTR: deep tendon reflex
dx: diagnosis
EC: enteric coated
ECG, EKG: electrocardiogram
elix: elixir
ER: extended release
ESR: erythrocyte sedimentation rate
ESRD: end-stage renal disease
ET: enterostomal therapist
FUO: fever of unknown origin
fx: fracture
g: gram
GI: gastrointestinal
gtt: drops
GU: genitourinary
Hb, Hgb: hemoglobin
HBV: hepatitis B virus
HCO_{3-}: bicarbonate
Hct: hematocrit
HCV: hepatitis C virus
HEPA: high-efficiency particulate air
HIV: human immunodeficiency virus
h/o: history of
HOB: head of bed
HR: heart rate
hs: at bedtime
HTN: hypertension
I&O: intake and output
ICP: intracranial pressure
ICU: intensive care unit

IDDM: insulin-dependent diabetes mellitus
IM: intramuscular
IPPB: intermittent positive-pressure breathing
IV: intravenous
JVD: jugular vein distention
K: potassium
KUB: kidney, ureter, bladder
kvo: keep vein open (run IV very slowly)
LLQ: left lower quadrant
LMP: last menstrual period
LOC: level of consciousness
lytes: electrolytes
MAP: mean arterial pressure
MCHC: mean corpuscular hemoglobin concentration
MCV: mean corpuscular volume
MI: myocardial infarction
MRI: magnetic resonance imaging
N: nitrogen
Na: sodium
NaCl: sodium chloride
neg: negative
NG: nasogastric
NPO: nothing by mouth
NSAIDs: nonsteroidal antiinflammatory drugs
O_2: oxygen
OD: right eye
OOB: out of bed
OR: operating room
OS: left eye
O.T.: occupational therapy
OTC: over the counter (medicine without prescription)
OU: both eyes
P: pulse
PACU: postanesthesia care unit
pc: after meals
PCA: patient-controlled analgesia
PE: physical education
PID: pelvic inflammatory disease
PMH: past medical history
PMI: point of maximum impulse
po: by mouth
postop: after surgery
preop: before surgery
prep: preparation
PRN: as needed
pt: patient
P.T.: physical therapy

PT: pothrombin time
PTT: partial thromboplastin time
PVD: peripheral vascular disease
q: each
qd: daily
q__h (fill in number of hours), e.g., q3h: every 3 hours
qid: four times a day
qod: every other day
qs: sufficient quantity
R: respirations
RA: rheumatoid arthritis
RBC: red blood cell
R/O: rule out (eliminate possibility of a condition)
ROM: range of motion
ROS: Review of systems
r/t: related to
RUQ: right upper quadrant
Rx: treatment
$\bar{s}$: without
sc (SQ): subcutaneous
sl (SL): sublingual
SOB: shortness of breath
sp gr: specific gravity
SR: sustained release
STAT: immediately
STD: sexually transmitted disease
supp: suppository
susp: suspension
sx: symptoms, signs
T: temperature
T&C: type and crossmatch
tab: tablet
TB: tuberculosis
TCDB: turn, cough, deep breathe
tid: 3 times a day
TPN: total parenteral nutrition
TPR: temperature, pulse, respirations
TURP: transurethral resection of prostate
UA: urinalysis
up ab lib: up as desired
URI: upper respiratory infection
US: ultrasound
UTI: urinary tract infection
VS: vital signs
VTBI: volume to be infused
WBC: white blood cell
WC: wheelchair
WNL: within normal limits
wt: weight

APPENDIX C

Nursing Diagnoses

(1999-2000) North American Nursing
Diagnosis Association (NANDA) and
Functional Health Patterns

NANDA-Approved Nursing Diagnoses 1999-2000

Activity intolerance
Activity intolerance, risk for
Adaptive capacity, decreased: intracranial
Adjustment, impaired
Airway clearance, ineffective
Anxiety
Anxiety, death
Aspiration, risk for
Body image disturbance
Body temperature, altered, risk for
Bowel incontinence
Breastfeeding, effective
Breastfeeding, ineffective
Breastfeeding, interrupted
Breathing pattern, inefffective
Cardiac output, decreased
Caregiver role strain
Caregiver role strain, risk for
Communication, impaired verbal
Community coping, ineffective
Community coping, potential for enhanced
Confusion, acute
Confusion, chronic
Constipation
Constipation, perceived
Constipation, risk for
Coping, defensive
Coping, family: potential for growth
Coping, ineffective family: compromised
Coping, ineffective family: disabling
Coping, ineffective individual
Decisional conflict (specify)
Denial, ineffective
Dentition, altered
Development, altered, risk for
Diarrhea

Disuse syndrome, risk for
Diversional activity deficit
Dysreflexia
Dysreflexia, autonomic, risk for
Energy field disturbance
Environmental interpretation syndrome, impaired
Failure to thrive, adult
Family processes, altered
Family processes, altered: alcoholism
Fatigue
Fear
Fluid volume deficit
Fluid volume deficit, risk for
Fluid volume excess
Fluid volume imbalance, risk for
Gas exchange, impaired
Grieving, anticipatory
Grieving, dysfunctional
Growth, altered, risk for
Growth and development, altered
Health maintenance, altered
Health-seeking behaviors (specify)
Home maintenance management, impaired
Hopelessness
Hyperthermia
Hypothermia
Incontinence, stress
Incontinence, total
Inconinence, urge
Incontinence, urinary, functional
Incontinence, urinary, reflex
Incontinence, urinary urge, risk for
Infant behavior, disorganized
Infant behavior, disorganized: risk for
Infant behavior, organized: potential for enhanced
Infant feeding pattern, ineffective

Infection, risk for
Injury, perioperative positioning: risk for
Injury, risk for
Knowledge deficit (specify)
Latex allergy
Latex allergy, risk for
Loneliness, risk for
Management of therapeutic regimen, community: ineffective
Management of therapeutic regimen, families: ineffective
Management of therapeutic regimen, individual: ineffective
Management of therapeutic regimen, individuals: ineffective
Memory, impaired
Mobility, impaired bed
Mobility, impaired physical
Mobility, impaired wheelchair
Nausea
Noncompliance (specify)
Nutrition, altered: less than body requirements
Nutrition, altered: more than body requirements
Nutrition, altered: risk for more than body requirements
Oral mucous membrane, altered
Pain
Pain, chronic
Parent/infant/child attachment, altered: risk for
Parental role conflict
Parenting, altered
Parenting, altered, risk for
Peripheral neurovascular dysfunction, risk for
Personal identity disturbance
Poisoning, risk for
Posttrauma syndrome
Posttrauma syndrome, risk for
Powerlessness
Protection, altered
Rape-trauma syndrome
Rape-trauma syndrome: compound reaction
Rape-trauma syndrome: silent reaction
Relocation stress syndrome
Role performance, altered
Self-care deficit, bathing/hygiene

Self-care deficit, dressing/grooming
Self-care deficit, feeding
Self-care deficit, toileting
Self-esteem, disturbance
Self-esteem, chronic low
Self-esteem, situational low
Self-mutilation, risk for
Sensory/perceptual alterations (specify) (visual, auditory, kinesthetic, gustatory, tactile, olfactory)
Sexual dysfunction
Sexuality patterns, altered
Skin integrity, impaired
Skin integrity, impaired, risk for
Sleep deprivation
Sleep pattern disturbance
Social interaction, impaired
Social isolation
Sorrow, chronic
Spiritual distress (distress of the human spirit)
Spiritual distress, risk for
Spiritual well-being, potential for enhanced
Suffocation, risk for
Surgical recovery, delayed
Swallowing, impaired
Thermoregulation, ineffective
Thought processes, altered
Tissue integrity, impaired
Tissue perfusion, altered (specify type) (renal, cerebral, cardiopulmonary, gastrointestinal, peripheral)
Trauma, risk for
Unilateral neglect
Urinary elimination, altered
Urinary retention
Ventilation, inability to sustain spontaneous
Ventilatory weaning response, dysfunction (DVWR)
Violence, risk for: directed at others
Violence, risk for: self-directed
Walking, impaired
Wheelchair transfer ability, impaired

Classification of Nursing Diagnoses by Functional Health Patterns

HEALTH PERCEPTION–HEALTH MANAGEMENT
Health-Seeking Behaviors (Specify)
Altered Health Maintenance
Ineffective Management of Therapeutic Regimen, Individual
Effective Management of Therapeutic Regimen, Individual
Ineffective Family Management of Therapeutic Regimen
Ineffective Community Management of Therapeutic Regimen
Noncompliance (Specify)
Risk for Infection
Risk for Injury
Risk for Trauma
Risk for Perioperative Positioning Injury
Risk for Poisoning
Risk for Suffocation
Altered Protection

Energy Field Disturbance
Risk for Altered Body Temperature

NUTRITIONAL–METABOLIC
Altered Nutrition: More than Body Requirements
Altered Nutrition: Risk for More than Body Requirements
Altered Nutrition: Less than Body Requirements
Ineffective Breastfeeding
Interrupted Breastfeeding
Effective Breastfeeding
Ineffective Infant Feeding Pattern
Impaired Swallowing
Risk for Aspiration
Altered Oral Mucous Membrane
Fluid Volume Deficit
Risk for Fluid Volume Deficit
Fluid Volume Excess
Risk for Impaired Skin Integrity

Modified from Gordon M: *Manual of nursing diagnosis, 1995-1996.* St Louis, 1995, Mosby.

Impaired Skin Integrity
Impaired Tissue Integrity
Ineffective Thermoregualtion
Hyperthermia
Hypothermia

ELIMINATION
Constipation
Colonic Constipation
Perceived Constipation
Diarrhea
Bowel Incontinence
Altered Urinary Elimination
Functional Incontinence
Reflex Incontinence
Stress Incontinence
Total Incontinence
Urge Incontinence
Urinary Retention

ACTIVITY–EXERCISE
Acivity Intolerance
Risk for Activity Intolerance
Fatigue
Impaired Physical Mobility
Risk for Disuse Syndrome
Self-Care Deficit, Bathing/Hygiene
Self-Care Deficit, Dressing/Grooming
Self-Care Deficit, Feeding
Self-Care Deficit, Toileting
Diversional Activity Deficit
Impaired Home Maintenance Management
Ventilatory Weaning Response, Dysfunctional
Inability to Sustain Spontaneous Ventilation
Ineffective Airway Clearance
Ineffective Breathing Pattern
Impaired Gas Exchange
Decreased Cardiac Output
Altered Tissue Perfusion (Renal, Cerebral, Cardiopulmonary,
    Gastrointestinal, Peripheral)
Dysreflexia
Disorganized Infant Behavior
Risk for Disorganized Infant Behavior
Potential for Enhanced Organized Infant Behavior
Risk for Peripheral Neurovascular Dysfunction
Altered Growth and Development

SLEEP–REST
Sleep-Pattern Disturbance
Anxiety
Energy Field Disturbance
Fear
Dysfunctional Grieving
Relocation Stress Syndrome
(See also Self-Perception–Self-Concept)

COGNITIVE–PERCEPTUAL
Pain
Chronic Pain
Sensory/Perceptual Alterations (Specify)
Unilateral Neglect
Knowledge Deficit (Specify)
Altered Thought Processes

Acute Confusion
Chronic Confusion
Impaired Environmental Interpretation Syndrome
Impaired Memory
Decisional Conflict (Specify)
Decreased Intracranial Adaptive Capacity

SELF-PRECEPTION–SELF-CONCEPT
Fear
Anxiety
Risk for Loneliness
Hopelessness
Powerlessness
Self-Esteem Disturbance
Chronic Low Self-Esteem
Situational Low Self-Esteem
Body Image Disturbance
Risk for Self-Mutilation
Personal Identity Disturbance

ROLE–RELATIONSHIP
Anticipatory Grieving
Dysfunctional Grieving
Altered Role Performance
Social Isolation
Impaired Social Interaction
Relocation Stress Syndrome
Altered Family Processes
Altered Family Processes: Alcoholism
Altered Parenting
Risk for Altered Parenting
Parental Role Conflict
Risk for Altered Parent Infant/Child Attachment
Caregiver Role Strain
Risk for Caregiver Role Strain
Impaired Verbal Communication
Risk for Violence

SEXUALITY–REPRODUCTION
Altered Sexuality Patterns
Sexual Dysfunction
Rape-Trauma Syndrome
Rape-Trauma Sundrome: Compound Reaction
Rape-Trauma Syndrome: Silent Reaction

COPING–STRESS TOLERANCE
Ineffective Coping (Individual)
Defensive Coping
Ineffective Denial, or Denial
Impaired Adjustment
Post-Trauma Response
Defensive Coping
Family Coping: Potential for Growth
Ineffective Family Coping: Compromised
Ineffective Family Coping: Disabling
Ineffective Individual Coping
Ineffective Community Coping
Potential for Enhanced Community Coping

VALUE–BELIEF
Spiritual Distress (Distress of Human Spirit)
Potential for Enhanced Spiritual Well-Being)

APPENDIX D

Norms for Common Laboratory Tests

SERUM: COMPLETE BLOOD COUNT

Hemoglobulin (Hgb)	Male: 13.5-18.0 g/dl	Female 12-16 g/dl
Hematocrit (Hct)	Male: 40%-54%	Female: 38%-47%
Red blood cells (RBCs)	Male: 4.6-6.2 million/mm^3	Female: 4.2-5.4 million/mm^3
Leukocytes (white blood cells, WBCs)	5000-10,000/mm^3	
Neutrophils	54%-75% (3000-7500/mm^3)	
Bands	3%-8% (150-700/mm^3)	
Eosinophils	1%-4% (50-400/mm^3)	
Basophils	0%-1% (25-100/mm^3)	
Monocytes	2%-8% (100-500/mm^3)	
Lymphocytes	25%-40% (1500-4500/mm^3)	
T lymphocytes	60%-80% of lymphocytes	
B lymphocytes	10%-20% of lymphocytes	
Platelets	150,000-450,000/mm^3	

SERUM: CLOTTING INDICES

Prothrombin (PT)	Male: 9.6-11.8 sec	Female 9.5-11.3 sec
Partial thromboplastin time (PTT)	30-45 sec	
Bleeding time		
Duke	1-3 min	
Ivy	3-6 min	
Template	3-6 min	
Closing time (Lee-White)	4-8 min	

SERUM: CHEMISTRY

Sodium (Na)	135-145 mEq/L
Potassium (K)	3.5-5.0 mEq/L
Chloride (Cl)	95-105 mEq/L
Bicarbonate (HCO$_{3-}$)	19-25 mEq/L
Total calcium	9-11 mg/dl *or* 4.5-5.5 mEq/L
Phosphorus/phosphate	2.4-4.7 mg/dl
Magnesium	1.8-3.0 mg/dl *or* 1.5-2.5 mEq/L
Glucose	70-110 mg/dl
Osmolality	285-310 mOsm/kg

LIVER FUNCTION TESTS

Aspartate aminotransferase (AST, SGOT) (see also cardiac)	Male: 8-46 U/L	Female: 7-34 U/L
Alanine aminotransferase (ALT, SGPT)	10-30 IU/ml	
Total bilirubin	0.3-1.2 mg/dl	
Conjugated	0.0-0.2 mg/dl	
Unconjugated (indirect)	0.2-0.8 mg/dl	
Alkaline phosphatase	20-90 U/L	

LIPIDS

Cholesteral	120-220 mg/100 ml
Total lipids	450-1000 mg/100 ml
Triglycerides	40-150 mg/ml

CARDIAC ENZYMES RELATED TO MYOCARDIAL INFARCTION

AST (SGOT; see also liver)	8-20 U/L (women slightly higher)	
Total creatine phosphokinase (CPK, creatine kinase)	Male: 12-70 U/ml	Female: 10-55 U/ml
CPK-MB (muscle/brain)	0%	
Lactate dehydrogenase (LDH)	45-90 U/L	

RENAL FUNCTION TESTS

Blood urea nitrogen (BUN)	6-20 mg/dl	
Creatinine	Male: 0.6-1.3 mg/dl	Female: 0.5-1.0 mg/dl
Uric acid	Male: 4.0-8.5 mg/dl	Female: 2.7-7.3 mg/dl

THYROID FUNCTION TESTS

TSH	$0.5-3.5 \mu U/ml$
T_3	25%-30%

ARTERIAL BLOOD GASES (ABGs)

pH	7.35-7.45
Oxygen partial pressure tension (P_{O_2})	80-100
Carbon dioxide partial pressure tension (P_{CO_2})	35-45 mm Hg
Bicarbonate (HCO_{3-})	22-26 mEq/L
O_2 saturation (arterial)	95%+
Base Excess	+2/−2

ROUTINE URINALYSIS

pH	4.5-8.0
Specific gravity	1.010-1.025
Protein	None
Glucose	None
Ketones	Negative
RBCs	<2
WBCs	0.4/low-power field (LPF)
Casts	None or occasional epithelial
Crystals	Negative
Bacteria	Negative

APPENDIX E
Height and Weight Table:

Weights for Persons 25 to 59 Years
According to Build*

Men					Women				
Height†		Small frame	Medium frame	Large frame	Height†		Small frame	Medium frame	Large frame
Feet	Inches				Feet	Inches			
5	2	128-134	131-141	138-150	4	10	102-111	109-121	118-131
5	3	130-136	133-143	140-153	4	11	103-113	111-123	120-134
5	4	132-138	135-145	142-156	5	0	104-115	113-126	122-137
5	5	134-140	137-148	144-160	5	1	106-118	115-129	125-140
5	6	136-142	139-151	146-164	5	2	108-121	118-132	128-143
5	7	138-145	142-154	149-168	5	3	111-124	121-135	131-147
5	8	140-148	145-157	152-172	5	4	114-127	124-138	134-151
5	9	142-151	148-160	155-176	5	5	117-130	124-141	137-155
5	10	144-154	151-163	158-180	5	6	120-133	130-144	140-159
5	11	146-157	154-166	161-184	5	7	123-136	133-147	143-163
6	0	149-160	157-170	164-188	5	8	126-139	136-150	146-167
6	1	152-164	160-174	168-192	5	9	129-142	139-153	149-170
6	2	155-168	164-178	172-197	5	10	132-145	142-156	152-173
6	3	158-172	167-182	176-202	5	11	135-148	145-159	155-176
6	4	162-176	171-187	181-207	6	0	138-151	148-162	158-179

Source of basic data *Build study*, Society of Actuaries and Association of Life Insurance Medical Directors of America, 1980. Copyright 1983 Metropolitan Life Insurance Company Statistical Bulletin.
*Indoor clothing weighing 5 pounds for men and 3 pounds for women.
†Shoes with 1-inch heels.

GLOSSARY

abduction   Movement of a limb away from the body.

abnormal reactive hyperemia Hyperemia over a pressure site lasting longer than 1 hour following removal of pressure; surrounding skin does not blanch.

absorption Passage of drug molecules into the blood. Factors influencing drug absorption include route of administration, ability of the drug to dissolve, and conditions at the site of absorption.

accessory muscles   Muscles in the thoracic cage that assist with respiration.

active transport   Movement of materials across the cell membrane by means of chemical activity that allows the cell to admit larger molecules than would otherwise be possible.

adaptation Process by which changes occur in any of a person's dimensions in response to stress.

adduction   Movement of a limb toward the body.

adventitious sounds Abnormal lung sounds heard with auscultation.

adverse reaction Harmful or unintended effect of a medication, diagnostic test, or therapeutic intervention.

afebrile Without fever.

afterload The resistance to left ventricular ejection.

AHCPR Agency for Health Care Policy and Research, which synthesizes research and develops standards of practice.

allergen Substance, usually a protein, that causes the formation of an antibody and reacts to initiate an allergic response.

Alzheimer's disease Disease of the brain parenchyma that causes a gradual and progressive decline in cognitive functioning.

analgesic Relieving pain; drug that relieves pain.

anaphylactic reaction Hypersensitive condition induced by contact with certain antigens.

angina pectoris Episodic chest pain caused most often by myocardial anoxia, resulting from atherosclerosis of the coronary arteries. Pain radiates down the inner aspect of the left arm and is often accompanied by feeling of suffocation and impending death.

angiography Radiographic visualization of internal anatomy of the heart and blood vessels after the introduction of a radiopaque contrast medium.

anorexia Lack or loss of appetite resulting in the inability to eat.

antibodies Immunoglobulins, essential to the immune system, that are produced by lymphoid tissue in response to bacteria, viruses, or other antigens.

anticipatory grief Grief response in which the person begins the grieving process before an actual loss.

antiembolic stockings   Elasticized stockings that prevent formation of emboli and thrombi, especially after surgery or during bed rest.

antipyretic Substance or procedure that reduces fever.

aphasia Abnormal neurological condition in which language function is defective or absent; related to injury to speech center in cerebral cortex, causing receptive or expressive aphasia.

apical pulse Heart beat taken with the bell or diaphragm of a stethoscope placed on the apex of the heart.

apnea Cessation of airflow through the nose and mouth.

apothecary system System of measurement; basic unit of weight is a grain. Weights derived from the grain are the gram, ounce, and pound. The basic measure for fluid is the minim. The fluidram, fluid ounce, pint, quart, and gallon are measures derived from the minim.

approximate To come close together, as in the edges of a wound.

asepsis Destruction or removal of germs or microorganisms.

asphyxia Decreased oxygen with or without excess of carbon dioxide in the body.

assessment First step of the nursing process; activities required in the first step are data collection, data validation, data sorting, and data documentation. The purpose is to gather information for health problem identification.

assimilation To become absorbed into another culture and to adopt its characteristics.

assistive personnel Category of health care providers such as nurse assistants or technicians who may be unlicensed and who have limited formal education. This individual is trained in basic client care and assists the registered nurse with client care. This may include activities of daily living, vital signs, assistance with meals, simple wound care, assisting with ambulation.

atelectasis Collapse of alveoli, preventing the normal respiratory exchange of oxygen and carbon dioxide.

atrioventricular (AV) node Portion of the cardiac conduction system located on the floor of the right atrium; it receives electrical impulses from the atrium and transmits them to the bundle of His.

auditory Related to, or experienced through, hearing.

auscultation Method of physical examination; listening to the sounds produced by the body, usually with a stethoscope.

auscultatory gap Disappearance of sound when obtaining a blood pressure; typically occurs between the first and second Korotkoff sounds.

autologous transfusion Collection of the client's blood for reinfusion after a surgical procedure.

autonomy Ability or tendency to function independently.

autopsy Postmortem examination performed to confirm or determine the cause of death.

autotransfusion Collection, anticoagulation, filtration, and reinfusion of blood from an active bleeding site.

bacteriuria Presence of bacteria in the urine.

bereavement Response to loss through death; a subjective experience that a person suffers after losing a person with whom there has been a significant relationship.

bioavailability Degree of activity or amount of an administered drug or other substance that becomes available for activity in the target tissue.

blanching Whitening of the skin from pressure, vasoconstriction, or hypotension.

bonding The parents' emotional tie to their child that usually develops soon after birth as a result of their interaction.

bone resorption Destruction of bone cells and release of calcium into the blood.

brachial pulse Rhythmic beating palpated over the brachial artery.

bradycardia Slower than normal heart rate; heart contracts fewer than 60 times per minute.

bradypnea An abnormally slow rate of breathing.

bronchoscopy Visual examination of the tracheal and bronchial tree using a flexible fiberoptic bronchoscope.

bruit Abnormal sound or murmur heard while auscultating an organ, gland, or artery.

buccal Of or pertaining to the inside of the cheek or the gum next to the cheek.

buffer Substance or group of substances that can absorb or release hydrogen ions to correct an acid-base imbalance.

bundle of His Portion of the cardiac conduction system that arises from the distal portion of the AV node and extends across the AV groove to the top of the intraventricular septum, where it divides into right and left bundle branches.

cachexia Malnutrition marked by weakness and emaciation, usually associated with severe illness.

carcinogen Substance or agent that causes the development or increases the incidence of cancer.

cardiac output Volume of blood expelled by the ventricles of the heart, equal to the amount of blood ejected at each beat, multiplied by the number of beats in the period of time used for computation (usually 1 minute).

carotid pulse Rhythmical beating palpated over the carotid artery.

carriers Animals or persons who harbor and spread disease-causing organisms but who do not become ill.

cathartics Drugs that act to promote bowel evacuation.

catheterization Introduction of a catheter into a body cavity or organ to inject or remove fluid.

cerumen Yellowish or brownish waxy secretion produced by sweat glands in the external ear.

channels Method used in the teaching-learning process to present content: visual, auditory, taste, smell. In the communication process, a method used to transmit a message: visual, auditory, touch.

charting by exception (CBE) A charting methodology in which data are entered only when there is an exception from what is normal or expected. Reduces time spent documenting in charting. It is a shorthand method for documenting normal findings and routine care.

circadian rhythm Repetition of certain physiological phenomena within a 24-hour cycle.

circulating nurse Assistant to the scrub nurse and surgeon whose role is to provide necessary supplies, dispose of soiled instruments and supplies, and keep an accurate count of instruments, needles, and sponges used.

circumduction Movement of the arm in full circle; includes all movements of the shoulder ball-and-socket joint.

collaboration The working together of health team members in the delivery of care to a client or group of clients.

colon Large intestine.

colonized Referring to the establishment of a mass of microorganisms, often nonpathogenic, in or on the body.

compliance Person's fulfillment of the prescribed course of treatment.

compress Soft pad of gauze or cloth used to apply heat, cold, or medications to the surface of a body part.

contaminated Process by which an object becomes unclean or unsterile.

contracture Permanent shortening of a muscle and the eventual shortening of associated ligaments and tendons.

core temperature Temperature of deep body tissues and organs.

crackles Fine bubbling sounds heard on auscultation of the lung; produced by air entering distal airways and alveoli, which contain serous secretions.

criteria Standards, principles, or requirements established for accomplishing or evaluating an activity or condition, such as formulating a nursing diagnosis.

culture Nonphysical traits, such as values, beliefs, attitudes, and customs, that are shared by a group of people and passed from one generation to the next.

cyanosis Bluish discoloration of the skin and mucous membranes caused by an excess of deoxygenated hemoglobin in the blood or a structural defect in the hemoglobin molecule.

death Cessation of life as indicated by the absence of heartbeat or respiration. Legally, death is total absence of activity in the brain and central nervous, cardiovascular, and respiratory systems.

débridement Removal of dead tissue from a wound.

defecation Passage of feces from the digestive tract through the rectum.

dehiscence Separation of a wound's edges, revealing underlying tissues.

dementia Irreversible mental state characterized by decreased intellectual function, changes in personality, impaired judgment, and often changes in affect as a result of permanently altered cerebral metabolism.

dermis Sensitive vascular layer of the skin directly below the epidermis composed of collagenous and elastic fibrous connective tissues that give the dermis strength and elasticity.

diaphoresis Secretion of sweat, especially profuse secretion associated with an elevated body temperature, physical exertion, or emotional stress.

diastole Time between contractions of the atria or the ventricles during which blood enters the relaxed chambers.

diffusion Movement of molecules from an area of high concentration to an area of lower concentration.

diplopia Double vision caused by an abnormality of the extraocular muscles or nerves that innervate the muscles.

disinfection Process of destroying all pathogenic organisms, except spores.

diuresis Increased rate of formation and excretion of urine.

dorsalis pedis pulse Rhythmical beating palpated over the dorsalis pedis artery.

dorsiflexion Flexion toward the back.

dyspnea Sensation of shortness of breath.

dysrhythmia Deviation from the normal pattern of the heartbeat.

dysuria Painful urination resulting from bacterial infection of the bladder and obstructive conditions of the urethra.

ecchymosis Discoloration of the skin or a bruise caused by leakage of blood into subcutaneous tissues as a result of trauma to underlying tissues.

edema Abnormal accumulation of fluid in interstitial spaces of tissues.

effluent Discharge or drainage.

egocentricity Regarding of the self as the center, object, and norm of all experience and having little regard for the needs, interests, ideas, and attitudes of others.

endogenous infections Infections produced within a cell or organism.

endorphins Naturally occurring neuropeptides composed of amino acids and secreted within the central nervous system to reduce pain.

endoscope Instrument used to visualize the interior of body organs and cavities.

endotracheal tube Artificial airway inserted into client's mouth or nose.

enteral nutrition (EN) Provision of nutrients through the gastrointestinal tract when the client cannot ingest, chew, or swallow food but can digest and absorb nutrients.

epidural infusion A type of nerve block anesthesia in which an anesthetic is intermittently or continuously injected into the lumbosacral region of the spinal cord.

epidermis Outer layer of the skin that has several thin layers of skin in different stages of maturation; shields and protects the underlying tissues from water loss, mechanical or chemical injury, and penetration by disease-causing microorganisms.

erythema Redness or inflammation of the skin or mucous membranes that is a result of dilation and congestion of superficial capillaries; sunburn is an example.

eschar Scab or dry crust that results from excoriation of the skin.

ethnocentrism Tendency of members of one cultural group to view the members of other cultural groups in terms of the standards of behavior, attitudes, and values of their own group.

euthanasia Deliberately bringing about the death of a person who has an incurable disease or condition, either actively, by administering a lethal drug, or passively, by withholding treatment and allowing the person to die.

evisceration Protrusion of visceral organs through a surgical wound.

exacerbations Increases in the seriousness of a disease or disorder as marked by greater intensity in signs or symptoms.

exogenous infection Infection originating outside an organ or part.

exophthalmos Abnormal protrusion of one or both eyes.

exudate Fluid, cells, or other substances that have been slowly discharged from cells or blood vessels through small pores or breaks in cell membranes.

febrile Pertaining to or characterized by an elevated body temperature.

feces Waste or excrement from the gastrointestinal tract.

fibrin Protein product formed from the action of thrombin on fibrinogen in the clotting process.

fissure Cleft or groove on the surface of an organ, often marking division of the organ into parts.

fistula Abnormal passage from an internal organ to the body surface or between two internal organs.

flatus Intestinal gas.

gait Manner or style of walking, including rhythm, cadence, and speed.

gingiva Gum of the mouth; a mucous membrane with supporting fibrous tissue that overlies the crowns of unerupted teeth and encircles the necks of those teeth that have erupted.

glomerulus Cluster or collection of capillary vessels within the kidney involved in the initial formation of urine.

granulation tissue Soft, pink, fleshy projections of tissue that form during the healing process in a wound not healing by primary intention.

gurgles Abnormal coarse sounds heard during auscultation of the lung; produced by air entering large mucus-containing airways. Also called *rhonchi.*

gustatory Pertaining to the sense of taste.

health Dynamic state in which individuals adapt to their internal and external environments so that there is a state of physical, emotional, intellectual, social, and spiritual well-being.

health behaviors Activities through which a person maintains, attains, or regains good health and prevents illness.

hematemesis Vomiting of blood indicating upper gastrointestinal bleeding.

hematoma Collection of blood trapped in the tissues of the skin or an organ.

hematuria Abnormal presence of blood in the urine.

hemolysis Breakdown of red blood cells and release of hemoglobin that may occur following administration of hypotonic intravenous solutions, causing swelling and rupture of erythrocytes.

hemoptysis Coughing up blood from the respiratory tract.

hemorrhoids Permanent dilation and engorgement of veins within the lining of the rectum.

hemostasis Termination of bleeding by mechanical or chemical means or by the coagulation process of the body.

hemothorax Accumulation of blood and fluid in the pleural cavity between the parietal and visceral pleurae.

hernias Protrusions of an organ through an abnormal opening in the muscle wall of the cavity that surrounds it.

hirsutism Excessive body hair in a masculine distribution caused by heredity, hormonal dysfunction, or medication.

homeostasis State of relative constance in the internal environment of the body, maintained naturally by physiological adaptive mechanisms.

hospice System of family-centered care designed to help terminally ill persons be comfortable and maintain a satisfactory lifestyle throughout the terminal phase of their illness.

hypercapnia Greater than normal amounts of carbon dioxide in the blood; also called *hypercarbia.*

hypercarbia Greater than normal amounts of carbon dioxide in the blood; also called *hypercapnia.*

hyperemia Redness over a pressure site lasting 1 hour or less after removal of pressure; surrounding skin does not blanch.

hyperextension A position of maximal extension of a joint.

hyperglycemia Elevated serum glucose levels.

hypertension Disorder characterized by an elevated blood pressure persistently exceeding 150/90 mm Hg.

hyperthermia Situation in which body temperature exceeds the set-point.

hypertonic Situation in which one solution has a greater concentration of solute than another solution; therefore the first solution exerts greater osmotic pressure.

hyperventilation Respiratory rate in excess of that required to maintain normal carbon dioxide levels in the body tissues.

hypervolemia Increase in the amount of fluid in the circulating blood volume.

hypoglycemia Reduced serum glucose levels.

hypotension Abnormal lowering of blood pressure, which is inadequate for normal perfusion and oxygenation of tissues.

hypothalamus Portion of the brain that activates, controls, and integrates the peripheral autonomic nervous system, endocrine processes, and many body functions, such as body temperature, sleep, and appetite.

hypothermia Abnormal lowering of body temperature below 35° C, (93° F) usually caused by prolonged exposure to cold.

hypotonic A situation in which one solution has a smaller concentration of solute than another solution; therefore the first solution exerts less osmotic pressure.

hypoventilation Respiratory rate insufficient to prevent carbon dioxide retention.

hypovolemia Abnormally low circulating blood volume.

hypoxia Inadequate cellular oxygenation that may result from a deficiency in the delivery or use of oxygen at the cellular level.

iatrogenic Caused by a treatment or diagnostic procedure.

idiosyncratic reactions Individual sensitivity to effects of a drug caused by inherited or other body constitution factors.

ileum Part of the small intestine.

immunity Quality of being insusceptible to or unaffected by a particular disease or condition.

induration Hardening of a tissue, particularly the skin, because of edema or inflammation.

infiltration Dislodging an intravenous catheter or needle from a vein into the subcutaneous space.

inflammation Protective response of body tissues to irritation or injury.

infusion Introduction of fluid into the vein, giving intravenous fluid over time.

inhalers Aerosol sprays, mists, or powders that penetrate lung airways, which the client inhales through the mouth.

injection Parenteral administration of medication; four major sites of injection: subcutaneous, intramuscular, intravenous, and intradermal.

insomnia Condition characterized by chronic inability to sleep or remain asleep through the night.

inspection Method of physical examination by which the client is visually and systematically examined for appearance, structure, function, and behavior.

instillation To cause to enter drop by drop, or very slowly.

integument Skin and its appendages: hair, nails, and sweat and sebaceous glands.

interstitial fluid Fluid that fills the spaces between most of the cells of the body and provides a substantial portion of the liquid environment of the body.

intonation Rise and fall in pitch of the voice in speech.

intracellular fluid Liquid within the cell membrane.

intractable pain Pain not easily relieved, such as that which occurs with some types of cancer.

intradermal Injection given between layers of the skin, into the dermis. Injections are given at a 5- to 15-degree angle.

intramuscular (IM) Injections given into muscle tissue. The intramuscular route provides a fast rate of absorption that is related to the muscle's greater vascularity. Injections are given at a 45- to 90-degree angle.

intrauterine Inside the uterus or womb.

intravascular Fluid contained within the vessels of the circulatory system.

intravenous (IV) Injection directly into the bloodstream. Action of the drug begins immediately when given intravenously.

inversion Movement of a limb by turning inward toward the body.

irrigation Process of washing out a body cavity or wounded area with a stream of fluid.

ischemia Decreased blood supply to a body part, such as skin tissue or to an organ such as the heart.

isolation Separation of a client from other clients to prevent the spread of infection or to protect the client from irritating environmental factors.

isometric Related to increased muscle tension without muscle shortening.

isotonic The situation in which two solutions have the same concentration of solute; therefore both solutions exert the same osmotic pressure.

jejunum Part of the small intestine.

kinesthetic Relating to perception of position of body parts, weight, and movement.

Korotkoff sounds Sounds heard during the taking of blood pressure using a sphygmomanometer and stethoscope.

laceration Torn, jagged wound.

lactation Process and period in which the mother produces milk for a child.

laryngospasm A sudden uncontrolled contraction of the laryngeal muscles, which in turn decreases airway size.

leukocyte White blood cell.

leukocytosis Abnormal increase in the number of circulating white blood cells.

leukoplakia Thick, white patches observed on oral mucous membranes.

lipids Compounds that are insoluble in water but soluble in organic solvents.

lymphocyte One type of leukocyte developing in the bone marrow; responsible for synthesizing antibodies and T cells that attack antigens.

maceration Softening and breaking down of skin from prolonged exposure to moisture.

macrophages Large phagocytic cells of the reticuloendothelial system.

malignant hyperthermia Autosomal dominant trait characterized by often fatal hyperthermia in affected people exposed to certain anesthetic agents.

malnutrition Any nutritional disorder such as unbalanced, insufficient, or excessive diet or impaired absorption, assimilation, or utilization of food.

masticate To chew or tear food with the teeth while it becomes mixed with saliva.

meconium First stools of a newborn; typically sticky, dark green or almost black, sterile, and odorless.

medical asepsis Procedures used to reduce the number of microorganisms and prevent their spread.

melena Abnormal black, sticky stool containing digested blood; indicative of gastrointestinal bleeding.

metabolism Aggregate of all chemical processes that take place in living organisms, resulting in growth, generation of energy, elimination of wastes, and other functions concerned with the distribution of nutrients in the blood after digestion.

metered-dose inhaler Device designed to deliver a measured dose of an inhalation drug.

micturition Urination; act of passing or expelling urine voluntarily through the urethra.

milliequivalent per liter (mEq/L) Number of grams of a specific electrolyte dissolved in 1 liter of plasma.

mobility Person's ability to move about freely.

multicultural nursing Framework for broadening nurses' understanding of health-related beliefs, practices, and issues that are part of the lived experiences of people from diverse cultural backgrounds.

murmurs Blowing or whooshing sounds created by changes in blood flow through the heart or by abnormalities in valve closure.

NANDA North American Nursing Diagnosis Association, organized in 1973, which formally identifies, develops, and classifies nursing diagnoses.

narcolepsy Syndrome involving sudden sleep attacks that a person cannot inhibit; uncontrollable desire to sleep may occur several times during a day.

narcotic Drug substance, derived from opium or produced synthetically, that alters perception of pain and that, with repeated use, may result in physical and psychological dependence.

nebulization Process of adding moisture to inspired air by the addition of water droplets.

necrotic Of or pertaining to the death of tissue in response to disease or injury.

nephrons Structural and functional units of the kidney containing renal glomeruli and tubules.

neurotransmitter Chemical that transfers the electrical impulse from the nerve fiber to the muscle fiber.

nitrogen balance Relationship between the nitrogen taken into the body, usually as food, and the nitrogen excreted from the body in urine and feces. Most of the body's nitrogen is incorporated into protein.

nosocomial infections Infections acquired during hospitalization or stay in a health care facility.

NPUAP National Pressure Ulcer Advisory Panel.

nutrients Foods that contain elements necessary for body function, including water, carbohydrates, proteins, fats, vitamins, and minerals.

nystagmus Involuntary, rhythmical movements of the eyes; the oscillations may be horizontal, vertical, rotatory, or mixed. May be indicative of vestibular, neurological, or vascular disease.

obesity Abnormal increase in the proportion of fat cells, mainly in the viscera and subcutaneous tissues of the body.

olfactory Pertaining to the sense of smell.

oncotic pressure The total influence of the protein on the osmotic activity of plasma fluid.

ophthalmic Drugs given into the eye, in the form of either eye drops or ointments.

organic brain syndrome Any psychological or behavioral abnormality associated with transient or permanent brain dysfunction caused by a disturbance of the physiological functioning of brain tissue.

orthopnea Abnormal condition in which a person must sit or stand up to breathe comfortably.

orthostatic hypotension Abnormally low blood pressure occurring when a person stands up.

osmolality Concentration of osmotic pressure of a solution expressed in osmoles or milliosmoles per kilogram of water.

osmoreceptors Receptors that are sensitive to fluid concentration in the blood plasma and regulate the secretion of antidiuretic hormone.

osmosis Movement of a pure solvent through a semipermeable membrane from a solution with a lower solute concentration to one with a higher solute concentration.

osmotic pressure Drawing power for water, which depends on the number of molecules in the solution.

ostomy Surgical creation of an artificial opening.

ototoxicity Having a harmful effect on the eighth cranial (auditory) nerve or the organs of hearing and balance.

oximeter, oximetry Device used to measure oxyhemoglobin in the blood.

oxygen saturation The amount of hemoglobin fully saturated with oxygen given as a percent value.

pain Subjective, unpleasant sensation caused by noxious stimulation of sensory nerve endings.

palliative Relating to treatment designed to relieve or reduce intensity of uncomfortable symptoms but not to produce a cure.

pallor Unnatural paleness or absence of color in the skin.

palpation Method of physical examination whereby the fingers or hands of the examiner are applied to the client's body for the purpose of feeling body parts underlying the skin.

palpitations Bounding or racing of the heart associated with normal emotions or a heart disorder.

pathogens Microorganisms capable of producing disease.

pathological fractures Fractures resulting from weakened bone tissue; frequently caused by osteoporosis or neoplasms.

perception Person's mental image or concept of elements in his or her environment, including information gained through the senses.

perfusion (1) Passage of a fluid through a specific organ or an area of the body; (2) therapeutic measure whereby a drug intended for an isolated part of the body is introduced via the bloodstream.

peripheral Pertains to the outside, surface, or surrounding area of an organ, structure, or field of vision.

PERRLA Acronym for "pupils equal, round, reactive to light, accommodative"; the acronym is recorded in the physical examination if eye and pupil assessments are normal.

petechiae Tiny purple or red spots that appear on skin as minute hemorrhages within dermal layers.

peristalsis Rhythmical contractions of the intestine that propel gastric contents through the length of the gastrointestinal tract.

pharmacokinetics Study of how drugs enter the body, reach their site of action, are metabolized, and exit from the body.

phlebitis Inflammation of a vein.

photophobia Abnormal sensitivity of the eyes to light.

pigmentation Organic material, such as melanin, that gives color to the skin.

placebo Dosage form that contains no pharmacologically active ingredients but may relieve pain through psychological effects.

plantar flexion Toe-down motion of the foot at the ankle.

pleural friction rub Adventitious lung sound caused by an inflamed parietal and visceral pleura rubbing together on inspiration.

pneumothorax Collection of air or gas in the pleural space.

popliteal pulse Pulse of the popliteal artery, palpated behind the knee.

posterior tibial pulse Pulse of the posterior tibial artery, palpated on the medial aspect of the ankle, just posterior to the prominence of the ankle bone.

postural drainage Use of positioning along with percussion and vibration to drain secretions from specific segments of the lungs and bronchi into the trachea.

postural hypotension Abnormally low blood pressure occurring when an individual assumes the standing posture; also called *orthostatic hypotension.*

preload Volume of blood in the ventricles at the end of diastole, immediately before ventricular contraction.

prescriptions Written directions for a therapeutic agent (e.g., medication, drugs).

pressure ulcer Inflammation, sore, or ulcer in the skin over a bony prominence.

primary intention Primary union of the edges of a wound, progressing to complete scar formation without granulation.

productive cough A sudden expulsion of air from the lungs that effectively removes sputum from the respiratory tract and helps clear the airways.

prolapse Falling, sinking, or sliding of an organ from its normal position or location in the body, such as a prolapsed uterus.

pronation Position of the hand in which the palm of the hand faces downward and backward.

prostaglandins Potent hormonelike substances that act in exceedingly low doses on target organs. They can be used to treat asthma and gastric hyperacidity.

protein Any of a large group of naturally occurring, complex, organic nitrogenous compounds. Each is composed of large combinations of amino acids containing the elements carbon, hydrogen, nitrogen, oxygen, usually sulfur, and occasionally phosphorus, iron, iodine, or other essential constituents of living cells. Protein is the major source of building material for muscles, blood, skin, hair, nails, and the internal organs.

proteinuria Presence in the urine of abnormally large quantities of protein, usually albumin. Persistent proteinuria is usually a sign of renal disease or renal complications of another disease, or hypertension or heart failure.

protocol Written and approved plan specifying the procedures to be followed during an assessment or in providing treatment.

ptosis Abnormal condition of one or both upper eyelids in which the eyelid droops, caused by weakness of the levator muscle or paralysis of the third cranial nerve.

ptyalin Digestive enzyme secreted by the salivary glands.

pulse deficit Condition that exists when the radial pulse is less than the ventricular rate as auscultated at the apex or seen on an electrocardiogram. The condition indicates a lack of peripheral perfusion for some of the heart contractions.

pulse pressure The difference between the systolic and diastolic pressures, normally 30 to 40 mm Hg.

pursed-lip breathing Prolonged expiration through pursed lips. Helpful with COPD.

pyrexia Abnormal elevation of the temperature of the body above 37° C (98.6° F) because of disease. Same as *fever.*

pyrogens Substances that cause a rise in body temperature, as in the case of bacterial toxins.

radial pulse Pulse of the radial artery palpated at the wrist over the radius. The radial pulse is the one most often taken.

radiation Method of temperature regulation used by the body to lower body temperature.

reactive hyperemia Condition characterized by an increased blood flow to part of the body, as in the inflammatory response, local relaxation of arterioles, or obstruction of the outflow of blood from an area.

receptive aphasia Abnormal neurological condition in which language function is defective because of an injury to certain areas of the cerebral cortex; specifically, language is not understood.

recommended daily allowances (RDAs) Suggested or recommended amounts of various nutrients used in planning diets.

reflex pain response Reflected, involuntary withdrawal of a body part away from a noxious or painful stimulus.

religious Relating to specific practices, rites, and rituals of one's professed religion.

reminiscence Recalling the past for the purpose of assigning new meaning to past experiences.

remissions Partial or complete disappearances of the clinical and subjective characteristics of chronic or malignant disease; remission may be spontaneous or the result of therapy.

renal calculi Calcium stones in the renal pelvis.

residual urine Volume of urine remaining in the bladder after a normal voiding; the bladder normally is almost completely empty after micturition.

respite care Short-term health services to the dependent older adult either in his or her home or in an institutional setting.

restraints Devices to aid in the immobilization of a client or client's extremity.

rhonchi Abnormal lung sound auscultated when the client's airways are obstructed with thick secretions.

rooting reflex Normal response of a newborn to move toward whatever touches around the mouth and to attempt to suck.

sebum Normal secretion of the sebaceous glands of the skin; when combined with sweat, forms a moist, oily, acidic film that protects the skin from drying.

sensory deficit Defect in the function of one or more of the senses, resulting in visual, auditory, or olfactory impairments.

sensory deprivation State in which stimulation to one or more of the senses is lacking, resulting in impaired sensory perception.

sensory overload State in which stimulation to one or more of the senses is so excessive that the brain disregards or does not meaningfully respond to stimuli.

serum half-life Time needed for excretion processes to lower the serum drug concentration by half.

sexual response cycle Phases of biological sexual response: excitement, plateau, orgasm, and resolution as defined by Masters and Johnson.

sexuality "A function of the total personality . . . concerned with the biological, psychological, sociological, spiritual and culture variables of life . . ." (Sex Information and Education Council of the United States, 1980).

shearing force Friction exerted when a person is moved or repositioned in bed by being pulled or allowed to slide down in bed.

shivering Process used by the body to raise body temperature.

sleep deprivation Condition resulting from a decrease in the amount, quality, and consistency of sleep.

sleep disorder Condition that interrupts the integrity of a normal sleep pattern, for example, the ability to fall or stay asleep.

sloughing Shedding of dead tissue cells.

socialization Process of being raised within a culture and acquiring the characteristics of the given group.

sterilization (1) Rendering a person unable to produce children; accomplished by surgical, chemical, or other means. (2) A technique for destroying microorganisms using heat, water, chemicals, or gases.

stoma Artificially created opening between a body cavity and the body's surface; for example, a colostomy, formed from a portion of the colon pulled through the abdominal wall.

stressor Any event, situation, or other stimulus encountered in a person's external or internal environment that necessitates change or adaptation by the person.

stroke volume Amount of blood ejected by the ventricles with each contraction.

sublingual Route of medication administration in which the medication is placed underneath the client's tongue.

supination Position of the hand in which the palm of the hand faces upward.

surgical asepsis Procedures used to eliminate any microorganisms from an area. Also called *sterile technique*.

synapse Region surrounding the point of contact between two neurons or between a neuron and an effector organ.

syncope A brief lapse in consciousness caused by transient cerebral hypoxia.

synergistic effect When two drugs act synergistically, the effect of the two drugs combined is greater than the effect that would be expected if the individual effects of the two drugs acting alone were added together.

systole Contraction of the heart, driving blood into the aorta and pulmonary arteries. The occurrence of systole is indicated by the first heart sound heard on auscultation and by the palpable apex beat.

tachycardia Rapid regular heart rate ranging between 100 and 150 beats per minute.

tachypnea Abnormally rapid rate of breathing.

tactile Relating to the sense of touch.

tactile fremitus Tremulous vibration of the chest wall during breathing that is palpable on physical examination.

teratogens Chemical or physiological agents that may produce adverse effects in the embryo or fetus.

territoriality Persistent attachment of a person to a specific area or space.

thermoregulation Internal control of body temperature.

thoracentesis Surgical perforation of the chest wall and pleural space with a needle for the aspiration of fluid or to obtain a specimen for diagnostic or therapeutic purposes.

threshold Point at which a person first perceives a painful stimulus as being painful.

thrombosis Abnormal vascular condition in which a thrombus develops within a blood vessel of the body.

thrombus Accumulation of platelets, fibrin, clotting factors, and the cellular elements of the blood attached to the interior wall of a vein or artery, sometimes occluding the lumen of the vessel.

tinnitus Ringing heard in one or both ears.

tolerance Point at which a person is not willing to accept pain of greater severity or duration.

toxic effect Effect of a medication that results in an adverse response.

trochanter roll Rolled towel support placed against the hips and upper leg to prevent external rotation of the legs.

turgor Normal resiliency of the skin caused by the outward pressure of the cells and interstitial fluid.

urticaria Itchy skin eruption characterized by transient wheals of varying shapes and sizes with well-defined erythematous margins and pale centers.

Valsalva maneuver Any forced expiratory effort against a closed airway, such as when an individual holds the breath and tightens the muscles in a concerted, strenuous effort to move a heavy object or to change positions in bed.

varicosities Abnormal conditions of a vein characterized by swelling and irregular shape or course.

vascular access device Catheters, cannulas, or infusion ports designed for long-term, repeated access to the vascular system.

vasoconstriction Narrowing of the lumen of any blood vessel, especially the arterioles and the veins in the blood reservoirs of the skin and abdominal viscera.

vasodilation Increase in the diameter of a blood vessel caused by inhibition of its vasoconstrictor nerves or stimulation of dilator nerves.

venipuncture Technique in which a vein is punctured transcutaneously by a sharp rigid stylet (e.g., butterfly needle), a cannula (e.g., angiocatheter that contains a flexible plastic catheter), or a needle attached to a syringe.

ventilation Respiratory process by which gases are moved into and out of the lungs.

vertigo Sensation of dizziness, or clients feel as though they are spinning.

virulence Very pathogenic or rapidly progressive condition.

vital signs Temperature, pulse, respirations, and blood pressure.

vitamins Organic compounds essential in small quantities for normal physiological and metabolic functioning of the body. With few exceptions, vitamins cannot be synthesized by the body and must be obtained from the diet or dietary supplements.

voiding The process of urinating.

wheezes Adventitious lung sound caused by a severely narrowed bronchus.

wound culture Specimen collected from a wound to determine the specific organism that is causing an infectious process.

Z-track injection A technique for injecting irritating preparations into muscle without tracking residual medication through sensitive tissues.

INDEX

A

AABB; *see* American Association of Blood Banks
Abbreviations and equivalents, 960-961
Abdomen
  breathing patterns and, 226
  comprehensive health assessment, 317-322
  postoperative pressure dressing, 511
  shift assessment, 269-273
  subcutaneous injection, 457
Abdominal binder, 596, 597-598
Abdominal pain
  comprehensive health assessment, 319
  enema administration and, 185, 188
  during peritoneal dialysis, 915
Abdominal reflex, 337
Abducens nerve, 333
Abduction, 341
  defined, 968
  finger, 626
  foot, 631
  hip, 620
  shoulder, 622
  thumb, 627
  wrist, 625
Abductor splint, 677
Abnormal reactive hyperemia, 968
Abrasion, 122, 579
Absorption, 404
  defined, 968
  intravenous, 711
  oral route, 422
  subcutaneous injection, 457
Acanthamoeba, 834
Accessory muscle, 968
Accident, 73, 74; *see also* Environmental safety
  prevention, discharge teaching, 918-922
Accommodation, 296
Accu-Check Easy, 369
Accu-Check III, 369
Accu-Check Instant, 369
Accu-Chek Advantage, 369
Accurate documentation, 15
Acetaminophen, 537
Acetylsalicylic acid
  heparin therapy, 459
  pain management, 537
Achilles reflex, 337
Acid-base imbalance, 864-868
Acid-fast bacillus smear, 50
Acidosis, 865, 866, 867
ACLS; *see* Advanced cardiac life support
Acne, 122
Activated partial thromboplastin time
  heparin therapy monitoring, 459
  shaving and, 136
Active listening, 34-35
  during interview, 38
Active range of motion
  assessment, 340
  exercise, 618
Active transport, 853, 968
Activities of daily living, 95-220
  activity and mobility promotion, 96-120
    assisted ambulation, 117-120
    bed to chair transfer, 107-112
    bed to chair transfer using mechanical lift, 112-115
    bed to stretcher transfer, 115-117
    moving and positioning clients in bed, 97-105
    nursing diagnoses, 96-97
    orthostatic hypotension, minimizing, 106-107

Activities of daily living–cont'd
  elimination, assisting with, 167-189
    enema administration, 185-189
    external catheter application, 181-184
    incontinence care, 177-181
    intake and output monitoring, 168-173
    nursing diagnosis, 167-168
    providing bedpan and urinal, 173-177
  hygiene promotion, 121-154
    bathing, complete, 123-129
    bedmaking, 147-153
    foot and nail care, 141-147
    hair care, 135-140
    nursing diagnosis, 122
    oral care, 130-135
  infant care, 103-220
    bathing, 212-215
    diaper changing, 214-218
    feeding, 206-211
    swaddling and mummy restraint, 218-220
    thermoregulation using radiant warmer, 204-206
  medications and, 417
  nutrition promotion, 155-166
    feeding dependent clients, 156-160
    impaired swallowing, assisting clients with, 160-162
    obtaining body weights, 163-166
  range of motion exercise for, 618
  sleep, 190-202
    comfort measures promoting, 191-195
    relaxation techniques, 195-202
Activity
  pressure ulcer formation and, 568, 569
  promotion; *see* Activity promotion
Activity intolerance, 96
  assistive devices, 661
  decreased cardiac output, 230
  heart and circulation assessment, 309
  oxygenation promotion, 727
  shift assessment, 256
Activity promotion, 96-120
  assisted ambulation, 117-120
  moving and positioning clients in bed, 97-105
  nursing diagnoses, 96-97
  orthostatic hypotension, minimizing, 106-107
  transfers, 107-117
    from bed to chair, 107-112
    from bed to chair using mechanical lift, 112-115
    from bed to stretcher, 115-117
    from bed to transfer, 115-117
Acuity system, 13
Acute confusion
  hot and cold therapies, 551
  neurologic function assessment, 328
Acute pain, defined, 530
Adaptation, defined, 968
Addiction, 406
Adduction
  assessment, 341
  defined, 968
  finger, 626
  foot, 631
  hip, 620
  shoulder, 622
  thumb, 627
  wrist, 625
Adenosine triphosphate, 853, 854
ADH; *see* Antidiuretic hormone
ADLs; *see* Activities of daily living
Admission patient profile form, 949

Adolescent, isolation precautions, 56
Adrenal gland atrophy in older adult, 864
Adrenalin; *see* Epinephrine
Advance directive
  Patient's Bill of Rights, 10
  resuscitation status, 869
Advanced cardiac life support, 870
Adventitious sounds
  defined, 968
  shift assessment, 263, 265, 266
Adverse reaction, defined, 968
Advil; *see* Ibuprofen
Advocate, nurse as, 3
AED; *see* Automatic external defibrillator
Aerobic culture, 357
Aerochamber, 439
Aerosol spray medication administration, 432
AFB; *see* Acid-fast bacillus
Afebrile, defined, 968
Affect
  neurologic function assessment, 330
  shift assessment, 257
AFO; *see* Ankle-foot orthosis
African American population
  hair care, 135
  infant care, 204
  physical contact, 256
Afterload, defined, 968
Age factors
  drug administration, 418-419
  isolation precautions, 56
  skin, 121
Agency for Health Care Policy and Research
  clinical practice, 3
  defined, 968
  pain management, 531, 532, 533
  pressure ulcer treatment, 577
  urinary incontinence, 167
Aging; *see* Geriatric considerations
Agonist, defined, 404, 405
AHA; *see* American Heart Association
AHCPR; *see* Agency for Health Care Policy and Research
Air bubble in syringe, 464
Air mattress, 602, 603-604
Airborne precautions, 55
Air-fluidized bed, 608-611
Air-mask-bag-unit, 870, 871, 874
Air-suspension bed, 605-608
Airway
  anesthesia complications, 504
  management
    endotracheal tube and tracheostomy care, 747-754
    noninvasive interventions, 735-739
    suctioning, 739-747
Airway clearance
  ineffective, 230
    cardiopulmonary resuscitation, 869-870
    laboratory and diagnostic testing, 345
    oxygenation promotion, 727
    shift assessment, 256
    surgery, 475
    thorax, lung and breast assessment, 299
  risk for ineffective
    newborn, 204
    surgery, 505
Airway obstruction, postoperative, 511
Alanine aminotransferase, 965
Alarm
  as communication aid, 29
  in restraint-free environment, 81
Albumin, 574, 578
Alcohol odor, 256

Aldosterone, 856
Alertness in postanesthesia recovery scoring system, 506
Aleve; *see* Naproxen sodium
Alkaline phosphatase, 965
Alkalosis, 865, 866, 867
Allergen, defined, 968
Allergic contact dermatitis, 429
Allergy
  anesthetic and antiseptic agents, 384, 398
  breath sounds and, 264
  drug, 405-406
    intravenous, 712, 719
  iodinated dye or shellfish, 376, 379, 380
  latex, 53, 65, 70, 429, 478, 479
  in peristomal skin damage, 799
  preoperative assessment, 478
  testing for, 469-472
  urinary catheterization and, 811
Alopecia, 135, 136
ALT; *see* Alanine aminotransferase
Altered body temperature
  pressure ulcers, 567
  risk for, 229-230
Altered bowel elimination, 791-808
  impaction removal, 792-794
  irrigating a colostomy, 803-807
  pouching an enterostomy, 794-802
Altered health maintenance
  discharge planning, 918
  personal hygiene, 122
  range of motion promotion, 617
  risk for
    communication and, 29
    perioperative, 505
Altered nutrition: less than body requirements, 156
  comprehensive health assessment, 317
  enteral nutrition, 776
  oral hygiene, 130
  pressure ulcers, 567
Altered nutrition: more than body requirements, 156, 317
Altered oral mucous membrane
  gastric intubation, 765
  nose, sinus, and mouth assessment, 288
  oral care, 130
  personal hygiene, 122
Altered peripheral tissue perfusion
  hot and cold therapies, 551
  pressure ulcers, 567
Altered protection, 415
Altered sexuality pattern, 322
Altered thought process
  neurologic function assessment, 327-328
  oxygenation promotion, 727
Altered tissue perfusion, 230
  cardiopulmonary resuscitation, 870
  perioperative, 505
  peripheral
    heart and circulation assessment, 309
    shift assessment, 256
Altered urinary elimination, 809-831
  continuous bladder irrigation, 825-827
  nursing diagnosis, 809
  suprapubic catheter, 828-830
  urinary catheterization, 810-818
  urinary diversions, 818-824
Alzheimer's disease, defined, 968
Ambu bag, 870, 871, 874
Ambularm monitoring device, 83-84
Ambulation
  assisted, 117-120
  assistive devices for, 659-681
    cane, crutches, and walker, teaching use of, 665-677
    for fall prevention, 662-665
    nursing diagnosis, 661
    orthotic device, caring for client with, 677-681
American Association of Blood Banks, 720
American Heart Association
  blood pressure documentation, 229
  cardiopulmonary resuscitation, 878

American Hospital Association Patient's Bill of Rights, 10-11
American Nurses Association, 2, 3, 4
Aminoglycosides, 712
Ammonia
  assessment of characteristic odor, 256
  blood, specimen collection and, 361
Amplitude of pulse, 226
Ampule, 451, 452-453, 455
ANA; *see* American Nurses Association
Anacin-3; *see* Acetaminophen
Anaerobic culture, 358
Analgesia
  epidural, 544-550
  patient-controlled, 511, 539-544
    ambulatory infusion pump with, 697
    flow sheet, 543
  postoperative, 511
Analgesic, 537
  cast application, 651
  defined, 968
  effects on sleep, 192
  elimination and, 174
  patient positioning and transfer, 99, 108, 115
  skin patch for administration, 431-432
  spinal traction procedure, 644
Anaphylactic reaction, 405, 406, 968
Anaprox; *see* Naproxen sodium
Aneroid sphygmomanometer, 229
Anesthesia
  complications, 504
  fires resulting from, 73
  local, for central venous line insertion, 891
  postoperative care, 506-512
Anesthetic
  aerosol, 384
  allergy, 384
  blood glucose and, 369
Anger
  effects on elimination, 167
  positive functions of, 42
  in potentially violent client, 42-44
Angina pectoris, defined, 968
Angiography, 376-379, 968
Angle of Louis, 311
Ankle
  range of motion
    assessment, 341
    exercise, 618, 630
  restraint, 87
Ankle-foot orthosis, 677, 678
Anorexia, defined, 968
Antagonist, defined, 404, 405
Antianginal ointment administration, 430-431
Antianxiety agents
  effects on sleep, 192, 194
  for pain management, 537
Antiarrhythmics, 231
Antibiotics
  intravenous administration, 712
  preoperative, 489
  teaching clients about side effects, 416-417
Antibodies, defined, 968
Anticipatory grief, defined, 968
Anticoagulant additive in blood specimen collection, 363
Anticoagulant therapy, shaving and, 136
Antidepressants, 192
Antidiuretic hormone, 856
Antiembolism stocking
  defined, 968
  preoperative application, 489
Antihistamine, 720
Antihypertensives
  effects on vital signs, 231
  hemodialysis and, 910
Antiinflammatory drugs
  effects on vital signs, 231
  heparin therapy and, 459
  for pain management, 533, 537
Antimicrobial agent for surgical hand scrub, 493, 494
Antipyretic, defined, 968

Antiseptic solution
  allergy, 384
  handwashing with, 51
Antithyroid agent, 459
Anus
  bathing of, 127
  surgery, rectal temperature in child and, 233
Anxiety
  casting, 648
  communication and, 29, 40-41
  discharge planning, 918
  effects on elimination, 167
  effects on vital signs, 231
  eye irrigation, 844
  gastrointestinal ostomy, 792
  intravenous therapy, 684
  laboratory and diagnostic testing, 345
  oxygenation promotion, 727
  pain, 532
  sleep and relaxation and, 191
  specialty beds, 601
  surgery, 475
  thoracentesis, 395
  thorax, lung and breast assessment, 299
  traction, 638
AORN; *see* Association of Operating Nurses
AP; *see* Assistive personnel
Aphasia
  communication with older adult and, 28, 34
  defined, 968
  receptive, 973
Apical pulse, 225-226
  comprehensive health assessment, 311-312
  defined, 968
  oximeter pulse rate and, 252, 253
  in pulse deficit, 235
  shift assessment, 266-269
APIE progress notes, 17
Apnea, 228, 236
  defined, 968
Apothecary system, 413, 960, 968
Appearance in neurologic function assessment, 330
Approximate, defined, 968
aPTT; *see* Activated partial thromboplastin time
Aquathermia pad, 556, 557
Arcus senilis, 299
Areola, 304
Arm
  massage, 200
  range of motion exercise, 624
  subcutaneous injection, 457
Arm board, intravenous, 692, 693
Armband for client identification, 9
  drug administration and, 411
Arterial blood gases
  acid-base imbalances, 864
  mechanical ventilation, 904
  normal values, 966
  oxygen therapy, 729, 733
Arterial carbon dioxide tension, 865-866
Arterial hemoglobin saturation
  acid-base imbalance, 865
  pulse oximetry measurement, 249-253
Arterial insufficiency, 275
Arterial oxygen saturation, 966
Arteriography, 376-379
Arteriosclerosis, blood pressure and, 228
Arteriovenous fistula for hemodialysis, 907-908, 909
Artery
  comprehensive health assessment, 314-315
  postoperative hemorrhage, 504
Arthritis, lumbar puncture and, 387
Artificial airway
  care of, 747-754
  communication and, 28
  suctioning, 507, 508, 740, 741, 742, 743-747
  teaching home care, 941-946
Artificial nail, surgical hand scrub and, 494
ASA; *see* Acetylsalicylic acid

Asepsis, 48; *see also* Infection control
  defined, 968
  injection administration, 447
  medical, 48, 971
  surgical, 48, 63-72, 492-493; *see also*
      Infection control
    continuous bladder irrigation, 825
    creating and maintaining a sterile field,
        64-68
    defined, 974
    dressing application, 589
    nursing diagnosis, 64
    perioperative nursing, 492-493
    sterile gloving, 69-72
Asian population
  infant care, 204
  physical contact, 256
Aspartate aminotransferase, 965, 966
Aspergum; *see* Aspirin
Aspiration, 383-396
  as anesthesia complication, 504
  during feeding, 161
  oral medication, 420
  risk for
    enteral nutrition, 776
    gastric intubation, 765
    laboratory and diagnostic testing, 345
    nutrition and, 156
    perioperative, 505
  in subcutaneous injection, 459
Aspiration tray, 383
Aspirin
  heparin therapy and, 459
  for pain management, 537
Assessment, 6, 7
  in change-of-shift report, 20
  comprehensive, 280-343
    abdomen, 317-322
    examination techniques, 281-283
    eyes and ears, 293-299
    general survey, 280
    genitalia and rectum, 322-327
    head, face, and neck, 283-288
    heart and circulation, 309-317
    musculoskeletal function, 339-343
    neurologic function, 327-338
    nose, sinuses, and mouth, 288-292
    thorax, lungs, and breasts, 299-308
  defined, 968
  drug therapy, 415
  licensed practical or vocational nurse's role
      in, 5
  nursing assessment form in, 6, 956-957
  preoperative, 476-479
  recording of, 12
  shift, 255-279
    abdomen, 269-273
    apical pulse, 266-269
    extremities and peripheral circulation,
        274-279
    general survey and integumentary inspec-
        tion, 257-262
    lung sounds, 262-266
    nursing diagnosis, 256
  standards of nursing practice and, 4
Assessment form, 6, 956-957
  preoperative, 477
Assimilation, defined, 968
Assisted ambulation, 117-120
Assistive devices for ambulation, 659-681
  cane, crutches, and walker, teaching use of,
      665-677
  for fall prevention, 662-665
  nursing diagnosis, 661
  orthotic device, caring for client with,
      677-681
Assistive personnel, 5
  active listening, 34
  defined, 968
Association of Operating Nurses
  sterile field, 63
  surgical hand scrub, 493
AST; *see* Aspartate aminotransferase

Atelectasis
  defined, 968
  during mechanical ventilation, 906
Athlete's foot, 142, 143
ATP; *see* Adenosine triphosphate
Atrioventricular node, defined, 968
Atrioventricular shunt, restraints and, 85
Atrophy
  adrenal gland, 864
  cutaneous, 261
Attention in neurologic function assessment,
    332
Audiotape change-of-shift report, 19
Auditory, defined, 968
Auditory nerve, 333
Auditory sensory/perceptual alterations, 832
  communication and, 29
  drug therapy, 415
  ear irrigation, 848-850
  eye and ear assessment, 293
  hearing aid client, caring for, 845-848
Auricle assessment, 297
Auscultation, 255, 282
  apical pulse
    comprehensive health assessment,
        311-312
    shift assessment, 226
  bowel sounds
    altered elimination and, 174
    comprehensive health assessment,
        319-320
    enema administration, 185
    enteral nutrition, 780, 783
    postoperative assessment, 515
    shift assessment, 270-272
  defined, 968
  Korotkoff sounds, 229, 230
  lung sounds
    intravenous therapy, 702
    mechanical ventilation, 904
    shift assessment, 262-266
Auscultatory gap, defined, 968
Autologous transfusion, 721, 968
Automatic external defibrillator, 877, 878
Autonomic nervous system, 191
Autonomy, defined, 968
Autopsy, 882, 968
Autotransfusion
  defined, 968
  postoperative, 754-764
AV; *see* Atrioventricular
Axillary crutch, 659, 660
Axillary temperature, 234, 240
  advantages and disadvantages, 224
  normal ranges, 223
  postanesthesia recovery scoring system, 506
  thermometer used for, 223

B

B lymphocyte, normal values, 965
Babinski's reflex, 337
Back
  bathing, 128
  subcutaneous injection, 457
Backrub for relaxation, 195-196, 201
Bacteria, urinary, 966
Bacteriuria, defined, 968
Balance scale, calibrated beam, 166
Balanced traction, 636
Balanced-suspension skeletal traction, 642
Baldness, 140
Balloon inflation for indwelling catheter,
    815, 816
Bandage application, 594-599
Bariatric bed, 601, 614-615
Barrier precautions, 48; *see also* Infection control
Base excess, normal values, 966
Basophils, normal values, 965
Bathing
  complete, 123-129
  infant, 203, 212-215
Bathing/hygiene self-care deficit, 122
  casting, 648
  nose, sinus and mouth assessment, 288

Bathing/hygiene self-care deficit,—cont'd
  oral hygiene, 130
  traction, 638
Bathroom, safety and, 77, 78
Bathtub, safety features, 77
Bayer Aspirin; *see* Aspirin
Beam balance scale, 166
Beard care, 136, 139
Bed, 601-616
  air-fluidized, 608-611
  air-suspension, 605-608
  bariatric, 614-615
  moving and positioning clients in, 97-105
  nursing diagnosis, 601
  pressure ulcer prevention, 576
  Rotokinetic, 611-613
  safety measures, 77, 79-80
  with support surface mattress, 602-605
  transfers; *see* Bed transfer
  weight-sensitive alarm placed under, 81, 82
Bed scale, 165
Bed transfer
  to chair, 107-112
    using mechanical lift, 112-115
  to stretcher, 115-117
Bedmaking, 147-153
Bedpan, 173-177
Bedroom, home hazard assessment, 78
Behavior
  health, 970
  manifestations during anxiety, 40-41
  neurologic function assessment, 330
  pain indicators, 534, 535
  shift assessment, 257
Behavioral restraint flow sheet, 90
Behind-the-ear hearing aid, 845
Bell
  as communication aid, 29
  for safety, 77, 79
Belt
  restraint, 86
  safety, 666, 668
  transfer, 107
Benign prostatic hyperplasia, 827
Bereavement, defined, 968
Beta blockers, 192
Bevel of needle, 447, 448
Bicarbonate, 864, 866
  normal values, 965, 966
Biceps reflex, 337
Bilevel positive airway pressure, 735
Bilirubin, normal values, 965
Bill of Rights, Patient's, 10-11
Binder application, 594-599
Bioavailability, defined, 968
Biochemical parameters in nutritional assess-
    ment, 155
Biofeedback for pain management, 532
Biopsy, liver, 383-396
Biot's respiration, 228
BiPAP; *see* Bilevel positive airway pressure
Bladder
  comprehensive health assessment, 317-322
  continuous irrigation, 825-827
  training for incontinence, 178
Blanket continuous suture, 524-525, 528
Blanket for client removal during fire, 75
Bleeding
  blood pressure and, 231
  in continuous bladder irrigation, 827
  during dialysis, 910
  enema administration and, 188
  from heparin therapy, 459
  postoperative, 504-505, 510, 511
Bleeding time, normal values, 965
Blood
  culture, 360-367
  normal values, 965-966
  specimen collection, 360-367
    during dialysis, 910
    through central venous lines, 896
  Standard Precautions, 49
  typing, 720, 721
  urine screening test, 370-371

Blood clot, 825
Blood glucose
    monitoring, 368
    normal values, 965
Blood pressure, 228-229, 230, 231-232,
        236-239, 241-242
    during assisted ambulation, 119
    bed to chair transfer and, 114
    blood transfusion and, 725
    during bronchoscopy, 392
    electronic, 245-249
    elevated; see Hypertension
    during endoscopy, 393, 395
    epidural analgesia and, 546
    normal ranges, 223
    in orthostatic hypotension, 106, 312
    in shift assessment, 257
Blood pressure cuff, 229, 246, 247-248
Blood transfusion, 720-725
    postoperative autotransfusion, 754-764
Blood urea nitrogen
    fluid imbalances, 858
    normal values, 966
Blood volume, 228
Blurred vision from contact lens, 838
Body
    alignment, patient positioning and, 97, 98
    movement in shift assessment, 257
Body cast, 649
Body fluid
    composition and distribution, 852-856
    imbalance
        etiologic factors, 8
        gastric intubation, 765
        intravenous therapy, 683
        monitoring, 857-859
        in monitoring intake and output, 168,
            171
        nursing diagnosis, 856-857
        perioperative, 505
        vital signs in, 230
    Standard Precautions, 49
Body hearing aid, 846
Body image disturbance
    gastrointestinal ostomy, 792
    musculoskeletal system assessment, 339
    oral hygiene, 130
    personal hygiene, 122
    urinary elimination, altered, 809
Body language, 26
Body lice, 136
Body mechanics, patient positioning and, 96,
        97
Body odor
    bathing for reduction, 121
    shift assessment, 255, 256
Body Substance Isolation, 48-49; see also
        Infection control
Body temperature, 222-225, 231, 232-234,
        239-240
    altered
        pressure ulcers, 567
        risk for, 229-230
    blood transfusion, 721, 725
    newborn
        bathing and, 212
        cold stress in, 205
    normal ranges, 222, 223
    during peritoneal dialysis, 915
    postanesthesia recovery scoring system, 506
    postoperative, 514
    regulation of; see Thermoregulation
    shift assessment, 257
    tympanic, 243-245
Body type in shift assessment, 257
Body weight
    fluid volume deficit, 856
    height and weight tables, 967
    monitoring intake and output, 168, 169
    obtaining, 163-166
    pressure ulcer formation, 578
    subcutaneous injection, 457, 461
    surgical wound healing, 517

Bonding, defined, 969
Bone marrow aspiration, 383-396
Bone resorption, defined, 969
Bone scan, 380-381
Bony prominence, massage and, 128
Bounding pulse, 226
Bowel elimination, 791-808
    impaction removal, 792-794
    irrigating a colostomy, 803-807
    pouching an enterostomy, 794-802
    pressure ulcer formation and, 572
    providing bedpan for, 173-177
Bowel incontinence, 168
Bowel sounds
    altered elimination, 174
    comprehensive health assessment, 319-320
    enema administration, 185
    enteral nutrition, 780
    postoperative assessment, 515
    shift assessment, 270-272
BP; see Blood pressure
BPH; see Benign prostatic hyperplasia
Brace, caring for client with, 677-681
Bracelet for client identification, 9
    drug administration and, 411
Brachial pulse
    comprehensive health assessment, 314, 315
    defined, 969
Braden Scale, 568, 569-570
Bradycardia, 226, 241, 969
Bradypnea, 228, 969
Braiding hair, 138
Brain scan, 380-381
Brain syndrome, organic, 972
Breast assessment, 299-308
Breast binder, 596, 598-599
Breast cancer, risk factors, 300-301
Breast self-examination, 306
    in older women, 308
Breastfeeding, 203, 206
    assisting with, 208-210
    bone scan and, 380
    as nursing diagnosis, 204
Breath sounds
    intravenous therapy, 702
    mechanical ventilation, 904
    shift assessment, 262-266
Breathing
    anesthesia complications, 504
    deep, preoperative teaching, 483
Breathing pattern
    ineffective, 230, 345
        cardiopulmonary resuscitation, 869
        comprehensive health assessment, 288,
            299
        oxygenation promotion, 727
        perioperative, 505
        shift assessment, 256
Bronchodilators
    for airway management, 735
    effects on vital signs, 231
Bronchoscopy, 383-396, 969
Bronchospasm as anesthesia complication, 504
Bruit, defined, 969
Bryant's traction, 636, 638
BSE; see Breast self-examination
BSI; see Body Substance Isolation
BSST; see Balanced-suspension skeletal trac-
        tion
BTE hearing aid; see Behind-the-ear hearing
        aid
Buccal, defined, 969
Buccal drug administration, 421, 427
Buck's traction, 636, 637, 639-641
Buffer, defined, 969
Buffer system, 864
BUN; see Blood urea nitrogen
Bundle of His, defined, 969
Bunion, 146
Burns
    fluid balance alteration, 855
    prevention in home, 921
Buttock, bathing of, 127

C

Cachexia, defined, 969
Caffeine
    effects on vital signs, 231
    sleep and, 193
Calcium
    imbalance, 859, 860, 861-863
    normal values, 965
Calculi, renal, 973
Calibrated beam balance scale, 166
Call bell
    as communication aid, 29
    for safety, 77, 79
Call light, 77
Callus, 141, 142, 143, 145
Canadian crutch, 659
Cancer
    breast, 300-301
    pulmonary, 264, 300
Candida, 799
Cane, 659, 660, 665-677
CAPD; see Continuous ambulatory peritoneal
        dialysis
Capillary, postoperative hemorrhage, 505
Capillary blood glucose test, 368
Capillary refill
    pulse oximetry site selection, 252
    shift assessment, 276
    skin traction and, 640
    vascular assessment, 314
    venous and arterial insufficiency, 275
Capsule medication, 412, 416, 424
    administration through feeding tube, 787,
        788
Carbon dioxide
    in acid-base balance, 864
    retention during oxygen therapy, 734
Carbon dioxide partial pressure, normal val-
        ues, 966
Carbonic acid, 864
Carcinogen, defined, 969
Cardiac arrest
    cardiopulmonary resuscitation for, 870-876
    code management, 877-882
Cardiac catheterization, 396-401
Cardiac dysrhythmia, 226
    as anesthesia complication, 504
    inhaled medication and, 441
    during peritoneal dialysis, 915
    suctioning induction of, 745, 747
Cardiac enzymes, normal values, 966
Cardiac output
    decreased, 230
        cardiopulmonary resuscitation, 870
        heart and circulation assessment, 309
        perioperative, 505
        shift assessment, 256
    defined, 969
Cardiac studies, 396-401
Cardiopulmonary resuscitation, 870-876
    code management, 877-882
    nursing diagnosis, 869
Cardiopulmonary resuscitation switch, 606
Cardiotonics, effects on vital signs, 231
Cardiovascular system
    cardiac studies, 396-401
    comprehensive health assessment, 309-317
    disease, blood pressure and, 231
Care of dying, 3
Caregiver, nurse as, 3
Caregiver role strain, 727
CareMaps, 3
Caries, 131
Carotid pulse
    comprehensive health assessment, 312
    in older adult, 317
    defined, 969
Carpuject injection system, 449, 450
Carrier, defined, 969
Cart
    medication, 408, 416
    resuscitation, 870, 871
Case management, 3, 13

Cast care, 648-658
    application, assessment, and care, 650-655
    nursing diagnosis, 648
    removal, 655-658
Casts, urinary, 966
Cathartic, defined, 969
Catheterization
    blood transfusion, 721
    defined, 969
    epidural, 544-550
    external, 181-184
    indwelling
        expected postoperative drainage, 505
        sterile urine specimen from, 346-347,
            351-352
    suprapubic, 828-830
    urinary, 810-818
        sterile urine specimen from, 346-347
        teaching home self-catheterization,
            932-936
CAVH; see Continuous arteriovenous hemofil-
    tration
CAVU; see Continuous arteriovenous ultrafil-
    tration
CBE; see Charting by exception
CBI; see Continuous bladder irrigation
CCPD; see Continuous cycling peritoneal dial-
    ysis
CDC; see Centers for Disease Control and
    Prevention
Cecostomy, 797
Centers for Disease Control and Prevention
    infusion tubing, changing of, 703
    isolation precautions, 48, 55
    needleless infusion lines, 712
    needle-stick prevention, 449
    postsurgical drainage collection, 521
    Standard Precautions, 49
    tuberculosis precautions, 49, 50
    wound infection, 566
Central nervous system, 504
Central venous lines, 889-897
Cephalosporin, 459
Certified nursing assistant, 5
Cerumen
    comprehensive health assessment, 297
    defined, 969
    ear drop administration and, 437
    older adult, 245
    removal, 848-850
Cervical collar, 677
Cervical traction, 636, 637, 639
Chair
    jacket restraint for client sitting in, 88
    pressure ulcer prevention, 576
    safety features, 77
    shower, 77
    sit in with crutches, 674
    transfer from bed to, 107-112
        using mechanical lift, 112-115
    weight-sensitive alarm placed under, 81, 82
Chair scale, 164-165
Change-of-shift report, 19-21
Changing diaper, 214-218
Channel, defined, 969
Charting, focus, 17
Charting by exception, 16, 969
Checklist, preoperative, 486
CheckMate Plus, 369
Cheek
    comprehensive health assessment, 291
    food found pocketed in, 162
Chemotherapy
    effects on hair, 135
    oral hygiene and, 130
    wound healing, delayed, 567
Chemstrip testing, 368-375
Chest
    compression in cardiopulmonary resuscita-
        tion, 875-876
    palpation, 301-302
    percussion, 282
Chest drainage systems, 754-764
Cheyne-Stokes respiration, 228

CHF; see Congestive heart failure
Child
    Bryant's traction, 636, 638
    cardiopulmonary resuscitation, 874, 875
    drug administration, 418, 428
        metered-dose inhalers, 441
    drug dosages, 411
    fluid volume deficit, 856
    isolation, 50
    lumbar puncture, 387, 396
    pain assessment, 533, 534
    point of maximal impulse location in, 266
    removal during fire, 75
    shift assessment, 279
    specimen collection, 259, 375
        blood, 367
        urine, 351
    temperature measurement, 233, 234
Children's Advil; see Ibuprofen
Chloride, normal values, 965
Choking, 160, 162
Cholecystography, oral, 376-379
Cholesterol, normal values, 966
Cholesterol intake, 158
Chronic confusion, 551
Chronic nonmalignant pain, defined, 530
Chronic obstructive pulmonary disease, 855
Chronic pain, 317, 532
Cigarette smoking
    breath sounds and, 264
    effects on vital signs, 231
    fire safety and, 73
Circadian rhythm, defined, 969
Circular bandage turn, 595
Circulating nurse, 492, 969
Circulation
    anesthesia complications, 504
    bathing for stimulation, 121
    comprehensive health assessment, 309-317
    delayed wound healing and, 567
    foot assessment and, 140
    postanesthesia recovery scoring system, 506
    shift assessment, 274-279
Circulation, sensation, and motion, 261
Circumcision, 214
Circumduction
    defined, 969
    hip, 620
    shoulder, 622
Civilian time, 15
Claustrophobia, 393
Clean glove, use, 53-54
Clean technique, 48; see also Infection control
Clean-voided urine specimen, 346, 349-350
Clear-liquid diet, 158
Client
    admission patient profile form, 949-953
    armband for identification, 9
    positioning
        airway management, 735, 736-737
        in bed, 97-105
        bone marrow aspiration, 386
        cardiopulmonary resuscitation, 872
        feeding, 158
        female genitalia assessment, 323
        liver biopsy, 390, 391
        lumbar puncture, 386-387
        lung auscultation, 264
        to minimize orthostatic hypotension,
            106-107
        paracentesis, 388
        pressure ulcer formation, 573-574
        rectal temperature measurement, 233
        shampooing of hair, 135, 137-138
        shift assessment, 257
        urinary catheterization, 811-812
    removal during fire, 75
    teaching; see Client teaching
Client advocate, nurse as, 3
Client teaching, 44-46
    communication and, 29
    discharge, 917-946
        home oxygen equipment, 936-940
        non-parenteral medication self-
            administration, 922-926

Client teaching—cont'd
    discharge—cont'd
        nursing diagnosis, 918
        risk assessment and accident prevention,
            918-922
        self-catheterization, 932-936
        self-injection, 926-931
        tracheostomy care, 941-946
    foot care, 145-146
    isolation precautions, 56
    medication administration, 416-417
    pain management, 532
    preoperative, 480-485
Clinitron bed, 608
Clinoril; see Sulindac
Clitoris assessment, 324
Closed chest drainage system, 754-764
Closed gloving, 497-501
Closed wound, 578
Cloth diaper, 215
Clotting; see Coagulation
Clotting time, normal values, 965
Clove-hitch restraint, 87
Coaching while feeding client, 162
Coagulation
    cardiac catheterization and, 398
    disseminated intravascular, 136
    flossing of teeth and, 134
    shaving and, 136
Code management, 877-882
Codeine sulfate, 537
Cognitive function, 417
Cold, therapeutic use, 551, 552, 559-563
    compress and ice bags, 559-562
    nursing diagnosis, 551
    pain management, 532
Cold stress in newborn, 205
Collaboration, defined, 969
Collagen, 566
Colon, defined, 969
Colonic constipation, 168
Colonized, defined, 969
Colonoscopy, 385
Color, skin, 259
Colostomy, 791, 797
    irrigation, 803-807
Comfort measures, 32-33
    newborn swaddling, 218
    postoperative, 510, 512-516
    promoting sleep, 190-202
Communication, 25-46
    active listening, 34-35
    aids in, 29
    with an anxious client, 40-41
    client teaching, 44-46
    comforting, 32-33
    cultural considerations, 26-28
    drug administration and, 407-412
    establishing therapeutic communication,
        29-31
    geriatric considerations, 28
    within health care team, 12-13
    impaired verbal
        hearing impairment, 833
        oxygenation promotion, 727
    interviewing, 36-39
    nursing diagnosis, 28-29
    verbally deescalating a potentially violent
        client, 42-44
Compartment syndrome
    after cast application, 654
    postoperative, 504, 511
Complete blood count, normal values, 965
Complete documentation, 15
Compliance, defined, 969
Comprehensive health assessment, 280-343
    abdomen, 317-322
    examination techniques, 281-283
    eyes and ears, 293-299
    general survey, 280
    genitalia and rectum, 322-327
    head, face, and neck, 283-288
    heart and circulation, 309-317
    musculoskeletal function, 339-343

Comprehensive health assessment–cont'd
  neurologic function, 327-338
  nose, sinuses, and mouth, 288-292
  thorax, lungs, and breasts, 299-308
Compress
  cold, 559-562
  defined, 969
  moist heat, 553-556
Computed tomography, 376-379
Computerized documentation system, 13
Computerized patient care summary, 14
Concentration in neurologic function assessment, 332
Confidentiality, 10, 16
Confusion
  hot and cold therapies, 551
  intravenous therapy, 702
  neurologic function assessment, 328
Congestive heart failure, 855
Conjugated bilirubin, 965
Conjunctiva, 297
Conjunctivitis, 833
Consent, signed
  angiography and computed tomography, 377
  bronchoscopy, magnetic resonance imaging and endoscopy, 384
  surgical, 487, 488
Constavac, 521-522
Constipation
  abdominal assessment, 317
  colonic, 168
  enteral nutrition, 776
  fecal impaction, 185, 792
  older adult, 327
  perceived, 168
  shift assessment, 256
Constrictors, effects on vital signs, 231
Contact dermatitis, 122
  allergic, 429
Contact lens client, caring for, 833-839
Contact precautions, 55
Contaminated, defined, 969
Contaminated linen, 49
Contaminated wound, 579
Continent urinary diversion, 818-824
Continuous ambulatory peritoneal dialysis, 912
Continuous arteriovenous hemofiltration, 912
Continuous arteriovenous ultrafiltration, 912
Continuous bladder irrigation, 825-827
Continuous cycling peritoneal dialysis, 912
Continuous passive motion machine, 632-635
Continuous positive airway pressure, 735, 738-739, 902
  to promote sleep, 193
Continuous suture, 524-525, 527-528
Contracture, defined, 969
Contrast media studies, 376-379
Controlled II substances, 417-419
Controlled Substances Act, 418
Contusion, 579
Convalescent phase, comfort measures in, 512-516
Conversion, drug, 412-413
COPD; see Chronic obstructive pulmonary disease
Coping
  ineffective
    communication and, 29
    gastrointestinal ostomy, 792
    oxygenation promotion, 727
    pain, 532
    surgery, 475
    urinary elimination, altered, 809
  strategies for anxious client, 41
Core temperature, 243, 969
Corn, 141, 142, 143, 145, 147
Cornea
  comprehensive health assessment, 297
  contact lenses and, 833-834
Corneal light reflex, 296
Cortisone, 168

Costal angle, 308
Costal spaces, 302
Costovertebral angle, 321
Cotton-tipped swab, 282
Cough
  airway management, 735, 738
  breath sounds and, 264, 265
  preoperative teaching, 483
  productive, 973
  in tuberculosis, 60
  while feeding client, 162
Coumadin
  dose calculation, 411
  shaving and, 136
Counselor, nurse as, 3
Countertraction, 636
CPAP; see Continuous positive airway pressure
CPK; see Creatine phosphokinase
CPM; see Continuous passive motion
CPR; see Cardiopulmonary resuscitation
Crab lice, 136
Cracked lip, 131
Crackles, 263, 265
  defined, 969
  during intravenous therapy, 702
  from Rotokinetic bed, 613
Cradle cap, 215
Cradle hold for breastfeeding, 208
Cramping, enema administration and, 188
Cranial nerves
  comprehensive health assessment, 284, 285, 295-296, 332, 333
  role in swallowing, 160
Cream medication, 430
  vaginal, 444
Creatine kinase, 966
Creatine phosphokinase, 966
Creatinine, 966
Crede's method, 178
Crepitus, 342
Criteria, defined, 969
Critical pathways, 3, 13
Crutch, 659-661, 665-677
Crutch palsy, 661
Cryoglobulins, 361
Crystals, urinary, 966
CSM; see Circulation, sensation, and motion
CT; see Computed tomography
Cuff, blood pressure, 229, 246, 247-248
Cultural considerations
  active listening, 36
  bathing, 124
  communication, 26-28, 34
  hair care, 135
  infant care, 204, 212
  shift assessment, 256
Culture, 346-359
  assessment, 347
  blood, 360-367
  defined, 969
  equipment, 346-347
  evaluation, 358-359
  implementation, 354-358
  planning, 347-348
Cup, specimen, 282
Current documentation, 15
Cyanosis
  defined, 969
  shift assessment, 259
Cycloplegics, 433

D

Dandruff, 136
DAR progress notes, 17
Darvon; see Propoxyphene hydrochloride
Darvon-N; see Propoxyphene napsylate
Data, subjective, 14
Database, interview, 36
Death
  care of body after, 882-885, 886
  defined, 969
  from falls, 73
Débridement, 577, 969

Decreased cardiac output, 230
  cardiopulmonary resuscitation, 870
  heart and circulation comprehensive assessment, 309
  perioperative, 505
  shift assessment, 256
Decubitus ulcer, 565
Deep breathing, preoperative teaching, 483
Deep palpation, 281
Deep tendon reflexes, 337, 338
Deep vein thrombosis, 126
Defecation; see also Bowel elimination
  defined, 969
  providing bedpan for, 173-177
Defensive stage of wound healing, 566
Defibrillation, 870, 877, 879-880
Dehiscence
  defined, 969
  surgical wound, 529
Dehydration
  blood pressure and, 231
  newborn, 211
  oral hygiene and, 130
Delegation, 3-5
  active listening, 34
Deltoid intramuscular injection, 464, 466
Dementia
  comprehensive health assessment, 330, 331
  defined, 969
Demerol; see Meperidine
Dental caries, 131
Dental-soft diet, 158
Denture care, 130, 131, 133
Department of Health and Human Services, 3
Dependence, drug, 406
Dependent client, 564-681
  assistive devices for ambulation, 659-681
    cane, crutches, and walker, teaching use of, 665-677
    for fall prevention, 662-665
    nursing diagnosis, 661
    orthotic device, caring for client with, 677-681
  cast care, 648-658
    application, assessment, and care, 650-655
    nursing diagnosis, 648
    removal, 655-658
  contact lens care, 833-839
  feeding, 156-160
  mattresses and beds, 601-616
    air-fluidized bed, 608-611
    air-suspension bed, 605-608
    bariatric bed, 614-615
    nursing diagnosis, 601
    Rotokinetic bed, 611-613
    support surface mattress, 602-605
  pressure ulcer and wound care management, 565-600
    binder and bandage application, 594-599
    dressing application, 585-591
    nursing diagnosis, 567
    pressure ulcer risk assessment and prevention strategies, 568-576
    pressure ulcer treatment, 577-585
    transparent dressing, changing, 592-594
  range of motion promotion, 617-635
    continuous passive motion machine, 632-635
    nursing diagnosis, 617
    range of motion exercise, 98, 618-633
  traction, 636-647
    nursing diagnosis, 638
    skeletal, 637-638, 642-646
    skin, 636, 637, 638, 639-641
Depression
  effects on hair, 135
  elimination and, 167
Depth of respiration, 226
Dermatitis, 122, 429
Dermis, defined, 969
Descending colostomy, 797

DHHS; *see* Department of Health and Human Services
Diabetes mellitus
 diet in, 158
 foot care, 140, 141
 management record, 954-955
 oral hygiene, 130
 soaking of feet, 126
 wound healing, 517, 567
Diagnosis, 6-8, 962-964
 in change-of-shift report, 20
 communication and, 28-29
 high-risk, 6
 infection control and, 50
 licensed practical or vocational nurse's role in, 5
 standards of nursing practice and, 4
Diagnosis-related groups, 3
Diagnostic studies, 383-396; *see also* Laboratory testing
Dialysate, 907, 911
Dialysis
 hemodialysis, 907-911
 peritoneal, 911-915
Diaper
 adult, 180
 changing, 214-218
Diaper rash, 215
Diaphoresis
 air-fluidized bed and, 608
 bathing and, 123
 defined, 969
 effects on hair, 135
Diaphragm, movement during inspiration and expiration, 226, 228
Diarrhea
 comprehensive health assessment of abdomen, 317
 enteral nutrition, 776
 fecal impaction, 185, 792
 infant, after feeding, 211
 as nursing diagnosis, 168
 pressure ulcer formation and, 572
 rectal temperature in child and, 233
 shift assessment, 256
Diascan-S, 369
Diastole, defined, 969
Diastolic blood pressure, 229
 defined, 228
 in orthostatic hypertension, 312
Diet, 155, 158; *see also* Nutrition
Dietitian, 155
Diffusion, 226, 853, 854
 defined, 969
 oxygen delivery and, 869
Dilaudid, 537
Dilutional hyponatremia, 860
Dimensional analysis for dosage calculation, 413, 414
Diplopia, defined, 969
Direct-question technique, 36
Discharge teaching, 917-946
 home oxygen equipment, 936-940
 non-parenteral medication self-administration, 922-926
 nursing diagnosis, 918
 risk assessment and accident prevention, 918-922
 self-catheterization, 932-936
 self-injection, 926-931
 tracheostomy care, 941-946
Disinfection
 contact lens, 836
 defined, 969
Disposable contact lens, 833
Disposable diaper, 215
Disposable glove
 application of, 57
 for physical examination, 282
 use, 53-54
Disposable injection unit, 449, 450
Disposable thermometer, 225, 226
Disseminated intravascular coagulation, 136

Distention
 abdominal
  comprehensive health assessment, 319
  shift assessment, 272
 neck vein, 313, 316
Distraction technique, 41, 44
Distress in shift assessment, 257
Distribution, drug, 404
Disuse syndrome, risk for, 96-97, 532
Diuresis, defined, 969
Diuretics
 blood glucose and, 369
 in blood transfusion, 720
Dizziness
 assistive device ambulation, 676
 orthostatic hypotension, 106, 107
Dobutamine
 code management, 881
 stress echocardiography, 396-401
Dobutrex; *see* Dobutamine
Documentation, 12-22
 change-of-shift report, 19-21
 communication within health care team and, 12-13
 computerized, 13
 confidentiality in, 16
 guidelines for effective, 13
 home health care, 16
 incident report, 21-22
 long-term care, 16
 medical records, 13, 14, 15
 medication error, 418
 reporting and recording guidelines, 13-16, 17-19
 sample forms, 949-959
 time of death, 882, 885, 886
Donor
 blood, 720
 organ/tissue, 882-883
Dopamine, 881
Dorsalis pedis pulse
 comprehensive health assessment, 314, 315
 defined, 969
 nonpalpable after angiography, 379
 shift assessment, 277
Dorsiflexion, 969
Dorsogluteal intramuscular injection, 464
Dosage
 calculation, 411, 413-415, 960
 intravenous administration, 711
Douche, vaginal, 445
Drain dressing, 586
Drainage
 bathing and, 123
 eye prosthesis, 842
 paracentesis site, 388
 postoperative, 504-505, 510
 postural, 973
 shift assessment, 262
 wound
  specimen collection, 345, 347, 354, 357
  surgical, 516, 517
  types, 567
Drainage devices
 chest, 754-764
 postoperative measuring and monitoring, 520-524
 restraints and, 85
Drape, sterile, 64
Dressing
 application, 585-591
  transparent, 592-594
 central venous lines, 889, 894-896
 intravenous therapy site, 690-691, 703, 704, 705-706, 710
 shift assessment, 262
 surgical, 511, 514
 changing, 518
Dressing change kit, sterile, 64, 65
Dressing/grooming self-care deficit
 casting, 648
 personal hygiene and, 122
 traction, 638
DRGs; *see* Diagnosis-related groups

Droplet precautions, 55
Dropper, scaled, 411
Drug administration, 404-419
 age factors, 418-419
 client and family teaching, 416-417, 922-926
 communication and transcription of orders, 407-412
 during dialysis, 910
 drug actions and, 404-407
 drug effects and, 404, 405
 generic *versus* trade name, 412
 injections, 447-473
  intradermal, 469-472
  intramuscular, 464-469
  nursing diagnosis, 451
  preparation, 451, 452-453, 454, 455, 456
  subcutaneous, 457-463
  syringes, 447-451
  teaching self-injection, 926-931
 intravenous, 711-720
 measurement systems, 413-415
 non-parenteral, 420-446
  eye and ear, 433-438
  metered-dose inhalers, 438-441
  oral, 422-428
  rectal and vaginal, 442-445
  topical, 429-433
 nursing process, 415-416
 physicians's order for, 406-407
 preparations for, 412-413
 routes of, 406, 407
 special handling of controlled II substances, 417-419
 through feeding tube, 787-790
Drug dependence, 406
Drug dosage
 calculation, 411, 413-415, 960
 intravenous administration, 711
Drug history
 in interview, 39
 preoperative assessment, 478
Drug label, 410, 412
Drugs
 administration; *see* Drug administration
 effects of, 404, 405
  on sleep, 192
  on vital signs, 231
 interactions, 406
 mild reactions to, 405
 neurologic function and, 328
 pharmacokinetics, 404-407
 tolerance and dependence, 406
 urine output and, 168
Dry dressing, 585-586, 590
Dry heat, 556-559
Dry skin, 122
 bathing and, 129
 newborn, 215
Dullness, 282
Dunlop's traction, 636, 637
Durable power of attorney, 10
Duragesic; *see* Fentanyl transdermal system
Duramorph; *see* Morphine
DVWR; *see* Dysfunctional ventilatory weaning response
Dying, care of, 3
Dysarthria, 35
Dysfunctional grieving, 870
Dysfunctional ventilatory weaning response, 727
Dyspnea, 226-228
 during assisted ambulation, 119
 in blood transfusion, 725
 defined, 969
 following allergy skin testing, 472
 respiration assessment and, 236
Dysrhythmia, 226
 as anesthesia complication, 504
 defined, 969
 inhaled medication and, 441
 during peritoneal dialysis, 915
 suctioning induction of, 745, 747
Dysuria, defined, 969

E

E tank oxygen source, 939-940
Ear
  assessment, 293-299
  cleansing, 294
    newborn, 213
  feeding tube measurement and, 778
  irrigation, 848-850
  medication instillation, 433-438
Ecchymosis
  defined, 969
  shift assessment, 259
ECF; *see* Extracellular fluid
ECG; *see* Electrocardiography
Echocardiography, dobutamine stress, 396-401
Ecotrin; *see* Aspirin
Eczema, 405
Edema
  after cast removal, 657
  defined, 969
  in fluid volume excess, 858
  laryngeal as anesthesia complication, 504
  shift assessment, 259, 276
  skeletal traction, 645, 646
Education; *see* Client teaching
Effective breast-feeding, 204
Effleurage massage, 199
Effluent, 791, 969
EGD; *see* Esophagogastroduodenoscopy
Egg-crate foam overlay, 602
Egocentricity, defined, 969
Elastic bandage, 594
Elbow, range of motion
  assessment, 341
  exercise, 618, 623
Electric heating pad, 557
Electrical fire, 73
Electrocardiography, 396-401
  during bronchoscopy, 392
  during endoscopy, 393, 395
Electrolyte imbalance, 856-857, 859-864
Electronic blood pressure measurement, 245-249
Electronic device for a restraint-free environment, 81-82, 83-84
Electronic scale for weighing infant, 166
Electronic thermometer, 223-225
Elimination, 167-189
  bowel, 791-808
    enema administration, 185-189
    impaction removal, 792-794
    irrigating a colostomy, 803-807
    pouching an enterostomy, 794-802
    pressure ulcer formation and, 572
  incontinence care, 177-181
  intake and output monitoring, 168-173
  nursing diagnosis, 167-168
  providing bedpan and urinal, 173-177
  urinary, 809-831
    catheterization in, 810-818
    continuous bladder irrigation, 825-827
    external catheter application, 181-184
    nursing diagnosis, 809
    suprapubic catheter, 828-830
    urinary diversions, 818-824
Elixir, 412
Embolism, fat, 646
Emergency call bell, 77
Emergency measures for life support, 869-887
  care of body after death, 882-885, 886
  code management, 877-882
  nursing diagnosis, 869-870
  resuscitation, 870-876
Emergency Nurses Association, 877
Emotional factors
  communication, 26
  elimination, 167
  interviewing, 36
Empathy in active listening, 34
Empirin; *see* Aspirin
Employment history, 919
EN; *see* Enteral nutrition
ENA; *see* Emergency Nurses Association

Endogenous infection, defined, 969
Endorphins
  defined, 969
  pain relief associated with imagery, 195
Endoscope, defined, 970
Endoscopy, 383-396
Endotracheal tube, 901-907
  defined, 970
  management, 747-754
    suctioning, 740, 742, 743-747
Enema administration, 185-189
Energy in postanesthesia recovery scoring system, 506
Enteral nutrition, 775-790
  defined, 970
  medication administration through feeding tube, 787-790
  nasogastric or nasointestinal intubation for, 776-781
  tube feeding administration, 781-787
Enteric-coated medication, 422
Enterostomy, 791
  pouching, 794-802
Environmental factors
  blood pressure measurement, 236, 237
  communication, 26
  pressure ulcer formation, 572
Environmental safety, 73-94
  accidents, 73, 74
  fire safety, 74, 75
  nursing diagnosis, 76
  radiation safety, 76
  radioactive materials, 92-94
  restraints, 76
    application, 85-89, 90
    designing a restraint-free environment, 81-84
  safety equipment and fall prevention, 76-81
  seizure precautions, 76, 91-92
Enzymes, cardiac, 966
Eosinophils, normal values, 965
Epidermis, defined, 970
Epidural analgesia flow sheet, 549
Epidural infusion, 544-550, 970
Epiglottitis, 359
Epinephrine, 881
Epithelial cell in wound healing, 566
Equipment
  isolation precaution, 56, 57-58
  safety, 76-81
Equivalents and abbreviations, 960-961
Erb's point, 311
Erythema
  defined, 970
  shift assessment, 259
Eschar, defined, 970
Esophagogastroduodenoscopy, 385
Esophagostomy, 797
Estrogen skin patch, 431-432
Ethical factors in medication error, 418
Ethnocentrism, defined, 970
Etiology statement in nursing diagnosis, 6
European American population, 204
Euthanasia, defined, 970
Evaluation, 7, 8
  in change-of-shift report, 20
  licensed practical or vocational nurse's role in, 5
  recording of, 12
  standards of nursing practice and, 4
Eversion, foot, 631
Evisceration, defined, 970
Exacerbation, defined, 970
ExacTech, 369
ExacTech RSG, 369
Examination; *see* Physical examination
Excedrin-IB; *see* Ibuprofen
Excretion
  bathing and, 123
  drug, 404
    intravenous, 711
    older adult, 419
  specimen collection, 344
  Standard Precautions, 49

Exercise
  effects on vital signs, 231
  incorporated into activities of daily living, 96, 97
  leg, preoperative teaching, 484
  pelvic floor, 178
  range of motion, 98, 618-633
    ankle, 630
    assessment, 618-619
    continuous passive motion machine, 632-635
    elbow, 623
    evaluation, 631
    fingers, 626
    forearm, 624
    hip, 628-629
    knee, 630
    neck, 620-621
    planning, 619
    shoulder, 621-622, 623
    thumb, 627
    wrist, 625
Exercise stress test, 396-401
Exogenous infection, defined, 970
Exophthalmos, defined, 970
Expected outcomes, 8
Expectoration, sputum culture from, 355-356
Expiration; *see* Respiration
Expressive aphasia, 28, 34
Extension, 341
  ankle, 630
  elbow, 623
  finger, 626
  foot, 631
  hip, 620
  knee, 630
  neck, 620
  shoulder, 621
  thumb, 627
  wrist, 625
External catheter application, 181-184
External fixation as skeletal fraction, 642
External genitalia
  assessment, 322-327
  cleansing, 127
    newborn, 214
External rotation, 341
  hip, 620
  shoulder, 622
Extracellular fluid, 852
Extraocular movement, 295
Extremity
  alarm attached to, 81, 83-84
  blood pressure measurement, 236-239, 241
  exercise, preoperative teaching, 484
  massage, 200
  deep vein thrombosis and, 126
  postoperative pressure dressing, 511
  principles for wrapping, 587
  range of motion
    assessment, 341
    exercise, 618, 624-627, 628-630
  restraint, 86, 87
  shift assessment, 274-279
  subcutaneous injection, 457
Exudate, defined, 970
Eye
  assessment, 293-299
  care of
    newborn, 213
    unconscious client, 125
  irrigation, 842-844
  medication administration in, 421, 433-438
Eye contact, cultural considerations, 26
Eye prosthesis, caring for client with, 839-842
Eye protection
  removal of, 59
  Standard Precautions, 49
Eyeglass hearing aid, 846

F

Face
  assessment, 283-288
  cleansing, 124
    newborn,, 213
Face shield
  application, 57
  Standard Precautions, 49
Facial nerve, 284, 333
Factual record or report, 13-14
Fainting in orthostatic hypotension, 106, 107
Falls
  during assisted ambulation, 119, 664
  prevention, 76-81
    discharge teaching, 920-921
    using assistive devices for ambulation, 662-665
  risk assessment, 73, 74
Family
  answering for client during interviewing, 39
  information in change-of-shift report, 20
  isolation precautions and, 56
  presence during code management, 877
  teaching medication administration, 416-417
Family coping, ineffective, 809
Family history, 478
Fat embolism, 646
Fatigue
  during assisted ambulation, 119
  in pain, 532
  sleep and relaxation and, 191
  in tuberculosis, 60
FDA; see Food and Drug Administration
Fear
  assistive devices, 661
  effects on elimination, 167
  infection control and, 50
  intravenous therapy, 684
  laboratory and diagnostic testing, 345
  oxygenation promotion, 727
  related to history of falling, 96
  specialty beds, 601
Febrile, defined, 970
Fecal impaction removal, 185, 792-794
Fecal incontinence, 167, 178
Feces
  assessment of characteristic odor, 256
  defined, 970
Feedback in communication, 25, 26
Feeding
  dependent clients, 156-160
  infant, 203, 206-211
Feeding self-care deficit, 156
Feeding tube, 775-790
  administration of feedings, 781-787
  medication administration through, 787-790
  nasogastric or nasointestinal intubation for, 776-781
  pressure ulcer formation and, 572
Feldene; see Piroxicam
Femoral artery, 314, 315
Fentanyl, 537, 544
Fentanyl transdermal system, 537
Fever, 239
  blood transfusion, 721, 725
  during dialysis, 911
  effects on hair, 135
  oral hygiene and, 130
  during peritoneal dialysis, 915
  postoperative, 514, 517
Fiber intake, 158
  bowel elimination and, 174
Fibrin, defined, 970
Fibroblast, 566
Figure eight bandage turn, 595
Filter needle, 449
Filtration, 853, 854
Finger, range of motion
  assessment, 341
  exercise, 618, 626

Fingernail
  handwashing for infection control, 52
  surgical hand scrub, 494
Fire extinguisher, 74
Fire safety, 73, 74, 75
  in home, 921
Fissure, defined, 970
Fistula
  arteriovenous for hemodialysis, 907-908, 909
  defined, 970
Fit test, respirator, 50
Five rights
  delegation, 5
  drug administration, 409-412
Fixation, external, 642
Flannel bandage, 594
Flash cards as communication aid, 29
Flatness, 282
Flatus, defined, 970
Flexion, 341
  ankle, 630
  elbow, 623
  finger, 626
  foot, 631
  hip, 620
  knee, 630
  neck, 620
  shoulder, 621
  thumb, 627
  wrist, 625
Floor, fall prevention and, 76, 921
Floor stock, drugs distributed as, 408
Florida pouch, 818
Flossing tooth, 134
Flow sheet, 14
  behavioral restraint, 90
  epidural analgesia, 549
  patient-controlled analgesia, 543
  preoperative education, 481
Fluid, composition and distribution of, 852-856
Fluid imbalance
  etiologic factors, 8
  gastric intubation, 765
  intake and output monitoring, 168, 171
  intravenous therapy, 683
  monitoring, 856, 857-859
  nursing diagnosis, 856-857
  perioperative, 505
  peritoneal dialysis, 915
  risk factors, 852
  vital signs in, 230
Fluid intake
  after gastroscopy, 395
  for airway management, 735
  body's regulation of, 855
  bowel elimination and, 174
  intake and output monitoring, 168, 169
  older adult
    urinary catheterization and, 818
    urinary diversion, 824
Fluid output, renal regulation of, 855
Fluid volume deficit
  etiologic factors, 8
  gastric intubation, 765
  intake and output monitoring, 168, 171
  intravenous therapy, 683
  monitoring of, 856, 857-859
  as nursing diagnosis, 856
  perioperative, 505
  risk factors, 852
  vital signs in, 230
Fluid volume excess
  intake and output monitoring, 168, 171
  intravenous therapy, 683
  monitoring, 858
  as nursing diagnosis, 856
  peritoneal dialysis, 915
  risk factors, 852
  vital signs in, 230
Foam, vaginal, 444
Foam replacement mattress, 602

Foam soap for handwashing, 50, 51
Focus charting, 17
Folstein's Mini-Mental State, 330, 331
Food
  drainage out of nose during feeding, 162
  effects on stoma output, 802
Food and Drug Administration, 85
Food Guide Pyramid, 155, 156
Food intake
  bowel elimination and, 174
  pressure ulcer formation and, 570
Foot
  care of, 141-147
  common problems, 142, 143
  massage, 200
Football hold for breastfeeding, 208
Footwear
  ambulation and, 662
  assessment, 141
Forearm, range of motion
  assessment, 341
  exercise, 624
Foreign body removal before cardiopulmonary resuscitation, 874
Foreskin
  comprehensive health assessment, 325
  external catheterization and, 183
  newborn, cleansing of, 214
Fork, tuning, 282, 283
Form, sample, 949-959
Formula feeding, 203, 210
Four-point crutch gait, 671
Fowler's position
  airway management, 735
  moving dependent client to, 97, 101
    minimizing orthostatic hypotension during, 106
Fracture, pathologic, 972
Friction injury, 570
  hydrocolloid for protection, 581
  patient positioning and, 98
Friction massage, 200
Frontal sinus, 289
Full-liquid diet, 158
Functional health patterns, 963-964
Functional incontinence, 167, 809
Fungal infection
  foot, 142, 143
  nail, 142, 143
  peristomal, 799
FVD; see Fluid volume deficit
FVE; see Fluid volume excess

G

Gag reflex
  oral hygiene and, 130
  oral medication and, 420
Gait
  comprehensive health assessment, 339
  crutch, 671-673
  defined, 970
  older adult, 343
Gait belt for assisted ambulation, 666, 668
Gallbladder, 317-322
Gas exchange, impaired, 230
  cardiopulmonary resuscitation, 870
  comprehensive health assessment, 299
  laboratory and diagnostic testing, 345
  oxygenation promotion, 727
Gas-permeable contact lens, 833
Gastric intubation, 765-774
  for enteral feeding, 776-781
  insertion of tube, 766-770
  irrigation, 770-772
  nursing diagnosis, 765
  postoperative care, 514
  removal of tube, 773-774
  specimen collection for Gastroccult testing, 373-374
Gastroccult test, 368-375
Gastrointestinal system
  comprehensive health assessment, 317-322
  shift assessment, 269-273

Gastrostomy tube
  characteristic output, 505, 797
  enteral feeding, 775
Gate control theory of pain, 190
Gauze bandage, 594
Gauze dressing, 586
  intravenous therapy site, 691, 703, 705
Gaze assessment, 295
GCS; see Glasgow Coma Scale
Gel pack, commercial, 560, 561
Gelatin capsule, administration through feeding tube, 788
General survey
  comprehensive health assessment, 280
  shift assessment, 257-262
Generalist, nurse as, 3
Generic name of drug, 410, 412
Genital self-examination, male, 325, 326
Genitalia
  assessment, 322-327
  cleansing, 127
    newborn, 214
Gerentologic considerations; see Geriatric considerations
Geri chair, 77
Geriatric considerations
  assisted ambulation, 119
    minimizing orthostatic hypotension during, 106, 107
  bathing, 121, 129
  bed to chair transfer, 111
    using mechanical lift, 115
  bedmaking, 153
  beds and mattresses, specialty, 605, 608, 611
  blood transfusion, 725
  cardiac studies, 401
  casting, 655, 658
  central venous lines, 897
  cerumen, 245
  communication, 28, 31
  comprehensive health assessment
    eyes and ears, 299
    genitalia and rectum, 327
    head, face and neck, 288
    heart and circulation, 317
    neurologic function, 338
    nose, sinuses and mouth, 292
    thorax, lungs and breasts, 308
  continuous bladder irrigation, 827
  contrast media studies, 379
  designing restraint-free environment, 81-84
  discharge planning
    oxygen therapy, 940
    risk assessment and accident prevention, 922
    self-administration of non-parenteral medication, 925
    self-catheterization, 936
    self-injection, 931
    tracheostomy care, 946
  ear irrigation, 850
  enema administration, 189
  falls, 73, 662, 665
  feeding, 160
  fluid imbalances, 859
  foot and nail care, 141, 146
  hair care, 140
  hearing aid care, 848
  heat and cold therapy, 557, 559, 562
  incontinence, 167, 181
  intake and output monitoring, 173
  intravenous therapy, 695, 702, 711
  isolation, 49-50
  lumbar puncture, 387, 396
  mechanical ventilation, 907
  medication administration, 418-419, 428
    intradermal injection for skin testing, 472
    intramuscular injection, 469
    metered-dose inhalers, 441
    subcutaneous injection, 463
  nasogastric intubation, 770, 787, 790
  nuclear imaging studies, 382
  oral hygiene, 134
  orthotic devices, 620

Geriatric considerations—cont'd
  ostomy, 802, 807
  oxygen therapy, 734
  pain management, 536, 539, 544
    epidural anesthesia, 549
  peritoneal dialysis, 915
  positioning of dependent client, 105
  pressure ulcers and wound care, 576, 585
  providing bedpan and urinal, 177
  pulse oximetry, 253
  range of motion exercise, 631, 635
  sleep, 195
  specimen collection, 359, 375
    blood, 367
  suctioning, 747
  surgery, 479
    postoperative care, 512
    preoperative physical preparation, 491
    preoperative teaching, 485
    suture and staple removal, 529
    wound care, 519
    wound drainage devices, 524
  surgical asepsis, 68
  thoracentesis, 390
  total parenteral nutrition, 900
  traction, 641, 646
  urinary catheterization, 818
    external, 184
  urinary diversion, 824
  verbal deescalation of potentially violent client, 44
  vital signs, 242
  wound healing, delayed, 567
Gingiva, defined, 970
Gingivitis, 131
Glasgow Coma Scale, 324
Glass thermometer, 223, 231, 240
Glaucoma, 294
Glomerulus, defined, 970
Glossopharyngeal nerve, 333
Gloving
  application of gloves, 57
  closed, 497-501
  correct sizing, 69
  disposable clean gloves in infection control, 53-54
  multiple versus single, 55
  for physical examination, 282
  removal of gloves, 59
  Standard Precautions, 49
  in standard protocols for nursing interventions, 9
  sterile, 69-72
Glucocorticoids, 856
Glucometer Elite, 369
Glucometer Encore, 369
Glucose
  normal values, 965, 966
  testing, 368-375
    urine screening for, 370-371
Gluteal reflex, 337
Goal in planning phase of nursing process, 8
Goggles, 57
Gowning
  client, intravenous therapy and, 703
  gloving and, 53
  removal of gown, 59
  Standard Precautions, 49
  sterile, 497-501
  surgical asepsis and, 64
Graft for hemodialysis, 907-908, 909
Gram positive organism, 517
Grand mal seizure, safety precautions, 76
Granulation tissue, defined, 970
Graphic sheet, 14
Graying of hair, 140
Grief
  anticipatory, 968
  dysfunctional, 870
Grip bar in bathroom, 77
Grooming; see Personal hygiene
GSE; see Genital self-examination
Guided imagery, 195, 198-199
Gums, 291

Gurgles, 263, 265, 970
Gustatory, defined, 970

H

Hair
  care of, 135-140
    newborn, 214
  common problems and related interventions, 136
  graying, 140
  loss, 135, 136
  preoperative removal, 490
  pubic, comprehensive health assessment, 323, 325
Halitosis, 131, 256
Halo traction, 642, 643
Hammer, reflex, 282, 283
Hand massage, 200
Handrails for fall prevention in home, 921
Handwashing, 50-52
  after removing gloves, 9
  Standard Precautions, 49
  surgical scrub, 493-497
  surgical wound care, 516
Hard contact lens, 833, 835-836, 837-838
Hard palate, 291
HBM; see Health-belief model
Hct; see Hematocrit
Head
  assessment, 283-288
  massage, 199
Head lice, 136
Head scarf for chemotherapy-related hair loss, 135
Headache
  during epidural analgesia, 548
  post spinal anesthesia, 509
  postpuncture, 388, 395
Head-tilt, chin-lift maneuver, 872, 873
Healing of incision, 516-517
Health, defined, 970
Health assessment
  comprehensive, 280-343
    abdomen, 317-322
    examination techniques, 281-283
    eyes and ears, 293-299
    general survey, 280
    genitalia and rectum, 322-327
    head, face, and neck, 283-288
    heart and circulation, 309-317
    musculoskeletal function, 339-343
    neurologic function, 327-338
    nose, sinuses, and mouth, 288-292
    thorax, lungs, and breasts, 299-308
  preoperative, 476-479
  shift assessment, 255-279
    abdomen, 269-273
    apical pulse, 266-269
    extremities and peripheral circulation, 274-279
    general survey and integumentary inspection, 257-262
    lung sounds, 262-266
    nursing diagnosis, 256
Health behavior, defined, 970
Health care
  long-term; see Long-term care
  trends in, 3
Health care proxy, 10
Health care team
  code management, 877-882
  communication within, 12-13
Health care worker
  body mechanics, patient positioning and, 96, 97
  tuberculosis skin testing for, 49
Health maintenance, 3
  altered
    discharge planning, 918
    personal hygiene, 122
    range of motion promotion, 617
  risk for altered
    communication and, 29
    perioperative, 505

Health promotion, 3
Health restoration, 3
Health teaching; *see* Client teaching
Health-belief model, 919
Health-seeking behaviors
　assistive devices, 661
　discharge planning, 918
　drug therapy, 415
　newborn, 204
　related to knowledge deficit, 29
Healthy People 2000, 3
Hearing aid client, caring for, 845-848
Hearing assessment, 293-299
Hearing loss in older adult, 28, 31, 35, 299
Heart
　cardiac studies, 396-401
　comprehensive health assessment, 309-317
　disease, blood pressure and, 231
Heart failure
　as anesthesia complication, 504
　congestive, fluid balance alteration in, 855
Heart murmur
　comprehensive health assessment, 312
　defined, 972
Heart rate
　comprehensive health assessment, 312
　target, exercise stress testing and, 396
Heart sounds, 226
　comprehensive health assessment, 311-312, 316
　shift assessment, 266-269
Heat, therapeutic use, 551-559
　dry, 556-559
　moist, 553-556
　nursing diagnosis, 551
　pain management, 532
Heat pack, commercial, 557-558
Heating pad, 557
Height, measurement of, 163
Height and weight table, 967
Heimlich maneuver, 874
Hematemesis, defined, 970
Hematocrit
　fluid imbalances, 858
　intake and output monitoring, 168, 169
　normal values, 965
　surgical wound healing and, 517
Hematoma, 710, 970
Hematuria, defined, 970
Hemiplegia, bed to chair transfer and, 108
Hemoccult test, 368-375
Hemodialysis, 907-911
Hemoglobin level
　after blood transfusion, 725
　normal values, 965
　surgical wound healing and, 517
Hemolysis, defined, 970
Hemophilia, shaving and, 136
Hemoptysis, defined, 970
Hemorrhage
　blood pressure and, 231
　in continuous bladder irrigation, 827
　during dialysis, 910
　enema administration and, 188
　from heparin therapy, 459
　postoperative, 504-505, 510, 511
Hemorrhoid
　defined, 970
　enema administration and, 185
　rectal suppository administration and, 443
Hemostasis
　defined, 970
　in wound healing, 566
Hemothorax, 754, 900, 970
Hemovac, 505, 520, 521-523
HEPA; *see* High-efficiency particulate air
Heparin
　intravenous administration, 712
　intravenous push and, 715, 718-719
　shaving and, 136
　subcutaneous injection, 457-463
　teaching self-injection, 926
Hepatic system, 317-322

Hernia
　defined, 970
　peristomal, 801
HFJV; *see* High-frequency jet ventilation
HFOV; *see* High-frequency oscillatory
　ventilation
HFPPV; *see* High-frequency positive-pressure
　ventilation
HICPAC; *see* Hospital Infection Control
　Practices Advisory Committee
High Fowler's position, 101, 106
High risk for impaired skin integrity, 8
High risk for injury
　etiologic factors, 8
　injection administration, 451
High-efficiency particulate air respirator, 49, 50, 60
High-fiber diet, 158
High-frequency jet ventilation, 902
High-frequency oscillatory ventilation, 902
High-frequency positive-pressure ventilation, 902
High-risk nursing diagnosis, 6
Hip, range of motion exercise, 618, 628-629
Hirsutism, 122, 970
Hispanic population
　infant care, 204
　physical contact, 256
History
　employment, 919
　in interview, 39
　nutritional assessment, 155
　preoperative assessment, 478
　sexual, 322
History form, 14
Hives, 405
Homan's sign
　comprehensive health assessment, 316
　shift assessment, 276, 278
Home care, 917-946
　ambulation
　　assisted, 119
　　assistive devices for, 677
　bathing, 129
　bed to chair transfer, 112
　　using mechanical lift, 115
　bedmaking, 153
　beds and mattresses, specialty, 605, 608, 611, 615
　blood transfusion, 725
　cardiac studies, 401
　casting, 655, 658
　continuous bladder irrigation, 827
　contrast media studies, 379
　documentation, 16
　drug safety, 417
　ear irrigation, 850
　enema administration, 189
　establishing therapeutic
　　communication, 31
　feeding of client, 160
　foot and nail care, 147
　gastric intubation, 770
　hearing aid care, 848
　hemodialysis, 911
　infant care, 207
　intake and output monitoring, 173
　intravenous therapy, 693, 702, 711
　liver biopsy, 391
　lumbar puncture, 387, 396
　mechanical ventilation, 907
　medication administration
　　intramuscular injection, 469
　　nasogastric intubation, 790
　　non-parenteral self-administration, 922-926
　　subcutaneous injection, 463
　nursing diagnosis, 918
　obtaining body weight, 166
　oral hygiene, 135
　orthotic devices, 620
　ostomy, 802, 807
　oxygen therapy, 734, 940

Home care—cont'd
　pain management, 539
　　epidural anesthesia, 550
　paracentesis, 389
　peritoneal dialysis, 915
　positioning of dependent client, 105
　potentially violent client, 44
　pressure ulcer and wound care, 576, 585, 591
　providing bedpan and urinal, 177
　pulse oximetry, 253
　range of motion exercise, 631, 635
　risk assessment and accident prevention, 918-922
　safety assessment, 77, 78
　shift assessment, 278
　sleep and relaxation, 195
　specimen collection, 367, 375
　suctioning, 747
　surgery
　　postoperative care, 512, 516
　　wound care, 519, 524
　surgical asepsis, 68
　teaching self-catheterization, 932-936
　teaching self-injection, 926-931
　total parenteral nutrition, 900
　tracheostomy, 941-946
　traction, 641, 646
　urinary catheterization, 184, 818
　　suprapubic, 830
　urinary diversion, 824
　urine collection, 351
　using home oxygen equipment, 936-940
　vital sign measurement, 243
Home maintenance management, impaired
　casting, 648
　discharge planning, 918
　intravenous therapy, 684
Homeostasis, defined, 970
Hopelessness
　laboratory and diagnostic testing, 345
　oxygenation promotion, 727
Hormones in body fluid regulation, 856
Hospice, defined, 970
Hospital bed
　safety measures, 77, 79-80
　weight-sensitive alarm placed under, 81, 82
Hospital Infection Control Practices Advisory
　Committee, 55
Hospital-acquired infection, 47
　during mechanical ventilation, 906
Household measurement of medication, 413, 960
Hoyer lift transfer, 112-115
Hub of needle, 447, 448
Human insulin, 457
Humidifier in oxygen therapy, 729
Hydrocolloid, 581, 583, 584
Hydromorphone hydrochloride, 537
Hydrothorax, 900
Hygiene, 121-154
　bathing, complete, 123-129
　bedmaking, 147-153
　endotracheal tube care, 749
　foot and nail care, 141-147
　hair care, 135-140
　intravenous therapy and, 703
　nursing diagnosis, 122
　oral care, 130-135
　　infant, 213
　shift assessment, 257
Hypercalcemia, 853, 860, 862
Hypercapnia, defined, 970
Hypercarbia, defined, 970
Hyperemia
　defined, 970
　reactive, 968, 973
Hyperextension, 341
　elbow, 623
　finger, 626
　hip, 620
　neck, 620
　shoulder, 622
　wrist, 625

Hyperextension, defined, 970
Hyperglycemia
  defined, 970
  insulin injections and, 458
  during total parenteral nutrition, 900
Hyperkalemia, 853, 860, 862
Hypermagnesemia, 853, 860, 863
Hypernatremia, 853, 860, 861
Hyperplasia, benign prostatic, 827
Hyperpnea, 228
Hyperresonance, 282
Hypersensitivity; see Allergy
Hypertension, 241, 248, 316
  as anesthesia complication, 504
  defined, 970
Hyperthermia, 229, 239
  during blood transfusion, 721, 725
  Celsius and Fahrenheit temperatures
    in, 223
  defined, 970
  during dialysis, 911
    peritoneal, 915
  effects on hair, 135
  fluid and electrolyte imbalances, 856
  malignant, 971
  newborn, 204
  older adult, 242
  oral hygiene and, 130
  postoperative, 514, 517
  pressure ulcers and, 567
Hypertonic, defined, 970
Hypertonic intravenous solution, 855
Hyperventilation, 228
  in acid-base imbalances, 866
  defined, 970
Hypervolemia, defined, 970
Hypnotics, 191, 192, 194
Hypocalcemia, 853, 860, 862-863
Hypoglossal nerve, 333
Hypoglycemia
  defined, 970
  insulin injections and, 458
  during total parenteral nutrition, 900
Hypokalemia, 853, 860, 861-862
  during peritoneal dialysis, 915
Hypomagnesemia, 853, 860, 863
Hyponatremia, 853, 859-861
Hypotension, 241, 248, 316
  as anesthesia complication, 504
  defined, 970
  during dialysis, 911
  epidural analgesia and, 546
  orthostatic
    defined, 972
    minimizing, 106-107
    from Rotokinetic bed, 613
    during vascular system assessment, 312
  postural, 973
Hypothalamus, defined, 970
Hypothermia, 229, 239
  Celsius and Fahrenheit temperatures
    in, 223
  defined, 971
  hot and cold therapies, 551
  in older adult, 242
  during peritoneal dialysis, 915
  postoperative, 511, 514
Hypotonic, defined, 971
Hypotonic intravenous solution, 855
Hypoventilation, 228
  as anesthesia complication, 504
  defined, 971
  in respiratory acidosis, 865
Hypovolemia
  as anesthesia complication, 504
  defined, 971
  postoperative, 511
Hypoxemia, 728, 865
  as anesthesia complication, 504
  from oxygen therapy in home, 940
Hypoxia, 865
  defined, 971
  oxygen therapy for, 728

I
Iatrogenic, defined, 971
Ibuprofen, 537
Ice bag, 559-562
ICF; see Intracellular fluid
ICN; see International Council of Nurses
Idiosyncratic reaction, 405, 971
Ileostomy, 791, 797, 803
Ileum, defined, 971
IM; see Intramuscular
Imagery, 195, 198-199, 532
Immobilization; see Restraint
Immobilized client, 564-681
  assistive devices for ambulation, 659-681
    cane, crutches, and walker, teaching use
      of, 665-677
    for fall prevention, 662-665
    nursing diagnosis, 661
    orthotic device, caring for client with,
      677-681
  cast care, 648-658
    application, assessment, and care, 650-655
    nursing diagnosis, 648
    removal, 655-658
  contact lens care, 833-839
  feeding, 156-160
  mattresses and beds, 601-616
    air-fluidized bed, 608-611
    air-suspension bed, 605-608
    bariatric bed, 614-615
    nursing diagnosis, 601
    Rotokinetic bed, 611-613
    support surface mattress, 602-605
  pressure ulcer and wound care management,
    565-600
    binder and bandage application, 594-599
    dressing application, 585-591
    nursing diagnosis, 567
    pressure ulcer risk assessment and preven-
      tion strategies, 568-576
    pressure ulcer treatment, 577-585
    transparent dressing, changing, 592-594
  range of motion promotion, 617-635
    continuous passive motion machine,
      632-635
    nursing diagnosis, 617
    range of motion exercise, 98, 618-633
  traction, 636-647
    nursing diagnosis, 638
    skeletal, 637-638, 642-646
    skin, 636, 637, 638, 639-641
Immobilizer, 677
Immunity, defined, 971
Immunization, 48
Immunosuppressive therapy, 567
Imodium, 572
Impaction removal, 185, 792-794
Impaired gas exchange, 230
  cardiopulmonary resuscitation, 870
  comprehensive health assessment, 299
  laboratory and diagnostic testing, 345
  oxygenation promotion, 727
Impaired home maintenance management
  casting, 648
  discharge planning, 918
  intravenous therapy, 684
Impaired memory, 328
Impaired physical mobility, 96
  assistive devices, 661
  casting, 648
  comprehensive health assessment
    musculoskeletal system, 339
    neurologic function, 328
  discharge planning, 918
  etiologic factors, 8
  hot and cold therapies, 551
  pain, 532
  perioperative, 505
  pressure ulcers, 567
  risk for, range of motion promotion, 617
  specialty beds, 601
  traction, 638

Impaired skin integrity
  casting, 648
  comprehensive health assessment
    genitalia and rectum, 322
    head, face, and neck, 283
  fluid and electrolyte imbalances, 856
  high risk for, 8
  hot and cold therapies, 551
  intravenous therapy, 683
  personal hygiene, 122
  pressure ulcers, 567
  risk for
    after death, 870
    gastrointestinal ostomy, 792
    neurologic function assessment, 328
    personal hygiene and, 122
    pressure ulcers, 567
    traction, 638
  shift assessment, 256
  specialty beds, 601
  urinary elimination, altered, 809
Impaired social interaction
  communication and, 29
  visual or hearing impairment, 833
Impaired swallowing, 160-162
  comprehensive health assessment, 283
  nutrition and, 156
  enteral, 776
Impaired tissue integrity
  hot and cold therapies, 551
  injection administration, 451
Impaired tissue perfusion, 451
Impaired verbal communication, 28-29
  hearing impairment, 833
  oxygenation promotion, 727
Implant
  preoperative assessment, 478
  radioactive, safety measures, 92
Implementation, 7, 8
  licensed practical or vocational nurse's role
    in, 5
  standards of nursing practice and, 4
Inability to sustain spontaneous ventilation,
  727
Incentive spirometer, 483
Incident report, 21-22
Incision
  care of, 516-519
  expected postoperative drainage, 505
  preoperative hair removal at site of, 490
Incontinence, 177-181, 809
  bathing and, 123
  external catheterization for, 181
  pressure ulcer formation and, 567, 568,
    572, 576
  types, 167-168
Incontinent urinary diversion, 818-824
Increased intracranial pressure, 231
Indiana pouch, 818
Individual coping, ineffective
  communication and, 29
  gastrointestinal ostomy, 792
  pain, 532
Indocin; see Indomethacin
Indocin SR; see Indomethacin
Indomethacin, 537
Induration, defined, 971
Indwelling catheter, 810, 815, 816
  expected postoperative drainage, 505
  sterile urine specimen from, 346-347,
    351-352
Ineffective airway clearance, 230
  cardiopulmonary resuscitation, 869-870
  comprehensive health assessment, 299
  laboratory and diagnostic testing, 345
  oxygenation promotion, 727
  risk for
    newborn, 204
    surgery, 505
  shift assessment, 256
  surgery, 475
Ineffective breast-feeding, 204

Ineffective breathing pattern, 230
  cardiopulmonary resuscitation, 869
  comprehensive health assessment
    nose, sinuses, and mouth, 288
    thorax, lungs and breasts, 299
  laboratory and diagnostic testing, 345
  oxygenation promotion, 727
  perioperative, 505
  shift assessment, 256
Ineffective coping
  communication and, 29
  gastrointestinal ostomy, 792
  oxygenation promotion, 727
  pain, 532
  surgery, 475
  urinary elimination, altered, 809
Ineffective management of therapeutic regimen
  discharge planning, 918
  drug therapy, 415
  intravenous therapy, 684
Ineffective thermoregulation, 230
  risk for, newborn, 204
Infant, 103-220
  bathing, 203, 212-215
  cardiopulmonary resuscitation, 874, 875
  diaper changing, 214-218
  feeding, 206-211
  fluid volume deficit, 856
  irregular respirations and apneic spells, 236
  radial or apical pulse, 225
  removal during fire, 75
  swaddling and mummy restraint, 218-220
  temperature measurement, 233, 234
  thermoregulation using radiant warmer,
    204-206
  urine collection, 351
  weighing of, 166
Infarction, myocardial, 966
Infection
  chain of, 47-48
  control of; *see* Infection control
  corneal, 833-834
  development after sterile technique, 71
  development after surgical aseptic tech-
    nique, 68
  endogenous, 969
  exogenous, 970
  foot, 142, 143
  head, face, and neck assessment, 283
  intravenous therapy site, 692, 703, 710
  nail, 142, 143
  nosocomial, 972
    during mechanical ventilation, 906
  peristomal, 799
  peritoneal dialysis site, 914
  resulting from epidural catheter, 546
  risk for
    comprehensive health assessment of geni-
      talia and rectum, 322
    discharge planning, 918
    infection control, 50
    intravenous therapy, 683
    laboratory and diagnostic testing, 345
    oxygenation promotion, 727
    perioperative, 505
    sterile technique, 64
    surgery, 475, 493
    traction, 638
    urinary elimination, altered, 809
    visual or hearing impairment, 833
  urinary tract, 830
  wound, 517, 566-567, 579
Infection control, 47-62
  caring for clients under isolation precau-
    tions, 55-59
  handwashing, 50-52
  injection administration, 447
  nursing diagnosis, 50
  sterile technique, 63-72
    creating and maintaining a sterile field,
      64-68
    nursing diagnosis, 64
    sterile gloving, 69-72

Infection control—cont'd
  surgical wound care, 516
  tuberculosis precautions, 60-62
  using disposable clean gloves, 53-54
Infectious disease through blood transfusion
  transmission, 720
Infiltration
  defined, 971
  intravenous therapy, 692, 710
Inflammation
  defined, 971
  in wound healing, 566
Infusion, defined, 971
Infusion container, changing of, 703, 704, 708,
  710
Infusion pump, feeding via, 785-786
Infusion tubing, changing of, 703, 704, 706,
  707, 710
Ingrown nail, 142, 143
Inhaler
  defined, 971
  metered-dose, 438-441, 971
Injection
  administration, 447-473
    intradermal, 469-472
    intramuscular, 464-469
    nursing diagnosis, 451
    preparation, 451, 452-453, 454, 455, 456
    subcutaneous, 457-463
    syringes, 447-451
    teaching self-injection, 926-931
  defined, 971
  Z-track, 974
Injection cap, 703
Injury
  high risk for
    etiologic factors, 8
    injection administration, 451
  risk for
    assistive devices, 661
    casting, 648
    comprehensive health assessment, 293,
      328, 339
    discharge planning, 918
    environmental safety, 76
    hot and cold therapies, 551
    intravenous therapy, 683
    laboratory and diagnostic testing, 345
    patient positioning and, 97
    surgery, 475
    visual or hearing impairment, 833
INS; *see* Intravenous Nurses Society
Insomnia, defined, 971
Inspection, 281
  defined, 971
  shift assessment, 255
Inspiration; *see* Respiration
Instillation, defined, 971
Instrument
  physical examination, 282-283
  sharp, Standard Precautions, 49
Insufficiency, arterial *versus* venous, 275
Insulin
  subcutaneous injection, 457-463
    syringes for, 447, 448
  teaching self-injection, 926
Intake and output monitoring, 168-173
  in fluid volume deficit, 856
  postoperative, 510, 511
Integument, 971; *see also* Skin
Intellectual function, 332
Intensive care unit, sleep-wake cycles in, 191
Intentional wound, 578
Intercom system, 77, 79
Intercostal space, 302
Intermittent peritoneal dialysis, 912
Intermittent urinary catheterization, 810
Internal rotation, 341
  hip, 620
  shoulder, 622
International Council of Nurses, 2
Interrupted suture, 524, 527
Interstitial fluid, defined, 971

Intervention
  in change-of-shift report, 20
  recording of, 12
  standard protocols, 9
Interviewing, 36-39
Intestine, 317-322
In-the-canal hearing aid, 845
In-the-ear hearing aid, 845
Intonation, defined, 971
Intracellular fluid, 852, 971
Intracranial pressure, increased, 231
Intractable pain, defined, 971
Intradermal injection, 407, 447, 469-472, 971
Intramuscular injection, 407, 447, 464-469
  defined, 971
  needles used for, 449
Intraocular disk medication, 433, 436
Intraoperative techniques, 492-502
  nursing diagnosis, 492-502
  sterile gowning and closed gloving, 497-501
  surgical hand scrub, 493-497
Intrauterine, defined, 971
Intravascular, defined, 971
Intravenous, defined, 971
Intravenous conscious sedation, 345
Intravenous maintenance record, 694-695
Intravenous Nurses Society, 683, 703
Intravenous Nursing Standards of Practice, 683
Intravenous piggyback, 716-717, 718-719
Intravenous pyelography, 376-379
Intravenous therapy, 407, 683-726
  abbreviations related to types of fluids, 960
  bathing and, 124
  blood transfusion, 720-725
  central venous lines for, 889-897
  flow rate regulation, 696-702
  insertion techniques, 684-695
  maintenance of site, 703-711
  medication administration, 711-720
  nursing diagnosis, 683-684
  restraints and, 85
  shift assessment, 260, 261
Intropin; *see* Dopamine
Intubation
  endotracheal, 747-754
  gastric, 765-774
    for enteral nutrition, 776-781
    inserting tube, 766-770
    irrigating tube, 770-772
    nursing diagnosis, 765
    removing tube, 773-774
  mechanical ventilation, 901-907
Inversion
  defined, 971
  foot, 631
Iodinated dye allergy, 376, 379, 380
IPD; *see* Intermittent peritoneal dialysis
Irrigation
  colostomy, 803-807
  continuous bladder, 825-827
  defined, 971
  ear, 848-850
  eye, 842-844
  nasogastric tube, 770-772
  vaginal, 445
Ischemia
  defined, 971
  in pressure ulcers, 565
  shift assessment, 274
Isolation
  caring for clients under, 55-59
  Centers for Disease Control and Prevention
    guidelines, 48
  defined, 971
  mercury-in-glass thermometers in, 231
  tuberculosis, 49, 60-62
Isometric, defined, 971
Isotonic, defined, 971
ITC hearing aid; *see* In-the-canal hearing aid
ITE hearing aid; *see* In-the-ear hearing aid
IV; *see* Intravenous
IVCS; *see* Intravenous conscious sedation
IVP; *see* Intravenous pyelography
IVPB; *see* Intravenous piggyback

J

Jacket restraint, 86, 88
Jackson-Pratt drain, 520, 522-523
Jaundice, 259
Jaw, role in swallowing, 160
Jaw-thrust maneuver, 872, 873
JCAHO; *see* Joint Commission on Accreditation of Healthcare Organizations
Jejunostomy enteral feeding tube, 775, 797
Jejunum, defined, 971
Jet ventilation, high-frequency, 902
Joint Commission on Accreditation of Healthcare Organizations
    evaluation, 8
    height-weight measurement, 163
Judgment in neurologic function assessment, 332
Jugular vein, 313

K

Kardex, 13, 14
Kegel's exercise, 178
Keratitis, corneal, 833-834
Ketones
    normal values, 966
    urine screening test, 370-371
Ketorolac tromethamine, 537
Kidney
    calculi, 973
    comprehensive health assessment, 317-322
    disease, blood pressure and, 231
    fluid output regulation by, 855
Kidney failure
    fluid balance alteration in, 855
    hemodialysis for, 907
Kinesthetic, defined, 971
Kirschner wire, 642
Kitchen, home hazard assessment, 78
Knee
    range of motion
        assessment, 341
        exercise, 618, 630
    total replacement, continuous passive motion machine, 632-635
Knowledge deficit
    assistive devices, 661
    casting, 648
    communication and, 29
    comprehensive health assessment
        genitalia and rectum, 322
        thorax, lungs and breasts, 299
    discharge planning, 918
    gastrointestinal ostomy, 792
    health-seeking behaviors related to, 29
    hot and cold therapies, 551
    infection control and, 50
    intravenous therapy, 683-684
    laboratory and diagnostic testing, 345
    surgery, 475
    visual or hearing impairment, 833
Knowledge level
    active listening and, 36
    influence on communication, 26
Kock pouch, 818
Korotkoff sounds, 229, 230, 971
Kussmaul respiration, 228
Kyphosis, 340, 343

L

Label, drug, 410, 412
Labia
    cleansing of, 127
        newborn, 214
        before urinary catheterization, 813-814
    comprehensive health assessment, 323, 324
    in older adult, 327
Laboratory testing, 344-403
    blood specimen collection, 360-367
    cardiac studies, 396-401
    contrast media studies, 376-379
    diagnostic studies, 383-396
        assessment, 384-385
        equipment, 383-384

Laboratory testing–cont'd
    diagnostic studies–cont'd
        evaluation, 395-396
        implementation, 386-394
        planning, 385
    fluid imbalances, 858
    normal values, 344-345, 965-966
    nuclear imaging studies, 380-381
    nursing diagnosis, 344
    in nutritional assessment, 155
    specimen collection, 346-359
        assessment, 347
        equipment, 346-347
        evaluation, 358-359
        implementation, 348-358
        planning, 347-348
    unit specimen testing, 368-375
Laceration, 579, 971
Lacrimal apparatus, 296
Lactate dehydrogenase, 966
Lactation, 971; *see also* Breastfeeding
Language in neurologic function assessment, 332
Laryngospasm
    as anesthesia complication, 504
    defined, 971
Larynx
    edema, as anesthesia complication, 504
    role in swallowing, 160
Lateral position, 97, 102
Latex allergy, 53, 65, 70, 429, 478, 479
LDH; *see* Lactate dehydrogenase
Leader, nurse as, 3
Learning needs, active listening and, 36
LED; *see* Light-emitting diode
Leg
    battery-operated alarm attached to, 81
    exercise, preoperative teaching, 484
    massage and deep vein thrombosis, 126
    range of motion
        assessment, 341
        exercise, 628-630
    restraint, 87
Legal factors, 345
Leukemia, shaving and, 136
Leukocyte
    defined, 971
    normal values, 965, 966
    in wound healing, 566
Leukocytosis, defined, 971
Leukoplakia, defined, 971
Level of consciousness
    epidural analgesia assessment, 546
    fluid imbalances, 858
    neurologic function assessment, 327, 329
    shift assessment, 257
Levophed; *see* Norepinephrine
Lice, 136
Licensed practical or vocational nurse, 5
Life support measures, 869-887
    care of body after death, 882-885, 886
    code management, 877-882
    nursing diagnosis, 869-870
    resuscitation, 870-876
Life-support equipment, magnetic resonance imaging and, 393
Lift, mechanical, 112-115
Light palpation, 281
Light-emitting diode, 249
Lightheadedness
    abdominal paracentesis, 395
    assistive device ambulation, 676
Lighting for safety, 767
Limb restraint, 87
Linen, Standard Precautions, 49
Lip
    comprehensive health assessment, 290
    cracked, 131
Lipids
    defined, 971
    normal values, 966
Liquid diet, 158
Liquid intake; *see* Fluid intake

Liquid medication, 412, 422, 425
    administration through feeding tube, 787-790
Liquid soap for handwashing, 50, 51
Listening, active, 34-35, 38
Lithotomy position, 323, 327
Liver
    biopsy, 383-396
    comprehensive health assessment, 317-322
Liver function tests, 965
Living will, 10
Local anesthesia for central venous line insertion, 891
Local anesthetic spray, 432
Lofstrand crutch, 659, 661
Logrolling to maintain neck and spinal alignment, 103
Lomotil, 572
Long-term care
    ambulation
        assisted, 119
        assistive devices for, 677
    bathing, 129
    bed to chair transfer, 112
        using mechanical lift, 115
    bedmaking, 153
    beds and mattresses, specialty, 605, 608, 611, 615
    blood transfusion, 725
    cardiac studies, 401
    casting, 655, 658
    central venous lines, 897
    continuous bladder irrigation, 827
    contrast media studies, 379
    documentation, 16
    ear irrigation, 850
    enema administration, 189
    establishing therapeutic communication, 31
    feeding of client, 160
    foot and nail care, 147
    gastric intubation, 770
    hearing aid care, 848
    hemodialysis, 911
    infant care, 207
    intake and output monitoring, 173
    intravenous therapy, 693, 702, 711
    isolation, 50
    liver biopsy, 391
    lumbar puncture, 387, 396
    mechanical ventilation, 907
    medication administration
        intramuscular injection, 469
        nasogastric intubation, 790
        subcutaneous injection, 463
    obtaining body weight, 166
    oral hygiene, 135
    orthotic devices, 620
    ostomy, 802, 807
    oxygen therapy, 734, 940
    pain management, 539
        epidural anesthesia, 550
    paracentesis, 389
    peritoneal dialysis, 915
    positioning of dependent client, 105
    potentially violent client, 44
    pressure ulcer and wound care, 576, 585, 591
    providing bedpan and urinal, 177
    pulse oximetry, 253
    range of motion exercise, 631, 635
    risk assessment and accident prevention, 922
    shift assessment, 278
    sleep and relaxation, 195
    specimen collection, 367, 375
    suctioning, 747
    surgery
        postoperative care, 512, 516
        wound care, 519, 524
    surgical asepsis, 68
    total parenteral nutrition, 900
    tracheostomy care, 946
    traction, 646

Long-term care–cont'd
    urinary catheterization, 818
        external, 184
        suprapubic, 830
    urinary diversion, 824
    urine collection, 351
    vital sign measurement, 243
Lordosis, 340
Lotion
    application after handwashing, 52, 53
    for massage, 199
    topical medication as, 421, 430, 432
Low-cholesterol diet, 158
Lower extremity
    battery-operated alarm attached to, 81
    blood pressure measurement, 241
    exercise, preoperative teaching, 484
    massage and deep vein thrombosis, 126
    range of motion
        assessment, 341
        exercise, 618, 628-630
    restraint, 87
    shift assessment, 275
    subcutaneous injection, 457
Low-fiber diet, 158
LPN/LVN; see Licensed practical or vocational
    nurse
Lubrication
    rectal temperature, 233
    urinary catheterization, 813
Luer-Lok syringe, 447, 448
Lumbar brace, 677
Lumbar puncture, 383-396
Lung
    acid-base balance and, 864
    comprehensive health assessment, 299-308
    perforation during thoracentesis, 390
    shift assessment, 262-266
Lung cancer
    risk factors, 300
    warning signs, 264
Lung sounds
    during intravenous therapy, 702
    in mechanical ventilation, 904
    shift assessment, 262-266
Lymph node, 286, 305
Lymphocyte
    defined, 971
    levels in pressure ulcer, 574, 578
    normal values, 965

M

Maceration, defined, 971
Macrophage
    defined, 971
    in wound healing, 566
Macule, 261
Magic slate as communication aid, 29
Magnesium
    imbalance, 859, 860, 863
    normal values, 965
Magnetic resonance imaging, 383-396
Mainz pouch, 818
Malignant hyperthermia, defined, 971
Malignant pain, defined, 530
Malnutrition
    clients at risk for, 155
    defined, 971
    effects on hair, 135
    pressure ulcer formation and, 574, 578
    wound healing, delayed, 567
Manager, nurse as, 3
MAR; see Medication administration record
Mask
    application of, 57
    oxygen therapy, 728, 732, 733
    pocket, 870, 871
    removal of, 59
    Standard Precautions, 49
    tuberculosis precautions, 60
Massage
    back
        during bathing, 128
        for relaxation, 195-196, 201

Massage–cont'd
    leg, deep vein thrombosis and, 126
    over bony prominences, 128
    pain management, 532
    for relaxation, 193, 195-196, 199-201
Masticate, defined, 971
Mattress, support surface, 601-605
Maturation stage of wound healing, 566
Maxillary sinus, 290
MDI; see Metered-dose inhaler
Mechanical diet, 158
Mechanical lift transfer, 112-115
Mechanical obstruction as anesthesia
    complication, 504
Mechanical ventilation, 901-907
Meconium, defined, 971
Mediastinal chest tube, 754-755
Medical asepsis, 48, 971; see also Infection
    control
Medical record, 13, 14, 15
Medicare, 16
Medicated powder, 432
Medication
    administration; see Medication
        administration
    effects of, 404, 405
        on sleep, 192
        on vital signs, 231
    interactions, 406
    mild reactions to, 405
    neurologic function and, 328
    pharmacokinetics, 404-407
    tolerance and dependence, 406
    urine output and, 168
Medication administration, 404-419
    age factors, 418-419
    client and family teaching, 416-417, 922-926
    communication and transcription of orders,
        407-412
    during dialysis, 910
    drug actions and, 404-407
    drug effects and, 404, 405
    generic versus trade name, 412
    injections, 447-473
        intradermal, 469-472
        intramuscular, 464-469
        nursing diagnosis, 451
        preparation, 451, 452-453, 454,
            455, 456
        subcutaneous, 457-463
        syringes, 447-451
        teaching self-injection, 926-931
    intravenous, 711-720
    measurement systems, 413-415
    non-parenteral, 420-446
        eye and ear, 433-438
        metered-dose inhalers, 438-441
        oral, 422-428
        rectal and vaginal, 442-445
        topical, 429-433
    nursing process, 415-416
    physicians's order for, 406-407
    preparations for, 412-413
    routes of, 406, 407
    special handling of controlled II substances,
        417-419
    through feeding tube, 787-790
Medication administration record, 408,
    409, 410
Medication card, 417
Medication cart, 408, 416
Medication error, 418, 428
Medication history
    in interview, 39
    preoperative assessment, 478
MediSense 2 Card, 369
MediSense 2 Pen, 369
MedStation, 408
Melena, defined, 971
Memory
    impaired, 328
    neurologic function assessment, 332

Mental function
    comprehensive health assessment, 327-338
    pressure ulcers and, 576
Meperidine
    effects on sleep, 192
    pain management, 537
mEQ/L; see Milliequivalent per liter
Mercury sphygmomanometer, 229
Mercury spill, 224
Mercury-in-glass thermometer, 223, 231, 240
Message in communication, 25
Metabolic acidosis, 865, 866, 867
Metabolic alkalosis, 865, 866
Metabolism
    defined, 971
    drug, 404
        intravenous, 711
        older adult, 419
        oral route, 422
Metallic objects, magnetic resonance imaging
    and, 393, 394
Metered-dose inhaler, 438-441, 971
Methicillin-resistant *Staphylococcus aureus*, 517
Metric system, 413, 960
MI; see Myocardial infarction
Micturition, 971; see also Urinary elimination
Midol-200; see Ibuprofen
Midstream urine specimen, 346, 349-350
Military time, 15
Milliequivalent per liter, 971
Milwaukee brace, 677
Mini-Mental State, Folstein's, 330, 331
Mitten restraint, 87
MMS; see Mini-Mental State
Mobility
    defined, 971
    impaired, 96
        assistive devices, 661
        casting, 648
        comprehensive health assessment,
            328, 339
        discharge planning, 918
        etiologic factors, 8
        hot and cold therapies, 551
        pain, 532
        perioperative, 505
        pressure ulcers, 567
        risk for, range of motion promotion, 617
        specialty beds, 601
        traction, 638
    pressure ulcer formation and, 568, 569
    promotion; see Mobility promotion
Mobility promotion, 96-120
    assisted ambulation, 117-120
    moving and positioning clients in bed,
        97-105
    nursing diagnoses, 96-97
    orthostatic hypotension, minimizing,
        106-107
    transfers, 107-117
        from bed to chair, 107-112
        from bed to chair using mechanical lift,
            112-115
        from bed to transfer, 115-117
Mode of transmission, isolation requirements
    and, 55
Moist dressing, 586
Moist heat, 553-556
Moisture, pressure ulcer formation and, 569
Molded splint, 677
Moleskin, 145, 147
Monitoring for environmental safety, 81-82,
    83-84
Monocytes
    normal values, 965
    in wound healing, 566
Montgomery ties, 590
Mood
    neurologic function assessment, 330
    shift assessment, 257
Morphine
    effects on sleep, 192
    epidural administration, 544
    pain management, 537

Mortality; *see* Death
Mortar and pestle, 425
Motor function
    comprehensive health assessment, 335-337
    self-administration of medication, 417
    shift assessment, 257
Motrin; *see* Ibuprofen
Motrin-IB; *see* Ibuprofen
Mouth
    assessment, 288-292
    care of, 130-135
        endotracheal intubation, 749
        newborn, 213
    postoperative suctioning, 507, 508
Mouth-to-mouth artificial respiration, 873-874
Moving client in bed, 97-105
MRI; *see* Magnetic resonance imaging
MRSA; *see* Methicillin-resistant *Staphylococcus
    aureus*
MS Contin; *see* Morphine
Mucositis prevention, 132-133
Mucous membrane
    drug administration through, 421
    oral
        altered, 122, 130, 288, 765
        comprehensive health assessment, 290
    Standard Precautions, 49
Multicultural nursing, defined, 972
Multistix reagent test strip, 368-375
Mummy restraint, 218-220
Murmur
    comprehensive health assessment, 312
    defined, 972
Muscle
    accessory, 968
    progressive relaxation, 195, 196-198
Muscle relaxants, 537
Muscle strength
    bed to chair transfer and, 108
    comprehensive health assessment, 342
    shift assessment, 275
Muscle weakness, 342
Musculoskeletal system, 339-343
Music for pain management, 532
Muslin bandage, 594
Mustache care, 136, 139
Musty odor, 256
Mydriatics, 433
Myocardial infarction, 966

N

N95 particulate respiratory mask, 50, 60
Nail
    care of, 141-147
    common problems, 142, 143
    handwashing for infection control, 52
    surgical hand scrub, 494
Nail angle, 314
Nail polish, surgical hand scrub and, 494
NANDA; *see* North American Nursing Diag-
    nosis Association
Naprosyn; *see* Naproxen
Naproxen, 537
Naproxen sodium, 537
Narcolepsy, defined, 972
Narcotic, 533
    administration, 426
    defined, 972
    effects on sleep, 192
    epidural catheterization, 544
Narrative note, 17
Nasal cannula for oxygen delivery, 728, 731
Nasogastric tube
    for enteral feeding, 776-781
    gastric specimen for Gastroccult testing,
        373-374
    insertion, 766-770
    irrigation, 770-772
    postoperative care, 514
    removal, 773-774
Nasointestinal feeding tube, 776-781
Nasopharyngeal culture, 354, 355
Nasotracheal suctioning, 739, 740, 742-743

National Council of State Boards of
    Nursing, 5
National Pressure Ulcer Advisory Panel, 972
Native American population
    infant care, 204
    physical contact, 256
Nausea
    from air suspension bed, 607
    from cold otic drop administration, 433
    postoperative, 515
Nebulization, defined, 972
Neck
    assessment, 283-288
    logrolling to maintain alignment, 103
    massage, 200
    newborn, cleansing of, 213
    postoperative pressure dressing, 511
    range of motion exercise, 618, 620-621
Neck vein distention, 313, 316
Necrotic, defined, 972
Necrotic tissue, removal, 581
Needle, 447-449
    disposal, 59
    intramuscular injections, 464
    recapping of, 450, 451
    Standard Precautions, 49
    subcutaneous injection, 457
    tuberculosis testing, 469
Needleless infusion line, 712
Needle-stick
    intravenous insertion and, 684
    prevention, 449-450, 451
Nephron, defined, 972
Neurologic system
    assessment, 327-338
    depression as anesthesia complication, 504
Neuromuscular blocking agents, 903
Neuropathy, external catheterization and, 184
Neurotransmitter, defined, 972
Neurovascular dysfunction, risk for peripheral
    casting, 648
    traction, 638
Neutrophils
    normal values, 965
    in wound healing, 566
Newborn, 103-220; *see also* Infant
    bathing, 212-215
    diaper changing, 214-218
    feeding, 206-211
    irregular respirations and apneic spells, 236
    radial or apical pulse, 225
    swaddling and mummy restraint, 218-220
    temperature measurement, 233, 234
    thermoregulation using radiant warmer,
        204-206
    urine collection, 351
Nicotine
    effects on vital signs, 231
    skin patch for administration, 431-432
Night sweats in tuberculosis, 60
Nipple, 304
Nipride; *see* Nitroprusside
Nitrogen balance, 972
Nitroglycerin
    code management, 881
    ointment administration, 430-431
    skin patch for administration, 431-432
Nitroprusside, 881
Nodule, 261
Noise
    blood pressure measurement and, 238
    sleep and, 191, 194
Nonantimicrobial soap for handwashing, 50,
    51
Noncompliance
    drug therapy, 415, 922
    older adult, 419
    intravenous therapy, 684
Non-Luer-Lok syringe, 447, 448
Nonnarcotic analgesics, 537
Non-parenteral medication administration,
    407, 420-446
    eye and ear, 433-438
    metered-dose inhalers, 438-441

Non-parenteral medication
        administration–cont'd
    oral, 422-428
    rectal and vaginal, 442-445
    teaching self-administration of, 922-926
    topical, 429-433
Nonpharmacologic pain management,
    533-536
Non-rapid eye movement sleep, 190
Nonrebreather mask for oxygen delivery, 728,
    733
Nonsteroidal antiinflammatory drugs
    heparin therapy and, 459
    for pain management, 533, 537
Nonverbal communication, 25, 26
Norepinephrine, 881
Normal saline
    blood transfusion, 722
    central venous lines, 890
    fluid and electrolyte imbalance, 855
    intravenous medication administration,
        714-715, 718-719
    nasogastric tube irrigation, 770-772
    suctioning, 740, 743
    urinary diversion postoperative care, 820
North American Nursing Diagnosis
    Association
    accepted nursing diagnoses of, 6-8, 962-964
    defined, 972
Nose
    assessment, 288-292
    feeding tube measurement, 778
    food and/or fluids draining out of during
        feeding, 162
    medication administration in, 421
    specimen collection, 345, 347, 354
Nosocomial infection, 47
    defined, 972
    during mechanical ventilation, 906
NPUAP; *see* National Pressure Ulcer Advisory
    Panel
NRC; *see* Nuclear regulatory Commission
NREM; *see* Non-rapid eye movement
NS; *see* Normal saline
Nuclear imaging studies, 380-381
    cardiac, 396-401
Nuclear Regulatory Commission, 76
Numeric Pain Intensity Scale, 534
Nuprin; *see* Ibuprofen
Nurse
    circulating, 492, 969
    licensed practical or vocational, 5
    perioperative, 492
    personal self-disclosure by, 29
    registered, 3-5
    roles of, 3
Nurse Practice Acts, 3, 5
Nursing, 2-23
    defined, 2
    delegation, 3-5
    documentation, 12-22
        change-of-shift report, 19-21
        communication within health care team
            and, 12-13
        confidentiality, 16
        home health care, 16
        incident report, 21-22
        long-term care, 16
        medical records in, 13, 14, 15
        reporting and recording guidelines, 13-16,
            17-19
    health care trends, 3
    multicultural, 972
    nursing process, 5-8
    professional nurse's role, 3
    standard protocols, 9-12
    standards of care, 3, 4
Nursing assessment form, 6, 956-957
Nursing assistant, certified, 5
Nursing diagnosis, 6-8, 962-964
    in change-of-shift report, 20
    communication, 28-29
    high-risk, 6

Nursing diagnosis—cont'd
　licensed practical or vocational nurse's role
　　in, 5
　standards of nursing practice and, 4
Nursing history form, 14
Nursing intervention, 9, 12
Nursing Kardex, 13, 14
Nursing practice, standards of, 3, 4
Nursing process, 5-8
　licensed practical or vocational nurse's role
　　in, 5
　medication administration and, 415-416
　standards of nursing practice versus, 4
Nutrient, defined, 972
Nutrition
　altered: less than body requirements, 156
　　comprehensive health assessment, 317
　　enteral nutrition, 776
　　oral hygiene, 130
　　pressure ulcers, 567
　altered: more than body requirements, 156
　　comprehensive health assessment, 317
　effects on stoma output, 802
　enteral, 775-790
　　defined, 970
　　medication administration through feed-
　　　ing tube, 787-790
　　nasogastric or nasointestinal intubation
　　　for, 776-781
　　tube feeding administration, 781-787
　newborn, 206-211
　pressure ulcer formation and, 570, 574, 576,
　　578
　promotion, 155-166
　　feeding dependent clients, 156-160
　　impaired swallowing, assisting clients
　　　with, 160-162
　　obtaining body weights, 163-166
　total parenteral, 898-900
　wound healing and, 517
　　delayed, 567
NVD; see Neck vein distention
Nystagmus, defined, 972

O

Obesity
　bariatric bed and, 614
　defined, 972
　pressure ulcer formation and, 578
　wound healing and, 517, 567
OBRA; see Omnibus Budget Reconciliation
Obstruction
　airway, postoperative, 511
　mechanical, as anesthesia complication, 504
　prostatic, external catheterization, 184
Obstructive sleep apnea, 735
Occupational Safety and Health Administra-
　tion
　needleless infusion lines, 712
　needle-stick prevention, 449
　tuberculosis precautions, 60
　Universal Precautions, 49
Oculomotor nerve, 333
Odor, body
　bathing for reduction, 121
　shift assessment, 255, 256
Ointment, topical medication as, 421, 430
　ocular, 435-436
Older adult; see Geriatric considerations
Olfaction in shift assessment, 255, 256
Olfactory, defined, 972
Olfactory nerve, 333
Omnibus Budget Reconciliation, 76
Oncotic pressure, defined, 972
One Touch Basic, 369
One Touch Profile, 369
Open wound, 578
Open-question technique, 36
Ophthalmic, defined, 972
Ophthalmoscope, 282-283
Opiates, 537
Opposition, thumb, 627
Optic nerve, 333

Oral cavity
　assessment, 288-292
　care of, 130-135
　　endotracheal intubation, 749
　　newborn, 213
　　postoperative suctioning, 507, 508
Oral change-of-shift report, 19
Oral cholecystography, 376-379
Oral medication administration, 407, 421,
　　422-428
　through feeding tube, 787-790
Oral mucous membrane
　altered
　　comprehensive health assessment, 288
　　gastric intubation, 765
　　oral care and, 130
　　personal hygiene and, 122
　comprehensive health assessment, 290
Oral temperature, 232-233, 240
　advantages and disadvantages, 224
　normal ranges, 223
　thermometer used for, 223
Organic brain syndrome, defined, 972
Organized documentation, 16
Organ/tissue donation, 882-883
Orientation in shift assessment, 257
Orientation phase of interviewing, 36, 37
Oropharyngeal suctioning, 739-743
Orthopnea, 228
　defined, 972
　lumbar puncture and, 387
Orthostatic hypotension
　defined, 972
　minimizing, 106-107
　from Rotokinetic bed, 613
　during vascular system assessment, 312
Orthotic device, caring for client with, 677-681
OSA; see Obstructive sleep apnea
Oscillatory ventilation, high-frequency, 902
Oscillometric blood pressure measurement,
　　245-249
Osmolality
　defined, 972
　normal values, 965
Osmoreceptor, defined, 972
Osmosis, 853, 854, 972
Osmotic pressure, 853, 972
Osteomyelitis, 646
Osteoporosis, 108
Ostomy
　defined, 972
　gastrointestinal
　　irrigating colostomy, 803-807
　　pouching an enterostomy, 794-802
　urinary, 818-824
Otoscope, 282, 283
Ototoxicity, defined, 972
Overflow incontinence, 178
Oximetry
　defined, 972
　pulse, 249-253
　　mechanical ventilation, 904
　　oxygen therapy, 729, 733
　　postoperative, 511
Oxycodone hydrochloride, 537
Oxygen concentrator, 936, 937
Oxygen partial pressure, 734
　acid-base imbalance, 865
　normal values, 966
Oxygen saturation
　defined, 972
　normal values, 966
　pulse oximetry measurement, 249-253
Oxygen therapy
　client teaching for home use, 936-940
　postoperative hypovolemia, 511
Oxygen toxicity during mechanical ventila-
　tion, 906
Oxygenation promotion, 727-764
　airway management
　　closed chest drainage systems, 754-764
　　endotracheal tube and tracheostomy care,
　　　747-754
Oxygenation promotion—cont'd

airway management—cont'd
　noninvasive interventions, 735-739
　suctioning, 739-747
nursing diagnosis, 727-764
oxygen administration, 728-734
　after endoscopy, 395
Oxymizer for oxygen delivery, 728

P

PaCO$_2$; see Arterial carbon dioxide tension
PACU; see Postanesthesia care unit
Pain
　abdominal
　　comprehensive health assessment, 319
　　enema administration and, 185, 188
　　during peritoneal dialysis, 915
　after nasogastric tube removal, 774
　autonomic nervous system response to, 191
　blood pressure and, 231
　casting, 648, 654
　chronic, 317, 532
　comprehensive health assessment, 317
　　eyes and ears, 293
　　heart and circulation, 309
　　musculoskeletal system, 339
　　nose, sinuses, and mouth, 288
　defined, 972
　effects on vital signs, 231
　elimination and, 174
　fecal impaction, 792
　foot, 140
　gate control theory of, 190
　hot and cold therapies, 551
　impaired mobility and, 97
　intractable, 971
　intravenous therapy, 684
　laboratory and diagnostic testing, 345
　physiologic and psychological responses,
　　534
　postoperative, 510, 511
　sensory nerve function assessment, 334
　shift assessment, 256
　shoulder, 915
　traction, 638
　types, 530
　urinary elimination, altered, 809
　venous and arterial insufficiency, 275
　visual or hearing impairment, 833
Pain management, 530-550
　epidural analgesia, 544-550
　nonpharmacologic, 533-536
　nursing diagnosis, 532
　patient-controlled analgesia, 539-544
　pharmacologic, 537-539
Pain scale, 533, 534
Palate, 291
Palliative, defined, 972
Pallor
　defined, 972
　shift assessment, 259
Palpation, 281
　defined, 972
　pulse, 225, 226
　shift assessment, 255
　systolic blood pressure, 242
Palpitation, defined, 972
Palsy, crutch, 669
Panadol; see Acetaminophen
Pancreas, 317-322
PaO$_2$; see Oxygen partial pressure
PAPR; see Powered air-purifier respirator
Papule, 261
Paracentesis, 383-396
Paralysis, overflow incontinence and, 178
Paraplegia, bed to chair transfer and, 108
Paregoric, 572
Parenteral drug administration, 407
Parent-infant attachment, 203, 204
Paresthesia
　epidural analgesia and, 546
　in venous and arterial insufficiency, 275
Partial agonist, defined, 404, 405
Partial rebreather mask for oxygen delivery,
　　728, 733

Partial thromboplastin time, 965
Passive motion, 340
Patch, transdermal, 431-432
Patellar reflex, 337
Pathogen, defined, 972
Pathologic fracture, defined, 972
Patient; see Client
Patient care summary, 14
Patient-controlled analgesia, 539-544
    ambulatory infusion pump with, 697
    flow sheet, 543
    postoperative, 511
Patient's Bill of Rights, 10-11
PCA; see Patient-controlled analgesia
Pco2; see Carbon dioxide partial pressure
Peak expiratory flow rate, 735, 738-739
Pedal pulses
    comprehensive health assessment, 314, 315
    nonpalpable after angiography, 379
    shift assessment, 277
Pediatric considerations
    Bryant's traction, 636, 638
    cardiopulmonary resuscitation, 874, 875
    drug administration, 418, 428
        metered-dose inhalers, 441
    drug dosages, 411
    fluid volume deficit, 856
    isolation, 50
    lumbar puncture, 387, 396
    pain assessment, 533, 534
    point of maximal impulse location, 266
    removal during fire, 75
    shift assessment, 279
    specimen collection, 259, 359, 375
        blood, 367
        urine, 351
    temperature measurement, 233, 234
Pediculosis, 136
PEEP; see Positive end-expiratory pressure
Pelvic belt traction, 636, 637
Pelvic floor exercise, 178
Penetrating wound, 579
Penis
    bathing of, 127
    comprehensive health assessment, 325
    external catheterization and, 181-183
    genital self-examination, 326
Penlight, 282
Penrose drain, 516, 517, 522-523
Pepto-Bismol, 572
Perceived constipation, 168
Perception
    defined, 972
    influence on communication, 26
Percocet; see Oxycodone hydrochloride
Percodan; see Oxycodone hydrochloride
Percussion, 281-282
Perforating penetrating wound, 579
Perforation, pulmonary, 390
Perfusion
    altered tissue, 230
        cardiopulmonary resuscitation, 870
        comprehensive health assessment, 309
        hot and cold therapies, 551
        perioperative, 505
        pressure ulcers, 567
        shift assessment, 256
    defined, 226, 972
    oxygen delivery and, 869
Perineum, washing of, 126-127
Periodontitis, 131
Perioperative nursing, 474-563
    heat and cold, therapeutic use of, 551-563
        cold compress and ice bags, 559-562
        dry heat, 556-559
        moist heat, 553-556
        nursing diagnosis, 551
    intraoperative techniques, 492-502
        nursing diagnosis, 493
        sterile gowning and closed gloving,
            497-501
        surgical hand scrub, 493-497
Perioperative nursing—cont'd
    pain management, 530-550

epidural analgesia, 544-550
    nonpharmacologic, 533-536
    nursing diagnosis, 532
    patient-controlled analgesia, 539-544
    pharmacologic, 537-539
postoperative care, 503-529
    comfort measures in convalescent phase,
        512-516
    drainage device monitoring and measur-
        ing, 520-524
    nursing diagnosis, 505
    in postanesthesia care unit, 506-512
    staple and suture removal, 524-529
    wound care, 516-519
preoperative phase, 475-491
    assessment, 476-479
    nursing diagnosis, 475
    physical preparation, 485-491
    teaching, 480-485
Peripheral, defined, 972
Peripheral artery assessment, 314-315
Peripheral circulation assessment, 274-279
Peripheral neurovascular dysfunction, risk for
    casting, 648
    traction, 638
Peripheral tissue perfusion, altered
    comprehensive health assessment, 309
    hot and cold therapies, 551
    pressure ulcers, 567
    shift assessment, 256
Peripheral vascular disease, 126
Peripherally inserted central catheter, 889,
    891-895
Peristalsis, defined, 972
Peritoneal dialysis, 911-915
Peritonitis, 914
PERRLA acronym, 972
Personal hygiene, 121-154
    bathing, complete, 123-129
    bedmaking, 147-153
    foot and nail care, 141-147
    hair care, 135-140
    nursing diagnosis, 122
    oral care, 130-135
    shift assessment, 257
Personal protective equipment, 48
Personal safety, potentially violent client
    and, 43
Personal space
    cultural considerations in
        communication, 26
    potentially violent client and, 43
        in home care or long-term care
            setting, 44
Petechiae
    defined, 972
    shift assessment, 259
Pétrissage massage, 200
pH
    acid-base imbalance, 865
    gastric intubation aspirate, 768
        tube placement and, 776
    gastrointestinal stoma output, 797
    normal values, 864, 966
    urine screening test, 370-371
Pharmacokinetics, 404-407, 972
Pharmacologic pain management, 537-539
Pharmacy, 407-408
Pharynx
    comprehensive health assessment, 291
    role in swallowing, 160
Phlebitis
    blood transfusion site, 724
    defined, 972
    intravenous therapy site, 691, 692, 710
Phosphate, normal values, 965
Phosphorus, normal values, 965
Photophobia, defined, 972
Physical activity
    pressure ulcer formation and, 568, 569
    promotion; see Physical activity promotion

Physical activity promotion, 96-120
    assisted ambulation, 117-120
    moving and positioning clients in bed,
        97-105
    nursing diagnoses, 96-97
    orthostatic hypotension, minimizing,
        106-107
    transfers, 107-117
        from bed to chair, 107-112
        from bed to chair using mechanical lift,
            112-115
        from bed to transfer, 115-117
Physical appearance
    neurologic function assessment, 330
    shift assessment, 257
Physical contact, cultural considerations, 256
Physical examination, 280-343
    abdomen, 317-322
    eyes and ears, 293-299
    general survey, 280
    genitalia and rectum, 322-327
    head, face, and neck, 283-288
    heart and circulation, 309-317
    musculoskeletal function, 339-343
    neurologic function, 327-338
    nose, sinuses, and mouth, 288-292
    nutritional assessment, 155
    postmortem, 882
    preoperative, 476-479
    shift assessment, 255-279
        abdomen, 269-273
        apical pulse, 266-269
        extremities and peripheral circulation,
            274-279
        general survey and integumentary inspec-
            tion, 257-262
        lung sounds, 262-266
        nursing diagnosis, 256
    techniques, 281-283
    thorax, lungs, and breasts, 299-308
Physical mobility, impaired, 96
    assistive devices, 661
    casting, 648
    comprehensive health assessment, 328, 339
    discharge planning, 918
    etiologic factors, 8
    hot and cold therapies, 551
    pain, 532
    perioperative, 505
    pressure ulcers, 567
    risk for, 617
    specialty beds, 601
    traction, 638
Physical preparation, preoperative, 485-491
Physical restraint; see Restraint
Physician's order for medication administra-
    tion, 406-412
PICC; see Peripherally inserted central catheter
PIE progress notes, 17
Pigmentation
    defined, 972
    pulse oximetry and, 250
Pill-crushing device, 425
Pin site in skeletal traction, 642, 643, 645
Piroxicam, 537
Pitting edema, 276
Placebo, defined, 972
Planning, 7, 8
    licensed practical or vocational nurse's role
        in, 5
    standards of nursing practice and, 4
Plantar flexion, defined, 972
Plantar reflex, 337
Plantar wart, 142, 143
Plasma protein, 711
Plaster of Paris cast, 648, 650, 651-652, 653
Platelet count
    after blood transfusion, 725
    normal values, 965
    rectal temperature in child and, 233
    shaving and, 136
Platform crutch, 661
Platform scale, 164

Pleural friction rub, 263, 972
Pleur-evac autotransfusion system, 762-763
PMI; *see* Point of maximal impulse
Pneumothorax, 754, 900, 906, 972
Po₂; *see* Oxygen partial pressure
Point of maximal impulse, 226, 266, 311-312, 317
Polypharmacy, 418
Popliteal pulse
comprehensive health assessment, 314, 315
defined, 972
Positioning
airway management, 735, 736-737
in bed, 97-105
bone marrow aspiration, 386
cardiopulmonary resuscitation, 872
feeding, 158
female genitalia assessment, 323
liver biopsy, 390, 391
lumbar puncture, 386-387
lung auscultation, 264
to minimize orthostatic hypotension, 106-107
paracentesis, 388
pressure ulcer formation, 573-574
rectal temperature, 233
shampooing of hair, 135, 137-138
shift assessment, 257
urinary catheterization, 811-812
Positive end-expiratory pressure, 902
Postanesthesia care unit, 503, 506-512
Postanesthesia recovery scoring system, 506
Posterior tibial pulse
comprehensive health assessment, 314, 315
defined, 972
Postmortem examination, 882
Postoperative bed, making of, 150
Postoperative care, 503-529
autotransfusions, 754-764
comfort measures in convalescent phase, 512-516
drainage device monitoring and measuring, 520-524
nursing diagnosis, 505
in postanesthesia care unit, 506-512
staple and suture removal, 524-529
wound care, 516-519
Postural drainage, defined, 973
Postural hypotension
defined, 973
minimizing, 106-107
Posture
comprehensive health assessment, 340
of nurse, potentially violent client and, 44
older adult, 343
shift assessment, 257
Potassium
imbalance, 859, 860, 861-862
normal values, 965
Pouching, enterostomy, 794-802
Powder
medicated, 432
reconstituting medication from, 455
Power of attorney, durable, 10
Powered air-purifier respirator, 60
Powerlessness
infection control, 50
sleep and relaxation, 191
surgery, 475
PPE; *see* Personal protective equipment
Precision Q.I.D., 369
Prednisone
body fluid balance and, 856
urine output and, 168
Preload, defined, 973
Preoperative assessment form, 477
Preoperative checklist, 486
Preoperative education flow sheet, 481
Preoperative nursing, 475-491
assessment, 476-479
nursing diagnosis, 475
physical preparation, 485-491
teaching, 480-485

Prescription, defined, 973
Pressure dressing, postoperative, 511
Pressure points, patient positioning and, 97, 98
Pressure ulcer, 565-585
defined, 973
nursing diagnosis, 567
risk assessment and prevention strategies, 568-576
treatment, 577-585
Prestige, 369
Primary intention, defined, 973
Privacy
bathing, 124
interview, 37
in Patient's Bill of Rights, 10
Probenecid, 459
Problem statement in nursing diagnosis, 6
Proctoscopy, 385
Productive cough, defined, 973
Professional nursing
delegation, 3-5
documentation, 12-22
change-of-shift report, 19-21
communication within health care team and, 12-13
confidentiality, 16
home health care, 16
incident report, 21-22
long-term care, 16
medical records in, 13, 14, 15
reporting and recording guidelines, 13-16, 17-19
health care trends, 3
nursing defined, 2
nursing process, 5-8
roles in, 2-23
standard protocols, 9-12
standards of care, 3, 4
Programmable hearing aid, 845
Progress notes, 17, 18
Progressive relaxation, 195, 532
Prolapse, defined, 973
Proliferative stage of wound healing, 566
Pronation, 341
defined, 973
forearm, 624
Propoxyphene hydrochloride, 537
Propoxyphene napsylate, 537
Prostaglandin, defined, 973
Prostatic hyperplasia, benign, 827
Prosthesis
eye, 839-842
preoperative assessment, 478
Prostrate obstruction, external catheterization and, 184
Protection, altered, 415
Protein
buildup on contact lens, 833
defined, 973
intravenous therapy and, 711
normal values, 966
urine screening test, 370-371
Proteinuria, defined, 973
Prothrombin time
normal values, 965
shaving and, 136
Protocol
defined, 973
for nursing intervention, 9-12
Proxy, health care, 10
Prudent diet, 158
Pruritus
bathing and, 123
drug allergy, 405
Pseudomonas aeruginosa, 834
PT; *see* Prothrombin time
Ptosis, defined, 973
PTT; *see* Partial thromboplastin time
Ptyalin, defined, 973
Pubic hair, 323, 325
Pulmonary cancer
risk factors, 300
warning signs, 264

Pulmonary system
acid-base balance and, 864
comprehensive health assessment, 299-308
perforation during thoracentesis, 390
shift assessment, 262-266
Pulse, 225-226, 227, 231-232, 234-235, 240-241
apical
defined, 968
shift assessment, 266-269
during assisted ambulation, 119
during bronchoscopy, 392
during endoscopy, 393, 395
normal ranges, 223
shift assessment, 257, 258, 276-277
in venous and arterial insufficiency, 275
Pulse deficit, 235, 973
Pulse oximetry, 249-253
in mechanical ventilation, 904
in oxygen therapy, 729, 733
postoperative, 511
Pulse pressure
defined, 973
normal ranges, 223
Pulse saturation, 249-253
Pupil, 295-296, 297
Pureed diet, 158
Pursed-lip breathing, defined, 973
Purulent wound drainage, 567
Pustule, 261
PVD; *see* Peripheral vascular disease
Pyelography, intravenous, 376-379
Pyramid cane, 659, 660
Pyrexia, defined, 973
Pyrogen, defined, 973

Q

Quad cane, 659, 660
Question phase of interviewing, 36, 37
Questran, 572

R

RACE acronym, 74
Radial pulse, 225, 226
comprehensive health assessment, 314, 315
defined, 973
oximeter pulse rate and, 252, 253
in pulse deficit, 235
weak or difficult-to-palpate, 240
Radiant warmer for infant thermoregulation, 204-206
Radiation
defined, 973
safety, 76
Radiation therapy
effects on hair, 135
oral hygiene and, 130
safety measures, 92-94
wound healing and, 517, 567
Radioactive material, safety measures, 92-94
Radiology for checking tube placement, 776
Rales, 263
Ram's horn nail, 142, 143
Random urine specimen, 346, 348
Range of motion, 617-635
bathing for promotion of, 121
comprehensive health assessment, 340-342
exercise for dependent client, 98, 618-633
ankle, 630
assessment, 618-619
continuous passive motion machine, 632-635
elbow, 623
evaluation, 631
fingers, 626
forearm, 624
hip, 628-629
knee, 630
neck, 620-621
planning, 619
shoulder, 621-622, 623
thumb, 627
wrist, 625

Range of motion—cont'd
    nursing diagnosis, 617
    older adult, 343
Rapid eye movement sleep, 190
RAS; *see* Reticular activating system
Rash, 122
    bathing and, 123
    diaper, 215
    drug allergy, 405
Rate of respiration, 226
RDA; *see* Recommended daily allowance
REACT; *see* Postanesthesia recovery scoring
        system
Reactive hyperemia, 973
Recapping of needle, 450, 451
Receiver in communication, 25
Receptive aphasia
    communication with older adult and, 28, 34
    defined, 973
Receptor site, 404
RECIPE acronym, 559
Reclining chair, 77
Recommended daily allowance, 973
Reconstruction stage of wound healing, 566
Recording, 17-19; *see also* Documentation
    for communication within health care team,
        12
    guidelines, 13-16
    medical record in, 13, 14, 15
    sample forms, 949-959
Recovery room, 506-512
Rectal temperature, 233-234, 240
    advantages and disadvantages, 224
    newborn bathing and, 212
    normal ranges, 223
Rectum, medication insertion, 421, 442-445
Recurrent bandage turn, 595
Red blood cells, normal values, 965, 966
Red reflex, 296
Reflex
    comprehensive health assessment, 337
    gag
        oral hygiene and, 130
        oral medication and, 420
    pupillary, 295-296
    rooting, 973
Reflex hammer, 282, 283
Reflex incontinence, 168, 809
Reflex pain response, defined, 973
Refocusing skill, 41
Registered nurse, 3-5
Reimbursement
    home health care documentation guide-
        lines, 16
    surgical procedure, 503
Relationships, influence on communication,
        26
Relaxation techniques, 195-202
    pain management, 532
Religious, defined, 973
Religious factors, 36
REM; *see* Rapid eye movement
Reminiscence, defined, 973
Remission, defined, 973
Renal failure
    fluid balance alteration in, 855
    hemodialysis for, 907
Renal system
    calculi, 973
    comprehensive health assessment, 317-322
    disease, blood pressure and, 231
    fluid output regulation by, 855
Reporting; *see also* Documentation
    change-of-shift report, 19-21
    for communication within health care team,
        12
    guidelines, 13-16
    incident, 21-22
    medication error, 418
Research, 11
Reservoir nasal cannula for oxygen delivery,
        731
Residual urine, defined, 973

Resonance, 282
Resorption, bone, 969
Respiration, 226-228, 231-232, 235-236, 241
    anesthesia complications, 504
    normal ranges, 223
    postanesthesia recovery scoring system, 506
    shift assessment, 257
Respirator
    application of, 57
    fit test, 50
    in tuberculosis precautions, 49, 50, 60
Respiratory acidosis, 865, 867
Respiratory alkalosis, 865, 866, 867
Respiratory arrest
    cardiopulmonary resuscitation, 870-876
    code management, 877-882
Respiratory rate, 226
    epidural analgesia assessment, 548
    postoperative, 511
Respiratory system
    acid-base balance and, 864
    comprehensive health assessment, 299-308
    epidural analgesia assessment, 546, 548
    postoperative depression, 511
    shift assessment, 262-266
Respite care, defined, 973
Restlessness during intravenous therapy, 702
Restraint, 76
    application, 85-89, 90
    defined, 973
    designing a restraint-free environment,
        81-84
    mummy, 218-220
    pediatric specimen collection, 359
Resuscitation, 870-876
    code management, 877-882
    nursing diagnosis, 869
Resuscitation cart, 870, 871
Retention, urinary, 317, 809
Retention catheter, 815
Reticular activating system, 536
Rh factor, 720
Rhinitis, 405
Rhonchi, 263, 973
Rhythm of respiration, 226
RICE acronym, 559
Rigid contact lens, 833, 835-836, 837-838
Ring, handwashing and, 51
Rinne test, 298
Risk assessment in home health management,
        918-922
Risk for altered body temperature, 229-230
Risk for altered health maintenance
    communication and, 29
    perioperative, 505
Risk for altered parent-infant attachment, 204
Risk for aspiration
    enteral nutrition, 776
    gastric intubation, 765
    laboratory and diagnostic testing, 345
    nutrition and, 156
    perioperative, 505
Risk for disuse syndrome, 96-97, 532
Risk for impaired physical mobility, 617
Risk for impaired skin integrity
    after death, 870
    comprehensive health assessment, 328
    gastrointestinal ostomy, 792
    personal hygiene and, 122
    pressure ulcers, 567
    shift assessment, 256
    traction, 638
Risk for ineffective airway clearance
    newborn, 204
    surgery, 505
Risk for ineffective thermoregulation, 204
Risk for infection
    comprehensive health assessment of geni-
        talia and rectum, 322
    discharge planning, 918
    infection control, 50
    intravenous therapy, 683
    laboratory and diagnostic testing, 345

Risk for infection—cont'd
    oxygenation promotion, 727
    perioperative, 505
    sterile technique, 64
    surgery, 475, 493
    traction, 638
    urinary elimination, altered, 809
    visual or hearing impairment, 833
Risk for injury
    assistive devices, 661
    casting, 648
    comprehensive health assessment
        eyes and ears, 293
        musculoskeletal system, 339
        neurologic function, 328
    discharge planning, 918
    environmental safety, 76
    hot and cold therapies, 551
    injection administration, 451
    intravenous therapy, 683
    laboratory and diagnostic testing, 345
    patient positioning and, 97
    surgery, 475
    visual or hearing impairment, 833
Risk for peripheral neurovascular dysfunction
    casting, 648
    traction, 638
Risk for violence: directed at others, 29
RN; *see* Registered nurse
Roles
    influence on communication, 26
    professional nurse, 3
    registered nurse, 3-5
ROM; *see* Range of motion
Rooting reflex, 973
Rotation, 341
    hip, 620
    neck, 621
    shoulder, 622
Rotokinetic bed, 601, 611-613
Routes of drug administration, 406, 407
Routine nursing assessment form, 956-957
Roxanol; *see* Morphine
Roxicodone; *see* Oxycodone hydrochloride
Running traction, 636

S

Sacrum, shearing force against, 98
Safety
    during bathing, 124
    drug, in home, 417
    environmental, 73-94
        accidents, 73, 74
        designing a restraint-free environment,
            81-84
        fire safety, 74, 75
        nursing diagnosis, 76
        radiation safety, 76
        for radioactive materials, 92-94
        restraints, 76, 85-89, 90
        safety equipment and fall prevention,
            76-81
        seizure precautions, 76, 91-92
    oxygen therapy, 730, 936
    potentially violent client, 43
    sensory alterations and, 832
    while obtaining body weights, 163
Safety belt for assisted ambulation, 666, 668
Safety grip bar in bathroom, 77
Saline
    blood transfusion, 722
    central venous lines, 890
    fluid and electrolyte imbalance, 855
    intravenous medication administration,
        714-715, 718-719
    nasogastric tube irrigation, 770-772
    suctioning, 740, 743
    urinary diversion postoperative care, 820
Sample forms, 949-959
Sanguineous wound drainage, 567
Sanitary pad, 180
SaO$_2$; *see* Arterial hemoglobin saturation
SASH acronym, 715

Scale for obtaining weight, 164-166
Scaled dropper, 411
Scalp
    comprehensive health assessment, 284
    massage, 199
Scarf for chemotherapy-related hair loss, 135
Scoliosis, 340
Scoop technique for recapping needle, 450, 451
Screening, blood donors, 720
Scrotum
    bathing of, 127
    comprehensive health assessment, 325
        in older adult, 327
    genital self-examination, 326
Scrub, hand, 493-497
Scrubs, 493
Sebum, defined, 973
Secretion
    retained and thick as anesthesia complication, 504
    Standard Precautions, 49
    suctioning of, 739-747
Sedation, intravenous conscious, 345
Sedatives
    mechanical ventilation, 903
    pain management, 537
    sleep promotion, 191
Seizure, safety precautions, 76, 91-92
Select GT, 369
Self-care deficit, 122
    altered elimination, 167
    casting, 648
    comprehensive health assessment, 288
    feeding, 156
    oral hygiene and, 130
    oxygenation promotion, 727
    personal hygiene and, 122
    traction, 638
Self-catheterization, 932-936
Self-examination
    breast, 306
        in older women, 308
    genital, male, 325, 326
Self-image, bathing for improvement of, 121
Semi-Fowler's position
    moving dependent client to, 101
        minimizing orthostatic hypotension during, 106
    oxygen therapy, 735
    paracentesis, 388
Semiprone position, 97, 103-104
Sender in communication, 25
Sensory deficit, defined, 973
Sensory deprivation, defined, 973
Sensory function
    comprehensive health assessment, 334, 335
    pressure ulcer formation and, 569
    self-administration of medication, 417
Sensory overload, defined, 973
Sensory/perceptual alterations, 832-851
    communication and, 29
    comprehensive health assessment of eyes and ears, 293
    contact lens client, caring for, 833-839
    discharge planning, 918
    drug therapy, 415
    ear irrigation, 848-850
    eye irrigation, 842-844
    eye prosthesis, caring for client with, 839-842
    hearing aid client, caring for, 845-848
    hot and cold therapies, 551
    nursing diagnosis, 832-833
Septicemia, postoperative, 517
Septum, 289
Sequential compression stocking, 489
Serosanguineous wound drainage, 567
Serous wound drainage, 567
Serum albumin, 574, 578
Serum glutamic oxaloacetic transaminase, 965
Serum glutamic pyruvic transaminase, 965
Serum half-life, defined, 973

Sexual history, 322
Sexual response cycle, defined, 973
Sexuality, defined, 973
Sexuality patterns, altered
    genitalia and rectum assessment, 322
    urinary elimination, altered, 809
Sexually transmitted disease, 322
    genital self-examination and, 326
SGOT; see Serum glutamic oxaloacetic transaminase
SGPT; see Serum glutamic pyruvic transaminase
Shaft of needle, 447, 448
Shampooing of hair, 135, 136, 137-138
    newborn, 214
Sharps
    one-hand disposal, 449, 450
    Standard Precautions, 49
Shaving of beard and mustache, 136, 139
Shearing force
    defined, 973
    patient positioning and, 98
    pressure ulcer formation and, 570
Shellfish allergy, 376, 379, 380
Shield
    application, 57
    radiation, 92, 93
    Standard Precautions, 49
Shift assessment, 255-279
    abdomen, 269-273
    apical pulse, 266-269
    extremities and peripheral circulation, 274-279
    general survey and integumentary inspection, 257-262
    lung sounds, 262-266
    nursing diagnosis, 256
Shivering, defined, 973
Shock
    anaphylactic, 405, 406
    blood pressure and, 231
Shoe, ambulation and, 662
Shortness of breath
    following thoracentesis, 395
    during intravenous therapy, 702
Shoulder
    pain during peritoneal dialysis, 915
    range of motion
        assessment, 341
        exercise, 618, 621-622, 623
Shower, safety features, 77
Shunt, atrioventricular, 85
Side effects of drugs, 405
    client teaching, 416-417
Side rail, 79-80, 663
Side-arm traction, 642, 643
Side-lying position, 102
Sigmoid colostomy, 791, 797
Sigmoidoscopy, 385
Signaling device for safety, 77
Signed consent
    angiography and computed tomography, 377
    bronchoscopy, magnetic resonance imaging and endoscopy, 384
    surgical, 487, 488
Silence, 26
    in active listening, 35
Sim's position
    moving dependent client to, 97, 103-104
    rectal temperature, 233
SIMV; see Synchronized intermittent mandatory ventilation
Sinus assessment, 288-292
Sitting position
    pressure points in, 98
    progressive muscle relaxation in, 196
Sitz bath moist heat therapy, 553
Skeletal traction, 637-638, 642-646
Skin
    after cast removal, 657
    age factors, 121

Skin—cont'd
    assessment
        during bathing, 121, 122
            pressure ulcer formation, 571, 572
        common problems and related interventions, 122
        dry, 122
            bathing and, 129
            newborn, 215
        incontinence and, 178
        irritation during external catheterization, 184
        newborn, care of, 212
        peristomal damage, 799, 801
        personal hygiene to maintain integrity, 121
        pigmentation, pulse oximetry and, 250
        shift assessment, 257-262
        Standard Precautions, 49
        temperature measurement, 224
        vascular assessment, 314
Skin color
    foot assessment, 140, 141
    shift assessment, 259
Skin integrity
    impaired
        casting, 648
        fluid and electrolyte imbalance, 856
        genitalia and rectum, 322
        head, face, and neck, 283
        hot and cold therapies, 551
        intravenous therapy, 683
        personal hygiene and, 122
        pressure ulcers, 567
        shift assessment, 256
        specialty beds, 601
        urinary elimination, altered, 809
    risk for impaired
        after death, 870
        gastrointestinal ostomy, 792
        neurologic function assessment, 328
        personal hygiene and, 122
        pressure ulcers, 567
        shift assessment, 256
        traction, 638
Skin lesion in shift assessment, 260, 261
Skin temperature, pressure ulcers and, 571, 573, 574
Skin testing
    intradermal injection for, 469-472
    tuberculosis for health care workers, 49, 60
Skin traction, 636, 637, 638, 639-641
Skin turgor in shift assessment, 260
Skull, 284
Sleep, 190-202
    comfort measures promoting, 191-195
    relaxation techniques and, 195-202
Sleep deprivation, defined, 973
Sleep disorder, defined, 973
Sleep pattern disturbance, 191
Sloughing, defined, 974
Small-bore feeding tube, 776-781
Smoking
    breath sounds and, 264
    effects on vital signs, 231
    fire safety and, 73
Sneezing following allergy skin testing, 472
Soaking, feet, 144
Soap for handwashing, 50, 51
SOAP progress notes, 17
Social communication, 29
Social interaction, impaired
    communication and, 29
    visual or hearing impairment, 833
Social isolation
    communication and, 29
    infection control and, 50
    visual or hearing impairment, 833
Socialization, defined, 974
Sociocultural factors, 26
Socioeconomic factors, 568
Sock care, 145

Sodium
  imbalance, 859-861
  normal values, 965
Sodium-potassium pump, 854
Sodium-restricted diet, 158
Soft contact lens, 833, 835, 837
Soft food diet, 158
Soft palate, 291
Solution, sterile, 67
Sound
  blood pressure measurement and, 238
  sleep and, 191, 194
Space
  influence on communication, 26
  potentially violent client and, 43
    in home care or long-term care setting, 44
Specific gravity
  fluid imbalances, 858
  in monitoring intake and output, 169, 171
  normal values, 966
Specimen collection, 344, 345, 346-359
  assessment, 347
  chest tube, 760
  during dialysis, 910
  equipment, 346-347
  evaluation, 358-359
  implementation, 348-358
    cultures, 354-358
    stool collection, 353-354
    urine collection, 348-353
  planning, 347-348
Specimen cup, 282
Speculum, vaginal, 282, 283
Speech in shift assessment, 257
Sphygmomanometer, 229, 282
Spill
  fall prevention and, 76
  mercury, 224
Spinal accessory nerve, 285, 333
Spinal anesthesia, 509
Spine
  comprehensive health assessment, 340
  logrolling to maintain alignment, 103
Spiral bandage turn, 595
Spiral-reverse bandage turn, 595
Spiritual factors, 36
Spirometer, incentive, 483-484
Splint, caring for client with, 677-681
Spo₂; see Pulse saturation
Sponge bath, 212
Sputum collection, 346-359
  assessment, 347
  equipment, 346-347
  implementation, 354, 355
  planning, 347-348
SQ; see Subcutaneous
Stairs
  climbing and descending with crutches, 673-674
  fall prevention in home, 920-921
Standard Precautions, 48, 49; see also Infection control
Standard protocols for nursing intervention, 9-12
Standards of care, 3, 4
Staphylococcus aureus
  methicillin-resistant, 517
  surgical wound infection, 517
Staple removal, 524-529
STAT, medication ordered, 411, 415
STD; see Sexually transmitted disease
Steinmann pin, 642
Sterile dressing change kit, 64, 65
Sterile field
  creating and maintaining, 64-68
  defined, 63
  dressing application, 589
Sterile gloving, 69-72
Sterile gowning, 497-501
Sterile solution, 67
Sterile technique, 48, 63-72; see also Infection control
  continuous bladder irrigation, 825
  creating and maintaining a sterile field, 64-68
  dressing application, 589

Sterile technique—cont'd
  nursing diagnosis, 64
  perioperative nursing, 492-493
  sterile gloving, 69-72
Sterile urine specimen from indwelling catheter, 346-347, 351-352
Sterilization, defined, 48, 974
Steristrip application, 524-529
Sternum compression in cardiopulmonary resuscitation, 875-876
Steroids
  body fluid balance and, 856
  effects on vital signs, 231
  wound healing and, 517, 567
Stethoscope, 282
  blood pressure measurement, 229
  pulse measurement, 226, 227
Stimulants, effects on sleep, 192
Stocking
  antiembolism
    defined, 968
    preoperative application, 489
  sequential compression, 489
Stoma, 791
  defined, 974
  pouching, 794-802
Stomach
  comprehensive health assessment, 317-322
  intubation, 765-774
    inserting tube, 766-770
    irrigating tube, 770-772
    nursing diagnosis, 765
    removing tube, 773-774
Stool collection, 346-359
  assessment, 347
  equipment, 346-347
  evaluation, 358-359
  Hemoccult test, 373
  implementation, 353-354
  planning, 347-348
Straight traction, 636
Straight-back chair, 77
Strength
  bed to chair transfer and, 108
  comprehensive health assessment, 342
  shift assessment, 275
Streptococcus faecalis, 517
Stress
  effects on hair, 135
  wound healing, delayed, 567
Stress incontinence, 167-168, 178, 809
Stress test, exercise, 396-401
Stressor, defined, 974
Stretcher
  safety concerns, 81
  transfer from bed to, 115-117
Stroke volume, defined, 974
Subclavian placement of central venous lines, 890-891
Subcutaneous injection, 407, 447, 449, 457-463
Subjective data, 14
Sublimaze; see Fentanyl
Sublingual, defined, 974
Sublingual drug administration, 407, 421, 427
Suctioning
  for airway management, 739-747
    in home, 941
    postoperative, 507, 508
  sputum specimen, 347, 356-357
Sulindac, 537
Superficial wound, 579
Supination, 341
  defined, 974
  forearm, 624
Supine position
  for airway management, 735
  moving dependent client to, 97, 104
Suppository drug administration, 407, 421, 442-445
Supraclavicular node, 286
Suprapubic catheter, 828-830
Supreme II, 369
Sure-Med Unit Dose Center, 408
SureStep, 369
Surface body temperature, 243
Surgery, 474-563

  fluid balance alteration after, 855
  intraoperative techniques, 492-502
    nursing diagnosis, 493
    sterile gowning and closed gloving, 497-501
    surgical hand scrub, 493-497
  preparing client for, 475-491
    nursing diagnosis, 475
    physical preparation, 485-491
    preoperative assessment, 476-479
    preoperative teaching, 480-485
Surgical asepsis, 48, 63-72; see also Infection control
  continuous bladder irrigation, 825
  creating and maintaining a sterile field, 64-68
  defined, 974
  dressing application, 589
  nursing diagnosis, 64
  perioperative nursing, 492-493
  sterile gloving, 69-72
Surgical bed, making of, 150
Surgical hand scrub, 493-497
Surgical wound
  dehiscence, 529
  expected postoperative drainage, 505
  infection, 566
  postoperative hemorrhage, 510
Suspension, 412
Suspension traction, 636
Suspension-based lotion, 432
Suture removal, 524-529
Swab, cotton-tipped, 282
Swaddling, 218-220
Swallowing
  impaired, 156, 160-162, 283, 776
  oral medication and, 420, 426
Swelling
  after cast removal, 657
  defined, 969
  in fluid volume excess, 858
  laryngeal as anesthesia complication, 504
  shift assessment, 259, 276
  skeletal traction, 645, 646
Swing carry, 75
Swing-through crutch gait, 673
Swing-to crutch gait, 673
Symbols, 960
Symptom, interviewing and, 38
Synapse, defined, 974
Synchronized intermittent mandatory ventilation, 902
Syncope, defined, 974
Synergistic effect, 406, 974
Synthetic cast, 648, 650, 651-652, 653
Syringe
  blood specimen collection, 360, 362-364
  disposal, 59
  ear irrigation, 848
  medication administration, 447-451
    intravenous, 713-715
  reuse in home setting, 463
  tuberculosis testing, 469
Syringe magnifier, 926
Syrup medication, 412
Systole, defined, 974
Systolic blood pressure, 229
  during assisted ambulation, 119
  defined, 228
  in orthostatic hypertension, 312
  palpation, 242
  patient positioning for measurement, 223

T

T lymphocytes, normal values, 965
T tube, 505
Tablet medication, 412, 416, 424
  administration through feeding tube, 788
Tachycardia, 226, 240
  blood transfusion, 725
  defined, 974
  intravenous therapy, 702
Tachypnea, 228
  defined, 974
  following thoracentesis, 395
Tactile, defined, 974

Tactile fremitus, defined, 974
Tactile sensory/perceptual alteration, 551
Tape measure, 282
Target heart rate, 396
T-binder, 596, 598
Teacher, nurse as, 3
Teaching, 44-46
    communication and, 29
    discharge, 917-946
        home oxygen equipment, 936-940
        non-parenteral medication self-adminis-
            tration, 922-926
        nursing diagnosis, 918
        risk assessment and accident prevention,
            918-922
        self-catheterization, 932-936
        self-injection, 926-931
        tracheostomy care, 941-946
    foot care, 145-146
    isolation precautions, 56
    medication administration, 416-417
    pain management, 532
    preoperative, 480-485
Telephone medication order, 407
Telfa gauze dressing, 586
Temperature
    body; see Body temperature
    of otic drops, 433
    in sensory nerve function assessment, 334
    skin, pressure ulcers and, 571, 573, 574
Temporal artery, 285
Temporomandibular joint, 285
Tempra; see Acetaminophen
Tenckhoff catheter, 912
TENS; see Transcutaneous electrical nerve
    stimulation
Teratogen, defined, 974
Termination phase of interviewing, 36, 39
Territoriality
    defined, 974
    influence on communication, 26
Testicle, 325
T-handle cane, 659, 660
Theo-Dur, 789
Therapeutic communication, establishing of,
    29-31
Therapeutic effects of drugs, 405
Thermometer, 223-225, 231, 240
    tympanic, 243
Thermoregulation
    defined, 974
    ineffective, 230
    newborn
        risk for ineffective, 204
        using radiant warmer, 204-206
    postoperative, 510
Thigh, subcutaneous injection in, 457
Third-space syndrome, 852
Thirst mechanism, 855
30-degree lateral position, 102
Thoracentesis, 383-396, 974
Thorax, 299-308
Thought content in neurologic function as-
    sessment, 332
Thought process
    altered
        neurologic function assessment, 327-328
        oxygenation promotion, 727
    neurologic function assessment, 332
Three-point crutch gait, 672
Threshold, defined, 974
Thrill, 310
Throat culture, 345, 347, 354-358
Thrombolytics, 459
Thrombosis
    deep vein, leg massage and, 126
    defined, 974
Thrombus, defined, 974
Thumb, range of motion
    assessment, 341
    exercise, 618, 627
Thyroid assessment, 286-287
Thyroid function tests, 966
Thyroid scan, 380-381

Thyroid-stimulating hormone, normal
    values, 966
Tibial pulse, 314, 315
Time
    cultural considerations in communication,
        28
    military versus civilian, 15
Tincture, 412
Tincture of benzoin, 749
Tinea pedis, 142, 143
Tinnitus, defined, 974
Tissue
    donation, 882-883
    impaired integrity
        hot and cold therapies, 551
        injection administration, 451
    shear injury during positioning, 98
Tissue perfusion, altered, 230
    cardiopulmonary resuscitation, 870
    heart and circulation assessment, 309
    hot and cold therapies, 551
    injection administration, 451
    perioperative, 505
    pressure ulcers, 567
    shift assessment, 256
Titralac tabs, 572
TMJ; see Temporomandibular joint
Toe, range of motion exercise, 618
Toenail
    care, 141-147
    common problems, 142, 143
Toileting self-care deficit
    altered elimination, 167
    casting, 648
Tolerance, 406, 974
Tongue
    comprehensive health assessment, 291
    cry, cracked, and coated, 131
    role in swallowing, 160
Tongue depressor, 282
Tonsil, 291
Tooth
    cleansing, 133, 134
    comprehensive health assessment, 291
    dental caries, 131
    flossing, 134
Toothbrush, 130
Topical medication administration, 407,
    420-421, 429-433
Toradol; see Ketorolac tromethamine
Total bilirubin, 965
Total calcium, 965
Total incontinence, 809
Total knee replacement, 632-635
Total lipids, 966
Total lymphocyte count, 574, 578
Total parenteral nutrition, 898-900
Touch
    anxious client, 41
    cultural considerations, 256
    in communication, 26
    sensory nerve function assessment, 334
Tourniquet
    blood specimen collection, 361
    intravenous insertion, 686
Toxic effect, 405
    defined, 974
    older adult, 419
    oxygen during mechanical ventilation, 906
TPN; see Total parenteral nutrition
Trachea, 285
Tracheostomy, 901-907
    care, 747-754
    communication and, 28
    suctioning, 740, 741, 742, 743-747
    teaching home care, 941-946
Traction, 636-647
    nursing diagnosis, 638
    skeletal, 637-638, 642-646
    skin, 636, 637, 638, 639-641
Trade name of drug, 410, 412
Transcutaneous electrical nerve stimulation,
    532
Transdermal patch, 431-432

Transfer
    from bed to chair, 107-112
        using mechanical lift, 112-115
    from bed to stretcher, 115-117
    safety concerns, 80-81
Transfer belt, 107
Transfusion, blood, 720-725
    postoperative autotransfusion, 754-764
Transillumination of sinuses, 290
Transparent dressing
    changing, 592-594
    intravenous therapy site, 690, 705
    for wound debridement, 581
Transport
    active, 853
    safety measures, 80-81
Transverse colostomy, 791, 797
Trapeze, 99, 100
Trauma; see Injury
Triceps reflex, 337
Tridil; see Nitroglycerin
Trigeminal nerve, 284, 333
Triglycerides, 966
Tripod cane, 659, 660
Trochanter, defined, 974
Trochlear nerve, 333
TSH; see Thyroid-stimulating hormone
Tub, safety features, 77
Tube feeding, 775-790
    administration of feedings, 781-787
    medication administration through, 787-790
    nasogastric or nasointestinal intubation for,
        776-781
    pressure ulcer formation and, 572
Tuberculosis
    skin testing
        for health care workers, 49, 60
        syringes for, 447, 448
    special precautions, 49, 60-62
Tubex injection system, 449, 450
Tumor, 261
Tuning fork test, 282, 283, 297-298
Tunneled epidural catheter, 544, 545
Turban for chemotherapy-related hair loss, 135
Turgor
    defined, 974
    shift assessment, 260
24-hour urine collection, 347, 352-353
Two-point crutch gait, 672
Two-point discrimination, 334
Tylenol; see Acetaminophen
Tylox; see Oxycodone hydrochloride
Tympanic temperature, 243-245
    advantages and disadvantages, 224
    normal ranges, 223
Tympany, 282

U

Ulcer
    cutaneous, 261
        in venous and arterial insufficiency, 275
    pressure, 565-585
        defined, 973
        nursing diagnosis, 567
        risk assessment and prevention strategies,
            568-576
        treatment, 577-585
Ulnar artery, 314, 315
Ultra+, 369
Umbilical cord site assessment, 212
Unconjugated bilirubin, 965
Unconscious client
    external catheterization, 181
    eye care, 125
    oral hygiene, 132
Unilateral neglect, 328
Unit dose system, 408
Unit specimen testing, 368-375
United States Department of Health and Hu-
    man Services, 3
United States Public Health Service's Agency
    for Health Care Policy and Research
    clinical practice guidelines, 3
    urinary incontinence, 167
Universal carry, 75

Universal Precautions, 49; *see also* Infection control
UP; *see* Universal Precautions
Upper extremity
  blood pressure measurement, 236-239
  massage, 200
  range of motion
    assessment, 341
    exercise, 618, 624-627
  subcutaneous injection, 457
Urethral orifice, 324
Urge incontinence, 168, 178, 809
Uric acid, normal values, 966
Urinal, 173-177
Urinary casts, normal values, 966
Urinary catheterization, 810-818
  sterile urine specimen from, 346-347
  suprapubic, 828-830
  teaching home self-catheterization, 932-936
Urinary diversion, 815, 818-824
Urinary elimination, 809-831
  continuous bladder irrigation, 825-827
  nursing diagnosis, 809
  providing bedpan or urinal for, 173-177
  suprapubic catheter, 828-830
  urinary catheterization, male and female, 810-818
  urinary diversions, 818-824
Urinary incontinence, 167
  client care, 177-178
  external catheterization for, 181
Urinary retention
  abdominal assessment, 317
  altered elimination, 167, 809
Urinary tract infection, 830
Urination; *see* Urinary elimination
Urine
  collection, 345, 346-359
    assessment, 347
    equipment, 346-347
    evaluation, 358-359
    implementation, 348-353
    planning, 347-348
  normal values, 966
  residual, 973
  screening test, 368-375
  stale, assessment of characteristic odor, 256
Urine output; *see also* Intake and output monitoring
  normal, 809
  postoperative, 510, 511
Urine specific gravity
  fluid imbalances, 858
  normal values, 966
Urticaria
  defined, 974
  drug allergy, 405
USDHHS; *see* United States Department of Health and Human Services

V

Vaccination, 48
VacuDrain, 521-522
Vacuum tube, 360-367
Vagina
  comprehensive health assessment of opening, 324
  medication insertion, 421, 442-445
  urinary catheter into, 817
Vaginal speculum, 282, 283
Vagus nerve
  function and assessment, 333
  stimulation, 792, 794
Valium, 192
Valsalva maneuver, defined, 974
Values, influence on communication, 26
Vancomycin, 712
Varicosities, defined, 974
Vascular access device, defined, 974
Vascular access for hemodialysis, 907, 909
Vascular disease, peripheral, 126
Vascular system assessment, 312-316
Vasoactive infusion, 880, 881

Vasoconstriction
  cold therapy to induce, 552
  defined, 974
Vasodilation
  blood pressure and, 231
  defined, 974
  heat application to produce, 552
Vasodilators, 231
Vastus lateralis intramuscular injection, 464, 465-466
Vein
  comprehensive health assessment, 313-314
  postoperative hemorrhage, 504-505
  selection for intravenous therapy, 686-687
    geriatric considerations, 695
Venipuncture, 360-367, 974
Venous insufficiency, 275
Ventilation
  defined, 226, 974
  inability to sustain spontaneous, 727
  mechanical, 901-907
  oxygen delivery and, 869
Ventrogluteal intramuscular injection, 464, 465
Venturi mask for oxygen delivery, 728, 732
Verbal coaching while feeding client, 162
Verbal communication, 25
  impaired
    hearing impairment, 833
    oxygenation promotion, 727
Verbal medication order, 407
Verbal report, 12
Verbally deescalating a potentially violent client, 42-44
Vertigo
  from cold otic drop administration, 433
  defined, 974
Vesicle, 261
Vial, 455
  drawing up medication from, 454
  insulin, 458
  mixing medications from, 456
Vibration in sensory nerve function assessment, 334
Violence, risk for: directed at others, 29
Violent client, 42-44
Virulence, defined, 974
Vision
  blurred from contact lens, 838
  comprehensive health assessment, 293-299
  older adult, 299
Visual sensory/perceptual alterations, 832
  communication and, 29
  comprehensive health assessment of eyes and ears, 293
  contact lens client, caring for, 833-839
  drug therapy, 415
  eye irrigation, 842-844
  eye prosthesis, caring for client with, 839-842
Vital signs, 222-254
  during assisted ambulation, 119
  blood pressure, 228-229, 230, 231-232, 236-239, 241-242
    electronic, 245-249
  blood transfusion, 721, 725
  chest tube drainage system, 759, 760
  defined, 974
  in fluid volume excess, 858
  nursing diagnosis, 229-230
  oxygen saturation measurement with pulse oximetry, 249-253
  postoperative assessment, 507, 514, 515
  pulse, 225-226, 227, 231-232, 234-235, 240-241
  respirations, 226-228, 231-232, 235-236, 241
  shift assessment, 257
  temperature, 222-225, 231, 232-234, 239-240
    tympanic, 243-245
Vital signs record, 958-959
Vitamins, defined, 974
Vocal emphasis of words, 26
Vocational nurse, 5
Voiding, defined, 974

Volume-cycled mechanical ventilation, 902
Vomiting
  infant, after feeding, 211
  postoperative, 515

W

Walker, 661, 665-677
Warfarin
  dose calculation, 411
  shaving and, 136
Wart, plantar, 142, 143
Water mattress, 604
Waterless chest drainage system, 755, 756, 758
Water-seal chest drainage system, 755, 756, 757-758
Weakness
  during assisted ambulation, 119
  comprehensive health assessment, 342
Weber's test, 298
Weighing client, 163-166
Weight
  fluid volume deficit, 856
  height and weight tables, 967
  intake and output monitoring, 168, 169
  obtaining, 163-166
  pressure ulcer formation and, 578
  subcutaneous injection and, 457, 461
  surgical wound healing and, 517
Weight loss in tuberculosis, 60
Weight-sensitive alarm, 81, 82
Wet-to-dry dressing, 586, 590
Wheal, 261
Wheelchair safety, 80-81
Wheezes, 263
  during assisted ambulation, 119
  defined, 974
  drug allergy, 405
Whirlpool moist heat therapy, 553
White blood cell
  normal values, 965, 966
  in wound healing, 566
Will, living, 10
Winged butterfly needle and catheter, 684, 685
Wong-Baker Faces Scale, 534
Working phase of interviewing, 36, 38-39
Worksheet, 14
Wound care, 565-600
  binder and bandage application, 594-599
  classifications, 578-579
  dehiscence, postsurgical, 529
  dressing application, 585-591
    transparent, 592-594
  nursing diagnosis, 567
  pressure ulcer
    risk assessment and prevention strategies, 568-576
    treatment, 577-585
  specimen collection, 345, 347, 354, 357
  surgical, 516-519
    expected postoperative drainage, 505
Wound culture, defined, 974
Wound healing, 517, 566, 567
Wrist
  range of motion
    assessment, 341
    exercise, 618, 625
  restraint, 87
Written report, 12

X

X-ray for checking tube placement, 776
Xyphoid process, 778

Y

Yankauer suctioning, 739-743

Z

Z-track injection, 464, 467, 974

INDEX OF SKILLS*

Abdomen, comprehensive health assessment, Skill 14.6, *317*

Abdomen, shift assessment, Skill 13.4, *266*

Accident prevention in home management, Skill 40.1, *918*

Acid-base imbalance, monitoring, Skill 37.3, *864*

Active listening, Skill 2.3, *34*

Airway management, endotracheal tube and tracheostomy care, Skill 31.4, *747*

Airway management, noninvasive intervention, Skill 31.2, *735*

Airway management, suctioning, Skill 31.3, *739*

Ambulation, assisted, Skill 6.6, *117*

Analgesia, epidural, Skill 22.4, *544*

Analgesia, patient-controlled, Skill 22.3, *539*

Anxious client, communication with, Skill 2.5, *40*

Apical pulse, shift assessment, Skill 13.3, *266*

Arteriography, Skill 15.4, *376*

Aspirations, assisting with, Skill 15.6, *383*

Assistive devices, ambulation, Skills 29.1 to 29.3, *662-677*

Auscultation, apical pulse, Skill 13.3, *266*

Auscultation, lung, Skill 13.2, *262*

Autotransfusion management, Skill 31.5, *754*

Bandage application, Skill 24.5, *594*

Bathing, complete, Skill 7.1, *123*

Bathing, infant, Skill 11.3, *212*

Bed, air-fluidized, Skill 25.3, *608*

Bed, air-suspension, Skill 25.2, *605*

Bed, bariatric, Skill 25.5, *614*

Bed, moving and positioning clients in, Skill 6.1, *97*

Bed, Rotokinetic, Skill 25.4, *611*

Bedmaking, Skill 7.5, *147*

Bedpan, providing, Skill 9.2, *173*

Binder application, Skill 24.5, *594*

Biopsy, liver, Skill 15.6, *383*

Bladder irrigation, continuous, Skill 35.3, *825*

Blood pressure, electronic, Skill 12.3, *245*

Blood pressure, Skill 12.1, *231*

Blood specimens, Skill 15.2, *360*

Blood transfusion, Skill 30.5, *720*

Body temperature, assessment, Skill 12.1, *231*

Body weight, obtaining, Skill 8.3, *163*

Bone marrow aspiration, assisting with, Skill 15.6, *383*

Bone scan, Skill 15.5, *380*

Brace, Skill 29.3, *677*

Brain scan, Skill 15.5, *380*

Breast assessment, Skill 14.4, *299*

Bronchoscopy, assisting with, Skill 15.6, *383*

Cane, teaching use, Skill 29.2, *665*

Cardiac assessment, Skill 14.5, *309*

Cardiac catheterization, Skill 15.7, *396*

Cardiac studies, Skill 15.7, *396*

Cast application, Skill 28.1, *650*

Cast removal, Skill 28.2, *655*

Catheter, external, Skill 9.4, *181*

Catheter, suprapubic, Skill 35.4, *828*

Catheterization, cardiac, Skill 15.7, *396*

Catheterization, urinary, male and female, Skill 35.1, *809*

Central venous lines, Skill 39.1, *889*

Change-of-shift report, Skill 1.3, *19*

Changing diaper, Skill 11.4, *215*

Chemstrip/Multistix testing, Skill 15.3, *368*

Chest drainage system, management, Skill 31.5, *754*

Circulation, comprehensive health assessment, Skill 14.5, *309*

Circulation, shift assessment, Skill 13.5, *274*

Closed chest drainage system, management, Skill 31.5, *754*

Code management, Skill 38.2, *877*

Cold compress, Skill 23.3, *559*

Colostomy, irrigation, Skill 34.3, *803*

Comfort measures, postoperative, Skill 21.2, *512*

Comfort measures, promoting sleep, Skill 10.1, *190*

Comforting, Skill 2.2, *32*

Communication with anxious client, Skill 2.5, *40*

Communication, therapeutic, Skill 2.1, *29*

Compress, cold, Skill 23.3, *559*

Computed tomography, Skill 15.4, *376*

Contact lens clients, caring for, Skill 36.1, *833*

Continuous passive motion machine, Skill 26.2, *632*

Contrast media studies, Skill 15.4, *376*

Convalescent phase care, Skill 21.2, *512*

Crutches, teaching use, Skill 29.2, *665*

Culture, blood, Skill 15.2, *360*

Culture, sputum, Skill 15.1, *346*

Death, care of body after, Skill 38.3, *882*

Diagnostic testing, Skills 15.1 to 15.7, *346-396*

Dialysis, peritoneal, Skill 39.5, *911*

Diaper changing, Skill 11.4, *215*

Dobutamine stress echocardiography, Skill 15.7, *396*

Drainage devices, postoperative monitoring and measuring, Skill 21.4, *520*

Drainage system, chest, management, Skill 31.5, *754*

Dressing, application, Skill 24.3, *585*

Dressing, transparent, changing, Skill 24.4, *592*

Ear assessment, Skill 14.3, *293*

Ear irrigation, Skill 36.5, *848*

Ear medication administration, Skill 17.3, *433*

Echocardiography, dobutamine stress, Skill 15.7, *396*

Electrocardiography, Skill 15.7, *396*

Electrolyte imbalance, monitoring, Skill 37.2, *859*

Electronic blood pressure, Skill 12.3, *245*

Endoscopy, assisting with, Skill 15.6, *383*

Endotracheal tube management, Skill 31.4, *747*

Enema administration, Skill 9.5, *185*

Enteral nutrition, Skills 33.1 to 33.3, *776-787*

Enterostomy, pouching, Skill 34.2, *794*

Epidural analgesia, Skill 22.4, *544*

Exercise, range-of-motion, Skill 26.1, *618*

Exercise stress test, Skill 15.7, *396*

External catheter, applying, Skill 9.4, *181*

Extremity, shift assessment, Skill 13.5, *274*

Eye assessment, Skill 14.3, *293*

Eye irrigation, Skill 36.3, *842*

Eye medication administration, Skill 17.3, *433*

Eye prosthesis, caring for, Skill 36.2, *839*

Face assessment, Skill 14.1, *283*

Fall prevention, Skill 5.1, *76* and Skill 29.1, *662*

Feeding dependent client, Skill 8.1, *156*

Feeding infant, Skill 11.2, *206*

Feeding tube, administration of feedings, Skill 33.2, *781*

Feeding tube, insertion, Skill 33.1, *775*

Feeding tube, medication administration, Skill 33.3, *787*

Fluid imbalance, monitoring, Skill 37.1, *857*

Foot care, Skill 7.4, *140*

Gastric intubation, Skills 32.1 to 32.3, *766-773*

Gastroccult testing, Skill 15.3, *368*

General survey, shift assessment, Skill 13.1, *257*

Genitalia assessment, Skill 14.7, *322*

Glove use, disposable clean, Skill 3.2, *53*

Gloving, closed, Skill 20.2, *497*

Gloving, sterile, Skill 4.2, *69*

Glucose testing, Skill 15.3, *368*

Gowning, sterile, Skill 20.2, *497*

Hair care, Skill 7.3, *135*

Hand scrub, surgical, Skill 20.1, *493*

Handwashing, Skill 3.1, *50*

Head assessment, Skill 14.1, *283*

Health assessment, Skills 14.1 to 14.9, *283-339*

Hearing aid client, caring for, Skill 36.4, *845*

Heart assessment, Skill 14.5, *309*

Heat, dry, Skill 23.2, *556*

Heat, moist, Skill 23.1, *553*

Hemoccult testing, Skill 15.3, *368*

Hemodialysis, Skill 39.4, *907*

Home management, Skills 40.1 to 40.6, *918-941*

Hoyer lift transfer, Skill 6.4, *112*

Hygiene promotion, Skills 7.1 to 7.5, *123-147*

Hypotension, orthostatic, minimizing, Skill 6.2, *106*

Ice bag, Skill 23.3, *559*

Impaction, removal, Skill 34.1, *792*

Incident report, Skill 1.4, *21*

Incontinent client, caring for, Skill 9.3, *177*

Infant bathing, Skill 11.3, *212*

Infant feeding, Skill 11.2, *206*

Infection control, Skills 3.1 to 3.4, *50-60*

Inhalers, metered-dose, Skill 17.4, *438*

Injection administration, Skills 18.1 to 18.3, *457-469*

Insulin injection, Skill 18.1, *457*

Intake and output monitoring, Skill 9.1, *168*

Integumentary inspection, shift assessment, Skill 13.1, *257*

Interviewing, Skill 2.4, *36*

Intradermal injection, Skill 18.2, *469*

Intramuscular injection, Skill 18.2, *464*

*Page numbers given indicate the beginning of Skill.